OKU 5

Orthopaedic Knowledge Update

Pediatrics

AAOS
American Academy of Orthopaedic Surgeons

OKU 5

Orthopaedic Knowledge Update

Pediatrics

EDITOR

Jeffrey E. Martus, MD, MS
Assistant Professor, Department of Orthopaedics and Rehabilitation
Monroe Carell Jr. Children's Hospital at Vanderbilt
Vanderbilt University Medical Center
Nashville, Tennessee

Developed by the Pediatric
Orthopaedic Society of North America

POSNA
PEDIATRIC ORTHOPAEDIC SOCIETY OF NORTH AMERICA

AAOS
AMERICAN ACADEMY OF
ORTHOPAEDIC SURGEONS

Staff

Ellen C. Moore, *Chief Education Officer*

Hans Koelsch, PhD, *Director, Department of Publications*

Lisa Claxton Moore, *Senior Manager, Book Program*

Kathleen Anderson, *Senior Editor*

Michelle Wild, *Associate Senior Editor*

Courtney Dunker, *Editorial Production Manager*

Abram Fassler, *Publishing Systems Manager*

Suzanne O'Reilly, *Graphic Designer*

Susan Morritz Baim, *Production Coordinator*

Karen Danca, *Permissions Coordinator*

Charlie Baldwin, *Digital and Print Production Specialist*

Hollie Muir, *Digital and Print Production Specialist*

Emily Douglas, *Page Production Assistant*

Genevieve Charet, *Editorial Coordinator*

Published 2016 by the
American Academy of Orthopaedic Surgeons
9400 West Higgins Road
Rosemont, IL 60018

Library of Congress Control Number:
2016947581
ISBN: 978-1-62552-548-2

Printed in the USA

Bone and Joint Initiative USA

Acknowledgments

Contributors

Joshua M. Abzug, MD
Assistant Professor
Director of Pediatric Orthopaedics
Director of University of Maryland Brachial Plexus Clinic
Deputy Surgeon-in-Chief, University of Maryland Children's Hospital
Vice Chair, Dean's Council for Pediatric Surgery
Department of Orthopaedics
University of Maryland Medical System
Baltimore, Maryland

Benjamin A. Alman, MD
Professor and Chair
Department of Orthopaedic Surgery
Duke University Medical Center
Durham, North Carolina

Alexandre Arkader, MD
Associate Professor
Department of Orthopaedic Surgery
The Children's Hospital of Philadelphia
Perelman School of Medicine at University of Pennsylvania
Philadelphia, Pennsylvania

Donald S. Bae, MD
Associate Professor
Department of Orthopaedic Surgery
Boston Children's Hospital
Harvard Medical School
Boston, Massachusetts

Jennifer J. Beck, MD
Assistant Professor
Department of Orthopaedic Surgery
Orthopaedic Institute for Children
University of California, Los Angeles
Los Angeles, California

James T. Beckmann, MD, MS
Orthopaedic Surgeon
Department of Sports Medicine
Saint Luke's Health System
Boise, Idaho

Clayton C. Bettin, MD
Instructor
Department of Orthopaedic Surgery and Biomedical Engineering
University of Tennessee - Campbell Clinic
Memphis, Tennessee

Richard E. Bowen, MD
Clinical Professor
Department of Pediatric Orthopaedic Surgery
Orthopaedic Institute for Children
David Geffen School of Medicine at University of California, Los Angeles
Los Angeles, California

Brian K. Brighton, MD, MPH
Pediatric Orthopaedic Surgeon
Department of Orthopaedic Surgery
Carolinas Healthcare System - Levine Children's Hospital
Charlotte, North Carolina

Robert B. Bryskin, MD
Director of Acute and Chronic Pain Management
Department of Anesthesiology and Critical Care
Nemours Children's Clinic
Jacksonville, Florida

Cordelia W. Carter, MD
Assistant Professor
Department of Orthopaedic Surgery
Yale University
New Haven, Connecticut

Pablo Castañeda, MD
Orthopaedic Surgeon
Department of Orthopaedic Surgery
Shriners Hospital for Children
Mexico City, Mexico

Johanna Chang, MD
Assistant Clinical Professor of Pediatrics
Department of Pediatrics
Division of Rheumatology, Allergy, and Immunology
University of California San Diego
San Diego, California

Robert H. Cho, MD
Chief of Staff
Department of Pediatric Orthopedic Surgery
Shriners Hospitals for Children
Los Angeles, California

Christopher Collins, MD
Fellow
Department of Pediatric Orthopedics
Orlando Regional Medical Center
Arnold Palmer Hospital for Children
Orlando, Florida

Lawson A.B. Copley, MD, MBA
Associate Professor of Orthopaedic Surgery
Department of Pediatric Orthopaedic Surgery
Texas Scottish Rite Hospital
Dallas, Texas

Jared William Daniel, MD
Clinical Fellow
Department of Orthopaedics - Pediatrics
The Hospital for Sick Children
Toronto, Ontario, Canada

Matthew B. Dobbs, MD
Professor
Department of Orthopaedic Surgery
Washington University School of Medicine
St. Louis, Missouri

Kathryn S. Doughty, MD, MPH, MS
Pediatric Orthopaedic Surgeon
Department of Orthopaedic Surgery
Shriners Hospital for Children
Los Angeles, California

Eric W. Edmonds, MD
Director of Orthopedic Research
Department of Orthopedic Surgery
Rady Children's Hospital San Diego
San Diego, California

John B. Emans, MD
Professor
Department of Orthopedic Surgery
Boston Children's Hospital
Harvard Medical School
Boston, Massachusetts

Corinna CD Franklin, MD
Pediatric Orthopaedic Surgeon
Shriners Hospital for Children
Philadelphia, Pennsylvania

Theodore J. Ganley, MD
Orthopedic Surgeon
Director, Sports Medicine and Performance Center
Division of Orthopedics
Children's Hospital of Philadelphia
Philadelphia, Pennsylvania

Michael Glotzbecker, MD
Assistant Professor, Harvard Medical School
Department of Orthopaedic Surgery
Boston Children's Hospital
Boston, Massachusetts

Charles A. Goldfarb, MD
Professor
Department of Orthopaedic Surgery
Washington University
St. Louis, Missouri

Dorothy K. Grange, MD
Professor
Department of Pediatrics
Washington University School of Medicine
St. Louis, Missouri

John J. Grayhack, MD, MS
Associate Professor
Department of Orthopaedic Surgery
Ann & Robert H. Lurie Children's Hospital of Chicago
Chicago, Illinois

Andrew J.M. Gregory, MD, FAAP, FACSM
Associate Professor of Orthopedics and Rehabilitation
Department of Sports Medicine
Vanderbilt University Medical Center
Nashville, Tennessee

Christina A. Gurnett, MD, PhD
Associate Professor
Department of Neurology
Washington University
St. Louis, Missouri

David H. Gutmann, MD, PhD
Donald O. Schnuck Family Professor
Department of Neurology
Washington University
St. Louis, Missouri

Gregory Hale, MD
Fellow
Department of Pediatric Orthopedic Surgery
Orlando Health
Orlando, Florida

Jennifer Harrington, MBBS, PhD
Pediatric Endocrinologist
Department of Pediatrics, Division of Endocrinology
Hospital for Sick Children
Toronto, Ontario, Canada

Daniel J. Hedequist, MD
Orthopedic Surgeon
Department of Orthopedics
Boston Children's Hospital
Harvard Medical School
Boston, Massachusetts

Jose Herrera-Soto, MD
Director, Pediatric Orthopedics
Department of Orthopedics
Arnold Palmer Hospital for Children
Orlando, Florida

Andrew W. Howard, MD, MSc, FRCSC
Pediatric Orthopaedic Surgeon
Department of Orthopaedic Surgery
Hospital for Sick Children
Toronto, Ontario, Canada

Christopher Iobst, MD
Surgeon
Department of Orthopedic Surgery
Nemours Children's Hospital
Orlando, Florida

Scott P. Kaiser, MD
Assistant Professor
Department of Orthopaedic Surgery
University of California, San Francisco
San Francisco, California

Erik C. King, MD
Associate Professor
Department of Orthopaedic Surgery
Ann & Robert H. Lurie Children's Hospital of Chicago
Chicago, Illinois

Joel Kolmodin, MD
Department of Orthopedic Surgery
The Cleveland Clinic Foundation
Cleveland, Ohio

Pamela Lang, MD
Clinical Fellow
Department of Pediatric Orthopaedic Surgery
Orthopaedic Institute for Children, University of California, Los Angeles
Los Angeles, California

A. Noelle Larson, MD
Associate Professor
Department of Orthopedic Surgery
Mayo Clinic
Rochester, Minnesota

David Lazarus, MD
Fellow
Department of Orthopaedics
Rady Children's Hospital
University of California San Diego School of Medicine
San Diego, California

Holly B. Leshikar, MD, MPH
Assistant Professor
Department of Pediatric Orthopaedic Surgery
University of California at Davis
Sacramento, California

Ying Li, MD
Assistant Professor
Department of Orthopaedic Surgery
C.S. Mott Children's Hospital, University of Michigan
Ann Arbor, Michigan

John F. Lovejoy III, MD
Orthopaedic Surgeon
Department of Orthopaedics and Sports Medicine
Nemours Children's Hospital
Orlando, Florida

Benjamin D. Martin, MD
Assistant Professor, Pediatric Orthopaedic Surgery
Division of Orthopaedic Surgery and Sports Medicine
Children's National Health System
Washington, DC

Douglas J. McDonald, MD, MS
Orthopedic Surgeon
Department of Orthopedics
Washington University
St. Louis, Missouri

Amy L. McIntosh, MD
Associate Professor
Department of Orthopedic Surgery
Texas Scottish Rite Hospital for Children
Dallas, Texas

Charles T. Mehlman, DO, MPH
Professor of Orthopaedic Surgery
Division of Orthopaedics, Department of Orthopaedic Surgery
Cincinnati Children's Hospital Medical Center
Cincinnati, Ohio

Matthew D. Milewski, MD
Assistant Professor
Elite Sports Medicine Division
Connecticut Children's Medical Center
Farmington, Connecticut

Firoz Miyanji, MD, FRCSC
Pediatric Orthopedic Surgeon
Department of Orthopedics
British Columbia Children's Hospital
Vancouver, British Columbia

Stephanie N. Moore, BS
Department of Pharmacology
Vanderbilt University
Nashville, Tennessee

Jose A. Morcuende, MD, PhD
Professor
Department of Orthopaedic Surgery
University of Iowa
Iowa City, Iowa

Ryan D. Muchow, MD
Assistant Professor
Lexington Shriners Hospital
University of Kentucky
Lexington, Kentucky

Matthew E. Oetgen, MD, MBA
Chief, Division of Orthopaedic Surgery and Sports Medicine
Children's National Health System
Washington, DC

J. Lee Pace, MD
Assistant Professor
Department of Orthopaedic Surgery
Children's Orthopaedic Center
Children's Hospital Los Angeles
Los Angeles, California

Nirav K. Pandya, MD
Assistant Professor
Department of Orthopaedic Surgery
University of California, San Francisco
San Francisco, California

Michael D. Partington, MD
Department of Pediatric Neurosurgery
Gillette Children's Specialty Healthcare
St. Paul, Minnesota

David A. Podeszwa, MD
Associate Professor
University of Texas Southwestern Medical Center
Texas Scottish Rite Hospital for Children
Dallas, Texas

Robert H. Quinn, MD
Chair and Professor
Department of Orthopaedic Surgery
University of Texas Health Science Center, San Antonio
San Antonio, Texas

Suhas Radhakrishna, MD
Assistant Professor of Pediatrics
Department of Pediatrics
Division of Allergy, Immunology, and Rheumatology
University of California San Diego School of Medicine
San Diego, California

Paul M. Saluan, MD
Director, Pediatric and Adolescent Sports Medicine
Department of Orthopaedic Surgery
The Cleveland Clinic Foundation
Cleveland, Ohio

Anthony A. Scaduto, MD
President and CEO
Department of Orthopaedic Surgery
Orthopaedic Institute for Children
Los Angeles, California

Brian P. Scannell, MD
Assistant Professor of Pediatric Orthopaedic Surgery
Department of Orthopaedic Surgery
Carolinas HealthCare System, Levine Children's Hospital
Charlotte, North Carolina

Jonathan G. Schoenecker, MD, PhD
Assistant Professor
Department of Orthopaedics
Vanderbilt University
Nashville, Tennessee

Mark A. Seeley, MD
Pediatric Orthopaedic Attending Surgeon
Department of Orthopaedic Surgery
Geisinger Medical Center
Danville, Pennsylvania

Apurva S. Shah, MD, MBA
Assistant Professor of Orthopaedic Surgery
Division of Orthopaedic Surgery
The Children's Hospital of Philadelphia
Philadelphia, Pennsylvania

Melinda S. Sharkey, MD
Assistant Professor of Orthopaedic Surgery
Department of Orthopaedics and Rehabilitation
Yale University
New Haven, Connecticut

Kevin G. Shea, MD
Orthopedic Surgeon
Department of Sports Medicine
St. Luke's Clinic
Boise, Idaho

Robert Sheets, MD
Clinical Professor of Pediatrics
Department of Pediatrics
University of California San Diego School of Medicine
San Diego, California

Eric D. Shirley, MD
Director of Sports Medicine
Department of Orthopaedic Surgery
Nemours Children's Specialty Care
Jacksonville, Florida

Mauricio Silva, MD
Medical Director
Department of Orthopaedic Surgery
Orthopaedic Institute for Children
Los Angeles, California

Brian Snyder, MD, PhD
Professor of Orthopaedic Surgery
Harvard Medical School
Orthopaedic Surgeon
Department of Orthopaedic Surgery
Boston Children's Hospital
Boston, Massachusetts

David D. Spence, MD
Assistant Professor
Department of Orthopaedic Surgery and Biomedical Engineering
University of Tennessee-Campbell Clinic
Memphis, Tennessee

Christopher Stutz, MD
Assistant Professor
Department of Orthopaedic Surgery
Texas Scottish Rite Hospital for Children
University of Texas Southwestern Medical School
Dallas, Texas

Michael D. Sussman, MD
Staff Surgeon, Former Chief of Staff
Shriners Hospital for Children
Portland, Oregon

Vineeta T. Swaroop, MD
Assistant Professor
Department of Orthopaedic Surgery
Northwestern University Feinberg School of Medicine
Chicago, Illinois

Mihir M. Thacker, MD
Pediatric Orthopedic Surgeon and Orthopedic Oncologist
Nemours Alfred I. duPont Hospital for Children
Associate Professor of Orthopedic Surgery and Pediatrics
Thomas Jefferson University
Wilmington, Delaware

Stephanie Thibaudeau, MD
Hand Surgery Fellow
Department of Orthopedic Surgery
University of Pennsylvania
Philadelphia, Pennsylvania

Rachel Mednick Thompson, MD
Fellow
Department of Orthopaedic Surgery
Texas Scottish Rite Hospital for Children
Dallas, Texas

Marc A. Tompkins, MD
Assistant Professor
Department of Orthopaedic Surgery
University of Minnesota - TRIA Orthopaedic Center
Minneapolis, Minnesota

Natasha Trentacosta, MD
Santa Monica Orthopaedic and Sports Medicine Group
Santa Monica, California

Ann E. Van Heest, MD
Professor
Department of Orthopaedic Surgery
University of Minnesota
Minneapolis, Minnesota

Janet L. Walker, MD
Professor
Department of Orthopaedic Surgery and Sports Medicine
University of Kentucky
Pediatric Orthopaedic Surgeon
Shriners Hospital for Children-Lexington
Lexington, Kentucky

Lindley B. Wall, MD
Assistant Professor
Department of Orthopedics
Washington University
St. Louis, Missouri

Amanda T. Whitaker, MD
Fellow
Department of Orthopaedic Surgery
Boston Children's Hospital
Boston, Massachusetts

Klane K. White, MD, MSc
Pediatric Orthopedic Surgeon
Assistant Professor
Department of Orthopaedics and Sports Medicine
Seattle Children's Hospital
University of Washington
Seattle, Washington

Theresa O. Wyrick, MD
Associate Professor
Department of Orthopedic Surgery
Arkansas Children's Hospital
Little Rock, Arkansas

Preface

The fifth edition of *Orthopaedic Knowledge Update: Pediatrics* is an extension of the previous editions of this series that focuses on musculoskeletal conditions in children and adolescents. This text is written for the experienced orthopaedic practitioner, not the superspecialist or the beginning student. The goal of *OKU: Pediatrics 5* is to describe the important developments in pediatric orthopaedics over the past 5 years, while providing core information for each topic. The editors and authors integrated new information with fundamental knowledge to provide an essential resource for the practicing general orthopaedic surgeon and pediatric subspecialist. The annotated reference list at the end of each chapter contains classic articles as well as updated references, with annotations provided for references published within the past 5 years.

This new edition contains some changes in the organization of the book compared with the fourth edition. In particular, a new section has been added entitled Neuromuscular, Metabolic, and Inflammatory Disorders. Chapters new to this edition include: Quality, Safety, and Value; Evidence-Based Quality and Outcomes Assessment in Pediatric Orthopaedics; Growth of the Musculoskeletal System; Orthopaedic-Related Syndromes; Medical Therapy in Pediatric Orthopaedics; Osteogenesis Imperfecta and Metabolic Bone Disease; Progressive Neuromuscular Disease in Childhood and Adolescence; Arthritis; and Child Abuse.

The quality of this book is directly related to the efforts of the section editors: Steven L. Frick, Benjamin A. Alman, Henry G. Chambers, Charles A. Goldfarb, Vishwas R. Talwalkar, James O. Sanders, and Jennifer M. Weiss. These individuals are leaders within the field of orthopaedics and worked hard to ensure that the content of this edition was complete, accurate, and high quality. The editors recruited expert authors who volunteered their time to contribute to this book. We are all indebted to the individual authors who spent many hours reviewing the literature and writing these excellent chapters.

The project would not have succeeded without the excellent work of the publications staff of the American Academy of Orthopaedic Surgeons. Special credit and thanks goes to the entire team and in particular to Michelle Wild, Lisa Claxton Moore, Genevieve Charet, and Kathleen Anderson. It has been a privilege to participate in this effort and I am grateful to Greg Mencio, Lori Karol, and the leadership of the Pediatric Orthopaedic Society of North America for the opportunity to be involved.

We hope that the readers find this book to be a useful resource in the management of children with musculoskeletal conditions. Suggestions to improve future editions would be appreciated.

Jeffrey E. Martus, MD, MS
Editor

Table of Contents

Preface xiii

Section 1: General

Section Editor:
Steven L. Frick, MD

Chapter 1
Quality, Safety, and Value
Brian K. Brighton, MD, MPH
Donald S. Bae, MD
Apurva S. Shah, MD, MBA. 3

Chapter 2
Evidence-Based Quality and Outcomes Assessment in Pediatric Orthopaedics
Kevin G. Shea, MD
Charles T. Mehlman, DO, MPH
Robert H. Quinn, MD
James T. Beckmann, MD, MS. 13

Chapter 3
Pediatric Anesthesia and Pain Management
Eric D. Shirley, MD
Robert B. Bryskin, MD. 25

Chapter 4
Musculoskeletal Infection
John F. Lovejoy III, MD
Lawson A. B. Copley, MD, MBA 35

Chapter 5
Benign and Malignant Musculoskeletal Neoplasms
Mihir M. Thacker, MD
Alexandre Arkader, MD 45

Chapter 6
Growth of the Musculoskeletal System
Christopher Iobst, MD
Brian P. Scannell, MD 59

Section 2: Basic Science

Section Editor:
Benjamin A. Alman, MD

Chapter 7
Genetics and Personalized Medicine
Christina A. Gurnett, MD, PhD
Dorothy K. Grange, MD
David H. Gutmann, MD, PhD
Douglas J. McDonald, MD, MS
Matthew B. Dobbs, MD 71

Chapter 8
Skeletal Dysplasias
Jose A. Morcuende, MD, PhD. 81

Chapter 9
Orthopaedic-Related Syndromes
Klane K. White, MD, MSc
Benjamin A. Alman, MD 99

Chapter 10
Medical Therapy in Pediatric Orthopaedics
Andrew W. Howard, MD, MSc, FRCSC
Stephanie N. Moore, BS
Jonathan G. Schoenecker, MD, PhD 107

Section 3: Neuromuscular, Metabolic, and Inflammatory Disorders

Section Editor:
Henry G. Chambers, MD

Chapter 11
Cerebral Palsy
Nirav K. Pandya, MD
Scott P. Kaiser, MD 123

Chapter 12
Myelomeningocele
Vineeta T. Swaroop, MD 137

Chapter 13
Arthrogrypotic Syndromes
Kathryn S. Doughty, MD, MPH, MS
Robert H. Cho, MD
Christopher Stutz, MD 153

Chapter 14
Osteogenesis Imperfecta and Metabolic Bone Disease
Jared William Daniel, MD
Jennifer Harrington, MBBS, PhD
Andrew W. Howard, MD, MSc, FRCSC. 165

Chapter 15
Progressive Neuromuscular Diseases in Childhood and Adolescence
Michael D. Sussman, MD 177

Chapter 16
Arthritis
Robert Sheets, MD
Johanna Chang, MD
Suhas Radhakrishna, MD 203

Section 4: Upper Extremity

Section Editor:
Charles A. Goldfarb, MD

Chapter 17
Congenital Upper Limb Differences
Lindley B. Wall, MD
Charles A. Goldfarb, MD 217

Chapter 18
Birth Brachial Plexus Palsy
Ann E. Van Heest, MD
Michael D. Partington, MD 227

Chapter 19
Congenital Transverse Deficiency of the Upper Limb
Apurva S. Shah, MD, MBA
Stephanie Thibaudeau, MD 235

Section 5: Lower Extremity

Section Editor:
Vishwas R. Talwalkar, MD

Chapter 20
Developmental Dysplasia of the Hip
Pablo Castañeda, MD. 245

Chapter 21
Slipped Capital Femoral Epiphysis and Femoroacetabular Impingement
Rachel Mednick Thompson, MD
David A. Podeszwa, MD. 259

Chapter 22
Legg-Calvé-Perthes Disease
Holly B. Leshikar, MD, MPH
Jonathan G. Schoenecker, MD, PhD 269

Chapter 23
Congenital Dislocations: Knee and Patella
Amy L. McIntosh, MD 283

Chapter 24
Tibial Deformities
Erik C. King, MD
John J. Grayhack, MD, MS. 289

Chapter 25
Congenital Disorders of the Foot
David D. Spence, MD
Clayton C. Bettin, MD 303

Chapter 26
Rotational and Angular Limb Deformity
Ryan D. Muchow, MD 315

Chapter 27
Limb-Length Discrepancy, Limb Deficiency, and Amputation
Janet L. Walker, MD. 323

Section 6: Spine

Section Editor:
James O. Sanders, MD

Chapter 28
Early-Onset Scoliosis and Congenital Spine Disorders
Michael Glotzbecker, MD
Daniel J. Hedequist, MD
John B. Emans, MD 339

Chapter 29
Adolescent Idiopathic Scoliosis
Matthew E. Oetgen, MD, MBA
Benjamin D. Martin, MD 351

Chapter 30
Neuromuscular Spine Deformity
Amanda T. Whitaker, MD
Brian Snyder, MD, PhD 365

Chapter 31
Kyphosis
Matthew E. Oetgen, MD, MBA 385

Chapter 32
Pediatric Cervical Spine Disorders
Firoz Miyanji, MD, FRCSC 395

Chapter 33
Back Pain, Disk Disease, Spondylolysis, and Spondylolisthesis
A. Noelle Larson, MD. 415

Section 7: Trauma

Section Editor:
Jeffrey E. Martus, MD, MS

Chapter 34
Pediatric Trauma Principles
Mauricio Silva, MD
Anthony A. Scaduto, MD 433

Chapter 35
Child Abuse
Brian K. Brighton, MD, MPH
Brian P. Scannell, MD 449

Chapter 36
Shoulder, Humerus, and Elbow
David Lazarus, MD
Eric W. Edmonds, MD 457

Chapter 37
Forearm, Wrist, and Hand
Joshua M. Abzug, MD
Theresa O. Wyrick, MD 473

Chapter 38
Pelvis, Hip, Femur, and Knee
Gregory Hale, MD
Christopher Collins, MD
Jose Herrera-Soto, MD 485

Chapter 39
Tibia, Ankle, and Foot
Ying Li, MD
Mark A. Seeley, MD 497

Chapter 40
Spine
Daniel J. Hedequist, MD
Michael Glotzbecker, MD. 509

Section 8: Sports-Related Topics

Section Editor:
Jennifer M. Weiss, MD

Chapter 41
Ligamentous Knee Injuries
Cordelia W. Carter, MD
Melinda S. Sharkey, MD 521

Chapter 42
Meniscal Tears in Children and Adolescents
Melinda S. Sharkey, MD
Cordelia W. Carter, MD 537

Chapter 43
Patellar Instability
Corinna CD Franklin, MD 545

Chapter 44
Osteochondritis Dissecans of the Knee and Elbow
Matthew D. Milewski, MD
Marc A. Tompkins, MD
Kevin G. Shea, MD
Theodore J. Ganley, MD. 555

Chapter 45
Shoulder Injuries
Natasha Trentacosta, MD
J. Lee Pace, MD 567

Chapter 46
Ankle Injuries
Joel Kolmodin, MD
Paul M. Saluan, MD 579

Chapter 47
Overuse Conditions
Jennifer J. Beck, MD
Pamela Lang, MD
Richard E. Bowen, MD. 591

Chapter 48
Pediatric and Adolescent Athletes: Special Considerations
Andrew J.M. Gregory, MD, FAAP, FACSM . . . 601

Index. 609

Section 1

General

SECTION EDITOR:
Steven L. Frick, MD

Chapter 1

Quality, Safety, and Value

Brian K. Brighton, MD, MPH Donald S. Bae, MD Apurva S. Shah, MD, MBA

Abstract

The concepts of healthcare quality, safety, and value have received increased attention in the current changing healthcare landscape. Improving patient outcomes, containing costs, and focusing on quality and safety provide value in orthopaedics. An understanding of quality measures and quality improvement methodology, as well using surgical simulation, implementing checklists, and engaging in a culture of safety, can improve the quality and safety of orthopaedic surgery.

Keywords: cost; quality; quality improvement; safety; value

Introduction

During the past decade, increased attention has been directed at providing high-quality care and improving patient safety and the value of patient care. Two reports published by the Institute of Medicine at the beginning of the 21st century raised the collective awareness of patients, payers, hospitals, and providers regarding the importance of quality, safety, and value in the practice of medicine.[1,2] To further this effort, the Pediatric Orthopaedic Society of North America (POSNA) implemented a "Quality, Safety, and Value Initiative" in 2011 to involve society members in providing leadership, education, and direction to discussions on quality, safety, and value taking place both locally and nationally.[3-5] Each concept—quality, safety, and value—will be discussed in this chapter, including specific applications to pediatric orthopaedic surgery.

Dr. Brighton or an immediate family member serves as a paid consultant to DePuy and serves as a board member, owner, officer, or committee member of the Pediatric Orthopaedic Society of North America and the American College of Surgeons. Dr. Bae or an immediate family member has stock or stock options held in Cempra, Johnson & Johnson, Kythera, and Vivus and serves as a board member, owner, officer, or committee member of the American Academy of Orthopaedic Surgeons, the American Society for Surgery of the Hand, and the Pediatric Orthopaedic Society of North America. Dr. Shah or an immediate family member serves as a board member, owner, officer, or committee member of the Pediatric Orthopaedic Society of North America and the American Society for Surgery of the Hand.

Quality

In the 1980s, the Ford Motor Company coined the marketing phrase, "Quality Is Job 1." Physicians would universally agree that their top priority is to provide the best possible care, but a challenging concept remains: "What defines quality?" The answer depends on who is answering the question and what is important to that individual. It also depends on who is defining quality and how the individual or organization is measuring it. Surgeons frequently refer to quality in the context of low infection, complication, and mortality rates or adherence to process measures and practice guidelines. Patients and families may view quality from the perspective of rate of recovery and return to function. The Institute of Medicine defined quality as the "degree to which health care services for individuals and populations increase the likelihood of desired outcomes and are consistent with current professional knowledge."[2] In addition, the Institute of Medicine outlined six specific aims for improving health care that are focused on delivering care that is safe, effective, patient centered, timely, efficient, and equitable. In the equation, *value = outcome/cost*, proposed by Porter,[6] quality is a composition of patient outcomes, safety, and patient experience. Improving the quality of care and patient outcomes provides an important opportunity to add value for a given cost.[7]

Quality Improvement

Quality improvement in health care is systematic, data-guided activities that are designed to bring about immediate positive change in the delivery of health care

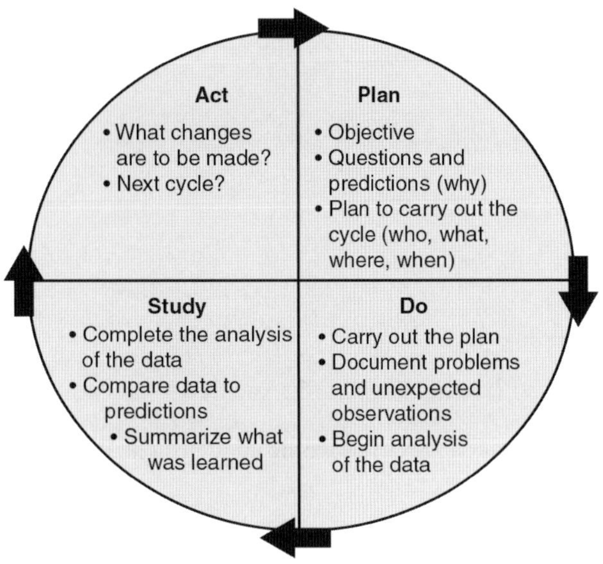

Figure 1 Illustration of the plan-do-study-act cycle for learning and improvement.

in particular settings.[8] Quality improvement methodology is used to incorporate new knowledge into clinical practice and apply this information to fix existing problems in care delivery. The aim is to become more effective, safe, and efficient and continually improve processes of care. Such methodologies and principles originally were designed and implemented in the manufacturing industry and have been applied to health care to provide a framework for improving patient care. Commonly used methodologies included Lean, Six Sigma, and the Model for Improvement.

Lean is a quality improvement methodology that evolved from the Toyota Production System, which was a framework to map out and preserve the processes of value and eliminate waste and inefficiency.[9] One hallmark of the Lean process is the standardization of processes to ensure consistency. The Lean approach requires an understanding of the process, including how the process is intended to work and variations in the process that have evolved across time. This methodology has been used in several healthcare settings to improve the surgical care of patients.[10]

Six Sigma also has its origins in the manufacturing industry. This approach relies on precise and accurate measurements of process and outcomes using the improvement process known by the acronym DMAIC (define, measure, analyze, improve, and control). The problem within a process is defined, any defects are measured, the cause of the defects are analyzed, the process performance is improved by removing the causes of the defects, and the process is controlled to ensure that the defects do not recur. The Six Sigma goal is to identify and reduce error rates to the six sigma level (<3.4 defects per million opportunities).[11] Examples of Six Sigma methodology can be seen in reducing medication administration errors and improving operating room efficiency.[10,12]

Lean Six Sigma is a combination of Lean and Six Sigma principles that is often applied in health care. It aims to improve care by incorporating the Lean principles of eliminating waste and improving efficiency and the Six Sigma approach of pursuing accuracy and effectiveness.

The Model for Improvement is another example of a quality improvement methodology that provides a framework for improving a process or a system.[13] The model contains four essential components: an aim, measurement, change ideas, and tests of change. The first three components are examined by three key questions: (1) What are we trying to accomplish? (2) How will we know that a change is an improvement? and (3) What changes can we make that will result in an improvement? The final component involves using a technique for rapid testing and learning from change known as the plan-do-study-act cycle (**Figure 1**). Using a series of small plan-do-study-act cycles, changes on a larger scale can be made to improve and sustain improved patient care across time.

Two recent publications reported on the experience of using quality improvement in pediatric orthopaedic surgery. A 2014 article described an education and training program instituted at Boston Children's Hospital to reduce cast saw injuries.[14] A 2015 article reported on the implementation of a multidisciplinary guideline for sedated MRI use for children with suspected musculoskeletal infections.[15] It was found that the sedated MRI approach led to improved diagnostic efficiency, with less scan time and fewer sequences needed, as well as improved rates of immediate surgical procedures performed while the children remained under continued anesthesia. Some clinical examples of the application of quality improvement methodology[14-19] are listed in **Table 1**.

Quality Indicators and Measures

Quality indicators refer to a set of clear, measurable items that are ideally related to outcome. Numerous public and private agencies have already begun to define, measure, and report on healthcare quality.[20,21] In a 2012 systematic review of the pediatric orthopaedic surgery literature, researchers found mortality, postoperative complications, reoperation, and readmission rates as the most commonly referenced quality indicators.[22]

Defining and measuring quality is essential to identify gaps in performance, make changes, and monitor

Table 1

Examples of the Application of Quality Improvement Methodology to Patient Care

Methodology	Example
Improving efficiency of processes (streamlining)	Improving operating room efficiency
Eliminating waste associated with the process (logistics)	MRI use in musculoskeletal infection
Reducing errors and adverse events (safety)	Eliminating cast saw injuries
Decreasing variation in choosing and using processes (utilization and standardization)	Best practice guidelines for high-risk spine surgery
Improving communication within the healthcare team (use of checklists)	Use of an intraoperative neuromonitoring checklist
Improving systematization of the process (care pathways)	Rapid recovery care pathways in adolescent idiopathic scoliosis
Maximizing health improvement (outcomes)	Patient-reported outcomes (PROMIS, PODCI)
Enhancing the patient's experience of care (satisfaction)	Patient satisfaction scores

PROMIS = Patient-Reported Outcomes Measurement Information System, PODCI = Pediatric Outcomes Data Collection Instrument.

Adapted with permission from Jevsevar DS: Health system perspective: Variation, costs, and physician behavior. *J Pediatr Orthop* 2015;35(5 suppl 1):S14-S19.

and compare long-term performance. Process measures require defined criteria that can be determined by nationally derived evidence-based guidelines, institutional guidelines, or consensus guidelines. These often serve as surrogates to define the quality of care and may include compliance with clinical care pathways or adherence to evidence-based guidelines, with limited effect on value. Measures of patient expectations, satisfaction, function, and patient-reported outcomes all can be used to measure outcomes, yet no universal set of outcomes measures exists to clearly define the quality of care being delivered. The ideal measures should be clearly defined, easily obtainable, and risk adjusted to discriminate among levels of quality. The concept of standardization of outcomes measures remains on the near horizon.[23]

Patient Safety

Beginning with the Institute of Medicine report "To Err Is Human: Building a Safe Health System,"[1] recognizing the magnitude and scope of preventable error and adverse events has led to the modern patient safety movement.[24] This movement has shifted focus away from individual errors because complications or adverse outcomes resulting from careless or technically incompetent providers are rare. Rather, current efforts aim to optimize care delivery systems, using principles such as standardization, simplification, reducing reliance on memory or experience, and crisis resource management.[24] Currently, patient safety is defined as the prevention and mitigation of harm caused by errors of omission or commission that are associated with health care, which involves the establishment of operational systems and processes that minimize the likelihood of errors and maximize the likelihood of intercepting them when they occur, before they reach the patient.

In pediatric orthopaedics, the first level of improving patient safety involves improving technical performance and minimizing technical error. Surgical simulation is an example of how performance may be improved through iterative, deliberate practice of surgery without patient risk.[25] Simulation training to improve technical performance has been used in several orthopaedic surgical disciplines, ranging from arthroscopy to complex spine surgery.[26-29] Although high-fidelity, virtual reality simulation trainers are available, effective training may be imparted with low-fidelity models focused on fundamental orthopaedic procedures. For example, recent publications highlight the use of a simple distal radius fracture cast model for improving both proficiency and safety in closed fracture treatment, cast application, and cast removal.[30,31]

In addition, the implementation of checklists has been an important measure to improve patient safety through error prevention. Most notably, the World Health Organization developed the Surgical Safety Checklist in 2008 as part of the Safe Surgery Saves Lives initiative. The checklist seeks to improve patient safety by promoting communication within surgical teams and minimizing the risk of preventable error. To this end, the checklist provides a list of safety checks to be taken before inducing anesthesia ("sign in"), just before incision ("time out"), and at the conclusion of each procedure ("sign out"). Although compliance with the checklist is still variable, prior investigations have suggested that this simple measure may prevent adverse events and improve patient outcomes.[32,33] Various checklists have been similarly introduced in several orthopaedic subspecialties, including implant arthroplasty, anterior cruciate ligament reconstruction, spine surgery, and hand surgery; future work in pediatric orthopaedics is underway.[16,34-36]

The Safety Culture

Perhaps the most important, yet most challenging and elusive, step toward improving patient safety is to create a culture of safety.[24,37] Pediatric orthopaedic care is a complex and ever-changing field, yet safety cultures have been effectively nurtured in other equally complex industries, such as aviation and manufacturing. Effective individuals and organizations create a culture of safety by (1) acknowledging that errors occur; (2) participating in nonjudgmental mechanisms to identify, understand, and own the root sources of error; (3) recognizing expertise from stakeholders regardless of hierarchy; and (4) embracing changes in practice to minimize errors and potential complications.[38] Prior studies of practicing orthopaedic surgeons have identified that surgeons are concerned about the safety climate in their work environments and are enthusiastic about promoting improved communication and procedural standardization to improve patient safety.[39] These attitudes serve as an important foundation, given the traditional hierarchal structure of surgery and its reliance on autonomous individual providers.

It is critical that this process involve all providers involved in patient care, including the practicing surgeon. Improvement in individual behavior—and a decrease in disruptive behavior—may not only improve team dynamics but also decrease medical error and adverse patient outcomes.[40] Several initiatives have been developed to assist in provider education and training. Team Strategies and Tools to Enhance Performance and Patient Safety (TeamSTEPPS), for example, was developed by the Agency for Healthcare Research and Quality as a comprehensive, evidence-based teamwork system.[41] By providing means for site assessment, team training, implementation, and sustainment of change, TeamSTEPPS can improve team-based behavior and, ultimately, patient safety. Prior application of TeamSTEPPS programs improved perceptions of teamwork and communication and positively influenced clinical performance (for example, nosocomial infection rates and time to successful extracorporeal membrane oxygenation cannulation) in pediatric intensive care units.[42,43] Similar team training may improve patient outcomes and create a sustainable culture of patient safety within pediatric orthopaedics.[44]

Future Directions

Despite widespread efforts to improve patient safety, challenges remain. Some errors, such as wrong-site surgery, seem more refractory to time-outs and other systematic protocols. Systems initiatives that were proven effective in smaller pilot studies have not been appreciated with widespread implementation and generalization. Changing technology, rapidly advancing surgical techniques, organizational silos of healthcare systems, and persistent reliance on individual surgeons to manage patient care likely represent some of the reasons for these challenges. The current reimbursement system in the United States may further add challenges. Providers are typically incentivized and rewarded based on volume, not value. Work is underway to understand variations in compliance with checklists and other safety measures to improve adoption of and adherence to these helpful tools. In addition, continued cultural shifts away from individual autonomy and toward collaborative systems are needed to maximize patient care and safety.

Value

For decades, healthcare expenditures in the United States and other developed countries have steadily risen. In the United States, healthcare costs have increased at a greater rate than the economy as a whole for 31 of the past 40 years and now constitute 17.4% of the gross domestic product.[45] This percentage is expected to reach 19.6% by 2024.[45] When considering regional variation in healthcare utilization and costs and also comparing healthcare delivery in other developed counties, it appears that $750 billion in healthcare expenditures are annually wasted in the United States.[46,47]

Health economists have suggested that competition of the wrong type is responsible for this staggering level of waste in the US healthcare system.[48] In healthy competitive markets, motivation to improve efficiency and quality generally results in productive innovation, improved service, and decreased costs. However, in the current healthcare economy, competition occurs at the wrong level and has a poor focus.[48] In this market, costs continue to rise without concomitant improvements in quality. Leading health economists have suggested that competition within the US healthcare sector is a "zero-sum" game, where value is divided through cost shifting between patients, payers, and providers. Cost shifting increases administrative expenses without net cost reduction or value creation. Value-based competition is lacking in the United States.

How Do We Define and Measure Value?

Value is defined as "the health outcomes achieved per dollar spent" to achieve those outcomes.[6] Most thought leaders emphasize that the health outcomes of interest to patients include both the quality of health care plus patient and family satisfaction. The value of health care is represented by the equation: *value = health outcomes + patient satisfaction/cost.*

One of the most difficult challenges in creating value-based competition is measuring value. Outcomes can be measured by a wide variety of quality metrics (patient-related outcome measures, function, and safety), and satisfaction can be measured by a wide variety of service metrics (patient satisfaction, convenience, timeliness, and communication). Although less attention has historically been paid to measuring cost, costs have received increasing scrutiny given the apparent deficiency of financial sophistication in many healthcare provider organizations. An investigation in 2013 demonstrated that only 10% to 45% of provider organizations could provide patients with cost estimates for a common orthopaedic surgical procedure such as total hip arthroplasty.[49]

How Do We Measure Patient Outcomes?

Patient-reported outcomes are important for assessing patient satisfaction and clinical outcomes. Most investigations suggest that self-assessed pain and function are closely associated with patient satisfaction. Some patient-reported outcome measures are generic and appropriate for use in a wide variety of conditions (for example, the Pediatric Quality of Life Inventory and the Child Health Questionnaire). Other patient-reported outcome measures are disease specific and focus on symptoms or side effects of a specific set of diseases, conditions, or treatments (for example, the Pediatric Outcomes Data Collection Instrument and the Scoliosis Research Society Questionnaire). Disease-specific patient-reported outcome measures tend to be more sensitive to treatment-related changes and may offer advantages when attempting to precisely measure healthcare value.[50]

The advent of computer adaptive testing appears to offer major advantages in determining patient-centered outcomes and satisfaction. The National Institutes of Health has funded the development of the Patient-Reported Outcomes Measurement Information System (PROMIS), a well-used set of computer-adaptive patient-reported outcome measures. PROMIS is a system of highly reliable, valid, flexible, precise, and responsive assessment tools that measure patient-reported health status. The use of PROMIS has increased in the measurement of musculoskeletal health outcomes. In 2014, researchers demonstrated that computerized adaptive testing using the PROMIS physical function item bank reduced testing burden and had a lower ceiling effect compared with a nonadaptive patient-reported outcome measure.[51] Several PROMIS physical function item banks have been validated for use in children.[52]

How Do We Measure Costs?

Most healthcare provider organizations measure costs using a cost-to-charge ratio or a relative value unit (RVU). In a cost-to-charge methodology, cost is estimated by multiplying charges set by the hospital charge master, which is a listing of every single procedure that a hospital can provide to its patients, by the cost-to-charge ratio. This type of methodology incorrectly assumes that each type of service consumes indirect costs in the same proportion; it tends to overallocate costs to some services and underallocate costs to others.

An RVU methodology can theoretically generate refined cost estimates. RVUs are estimates of the relative time, complexity, and value of a service; they are used to more accurately allocate costs to individual procedures and activities. In theory, RVUs can accurately reflect real costs; however, in practice, the allocation methodologies tend to be imprecise. This lack of granularity often leads to unintended cost distortions. It may be possible to improve cost estimates using RVUs with rigorous methodology.

These cost-measurement approaches have obscured value in health care and have led to cost reduction efforts that are incremental, ineffective, and occasionally counterproductive. Most healthcare organizations measure and accumulate costs according to departments, physician specialties, or discrete service lines—a reflection of internal organization and the financing of care. Costs, like outcomes, should instead be measured according to the patient and distributed across the entire care cycle. This type of cost accounting methodology could enable truly structural cost reduction by eliminating non–value-added services, improving capacity utilization, shortening cycle times, providing services in more efficient settings, and so forth.

In 2004, a new accounting technique, time-driven activity-based costing (TDABC), was introduced and has since gained popularity in leading healthcare organizations.[53,54] TDABC assigns costs based on the specific resource time each service or product requires and the unit cost of supplying capacity (labor, equipment, space): *resource cost = cost rate × time*. The total cost is the sum of each resource cost: $(\text{cost rate}_A \times \text{time}_A) + (\text{cost rate}_B \times \text{time}_B)$ and so on.

Recent data suggest that TDABC may more accurately reflect costs in orthopaedic surgery than cost-to-charge or RVU methodologies.[55] An investigation published in 2016 suggests that traditional accounting systems that use cost-to-charge or RVU methodologies may overestimate costs associated with many surgical procedures. TDABC appears to provide the granularity required to identify cost-reduction and value-improvement strategies.[54]

The measurement of value is the first step in improving value delivery in health care. Organizations that are able to precisely measure value, effectively eliminate practice pattern variations, and establish efficient clinical pathways will be best positioned to survive ongoing payment reform (for example, pay for performance, payment bundling, and accountable care organizations). The American Academy of Orthopaedic Surgeons has advocated the use of evidence-based clinical practice guidelines, which are systematically developed statements designed to support provider decision making in specific clinical scenarios. Such guidelines are based on available scientific evidence and attempt to reduce practice pattern variations and improve patient outcomes.

Standardized clinical assessment and management plans (SCAMPs) represent a promising adjunct to clinical practice guidelines.[56] A SCAMP is a flexible guideline that is designed to reduce practice variability while still permitting physicians the opportunity to exercise clinical judgment and offer treatment that is specific to a patient's clinical situation or personal preferences. SCAMP pathways are designed as decision trees that provide guidance based on the particular clinical scenario, such that management is individualized to the specific condition and patient. The first SCAMPs were developed and implemented at Boston Children's Hospital in 2009. Many features of SCAMPs are similar to the evidence-based care process models developed at the Intermountain Healthcare System in Utah.[57] In concept, either SCAMPS or evidence-based care process models could be seamlessly shared across provider organizations, resulting in rapid dissemination of actionable information. The transferability of these decision-support tools could permit provider organizations not initially involved in the design or implementation to rapidly reduce variation and create value.

Summary

To improve value in pediatric orthopaedic surgery, there must be increased focus on improving outcomes and containing expenditures. Continuous quality measurement and rapid process change are critical aspects of any value improvement model. Although great challenges exist in outcome measurement, cost measurement, and the sharing of best practices across provider organizations, medical organizations, including POSNA, have taken a leadership role in uniting efforts across provider organizations.

Key Study Points

- Quality in orthopaedic surgery often refers to process measures, patient-reported outcomes, patient experience, or patient safety measures.
- Quality improvement is a data-driven process using methods such as the Model for Improvement, Lean methodology, or Six Sigma to improve care in a particular setting.
- Patient safety is at the core of quality in health care, and activities such as the use of checklists, surgical simulation, and creating a safety culture are examples of methods to prevent harm and reduce errors.
- Value, although difficult to measure, is best thought of as a patient outcome or level of satisfaction achieved per unit of money spent to achieve said outcome.

Annotated References

1. Kohn LT, Corrigan J, Donaldson MS: *To Err Is Human: Building a Safer Health System* .Washington, DC, National Academy Press, 2000.

2. Institute of Medicine (U.S.): *Committee on Quality of Health Care in America: Crossing the Quality Chasm: A New Health System for the 21st Century* .Washington, DC, National Academy Press, 2001.

3. Glotzbecker MP, Wang K, Waters PM, et al: Quality, safety, and value in pediatric orthopaedic surgery. *J Pediatr Orthop* 2015; August 29 [Epub ahead of print].

   The authors reflect on the POSNA Quality, Safety, and Value Initiative by defining quality, safety, and value; describing how they are measured; and discussing the principles of quality improvement. Level of evidence: V.

4. McCarthy JJ, Alessandrini EA, Schoettker PJ: POSNA quality, safety, value initiative 3 years old and growing strong: POSNA precourse 2014. *J Pediatr Orthop* 2015;35(5suppl 1):S5-S8.

   The difference between traditional research techniques and quality improvement techniques are discussed. Current efforts, projects, and directions for the POSNA Quality, Safety, and Value Initiative also are presented. Level of evidence: V.

5. Waters PM, Flynn JM: POSNA Quality Safety Value Initiative: From vision to implementation to early results. *J Pediatr Orthop* 2015;35(5 suppl 1):S43-S44.

The authors review POSNA's Quality, Safety, and Value Initiative and the details and implementation of its mission statement. Level of evidence: V.

6. Porter ME: What is value in health care? *N Engl J Med* 2010;363(26):2477-2481.

7. Shore BJ, Murphy RF, Hogue GD: Quality, safety, value: From theory to practice management what should we measure? *J Pediatr Orthop* 2015;35(5suppl 1):S61-S66.

   The current state of patient-reported outcome measures within pediatric orthopaedics as it relates to value, cost, and outcomes is presented. Specific examples of both general pediatric-reported outcome measures and disease-specific outcome measures are discussed, along with a hierarchy of measures. Level of evidence: V.

8. Baily MA, Bottrell M, Lynn J, Jennings B; Hastings Center: The ethics of using QI methods to improve health care quality and safety. *Hastings Cent Rep* 2006;36(4):S1-S40.

9. *Going Lean in health care*: IHI Innovation Series white paper. Cambridge, MA, Institute for Healthcare Improvement, 2005. Available at: https://www.entnet.org/sites/default/files/GoingLeaninHealthCareWhitePaper-3.pdf. Accessed April 15, 2016.

10. Mason SE, Nicolay CR, Darzi A: The use of Lean and Six Sigma methodologies in surgery: A systematic review. *Surgeon* 2015;13(2):91-100.

    This article systematically reviews the literature aimed at exploring the use of Lean and Six Sigma quality improvement methodologies in the outpatient and perioperative periods and inpatient surgical settings. Level of evidence: III.

11. Liberatore MJ: Six Sigma in healthcare delivery. *Int J Health Care Qual Assur* 2013;26(7):601-626.

    The author comprehensively reviews and assesses the Six Sigma healthcare literature, focusing on application, process changes initiated, and outcomes, including improvements in process metrics, cost, and revenue. Level of evidence: III.

12. Cima RR, Brown MJ, Hebl JR, et al: Use of Lean and Six Sigma methodology to improve operating room efficiency in a high-volume tertiary-care academic medical center. *J Am Coll Surg* 2011;213(1):83-92, discussion 93-94.

    The Mayo Clinic experience with the use of Lean and Six Sigma methodologies is outlined. Improved efficiency and financial performance across the clinic's operating rooms was shown. Level of evidence: III.

13. Langley GJ: *The Improvement Guide: A Practical Approach to Enhancing Organizational Performance* ,ed 2. San Francisco, CA, Jossey-Bass, 2009, pp 13-25.

14. Shore BJ, Hutchinson S, Harris M, et al: Epidemiology and prevention of cast saw injuries: Results of a quality improvement program at a single institution. *J Bone Joint Surg Am* 2014;96(4):e31.

    The Boston Children's Hospital quality improvement experience with cast saw injuries and the use of an education and training program decreased the prevalence of cast saw injuries. Level of evidence: III.

15. Mueller AJ, Kwon JK, Steiner JW, et al: Improved magnetic resonance imaging utilization for children with musculoskeletal infection. *J Bone Joint Surg Am* 2015;97(22):1869-1876.

    Diagnostic efficiency, therapeutic consistency, and patient safety related to MRI use in pediatric patients with musculoskeletal infection improved across time with the implementation of multidisciplinary guidelines and continuous process improvement methodology. Level of evidence: III.

16. Vitale MG, Riedel MD, Glotzbecker MP, et al: Building consensus: Development of a best practice guideline (BPG) for surgical site infection (SSI) prevention in high-risk pediatric spine surgery. *J Pediatr Orthop* 2013;33(5):471-478.

    This consensus-based best practice guideline has 14 recommendations for the prevention of surgical site infections in high-risk pediatric patients undergoing spine surgery. Level of evidence: V.

17. Healey T, El-Othmani MM, Healey J, Peterson TC, Saleh KJ: Improving operating room efficiency, part 1: General managerial and preoperative strategies. *JBJS Rev* 2015;3(10):e3.

    The use of quality improvement methodology and checklists are two examples of general managerial strategies for improving operating room efficiency. Optimizing patient safety and complication prevention, scheduling and allocating operating room time, reducing preoperative delays, and improving operating room start times are all examples of strategies for improving operating room efficiency.

18. Healey T, Peterson TC, Healey J, El-Othmani MM, Saleh KJ: Improving operating room efficiency, part 2: Intraoperative and postoperative strategies. *JBJS Rev* 2015;3(10):e4.

    Intraoperative and postoperative strategies for improving operating room efficiency, including perioperative briefings and the concept of parallel processing, are discussed.

19. Vitale MG, Skaggs DL, Pace GI, et al: Best practices in intraoperative neuromonitoring in spine deformity surgery: Development of an intraoperative checklist to optimize response. *Spine Deform* 2014;2(5):333-339.

    This article presents a consensus-based best practice guideline and intraoperative checklist for neuromonitoring alerts during spine surgery. Level of evidence: V.

20. Black KP, Armstrong AD, Hutzler L, Egol KA: Quality and safety in orthopaedics: Learning and teaching at the same time. AOA critical issues. *J Bone Joint Surg Am* 2015;97(21):1809-1815.

    Resident education within the areas of quality and safety are essential for both current and future residents. Scale and knowledge acquisition in these domains is the responsibility of academic leaders of accredited orthopaedic surgery residency programs.

21. Bumpass DB, Samora JB, Butler CA, Jevsevar DS, Moffatt-Bruce SD, Bozic KJ: Orthopaedic quality reporting: A comprehensive review of the current landscape and a roadmap for progress. *JBJS Rev* 2014;2(8):e5.

    The complex landscape of healthcare quality measures is summarized in this overview of key public and private stakeholders guiding the measurement and reporting of healthcare quality.

22. Kennedy A, Bakir C, Brauer CA: Quality indicators in pediatric orthopaedic surgery: A systematic review. *Clin Orthop Relat Res* 2012;470(4):1124-1132.

    This article presents the most commonly reported quality indicators in pediatric orthopaedic surgery, including mortality, reoperation rates, readmission rates, and various patient-centered quality indicators. Level of evidence: III.

23. Porter ME, Larsson S, Lee TH: Standardizing patient outcomes measurement. *N Engl J Med* 2016;374(6):504-506.

    This article presents the International Consortium for Health Outcomes Measurement working group approach to the standardization of outcomes measures.

24. Leape LL: Patient safety in the era of healthcare reform. *Clin Orthop Relat Res* 2015;473(5):1568-1573.

    A recognized leader in the field of patient safety, the author provides his perspective on the barriers to safe patient care, as well as steps the individual orthopaedic surgeon can take to improve the culture of safety. Level of evidence: V.

25. Bae DS: Simulation in pediatric orthopaedic surgery. *J Pediatr Orthop* 2015;35(5 suppl 1):S26-S29.

    The current state of simulation training in pediatric orthopaedic surgery is described in this recent review article. Level of evidence: V.

26. Rambani R, Ward J, Viant W: Desktop-based computer-assisted orthopedic training system for spinal surgery. *J Surg Educ* 2014;71(6):805-809.

    Training with a simulated computer-navigation system improved time-to-task completion and accuracy in this study of pedicle screw insertion. Level of evidence: II.

27. Howells NR, Gill HS, Carr AJ, Price AJ, Rees JL: Transferring simulated arthroscopic skills to the operating theatre: A randomised blinded study. *J Bone Joint Surg Br* 2008;90(4):494-499.

28. Butler A, Olson T, Koehler R, Nicandri G: Do the skills acquired by novice surgeons using anatomic dry models transfer effectively to the task of diagnostic knee arthroscopy performed on cadaveric specimens? *J Bone Joint Surg Am* 2013;95(3):e15(1-8).

    Surgical trainees who were first trained on dry knee models performed better than those who did not have any prior simulated training on a cadaver knee arthroscopy model. Level of evidence: II.

29. Gottschalk MB, Yoon ST, Park DK, Rhee JM, Mitchell PM: Surgical training using three-dimensional simulation in placement of cervical lateral mass screws: A blinded randomized control trial. *Spine J* 2015;15(1):168-175.

    Simulated lateral cervical mass screw placement improved performance and safety in cadaver models compared with those trainees who did not have additional simulation training. Level of evidence: II.

30. Moktar J, Popkin CA, Howard A, Murnaghan ML: Development of a cast application simulator and evaluation of objective measures of performance. *J Bone Joint Surg Am* 2014;96(9):e76.

    The authors describe a casting simulation model and performance measurement instrument that has high reliability and validity for short-arm cast application in orthopaedic providers of varying experience. Level of evidence: II.

31. Brubacher JW, Karg J, Weinstock P, Bae DS: A novel cast removal training simulation to improve patient safety. *J Surg Educ* 2016;73(1):7-11.

    A novel simulation model is presented to assess competency and enhance performance in cast application and removal, with an emphasis on monitoring temperatures during cast saw use. Level of evidence: II.

32. Panesar SS, Noble DJ, Mirza SB, et al: Can the surgical checklist reduce the risk of wrong site surgery in orthopaedics? Can the checklist help? Supporting evidence from analysis of a national patient incident reporting system. *J Orthop Surg Res* 2011;6:18.

    A review of 133 actual or near-miss wrong-site surgeries identified in the National Reporting and Learning Service database revealed that using the World Health Association Surgical Safety Checklist could have prevented approximately 20% of the wrong-site procedures. Level of evidence: IV.

33. Patel J, Ahmed K, Guru KA, et al: An overview of the use and implementation of checklists in surgical specialties: A systematic review. *Int J Surg* 2014;12(12):1317-1323.

    In a systematic review of 16 studies, use of the World Health Association Surgical Safety Checklist resulted in substantial improvements in patient outcomes across surgical subspecialties. Level of evidence: III.

34. van Eck CF, Gravare-Silbernagel K, Samuelsson K, et al: Evidence to support the interpretation and use of the Anatomic Anterior Cruciate Ligament Reconstruction Checklist. *J Bone Joint Surg Am* 2013;95(20):e153.

    A checklist for surgical anterior cruciate ligament reconstruction was developed; preliminary testing of its reliability, validity, and consistency was performed. Level of evidence: II.

1: General

35. Rosenberg AD, Wambold D, Kraemer L, et al: Ensuring appropriate timing of antimicrobial prophylaxis. *J Bone Joint Surg Am* 2008;90(2):226-232.

36. Cobb TK: Wrong site surgery: Where are we and what is the next step? *Hand (N Y)* 2012;7(2):229-232.

    The author presents a review of universal protocol and advocates for additional measures to avoid wrong-site surgery.

37. Morello RT, Lowthian JA, Barker AL, McGinnes R, Dunt D, Brand C: Strategies for improving patient safety culture in hospitals: A systematic review. *BMJ Qual Saf* 2013;22(1):11-18.

    The authors present a systematic review of 21 studies and point to evidence regarding the efficacy of leadership "walk-arounds" and unit-based programs in improving a culture of patient safety. Level of evidence: III.

38. Weick KE, Sutcliffe KM: Managing the Unexpected: Assuring High Performance in an Age of Complexity. University of Michigan Business School management series. San Francisco, CA, Jossey-Bass, 2001.

39. Janssen SJ, Teunis T, Guitton TG, Ring D, Herndon JH: Orthopaedic surgeons' view on strategies for improving patient safety. *J Bone Joint Surg Am* 2015;97(14):1173-1186.

    In surveys of members of the Science of Variation Group and Ankle Platform, 18% of responses implied a lack of a climate of patient safety. Despite these concerning findings, a high rate of enthusiasm exists for improving communication, standardization, and safety.

40. Rosenstein AH, O'Daniel M: A survey of the impact of disruptive behaviors and communication defects on patient safety. *Jt Comm J Qual Patient Saf* 2008;34(8):464-471.

41. TeamSTEPPS: Strategies and Tools to Enhance Performance and Patient Safety. September 2015. Agency for Healthcare Research and Quality. Available at: http://www.ahrq.gov/professionals/education/curriculum-tools/teamstepps/index.html.Accessed April 14, 2016.

    This website presents a comprehensive set of ready-to-use materials and a training curriculum to successfully integrate teamwork principles to enhance performance and patient safety.

42. Mayer CM, Cluff L, Lin WT, et al: Evaluating efforts to optimize TeamSTEPPS implementation in surgical and pediatric intensive care units. *Jt Comm J Qual Patient Saf* 2011;37(8):365-374.

    After a 2.5-hour TeamSTEPPS training program was provided to intensive care unit staff, observed team performance improved in areas of time for extracorporeal membrane oxygenation cannulation placement and response time for code teams. The rate of nosocomial infections remained below the upper control limit for 7 of the 8 months after training. Level of evidence: II.

43. Brodsky D, Gupta M, Quinn M, et al: Building collaborative teams in neonatal intensive care. *BMJ Qual Saf* 2013;22(5):374-382.

    A multidisciplinary TeamSTEPPS workshop resulted in improved communication, situational awareness, support, and satisfaction among providers in a neonatal intensive care unit. Level of evidence: II.

44. Weaver SJ, Dy SM, Rosen MA: Team-training in healthcare: A narrative synthesis of the literature. *BMJ Qual Saf* 2014;23(5):359-372.

    The authors reviewed the literature on team-training interventions in acute care settings. The literature suggests that team training results in improved healthcare team processes and patient outcomes. Level of evidence: V.

45. Keehan SP, Cuckler GA, Sisko AM, et al: National health expenditure projections, 2014-24: Spending growth faster than recent trends. *Health Aff (Millwood)* 2015;34(8):1407-1417.

    This article projects anticipated growth in healthcare expenditures in the United States from 2014 to 2024 at 5.8%, reflecting the Affordable Care Act's coverage expansions, faster economic growth, and population aging. It describes the health sector's share of the US gross domestic product (17.4% in 2013, projected at 19.6% in 2024). Level of evidence: IV.

46. Farrell DJ, Kocher B, Lovegrove N, Melhem F, Mendonca L, Parish B: *Accounting for the Cost of US Health Care: A New Look at Why Americans Spend More* .Washington, DC, McKinsey Global Institute, 2008.

47. Wennberg JE, Fisher ES, Skinner JS: Geography and the debate over Medicare reform. *Health Aff (Millwood)* 2002;(suppl web exclusives):W96-114.

48. Porter ME, Teisberg EO: Redefining competition in health care. *Harv Bus Rev* 2004;82(6):64-76, 136.

49. Rosenthal JA, Lu X, Cram P: Availability of consumer prices from US hospitals for a common surgical procedure. *JAMA Intern Med* 2013;173(6):427-432.

    The authors present the results of a prospective investigation of whether pricing data for a common elective surgical procedure—total hip arthroplasty—could be obtained from 100 randomly selected hospitals across the United States as well as the top 20 hospitals according to the *US News and World Report* rankings. They found it difficult to obtain price information for total hip arthroplasty and observed wide variations in quoted prices.

50. Wiebe S, Guyatt G, Weaver B, Matijevic S, Sidwell C: Comparative responsiveness of generic and specific quality-of-life instruments. *J Clin Epidemiol* 2003;56(1):52-60.

51. Hung M, Stuart AR, Higgins TF, Saltzman CL, Kubiak EN: Computerized adaptive testing using the PROMIS Physical Function Item Bank reduces test burden with less ceiling effects compared with the Short Musculoskeletal

Function Assessment in orthopaedic trauma patients. *J Orthop Trauma* 2014;28(8):439-443.

This article directly compares the Short Musculoskeletal Function Assessment to the PROMIS Physical Function Computer Adaptive Test in orthopaedic trauma patients. The PROMIS test required less than one-tenth the amount of time for patients to complete compared with the Short Musculoskeletal Function Assessment while achieving equally high reliability and lower ceiling effects. Level of evidence: II.

52. Waljee JF, Carlozzi N, Franzblau LE, Zhong L, Chung KC: Applying the Patient-Reported Outcomes Measurement Information System to assess upper extremity function among children with congenital hand differences. *Plast Reconstr Surg* 2015;136(2):200e-207e.

    This article compares the PROMIS Pediatric Upper Extremity item bank to the Pediatric Outcomes Data Collection Instrument; the Michigan Hand Outcomes Questionnaire; and the Disabilities of the Arm, Shoulder and Hand questionnaire in children with congenital hand differences. PROMIS was found to highly correlate with self-reported function and functional assessment in children with congenital hand differences. Level of evidence: II.

53. Kaplan RS, Anderson SR: Time-driven activity-based costing. *Harv Bus Rev* 2004;82(11):131-138, 150.

54. Kaplan RS, Witkowski M, Abbott M, et al: Using time-driven activity-based costing to identify value improvement opportunities in healthcare. *J Healthc Manag* 2014;59(6):399-412.

    This article highlights the use of TDABC to identify value improvement opportunities in several healthcare provider organizations. Level of evidence: III.

55. Akhavan S, Ward L, Bozic KJ: Time-driven activity-based costing more accurately reflects costs in arthroplasty surgery. *Clin Orthop Relat Res* 2016;474(1):8-15.

    This article compares the accuracy of TDABC with traditional accounting techniques in total joint arthroplasty at a single institution. Level of evidence: III.

56. Shah AS, Waters PM, Bozic KJ: Orthopaedic healthcare worldwide: Standardized clinical assessment and management plans. An adjunct to clinical practice guidelines. *Clin Orthop Relat Res* 2015;473(6):1868-1872.

    This article reviews the potential value of SCAMPs by making a direct comparison to clinical practice guidelines. Level of evidence: III.

57. Byington CL, Reynolds CC, Korgenski K, et al: Costs and infant outcomes after implementation of a care process model for febrile infants. *Pediatrics* 2012;130(1):e16-e24.

    The authors review the effect of an evidence-based care process model at Intermountain Healthcare System in Utah on health outcomes and cost in well-appearing febrile infants. Level of evidence: III.

Chapter 2

Evidence-Based Quality and Outcomes Assessment in Pediatric Orthopaedics

Kevin G. Shea, MD Charles T. Mehlman, DO, MPH Robert H. Quinn, MD James T. Beckmann, MD, MS

1: General

Abstract

Evidence-based clinical practice guidelines, appropriate use criteria, outcome measures, and patient-reported outcome measures are critical tools to ensure the best clinical care for patients. These guidelines, criteria, and measures will be increasingly integrated into care pathways.

Keywords: appropriate use criteria (AUC); computerized adaptive testing; evidence-based clinical practice guidelines; outcome measures; Patient Reported Outcome Measurement Information System (PROMIS)

Dr. Shea or an immediate family member serves as an unpaid consultant to Clinical Data Solutions and SourceTrust and serves as a board member, owner, officer, or committee member of the Pediatric Orthopaedic Society of North America, Pediatric Research in Sport Medicine, and Research for Osteochondritis Dissecans of the Knee. Dr. Mehlman or an immediate family member serves as an unpaid consultant to Stryker and serves as a board member, owner, officer, or committee member of the American Academy of Orthopaedic Surgeons, the Pediatric Orthopaedic Society of North America, and the Scoliosis Research Society. Dr. Quinn or an immediate family member has received research or institutional support from the Musculoskeletal Transplant Foundation and serves as a board member, owner, officer, or committee member of American Academy of Orthopaedic Surgeons, the American Orthopaedic Association, the Musculoskeletal Tumor Society and the Wilderness Medical Society. Neither Dr. Beckmann nor any immediate family member has received anything of value from or has stock or stock options held in a commercial company or institution related directly or indirectly to the subject of this chapter.

Introduction

Critical analysis of clinical care can lead to answers to a wide variety of clinical questions.[1-3] Pierre Charles Alexandre Louis, a French physician, applied the numerical method (early biostatistics) and helped end the practice of bloodletting.[4] The teachings and "end result idea" advocated by American surgeon Ernest Amory Codman influenced generations of outcomes researchers and inspired the American College of Surgeons and the Joint Commission for the Accreditation of Healthcare Organizations.[5] Randomized clinical trials and prospective study designs may produce the highest quality/lowest bias evidence; these types of studies, along with other forms of evidence, guide clinical care decisions.

It is important for orthopaedic surgeons to review the use of evidence for clinical care, with an emphasis on evidence-based clinical practice guidelines (CPGs), appropriate use criteria (AUC), and outcome measures, including those from the Patient Reported Outcome Measurement Information System (PROMIS) and computerized adaptive testing.

Clinical Practice Guidelines and Systematic Reviews

The Institute of Medicine has called for the increased use of CPGs to reduce practice variation, improve quality of care, and decrease inefficiencies.[6-8] A CPG is a "systematically developed statement to assist practitioner and patient decisions about appropriate health care for one or more specific clinical circumstances."[7,8]

Historically, guidelines have been based on the consensus of expert groups, but consensus guidelines have several potential limitations: (1) Many guidelines do not consider all evidence; (2) Evidence integration and quality ranking may be flawed; (3) There may be a lack of transparency about conflicts of interest; (4) Results may

Table 1

Institute of Medicine Standards for Evidence-Based Clinical Practice Guidelines

Transparency
Management of conflicts of interest
Composition of the guideline group
Standards for systematic reviews
Establishing evidence foundations for and rating strength of recommendations
Standard form for the articulation of the recommendations
External review
Updating

not be reproducible by other groups. To address these limitations, the American Academy of Orthopaedic Surgeons (AAOS) guidelines are based on a systematic review of the literature and follow a rigorous, transparent, and reproducible methodology that meets all of the Institute of Medicine standards for developing trustworthy guidelines[9] (**Table 1**).

Two groups are required to develop CPGs. Clinical content experts develop patient, intervention, comparison, and outcome (PICO) questions. Experts in the field of evidence analysis review the literature comprehensively, rank the quality and bias of the articles, and ensure that the evidence review is transparent, reproducible, reviewed by others, and updated.

Overview: AAOS Guideline and Systematic Review Process

For topics in which the published evidence contains a broad range of high-level/low-bias evidence, the CPG is an appropriate analysis. In cases in which the published evidence is not as robust to support a full CPG, a systematic review may be the best analysis. The AAOS addresses bias beginning with the selection of CPG and systematic review work group members, who function as the clinical content experts. Applicants with financial conflicts of interest related to the CPG or systematic review topic cannot participate if the conflict occurred within 1 year of the start date of the CPG or systematic review development, or if an immediate family member has a relevant financial conflict. In addition, all CPG or systematic review development group members sign an attestation form agreeing to remain free of relevant financial conflicts for 1 year following the publication of the CPG or the systematic review.

Physician and clinician groups (clinical experts) prepare CPGs and systematic reviews with the assistance of the AAOS Evidence-Based Medicine unit in the Department of Research and Scientific Affairs (expert evidence methodologists). As the physician experts, the CPG or systematic review work group defines the scope of the CPG or systematic review by creating PICO questions that direct the literature search. The medical librarian creates and executes the search(es). The supporting group of expert methodologists reviews all abstracts, reviews pertinent full-text articles, and evaluates the quality of studies meeting the inclusion criteria. They also abstract, analyze, interpret, and summarize the relevant data for each PICO question and prepare the initial draft for the final work group meeting.

After completion of the systematic reviews, physician CPG work groups meet in person to participate in a 3-day meeting to develop the recommendations. To complete their charges, the physician experts and methodologists evaluate and integrate all material to develop the final recommendations. The final recommendations and rationales are edited, written, and voted on. The CPG or systematic research work group may approve additional edits to the rationales via subsequent webinar meetings. The draft CPG or systematic review recommendations and rationales receive final review by the methodologists to ensure consistency with the data. The draft is then completed and submitted for peer review and/or submitted to a musculoskeletal journal for publication.

After peer review and editing, the CPG or systematic review draft is distributed for public commentary. Thereafter, the AAOS Committee on Evidence-Based Quality and Value, AAOS Council on Research and Quality, and the AAOS Board of Directors sequentially approve the draft CPG or systematic review. All AAOS CPGs are reviewed and updated or retired every 5 years in accordance with the criteria of the National Guideline Clearinghouse. The process of AAOS CPG or systematic review development incorporates the benefits from clinical physician expertise and the statistical knowledge and interpretation of methodologists without conflict. The process also includes an extensive review process offering the opportunity for more than 200 clinical physician experts to provide input before publication. This process minimizes bias, enhances transparency, and ensures the highest level of accuracy for interpretation of the evidence.

The language used in the recommendations is based on the quality of the evidence, and a star system is used for ranking the strength of the recommendation (more stars = greater strength; **Table 2**).

The AAOS has developed 18 evidence-based Clinical Practice Guidelines since 2007, and 6 have direct clinical

Table 2

AAOS Clinical Practice Guideline Strength of Recommendation Language

Strength of Recommendation Descriptions

Strength	Overall Strength of Evidence	Description of Evidence Strength	Strength Indication Visual (Star Rating)
Strong	Strong	Evidence from two or more high-strength studies with consistent findings for recommending for or against the intervention.	☆☆☆☆
Moderate	Moderate	Evidence from two or more moderate-strength studies with consistent findings, or evidence from a single high-quality study for recommending for or against the intervention.	☆☆☆
Limited	Low-strength evidence of conflicting evidence	Evidence from two or more low-strength studies with consistent findings or evidence from a single study for recommending for or against the intervention or diagnostic test, or the evidence is insufficient or conflicting and does not allow a recommendation for or against the intervention.	☆☆
Consensus	No evidence	There is no supporting evidence. In the absence of reliable evidence, the work group is making a recommendation based on their clinical opinion. Consensus recommendations can only be created when not establishing a recommendation could have catastrophic consequences.	☆

AAOS = American Academy of Orthopaedic Surgeons

Reproduced from the American Academy of Orthopaedic Surgeons: *Clinical Practice Guidelines*. Rosemont, IL, American Academy of Orthopaedic Surgeons, 2016. http://www.aaos.org/cpg/?ssopc=1.

applicability to pediatric and adolescent care (**Table 3**). These guidelines can be accessed through the OrthoGuidelines website; a free mobile application is available.[10]

Appropriate Use Criteria

The randomized clinical trial serves as the gold standard for clinical research, but these trials are complicated, expensive, and time- and labor-intensive. Because they are performed under ideal circumstances, the results are not always generalizable. In many technical fields, including orthopaedic surgery, randomized clinical trials are complex (thereby limiting their construction and recruitment), may not have broad external applicability, or simply are not available. CPGs rely on higher-level evidence, but in many fields, that higher-level evidence may be lacking. In areas in which the evidence base is less robust, AUC may be especially valuable. In 1986, a method was introduced for the detailed assessment of the appropriateness of medical technologies based on the concept that synthesizing expert medical opinion could simultaneously incorporate the knowledge gained from randomized clinical trials with that of clinical experience.[11] Expert panels were asked to rate the appropriateness of different interventions where "appropriate was defined to mean that the expected health benefit (that is, increased life expectancy, relief of pain, reduction in anxiety, improved functional capacity)...exceeded the expected negative consequences (that is, mortality, morbidity, anxiety of anticipating the procedure, pain produced by the procedure, time lost from work) by a sufficiently wide margin that the procedure was worth doing [exclusive of cost]." This early concept developed into the RAND/UCLA Appropriateness Method, which was developed by the RAND corporation and clinicians at the University of California at Los Angeles as an instrument primarily designed to measure the overuse and underuse of medical and surgical procedures.[12,13]

Table 3

Published AAOS Clinical Practice Guidelines

Achilles Tendon Rupture	Osteoarthritis of the Knee (Arthroplasty/Surgical Management)
Anterior Cruciate Ligament Injuries[a]	Osteochondritis Dissecans[a]
Carpal Tunnel Syndrome: Diagnosis	Pediatric Developmental Dysplasia of the Hip in Infants up to Six Months of Age: Detection and Management[a]
Carpal Tunnel Syndrome: Treatment	Pediatric Diaphyseal Femur Fractures[a]
Distal Radius Fractures	Pediatric Supracondylar Humerus Fractures[a]
Glenohumeral Joint Arthritis	Periprosthetic Joint Infections
Hip Fractures in the Elderly	Rotator Cuff Problems
Orthopaedic Implant Infection in Patients Undergoing Dental Procedures: Prevention[a]	Symptomatic Osteoporotic Spinal Compression Fractures
Osteoarthritis of the Knee (Non-arthroplasty)	Venous Thromboembolic Disease: Prevention

AAOS = American Academy of Orthopaedic Surgeons

[a] Guideline is applicable to pediatric and adolescent care.

Reproduced from the American Academy of Orthopaedic Surgeons: *Clinical Practice Guidelines*. Rosemont, IL, American Academy of Orthopaedic Surgeons, 2016. http://www.aaos.org/cpg/?ssopc=1.

Whereas a CPG indicates, based on best evidence, if a given intervention is associated with a desirable outcome, the AUC indicates when (that is, in what specific clinical situation) the same intervention is best applied. The purpose of the AUC is to help determine the appropriateness of CPG recommendations for the heterogeneous patient populations routinely seen in practice. The best available scientific evidence is synthesized with collective expert opinion on topics where gold standard, randomized clinical trials are not available or are inadequately detailed for identifying distinct patient types. When there is evidence corroborated by consensus that expected benefits substantially outweigh potential risks, exclusive of cost, a procedure is determined to be appropriate. The AAOS uses the RAND/UCLA Appropriateness Method. The process includes the following steps: reviewing the results of the evidence analysis, compiling a list of clinical vignettes, and having an expert panel composed of representatives from multiple medical specialties determine the appropriateness of each of the clinical indications for treatment; classification is stratified as appropriate, may be appropriate, or is rarely appropriate.

In 2014, the AAOS completed and published two AUC documents relevant to pediatric orthopaedic surgery: one addressing the management of pediatric supracondylar humerus fractures[14] and one on pediatric supracondylar fractures with vascular injury.[15] These follow the CPG on the treatment of pediatric supracondylar humerus fractures published by the AAOS in 2011.[16]

In developing an AAOS AUC document (and in keeping with the RAND/UCLA Appropriateness Method), the AAOS first assembles a writing panel made up of orthopaedic specialists who have expertise in treating the specific condition. The panel follows the following guiding principles: Patient scenarios must include a broad spectrum of patients who may be eligible for treatment of pediatric supracondylar humerus fractures (comprehensive). Patient indications must classify patients into a unique scenario (mutually exclusive). Patient indications must consistently classify similar patients into the same scenario (reliable, valid indicators).

The writing panel develops the scenarios by categorizing patients in terms of indications evident during the clinical decision-making process. These scenarios rely on definitions and general assumptions, mutually agreed on by the writing panel during the development of the scenarios. These definitions and assumptions are necessary to provide consistency in the interpretation of the clinical scenarios among experts voting on the scenarios and readers using the final criteria. The writing panel then organizes these indications into a matrix of clinical scenarios that address all combinations of the classifications.

When the work of the writing panel is completed, a separate independent voting panel is formed, composed of approximately 50% specialists and 50% nonspecialists (a

Table 4

Interpreting the Nine-Point Appropriateness Scale

Rating	Explanation
7-9	**Appropriate:** Appropriate for the indication provided, meaning treatment is generally acceptable and is a reasonable approach for the indication and is likely to improve the patient's health outcome or survival.
4-6	**May Be Appropriate:** Uncertain for the indication provided, meaning treatment may be acceptable and may be a reasonable approach for the indication, but with uncertainty implying that more research and/or patient information is needed to further classify the indication.
1-3	**Rarely Appropriate:** Rarely an appropriate option for management of patients in this population because of the lack of a clear benefit/risk advantage; rarely an effective option for individual care plans; exceptions should have documentation of the clinical reasons for proceeding with this care option (that is, procedure is not generally acceptable and is not generally reasonable for the indication).

Reproduced from the American Academy of Orthopaedic Surgeons: *Clinical Practice Guidelines*. Rosemont, IL, American Academy of Orthopaedic Surgeons, 2016. http://www.aaos.org/cpg/?ssopc=1.

Table 5

Defining Agreement and Disagreement for Appropriateness Ratings

	Disagreement	Agreement
Panel size	Number of panelists rating in each extreme (1-3 and 7-9)	Number of panelists rating outside the three-point region containing the median (1-3, 4-6, 7-9)
8, 9, 10	≥3	≤2
11, 12, 13	≥4	≤3
14, 15, 16	≥5	≤4

Reproduced from the American Academy of Orthopaedic Surgeons: *Appropriate Use Criteria*. Rosemont, IL, American Academy of Orthopaedic Surgeons. Accessed Dec., 2015. http://www.aaos.org/Quality/Appropriate_Use_Criteria_(AUC)/Appropriate_Use_Criteria/.

specialist is defined as an orthopaedic surgeon who treats the condition addressed in the AUC that is under study). The panel uses a modified Delphi process to determine appropriateness ratings. The objective of this process is not to force consensus, but rather to determine whether discrepancies in the ratings are the result of actual clinical disagreement over the use of a procedure. The appropriateness of each scenario is rated as shown in **Table 4**. Following the final (second) round of voting, the final levels of appropriateness are determined as shown in **Tables 5** and **6**. Web-based AUC applications are available at the AAOS website. An example of the AUC application for pediatric supracondylar humerus fractures[17] is shown in **Figure 1**. The RAND/UCLA Appropriateness Method has now been used and studied in many procedural disciplines beyond orthopaedic surgery and found to be reliable.

Outcomes Assessment

Outcomes assessment is important.[18] Ernest Codman is often referred to as the father of outcomes research because of his common-sense notion that every hospital should follow every patient it treats long enough to determine whether or not the treatment has been successful. If treatment is unsuccessful, Codman advocated that the reason for the failure should be determined to preventing similar failures in the future.[19] Modern outcomes assessment in pediatric orthopaedics is dependent on the interrelated concepts of validity (measuring what we intend to measure), reliability (measuring it in a reproducible fashion), responsiveness to change (detecting true improvement or worsening), and minimum clinically important difference (MCID; measuring differences that are important to patients and parents).[20] Collectively, these traits of outcome instruments are referred to as psychometrics or psychometric properties. These same principles apply to both traditional clinician measured parameters (for example, radiographic angles, joint range of motion) and patient-generated measures (both general and disease-specific, health-related quality-of-life instruments).

Validity has several dimensions that must be considered.[21] The simplest is face validity, which amounts to passing the so-called "sniff test" or "duck test." For example, using the Scoliosis Research Society (SRS)-22 questionnaire as the main outcome measure for a study of pediatric phalangeal neck fractures has no face validity.

Content validity relates to the fact that questions or measurements pertinent to the thing being assessed are appropriately included. The content validity of the Early Onset Scoliosis Questionnaire was established via a process that created questions based on recorded interviews focusing on factors that are important to parents.[22]

1: General

Table 6

Interpreting Final Ratings of Criteria

Level of Appropriateness	Description
Appropriate	Median panel rating between 7-9 and no disagreement
May be appropriate	Median panel rating between 4-6 or Median panel rating 1-9 with disagreement
Rarely appropriate	Median panel rating between 1-3 and no disagreement

Adapted from Fitch K, Bernstein SJ, Aguilar MD: *The Rand/UCLA Appropriateness Method User's Manual.* Santa Monica, CA, The Rand Corporation, 2001.

Construct validity refers to how consistent the new test or questionnaire seems to be when compared with existing tools that measure similar things. When the Muscular Dystrophy Spine Questionnaire was being developed, its construct validity was established by comparing it to two other established instruments (the Activity Scale for Kids and the Pediatric Outcome Data Collection Questionnaire).[23]

Criterion validity relates specifically to how well the new measure correlates with an established gold standard (if one exists). In a recent study of a new shoulder instability scale, the authors tested its criterion validity by comparing it to the Rowe anterior shoulder instability scale.[24]

The types of reliability commonly assessed are interrater reliability (two or more raters) and intrarater reliability (the same rater on different occasions).[25] Moreover, these types of reliability may involve either continuous or categoric variables. The key aspect of statistical methods aimed at assessing reliability is that they control for chance agreement. The intraclass correlation coefficient (ICC) is most commonly used for continuous variables, whereas the kappa coefficient (also known as the Cohen kappa) is usually used for categoric variables.[26] Interpretation of reliability data is similarly dictated by the type of data being analyzed (**Tables** 7 and 8).

The concept of responsiveness to change relates to whether the measuring instrument is appropriately able to detect improvement or worsening after a treatment intervention. Ceiling and floor effects play an important role in the responsiveness of a questionnaire. An example of the ceiling effect is when all students taking an examination get an "A" because the test was too easy. An example of the floor effect is when another group of students all get an "F" because the test was too hard. It may seem obvious to clinicians, but it also has been shown that retrospective methods of evaluating responsiveness to change are of little value because they consistently provide overestimates.[27] Responsiveness to change is directly related to effect size.[28]

Effect size refers to the inherent difference in statistically significant and clinically significant outcomes.[29,30] Estimates of the proportion of patients benefiting from a treatment based on effect size and so-called anchor-based approaches such as the MCID have been shown to perform equivalently.[31] The MCID (also known as a minimum important difference) is attractive because it reflects the importance of the patient.[32,33] When the MCID following scoliosis surgery (as measured by the SRS-22 questionnaire) was assessed, there was a large change in the appearance domain, but minimal change (within measurement error) was noted in the activity domain.[34] It is important to keep in mind that some trials may demonstrate a statistically significant difference in treatment outcome, but the difference may not be meaningful or perceptible to patients. Designing studies to assess MCID insures outcomes are meaningful to patients.

A growing number of orthopaedic researchers are improving instrument development using Rasch analysis. These analytic methods have been applied in a wide variety of fields besides health care, including education, psychology, marketing, and economics.[35] Rasch analysis is a form of item response theory that mathematically models question difficulty and examiner aptitude. Recently, the Pediatric Outcomes Data Collection Instrument was subjected to Rasch analysis for cerebral palsy patients with Gross Motor Function Classification System levels 1 through 3. This process identified several redundant items as well as ceiling effect in all domains except the sports/physical function domain.[35]

Patient Outcomes: PROMIS, Computerized Adaptive Testing

The National Institutes of Health has funded the development of PROMIS to address deficiencies associated with legacy instruments. The PROMIS marks a new paradigm for measuring patient-reported outcomes that is made possible through computerized adaptive testing. Instead of administering a fixed set of questions that are indivisibly validated (classic test theory),[36] computerized adaptive testing uses computer algorithms to dynamically administer only the most informative questions based on that individual's previous responses from a large question bank until a prespecified level of precision is met. This method paradoxically allows for maximal measurement precision through the fewest possible number

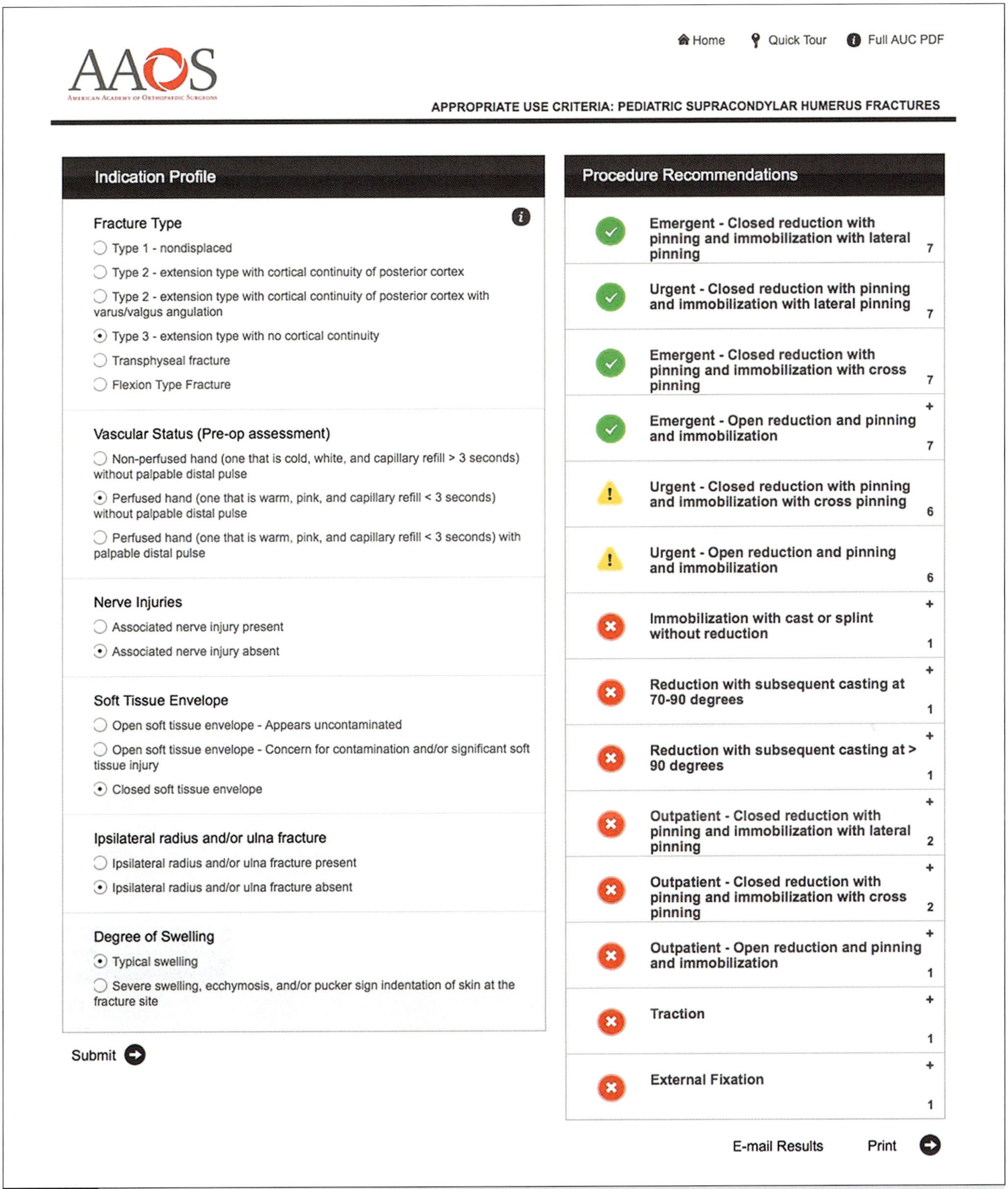

Figure 1 Image shows an example of the AAOS Appropriate Use Criteria for pediatric supracondylar humerus fractures. (Reproduced from the American Academy of Orthopaedic Surgeons: *Appropriate Use Criteria on Pediatric Supracondylar Humerus Fractures: Treatment.* Rosemont, IL, American Academy of Orthopaedic Surgeons, 2012. http://www.aaos.org/Quality/Appropriate_Use_Criteria_(AUC)/Appropriate_Use_Criteria/.)

Table 7

Fleiss Criteria (Typically Used for Continuous Variables)

ICC ≥ 0.75 = excellent

ICC ≥ 0.40 and <0.75 = fair to good

ICC <0.40 = poor

ICC = intraclass correlation coefficient

Adapted with permission from Fleiss J, Levin B, Paik MC: *Statistical Methods for Rates and Proportions*, ed 2. New York, NY, 1981, pp 1-800.

Table 8

Criteria of Landis and Koch (Typically Used for Categoric Variables)

<0 = less than chance agreement

0.01 to 0.20 = slight agreement

0.21 to 0.40 = fair agreement

0.41 to 0.60 = moderate agreement

0.61 to 0.80 = substantial agreement

0.81 to 0.99 = almost perfect agreement

Adapted with permission from Landis JR, Koch GC: The measurement of observer agreement for categorical data. *Biometrics* 1977;33(1):159-174.

of administered questions (typically only 3 to 5 per domain).[37,38] Pediatric-specific question banks are available for various domains, including physical function, pain, anxiety, and depression.[39]

Reported benefits of computerized adaptive testing include reduced completion time that lowers the responder burden of the patient;[40,41] increases measurement precision with reduction of ceiling and floor effects;[42-44] and has the ability to add or subtract questions from the item bank without the need to re-create and validate an entirely new scale. The psychometric properties of computerized adaptive testing have outperformed legacy scales in adult orthopaedic patients.[40,42,43,45,46] Studies consistently show high correlation between the PROMIS and traditional instruments, but the PROMIS has increased reliability, decreased test length, and less unexplained variance in baseline studies. However, the responsiveness, or the ability of the PROMIS to detect change after treatment, has not been thoroughly evaluated in orthopaedic patients,[46] and will be an important research focus in the future.

The PROMIS has similarly been applied to pediatric orthopaedic patients to address the current limitations of existing instruments. The PROMIS can be used to assess multiple domains in pediatric patients, of which the most pertinent domains for pediatric orthopaedic patients include physical function, pain interference, anxiety, depression, and global health. The physical function domain may be scored singularly or broken into mobility (23-item question bank) and upper extremity (29-item question bank) domains that share approximately 35% common variance.[47] The PROMIS has shown good reliability in pediatric patients from 8 to 17 years of age, whether completed by the child or for the child by a parent.[48,49] In addition, fewer children require parental assistance to complete the survey compared with legacy scales.[50,51]

The psychometric properties of computerized adaptive testing in pediatric orthopaedic patients have not been extensively researched, but have been compared with legacy scales in certain patient populations. PROMIS pediatric measures of general health have been shown to have excellent convergent and discriminant validity with the KIDSCREEN-10 and the Pediatric Quality of Life (PedsQL)-15.[52] In pediatric patients with congenital hand deformities, the PROMIS was found to correlate with the Disabilities of the Arm, Shoulder and Hand score and the Pediatric Outcomes Data Collection Instrument, but was only mildly correlated with the Michigan Hand Questionnaire.[50] In children with cerebral palsy, the PROMIS physical function mobility portion showed good correlation with patient and parent assessments of mobility, but was less responsive to treatment than legacy scales (the Pediatric Outcomes Data Collection Instrument, the Functional Assessment Questionnaire, the Shriners Hospitals for Children with Cerebral Palsy Computer-Adapted Testing Battery) and did not distinguish between Gross Motor Function Measures as well as other instruments.[53,54] The investigators concluded that item-bank expansion may be needed before mobility computerized adaptive testing is applied to patients with cerebral palsy.

Pediatric orthopaedic surgeons should be aware of the PROMIS because it is likely that it will be used as a patient-reported outcome measure in the future. The number of scientific articles assessing or using PROMIS has increased exponentially in the past 10 years from 16 in 2005 to more than 150 in 2015. The measurement properties of the PROMIS appear favorable in adult orthopaedic patients across multiple specialties, but it is not known if they will translate into similar results in pediatric orthopaedic patients.

Summary

Better outcomes for patients are based on evidence-based CPGs, appropriate use criteria, outcome measures, and the PROMIS.

Key Study Points

- Evidence-based CPGs inform patients and clinicians if a given intervention is associated with a desirable outcome.
- AUC documents indicate when (that is, in what specific clinical circumstance) the same intervention is best applied.
- Outcome measure assessments are dependent on the interrelated concepts of validity, reliability, responsiveness to change, and MCID.
- In addition to clinical measures that matter to clinicians, patient-reported outcome measures include variables that are important to patients. An increased emphasis on patient-reported outcome measures and computerized adaptive testing allow clinicians to better understand the effects of interventions on patients.

Annotated References

1. Farrokhyar F, Karanicolas PJ, Thoma A, et al: Randomized controlled trials of surgical interventions. *Ann Surg* 2010;251(3):409-416.

2. Ioannidis JP: Why most published research findings are false. *PLoS Med* 2005;2(8):e124.

3. Ioannidis JP: How to make more published research true. *PLoS Med* 2014;11(10):e1001747.

   To produce more true research, the author argues that many things must be done, including improvements in study design standards, the use of more stringent statistical thresholds, and the use of standardized definitions and analyses.

4. Morabia A: P. C. A. Louis and the birth of clinical epidemiology. *J Clin Epidemiol* 1996;49(12):1327-1333.

5. Mallon WJ: E. Amory Codman, surgeon of the 1990s. *J Shoulder Elbow Surg* 1998;7(5):529-536.

6. Institutes of Medicine: *Crossing the Quality Chasm: A New Health System for the 21st Century.* Washington, DC, The National Academies Press, 2001, p 360.

7. National Institutes of Health: *Health Technology Assessment (HTA) 101: Glossary.* Available at: http://www.nlm.nih.gov/nichsr/hta101/ta101014.html. Accessed August 27, 2011.

   Terms applicable to healthcare measurements are defined.

8. Institutes of Medicine: *Clinical Practice Guidelines: Directions for a New Program.* Washington, DC, The National Academies Press, 1990, p 168.

9. The National Academies of Sciences: Engineering, Medicine: *Clinical Practice Guidelines We Can Trust.* 2011. Available at: http://www.nationalacademies.org/hmd/Reports/2011/Clinical-Practice-Guidelines-We-Can-Trust.aspx. Accessed April 5, 2016.

   Standards for developing trustworthy CPGs are detailed.

10. OrthoGuidelines website of the American Academy of Orthopaedic Surgeons. Available at: http://www.orthoguidelines.org/. Accessed April 5, 2016.

    This website is an online information resource that provides up-to-date treatment guidelines to orthopaedic surgeons and professionals.

11. Brook RH, Chassin MR, Fink A, Solomon DH, Kosecoff J, Park RE: A method for the detailed assessment of the appropriateness of medical technologies. *Int J Technol Assess Health Care* 1986;2(1):53-63.

12. Fitch K, Bernstein SJ, Aguilar MD, et al: *The RAND/UCLA Appropriateness Method User's Manual* .Santa Monica, CA, RAND Corporation, 2001.

13. Lawson EH, Gibbons MM, Ko CY, Shekelle PG: The appropriateness method has acceptable reliability and validity for assessing overuse and underuse of surgical procedures. *J Clin Epidemiol* 2012;65(11):1133-1143.

    The findings support the use of the appropriateness method to assess variation in the rates of the procedures studied by identifying overuse and underuse.

14. American Academy of Orthopaedic Surgeons: *Appropriate Use Criteria for the Management of Pediatric Supracondylar Humerus Fractures.* Rosemont, IL, American Academy of Orthopaedic Surgeons, 2014. Available at: http://www.aaos.org/research/Appropriate_Use/PSHF_AUC.pdf.

    The AAOS developed this AUC to determine appropriateness of various healthcare services for pediatric supracondylar fractures.

15. American Academy of Orthopaedic Surgeons: *Appropriate Use Criteria for the Management of Pediatric Supracondylar Humerus Fractures With Vascular Injury.* Rosemont, IL, American Academy of Orthopaedic Surgeons, June 2015. Available at: http://www.aaos.org/research/Appropriate_Use/PSHF_Vascular_Injury_AUC.pdf.

    The AAOS developed this AUC to determine appropriateness of various healthcare services for pediatric supracondylar fractures with vascular injury.

16. American Academy of Orthopaedic Surgeons: *Clinical Practice Guideline on the Treatment of Supracondylar Humerus Fractures.* Available at: http://www.aaos.org/research/guidelines/SupracondylarFracture/SupConFullGuideline.pdf. 2011.

This CPG was developed by an AAOS physician volunteer group and is based on a systematic review of the current scientific and clinical information and accepted approaches to treatment and/or diagnosis. The CPG is not intended to be a fixed protocol. The clinician's independent medical judgment, given the individual patient's clinical circumstances, should always determine patient care and treatment.

17. Appropriate use criteria for pediatric supracondylar humerus fractures: Application. Available at: http://www.orthoguidelines.org/go/auc/auc.cfm?auc_id=224922. Accessed April 5, 2016.

    This application provides procedure recommendations based on an individualized condition profile completed by the clinician. The AUC provides a general outline for the evaluation of numerous clinical scenarios encountered by clinicians that care for patients with pediatric supracondylar humerus fractures.

18. Poolman RW, Struijs PA, Krips R, et al: Reporting of outcomes in orthopaedic randomized trials: Does blinding of outcome assessors matter? *J Bone Joint Surg Am* 2007;89(3):550-558.

19. Brand RA: Ernest Amory Codman, MD, 1869-1940. *Clin Orthop Relat Res* 2009;467(11):2763-2765.

20. Mehlman CT: Clinical epidemiology, in Kj K, ed: *Orthopaedic Knowledge Update 7*. Rosemont, IL, American Academy of Orthopaedic Surgeons, 2002, pp 79-83.

21. Greenfield ML, Kuhn JE, Wojtys EM: A statistics primer: Validity and reliability. *Am J Sports Med* 1998;26(3):483-485.

22. Corona J, Matsumoto H, Roye DP, Vitale MG: Measuring quality of life in children with early onset scoliosis: Development and initial validation of the Early Onset Scoliosis Questionnaire. *J Pediatr Orthop* 2011;31(2):180-185.

    The Early Onset Scoliosis Questionnaire reflects quality of life and caregiver burden in the population of patients with early-onset scoliosis. The questionnaire will expand options for outcome assessment in this unique population.

23. Wright JG, Smith PL, Owen JL, Fehlings D: Assessing functional outcomes of children with muscular dystrophy and scoliosis: The Muscular Dystrophy Spine Questionnaire. *J Pediatr Orthop* 2008;28(8):840-845.

24. Weinstein SL, Dolan LA, Wright JG, Dobbs MB: Effects of bracing in adolescents with idiopathic scoliosis. *N Engl J Med* 2013;369(16):1512-1521.

    Bracing substantially decreased the progression of high-risk curves to the threshold for surgery in patients with adolescent idiopathic scoliosis. The benefit increased with longer hours of brace wear. Level of evidence: II.

25. Karanicolas PJ, Bhandari M, Kreder H, et al; Collaboration for Outcome Assessment in Surgical Trials (COAST) Musculoskeletal Group: Evaluating agreement: Conducting a reliability study. *J Bone Joint Surg Am* 2009;91(suppl 3):99-106.

26. Viera AJ, Garrett JM: Understanding interobserver agreement: The kappa statistic. *Fam Med* 2005;37(5):360-363.

27. Norman GR, Stratford P, Regehr G: Methodological problems in the retrospective computation of responsiveness to change: The lesson of Cronbach. *J Clin Epidemiol* 1997;50(8):869-879.

28. Norman GR, Wyrwich KW, Patrick DL: The mathematical relationship among different forms of responsiveness coefficients. *Qual Life Res* 2007;16(5):815-822.

29. Middel B, van Sonderen E: Statistical significant change versus relevant or important change in (quasi) experimental design: Some conceptual and methodological problems in estimating magnitude of intervention-related change in health services research. *Int J Integr Care* 2002;2:e15.

30. Streiner DL, Norman GR: Mine is bigger than yours: Measures of effect size in research. *Chest* 2012;141(3):595-598.

    The authors explain the various indices of effect sizes: how they are calculated, what they mean, and how they are interpreted.

31. Norman GR, Sridhar FG, Guyatt GH, Walter SD: Relation of distribution- and anchor-based approaches in interpretation of changes in health-related quality of life. *Med Care* 2001;39(10):1039-1047.

32. Schünemann HJ, Guyatt GH: Commentary: Goodbye M(C)ID! Hello MID, where do you come from? *Health Serv Res* 2005;40(2):593-597.

33. Jevsevar DS, Sanders J, Bozic KJ, Brown GA: An introduction to clinical significance in orthopaedic outcomes research. *JBJS Rev* 2015. Available at: http://reviews.jbjs.org/content/3/5/e2. Accessed April 5, 2016.

34. Carreon LY, Sanders JO, Diab M, Sucato DJ, Sturm PF, Glassman SD; Spinal Deformity Study Group: The minimum clinically important difference in Scoliosis Research Society-22 appearance, activity, and pain domains after surgical correction of adolescent idiopathic scoliosis. *Spine (Phila Pa 1976)* 2010;35(23):2079-2083.

35. Seok Park M, Youb Chung C, Min Lee K, et al: Rasch analysis of the pediatric outcomes data collection instrument in 720 patients with cerebral palsy. *J Pediatr Orthop* 2012;32(4):423-431.

    The sports/physical function domain of the Pediatric Outcomes Data Collection Instrument generally satisfies the requirements of Rasch item response theory and is an appropriate measure of function in patients with cerebral palsy. Level of evidence: II.

36. Hudak PL, Amadio PC, Bombardier C; The Upper Extremity Collaborative Group (UECG): Development of an upper extremity outcome measure: The DASH

(disabilities of the arm, shoulder and hand). *Am J Ind Med* 1996;29(6):602-608.

37. Chakravarty EF, Bjorner JB, Fries JF: Improving patient reported outcomes using item response theory and computerized adaptive testing. *J Rheumatol* 2007;34(6):1426-1431.

38. Hung M, Clegg DO, Greene T, Saltzman CL: Evaluation of the PROMIS physical function item bank in orthopaedic patients. *J Orthop Res* 2011;29(6):947-953.

    A single physical function dimension accounts for most of the item variance in the physical function item bank. This suggests that the items are predominantly measuring a single construct.

39. Cella D, Riley W, Stone A, et al; PROMIS Cooperative Group: The Patient-Reported Outcomes Measurement Information System (PROMIS) developed and tested its first wave of adult self-reported health outcome item banks: 2005-2008. *J Clin Epidemiol* 2010;63(11):1179-1194.

40. Hung M, Stuart AR, Higgins TF, Saltzman CL, Kubiak EN: Computerized adaptive testing using the PROMIS physical function item bank reduces test burden with less ceiling effects compared with the Short Musculoskeletal Function Assessment in orthopaedic trauma patients. *J Orthop Trauma* 2014;28(8):439-443.

    Administered by electronic means, PROMIS physical function computerized testing required less than 10% of the amount of time for patients to complete compared with the Short Musculoskeletal Function Assessment questionnaire; equally high reliability and less ceiling effect were achieved.

41. Hung M, Nickisch F, Beals TC, Greene T, Clegg DO, Saltzman CL: New paradigm for patient-reported outcomes assessment in foot & ankle research: Computerized adaptive testing. *Foot Ankle Int* 2012;33(8):621-626.

    A paradigm shift to broader use of PROMIS-based computerized adaptive testing should improve precision and reduce patient burden using patient-reported outcome measurements in foot and ankle research.

42. Beckmann JT, Hung M, Bounsanga J, Wylie JD, Granger EK, Tashjian RZ: Psychometric evaluation of the PROMIS physical function computerized adaptive test in comparison to the American Shoulder and Elbow Surgeons score and Simple Shoulder Test in patients with rotator cuff disease. *J Shoulder Elbow Surg* 2015;24(12):1961-1967.

    The measurement properties of PROMIS physical function computerized testing compared favorably with the American Shoulder and Elbow Surgeons score and the Simple Shoulder Test, and required the completion of fewer questions.

43. Tyser AR, Beckmann J, Franklin JD, et al: Evaluation of the PROMIS physical function computer adaptive test in the upper extremity. *J Hand Surg Am* 2014;39(10):2047-2051.e4.

    The psychometric characteristics of the PROMIS physical function computerized testing instrument compared favorably with the Disabilities of the Arm, Shoulder and Hand instrument in a tertiary upper extremity practice.

44. Hung M, Hon SD, Franklin JD, et al: Psychometric properties of the PROMIS physical function item bank in patients with spinal disorders. *Spine (Phila Pa 1976)* 2014;39(2):158-163.

    The PROMIS physical function item bank adequately addressed outcomes of patients with spinal disorders because reliabilities were excellent, minimal ceiling/floor effect existed, and item bias was limited.

45. Hung M, Baumhauer JF, Brodsky JW, et al; Orthopaedic Foot & Ankle Outcomes Research (OFAR) of the American Orthopaedic Foot & Ankle Society (AOFAS): Psychometric comparison of the PROMIS physical function CAT with the FAAM and FFI for measuring patient-reported outcomes. *Foot Ankle Int* 2014;35(6):592-599.

    The authors reported that physical function, computerized adaptive testing instrument performed best in terms of reliability, responsiveness, and efficiency in this broad sample of foot and ankle patients.

46. Hunt KJ, Alexander I, Baumhauer J, et al; OFAR (Orthopaedic Foot and Ankle Outcomes Research Network): The Orthopaedic Foot and Ankle Outcomes Research (OFAR) network: Feasibility of a multicenter network for patient outcomes assessment in foot and ankle. *Foot Ankle Int* 2014;35(9):847-854.

    The Orthopaedic Foot and Ankle Outcomes Research network was able to enroll large numbers of patients in a short enrollment period for this preliminary study of the organization's ability to collect and measure patient-reported outcomes data. The data were easily aggregated and analyzed.

47. Hays RD, Spritzer KL, Amtmann D, et al: Upper-extremity and mobility subdomains from the Patient-Reported Outcomes Measurement Information System (PROMIS) adult physical functioning item bank. *Arch Phys Med Rehabil* 2013;94(11):2291-2296.

    Upper extremity and mobility subdomains from PROMIS shared approximately 35% of the variance in common, and produced comparable scores, whether calibrated separately or together.

48. Varni JW, Thissen D, Stucky BD, et al: Item-level informant discrepancies between children and their parents on the PROMIS pediatric scales. *Qual Life Res* 2015;24(8):1921-1937.

    The authors reported that parent-child item-level discrepancies were lower for more objective or visible items than for items measuring internal states or less observable items when measuring latent variables such as peer relationships and fatigue.

49. Irwin DE, Gross HE, Stucky BD, et al: Development of six PROMIS pediatrics proxy-report item banks. *Health Qual Life Outcomes* 2012;10:22.

The initial calibration data for six PROMIS pediatric proxy-report item banks were provided by a diverse set of caregivers of children with a variety of common chronic illnesses and racial and ethnic backgrounds.

50. Waljee JF, Carlozzi N, Franzblau LE, Zhong L, Chung KC: Applying the Patient-Reported Outcomes Measurement Information System to assess upper extremity function among children with congenital hand differences. *Plast Reconstr Surg* 2015;136(2):200e-207e.

The PROMIS is highly correlated with both functional assessment and self-reported function among children with congenital hand differences.

51. Tucker CA, Bevans KB, Teneralli RE, Smith AW, Bowles HR, Forrest CB: Self-reported pediatric measures of physical activity, sedentary behavior, and strength impact for PROMIS: Item development. *Pediatr Phys Ther* 2014;26(4):385-392.

The authors found that semistructured interview methods provided valuable information about children's perspectives and the ways children recall previous activities.

52. Forrest CB, Tucker CA, Ravens-Sieberer U, et al: Concurrent validity of the PROMIS pediatric global health measure. *Qual Life Res* 2016;25(3):739-751.

The PROMIS pediatric global health-7 measure summarizes a child's physical, mental, and social health into a single score.

53. Mulcahey MJ, Haley SM, Slavin MD, et al: Ability of PROMIS pediatric measures to detect change in children with cerebral palsy undergoing musculoskeletal surgery. *J Pediatr Orthop* 2015.

PROMIS measures were less able to detect changes in children undergoing musculoskeletal surgery than other measures.

54. Kratz AL, Slavin MD, Mulcahey MJ, Jette AM, Tulsky DS, Haley SM: An examination of the PROMIS pediatric instruments to assess mobility in children with cerebral palsy. *Qual Life Res* 2013;22(10):2865-2876.

Results support the convergent and discriminant validity of the pediatric PROMIS Mobility Short Form in children with cerebral palsy.

Chapter 3

Pediatric Anesthesia and Pain Management

Eric D. Shirley, MD   Robert B. Bryskin, MD

Abstract

Appropriate planning for anesthesia and pain management is a critical component of orthopaedic surgery. In the setting of forearm fracture reductions, both conscious sedation and intravenous regional anesthesia are safe and effective options. For infants who may require surgery, it is important to discuss the potential and uncertain risk of anesthetic neurotoxicity. Considerations during spine surgery include the preservation of neuromonitoring signals, fluid balance, and hemostasis with or without antifibrinolytics. Perioperative and postoperative analgesia benefits from a multimodal strategy that addresses pain and muscle spasms while preventing increases in complications, such as bleeding or nonunion.

Keywords: anesthetic neurotoxicity; antifibrinolytics; conscious sedation; regional anesthesia

Introduction

Anesthesia and pain management options for the pediatric orthopaedic population include conscious sedation, regional and general anesthesia, and pharmacologic agents. These options must be used judiciously—alone or in combination—to optimize patient comfort. It is important to address recent research and intervention advancements in terms of fracture management, neonatal considerations, spine surgery, and postoperative pain control.

Dr. Shirley or an immediate family member has stock or stock options held in Depomed and serves as a board member, owner, officer, or committee member of the Jacksonville Sports Medicine Program and the Pediatric Orthopaedic Society of North America. Neither Dr. Bryskin nor any immediate family member has received anything of value from or has stock or stock options held in a commercial company or institution related directly or indirectly to the subject of this chapter.

Pain Management: Fracture Manipulation

Forearm and wrist fractures are common injuries in the pediatric population. Although open reduction and internal fixation is often not required, displaced or angulated fractures often require closed reduction. Closed reduction may be performed under either general anesthesia or by means of conscious sedation using agents such as ketamine or nitrous oxide. These agents may be used alone because the addition of a hematoma block to conscious sedation for distal forearm fractures does not decrease pain or sedation time.[1]

The optimal setting for forearm fracture reduction remains unclear. Although closed reduction under general anesthesia in the operating room provides excellent sedation with muscle relaxation, the potential disadvantages include cost, efficiency, and access. Conversely, conscious sedation in the emergency department often may be done immediately and at a lower cost but can negatively affect the efficiency of the emergency department. A 2012 study compared nonphyseal forearm fractures reduced in the emergency department under conscious sedation using nitrous oxide with those reduced in the operating room under general anesthesia.[2] Orthopaedic residents performed the reductions in both groups. No substantial differences in the quality of reduction or the long-arm plaster casts could be found, but the rate of repeat manipulation was substantially higher in fractures reduced in the emergency department compared with the operating room (32% versus 11%, respectively). The study authors proposed that the higher failure rate in the emergency department was the result of treating a larger number of unstable fracture patterns, which subsequently required immediate reduction in that setting. Highly unstable fractures brought to the operating room for manipulation that underwent immediate internal fixation were excluded from the study.

Reductions in the emergency department also may be performed under intravenous regional anesthesia (Bier block). The block is performed by placing an intravenous line in the affected limb, inflating a brachial tourniquet, and then administering diluted lidocaine.[3] In 2014, a group of researchers compared two groups of pediatric patients undergoing reduction and long-arm cast application for displaced forearm fractures: 600 patients were treated with intravenous regional anesthesia (using a lidocaine dose of 3.33 mg/kg of body weight), and 645 patients were treated with conscious sedation (using ketamine and propofol).[3] The method of analgesia was determined by the orthopaedic resident at the time of treatment. The use of intravenous regional anesthesia was associated with a shorter time from procedure initiation to discharge (47 minutes versus 102 minutes, respectively) and lower cost ($4,956 versus $6,313, respectively). Neither group had complications, such as compartment syndrome, that required readmission.

Anesthetic Neurotoxicity and the Developing Brain

Selected pediatric orthopaedic conditions may require surgical treatment during infancy. The risks of general anesthetic neurotoxicity and subsequent learning deficits have been documented in animal[4,5] and retrospective human[6,7] studies. However, these studies are limited by many factors, including the confounding effects of surgery and pathology. To coordinate additional research efforts regarding the risks of general anesthesia on the developing brain, the FDA, with assistance from the International Anesthesia Research Society, established SmartTots (Strategies for Mitigating Anesthesia-Related (Neuro) Toxicity in Tots) in 2011. The General Anesthesia Compared to Spinal Anesthesia trial, which was facilitated by SmartTots in 2015, prospectively randomized 700 infants younger than 60 weeks to receive general or regional anesthesia for inguinal hernia repair.[8] The median duration of surgery in both groups was approximately 1 hour. At age 2 years, evidence did not indicate that exposure to less than 1 hour of general anesthesia in infancy increased the risk of adverse neurodevelopment outcomes. Subsequent neurodevelopmental outcomes will be assessed when these children reach age 5 years.

The Pediatric Anesthesia and NeuroDevelopment Assessment prospective study, also facilitated by SmartTots, is currently in progress.[9] This study is following for 8 to 15 years 500 twin-sibling pairs who are discordant in their exposure to anesthesia. Based on the currently available data, SmartTots has released a consensus statement about studies suggesting that cognitive deficits may occur in children after early exposure to anesthesia.[10] The statement also acknowledges the limitations of these studies, concluding that further research is needed to confirm the cognitive risk of anesthetics and whether the risk is large enough to outweigh the benefits of a proposed procedure.

Anesthetic Considerations: Spine Surgery

Surgery for spinal deformities presents unique anesthetic challenges, such as the preservation of signals for neuromonitoring, fluid management, and bleeding. The complexity of these issues is greater in patients with neuromuscular conditions or those undergoing procedures requiring osteotomies. Recent research has evaluated the use of antifibrinolytics and pharmacologic agents to assist in total intravenous anesthesia.

Antifibrinolytics

Minimizing perioperative blood loss is a priority for avoiding transfusion risks, such as disease transmission, transfusion reaction, and increased risk of infection. Traditional methods of hemostasis include meticulous surgical technique, hypotensive anesthesia, muscle paralysis, acute hemodilution, and the use of cell salvage systems. According to the Pediatric Health Information Systems database for US children's hospitals, the median rates of transfusion for idiopathic and neuromuscular scoliosis are 24% and 43%, respectively.[11] Patients with neuromuscular scoliosis may have underlying coagulopathy from poor nutritional status, seizure medications, platelet abnormalities, and the depletion of clotting factors.[12] Fusion for neuromuscular scoliosis also has a higher risk of blood loss because it usually includes more fusion levels.

Antifibrinolytics, such as aprotinin, epsilon-aminocaproic acid (EACA), and tranexamic acid (TXA), have been used to minimize blood loss during cardiac surgery, total joint arthroplasty, and spine surgery. In 2007, the FDA stopped the production of aprotinin because of its higher morbidity and mortality rates in adults undergoing cardiac surgery.[13] EACA and TXA appear to be safe and have a low risk of adverse events.[14] Both EACA and TXA are synthetic derivatives that block lysine binding sites on plasminogen to impede blood clot degradation. Although a Cochrane systematic review concluded that these medications decrease blood loss in scoliosis surgery,[15] whether these medications decrease transfusion requirements is more difficult to determine because of variations in surgical technique, the use of cell salvage systems and/or autologous blood, and other postoperative management protocols.

The most pronounced effects of antifibrinolytics on blood loss are seen in spinal fusion for patients with neuromuscular scoliosis. In a randomized trial of TXA versus placebo, researchers found that using TXA resulted in a 40% reduction in blood loss in patients with neuromuscular scoliosis but no reduction in patients with idiopathic scoliosis.[16] In a retrospective study of EACA versus placebo in patients with different types of neuromuscular scoliosis, other researchers found that EACA reduced intraoperative blood loss and blood transfusion requirements in 62 patients compared with 34 historical control subjects.[17]

Other studies involving antifibrinolytics in neuromuscular scoliosis have focused on a single underlying diagnosis. In a retrospective multicenter study of patients with cerebral palsy, researchers found a mean blood loss of 1,684 mL in 44 patients receiving antifibrinolytics compared with 2,685 mL in 40 patients not treated with antifibrinolytics.[14] Although patients receiving antifibrinolytics had fewer transfusions with cell salvage blood, the total transfusion requirements did not decrease. In patients with muscular dystrophy undergoing spinal fusion, other researchers found that the use of TXA was associated with a decrease in both blood loss and transfusions.[18]

Vertebral column resection procedures also have the potential for increased blood loss. In 2012, a group of researchers retrospectively reviewed 147 patients younger than 21 years who underwent vertebral column resection at multiple centers.[19] The estimated blood loss percentage of blood volume per vertebral level removed was substantially lower in patients receiving TXA (30%) or aprotinin (32%) compared with those not receiving antifibrinolytics (52%). In addition, the volume of blood products transfused (divided by total blood volume) was substantially lower in patients receiving TXA (16%) than in those not receiving antifibrinolytics (32%). TXA was associated with an estimated 42% decrease in intraoperative blood loss during these procedures.

The effect of antifibrinolytics is less pronounced in surgery for idiopathic scoliosis. One group of researchers prospectively randomized 125 patients with idiopathic scoliosis to receive TXA, EACA, or saline.[20] Both TXA and EACA decreased intraoperative and total blood losses without a difference in transfusion rate compared with the control group. Another group of researchers compared the use of TXA in 43 patients to 63 control patients in surgery for idiopathic scoliosis.[21] Blood loss (613 mL versus 1,079 mL, respectively) and intraoperative transfusion volume (258 mL versus 377 mL, respectively) were substantially lower in patients receiving TXA.

In direct comparisons, TXA tends to be favored over EACA. TXA is up to 10 times more potent in vitro than EACA,[22] has a longer half-life, and costs less. A prospective study in 2014 compared the two agents in patients with idiopathic or neuromuscular scoliosis.[23] TXA was associated with a lower transfusion requirement, less alteration in clotting studies, and a trend toward less blood loss. In patients with idiopathic scoliosis, TXA and EACA were found to be equally effective at reducing intraoperative blood loss, but TXA was more effective at reducing postoperative drainage and total blood loss.[20] In patients with cerebral palsy, TXA was more effective than EACA in decreasing blood loss.[14]

Pharmacologic Agents

Pharmacologic agents given during spinal deformity surgery must not interfere with neuromonitoring. Dexmedetomidine, a selective alpha-2 adrenoreceptor agonist with anesthetic and analgesic properties, has emerged as an effective adjuvant to total intravenous anesthesia for such cases. Its advantages include reduced intraoperative and postoperative analgesia requirements, shorter length of postoperative mechanical ventilation times, and a lower incidence of agitation and delirium.[24] When given during spine surgery, it provides hemodynamic stability, does not suppress evoked potentials, attenuates opioid-induced hyperalgesia, allows early neurologic assessment, and reduces analgesic needs postoperatively.[25,26]

Gabapentin, an agent commonly used to treat neuropathic pain, also may assist with postoperative analgesia by decreasing narcotic requirements. A prospective study in 2010 randomized 59 patients undergoing spinal fusion for idiopathic scoliosis to receive gabapentin (15 mg/kg of body weight preoperatively and 5 mg/kg of body weight every 8 hours for 5 days postoperative) or a placebo.[27] In the gabapentin group, total morphine consumption during the first 48 hours was substantially lower, and pain scores were significantly lower in the recovery room and the morning after surgery. The study authors advocated the use of gabapentin for 48 hours postoperatively. In another study, researchers found that a single preoperative dose of gabapentin (600 mg) before idiopathic scoliosis surgery was not associated with a substantial decrease in pain scores or total morphine consumption compared with placebos.[28] However, these authors suggested that their dose may have been too small to achieve a benefit.

Perioperative and Postoperative Pain Management

Pain management goals include relieving pain, decreasing the length of stay, allowing return to preoperative levels of activity, and creating minimal adverse side effects. Adequate postoperative pain control is essential to meet expectations and achieve an acceptable patient experience. Recent literature has focused on advanced regional anesthesia techniques and evaluating the adverse effects of pharmacologic agents such as ketorolac.

Regional Anesthesia

Regional anesthesia for pediatric patients has seen substantial development in recent years, including further evaluation of potential complications from performing regional anesthesia under general anesthesia in children. The French Language Society of Pediatric Anesthesiologists prospectively evaluated more than 30,000 regional blocks performed in 47 institutions between November 2005 and October 2006.[29] The overall rate of complications was 1.2 per 1,000 children, and none of the complications resulted in long-term effects. In another study, the Pediatric Regional Anesthesia Network prospectively evaluated more than 53,000 cases of regional anesthesia performed between 2007 and 2012 in the United States.[30] The risk of neurologic complications was 8.3 per 1,000 in sedated patients, 3.4 per 1,000 in awake patients, 2.4 per 1,000 under general anesthesia with neuromuscular blockade, and 0.62 per 1,000 under general anesthesia without neuromuscular blockade. The European Society of Regional Anesthesia and the American Society of Regional Anesthesia and Pain Medicine Joint Committee issued a practice advisory that concluded that the practice of pediatric regional anesthesia under general anesthesia or deep sedation is associated with acceptable safety and should be viewed as the standard of care.[31]

Continuous peripheral nerve blocks remain an option for postoperative analgesia in pediatric patients. These blocks can extend the duration of postoperative analgesia, reduce the need for postoperative admissions for pain control, and decrease the use of intravenous opioid analgesics.[32] The feasibility of continuous peripheral nerve blocks to provide postoperative analgesia for pediatric ambulatory procedures has been explored in two large studies.[33,34] With 410 and 1,285 procedures in pediatric orthopaedic patients, these studies showed failure rates (6.9% and 1.9%, respectively) and complication rates (14.4% and 5%, respectively) comparable with those in the adult population. Most of the complications were minor and did not require medical interventions; none resulted in permanent neurologic injury. These studies support the use of continuous peripheral nerve blocks in pediatric hospitals under the careful supervision of a dedicated team performing placement and follow-up.

Femoral nerve block is a common regional anesthetic for knee surgery. In 2015, a group of researchers evaluated strength and return to sports in pediatric patients receiving a femoral nerve block for anterior cruciate ligament (ACL) reconstruction.[35] The fast isokinetic extension strength deficit was significantly higher and meeting return-to-play criteria at 6 months was significantly lower in pediatric patients treated with a nerve block compared with patients who were not treated with a nerve block (17.6% versus 11.2% [$P = 0.01$] and 67.7% versus 90.2% [$P = 0.002$], respectively). Although definitive recommendations cannot be made, the need for a motor-sparing regional anesthesia technique has been identified.

The ultrasound-guided adductor canal block is a novel technique that allows selective sensory nerve blockade, including the saphenous nerve, the medial femoral cutaneous nerve, the articular branches of the obturator nerve, and the nerve to the vastus medialis (sensory/motor) (**Figure 1**). With larger injection volumes, this block may allow sciatic nerve blockade to spread to the popliteal fossa.[36] In patients undergoing ACL reconstruction with patellar tendon autograft, the adductor canal block provided similar postoperative analgesia and narcotic consumption as a femoral nerve block.[37] Therefore, with its analgesic potency, preserved muscle strength, and favorable side-effect profile, adductor canal block (single shot or continuous) may emerge as a preferred regional technique after pediatric ACL reconstruction.

The concern that regional anesthesia delays the diagnosis of acute compartment syndrome with irreversible neuronal death, myonecrosis, and limb loss remains controversial. This concern is primarily based on traditional paradigms taught during training. In addition, isolated case reports, such as the development of compartment syndrome in two patients who were treated with epidural catheters after pelvic and femoral osteotomies,[38] contribute to these concerns. However, all forms of pain control, including opioid-based analgesics, have been implicated in the delayed diagnosis of compartment syndrome but have no convincing evidence of causation. A joint committee from the European Society of Regional Anesthesia and the American Society of Regional Anesthesia and Pain Medicine found no evidence-based data that the use of regional anesthesia increases the risk for acute compartment syndrome or delays its diagnosis in children and issued best-practice rules for this setting[31] (**Table 1**).

Postoperative Analgesia

Providing adequate pain control starts before surgery by setting realistic expectations, and perioperative care requires a well-coordinated team approach. In addition to providing the correct analgesic dose, it also is important that the medication be administered at the correct time. For example, a study reported that only 20% of

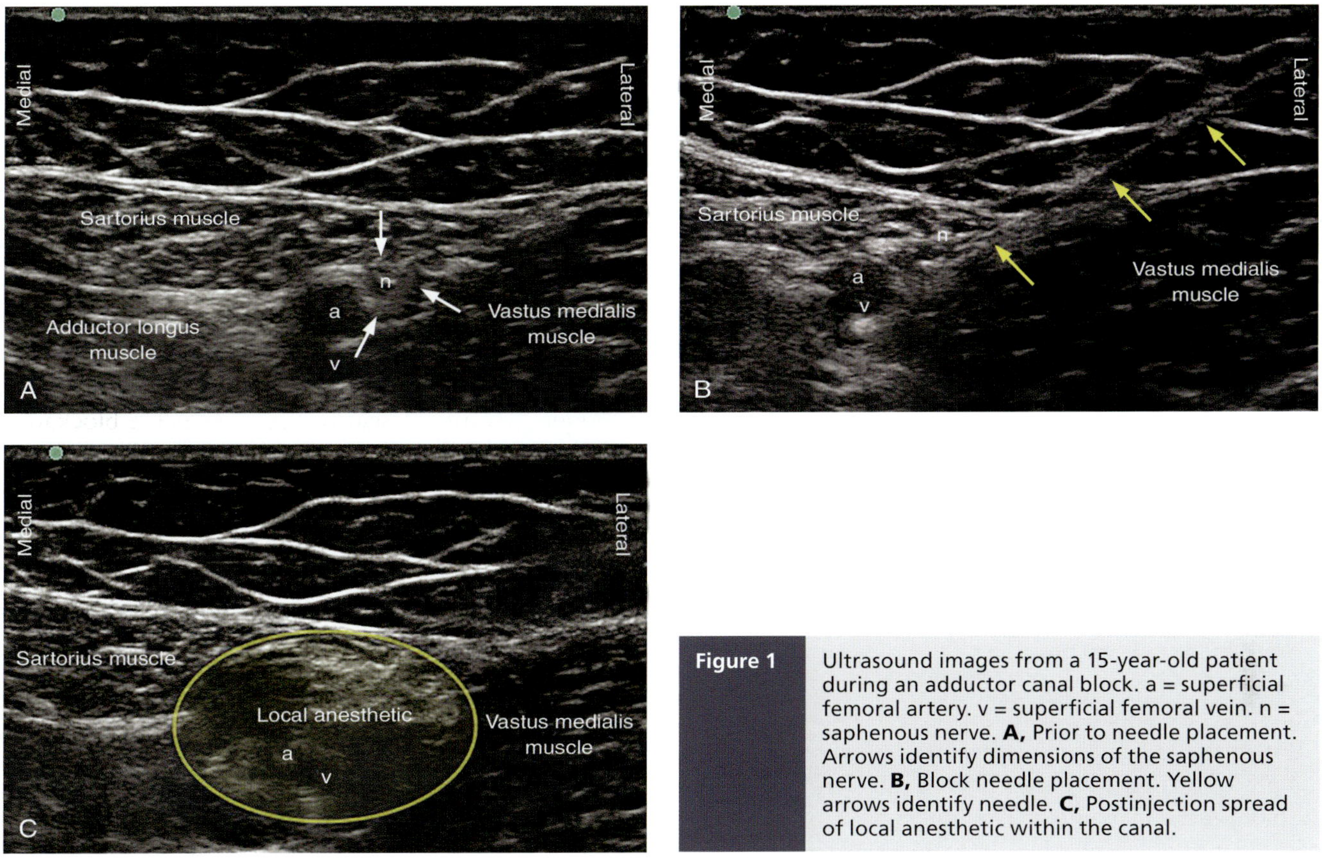

Figure 1 Ultrasound images from a 15-year-old patient during an adductor canal block. a = superficial femoral artery. v = superficial femoral vein. n = saphenous nerve. **A,** Prior to needle placement. Arrows identify dimensions of the saphenous nerve. **B,** Block needle placement. Yellow arrows identify needle. **C,** Postinjection spread of local anesthetic within the canal.

patients with presumed long-bone limb fractures received intravenous opioids within 45 minutes of arrival at the emergency department.[39] Postoperative analgesic options include opioids, benzodiazepines, and NSAIDs.

Opioids are the most powerful analgesics. They can be administered by injection or a patient-controlled analgesia pump in patients 6 years and older with normal cognitive function and by proxy (for example, a nurse) in children younger than 6 years.[40] Oral opioids such as oxycodone, hydrocodone, and codeine (in order of increasing potency) also may be prescribed. However, adverse side effects such as pruritus, drowsiness, respiratory depression, urinary retention, nausea, ileus, and constipation can be problematic. In addition, the efficacy of codeine is compromised in nearly 50% of patients because of cytochrome P450-metabolizing enzyme 2D6 phenotypes, resulting in a decreased ability to convert codeine to its active metabolite.[41]

Addressing postoperative muscle spasms or pain with benzodiazepines after surgery in patients with fractures or neuromuscular conditions is beneficial in achieving adequate pain relief. Although benzodiazepines cannot be used alone, they can be added to limit the adverse side effects of opioids.[42] Patients receiving opioids and benzodiazepines should be monitored for respiratory depression.

NSAIDs decrease prostaglandin production by inhibiting cyclooxygenase. Adverse side effects include renal impairment, gastritis, and reversible platelet dysfunction. Ketorolac may be administered intravenously for postoperative pain management in the first 72 hours.[42] Although concerns about adverse effects on osseous healing have been raised, they have not been substantiated in pediatric patients. A group of researchers found no increase in pseudarthrosis or other complications in 158 patients who received ketorolac after spinal fusion for idiopathic scoliosis.[43] Another group of researchers identified no occurrence of delayed union, malunion, or bleeding complications in 221 surgical pediatric fractures;[44] in another study, they also found that ketorolac did not appear to inhibit osteotomy healing.[45]

Additional research may provide further support for other analgesics. Intravenous acetaminophen was introduced in the United States in 2011 for postoperative anesthesia after its efficacy and safety was demonstrated in international settings.[46,47] Further studies are expected regarding its use after pediatric orthopaedic procedures. Liposomal bupivacaine uses a multivesicular liposomal vehicle to provide increased stability and extended drug release. Systemic levels of bupivacaine may persist for 96 hours. Although this agent is used in adult patients,

Table 1

Best Practice Rules for Guiding the Application of Perioperative Regional Anesthesia in Children at Risk for Compartment Syndrome

1	Use dilute local anesthetics (0.1% to 0.25% bupivacaine or ropivacaine) for single-shot peripheral and neuraxial blocks because they are less likely than more concentrated solutions to mask ischemic pain and/or produce muscle weakness.
2	Limit local anesthetic concentration to 0.1% for continuous infusions.
3	Restrict volume and concentration in sciatic catheters in patients undergoing lower leg surgeries or other high-risk surgeries for compartment syndrome.
4	Use local anesthetic additives cautiously because they can increase the duration and/or density of the block.
5	Exercise a high index of clinical suspicion in patients at risk for compartment syndrome to allow the early detection of potential signs.
6	Urgently assess compartment pressure measurements if compartment syndrome is suspected.

Reproduced with permission from Ivani G, Suresh S, Ecoffey C, et al: The European Society of Regional Anesthesia and Pain Therapy and the American Society of Regional Anesthesia and Pain Medicine Joint Committee Practice Advisory on Controversial Topics in Pediatric Regional Anesthesia. *Reg Anesth Pain Med* 2015;40:526-532.

bupivacaine has not been studied in patients younger than 18 years and, therefore, cannot be recommended for use in the pediatric population. Further study is required because pediatric patients may be uniquely predisposed to bupivacaine overdose secondary to a decrease in hepatic function and plasma protein production.[48]

Summary

Numerous advances have been made in pediatric anesthesia and pain management. Both conscious sedation and intravenous regional anesthesia have demonstrated safety and efficacy during closed reduction of fractures. It remains critical to identify the risks of anesthetic neurotoxicity in infants, and these risks require additional evaluation. Future research also will help refine the indications for antifibrinolytics and regional anesthetic techniques in pediatric patients. Postoperative analgesia continues to consist of a multimodal strategy that addresses pain and muscle spasms while preventing increases in complications, such as bleeding or nonunion. Further research may identify additional pharmacologic agents that are helpful in this setting.

Key Study Points

- Closed reduction of fractures in the emergency department under conscious sedation or Bier block represents a safe alternative to general anesthesia in the operating room.
- Antifibrinolytics decrease bleeding in pediatric spine deformity surgery, particularly for patients with neuromuscular scoliosis or those undergoing vertebral column resection.
- Ketorolac is safe for use in pediatric patients after surgery for spinal deformity, fractures, and osteotomies.

Annotated References

1. Constantine E, Tsze DS, Machan JT, Eberson CP, Linakis JG, Steele DW: Evaluating the hematoma block as an adjunct to procedural sedation for closed reduction of distal forearm fractures. *Pediatr Emerg Care* 2014;30(7):474-478.

   A randomized trial of 90 patients with forearm fracture found that adding a hematoma block to conscious sedation with ketamine did not result in decreased pain scores, sedation time, or the total ketamine dose. Level of evidence: I.

2. McKenna P, Leonard M, Connolly P, Boran S, McCormack D: A comparison of pediatric forearm fracture reduction between conscious sedation and general anesthesia. *J Orthop Trauma* 2012;26(9):550-555, discussion 555-556.

   This retrospective review found a higher rate of failure for forearm fractures reduced in the emergency department compared with the operating room. Level of evidence: III.

3. Aarons CE, Fernandez MD, Willsey M, Peterson B, Key C, Fabregas J: Bier block regional anesthesia and casting for forearm fractures: Safety in the pediatric emergency department setting. *J Pediatr Orthop* 2014;34(1):45-49.

   This retrospective study found that Bier block regional anesthesia for forearm fractures was associated with a lower time to discharge and a lower cost compared with procedural sedation. Level of evidence: III.

4. Brambrink AM, Evers AS, Avidan MS, et al: Isoflurane-induced neuroapoptosis in the neonatal rhesus macaque brain. *Anesthesiology* 2010;112(4):834-841.

5. Jevtovic-Todorovic V, Hartman RE, Izumi Y, et al: Early exposure to common anesthetic agents causes widespread

neurodegeneration in the developing rat brain and persistent learning deficits. *J Neurosci* 2003;23(3):876-882.

6. Flick RP, Katusic SK, Colligan RC, et al: Cognitive and behavioral outcomes after early exposure to anesthesia and surgery. *Pediatrics* 2011;128(5):e1053-e1061.

   A matched cohort study identified that multiple exposures to surgery and anesthesia before age 2 years were a substantial risk factor for the development of learning disabilities. Level of evidence: III.

7. Wilder RT, Flick RP, Sprung J, et al: Early exposure to anesthesia and learning disabilities in a population-based birth cohort. *Anesthesiology* 2009;110(4):796-804.

8. Davidson AJ, Disma N, de Graaff JC, et al; GAS consortium: Neurodevelopmental outcome at 2 years of age after general anaesthesia and awake-regional anaesthesia in infancy (GAS): An international multicentre, randomised controlled trial. *Lancet* 2016;387(10015):239-250.

   A multicenter randomized trial of 700 infants examined the neurologic effects of anesthesia in children undergoing inguinal hernia repair under general anesthesia compared with awake regional anesthesia. No differences in neurodevelopment outcomes were found at age 2 years. Level of evidence: I.

9. Miller TL, Park R, Sun LS: Report of the fourth PANDA symposium on "Anesthesia and Neurodevelopment in Children." *J Neurosurg Anesthesiol* 2014;26(4):344-348.

   This symposium report evaluates evidence for anesthesia neurotoxicity and discusses approaches to research. The Pediatric Anesthesia and NeuroDevelopment Assessment symposium has become a platform for reviewing current preclinical and clinical data related to anesthetic neurotoxicity, discussing relevant considerations in study design and approaches to future research among clinicians and researchers, and engaging key stakeholders in this controversial public health topic. Level of evidence: V.

10. *SmartTots: Consensus statement on the use of anesthetic and sedative drugs in infants and toddlers.* Available at: http://smarttots.org/about/consensus-statement/. Published October 2015. Accessed January 17, 2016.

    This advisory statement for providers and families discusses the potential risks of anesthesia in children. Level of evidence: V.

11. McLeod LM, French B, Flynn JM, Dormans JP, Keren R: Antifibrinolytic use and blood transfusions in pediatric scoliosis surgeries performed at US children's hospitals. *J Spinal Disord Tech* 2015;28(8):E460-E466.

    A retrospective cohort study used the Pediatric Health Information Systems database to determine the effects of antifibrinolytics on blood transfusions and concluded that the effects of these agents when used outside of clinical trials are unclear. Level of evidence: III.

12. Brenn BR, Theroux MC, Dabney KW, Miller F: Clotting parameters and thromboelastography in children with neuromuscular and idiopathic scoliosis undergoing posterior spinal fusion. *Spine (Phila Pa 1976)* 2004;29(15):E310-E314.

13. Mangano DT, Miao Y, Vuylsteke A, et al: Mortality associated with aprotinin during 5 years following coronary artery bypass graft surgery. *JAMA* 2007;297(5):471-479.

14. Dhawale AA, Shah SA, Sponseller PD, et al: Are antifibrinolytics helpful in decreasing blood loss and transfusions during spinal fusion surgery in children with cerebral palsy scoliosis? *Spine (Phila Pa 1976)* 2012;37(9):E549-E555.

    A multicenter retrospective review of patients with cerebral palsy undergoing posterior spinal fusion found that antifibrinolytics significantly decreased intraoperative blood loss without differences in total transfusion. Level of evidence: IV.

15. Tzortzopoulou A, Cepeda MS, Schumann R, Carr DB: Antifibrinolytic agents for reducing blood loss in scoliosis surgery in children. *Cochrane Database Syst Rev* 2008;3:CD006883.

16. Sethna NF, Zurakowski D, Brustowicz RM, Bacsik J, Sullivan LJ, Shapiro F: Tranexamic acid reduces intraoperative blood loss in pediatric patients undergoing scoliosis surgery. *Anesthesiology* 2005;102(4):727-732.

17. Thompson GH, Florentino-Pineda I, Poe-Kochert C, Armstrong DG, Son-Hing J: Role of Amicar in surgery for neuromuscular scoliosis. *Spine (Phila Pa 1976)* 2008;33(24):2623-2629.

18. Shapiro F, Zurakowski D, Sethna NF: Tranexamic acid diminishes intraoperative blood loss and transfusion in spinal fusions for Duchenne muscular dystrophy scoliosis. *Spine (Phila Pa 1976)* 2007;32(20):2278-2283.

19. Newton PO, Bastrom TP, Emans JB, et al: Antifibrinolytic agents reduce blood loss during pediatric vertebral column resection procedures. *Spine (Phila Pa 1976)* 2012;37(23):E1459-E1463.

    A multicenter review found that blood loss during vertebral column resection was variable and often greater than the patient's blood volume. TXA decreased intraoperative blood loss and the need for transfusion. Level of evidence: IV.

20. Verma K, Errico T, Diefenbach C, et al: The relative efficacy of antifibrinolytics in adolescent idiopathic scoliosis: A prospective randomized trial. *J Bone Joint Surg Am* 2014;96(10):e80.

    A prospective randomized trial compared TXA, EACA, and placebo for idiopathic scoliosis. Both antifibrinolytics decreased blood loss but not the transfusion rate. Level of evidence: I.

21. Yagi M, Hasegawa J, Nagoshi N, et al: Does the intraoperative tranexamic acid decrease operative blood loss during posterior spinal fusion for treatment of adolescent idiopathic scoliosis? *Spine (Phila Pa 1976)* 2012;37(21):E1336-E1342.

1: General

A retrospective study of TXA found a substantial decrease in both blood loss and transfusions in patients with idiopathic scoliosis. Level of evidence: IV.

22. Lecker I, Wang DS, Romaschin AD, Peterson M, Mazer CD, Orser BA: Tranexamic acid concentrations associated with human seizures inhibit glycine receptors. *J Clin Invest* 2012;122(12):4654-4666.

    This study demonstrated that TXA and EACA are competitive antagonists of glycine receptors in mice.

23. Halanski MA, Cassidy JA, Hetzel S, Reischmann D, Hassan N: The efficacy of Amicar versus tranexamic acid in pediatric spinal deformity surgery: A prospective, randomized, double-blinded pilot study. *Spine Deform* 2014;2:191-197.

    A prospective study of antifibrinolytics in posterior spine fusion found that TXA resulted in lower allogenic transfusions and a trend toward lower blood loss compared with Amicar. Level of evidence: I.

24. Pan W, Wang Y, Lin L, Zhou G, Hua X, Mo L: Outcomes of dexmedetomidine treatment in pediatric patients undergoing congenital heart disease surgery: A meta-analysis. *Paediatr Anaesth* 2016;26(3):239-248.

    This article is a systematic review of the perioperative use of dexmedetomidine in children undergoing congenital heart disease surgery. Level of evidence: V.

25. Bekker A, Haile M, Kline R, et al: The effect of intraoperative infusion of dexmedetomidine on the quality of recovery after major spinal surgery. *J Neurosurg Anesthesiol* 2013;25(1):16-24.

    This study found that dexmedetomidine infusion used during multilevel spinal fusions moderately improved the quality of recovery, possibly reduced fatigue, and decreased the stress response. Level of evidence: I.

26. Hwang W, Lee J, Park J, Joo J: Dexmedetomidine versus remifentanil in postoperative pain control after spinal surgery: A randomized controlled study. *BMC Anesthesiol* 2015;15(1):21.

    A randomized trial found that the use of dexmedetomidine as an adjuvant to propofol-based total intravenous anesthesia improved pain control, decreased the requirement for rescue analgesics, and decreased the occurrence of postoperative nausea and vomiting compared with remifentanil. Level of evidence: I.

27. Rusy LM, Hainsworth KR, Nelson TJ, et al: Gabapentin use in pediatric spinal fusion patients: A randomized, double-blind, controlled trial. *Anesth Analg* 2010;110(5):1393-1398.

28. Mayell A, Srinivasan I, Campbell F, Peliowski A: Analgesic effects of gabapentin after scoliosis surgery in children: A randomized controlled trial. *Paediatr Anaesth* 2014;24(12):1239-1244.

    A randomized controlled trial found that a single preoperative gabapentin dose did not result in substantial decreases in pain scores or opioid consumption after idiopathic scoliosis surgery. Level of evidence: I.

29. Ecoffey C, Lacroix F, Giaufre E, Orliaquet G, Courreges P,Association des Anesthesistes Reanimateurs Pediatriques d'Expression Francaise (ADERPEF):Epidemiology and morbidity of regional anesthesia in children: A follow up one-year prospective survey of the French Language Society of Pediatric Anesthesiologists (ADARPEF). *Paediatr Anaesth* 2010;20:1061-1069.

30. Taenzer AH, Walker BJ, Bosenberg AT, et al: Asleep versus awake: Does it matter? Pediatric regional block complications by patient state: A report from the Pediatric Regional Anesthesia Network. *Reg Anesth Pain Med* 2014;39(4):279-283.

    An analysis of more than 50,000 pediatric regional anesthesia blocks demonstrated that the practice of placing regional blocks in pediatric patients under general anesthesia is as safe as placement in sedated and awake patients. Level of evidence: IV.

31. Ivani G, Suresh S, Ecoffey C, et al: The European Society of Regional Anaesthesia and Pain Therapy and the American Society of Regional Anesthesia and Pain Medicine Joint Committee practice advisory on controversial topics in pediatric regional anesthesia. *Reg Anesth Pain Med* 2015;40(5):526-532.

    This practice advisory established the performance of regional anesthesia in pediatric patients under general anesthesia or sedation as the standard of care. Level of evidence: V.

32. Dadure C, Capdevila X: Continuous peripheral nerve blocks in children. *Best Pract Res Clin Anaesthesiol* 2005;19(2):309-321.

33. Visoiu M, Joy LN, Grudziak JS, Chelly JE: The effectiveness of ambulatory continuous peripheral nerve blocks for postoperative pain management in children and adolescents. *Paediatr Anaesth* 2014;24(11):1141-1148.

    A retrospective report of 410 ambulatory patients with continuous peripheral nerve blocks from a single academic center demonstrated efficacy in 93.1% of the patients and complication rate of 14.4%. None resulted in permanent neurologic injury. Level of evidence: IV.

34. Gurnaney H, Kraemer FW, Maxwell L, Muhly WT, Schleelein L, Ganesh A: Ambulatory continuous peripheral nerve blocks in children and adolescents: A longitudinal 8-year single center study. *Anesth Analg* 2014;118(3):621-627.

    An audit of 1,285 children with ambulatory continuous peripheral nerve blocks demonstrated rates of catheter problems (4.2%) and catheter failure rates (1.9%) similar to those in adult studies. Level of evidence: IV.

35. Luo TD, Ashraf A, Dahm DL, Stuart MJ, McIntosh AL: Femoral nerve block is associated with persistent strength deficits at 6 months after anterior cruciate ligament

reconstruction in pediatric and adolescent patients. *Am J Sports Med* 2015;43(2):331-336.

A retrospective review of pediatric patients who underwent ACL reconstruction found that those treated with a femoral nerve block were more likely to experience deficit at 6 months with respect to fast isokinetic extension strength and were delayed in meeting clearance to return to sports. Level of evidence: III.

36. Gautier PE, Hadzic A, Lecoq JP, Brichant JF, Kuroda MM, Vandepitte C: Distribution of injectate and sensory-motor blockade after adductor canal block. *Anesth Analg* 2016;122(1):279-282.

    A study that assessed local anesthetic spread and sensory-motor block following adductor canal nerve block for knee surgery found spread of injectate to the popliteal fossa, resulting in sensory block of the sciatic nerve.

37. Chisholm MF, Bang H, Maalouf DB, et al: Postoperative analgesia with saphenous block appears equivalent to femoral nerve block in ACL reconstruction. *HSS J* 2014;10(3):245-251.

    A randomized trial that compared analgesic quality in patients undergoing ACL reconstruction with patellar tendon autograft identified no differences in pain scores between femoral and adductor nerve blocks. Level of evidence: I.

38. Dunwoody JM, Reichert CC, Brown KL: Compartment syndrome associated with bupivacaine and fentanyl epidural analgesia in pediatric orthopaedics. *J Pediatr Orthop* 1997;17(3):285-288.

39. Iyer SB, Schubert CJ, Schoettker PJ, Reeves SD: Use of quality-improvement methods to improve timeliness of analgesic delivery. *Pediatrics* 2011;127(1):e219-e225.

    A quality improvement study described improvement in delays of providing opioids to patients with apparent long-bone fractures in the emergency department. Level of evidence: IV.

40. Monitto CL, Greenberg RS, Kost-Byerly S, et al: The safety and efficacy of parent-/nurse-controlled analgesia in patients less than six years of age. *Anesth Analg* 2000;91(3):573-579.

41. Ali S, Drendel AL, Kircher J, Beno S: Pain management of musculoskeletal injuries in children: Current state and future directions. *Pediatr Emerg Care* 2010;26(7):518-524, quiz 525-528.

42. Nowicki PD, Vanderhave KL, Gibbons K, et al: Perioperative pain control in pediatric patients undergoing orthopaedic surgery. *J Am Acad Orthop Surg* 2012;20(12):755-765.

    This article reviews the pharmacology of pediatric pain management options after orthopaedic surgery. Level of evidence: V.

43. Sucato DJ, Lovejoy JF, Agrawal S, Elerson E, Nelson T, McClung A: Postoperative ketorolac does not predispose to pseudoarthrosis following posterior spinal fusion and instrumentation for adolescent idiopathic scoliosis. *Spine (Phila Pa 1976)* 2008;33(10):1119-1124.

44. Kay RM, Directo MP, Leathers M, Myung K, Skaggs DL: Complications of ketorolac use in children undergoing operative fracture care. *J Pediatr Orthop* 2010;30(7):655-658.

45. Kay RM, Leathers M, Directo MP, Myung K, Skaggs DL: Perioperative ketorolac use in children undergoing lower extremity osteotomies. *J Pediatr Orthop* 2011;31(7):783-786.

    A retrospective review found that pediatric patients receiving ketorolac after osteotomy surgery had no increase in osseous or soft-tissue complications. Level of evidence: III.

46. Shastri N: Intravenous acetaminophen use in pediatrics. *Pediatr Emerg Care* 2015;31(6):444-448, quiz 449-450.

    This article reviews the pharmacology, indications, and risks of intravenous acetaminophen in pediatric patients. Level of evidence: V.

47. Baley K, Michalov K, Kossick MA, McDowell M: Intravenous acetaminophen and intravenous ketorolac for management of pediatric surgical pain: A literature review. *AANA J* 2014;82(1):53-64.

    This article reviews the literature regarding the use of intravenous ketorolac and intravenous acetaminophen in the pediatric surgical setting. Level of evidence: V.

48. Golembiewski J, Dasta J: Evolving role of local anesthetics in managing postsurgical analgesia. *Clin Ther* 2015;37(6):1354-1371.

    A literature review found that including liposome bupivacaine in a multimodal analgesic regimen can reduce total opioid consumption and the length of stay. Level of evidence: V.

1: General

Chapter 4

Musculoskeletal Infection

John F. Lovejoy III, MD   Lawson A. B. Copley, MD, MBA

Abstract

Pediatric musculoskeletal infections continue to be a challenging problem for orthopaedic surgeons. The clinical presentation of these infections is highly variable, with a continuum of disease that ranges from very mild to life threatening. The diversity of locations potentially involved and the wide range of severity further complicate the process of determining a diagnosis. A recent trend to address these issues is the use of a multidisciplinary approach. This includes involvement of emergency department physicians, hospitalists, pediatricians, infectious disease specialists, radiologists, and pathologists. The key leader in this effort must be the orthopaedic surgeon. The expertise of the orthopaedic surgeon leads to less resource utilization and more timely interventions, whether choosing the correct study, determining the differential diagnoses, or performing the definitive treatment. To improve outcomes for children with suspected bone, joint, and soft-tissue infections, orthopaedic surgeons must remain up to date with current trends in the diagnosis and treatment of these infections and play an early, active leadership role within multidisciplinary teams.

Keywords: abscess; chronic recurrent multifocal osteomyelitis (CRMO); infections; methicillin-resistant Staphylococus aureus (MRSA); musculocutaneous infection; osteomyelitis

Dr. Lovejoy or an immediate family member serves as a board member, owner, officer, or committee member of the Pediatric Orthopaedic Society of North America. Dr. Copley or an immediate family member serves as an unpaid consultant to Epic and serves as a board member, owner, officer, or committee member of the Pediatric Orthopaedic Society of North America.

Introduction

Pediatric musculoskeletal infections can be acute or chronic and present with a wide range of severity. Infections can be superficial (septic bursitis, abscess, cellulitis, fasciitis, lymphangitis, and lymphadenitis) or deep (osteomyelitis, septic arthritis, and pyomyositis). Any soft tissue or bone is susceptible to infection. The initial presentation of children with a pediatric musculoskeletal infection is highly variable and necessitates a careful physical examination, laboratory studies, and appropriate imaging to establish the diagnosis and clarify the anatomic location and extent of disease. After a diagnosis is established, a treatment algorithm should be used to facilitate rapid and timely resolution of the infection. The likelihood, severity, and difficulty of treating infections is increased with the presence of implanted hardware.[1] The recent trend toward establishing clinical practice guidelines is an effort to reduce variation in care and improve short- and intermediate-term outcomes for these conditions.[1-3] In addition, efforts to reduce the costs of care while maintaining care quality have yielded treatment algorithms with early transitions from intravenous to oral antibiotics and shortened lengths of hospital stays.[4-6] These treatment algorithms vary greatly as a function of the severity of disease, the patient's response to therapy, and the need for surgical intervention.[7-9] Because recent literature indicates that variations in clinical evaluation and treatment of these conditions exist regionally and internationally,[1,7,10-14] no algorithm has been universally accepted.

It is important that the orthopaedic surgeon be mindful of the many conditions (such as neoplasms, inflammatory disorders, and trauma), that can mimic the clinical presentations of soft-tissue, joint, and bone infections. For example, early in the course of the patient's disease, the orthopaedic surgeon must distinguish benign and self-limited processes such as transient synovitis from serious and life-threatening disorders such as leukemia or Ewing sarcoma.[3] Early involvement of an orthopaedic surgeon often leads to less resource utilization (fewer laboratory and imaging studies) if the clinical scenario suggests a benign, self-limited problem (such as transient synovitis) or an orthopaedic problem (such as a fracture in a child with spina bifida) rather than an infectious problem. To improve outcomes for children with suspected bone, joint, and soft-tissue infections, orthopaedic surgeons should play an early, active leadership role within multidisciplinary teams.[3,15]

A Continuum of Disease

Musculoskeletal infections in children can occur in isolation, can be contiguous with other structures, can be multifocal, or can be part of a disseminated infection.[1,3,15-18] Because pediatric musculoskeletal infections can be complex and have life- or limb-threatening complications, an early, accurate, complete diagnosis is a priority.

Recent studies suggest that infections involving different tissue types behave differently according to the primary tissue of involvement, within a relative descending hierarchy from bone to joint to muscle to soft tissue.[1,18] Children with osteomyelitis in isolation or those who have osteomyelitis associated with septic arthritis have higher rates of bacteremia at presentation than do children with isolated septic arthritis.[18] Children with osteomyelitis require longer hospital stays and antibiotic treatment of longer durations than do children with isolated septic arthritis.[1,2,16,19] Children with osteomyelitis are susceptible to adverse outcomes from their infections, including physeal arrest, osteonecrosis, pathologic fracture, and deformity.[1,7,14,16] In contrast to children with osteomyelitis, children with skin and skin structure infections have a negligible rate of bacteremia and require the shortest duration of treatment.[18]

Osteomyelitis

Evaluation

The clinical assessment of a child with osteomyelitis often reveals bone tenderness that is most pronounced over the epicenter of the disease. However, because increased pressure within the bone will be disseminated more widely, it is helpful to evaluate for tenderness of the bone away from the site of the complaint. This helps to differentiate other causes of local tissue inflammation and swelling such as cellulitis, bursitis, or even septic arthritis in which there appears to be local bone tenderness adjacent to the joint.

Plain radiographs should be obtained for any possible infection to assess for other causes of symptoms (for example, fracture or neoplasm) and for obvious radiographic changes that may occur in advanced disease (for example, lytic lesions, cortical erosions, sequestrum, or involucrum). These radiographic changes require time to develop and imply that the bone architecture has been substantially affected by the underlying process. Typically, a loss of approximately one-third of the local bone mineral density must occur before it is apparent on a plain radiograph. The most important initial plain radiographic finding in children with early presentation of acute hematogenous osteomyelitis is deep soft-tissue swelling.

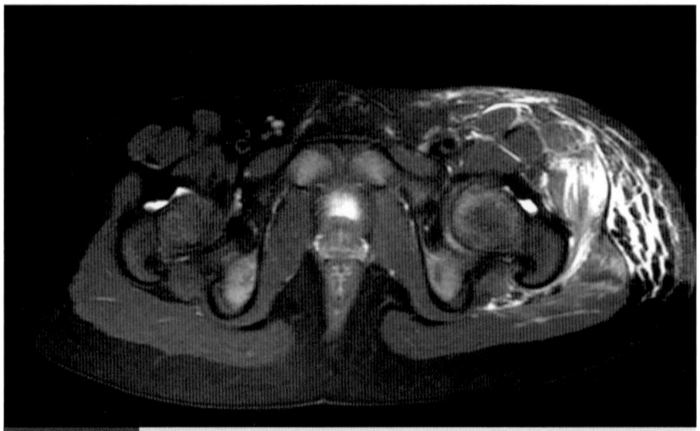

Figure 1 MRI from a patient with hip pyomyositis shows extensive edema within the musculature of the proximal left thigh.

MRI is an accurate and reliable imaging study to determine the anatomic and spatial extent of bone, joint, and soft-tissue infection (**Figure 1**). The use of MRI to assess suspected bone, joint, and soft-tissue infections often provides a more complete understanding of the primary and contiguous tissues involved in the infection, as well as a determination of the presence and size of abscesses that may require surgical drainage.[3,9,18,19] Institutions are reporting an increased rate of MRI use to evaluate children with suspected musculoskeletal infection.[7] Challenges to obtaining MRIs include cost and the need for sedation or anesthesia in younger children. In many busy pediatric centers, there are logistical challenges to obtaining MRI studies in a timely manner. Rapid image acquisition protocols can allow coronal screening MRI from the lumbar spine to the ankles with a minimal need for sedation. Evidence suggests that multispecialty coordination of the care of a child who has been sedated for MRI with continuation of anesthesia for immediate surgery can improve the efficiency of scanning and result in less scanning time, better coordination and timing of surgical intervention, and an overall shorter total length of hospitalization.[3]

Clinical Practice Guideline

Children with bone and joint infections have benefitted from the development and implementation of clinical guidelines to reduce variations in care.[1,2] The development of such guidelines for conditions such as osteomyelitis has led to improvements in the use of antibiotics, greater consistency in the acquisition of culture material from the site of infection, a reduction in the time to obtain appropriate diagnostic imaging, and a trend toward reduction in the length of hospitalization[2] (**Figure 2**).

Severity of Illness

Determining the severity of illness for children with acute hematogenous osteomyelitis may help clinicians stratify children objectively based on their clinical and laboratory presentations.[15] Severity of illness determinations for children may also improve the study of disease cohorts that differ chronologically, geographically, or therapeutically, without being subjected to misleading assumption about fundamental population differences caused by the relative severity of the underlying disease.[15] Recent comparative studies indicate that children with osteomyelitis caused by methicillin-resistant *Staphylococus aureus* (MRSA) may be more ill than children with osteomyelitis caused by methicillin-sensitive *S aureus* (MSSA).[8,10-12,14-16] In an effort to anticipate which children will have confirmed MRSA infections before the culture results are available, a prediction algorithm has been created.[10] However, the use of such algorithms has not been confirmed in other communities, some of which have a higher incidence of MRSA osteomyelitis.[11]

Treatment

Antibiotic Therapy

A challenge in the diagnosis and management of suspected bone, joint, and soft-tissue infections is choosing the most appropriate time for antibiotic administration. In stable patients, it is reasonable to withhold antibiotics until cultures are collected, thereby maximizing the sensitivity of the cultures obtained. In unstable patients, such as those showing signs of hemodynamic instability or signs of sepsis, early empiric antibiotic therapy should be considered before obtaining cultures.[18] In all patients, blood cultures should be obtained and laboratory tests performed (including a complete blood count with differential, erythrocyte sedimentation rate [ESR], and C-reactive protein [CRP] level), and antibiotics should not be administered until a blood culture is obtained.[18]

Empiric antibiotic therapy should be chosen based on several considerations: the age of the patient (for example, group B streptococcal osteomyelitis is common is young infants, but rare in older children; *Kingella kingae* is most common in children younger than 4 years), the presumed mode of infection (hematogenous spread or penetrating injury), underlying chronic diseases (for example, sickle cell disease or primary immunodeficiency), and local epidemiology and antimicrobial susceptibilities of the most likely pathogens.[1,7,10,12,15] In recent years, community-acquired MRSA has been responsible for a high proportion of culture-positive bone, joint, and soft-tissue infections, leading to increased use of vancomycin and clindamycin instead of the cephalosporin drugs used when methicillin-sensitive staphylococcal infections predominated.[11,12,14,16] Because antimicrobial susceptibilities of bacterial pathogens, most notably *S aureus*, vary widely, clinicians should monitor antibiotic resistance patterns within their communities, thereby ensuring optimal empiric therapy.[1,7,15,18]

Recommendations for the administration route and duration of antibiotic treatment of acute hematogenous osteomyelitis have changed substantially in recent years.[4,5,13] Historically, the standard practice was to administer intravenous antibiotics in the hospital for 4 to 6 weeks. With the advent of peripherally inserted central catheters, placement of the catheter and a short course of in-hospital administered antibiotics followed by a course of parenteral antibiotics administered at home has become the normal protocol.

Oral therapy after a course of intravenous antibiotics has also become common. Many children are managed effectively with a limited course of intravenous antibiotics, followed by 3 to 5 weeks of oral therapy.[4,5,13] Oral antibiotics with good bioavailability to susceptible infecting organisms offer flexibility with respect to the route of administration. Sequential parenteral to oral antibiotic therapy is considered safe and effective and should be used whenever there are no contraindications (such as malabsorption or risk of noncompliance), or when antibiotic resistance of the causative organism necessitates the use of a parenteral antimicrobial agent.

Antimicrobial therapy is finished when the prescribed course is completed, there are no physical examination findings suggesting inflammation, and inflammatory markers have normalized. If, at the completion of the planned antibiotic course of treatment, physical examination findings of inflammation persist, or if inflammatory indices remain elevated, antibiotic treatment should be continued with clinical and laboratory reassessment every 1 to 2 weeks until examination and laboratory findings normalize. If there is not a trend toward improvement, consideration should be given to evaluating the patient for a residual focus of infection (such as an abscess or sequestrum), which may be preventing resolution of the infection. Failure to improve or resolve the inflammatory indices is a sign of treatment failure, and the clinician should consider repeat MRI and possible repeat incision and débridement with new culture acquisition to ensure that the initially selected antibiotic remains the correct choice.[3]

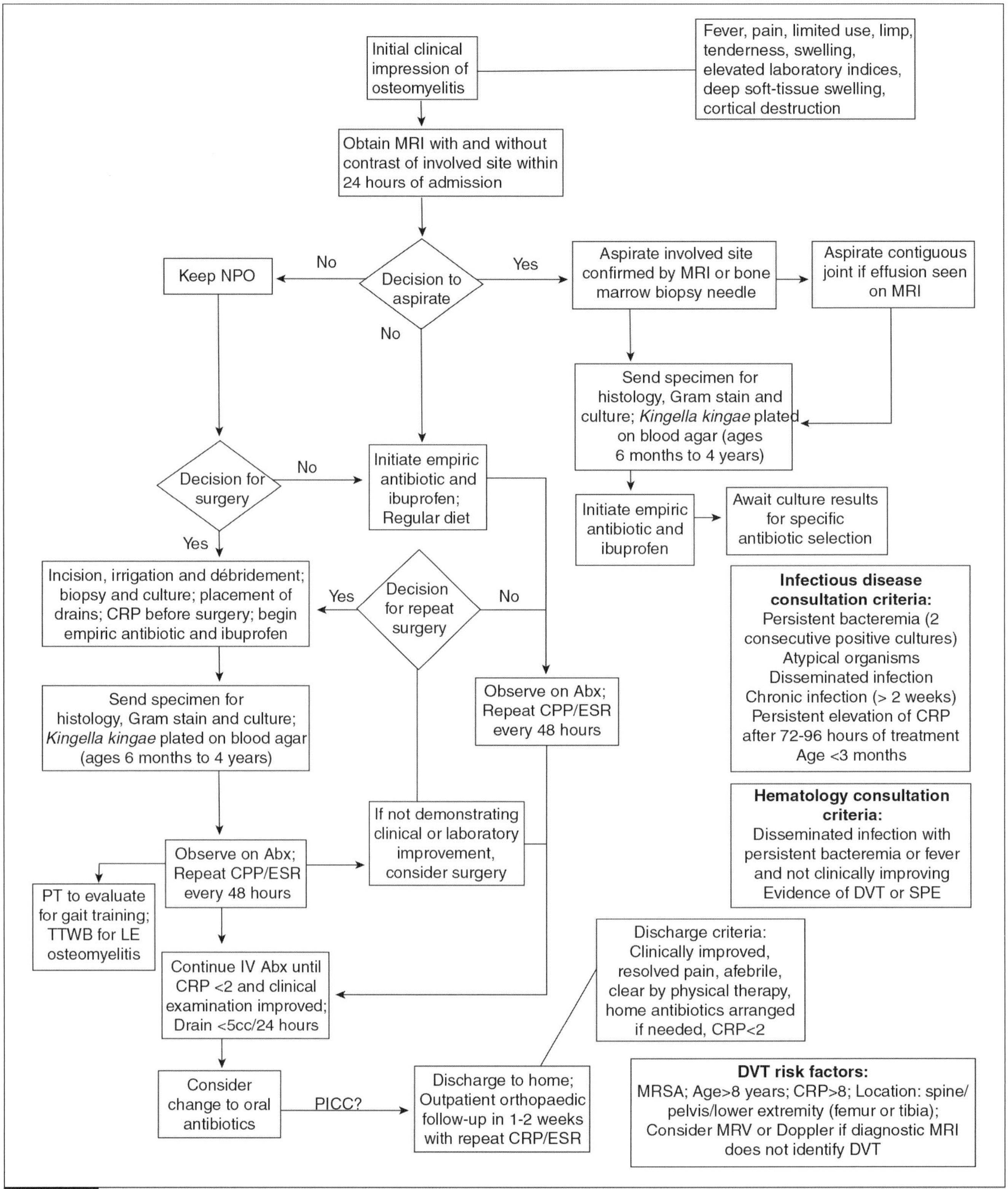

Figure 2 Flowchart of the Children's Medical Center of Dallas guideline for the evaluation and treatment of children with suspected osteomyelitis. Abx = antibiotics, CRP = C-reactive protein level, DVT = deep vein thrombosis, ESR = erythrocyte sedimentation rate, IV = intravenous, LE = lower extremity, MRSA = methicillin-resistant *Staphylococcus aureus*, MRV = magnetic resonance venography, NPO = nothing by mouth, PICC = peripherally inserted catheter, PT = physical therapist, SPE = septic pulmonary embolism, TTWB = toe-touch weightbearing. (Reproduced with permission from Copley LA, Kinsler MA, Gheen T, Shar A, Sun D, Browne R: The impact of evidence-based clinical practice guidelines applied by a multidisciplinary team for the care of children with osteomyelitis. *J Bone Joint Surg Am* 2013;95[8];686-693.)

Children receiving vancomycin for serious MRSA infections should have laboratory monitoring of vancomycin trough and serum creatinine levels assessed on a periodic basis. Some antibiotics, such as clindamycin, have excellent oral bioavailability and do not require routine serum concentration monitoring.

Surgical Intervention

There is a dearth of evidence guiding the indications and methods for surgical intervention for children with osteomyelitis.[7,8] The clinician should determine whether surgery is necessary for children with osteomyelitis on the basis of clinical, laboratory, and imaging data. Although there is no clear guidance in the literature on this subject, surgery is generally indicated for children with osteomyelitis who demonstrate hemodynamic compromise consistent with septic shock or who have imaging findings consistent with drainable abscesses (intraosseous, subperiosteal, or extraperiosteal) that will not likely resolve with antibiotic treatment alone[7,8] (**Figure 3**). New evidence suggests that, in children with osteomyelitis, the degree of illness at presentation predicts the need for repeat surgery.[8,14] Children who have mild illness are unlikely to require surgery, whereas children with severe illness (characterized by markedly elevated inflammatory markers; recurring febrile days on antibiotics; and evident disseminated disease, including deep vein thrombosis, septic pulmonary emboli, or pneumonia) are more likely to require surgery and may require more than one surgical procedure to resolve the infection.[8] In the era of MRSA, there appears to be a higher incidence of abscess formation, which may be responsible for a higher rate of surgical intervention for children with osteomyelitis.[10,14-16]

The literature also lacks data to guide the decision for which surgical procedure(s) to perform for osteomyelitis. Choices for the surgical treatment of osteomyelitis include drainage of subperiosteal abscesses; drilling of the bone; and incision of bone cortex, with irrigation and débridement of infected cancellous bone. Surgical decompression of infected bone has the potential benefit of reducing intraosseous pressure that may result in diminished perfusion and antibiotic delivery to the site of infection. In all drainage procedures, care should be taken to avoid injury to the growth plate and perichondrial ring. Surgical approach planning should incorporate a review of advanced imaging, taking into account all foci of infection. Adjacent or contiguous abscess should be drained at the time of bone decompression. Involvement of adjacent joints in children with acute osteomyelitis may occur at a higher rate than initially anticipated.[1,17,19] Recent studies suggest methods to help anticipate contiguous disease.[17-20]

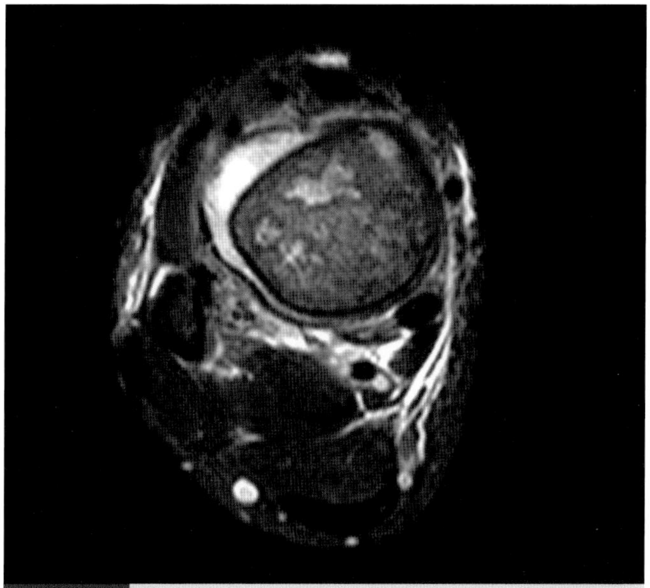

Figure 3 MRI shows tibial osteomyelitis with a subperiosteal abscess and extensive soft-tissue edema.

Revision Surgery

If the child does not demonstrate satisfactory clinical or laboratory improvement within 72 to 96 hours after surgical débridement, consideration should be given to repeat irrigation and débridement. Additional imaging is of limited use unless a previously unaddressed focus of infection is suspected. Caution should be exercised in interpreting postoperative MRI scans, which will often appear to show a worsening condition as the infection progresses through its normal course.[3]

Chronic Recurrent Multifocal Osteomyelitis

Evaluation

Chronic recurrent multifocal osteomyelitis (CRMO) or chronic nonbacterial osteomyelitis is a self-limiting disease of variable course and location. Although poorly understood, a genetic predisposition is hypothesized.[21] CRMO presents primarily in late childhood and adolescence with a female to male ratio of 4:1. Initial presentation ranges from mild conditions to severe acute conditions with chronic pain and swelling of the involved area. CRMO may be associated with other inflammatory diseases.[22,23] The diagnosis of CRMO is based on the patient history and physical examination, radiographic, and laboratory findings. Compared with acute bacterial osteomyelitis, patients with CRMO present with a more gradual onset, often with pain relieved by NSAIDs, and without a history of systemic infection or symptoms (such as fever). Although the ESR is often mildly elevated at presentation, both the ESR and the CRP level are inconsistent and do not correlate with the initial clinical presentation or with the clinical course.[22,23] Patients with CRMO typically have normal white blood cell (WBC) counts and, importantly, multiple bone lesions are typically seen on imaging studies. Management for some patients involves biopsy, débridement, obtaining cultures, and irrigation of the surgical field. Pathologic assessment of biopsy specimens typically shows chronic fibrotic and inflammatory changes, and cultures in patients with CRMO are generally sterile. Making a diagnosis of CRMO is challenging, and it is often a diagnosis of exclusion.

Treatment

Treatment of CRMO is challenging. Because of the difficulty in distinguishing CRMO from acute osteomyelitis, most patients receive a trial of antibiotic therapy. Importantly, pain in patients with CRMO generally responds well to NSAIDs, activity modification, and immobilization.

Septic Arthritis

Evaluation

Neonates are at high risk of bone, joint, and deep soft-tissue infections with both community-acquired and hospital-acquired pathogens. *Streptococcus agalactiae* (group B *Streptococcus*) infection is a common cause of osteomyelitis, septic arthritis, and pyomyositis in infants. For many reasons, most notably treatment using invasive lines and catheters, neonates are also at high-risk for infections with hospital-acquired pathogens, including MRSA; multidrug-resistant gram-negative rods; and *Candida* species, most often *Candida albicans* and *Candida parapsilosis*.

Although most neonates who experience infectious complications of treatment do so while in the hospital, neonates who are otherwise healthy may present with bone, joint, and deep muscle infections weeks after discharge. The immature immune system of neonates may result in a nonclassic presentation such as lack of fever or normal inflammatory markers and less than expected pain. Neonates with musculoskeletal infections often present with pseudoparalysis as the only sign. After one site of musculoskeletal infection is found, a diligent search for other sites is indicated (perhaps including ultrasound or other imaging given the difficulty of a physical examination) because up to 40% of neonates have multifocal musculoskeletal infections.

At all ages past early infancy, the most common cause of musculoskeletal infection is *S aureus*;[1,7,18] however, it should be noted that septic arthritis caused by *K kingae* is common in children 6 months to 4 years of age. Septic arthritis caused by *Streptococcus pneumoniae* can occur, most frequently in unimmunized children, but can also be caused by nonvaccine serotypes in fully immunized children.[18,24-27]

A challenge in the assessment of children with suspected septic arthritis is recognition of the risk factors for and clinical features of osteomyelitis in the adjacent bones. The pathophysiology of concurrent infections of bone and joint are incompletely understood. It has been theorized that there are vascular channels that traverse the physis in neonates and remain open until approximately 18 months of age. Beyond that age group, it is surmised that bacteria enter the metaphyseal circulation and then leave the bloodstream in the area adjacent to the physis where the circulatory pattern makes a 180° turn. Because the blood vessels in that area are relatively more permeable and the blood flow is more sluggish, a permissive environment for bacterial seeding is created.

The role of minor trauma preceding the event of infection has been identified as a trend in some children, but most of these infections appear to evolve spontaneously.[28] Joints with intracapsular metaphyses, such as the proximal humerus and proximal femur, are most susceptible to the development of adjacent osteomyelitis. To evaluate young children with septic arthritis and possible adjacent osteomyelitis, advanced imaging should be considered.[17,29] However, in the specific case of hip pyarthrosis, advanced imaging after ultrasound assessment may be less valuable.[20]

Confirmation of the diagnosis of septic arthritis is also challenging because of the low rate of successful bacterial isolation from joint fluid. One recent study of children who had suspected septic arthritis based on clinical findings reported a positive culture rate of only 35%.[18] Because it is sufficiently difficult to grow bacteria from joint fluid, supplemental methods may be used.[24,29] In attempts to increase the sensitivity and improve the identification of organisms infecting joints, the use of polymerase chain reaction amplifying bacterial DNA sequences in joint fluid is being investigated. Because this method is currently experimental, polymerase chain reaction assessment of joint fluid is neither standardized nor widely available.[24,25]

To make a diagnosis of septic arthritis in children, clinicians often use supplemental laboratory tests, including chemical and cellular analysis of the joint fluid, peripheral WBC count, serum ESR, and serum CRP level.[30] Infected joints typically present with cell counts greater than 40,000 nucleated cells/mL, of which more than 75% are neutrophils. Patients with infected joints typically have elevated peripheral WBC counts greater than 12,000 cells/mL, serum C-reactive protein levels greater than 2 mg/dL, and an initial ESR greater than 40 mm/hr. Improvements in these inflammatory markers after surgery and antibiotic administration support a diagnosis of acute septic arthritis.

Surgical Treatment

Septic arthritis may be treated surgically with either arthrotomy or arthroscopy, depending on the surgeon's level of comfort with these techniques.[27] Arthroscopic drainage has been found to be safe and effective in a wide variety of joints, including the hip, knee, ankle, shoulder, elbow, and wrist. Minimal soft-tissue disruption, a shorter hospital stay, and improved visualization of the joint space are reported as potential advantages of arthroscopy.[31]

Advanced imaging may be required if expected clinical and laboratory improvements are not demonstrated within the first 3 to 4 days after joint irrigation and drainage.[20] Particularly for presumed septic arthritis of the hip, pericapsular pyomyositis may mimic the classic clinical presentation of hip sepsis and should be suspected. In children in whom expected clinical and laboratory improvements are not seen, the possibilities of contiguous osteomyelitis and abscess should be considered. If repeat imaging does not discover an infectious explanation for the failure to improve, mimickers of septic arthritis such as leukemia should be considered. Patients with leukemia who present with musculoskeletal symptoms are frequently anemic. Recognition of contiguous osteomyelitis in patients with septic arthritis is particularly important for patients with pyarthrosis, especially in joints where the metaphysis is predominantly intracapsular, such as the shoulder or the hip.

Antibiotic Treatment

For most patients with proven or suspected septic arthritis, therapy is initiated with antistaphylococcal parenteral antibiotics. After culture results are obtained and there is a demonstrable decline in systemic inflammatory markers (for example, CRP level and ESR) patients may be transitioned to high-dose oral antibiotics.[32] If the patient evaluation suggests that the infection is isolated septic arthritis, antibiotics are typically given for 2 to 3 weeks. If there is concern for adjacent osteomyelitis, either because of the patient's young age or radiographic findings, a longer course of antibiotic therapy, often 4 to 8 weeks, is recommended.

Lyme Arthritis in Children

Lyme arthritis may be difficult to differentiate from acute septic arthritis in children.[33-35] One study reported that there were no substantial differences in the synovial fluid WBC count, absolute neutrophil count, and percentage of segmented neutrophils in children with proven septic arthritis caused by pyogenic bacteria and children presenting with acute knee monoarthritis in Lyme endemic areas.[33] It was also found that no child with a peripheral absolute neutrophil count of less than 10,000 cells/mL and an ESR of less than 40 mm/hr had septic arthritis.[34] In Lyme endemic areas, the presentation of a child with an acutely swollen knee is more likely to be Lyme arthritis than bacterial septic arthritis.[35]

Lyme arthritis in children has an excellent prognosis after oral antibiotic treatment for approximately 4 weeks. Children with antibiotic-refractory disease respond well to NSAIDs, intra-articular steroid injection, or immune-modulatory drugs. Chronic arthritis, joint deformities, and recurrent infection usually do not develop in children with Lyme arthritis.

Pyomyositis

Evaluation and Treatment

Primary muscle infections are less common than infections of bones or joints. Children with suspected pyomyositis should be evaluated urgently for bacteremia (in children with pyomyositis, the rate of initial bacteremia is approximately 15%),[18] for the possibility of necrotizing fasciitis, and for compartment syndrome. When an abscess develops within the muscle, surgical drainage is often needed for timely resolution. MRI is often required for the definitive diagnosis of pyomyositis and the assessment for surgical intervention. The identification of pyomyositis as a contiguous process related to adjacent osteomyelitis or septic arthritis is often challenging. Careful evaluation of MRI to look for substantial intramuscular inflammation is necessary and sufficient to make a diagnosis of pyomyositis.

Summary

Children with musculoskeletal infections require careful evaluation to determine their specific diagnoses, relative severity of illness, and appropriate treatment. Although bone, joint, and muscle infections are common, it is important to consider other conditions that might mimic the diverse clinical and laboratory presentations of bone, joint, and deep soft-tissue infections. Evidence-based clinical pathways, improved communication between members of the healthcare team, and coordination of care can improve short- and intermediate-term clinical outcomes and reduce the length of hospital stay. Such evidence-based clinical practice guidelines are now emerging and merit clinical and economic evaluation.

Key Study Points

- Clinical and laboratory parameters appear to correlate with severity of illness and permit objective differentiation of children with acute hematogenous osteomyelitis who may be separated chronologically, geographically, or therapeutically.
- Clinical practice guidelines may be implemented in large pediatric medical centers and lead to better short- and intermediate-term outcomes.
- Improved use of MRI with sedation through a careful pre-MRI evaluation and interdisciplinary communication results in shortened MRI duration, a reduced rate of preliminary scanning, and a shortened period of hospitalization.

Annotated References

1. Gafur OA, Copley LA, Hollmig ST, Browne RH, Thornton LA, Crawford SE: The impact of the current epidemiology of pediatric musculoskeletal infection on evaluation and treatment guidelines. *J Pediatr Orthop* 2008;28(7):777-785.

2. Copley LA, Kinsler MA, Gheen T, Shar A, Sun D, Browne R: The impact of evidence-based clinical practice guidelines applied by a multidisciplinary team for the care of children with osteomyelitis. *J Bone Joint Surg Am* 2013;95(8):686-693.

   The authors describe an evidence-based, clinical practice guideline that was implemented by a multidisciplinary team. Improvement occurred with regard to the timing of initial MRI and the improved rate of administration of appropriate empiric antibiotic. There was a trend toward shorter hospitalization. Level of evidence: III.

3. Mueller AJ, Kwon JK, Steiner JW, et al: Improved magnetic resonance imaging utilization for children with musculoskeletal infection. *J Bone Joint Surg Am* 2015;97(22):1869-1876.

   This study demonstrates improvements in MRI scan duration, body areas imaged, and rate of acquisition after the use of a family-centered approach to care with interdisciplinary communication and coordination of the sedated MRI process. Level of evidence: II.

4. Zaoutis T, Localio AR, Leckerman K, Saddlemire S, Bertoch D, Keren R: Prolonged intravenous therapy versus early transition to oral antimicrobial therapy for acute osteomyelitis in children. *Pediatrics* 2009;123(2):636-642.

5. Jagodzinski NA, Kanwar R, Graham K, Bache CE: Prospective evaluation of a shortened regimen of treatment for acute osteomyelitis and septic arthritis in children. *J Pediatr Orthop* 2009;29(5):518-525.

6. Keren R, Shah SS, Srivastava R, et al; Pediatric Research in Inpatient Settings Network: Comparative effectiveness of intravenous vs oral antibiotics for postdischarge treatment of acute osteomyelitis in children. *JAMA Pediatr* 2015;169(2):120-128.

   The authors retrospectively reviewed 2,060 children treated for osteomyelitis. Oral antibiotics were administered to 48.7% of the patients and 52.3% were treated with intravenous antibiotics via a peripherally inserted central catheter line. The patients treated with the intravenous antibiotics had a 14.6% greater chance of a return visit to the emergency department or rehospitalization.

7. Street M, Puna R, Huang M, Crawford H: Pediatric acute hematogenous osteomyelitis. *J Pediatr Orthop* 2015;35(6):634-639.

   A 10-year series of 813 children with acute hematogenous osteomyelitis in New Zealand was reviewed for local epidemiology and outcomes. MSSA was the most common culture organism. MRSA occurred in 2% of the patients. Most of the children had minimally severe complications after approximately 6 weeks of combined antibiotic treatment with flucloxacillin followed by amoxicillin clavulanate. The rate of surgical intervention was 44%. Level of evidence: IV.

8. Tuason DA, Gheen T, Sun D, Huang R, Copley L: Clinical and laboratory parameters associated with multiple surgeries in children with acute hematogenous osteomyelitis. *J Pediatr Orthop* 2014;34(5):565-570.

   Children with osteomyelitis were stratified according the number of surgeries that they underwent during treatment. Objective laboratory and clinical parameters available early during the course of treatment were identified by regression analysis to substantially differentiate children who underwent zero, one, or multiple surgeries. Level of evidence: III.

9. Menge TJ, Cole HA, Mignemi ME, et al: Medial approach for drainage of the obturator musculature in children. *J Pediatr Orthop* 2014;34(3):307-315.

   The authors define a unique surgical approach that addresses a difficult problem that may exist in pelvic osteomyelitis with adjacent pyomyositis of the obturator internus and inner pelvic abscess. When this condition is associated with septic arthritis of the hip, the medial approach allows both problems to be addressed through a single surgical approach. Level of evidence: IV.

10. Ju KL, Zurakowski D, Kocher MS: Differentiating between methicillin-resistant and methicillin-sensitive Staphylococcus aureus osteomyelitis in children: An evidence-based clinical prediction algorithm. *J Bone Joint Surg Am* 2011;93(18):1693-1701.

    A clinical prediction algorithm was proposed to identify children with MRSA osteomyelitis from those with MSSA. Risk factors include temperature greater than 38°C, WBC greater than 12,000 cells/μL, hematocrit value less than 34%, and CRP level greater than 13 mg/L. All four predictors were present in 92% of the children with MRSA. Limitations of this study included the identification of only 11 children with MRSA osteomyelitis over a 10-year period. Level of evidence: IV.

11. Wade Shrader M, Nowlin M, Segal LS: Independent analysis of a clinical predictive algorithm to identify methicillin-resistant Staphylococcus aureus osteomyelitis in children. *J Pediatr Orthop* 2013;33(7):759-762.

    This study, performed in an MRSA endemic environment, showed that a previously reported clinical predication algorithm had a relatively poor diagnostic performance. The percentages of children with MRSA osteomyelitis were the same whether one or four risk factors were present. Level of evidence: III.

12. Saavedra-Lozano J, Mejías A, Ahmad N, et al: Changing trends in acute osteomyelitis in children: Impact of methicillin-resistant Staphylococcus aureus infections. *J Pediatr Orthop* 2008;28(5):569-575.

13. Peltola H, Pääkkönen M, Kallio P, Kallio MJ; Osteomyelitis-Septic Arthritis Study Group: Short- versus long-term antimicrobial treatment for acute hematogenous osteomyelitis of childhood: Prospective, randomized trial on 131 culture-positive cases. *Pediatr Infect Dis J* 2010;29(12):1123-1128.

14. Sarkissian EJ, Gans I, Gunderson MA, Myers SH, Spiegel DA, Flynn JM: Community-acquired methicillin-resistant Staphylococcus aureus musculoskeletal infections: Emerging trends over the past decade. *J Pediatr Orthop* 2016;36(3):323-327.

    The authors report a threefold increase in community-acquired MRSA musculoskeletal infections. These infections were associated with a higher incidence of complications during inpatient management, with multiple surgical procedures and longer inpatient hospitalization. Level of evidence: II.

15. Copley LA, Barton T, Garcia C, et al: A proposed scoring system for assessment of severity of illness in pediatric acute hematogenous osteomyelitis using objective clinical and laboratory findings. *Pediatr Infect Dis J* 2014;33(1):35-41.

    Objective clinical and laboratory data obtained within the first several days of hospitalization were used to construct a severity of illness scoring system to serve as a useful way to categorize children with acute hematogenous osteomyelitis by severity. The scoring system was then internally validated with evidence that severity of illness scoring significantly differentiates children on the basis of causative organism, length of hospitalization, number of surgeries, and complications.

16. Hawkshead JJ III, Patel NB, Steele RW, Heinrich SD: Comparative severity of pediatric osteomyelitis attributable to methicillin-resistant versus methicillin-sensitive Staphylococcus aureus. *J Pediatr Orthop* 2009;29(1):85-90.

17. Monsalve J, Kan JH, Schallert EK, Bisset GS, Zhang W, Rosenfeld SB: Septic arthritis in children: Frequency of coexisting unsuspected osteomyelitis and implications on imaging work-up and management. *AJR Am J Roentgenol* 2015;204(6):1289-1295.

    This study suggests a high rate of unrecognized osteomyelitis in children with septic arthritis (68% of those categorized as having septic arthritis before imaging). The authors recommend using MRI in all cases of suspected musculoskeletal infection and ensuring that the adjacent joint is visualized. Level of evidence: III.

18. Section J, Gibbons SD, Barton T, Greenberg DE, Jo CH, Copley LA: Microbiological culture methods for pediatric musculoskeletal infection: A guideline for optimal use. *J Bone Joint Surg Am* 2015;97(6):441-449.

    Culture methods and outcomes of children with a variety of musculoskeletal infections were compared across three different time periods. Rates of positive blood cultures and deep-tissue cultures were assessed by diagnosis and previous antibiotic exposure. The highest rates of bacteremia were noted for children with osteomyelitis. The lowest infection-site culture-positive rate was noted among children with septic arthritis. Anaerobic, fungal, and acid-fast bacteria cultures were not helpful in guiding treatment except in cases of suspected penetrating inoculation, immunocompromise, or failed primary treatment. A guideline is proposed for both superficial and deep infections. Level of evidence: III.

19. Rosenfeld S, Bernstein DT, Daram S, Dawson J, Zhang W: Predicting the presence of adjacent infections in septic arthritis in children. *J Pediatr Orthop* 2016;36(1):70-74.

    Patient age, CRP level, duration of symptoms, platelet count, and absolute neutrophil count were found to provide guidance for determining the probability of contiguous disease. Patients with multiple risk factors should have a preoperative MRI. Level of evidence: III.

20. Laine JC, Denning JR, Riccio AI, Jo C, Joglar JM, Wimberly RL: The use of ultrasound in the management of septic arthritis of the hip. *J Pediatr Orthop B* 2015;24(2):95-98.

    This study followed a guideline that children with clinical and ultrasound findings suggesting isolated septic arthritis were treated as having septic arthritis until proven otherwise by a failure to show clinical and laboratory improvement. Supplemental MRI was rarely needed. Level of evidence: IV.

21. Golla A, Jansson A, Ramser J, et al: Chronic recurrent multifocal osteomyelitis (CRMO): Evidence for a susceptibility gene located on chromosome 18q21.3-18q22. *Eur J Hum Genet* 2002;10(3):217-221.

22. Huber AM, Lam PY, Duffy CM, et al: Chronic recurrent multifocal osteomyelitis: Clinical outcomes after more than five years of follow-up. *J Pediatr* 2002;141(2):198-203.

23. Kaiser D, Bolt I, Hofer M, et al: Chronic nonbacterial osteomyelitis in children: A retrospective multicenter study. *Pediatr Rheumatol Online J* 2015;13:25.

    The authors noted a mean age of 9.5 years, a 3:1 female to male ratio, and an average delay in diagnosis of 8 months in patients with chronic nonbacterial osteomyelitis. They found no correlation between clinical presentation and positive laboratory tests. Most patients were treated with antibiotics (46%) and NSAIDs (90%). Chronic disease developed in 67.5% of the patients.

24. Carter K, Doern C, Jo CH, Copley LA: The clinical usefulness of polymerase chain reaction as a supplemental diagnostic tool in the evaluation and the treatment of children with septic arthritis. *J Pediatr Orthop* 2016;36(2):167-172.

    Polymerase chain reaction was found to be a useful tool to supplement blood and joint fluid culture findings and improve the rate of positive identification of a causative bacterial organism among children with septic arthritis. Level of evidence: II.

25. Williams N, Cooper C, Cundy P: Kingella kingae septic arthritis in children: Recognising an elusive pathogen. *J Child Orthop* 2014;8(1):91-95.

    A high level of suspicion for septic arthritis should be maintained for children between the age of 6 months and 4 years. Polymerase chain reaction techniques should be encouraged to increase the rate of positive confirmation of the *K kingae* bacteria. Level of evidence: IV.

26. Basmaci R, Lorrot M, Bidet P, et al: Comparison of clinical and biologic features of Kingella kingae and Staphylococcus aureus arthritis at initial evaluation. *Pediatr Infect Dis J* 2011;30(10):902-904.

    This study compared children with *S aureus* and children with *K kingae* septic arthritis. The children with *K kingae* septic arthritis were younger, had shorter hospitalizations, and fewer adverse events. Interestingly, the two groups did not otherwise differ with respect to synovial fluid cell count or inflammatory markers. Level of evidence: III.

27. Ceroni D, Belaieff W, Cherkaoui A, et al: Primary epiphyseal or apophyseal subacute osteomyelitis in the pediatric population: A report of fourteen cases and a systematic review of the literature. *J Bone Joint Surg Am* 2014;96(18):1570-1575.

    Primary epiphyseal osteomyelitis is a rare condition that should raise suspicion of possible *K kingae* osteomyelitis in children of an appropriate age. An organism-specific, real-time polymerase chain reaction assay markedly improves the rate of identification of the causative bacteria.

28. Morrissy RT, Haynes DW: Acute hematogenous osteomyelitis: A model with trauma as an etiology. *J Pediatr Orthop* 1989;9(4):447-456.

29. Montgomery CO, Siegel E, Blasier RD, Suva LJ: Concurrent septic arthritis and osteomyelitis in children. *J Pediatr Orthop* 2013;33(4):464-467.

    A closer evaluation is recommended for patients in certain age groups with septic arthritis in certain anatomic locations. There is a higher risk for contiguous infection, particularly in patients younger than 4 months and those between 13 and 20 years of age with septic arthritis of the shoulder. Supplemental advanced imaging is recommended in those groups. Level of evidence: III.

30. Caird MS, Flynn JM, Leung YL, Millman JE, D'Italia JG, Dormans JP: Factors distinguishing septic arthritis from transient synovitis of the hip in children. A prospective study. *J Bone Joint Surg Am* 2006;88(6):1251-1257.

31. Thompson RM, Gourineni P: Arthroscopic treatment of septic arthritis in very young children. *J Pediatr Orthop* 2015.

    A single portal inflow and outflow arthroscopic technique was shown to be safe and effective in a series of 24 children age 3 weeks to 6 years. In addition, the technique allowed improved joint visualization and minimal soft-tissue dissection. Level of evidence: IV.

32. Chou AC, Mahadev A: The use of C-reactive protein as a guide for transitioning to oral antibiotics in pediatric osteoarticular infections. *J Pediatr Orthop* 2016;36(2):173-177.

    Conversion to oral antibiotic therapy and hospital discharge was guided by the combination of clinical improvement with a specific reduction in CRP level by 50% over 4 days. A persistently elevated CRP level was associated with adverse outcomes. Level of evidence: IV.

33. Deanehan JK, Nigrovic PA, Milewski MD, et al: Synovial fluid findings in children with knee monoarthritis in Lyme disease endemic areas. *Pediatr Emerg Care* 2014;30(1):16-19.

    Synovial fluid results are not sufficient to differentiate Lyme arthritis from septic arthritis. Other clinical and laboratory indicators are required to guide treatment. Level of evidence: III.

34. Deanehan JK, Kimia AA, Tan Tanny SP, et al: Distinguishing Lyme from septic knee monoarthritis in Lyme disease-endemic areas. *Pediatrics* 2013;131(3):e695-e701.

    Children with knee monoarthritis may be safely distinguished from those who probably have septic arthritis using laboratory criteria. This may avoid the need for diagnostic arthrocentesis in most low-risk cases. Level of evidence: III.

35. Tory HO, Zurakowski D, Sundel RP: Outcomes of children treated for Lyme arthritis: Results of a large pediatric cohort. *J Rheumatol* 2010;37(5):1049-1055.

Chapter 5

Benign and Malignant Musculoskeletal Neoplasms

Mihir M. Thacker, MD   Alexandre Arkader, MD

Abstract

Malignant bone and soft-tissue tumors in children are far less common than benign lesions. Most orthopaedic surgeons, as well as primary care practitioners, are frequently unfamiliar with these conditions. This can lead to inappropriate workup, delayed diagnoses, and, in some instances, improper initial treatment. It is helpful to be familiar with the principles of clinical and imaging evaluations of bone and soft-tissue lesions in children, along with the genetic syndromes that predispose children to tumor development. It is important to be knowledgeable about recent advances for imaging and treatment of the most common benign and malignant tumors in children.

Keywords: benign lesion; bone tumor; Ewing sarcoma; malignant tumor; osteosarcoma; sarcoma; soft-tissue tumor; rhabdomyosarcoma

Introduction

Cancer is the main cause of death from disease during childhood. Fortunately, most bone and soft-tissue tumors in children are benign. The correct and prompt diagnosis of these lesions can be challenging, leading to unnecessary stress and anxiety for families and patients. Understanding the steps in making a diagnosis and managing this broad group of conditions may allow early appropriate treatment, improving the child's prognosis and outcome.

In this chapter, the principles of approaching bone and soft-tissue lesions in children and the most common genetic syndromes that predispose children to the development of tumors are discussed. The chapter also focuses on recent advances in the treatment and prognosis for the most common benign and malignant lesions.

Dr. Thacker or an immediate family member has received nonincome support (such as equipment or services), commercially-derived honoraria, or other non–research-related funding (such as paid travel) from Biomarin and serves as a board member, owner, officer, or committee member of the Pediatric Orthopaedic Society of North America. Dr. Arkader or an immediate family member serves as an unpaid consultant to Orthopediatrics SAB.

Genetic Syndromes With an Increased Risk for Neoplasia

Li-Fraumeni Syndrome

Li-Fraumeni syndrome is a rare autosomal dominant familial disorder that increases the risk for the development of several types of cancer, particularly in children and young adults. The hallmark of the syndrome is germline alterations of the *TP53* tumor suppressor gene; however, a smaller percentage of patients have inactivation of the *CHEK2* suppressor gene. Up to 10% of children with sporadic rhabdomyosarcoma or osteosarcoma carry germline *TP53* mutations; clinically, these patients tend to be younger and have poorer outcomes.[1]

Beckwith-Wiedemann Syndrome

Beckwith-Wiedemann syndrome is a rare congenital overgrowth syndrome, with an incidence of 1 in 14,000 births. It occurs predominantly with a sporadic inheritance pattern; however, autosomal dominance with variable expression is possible. The responsible gene is located at 11p15.5, and the risk of recurrence in the same family is as high as 20%.

A diagnosis is usually made after birth based on the clinical features, including neonatal hypoglycemia and accelerated bone maturation, which is demonstrated by gigantism, metaphyseal flaring, and narrowing of the diaphysis. Patients may also present with craniofacial features, renal/endocrine involvement, abdominal wall defects, polycythemia, and cardiovascular anomalies. There is an increased risk of malignancy (approximately 7%), particularly for embryonal tumors such as Wilms tumor, rhabdomyosarcoma, and neuroblastoma.[2] It is recommended that patients be monitored with serial ultrasounds of the pelvis and abdomen at 3- to 4-month intervals for the first 4 years of life.[2]

McCune-Albright Syndrome

McCune-Albright syndrome is characterized by the classic triad of polyostotic fibrous dysplasia, café au lait spots, and endocrinopathies (precocious puberty being the most common).

The etiology of fibrous dysplasia has been linked to an activating mutation in the *GNAS* gene (located on 20q13.2-13.3) that encodes the Gsα protein. The result is failure of maturation from woven to lamellar bone, with a subsequent decrease in the mechanical strength of the affected bone; this leads to pain, fractures, and angular deformities.

The polyostotic form of this syndrome is less common but more severe, has the tendency to involve one side more severely, and causes deformities and limb-length discrepancies. Any bone may be involved, and craniofacial involvement occurs in 50% of patients.

McCune-Albright syndrome is associated with a 1% to 4% incidence of malignant degeneration, most commonly to osteosarcoma, fibrosarcoma, chondrosarcoma, and malignant fibrous histiocytoma. Malignant degeneration should be suspected if there is an increase in pain and a radiographically detected interval growth of the lesion, especially with a new associated soft-tissue mass. The use of radiation therapy to treat primary lesions (no longer recommended) increases the risk of malignancy.[3]

Ollier Disease and Maffucci Syndrome

Both Ollier disease and Maffucci syndrome represent a spectrum of the same disease and are characterized by the presence of multiple enchondromas, typically in a unilateral pattern and associated with deformities. There is no evidence of a hereditary component, and the conditions affect both sexes and all races.

The risk of malignant degeneration with Ollier disease is approximately 5% to 30% by age 40 years (the risk of malignant degeneration of a solitary enchondroma is 1% or less). Increased growth of a lesion that is associated with pain is a cause for suspicion, especially in skeletally mature patients. Although no consensus exists on the best method to monitor these lesions, it is generally agreed that MRI is the first modality that should be used. Bone scans and positron emission tomography (PET) can be used to assess the level of activity within the lesion, but false positivity is an issue.[4]

The association of multiple enchondromas and multiple hemangiomas involving the soft tissues and other viscera characterizes Maffucci syndrome. This condition presents with a higher risk for malignant degeneration (approximately 50%; most commonly into chondrosarcoma or angiosarcoma), particularly among pelvic lesions.[4]

Multiple Hereditary Exostoses

Multiple hereditary exostoses is an autosomal dominant condition with a 96% penetrance rate. There are two main genes linked to the disease, *EXT1* located on 8q24.1 (responsible for approximately 50% of the cases), and *EXT2* located on 11p13 (seen in 30% of the patients). Both genes are suppressor genes that are responsible for regulating chondrocyte maturation and differentiation and are absent in this condition.

Clinical features include multiple osteochondromas, short stature, angular deformities, pain, and limited motion. The rate of secondary malignant degeneration varies from 1% to 20% depending on the series (most recently 2.7%), and occurs after the third decade of life. Lesions in the axial skeleton more frequently become malignant.[5]

Screening for possible malignant degeneration should be done on a case-by-case basis. Enlarged lesions seen after skeletal maturity should raise suspicion and should be screened with MRI. A cartilaginous cap larger than 2 cm in adults is highly suspicious for malignancy, and lesion excision is generally recommended.[6]

Hereditary Retinoblastoma

Retinoblastoma is a malignant tumor of the embryonic neural retina and is the most common intraocular malignancy in children with an annual incidence of 1 in 18,000 live births per year.

The hereditary form (40% of all patients) is caused by deletions in the *Rb1* suppressor gene. In 10% of patients, there is a family history of retinoblastoma. Sixty percent of cases are bilateral, and there is increased risk (approximately 50%) of a second malignancy (most commonly osteosarcoma).[7]

Patient Workup

Imaging

After a thorough clinical evaluation has been completed, imaging modalities are critical for further workup of patients with bone and soft-tissue tumors. Plain radiographs are the best diagnostic imaging modality to establish a differential diagnosis for bone tumors and may be diagnostic in many instances (**Table 1**). The clinician

Table 1

Differential Diagnoses of Bone Lesions

	Single Lesion		Multiple Lesions	
Where is it?	Epiphysis	Chondroblastoma, GCT, Clear cell CHSA, Brodie abscess, Trevor disease (DEH)	Osseous	Bone islands (osteopoikilosis), melorheostosis, multifocal osteosarcoma
	Metaphysis	Most tumors		
	Diaphysis	Fibrous dysplasia, Ewing sarcoma, osteofibrous dysplasia/ adamantinoma, LCH, leukemia/lymphoma, osteoid osteoma		
What is it doing to the bone?	Sclerotic		Chondroid	Multiple osteochondromatosis, Trevor disease (DEH), Ollier disease, Maffucci syndrome
	Lucent			
What is the bone doing to it?	Zone of transition (margin)	Biologic behavior: narrow/geographic, less aggressive	Fibrous	Polyostotic fibrous dysplasia, multiple NOFs
	Periosteal reaction	Onion skin, sunburst, buttress type (solid)		
Is there any identifiable matrix mineralization pattern?	Cloud-like	Osseous	Miscellaneous	LCH, leukemia, lymphoma, brown tumors
	Rings, arcs, stipples	Chondroid		
	Ground glass	Fibro-osseous		

CHSA = chondrosarcoma, DEH = dysplasia epiphysealis hemimelica, GCT = giant cell tumor, LCH = Langerhans cell histiocytosis, NOF = nonossifying fibroma, OFD = osteofibrous dysplasia.

should evaluate the anatomic location of the lesion (for example, which bone and which part of the bone), the zone of transition, the mineralization pattern, and the presence or absence of a soft-tissue extension. Radiographs of soft-tissue masses may reveal the presence of phleboliths (in a vascular malformation), extrinsic compression of the bone (in slow-growing lesions), or bone invasion (in aggressive lesions). Ultrasound is extremely useful for differentiating between solid and cystic lesions, as well as for the evaluation of vascular lesions. Bone scans are essential for staging malignant bone lesions (such as osteosarcoma and Ewing sarcoma) and also for the evaluation of metastatic disease.

MRI has become standard for the diagnosis and evaluation of the local extent of most bone and soft-tissue lesions (with the notable exception of osteoid osteomas, which are better evaluated with a fine-cut CT scan). Full-body MRI is being increasingly used for screening in infantile myofibromatosis and Langerhans cell histiocytosis, and its use is being evaluated in soft-tissue sarcomas, although it is not as reliable as CT in detecting pulmonary metastases. Full-body MRI seems to be better for detecting lymph node and osseous involvement.

The role of PET continues to evolve. It has become standard in the staging of lymphomas and melanomas (in adults). PET scans are being used with increasing frequency to stage other tumors and predict the response to chemotherapy (potentially guiding the selection of proper margins of resection). PET is also being used to try to differentiate between plexiform neurofibromas and malignant peripheral nerve sheath tumors, although PET has higher sensitivity than specificity in this setting.

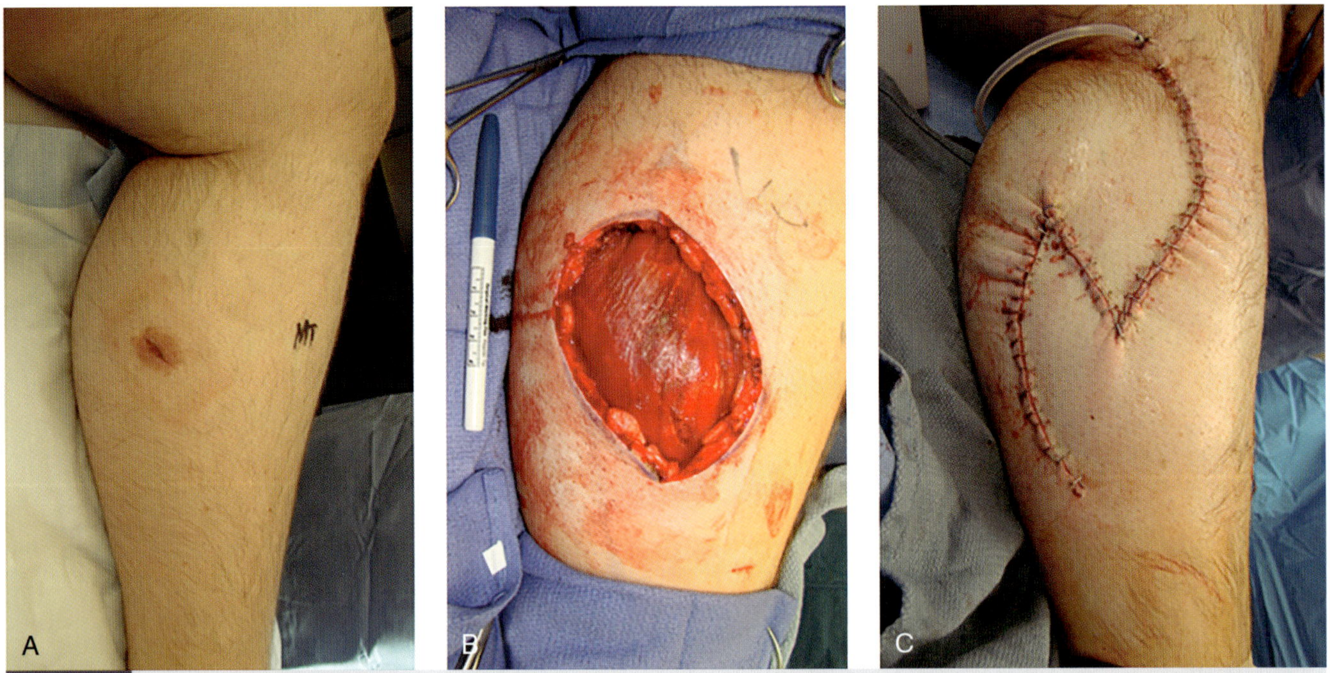

Figure 1 Clinical photographs showing an inappropriately performed biopsy. The incision is obliquely oriented on the calf (**A**), necessitating wide resection of the entire biopsy tract (**B**), and local flaps were used for coverage after definitive resection (**C**).

Imaging is nonspecific for soft-tissue tumors (except for lipomas, which can be reliably diagnosed on MRI), and biopsy becomes more critical in establishing a definitive diagnosis.

Biopsy Principles

Biopsy is an essential step in the diagnosis of many bone and soft-tissue lesions; however, there are risks associated with inappropriately performed biopsies. The Musculoskeletal Tumor Society has reported that biopsy has an 18% rate of diagnostic error and a 19% complication rate.[8] The definitive surgical procedure often needs to be modified as a result of an inappropriately performed biopsy, which can lead to a more complex resection and sometimes amputation (Figure 1). Biopsy-related complications are five times more common when the procedure is performed at a community or referring hospital compared with a tertiary care center.

Controversy still persists regarding the optimal biopsy modality. Core needle biopsy has a lower risk of contamination and cost compared with open incisional biopsy. The use of image guidance increases the accuracy of percutaneous biopsies, while reducing the risk of complications.[9]

For bone biopsy, planning should take into consideration the definitive surgery and the presence of a soft-tissue mass that may be more accessible than the bone. In general, for a soft-tissue biopsy, the most direct approach to the tumor is the preferred strategy.

Other strategies while planning a biopsy include reviewing the optimal location with the pathologist and radiologist because, in some instances, a second, more accessible lesion can be identified. For open biopsy, a longitudinal incision should be made without raising flaps. Meticulous homeostasis is essential to prevent the spread of tumor cells, thus limiting the size of the eventual resection to obtain clean margins. Obtaining an intraoperative frozen section is important to ensure adequate sampling, and specimens also should be sent for culture. Biopsy principles are outlined in Table 2. Routine use of immunohistochemistry has made it much easier to identify and classify tumors. The detection of specific mutations within tumor cells may determine the prognosis and even help target specific treatments.

Benign Bone Tumors

Benign bone tumors are very common and most frequently discovered incidentally. It is important for the evaluating physician to be familiar with the pathogenesis and prognosis for each skeletal lesion to guide the workup and treatment. The treatment of benign bone lesions depends on the natural history of the lesion, the risk of tumor progression, the risk of pathologic fracture, and the current symptoms of the patient. Most benign active or aggressive bone lesions are treated surgically, although other modalities may be used in certain situations.

Osteoid Osteomas

Osteoid osteomas are characterized by night pain that is classically relieved by NSAIDs. In the past, these lesions were treated with surgical excision of the nidus (**Figure 2**). Radiofrequency ablation is now the standard treatment of osteoid osteoma and also has achieved some success in the treatment of chondroblastoma. Percutaneous image-guided laser photocoagulation has been used in spinal osteoid osteoma with good results. Special thermal protection techniques for the neural structures should be used if the nidus is within 1 to 2 cm of neural structures or in the absence of a protective cortex.[10]

Table 2

Principles of Biopsy of Bone and Soft-Tissue Tumors

- The biopsy should be performed at the site of definitive treatment whenever possible.
- Review clinical and radiographic findings with radiologist and pathologist before the biopsy.
- Use a tourniquet but avoid expressive exsanguination (Esmarch bandage).
- Use shortest possible incision, longitudinally placed, along the line of definitive resection.
- Minimize soft-tissue dissection and contamination by dissecting through muscle, taking the most direct route feasible to the tumor.
- Biopsy the advancing edge of the tumor, obtaining adequate lesional tissue (use of frozen section).
- Obtain good hemostasis before closure, with use of a drain (brought out in line with the incision) as needed.
- Sutures should be placed close to the skin edge to minimize amount of skin to be excised at definitive resection.

Bone Cysts

Unicameral bone cysts are cystic lesions found in the metaphyses of long bones, most commonly in the proximal humerus (approximately 60%), proximal femur (approximately 30%), and the os calcis (typically under the angle of Gissane). These lesions cause thinning of the bone and may result in a pathologic fracture, often with the "fallen leaf/fragment" sign (**Figure 3**). Treatment of unicameral bone cysts remains controversial.[11] There is a prospective multicenter study currently underway (the Simple Bone Cysts in Kids [SBocK] clinical trial) that is evaluating the role of cyst perforation versus perforation and injection; results are not yet available.

Aneurysmal bone cysts may be primary or secondary to another underlying lesion. These lesions can be quite aggressive. Nodular enhancement of the cyst wall on postcontrast MRI as well as a lack of a peripheral rim of bone should raise suspicion for a possible telangiectatic osteosarcoma (**Figure 4**). The possibility of a secondary aneurysmal bone cyst must be considered, especially if it is in an epiphyseal location. The treatment of aneurysmal

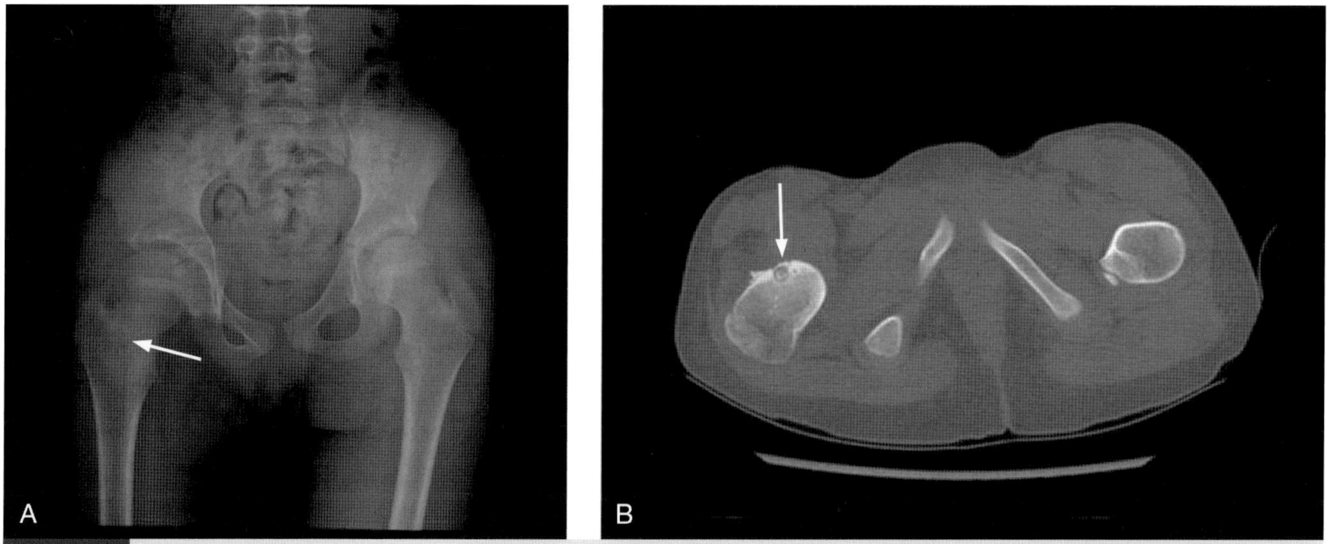

Figure 2 Imaging studies from a 10-year-old girl who presented with right hip pain. **A,** AP radiograph demonstrates a lucent lesion in the intertrochanteric region with a sclerotic focus within it (arrow) and surrounding reactive new bone. **B,** CT scan demonstrates a cortically-based nidus (arrow) that is suggestive of an osteoid osteoma.

bone cysts is primarily surgical, with aggressive curettage (with or without the use adjuvant therapy). For aneurysmal bone cysts, especially those in surgically challenging locations, repeated embolization or injection of doxycycline foam has been used with moderate success.[12]

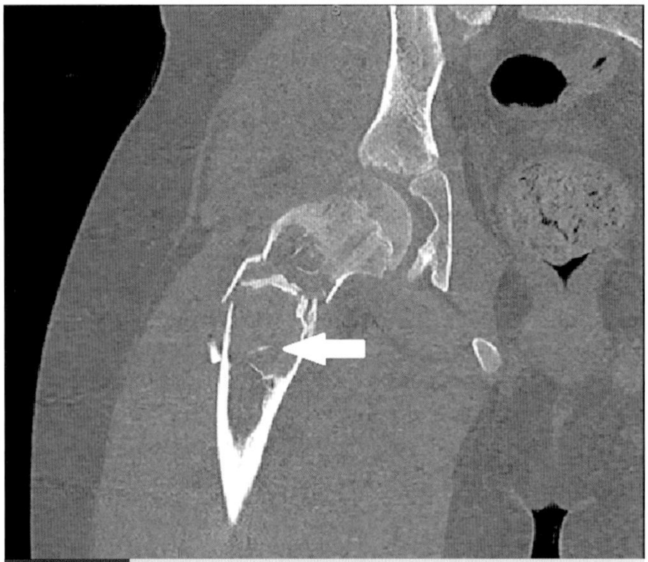

Figure 3 Coronal CT section shows a fracture through a proximal femoral unicameral bone cyst with a "fallen leaf/fragment" sign (arrow).

Chondroid Lesions

Osteochondromas are the most common chondroid lesions. These lesions may be single or multiple. Symptoms may be related to pressure or irritation of surrounding structures, fracture, limitation of motion, growth abnormality, or a rare malignant transformation (more likely in multiple osteochondromas). Mutations of the *EXT1* and *EXT2* genes result in disordered cartilage growth and account for most cases of multiple hereditary osteochondromatosis. These mutations are inherited in an autosomal dominant fashion. Given the increased appreciation of spinal osteochondromas, it is important to screen these patients for occipital headaches and neck and back pain and perform a thorough neurologic examination.

Chondroblastomas are the most common epiphyseal benign bone lesions in skeletally immature patients and typically cause pain. MRI will demonstrate characteristic perilesional edema around the lesion (**Figure 5**). Approximately one-third of these lesions will be associated with secondary aneurysmal bone cysts. Treatment is usually extended curettage and grafting, but there are recent reports of successful use of radiofrequency ablation.[13]

Fibrous Dysplasia

Fibrous dysplasia results from a nonheritable missense mutation of the alpha subunit of the G-protein (*GNAS1* mutation). Approximately 80% of patients have monostotic

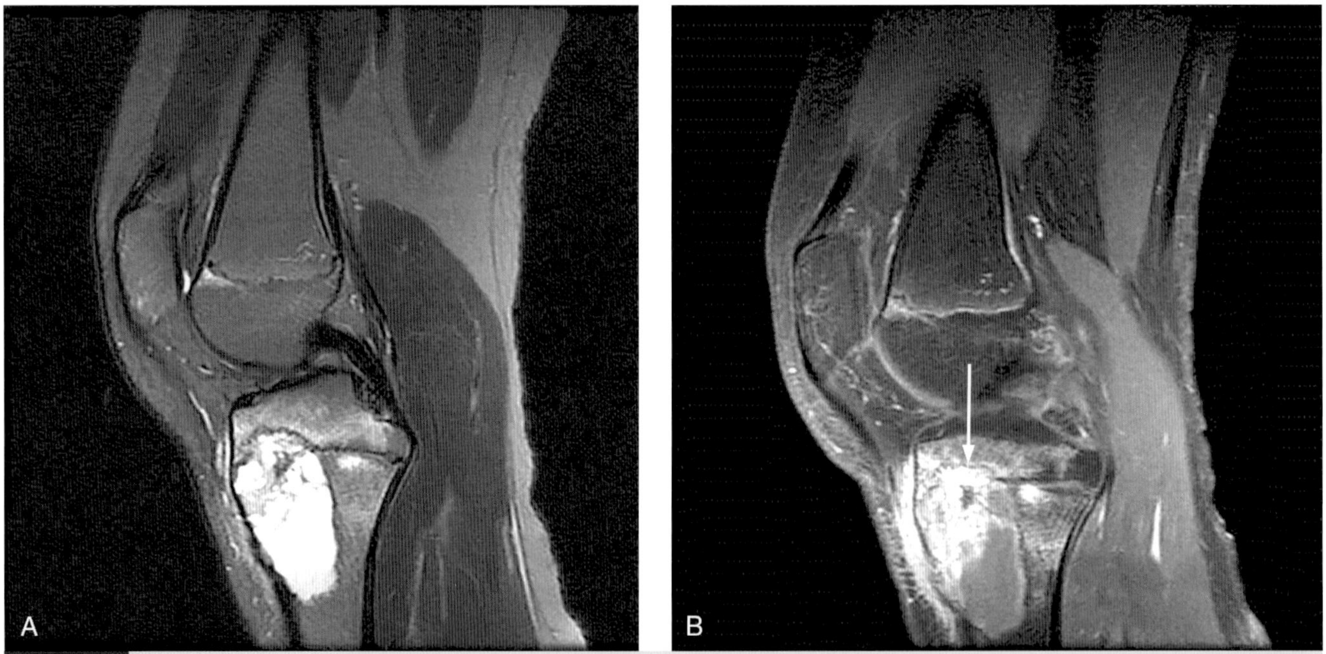

Figure 4 **A,** T2-weighted MRI of a proximal tibial cystic lesion with multiple fluid levels is suggestive of an aneurysmal bone cyst. **B,** T1-weighted MRI with nodular enhancement (arrow) with contrast raises suspicion of a telangiectatic osteosarcoma, which was the diagnosis in this case based on the biopsy.

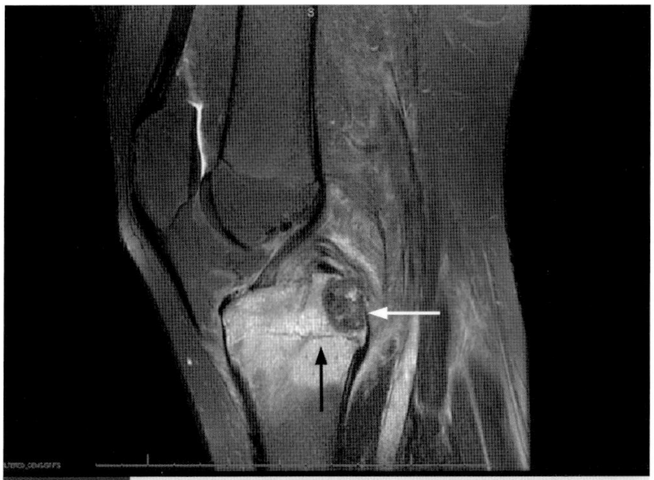

Figure 5 Proximal tibial epiphyseal lesion, with hypointense signal on a T2-weighted MRI sequence (white arrow) with characteristic perilesional edema (black arrow), is suggestive of a chondroblastoma.

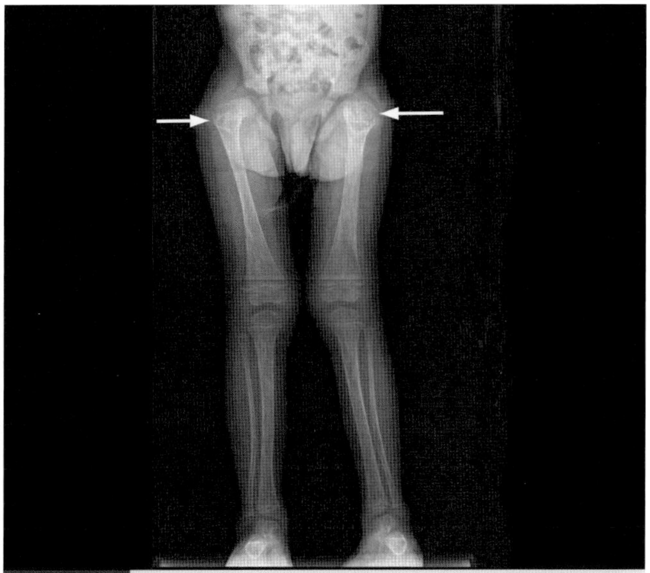

Figure 6 Radiograph from a child (age, 2 years and 9 months) with polyostotic fibrous dysplasia with bilateral coxa vara (arrows).

involvement and 20% have polyostotic involvement. The combination of polyostotic fibrous dysplasia, café au lait spots with jagged or irregular (coast of Maine) borders, and endocrinopathy is referred to as McCune-Albright syndrome. Indications for treatment in fibrous dysplasia include pain, fracture and deformity (especially in the proximal femur-shepherd crook deformity; **Figure 6**). Because there is a high rate of bone graft resorption in fibrous dysplasia, bulk allografts seem to offer the best resistance. Intramedullary fixation is preferred in patients with more extensive diaphyseal involvement.

The use of diphosphonates in polyostotic fibrous dysplasia remains controversial and is associated with reduction of biologic markers of bone turnover, improved bone mineral density, and improved radiographic appearance. Improvement in pain and function is not as clear.[14]

Langerhans Cell Histiocytosis

Langerhans cell histiocytosis is a disorder caused by clonal proliferation of CD1a+/CD207+ cells. Recent studies have identified MAPK pathway mutations in most patients with this lesion with *BRAF* V600E mutations in approximately 50% of patients and *MAP2K1* mutations in approximately 25% of the patients.[15] *BRAF* V600E mutations are associated with some increased risk of recurrence but do not affect overall survival. Treatment is risk stratified. Single-site involvement is usually treated locally, but multiple-site involvement, especially with involvement of the liver, spleen, lung, or hematopoietic system (high-risk organs), is treated more aggressively with chemotherapy. BRAF enzyme inhibitors (such as vemurafenib) have been used with some success.[16]

Malignant Bone Tumors

Osteosarcoma

Osteosarcoma is the most common primary bone sarcoma. It has two peak periods of incidence: during adolescence (>60% in the second decade of life) and during the sixth decade of life (often in Paget disease of bone). Although a genetic predisposition has been described, no constant genetic aberration has been identified.

Pain is the most common presenting symptom and is often associated with the presence of a firm, nonmobile mass. Pathologic fracture may occur in up to 10% of patients, and constitutional symptoms are usually a late sign. Most osteosarcomas occur around the knee (60%) or the shoulder.[17]

Radiographically, osteosarcoma is usually a destructive, poorly marginated blastic or mixed blastic-lytic lesion, arising in the metaphysis of long bones (**Figure 7**). Codman triangle and sunburst patterns of periosteal reaction are usually seen. MRI with and without contrast shows a heterogeneous-appearing mass with increased signal intensity on T2-weighted sequences and enhancement with gadolinium. There is typically a soft-tissue component to the bone tumor. Staging includes MRI of the entire affected bone (to look for skip lesions), a full-body bone scan, and a CT scan of the chest.

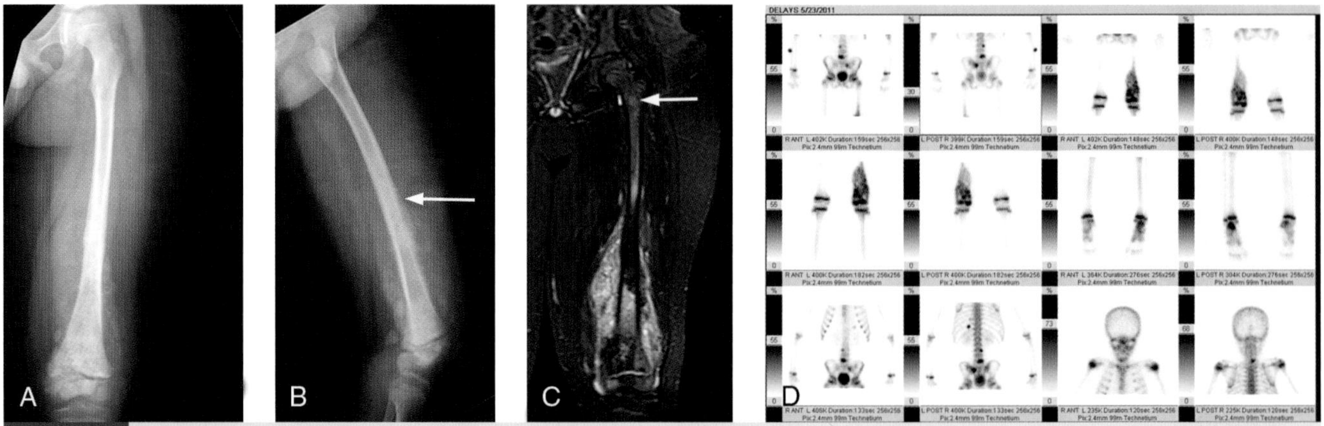

Figure 7 Images from a 9-year-old child with thigh pain and a mass. **A,** Radiograph shows moth-eaten appearance of the distal femur, with a poorly defined sclerotic lesion in the metaphysis and distal diaphysis and mineralization in the soft tissue. **B,** Radiograph shows a Codman triangle (arrow) created by the tumor, elevating the periosteum. **C,** MRI shows extensive involvement of the femur with a large soft-tissue mass as well as a skip lesion (arrow) in the proximal femoral metaphysis. **D,** A full-body bone scan shows multiple osseous metastatic lesions.

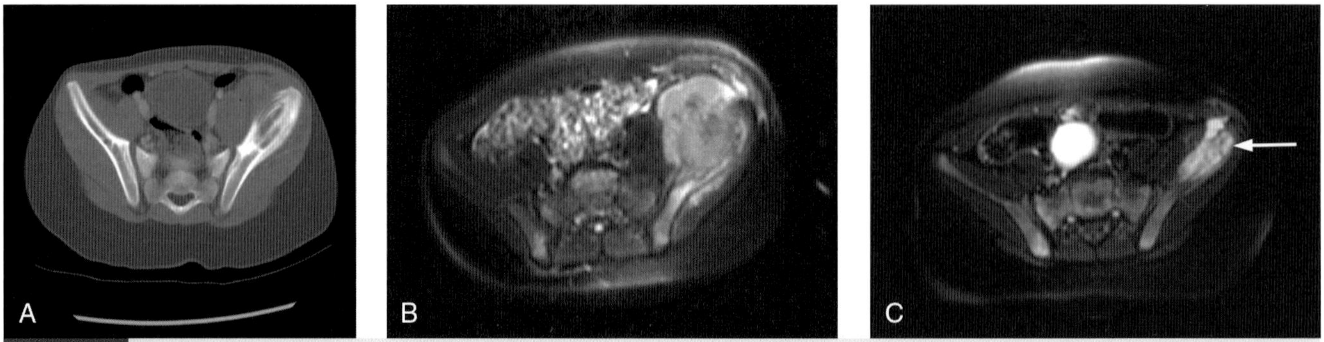

Figure 8 Images from a 6-year-old child with a left-sided pelvic mass. **A,** Axial cut CT shows a soft-tissue mass on the inner table and a lytic lesion in the left ilium with a lamellated periosteal reaction (onion skin). T2-weighted MRIs before chemotherapy (**B**) and after chemotherapy (**C**) show substantial shrinkage of the soft-tissue component. This response is fairly typical in Ewing sarcoma.

The treatment of osteosarcoma is multimodal, including neoadjuvant (presurgery) and adjuvant (postoperative) chemotherapy; most protocols use a combination of doxorubicin, ifosfamide, cisplatinum, and high-dose methotrexate. Local control is achieved with resection via limb salvage (90% of patients) or amputation. The overall survival rate for patients with localized disease is approximately 70% at 5 years, which has improved from the zero to 30% survival rates during the era before chemotherapy.[18]

A poor prognosis is associated with an axial location, a large tumor (>8 cm), the presence of metastases or skip lesions at presentation (approximately 20% of cases, with most of these lesions in the lungs), a less than 90% tumor necrosis rate after chemotherapy, and a highly elevated alkaline phosphatase level at diagnosis (greater than 3 times the normal level).

Ewing Sarcoma

Ewing sarcoma is in the family of primitive neuroectodermal tumors and is the second most common primary bone tumor in children. Although the cell of origin is unknown, it is characterized by a recurrent 11:22 translocation and the presence of the *EWS-FLI1* gene.

Similar to osteosarcoma, Ewing sarcoma often occurs around the knee and shoulder. However, it has a higher propensity to involve the axial skeleton. Ewing sarcoma is more common than osteosarcoma in the first decade of life, but in the second decade of life, osteosarcoma becomes approximately three times as common.

Clinically, Ewing sarcoma can present with constitutional symptoms in addition to the classic signs of pain and a palpable mass, and it thus may mimic infection. On imaging, Ewing sarcoma is often associated with a very large soft-tissue mass, and it classically arises from

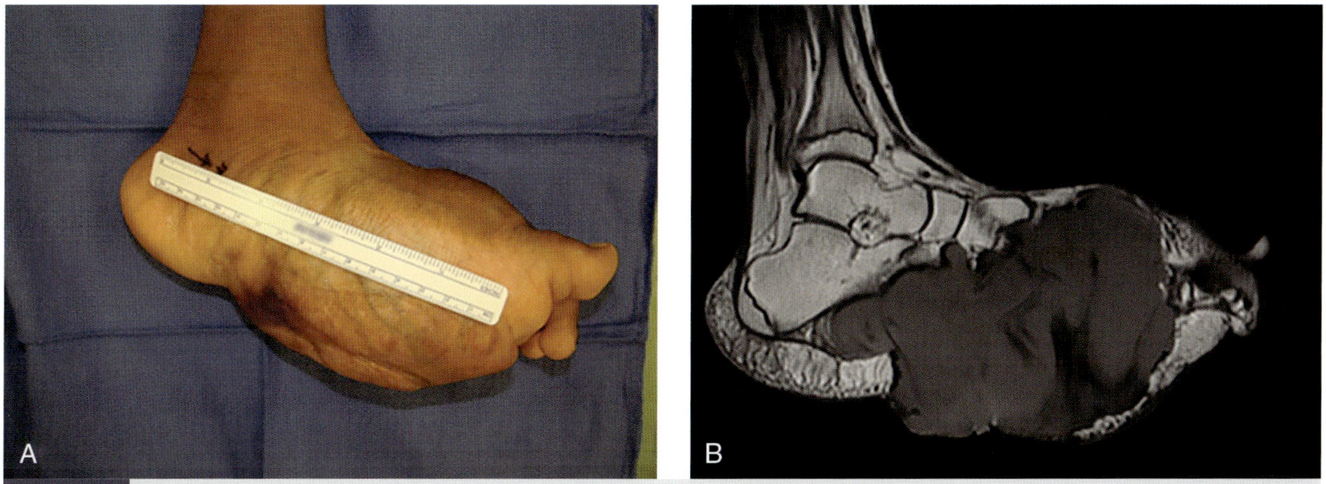

Figure 9 **A,** Clinical photograph of the foot of a 13-year-old patient with aggressive fibromatosis. MRI shows that the lesion invades the soft tissues and extends from the dorsum to the plantar aspect of the foot and fungates through the bottom of the foot.

the diaphysis instead of the metaphysis. There is no bone production. Onion skin (lamellated) periosteal reaction may be seen but is not diagnostic (**Figure 8**). Staging is similar to that performed for osteosarcoma, but additionally includes a bone marrow biopsy.

The treatment of Ewing sarcoma is also multimodal, with neoadjuvant and adjuvant chemotherapy. In contrast to osteosarcoma, radiation therapy is also an alternative to surgery for local control, but it has its own set of complications, especially in a growing child.[19] Some described complications include growth disturbance, neurologic compromise, contracture, pathologic fracture, and secondary sarcoma. Radiation therapy may also be used in patients with close or positive tumor margins.

Benign Soft-Tissue Tumors

Lipoma and Lipoblastoma

Lipomas are the most common mesenchymal soft-tissue tumors. They are composed of mature white adipocytes, and most lipomas have a recurrent chromosomal aberration at 12q. These tumors have no malignant potential. Approximately 5% of lipomas are related to a familial predisposition. Most patients present with a painless mass and are adults past the fourth decade of life. MRI is diagnostic for lipomas with uniform fatty signal (hyperintense on both T1- and T2-weighted MRIs) with uniform and complete suppression on fat-suppression sequences.

Lipoblastomas are characterized by nodules of adipose and myxoid tissue, which are demarcated by bands of fibrous tissue. Although they can be localized and clinically similar to lipomas, lipoblastomas also can present in a diffuse form that infiltrates surrounding muscles and soft tissues. These are exclusively tumors of infancy (most patients are younger than 3 years), with trunk and limb involvement occurring at similar incidences. The diffuse form is also known as lipoblastomatosis, and it has a 10% to 20% recurrence rate, with axial involvement being common.[20] The treatment of these lesions varies from observation alone to surgical resection.

Desmoid Tumors and Fibromatosis

Desmoid tumors and fibromatosis represent a benign fibroblastic proliferation with an infiltrative growth pattern. These lesions have a high recurrence rate and no metastatic potential. These lesions can be superficial (fibromatosis) or deep (aggressive fibromatosis or desmoid tumors). The superficial form is mostly limited to the fascia and includes Dupuytren (palmar), Ledderhose (plantar), and Peyronie disease (penile), or digital fibromatosis. Desmoid tumors can occur in a limb or in abdominal and retroperitoneal regions.

Although the etiology of these lesions is unknown, they have been associated with epilepsy, diabetes, and alcoholism in adults. A family history of the lesion may also exist.

Clinically, the disease starts as a painless firm mass (especially the superficial form). The rate of progression is variable, with some deep lesions being quite infiltrative. MRI demonstrates an irregular mass with poorly defined borders (unlike most other soft-tissue masses) and a variable degree of hypointense signal (depending on the degree of fibrosis) (**Figure 9**). WNT/beta catenin (*CTNNB1*) mutations have been identified in these tumors. The *S45F* mutation has been associated with very rapid recurrence, and identification of this mutation may suggest use of nonsurgical modalities.[21]

Surgical resection is the mainstay of treatment. Although nonsurgical treatments with NSAIDs, tamoxifen, methotrexate, vinblastine, and sorafenib have been described, the results are inconsistent and frequently temporary. The two main concerns with this condition are the high recurrence rate and the potential for infiltration of surrounding tissues.[22] With improvement in the understanding of the pathogenesis of desmoid tumors and fibromatosis (involvement of the WNT/beta catenin pathway and Notch signaling), targeted medical treatments are being explored.[23]

Peripheral Nerve Tumors

The most common peripheral nerve tumors are neuromas, schwannomas, and neurofibromas. Neuromas are a result of a trauma and are a nonneoplastic proliferation. These tumors are most commonly seen after amputation.

Schwannomas are encapsulated nerve sheath tumors. Although they are more common between the ages of 20 and 50 years, they may occur in children. The most common locations are the head, the neck, and flexor surfaces. Schwannomas are usually solitary and sporadic lesions and are rarely associated with neurofibromatosis type 2. The risk of malignant degeneration is minimal. Histology reveals characteristic Antoni A and Antoni B areas with nuclear palisading (Verocay bodies).

Neurofibromas can be isolated or associated with neurofibromatosis type 1. Neurofibromas are usually painless, superficial, slow-growing lesions generally involving small nerves. These are more difficult to separate from the parent nerve at surgery compared with schwannomas. The diffuse/plexiform form is associated with neurofibromatosis type 1. These lesions can degenerate into malignant peripheral nerve sheath tumor and warrant monitoring.[24]

Giant Cell Tendon Sheath Tumors and Pigmented Villonodular Synovitis

Giant cell tendon sheath tumors and pigmented villonodular synovitis (PVS) are tumors of the synovium and can be localized or diffuse. Increased levels of colony stimulating factor-1 have been demonstrated in these tumors. This attracts macrophages that have a receptor for colony stimulating factor-1 and induce inflammation and consequent joint damage. Giant cell tendon sheath tumors often involve the limbs and present as a painless growing mass, whereas PVS can be intra-articular, with the knee as the most common location, or extra-articular. PVS is often diffuse, and patients have recurrent joint swelling and pain.

These lesions characteristically present as low signal on both T1- and T2-weighted MRIs. Gradient-recalled echo imaging highlights the presence of hemosiderin, which results in the typical "blooming" artifact.

The mainstay of treatment is surgical resection, although there are studies researching the use of chemotherapy (such as tyrosine kinase inhibitor).[25] The local recurrence risk (approximately 20%) in patients with diffuse PVNS is much higher than in patients with localized disease in whom surgery is often curative and has a very low recurrence rate.[26]

Table 3

Cytogenetic Abnormalities in Some Common Tumors

Tumor	Cytogenetic Abnormality
Embryonal rhabdomyosarcoma	Loss of heterozygosity at 11p15
Alveolar rhabdomyosarcoma	t(2;13)(q35;q14) or t(1;13)(q36;q14) or 25% to 40% of cases without either
Synovial sarcoma	t(X;18)(p11;q11)
Infantile fibrosarcoma	t(12;15)(9p13;q25)
Epithelioid sarcoma-proximal	22q11.2 alterations
Alveolar soft-part sarcoma	(der17)(x;17)(p11.2;q25)
Myxoid liposarcoma	t(12;16)(q13;11) and t(2;22)(q13;q12)
Extraskeletal myxoid chondrosarcoma	t(9;22)(q22;q12) or t(9;17)(q22;q12) or t(9;15)(q22;q21)
Extraskeletal Ewing sarcoma	t(11;22)(q24;q12) and other less common variants

Malignant Soft-Tissue Tumors

Pediatric soft-tissue sarcomas account for 7% of all childhood tumors. The clinical presentation of soft-tissue sarcomas may be somewhat misleading because they often present as painless soft-tissue masses with a variable growth rate. Some tumors, such as infantile fibrosarcoma, may be present at birth and can be mistaken for vascular lesions. A careful clinical evaluation (including transillumination) can often help differentiate solid from cystic lesions. Many soft-tissue sarcomas are associated with characteristic cytogenetic abnormalities (**Table 3**).

Rhabdomyosarcoma

Rhabdomyosarcoma accounts for 50% of the soft-tissue sarcomas in children from birth to 14 years of age. The prevalence of rhabdomyosarcoma is approximately 4.5 per 1 million individuals.[27] Approximately 20% of rhabdomyosarcomas affect the limbs. Embryonal and alveolar are the two main types of rhabdomyosarcoma. Alveolar rhabdomyosarcoma is more common in the limbs and is usually seen in older children (5 to 15 years of age). Lymph node involvement is also more common in patients with alveolar rhabdomyosarcoma. Translocations (*PAX3-FOXO1*, *PAX7-FOXO1*) are seen in most patients with alveolar rhabdomyosarcoma. The prognosis of patients with embryonal rhabdomyosarcoma, nontranslocation-associated alveolar rhabdomyosarcoma, and alveolar rhabdomyosarcoma with *PAX7-FOXO1* translocation is better than for those with *PAX3-FOXO1* translocation. Staging includes MRI of the local area (including lymph nodes), bone marrow biopsies, and CT of the chest. The role of PET-CT combination imaging or a full-body MRI for staging and estimating the response to chemotherapy is being investigated. Treatment is risk stratified and usually is a combination of multiagent chemotherapy, with surgery with or without radiation therapy for local control.

Nonrhabdomyosarcoma Soft-Tissue Sarcomas

Nonrhabdomyosarcoma soft-tissue sarcomas are less common and comprise a heterogeneous group of malignancies. Synovial sarcoma, malignant peripheral nerve sheath tumors, and fibrosarcomas are among the more common nonrhabdomyosarcoma soft-tissue sarcomas in the pediatric population.

Synovial Sarcoma

Synovial sarcoma is the second most common soft-tissue sarcoma in children and young adults. The name is misleading because the cell of origin is not a synovial cell, and a joint is involved in only 0.5% to 5% of patients; however, it frequently occurs close to joints. The lower extremity is the most common location (especially the knee and the ankle) (**Figure 10**). Histologically, the tumor may be monophasic with spindle cells (fibrous) or epithelial variants, or biphasic with epithelial and spindled areas. These lesions often have the characteristic X:18 translocation with fusion of the *SYT* gene on chromosome 18 to the *SSX* genes on the X chromosome. Surgery is the mainstay of treatment, with radiation also useful in decreasing local recurrence. The role of chemotherapy is still unclear.

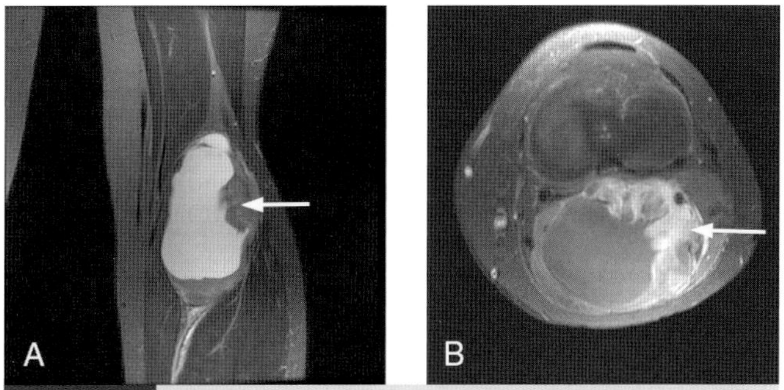

Figure 10 Images from a 17-year-old patient with synovial sarcoma in the popliteal fossa that presented with deep vein thrombosis secondary to mass effect and invasion of the popliteal vein. The lesion is complex with cystic as well as solid components (arrows) on both coronal (**A**) and axial (**B**) MRI.

Malignant Peripheral Nerve Sheath Tumors

The diagnosis of 10% to 20% of malignant peripheral nerve sheath tumors is made in the first two decades of life. The lifetime risk of these tumors in patients with neurofibromatosis type 1 is 2% to 10% higher in patients younger than 30 years. In contrast to adults, fewer than 50% of malignant peripheral nerve sheath tumors in children arise in the setting of neurofibromatosis type 1. Radiation is also a risk factor for the development of malignant peripheral nerve sheath tumors. The clinical presentation is a progressively enlarging soft-tissue mass, with pain or neurologic symptoms frequently absent. Treatment is primarily wide surgical excision, because chemotherapy and radiation have limited efficacy. The prognosis is poor, with a 5-year survival rate of 38% to 51%.

Summary

Appropriate workup of pediatric bone and soft-tissue tumors includes a thorough clinical evaluation, judicious use of imaging studies, and a well planned and executed biopsy (when needed). Making the correct diagnosis and knowing the natural history of a particular tumor helps the physician to devise the most appropriate treatment plan. With improved understanding of the mechanisms involved in tumorigenesis, new therapeutic targets are being identified. Improved imaging with better interpretation of the response to neoadjuvant treatment may help determine the best surgical margins. Newer surgical techniques such as intraoperative navigation will help improve the ability of surgeons to obtain appropriate margins. Improvements in metallurgy and tailoring implants to the resection with improved efficacy using computerized planning should help improve reconstruction outcomes. Future innovations should improve the care of children with bone and soft-tissue tumors.

Key Study Points

- The differential diagnosis of a tumor or lesion is driven primarily by the age of the patient and the location of the tumor.
- Radiographs are extremely useful in the evaluation of osseous lesions and often may be diagnostic by themselves.
- Soft-tissue sarcomas may not have substantial pain associated with them (at least in the initial stages), grow centrifugally, and push rather than invade the surrounding tissues (hence, are well circumscribed) leading to diagnostic confusion with benign lesions.
- Imaging is less often diagnostic in soft-tissue tumors compared with osseous tumors, and biopsy is needed much more frequently in the evaluation of soft-tissue tumors.
- Osteosarcoma and rhabdomyosarcoma are the most common bone and soft-tissue sarcomas, respectively, in children (alveolar rhabdomyosarcoma is more common than embryonal rhabdomyosarcoma in the extremities).

Annotated References

1. Mirabello L, Yeager M, Mai PL, et al: Germline TP53 variants and susceptibility to osteosarcoma. *J Natl Cancer Inst* 2015;107(7):djv101.

   The authors evaluated 765 patients with osteosarcoma. They found 9.5% of *TP53* mutations in patients younger than 30 years and none in patients older than 30 years. Level of evidence: II.

2. DeBaun MR, Tucker MA: Risk of cancer during the first four years of life in children from The Beckwith-Wiedemann Syndrome Registry. *J Pediatr* 1998;132(3 pt 1):398-400.

   This study of tumors in children with Beckwith Wiedemann syndrome found a high overall prevalence of cancer (13 of 185 patients) in the first 4 years of life. The most common tumors were Wilms tumor, nephroblastoma, and hepatoblastoma. The relative risk was increased in children with hemihypertrophy. Level of evidence: II.

3. Qu N, Yao W, Cui X, Zhang H: Malignant transformation in monostotic fibrous dysplasia: Clinical features, imaging features, outcomes in 10 patients, and review. *Medicine (Baltimore)* 2015;94(3):e369.

   The authors discuss malignant transformation in monostotic fibrous dysplasia. Level of evidence: III.

4. Verdegaal SH, Bovée JV, Pansuriya TC, et al: Incidence, predictive factors, and prognosis of chondrosarcoma in patients with Ollier disease and Maffucci syndrome: An international multicenter study of 161 patients. *Oncologist* 2011;16(12):1771-1779.

   The authors of an international multicenter study of 144 patients with Ollier disease and 17 with Maffucci syndrome found a prevalence of chondrosarcoma of approximately 40% in this population. Patients with multiple enchondromas in the hand and feet had approximately a 15% prevalence compared with 46% in those with involvement of the long bones and pelvis. Level of evidence: III.

5. Czajka CM, DiCaprio MR: What is the proportion of patients with multiple hereditary exostoses who undergo malignant degeneration? *Clin Orthop Relat Res* 2015;473(7):2355-2361.

   The authors report the results of a social media–based questionnaire sent to patients with multiple osteochondromas. The proportion of respondents who experienced malignant transformation was 2.7% (21 of 757 respondents) at a mean age of 28.6 years (± 9.3 years). The most common sites of malignant change from benign exostoses included the pelvis (8 of 21 respondents) and scapula (4 of 21 respondents). Level of evidence: IV.

6. Bernard SA, Murphey MD, Flemming DJ, Kransdorf MJ: Improved differentiation of benign osteochondromas from secondary chondrosarcomas with standardized measurement of cartilage cap at CT and MR imaging. *Radiology* 2010;255(3):857-865.

7. Ren W, Gu G: Prognostic implications of RB1 tumour suppressor gene alterations in the clinical outcome of human osteosarcoma: A meta-analysis. *Eur J Cancer Care (Engl)* 2015.

   A meta-analysis of 491 patients demonstrated that loss of *RB1* gene function results in increased metastatic and mortality rates for patients with osteosarcoma and a substantial reduction in the histologic response of osteosarcoma to chemotherapy. Level of evidence: I.

8. Mankin HJ, Mankin CJ, Simon MA; Members of the Musculoskeletal Tumor Society: The hazards of the biopsy, revisited. *J Bone Joint Surg Am* 1996;78(5):656-663.

9. Skrzynski MC, Biermann JS, Montag A, Simon MA: Diagnostic accuracy and charge-savings of outpatient core needle biopsy compared with open biopsy of musculoskeletal tumors. *J Bone Joint Surg Am* 1996;78(5):644-649.

10. Tsoumakidou G, Thénint MA, Garnon J, Buy X, Steib JP, Gangi A: Percutaneous image-guided laser photocoagulation of spinal osteoid osteoma: A single-institution series. *Radiology* 2016;278(3):936-943.

The authors report on 58 patients with spinal osteoid osteomas treated at a single institution. Recurrences (5.3% of the patients) were successfully treated with laser photocoagulation. In osteoid osteomas with less than 8 to 10 mm of surrounding cortical bone, thermal protection techniques were recommended by the authors. Level of evidence: I.

11. Kadhim M, Thacker M, Kadhim A, Holmes L Jr: Treatment of unicameral bone cyst: Systematic review and meta analysis. *J Child Orthop* 2014;8(2):171-191.

 The meta-analysis of various treatment modalities for unicameral bone cysts suggested improved outcomes for active interventions versus conservative treatment. The success of various treatment outcomes is discussed. Level of evidence: V.

12. Shiels WE II, Beebe AC, Mayerson JL: Percutaneous doxycycline treatment of juxtaphyseal aneurysmal bone cysts. *J Pediatr Orthop* 2016;36(2):205-212.

 This study of 16 patients with juxtaphyseal aneurysmal bone cysts treated with doxycycline foam demonstrated a recurrence rate of 6%. All patients needed multiple injections (2 to 14 injections) for their treatment. Level of evidence: IV.

13. Xie C, Jeys L, James SL: Radiofrequency ablation of chondroblastoma: Long-term clinical and imaging outcomes. *Eur Radiol* 2015;25(4):1127-1134.

 The authors report a 12% recurrence rate in 25 patients with chondroblastoma treated with radiofrequency ablation. These results are equivalent to those of open surgical treatment.

14. Boyce AM, Kelly MH, Brillante BA, et al: A randomized, double blind, placebo-controlled trial of alendronate treatment for fibrous dysplasia of bone. *J Clin Endocrinol Metab* 2014;99(11):4133-4140.

 Forty patients with polyostotic fibrous dysplasia were treated with 6-month cycles of alendronate. The authors found alendronate treatment led to a reduction in the bone resorption marker NTX-telopeptides and improvement in areal bone mineral density but had no substantial effect on serum osteocalcin, pain, or functional parameters. Level of evidence: I.

15. Berres ML, Lim KP, Peters T, et al: BRAF-V600E expression in precursor versus differentiated dendritic cells defines clinically distinct LCH risk groups. *J Exp Med* 2014;211(4):669-683.

 The authors found that that patients with active, high-risk Langerhans cell histiocytosis carried BRAF-V600E in the hematopoietic cell progenitors in the bone marrow, whereas the mutation was restricted to lesional dendritic cells in low-risk patients. They postulate that Langerhans cell histiocytosis should be classified as myeloid neoplasia and that high-risk Langerhans cell histiocytosis arises from somatic mutation of a hematopoietic progenitor, whereas low-risk disease arises from somatic mutation of tissue-restricted precursor dendritic cells. Level of evidence: II.

16. Haroche J, Cohen-Aubart F, Emile JF, et al: Dramatic efficacy of vemurafenib in both multisystemic and refractory Erdheim-Chester disease and Langerhans cell histiocytosis harboring the BRAF V600E mutation. *Blood* 2013;121(9):1495-1500.

 BRAF V600E gain-of-function mutations have been observed in 57% of cases of Langerhans cell histiocytosis. The authors treated three patients with refractory Erdheim-Chester disease and Langerhans cell histiocytosis with vemurafenib, a mutated BRAF inhibitor, and reported substantial and rapid clinical and biologic improvement. Level of evidence: IV.

17. Cates JM: Pathologic fracture a poor prognostic factor in osteosarcoma: Misleading conclusions from meta-analyses? *Eur J Surg Oncol* 2016; Jan 29 [Epub ahead of print].

 The authors of this multivariable survival analysis of 131 patients with high-grade osteosarcoma of the extremity long bones concluded that pathologic fracture was not an important prognostic factor for osteosarcoma of the limbs.

18. Luetke A, Meyers PA, Lewis I, Juergens H: Osteosarcoma treatment: Where do we stand? A state of the art review. *Cancer Treat Rev* 2014;40(4):523-532.

 The authors review the current state of the art of systemic therapy for osteosarcoma and focus on the experiences of cooperative osteosarcoma groups. Level of evidence: V.

19. Biswas B, Rastogi S, Khan SA, et al: Outcomes and prognostic factors for Ewing-family tumors of the extremities. *J Bone Joint Surg Am* 2014;96(10):841-849.

 In a study of 158 patients with Ewing sarcoma of the extremities, the authors found radiation to be less effective for local control compared with surgery despite similar histologic response rates to neoadjuvant chemotherapy. They also found that a white blood cell count of 11×10^9/L or more was associated with a worse prognosis in these patients. Level of evidence: IV.

20. Coffin CM, Lowichik A, Putnam A: Lipoblastoma (LPB): A clinicopathologic and immunohistochemical analysis of 59 cases. *Am J Surg Pathol* 2009;33(11):1705-1712.

21. Colombo C, Miceli R, Lazar AJ, et al: CTNNB1 45F mutation is a molecular prognosticator of increased postoperative primary desmoid tumor recurrence: An independent, multicenter validation study. *Cancer* 2013;119(20):3696-3702.

 In a study of 179 patients with desmoid fibromatosis treated primarily with surgery, the authors found primary, completely resected, sporadic desmoid tumors with the *S45F* mutation have a greater tendency for local recurrence. They found an estimated 5-year relapse-free survival rate of 91% in the patients without the mutation versus 41% in the patients with the mutation. Level of evidence: IV.

22. Garbay D, Le Cesne A, Penel N, et al: Chemotherapy in patients with desmoid tumors: A study from the French Sarcoma Group (FSG). *Ann Oncol* 2012;23(1):182-186.

1: General

In a study of various chemotherapy regimens for desmoid tumors, the authors found anthracycline-containing regimens appear to be associated with a higher response rate.

23. Shang H, Braggio D, Lee YJ, et al: Targeting the Notch pathway: A potential therapeutic approach for desmoid tumors. *Cancer* 2015;121(22):4088-4096.

    The authors discuss Notch expression in desmoid tumors and reports that the use of a notch pathway inhibitor resulted in decreased cell growth, invasion, and cell migration. Level of evidence: IV.

24. Varan A, Şen H, Aydın B, Yalçın B, Kutluk T, Akyüz C: Neurofibromatosis type 1 and malignancy in childhood. *Clin Genet* 2016;89(3):341-345.

    In this study, non-neurofibroma neoplasms developed in 26 of 473 patients (5%) with neurofibromatosis type 1. These included 12 soft-tissue tumors (6 malignant peripheral nerve sheath tumors, 5 rhabdomyosarcomas, and 1 malignant fibrous histiocytoma), 11 brain tumors (6 low-grade gliomas, 3 high-grade gliomas, and 2 medulloblastomas), 2 neuroblastomas, and 1 non-Hodgkin lymphoma. Level of evidence: IV.

25. Cassier PA, Gelderblom H, Stacchiotti S, et al: Efficacy of imatinib mesylate for the treatment of locally advanced and/or metastatic tenosynovial giant cell tumor/pigmented villonodular synovitis. *Cancer* 2012;118(6):1649-1655.

    Because metastatic tenosynovial giant cell tumor and PVS express CFS1, the authors used imatinib (a CSF1R antagonist) to treat patients with these locally advanced or metastatic tumors. Good symptom relief was reported in 16 of 22 patients (73%) in the study. However, the medication had to be discontinued in 6 of 22 patients because of toxicity. Level of evidence: IV.

26. Mollon B, Lee A, Busse JW, et al: The effect of surgical synovectomy and radiotherapy on the rate of recurrence of pigmented villonodular synovitis of the knee: An individual patient meta-analysis. *Bone Joint J* 2015;97-B(4):550-557.

    In a meta-analysis of 35 observational studies of PVNS around the knee that included 630 patients, the authors reported a local recurrence rate of 21.8% in patients with diffuse PVNS. Weak evidence suggested a lower recurrence rate with open synovectomy, arthroscopic anterior and open posterior synovectomy for the knee, and the use of postoperative radiation therapy.

27. Ognjanovic S, Linabery AM, Charbonneau B, Ross JA: Trends in childhood rhabdomyosarcoma incidence and survival in the United States, 1975-2005. *Cancer* 2009;115(18):4218-4226.

Chapter 6

Growth of the Musculoskeletal System

Christopher Iobst, MD   Brian P. Scannell, MD

Abstract

Growth is unique in pediatric patients compared with adult patients. Growth is a complex and well-synchronized phenomenon. It is important that orthopaedic surgeons who care for children have a good understanding of normal growth to better address deviations from normal that can result in progressive deformity, impaired function, or future pain.

Keywords: bone age; growth; peak height velocity; skeletal maturity

Introduction

Growth is unique in pediatric care compared with adult care. Because growth is a complex and well-synchronized phenomenon,[1] orthopaedic surgeons who care for children should understand what normal growth is to better address deviations from normal that can result in progressive deformity, impaired function, or pain.

Growth is divided into two areas: microgrowth and macrogrowth.[2] Microgrowth occurs at the cellular level in the growth plate. Macrogrowth is the total effect of microgrowth and allows for changes in height, weight, and body proportion. From birth through adulthood, height increases 350% and weight increases 20-fold.[3]

Dr. Iobst or an immediate family member is a member of a speakers' bureau or has made paid presentations on behalf of Smith & Nephew and serves as a paid consultant to Ellipse Technologies and Orthofix. Neither Dr. Scannell nor any immediate family member has received anything of value from or has stock or stock options held in a commercial company or institution related directly or indirectly to the subject of this chapter.

Normal Growth

Height

It is important to document the standing height of children at regular physician visits. Standing height is the composition of sitting height (trunk) and subischial height (lower limbs).[3] Each component grows at different rates and times. A child's overall standing height increases rapidly from birth to age 5 years. It then slows down until beginning another rapid increase during puberty.[3] At age 2 years, a child's standing height is approximately 50% of his or her adult height; at puberty, a child's standing height is approximately 86% of adult height.

In the same manner as standing height, sitting height can be measured supine in young children. Sitting height has been used to anticipate the onset of puberty. In an average population, puberty starts when the sitting height is approximately 75 cm in girls and 78 cm in boys. At 84 cm of sitting height, 80% of girls have reached menarche.[2]

Subischial height is determined by subtracting the sitting height from the standing height.[2] Over time, the subischial height contributes a far greater growth percentage in height than does the sitting height.[2] In a newborn, the proportion of sitting height to subischial height is 65:35. At skeletal maturity, this ratio is 52:48. Thus, as children age, a much higher percentage of growth occurs in the lower limbs compared with growth in the trunk.[3]

Weight

Similar to height, weight gain is not constant. The average male weighs 10 kg at age 1 year, 20 kg at age 5 years, 30 kg at age 10 years, and 60 kg at age 17 years.[2,4] Weight nearly doubles from ages 10 to 17 years during puberty.[3] These estimates are from studies several decades ago, but newer studies suggest that children and adolescents are heavier than previously thought.[5] The National Center for Health Statistics in 2015 documented an obesity rate of 17.5% in children aged 3 to 19 years in the United States.[6]

Body Mass Index

The body mass index is an estimate of body fat based on weight and height. It is calculated by taking a person's weight and dividing it by the person's height squared (kg/m^2). Because the body composition of children is different from that of adults, the body mass index is calculated based on both age and sex. Normal or healthy weight is the 5th percentile to less than the 85th percentile for children of the same age and sex. Overweight is defined as being in the 85th percentile to less than the 95th percentile for children of the same age and sex. Obesity is defined as greater than the 95th percentile.

Chronologic Growth

Within the first year of life, growth in both sitting height and subischial limb length substantially accelerates. This higher rate of growth commonly continues until approximately age 5 years.[3] During the first 5 years of life, the proportions of growth change as the cephalic end becomes relatively smaller compared with increases seen in subischial limb length.

From 5 years to the onset of puberty, the growth rate markedly decelerates. On average, standing height increases 5.5 cm/yr.[3] Approximately two-thirds of growth occurs in the lower limbs, and one-third occurs in the sitting height. The trunk grows at a slower rate than the lower limbs, thus altering the body's proportions.[4]

Acceleration of growth velocity characterizes the beginning of puberty, which occurs at approximately age 10 years in girls and 12 years in boys. During puberty, standing height increases approximately 1 cm/mo, with more growth occurring in the trunk compared with the subischial limbs. The four main characteristics of puberty are as follows: (1) dramatic increase in stature; (2) changing proportions of the upper and lower body; (3) change in overall morphology, including fat distribution, shoulder width, and pelvic diameter; and (4) the development of secondary sexual characteristics (testicular growth, breast buds).[3]

Puberty and Peak Height Velocity

The exact onset of puberty and a determination of future growth can be difficult. It requires assessing the following: bone age, the Tanner classification of secondary sexual characteristics, height changes, the onset of menstruation, and the Risser sign. The issue with using menstruation onset and the Risser sign in isolation is that they typically occur later in puberty.[2]

Growth has two primary phases during puberty (**Figure 1**). The first phase is the ascending phase of the growth velocity curve. This phase lasts approximately 2 years; during this phase, the peak height velocity (PHV), or the maximum growth rate, occurs. PHV occurs between 13 and 15 years of bone age (according to Greulich and Pyle[7]) in boys and 11 to 13 years of bone age in girls.[3] Determining whether children are in the ascending phase of the growth velocity curve can be difficult, but it can be accomplished with serial height measurements. Height commonly increases at least 8 cm/yr during PHV. As seen on radiographs, the triradiate cartilage commonly closes about halfway through the ascending phase. The Risser sign is not very useful in determining PHV because most patients have a Risser grade of 0 during this phase (**Figure 1**). In girls with idiopathic scoliosis, the PHV was correlated with a Risser grade of 0 and open triradiate cartilage.[8]

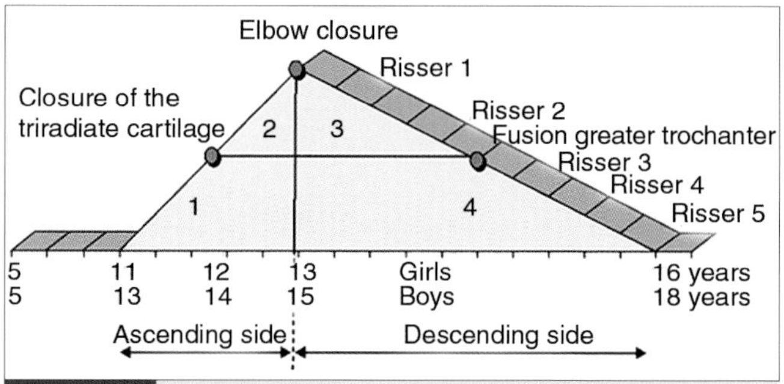

Figure 1 Illustration of a pubertal growth diagram that shows ascending and descending growth phases with corresponding radiographic findings. (Reproduced with permission from Diméglio A: Growth in pediatric orthopaedics, in Morrissey RT, Weinstein SL, eds: *Lovell and Winter's Pediatric Orthopaedics*, ed 6. Philadelphia, PA, Lippincott Williams and Wilkins, 2006, p 52.)

The second phase is the descending phase of the growth velocity curve (**Figure 1**). During this phase, the growth rate slows, children are becoming more skeletally mature (elbow physis closure and Risser progression), and girls commonly begin menarche. Using the Sauvegrain method, the olecranon apophysis typically closes near the beginning of the descending phase.[4] Menarche occurs after closure of this apophysis in girls, but this can be variable.[3] Girls experience menarche variably according to the Risser grades: 42% before Risser grade 1, 31% at Risser grade 1, 13% at Risser grade 2, 8% at Risser grade 3, and 5% at Risser grade 4.[9]

Spine Growth

Growth of the Spinal Column

The overall development of the spine includes both longitudinal (vertical) and axial growth. The spine is approximately 60% of sitting height. The overall height of the spine nearly triples between birth and adulthood, with peak growth rates in the first 5 years of life and again during puberty.[3,4]

Growth of the spinal canal occurs at each vertebral level through essentially three primary ossification centers: the posterior spinous process synchondrosis and two neurocentral synchondroses at the junction of each pedicle and vertebral body. The diameter of the canal reaches adult size sometime between ages 6 and 8 years.[10-12] In addition, spinal growth occurs at each vertebral level at the ring apophysis (two per vertebral body) to contribute to longitudinal growth. The posterior elements also contribute to longitudinal growth.[13]

The cervical spine will grow approximately 9 cm from birth to adulthood, reaching an adult length of 12 to 13 cm, and is approximately 15% of sitting height.[3] Two-thirds of this growth occurs by age 5 years, and the remaining growth occurs during puberty. All vertebral body growth occurs as previously discussed, with the exception of C1 (atlas) and C2 (axis). C1 is unique because the primary anterior ossification center is present in less than 20% of neonates.[14] The anterior ossification center typically develops between 9 and 12 months, and two neurocentral synchondroses are formed with the posterior ossification centers.[13] C2 is unique because it involves the dens. The dens is more similar to a long bone, with a cartilaginous epiphysis at each end.

The thoracic spine will grow approximately 18 cm from birth to adulthood, reaching an adult length of approximately 28 cm in men and 26 cm in women.[4] It comprises approximately 30% of sitting height. Similar to the cervical spine, a growth spurt occurs from birth to age 5 years and again during puberty. The posterior components of the spine grow at a faster rate than the anterior counterparts.[3] By knowing and understanding the growth of the thoracic spine, it is possible to calculate the effect of a thoracic fusion on final height.[3,4]

The lumbar spine will grow approximately 9 cm from birth to adulthood, reaching an adult length of 16 cm in men and 15.5 cm in women. It comprises approximately 18% of sitting height.[3,4] Growth of the vertebral elements occurs in reverse from the thoracic spine; the anterior elements grow at a faster rate than the posterior elements.[3]

Scoliosis and Spine Growth

A close relationship has been demonstrated to exist between increased height and scoliosis progression.[15] Curve progression markedly increases at the time of adolescent growth spurts for idiopathic and neuromuscular curves. In addition, curve progression slows or ceases when skeletal maturity is achieved.

Studies have attempted to look at the natural history of curve progression during puberty. In the ascending phase of the growth diagram, any spinal curvature increasing by 1°/mo or 12°/yr is likely to be progressive and require treatment. Any curve increase of less than 0.5°/mo is mild and less likely to need treatment.[4] Female patients with a curve of less than 30° at the time of PHV were demonstrated to have only a 4% chance of progression to a surgical range.[16] However, female patients with a curve greater than 30° at the time of PHV had an 84% chance of requiring surgical intervention. This risk of progression appears similarly in males, with nearly a 100% chance of progression to surgical range with curves greater than 30° at PHV.[17]

Table 1

Risk of Curve Progression (5° or More)

	20° Curve	30° Curve
Risser grade 0	30%	100%
Risser grade 1	10%	60%
Risser grade 2	2%	30%

Even in the descending phase of the growth diagram, the risk for scoliosis progression is present. The Risser grades are not the best indicators of risk progression; however, based on previous literature,[18-21] they can be used to predict progression (**Table 1**). Some authors recommend using radiographs of the hand to determine skeletal age. One group of researchers found that curve acceleration most closely correlated with the Tanner-Whitehouse-III scoring system for hand radiographs.[22] This scoring system provides better maturity and prognosis determination during adolescence.

Arthrodesis for scoliosis often is required before skeletal maturity. For some patients undergoing surgery, the risk for a crankshaft phenomenon secondary to remaining growth of the spine is present. The crankshaft phenomenon was first described in 1989 and occurs when a solid posterior arthrodesis is performed while growth remaining anteriorly produces rotation of the spine or trunk with progression of the spinal curvature.[23] Patients at Tanner stage 1 with open triradiate cartilage have the greatest risk for the crankshaft phenomenon. Another group of researchers observed crankshaft deformities in 10 of 23 patients who had open triradiate cartilage but only 1 of 20 patients with closed triradiate cartilage.[24] The strongest predictor of the crankshaft phenomenon appears to be when arthrodesis is performed in the setting of open triradiate cartilage before or during PHV.[25] Ultimately, understanding the growth of the spine can help determine treatment and the timing of treatment of patients with scoliosis.

Growth Remaining

In discussing growth, it is important to not only ascertain how much total growth a child will accrue but also determine how much growth is remaining for a child at a particular point in time. This information often is necessary when determining treatment strategies for patients who are skeletally immature and have limb-length discrepancy (LLD) or an angular deformity. Traditionally, the three most widely used methods of determining the amount of growth remaining were the arithmetic method, the Anderson-Green-Messner growth-remaining charts, and the Moseley straight-line method. The arithmetic method states that girls cease growing at age 14 years and boys at age 16 years.[26] This method also assumes a yearly growth rate of 0.375 inches from the distal femoral physis and 0.25 inches from the proximal tibial physis. Growth remaining at each physis can be calculated by multiplying the number of years of growth remaining by the amount of growth expected from each physis. This simplistic approach is a quick method that can be used in the clinic and does not require graphs or complex computations.

In 1969, growth-remaining graphs were published to determine the amount of growth remaining in the femur and the tibia until skeletal maturity was reached.[27] Using these growth data, a straight-line graph method was created in 1977 to predict LLD in a lower extremity and the amount of growth remaining.[28] Both methods require a child's skeletal age and a determination of the growth percentile of the patient. In addition, the straight-line method requires a special graph and a minimum of three measurements. One important concern with both the growth-remaining charts and the straight-line method is that they are based on a population of children living under conditions different than those experienced by the current population of children. Because growth data can be affected by regional, racial, ethnic, and generational differences, it may not be possible to extrapolate these methods to the current population of children and expect accurate predictions.

The multiplier method is an alternative method for assessing the amount of growth remaining.[29-34] Lower limb growth is thought to follow a biologic constant based on age and sex. Children of all generations and ethnic backgrounds grow the same percentage of their limb length at the same age. The multiplier method characterizes the pattern of normal human growth by using an age- and sex-specific coefficient. The multiplier for each age and sex is a measure of the percentage of growth remaining. The multiplier method is, therefore, viewed as a universal method for predicting lower limb length because it is independent of percentile, regional, racial, ethnic, and generational differences in growth data. The multiplier values for boys and girls differ from each other only because growth in boys continues for approximately 2.25 years longer than growth in girls. The patterns of the multipliers are otherwise the same.

To predict limb or bone length, the current limb or bone length is multiplied by the current age multiplier to obtain the predicted limb or bone length at maturity. Lower limb length, upper limb length, total height, foot length, and foot height have each been characterized by the multiplier method.[29-34] Predictions are based on a single radiograph obtained at any age for congenital conditions and two radiographs obtained at any age for developmental conditions. The multiplier method provides a simple, rapid method of predicting remaining growth. It is especially valuable when attempting to evaluate the growth pattern of a patient without previous radiographs or a very young patient with few previous radiographs. In these situations, the multiplier method provides a concise way of providing information and guidance to families who want to know the predicted LLD at skeletal maturity to allow for long-term treatment planning.

Relying on chronologic age to estimate the amount of growth remaining may lead to errors. Chronologic age has been found to correspond to skeletal age within a 6-month range in only 49% of boys and 51% of girls.[2] Chronologic age is superior to skeletal age for predicting ultimate limb length before the adolescent growth spurt but is inferior once the growth spurt begins.[35] Therefore, skeletal age is preferable for making predictions in adolescents. With the multiplier method, the multiplier corresponding to skeletal age can be used rather than the multiplier corresponding to chronologic age.

Even though various mathematical formulas have been designed to capture the complexity of growth, it is unwise to rely solely on these equations. When attempting to understand the growth dynamics of a patient, the ideal approach should use multiple methods that complement each other. For example, checking the Anderson-Green-Messner growth-remaining chart in addition to the arithmetic method or the multiplier method is better than using only one method. If the different methods agree with each other, then the probability exists that the calculations are reliable. If, however, the calculations produce widely disparate results, then further investigation may be necessary. Combining these methods with an evaluation of a child's Tanner stages and annual growth velocity can further refine the accuracy of prediction. In the best-case scenario, the clinician should accumulate multiple, meticulous, lower limb measurements while continuously monitoring the onset of puberty (acceleration of the annual lower limb growth velocity, the onset

Table 2

Description of Radiographic Criteria Used to Determine Skeletal Age in Males Aged 12.5 to 16 Years and Females Aged 10 to 14 Years, According to the Shorthand Bone Age Assessment Method

Criterion	Males (Years)	Females (Years)
Appearance of the hook of hamate ossific nucleus	12.5	10
Appearance of the thumb sesamoid ossific nucleus	13	11
Proximal aspect of the distal radius epiphysis has extended to meet the maximum width of the distal width of the distal aspect of distal radius metaphysis but has not yet begun to cap	13.5	
Capping of the distal radius epiphysis	14	12
Closure of the thumb distal phalanx physis	15	13
Closure of the index finger distal phalanx physis	15.5	13.5
Closure of the index finger proximal phalanx physis	16	14

of Tanner stages, double ossification of the olecranon, and ossification of the sesamoid of the thumb).[36] The beginning of puberty corresponds to 11 years of skeletal age in girls and 13 years of skeletal age in boys.[37]

Skeletal Maturity

Similar to the growth remaining predictions, the bone age assessment of children is influenced by sex, race, nutrition status, living environment, and social resources.[38] Different methods for determining skeletal age have been described, using hand, elbow, foot, knee, or pelvic radiographs.[39] Accurate measurements of skeletal maturity should yield better growth remaining predictions, but the optimal method or a combination of methods for assessing skeletal maturity remains controversial. *The Radiographic Atlas of the Hand and Wrist* is the most common tool for evaluating bone age, and many practitioners consider it the preferred method.[7] However, this method has known weaknesses that limit its effectiveness. It relies on the subjective analysis of subtle morphologic changes described within the atlas and has long intervals between reference standards, especially during the critical pubertal growth period. The standards for 11.5 and 12.5 years of skeletal age in girls and 14.5 years of skeletal age in boys are absent. Furthermore, training in the technique is required to become proficient, and access to the atlas in hard copy form is necessary for its use.

The shorthand bone age assessment is an abridged method of bone age assessment based on the basic principles of the Greulich and Pyle method (also known as the atlas method).[39] It allows the assessment of skeletal maturity in males aged 12.5 to 16 years and females aged 10 to 14 years (**Table 2**). The relatively simple set of radiographic criteria for interpreting skeletal age can be easily referenced in tabular form or committed to memory. The shorthand assessment method has been shown to have high intraobserver and interobserver reliability and can be quickly mastered by practitioners at all levels of training. Because it is derived from the Greulich and Pyle method, the shorthand bone age has some limitations. For example, skeletal half-age determinations such as 12.5 and 15.5 years in females and 14.5 years in both males and females are not included in the shorthand bone age. In addition, similar to the Greulich and Pyle method, the shorthand bone age depends on the patient having a normal left-hand radiograph, which may not be applicable for patients with skeletal dysplasias affecting the left hand or other hand abnormalities. In such cases, a method of skeletal age determination using radiographs of other body parts should be used.

To address these limitations, other methods of bone age estimation have been proposed as alternatives to the Greulich and Pyle method or the shorthand bone age. The Sauvegrain method uses changes in the radiographic appearance of the ossification centers of the elbow to determine skeletal age.[40] The elbow undergoes regular morphologic changes at the epiphysis ossification centers that are clearly identifiable before and during puberty. For this reason, elbow radiographs are helpful to study skeletal age near and during the adolescent growth spurt. Elbow radiographs should be obtained between 10 and 13 years of skeletal age in girls and between 12 and 15 years of skeletal age in boys. In younger children, elbow radiographs cannot be used to assess skeletal age because the elbow is still mainly cartilaginous, and the ossification centers do not yet show any remarkable morphologic characteristics.

The Sauvegrain method is based on a 27-point scoring system of four anatomic landmarks: the lateral condyle/epicondyle, the trochlea, the olecranon apophysis, and

Table 3

Modified Sauvegrain Method for Skeletal Age

	Males (Years)	Females (Years)
Two ossification centers at the level of the olecranon apophysis	13	11
Half-moon shape of the olecranon apophysis	13.5	11.5
Rectangular shape of the olecranon apophysis	14	12
Beginning of fusion of the olecranon apophysis	14.5	12.5
Complete fusion of the olecranon apophysis	15	13

the proximal radial epiphysis. Skeletal age is determined by summing the individual scores of each landmark to arrive at a total score. The score is then plotted on a graph (separate graphs for girls and boys), which gives the corresponding skeletal age. A score of 26 or higher indicates that a child has passed PHV.

In 2005, a group of researchers simplified the original Sauvegrain method by condensing the method from evaluating four different ossification centers in the elbow to one ossification center.[41] These researchers demonstrated that the morphology of the olecranon apophysis on lateral radiographs goes through five distinct and characteristic appearances (**Table 3**). It allows skeletal age to be determined in regular 6-month intervals in girls aged 11 to 13 years and boys aged 13 to 15 years. Furthermore, the learning curve of this simplified method is short. Studies have shown that this modified Sauvegrain method is reliable and accurate.[41-43] Clinically, the maturation of the olecranon is relevant because it occurs during the pubertal growth spurt, when the Risser grade is still 0. During this phase of accelerated growth, the information obtained from the olecranon apophyseal lines complements the assessment of the triradiate cartilage, and it helps identify patients who are skeletally immature. Closure of the epiphyses at the elbow indicates the end of the accelerated growth spurt, when the adolescent is entering the decelerating phase of pubertal growth.

As another alternative to the Greulich and Pyle method, a group of researchers presented a method of digital (phalangeal) skeletal age assessment derived from the Tanner-Whitehouse III method.[44] This technique is based on a radiologic analysis of the metacarpals and fingers on AP hand radiographs. The simplified digital method is useful from the prepubertal growth period to skeletal maturity. It divides this period into eight stages and includes several markers before Risser grade 1. The eight stages are as follows: Stages 1 and 2 correspond to the prepubertal period, stages 3 and 4 correspond to the pubertal growth spurt (Risser grade of 0), and stages 5 to 8 cover the period from Risser grade 1 to 5, when full skeletal maturity has occurred. Although this technique is less detailed than the modified Sauvegrain method during the 2-year phase of accelerated growth, the digital method can be combined with the Sauvegrain method to cover every Risser grade until skeletal maturity.

Each method has its own strengths and weaknesses. The proper strategy should be to take advantage of each method's strengths and apply it at the proper time. For example, a lateral elbow radiograph may be more effective than a hand radiograph when assessing skeletal maturity during puberty. A hand radiograph is preferable before puberty and from Risser grade 1 to skeletal maturity. A combination of both methods adequately covers the gap between elbow fusion and Risser grade 1 because one complements the other.

Because many of the commonly used methods of skeletal age assessment are associated with some intraobserver and interobserver variability, there may be a future role for automated bone age assessment. Evidence shows that using computer software to evaluate radiographs for skeletal age may be faster and more accurate than subjective readings by radiologists.[38] The software also may allow an evaluation that is applicable across different racial and ethnic groups. At this time, however, automated techniques require further testing before they can be considered as a valid alternative to current methods.

Angular Correction

Gradual correction of angular deformity by asymmetric physeal suppression is an attractive option in growing children. Creating a tether on the convex side of the physis allows subsequent growth from the opposite side of the physis to correct the angular deformity. However, when using this method, the chosen physis must retain enough viable growth potential to successfully respond to growth guidance. Percutaneous hemiepiphyseal drilling, hemiepiphyseal stapling, hemitransphyseal screws, and tension-band plating are the most commonly used techniques. With the exception of percutaneous hemiepiphyseal drilling, these methods are potentially reversible and minimally invasive in nature. After angular correction has been achieved, the tethering device (staple, screw, plate) may be removed, and normal linear growth should resume. However, the response of the physis can be unpredictable after the removal of a tethering device. Recurrence of deformity as a rebound effect (accelerated growth on the side of the physis that was temporarily restrained) is known to occur in some patients.[45]

Determining the appropriate timing of hemiepiphysiodesis is one of the most difficult aspects of using guided growth to correct angular deformity. Incorrect timing can lead to either overcorrection or undercorrection. When planning to use any of these techniques, the surgeon should consider the magnitude of the deformity and the amount of remaining growth available. In general, the speed of angular correction is a function of two variables: the growth rate of the physis and the distance from the tether to the far edge of the growth plate (the narrower the width of the physis, the faster the rate of correction will be).[46] The rate of correction, however, also is known to be influenced by the age and sex of the patient, the surgical method used (staples, transphyseal screws, or flexible plate), etiology, and the location of the physis being treated.

In 1985, a technique for determining the timing of hemiepiphysiodesis was published.[46] Data were incorporated from the Anderson-Green-Messer growth remaining chart, skeletal age, and physeal width for development of a chart guiding angular deformity versus growth remaining for coronal plane deformities about the knee. Based on these data, correction was estimated at 7° per year following distal femoral hemiepiphysiodesis and 5° per year in the proximal tibia. This chart is helpful when applied to a patient with a normally functioning physis. However, when considering patients with abnormal physes, such as in skeletal dysplasias and Blount disease, the chart is less reliable.

Further studies on guided growth, however, have provided additional guidelines.[45,47-51] For example, the rate of improvement in mechanical axis alignment that is derived from the tibial segment is slower than that from the femoral segment. The correction rates of coronal angular deformity at the distal femur range from 0.56°/mo to 1.0°/mo and range from 0.36°/mo to 0.82°/mo at the proximal tibia.[45,47-51] The fastest rates of correction are achieved in two instances: (1) when the distal femoral and proximal tibial physes are treated concurrently and (2) when the technique is used in children younger than 10 years. One study reported that the overall rates of correction for children younger than 10 years was 1.4°/mo and 0.6°/mo for children older than 10 years.[50] A 2012 study of valgus deformity found that in boys 14 years or younger and girls 12 years or younger, the rates of correction at the distal femur, the proximal tibia, and the distal tibia were 0.71°/mo (8.5°/yr), 0.40°/mo (4.8°/yr), and 0.48°/mo (5.8°/yr), respectively.[51] In older children, the rates of correction at the distal femur, the proximal tibia, and the distal tibia were 0.39°/mo (4.7°/yr), 0.29°/mo (3.5°/yr), and 0.48°/mo (5.8°/yr), respectively.[51] Measuring the rates of correction per month allows the surgeon to estimate the overall treatment time. Visual appreciation of the effect of gradual correction usually does not occur until near the end of the treatment period. Consequently, providing the patient and parents with counseling about the expected time needed for correction will help diffuse any anxiety over what may initially appear to be a lack of improvement.

Smartphone Applications

Two free smartphone apps (Multiplier, Paley Growth) have been developed to help the clinician make growth assessments quickly and conveniently. The equations for limb-length inequality can be complicated and are prone to arithmetic errors when computed manually. With smartphone apps, the user simply enters the patient's sex and age and the direct measurements from the limb-length study. All calculations and predictions are then processed by the app. Such apps allow faster and more accurate determination of the timing of epiphysiodesis compared with traditional methods.[52] For example, the Multiplier has multiple platforms that allow a comprehensive evaluation of growth. The formulas and tables available in the Multiplier include calculating LLD at maturity (congenital and developmental), growth remaining (femur, tibia, and entire leg), and bone length at maturity for both the upper and lower limbs. Functions also are available for calculating the timing of both epiphysiodesis and angular correction. In addition, the Multiplier contains helpful supplemental information, such as the standard deformity measurements of the lower limbs and the foot, the Sauvegrain bone age method, the shorthand bone age assessment method, height and growth charts from the Centers for Disease Control and Prevention, oblique plane deformity calculation, and multiplier tables and formulas. Having a comprehensive wealth of information at the click of a button allows the clinician to provide practical information to the patient and his or her family in a quick and accurate manner.

Reversible Growth Arrest

With the advent of tension-band plating to achieve guided growth of angular deformities in patients who are skeletally immature, some surgeons have attempted to apply this technique to reversible epiphysiodesis.[53-56] By implanting tension band plates on both the medial and lateral sides of the physis, it is theoretically possible to slow longitudinal physeal growth without damaging the physis. Physeal growth would then resume after the plates are removed. The need for accurate prediction would be less critical because the plates could be removed after equality in leg length has been obtained. This technique would allow surgeons to treat LLDs at a younger age, not necessarily according to the age of maturity. The correction also could potentially be performed more than once during a child's growth period.

Although reversible epiphysiodesis in an animal model was successful by using tension-band plating, the duration that a physis may be tethered with the expectation of growth after implant removal remains unknown.[53] The resumption of growth after the removal of medial and lateral tension-band plates has not yet been clinically demonstrated in the literature. Other concerns with the technique include creating an angulation by asymmetric growth retardation if the screws do not reach maximum splay at the same time. In addition, the eight-Plate (Orthofix) seems to allow for central physeal growth.[54] The current recommendation is that surgeons use the "2-year rule," which states that it is safe to leave tethering over a physis for up to 2 years in a growing child before permanent epiphysiodesis takes place.[53]

Summary

It is important to understand the pattern of normal growth. Management decisions for pediatric orthopaedic conditions can be guided by knowing the expected growth rate of a child. Estimating growth remaining and skeletal maturity, however, is still not an exact science. Using multiple complementary methods to calculate these parameters will help to decrease the chance of error.

Key Study Points

- Knowledge of PHV can be used to guide decision making in children with scoliosis.
- The multiplier method is independent of percentile, regional, racial, ethnic, and generational differences in growth data.
- When assessing bone age, a hand radiograph is preferable before puberty and from Risser grade 1 to skeletal maturity. A lateral elbow radiograph should be obtained during puberty.

Annotated References

1. Buckwalter JA, Ehrlich MG, Sandell LJ, Trippel SB, eds: *Skeletal Growth and Development: Clinical Issues and Basic Science Advances.* Rosemont, IL, American Academy of Orthopaedic Surgeons, 1997, p 577.

2. Diméglio A: Growth in pediatric orthopaedics. *J Pediatr Orthop* 2001;21(4):549-555.

3. Diméglio A: *Growth in pediatric orthopaedics* , in Morrissey, RT, Weinstein, SL, eds: *Lovell and Winter's Pediatric Orthopaedics,* ed 6. Philadelphia, PA, Lippincott Williams and Wilkins, 2006, pp 35-63.

4. Diméglio A: *La croissance en orthopedie* . Montpellioer, France: Sauramps Medical, 1987.

5. Adair LS: Child and adolescent obesity: Epidemiology and developmental perspectives. *Physiol Behav* 2008;94(1):8-16.

6. Carroll MD, Navaneelan T, Bryan S, Ogden C: Prevalence of obesity among children and adolescents in the United States and Canada. National Center for Health Statistics Data Brief, Volume 211. Available at: http://www.cdc.gov/nchs/data/databriefs/db211.htm. Accessed March 11, 2016.

   This online article discusses the prevalence of obesity in children in the United States and Canada. Both countries have seen a substantial increase in obesity in the past 30 years.

7. Greulich WW, Pyle SI: *Radiographic Atlas of Skeletal Development of the Hand and Wrist,* ed 2. Stanford, CA, Stanford University Press, 1959.

8. Sanders JO, Browne RH, Cooney TE, Finegold DN, McConnell SJ, Margraf SA: Correlates of the peak height velocity in girls with idiopathic scoliosis. *Spine (Phila Pa 1976)* 2006;31(20):2289-2295.

9. Needlman RD: Growth and development, in Behrman RE, ed: *Nelson Textbook of Pediatrics,* ed 16. Philadelphia, PA, WB Saunders, 2000, pp 23-65.

10. Ford DM, McFadden KD, Bagnall KM: Sequence of ossification in human vertebral neural arch centers. *Anat Rec* 1982;203(1):175-178.

11. Hinck VC, Hopkins CE, Clark WM: Sagittal diameter of the lumbar spinal canal in children and adults. *Radiology* 1965;85(5):929-937.

12. Yousefzadeh DK, El-Khoury GY, Smith WL: Normal sagittal diameter and variation in the pediatric cervical spine. *Radiology* 1982;144(2):319-325.

13. Labrom RD: Growth and maturation of the spine from birth to adolescence. *J Bone Joint Surg Am* 2007;89(suppl 1):3-7.

14. Ogden JA: Radiology of postnatal skeletal development: XI. The first cervical vertebra. *Skeletal Radiol* 1984;12(1):12-20.

15. Duval-Beaupere G: Pathogenic relationship between scoliosis and growth, in Zorab PA, ed: *Scoliosis and Growth* .Edinburgh, Scotland, Churchill Livingstone, 1971, pp 58-64.

16. Little DG, Song KM, Katz D, Herring JA: Relationship of peak height velocity to other maturity indicators in idiopathic scoliosis in girls. *J Bone Joint Surg Am* 2000;82(5):685-693.

17. Song KM, Little DG: Peak height velocity as a maturity indicator for males with idiopathic scoliosis. *J Pediatr Orthop* 2000;20(3):286-288.

18. Bunch WH, Dvonch VM: Pitfalls in the assessment of skeletal immaturity: An anthropologic case study. *J Pediatr Orthop* 1983;3(2):220-222.

19. Bunnell WP: The natural history of idiopathic scoliosis before skeletal maturity. *Spine (Phila Pa 1976)* 1986;11(8):773-776.

20. Lonstein JE, Carlson JM: The prediction of curve progression in untreated idiopathic scoliosis during growth. *J Bone Joint Surg Am* 1984;66(7):1061-1071.

21. Perdriolle R, Vidal J: Thoracic idiopathic scoliosis curve evolution and prognosis. *Spine (Phila Pa 1976)* 1985;10(9):785-791.

22. Sanders JO, Browne RH, McConnell SJ, Margraf SA, Cooney TE, Finegold DN: Maturity assessment and curve progression in girls with idiopathic scoliosis. *J Bone Joint Surg Am* 2007;89(1):64-73.

23. Dubousset J, Herring JA, Shufflebarger H: The crankshaft phenomenon. *J Pediatr Orthop* 1989;9(5):541-550.

24. Sanders JO, Herring JA, Browne RH: Posterior arthrodesis and instrumentation in the immature (Risser-grade-0) spine in idiopathic scoliosis. *J Bone Joint Surg Am* 1995;77(1):39-45.

25. Sanders JO, Little DG, Richards BS: Prediction of the crankshaft phenomenon by peak height velocity. *Spine (Phila Pa 1976)* 1997;22(12):1352-1356, discussion 1356-1357.

26. Menelaus MB: Correction of leg length discrepancy by epiphysial arrest. *J Bone Joint Surg Br* 1966;48(2):336-339.

27. Anderson M, Green WT, Messner MB: Growth and predictions of growth in the lower extremities. *J Bone Joint Surg Am* 1963;45:1-14.

28. Moseley CF: A straight-line graph for leg-length discrepancies. *J Bone Joint Surg Am* 1977;59(2):174-179.

29. Paley D, Bhave A, Herzenberg JE, Bowen JR: Multiplier method for predicting limb-length discrepancy. *J Bone Joint Surg Am* 2000;82(10):1432-1446.

30. Paley J, Talor J, Levin A, Bhave A, Paley D, Herzenberg JE: The multiplier method for prediction of adult height. *J Pediatr Orthop* 2004;24(6):732-737.

31. Aguilar JA, Paley D, Paley J, et al: Clinical validation of the multiplier method for predicting limb length at maturity, part I. *J Pediatr Orthop* 2005;25(2):186-191.

32. Aguilar JA, Paley D, Paley J, et al: Clinical validation of the multiplier method for predicting limb length discrepancy and outcome of epiphysiodesis, part II. *J Pediatr Orthop* 2005;25(2):192-196.

33. Lamm BM, Paley D, Kurland DB, Matz AL, Herzenberg JE: Multiplier method for predicting adult foot length. *J Pediatr Orthop* 2006;26(4):444-448.

34. Paley D, Gelman A, Shualy MB, Herzenberg JE: Multiplier method for limb-length prediction in the upper extremity. *J Hand Surg Am* 2008;33(3):385-391.

35. Sanders JO, Howell J, Qiu X: Comparison of the Paley method using chronological age with use of skeletal maturity for predicting mature limb length in children. *J Bone Joint Surg Am* 2011;93(11):1051-1056.

Although the multiplier method, which is based on chronologic age, provides reasonable estimates of ultimate limb length for most patients, the use of skeletal maturity determinations appears to provide better predictions of mature limb length during adolescence.

36. Kelly PM, Diméglio A: Lower-limb growth: How predictable are predictions? *J Child Orthop* 2008;2(6):407-415.

37. Canavese F, Charles YP, Dimeglio A, et al: A comparison of the simplified olecranon and digital methods of assessment of skeletal maturity during the pubertal growth spurt. *Bone Joint J* 2014;96-B(11):1556-1560.

The simplified olecranon and digital methods are equally reliable in assessing skeletal maturity. The olecranon method offers detailed information during the pubertal growth spurt, whereas the digital method is equally accurate but less detailed, making it more useful after the pubertal growth spurt after the olecranon has ossified.

38. De Sanctis V, Soliman AT, Di Maio S, Bedair S: Are the new automated methods for bone age estimation advantageous over the manual approaches? *Pediatr Endocrinol Rev* 2014;12(2):200-205.

Automated bone age software is being developed to improve the accuracy of determining radiographic bone age.

39. Heyworth BE, Osei DA, Fabricant PD, et al: The shorthand bone age assessment: A simpler alternative to current methods. *J Pediatr Orthop* 2013;33(5):569-574.

The shorthand method uses a single, univariable criterion for each age rather than a multivariable subjective comparison to a radiographic atlas. The study results are comparable or superior to previous reports that have investigated the validity and the reliability of other skeletal age assessment tools. The shorthand bone age assessment tool offers a simple and efficient alternative to current methods. Level of evidence: III.

40. Sauvegrain J, Nahum H, Bronstein H: Study of bone maturation of the elbow [French]. *Ann Radiol (Paris)* 1962;5:542-550.

41. Diméglio A, Charles YP, Daures JP, de Rosa V, Kaboré B: Accuracy of the Sauvegrain method in determining skeletal age during puberty. *J Bone Joint Surg Am* 2005;87(8):1689-1696.

42. Charles YP, Diméglio A, Canavese F, Daures JP: Skeletal age assessment from the olecranon for idiopathic scoliosis at Risser grade 0. *J Bone Joint Surg Am* 2007;89(12):2737-2744.

43. Hans SD, Sanders JO, Cooperman DR: Using the Sauvegrain method to predict peak height velocity in boys and girls. *J Pediatr Orthop* 2008;28(8):836-839.

44. Sanders JO, Khoury JG, Kishan S, et al: Predicting scoliosis progression from skeletal maturity: A simplified classification during adolescence. *J Bone Joint Surg Am* 2008;90(3):540-553.

45. Lykissas MG, Jain VV, Manickam V, Nathan S, Eismann EA, McCarthy JJ: Guided growth for the treatment of limb length discrepancy: A comparative study of the three most commonly used surgical techniques. *J Pediatr Orthop B* 2013;22(4):311-317.

The authors reported that epiphysiodesis for LLD can be effectively performed with staples, tension-band plates, or percutaneous transphyseal screws.

46. Bowen JR, Leahey JL, Zhang ZH, MacEwen GD: Partial epiphysiodesis at the knee to correct angular deformity. *Clin Orthop Relat Res* 1985;198:184-190.

47. Castañeda P, Urquhart B, Sullivan E, Haynes RJ: Hemiepiphysiodesis for the correction of angular deformity about the knee. *J Pediatr Orthop* 2008;28(2):188-191.

48. Wiemann JM IV, Tryon C, Szalay EA: Physeal stapling versus 8-plate hemiepiphysiodesis for guided correction of angular deformity about the knee. *J Pediatr Orthop* 2009;29(5):481-485.

49. Shin SJ, Cho TJ, Park MS, et al: Angular deformity correction by asymmetrical physeal suppression in growing children: Stapling versus percutaneous transphyseal screw. *J Pediatr Orthop* 2010;30(6):588-593.

50. Ballal MS, Bruce CE, Nayagam S: Correcting genu varum and genu valgum in children by guided growth: Temporary hemiepiphysiodesis using tension band plates. *J Bone Joint Surg Br* 2010;92(2):273-276.

51. Sung KH, Ahn S, Chung CY, et al: Rate of correction after asymmetrical physeal suppression in valgus deformity: Analysis using a linear mixed model application. *J Pediatr Orthop* 2012;32(8):805-814.

Asymmetric physeal suppression with staples, percutaneous transphyseal screws, and the permanent method are effective methods for treating valgus deformity in growing children. The rate of correction at the distal femur is slower in older children and faster in the proximal tibia in the screw group. Level of evidence: III.

52. Wagner P, Standard SC, Herzenberg JE: Abstract: Evaluation of a mobile application for multiplier method growth and epiphysiodesis predictions. *ILLRS Congress, Miami 2015.* Montreal, Canada, Limb Lengthening and Reconstruction Society of North America, 2015, p 141.

Using a mobile application was simpler, faster, and more accurate than traditional multiplier method calculations.

53. Gottliebsen M, Møller-Madsen B, Stødkilde-Jørgensen H, Rahbek O: Controlled longitudinal bone growth by temporary tension band plating: An experimental study. *Bone Joint J* 2013;95-B(6):855-860.

Temporary epiphysiodesis can be obtained by using tension band plating. The technique is not yet in common clinical practice, but it might avoid the need for the accurate timing of epiphysiodesis.

54. Lauge-Pedersen H, Hägglund G: Eight plate should not be used for treating leg length discrepancy. *J Child Orthop* 2013;7(4):285-288.

When applied both medially and laterally in a symmetric manner at the proximal tibial physis, the eight-Plate does not significantly reduce growth.

55. Stewart D, Cheema A, Szalay EA: Dual 8-plate technique is not as effective as ablation for epiphysiodesis about the knee. *J Pediatr Orthop* 2013;33(8):843-846.

Physeal ablation is a substantially superior treatment compared with dual eight-Plates for epiphysiodesis. Despite the theoretic advantages of eight-Plates for performing epiphysiodesis about the knee, this study did not recommend the use of medial and lateral eight-Plates to effect epiphysiodesis. Level of evidence: III.

56. Siedhoff M, Ridderbusch K, Breyer S, Stucker R, Rupprecht M: Temporary epiphysiodesis for limb-length discrepancy: 8- to 15-year follow-up of 34 children. *Acta Orthop* 2014;85:626-632.

Temporary epiphysiodesis is an effective and safe option for the treatment of LLD. The timing of the procedure must be chosen according to the remaining growth available, thus facilitating full correction of LLD.

Section 2

Basic Science

SECTION EDITOR:
Benjamin A. Alman, MD

Chapter 7

Genetics and Personalized Medicine

Christina A. Gurnett, MD, PhD Dorothy K. Grange, MD David H. Gutmann, MD, PhD

Douglas J. McDonald, MD, MS Matthew B. Dobbs, MD

Abstract

Physicians are striving to develop treatment and prevention strategies that can be targeted to meet a patient's unique genetic and environmental milieu. Genetic advances that facilitate comprehensive and inexpensive genome-wide testing are largely driving personalized medicine. Rich opportunities exist for developing personalized treatment approaches for pediatric orthopaedic disorders. It is helpful to be aware of the latest advances in genetic technology and pharmacogenetics, the new discoveries of somatic mutations in bone cancers and segmental overgrowth syndromes, and the new insights into the etiology of clubfoot and adolescent idiopathic scoliosis.

Keywords: personalized medicine; pharmacogenetics; segmental overgrowth; somatic mutation

Dr. Gurnett or an immediate family member has received royalties from D-Bar Enterprises; serves as a paid consultant to D-Bar Enterprises; and serves as a board member, owner, officer, or committee member of the Association of Bone and Joint Surgeons. Dr. Grange or an immediate family member has received research or institutional support from Biomarin Pharmaceuticals and Edimer Pharmaceuticals. Dr. McDonald or an immediate family member serves as a board member, owner, officer, or committee member of the Musculoskeletal Tumor Society. Dr. Dobbs or an immediate family member has received royalties from D-Bar Enterprises; serves as a paid consultant to D-Bar Enterprises; and serves as a board member, owner, officer, or committee member of the Association of Bone and Joint Surgeons and the Orthopaedic Research and Education Foundation. Neither Dr. Gutmann nor any immediate family member has received anything of value from or has stock or stock options held in a commercial company or institution related directly or indirectly to the subject of this chapter.

Introduction

In January 2015, President Barack Obama launched a new $215 million initiative to advance the research and implementation of "precision" medicine.[1] Personalized medicine promises to (1) deliver pharmaceutical agents with minimal toxicity and optimal efficacy and (2) guide treatment and preventive interventions informed by a patient's unique biology. Abandoning a one-size-fits-all approach to health care will require more research into the genetic and environmental factors that influence disease presentations and surgical outcomes for pediatric orthopaedic conditions. This chapter highlights recent advances in genetic technology and new insights into rare and common pediatric orthopaedic disorders that will pave the way for personalized medicine in the next decade.

Comprehensive Genetic Profiling

The first wave of genetic and genomic discoveries followed the development of microarray technology, which facilitated the simultaneous ascertainment of an extremely large number (often >1 million) of known single nucleotide polymorphic genotypes (**Table 1**). Microarray technology also allows the identification of genomic abnormalities, including microdeletions and microduplications of small chromosomal regions that are too small to be viewed microscopically, on a routine karyotype.[2] Single nucleotide polymorphisms (SNPs) are informative for some disorders because a plethora of genome-wide association studies (GWASs), mostly for common and complex diseases, have yielded SNPs or groups of SNPs that increase the risk for complex human diseases.[3] Genetic risk factors for common diseases identified through GWASs are mostly associated with a small to modest increase in risk, increasing the odds ratio from 1.0 to approximately 1.1 to 1.4. These SNPs are typically variants that are present in approximately 5% to 40% of the population, and the variants may be either protective or risk alleles. Although most of these genetic risk factors are not highly predictive

Table 1

Common Genetic Terms

Term	Definition and Characteristic
Complex genetic disease	A disorder caused by multiple genetic variations in a single individual.
De novo	Arising newly in the genome in either somatic cells or the germline, germline de novo mutations can be identified by sequencing unaffected parents and the affected child, whereas somatic de novo mutations can be detected by paired sequencing of normal and abnormal tissues.
DNA variant	Differences in DNA between individuals.
Genetic association	DNA sequence variants that are more common in a group of patients compared with a control group.
Germline mutation	A mutation that occurs in the ova or the sperm before fertilization.
Mendelian genetic disorder	A genetic disorder that is caused by a single genetic variation and is highly heritable.
Microdeletion/microduplication	A small deletion or duplication of DNA that is undetectable under the microscope but detectable with other methods.
Mosaic	Differences in genetic composition between different cells in an organism result from a somatic mutation.
Pharmacogenetic variant	A genetic variant that influences a drug response, by either altering drug absorption, distribution, metabolism, or the drug target.
Segmental overgrowth syndrome	One of many syndromes that results from abnormal growth of a region of the body.
Single nucleotide polymorphism (SNP)	A variant that consists of a change of one nucleotide between individuals. The term often is used to indicate a common SNP that is present in more than 1% and up to 5% of the population.
Somatic mutation	A mutation during cell division that occurs at any time after fertilization. Depending on the temporal and spatial patterns of the mutational event, these mutations may cause cancer or congenital malformations.
Ultrarapid metabolizer	An individual who has a genetic variant that results in better metabolism of a prodrug into the active drug.

of disease within a single individual, collectively they provide an understanding of the pathways involved and the overall landscape of a single disease in terms of how much disease risk is predicted by common versus rare genetic variants.

The investigation of de novo variants, defined as mutations that are present in an affected child but not the unaffected parents, has made possible extensive new genetic discoveries for patients with rare genetic diseases. De novo variants may arise in two places: (1) the germline (the ova or the sperm), where they would then be incorporated into all cells in the developing fetus, or (2) in somatic cells during cell division, where they would be present only in a subset of cells depending on the location and timing of the mutational event. De novo germline mutations play an important role in the causality of diseases and are associated with reduced life expectancy and/or diminished reproductive fitness, which often occurs in children with severe autism or developmental disabilities.[4] Whole genome sequencing studies of healthy trios (a healthy child and both healthy parents) estimate that the germline mutation rate is approximately 1.0×10^{-8}, which results in 10 to 20 de novo coding sequence variants per child.[5] Although all human genomes harbor de novo variants, most do not negatively affect the coding genes. Congenital disorders occur when de novo mutations deleteriously affect genes that are important for development. Because more germ cell divisions occur in males than in females, most de novo missense mutations arise on paternally derived chromosomes. The male germline accumulates mutations during normal aging, such that approximately twice as many de novo mutations are present in the child of a 40-year-old father compared with the child of a 20-year-old father. As a consequence of recent de novo gene discovery for children with presumed genetic disease, exome sequencing of trios is rapidly becoming a first-line test for children with severe cognitive and developmental disabilities and results in a diagnosis in nearly 50% of all patients. This approach is useful to study severe, sporadic disorders that arise without any family history of the disorder.

In addition to revealing the cause of a disease for which clinical diagnostic exome sequencing is performed, comprehensive gene sequencing often reveals mutations in disease genes that are found incidentally because all genes are sequenced in this test. In 2013, the American College of Medical Genetics compiled a list of 56 disease genes that are clinically actionable because treatments are available and routinely used to prevent or reduce the severity of a disorder.[6] Information on mutations in clinically actionable genes are typically provided to the patient, even when they are found incidentally; however, during the genetic testing consent process, some patients may opt not to learn about possible mutations. Clinically actionable disease genes include the breast cancer genes *BRCA1* and *BRCA2*, along with several genes responsible for disorders frequently encountered in orthopaedic clinics, including Marfan syndrome and Loeys-Dietz syndrome, because the cardiac manifestations of these syndromes can be prevented with early diagnosis. As comprehensive genetic testing becomes routine, it is likely that patients with clinically actionable disease gene mutations will receive an earlier diagnosis, which will provide additional opportunities for improvements in care.

High-coverage next-generation sequencing is revealing a major role for somatic mutations in the pathogenesis of both developmental disorders and cancer.[7] The mutation rate in somatic cells is estimated to be 4 to 25 times higher than in the germline cells; therefore, dividing cells accumulate a high burden of mutations during the course of a lifetime, which contributes to the development of cancer.[5] Likewise, somatic mutations occurring during development contribute to the pathogenesis of congenital malformations and overgrowth syndromes. Somatic mutations contribute to a mosaic phenotype in which only a fraction of all cells contain the disease mutation, resulting in differentially affected tissues and organs. In these heterogeneous and mosaic disorders, the resultant phenotype is highly dependent on the spatial and temporal course of mutagenesis.

Pharmacogenetic Variability in Codeine Metabolism

Pharmacogenetic testing to reduce the frequency of adverse drug events is moving quickly to the clinic. Such testing includes evaluating the metabolism of cancer drugs, carbamazepine, and warfarin.[8] Of particular interest to orthopaedic surgeons are data regarding codeine, a commonly prescribed opioid. Codeine and other opioids, such as tramadol, hydrocodone, and oxycodone, are metabolized to morphine in the liver by means of the cytochrome P450 CYP2D6 enzyme. Individuals who are ultrarapid metabolizers make up 1% to 2% of the general population and are at higher risk for toxicity.[9] In 2006, the death of a breast-fed infant by a mother taking codeine, who was an ultrarapid metabolizer, was attributed to opioid toxicity secondary to morphine secretion into breast milk.[10] Even at normal codeine dosages, deaths in children undergoing a tonsillectomy or an adenoidectomy have been attributed to CYP2D6 polymorphisms leading to ultrarapid metabolism,[9] resulting in an FDA warning against codeine use for postoperative pain for tonsillectomies or adenoidectomies.[11] Although the FDA did not comment on the use of codeine for pain control in other situations, some pediatric hospitals have completely removed codeine from their pharmacopeia. Individuals who are ultrarapid metabolizers are at high risk for life-threatening respiratory depression or signs of overdose, including sleepiness, confusion, and shallow breathing, even at approved doses, particularly combined with airway swelling from surgery or infection. Because these CYP2D6 variants have lesser roles in the metabolism of other opioids, the primary concerns have been with codeine. Carrier frequency of ultrarapid metabolizer variants varies by ethnicity and, for example, is approximately 4% in Caucasians in North America, 10% in Greece and Portugal, 20% in Saudi Arabia, and 30% in Ethiopia. Some CYP2D6 polymorphisms also can reduce the conversion to morphine and result in poor analgesic response. Poor metabolizer polymorphisms are present in 6% to 10% of Caucasian Americans, 3% to 6% of Mexican Americans, 2% to 5% of African Americans, and 1% of Asian Americans. Genetic testing for CYP2D6 polymorphisms to identify individuals who are ultrarapid or poor metabolizers is available but typically takes days to weeks to obtain; therefore, testing needs to be performed well in advance of codeine administration. Genetic testing has not yet been advocated for other types of opioid anesthetics.

Somatic Mutations in Ewing Sarcoma and Osteosarcoma

Germline and somatic mutations play a role in cancer pathogenesis, but the relative contributions of each and the specific genes involved differ substantially among tumor types.[12] Recent data suggest that approximately 8% of pediatric cancers are associated with a germline mutation in a known inherited cancer predisposition gene.[13] Although relatively rare cancers (representing 6% to 8% of all primary malignant bone tumors), Ewing

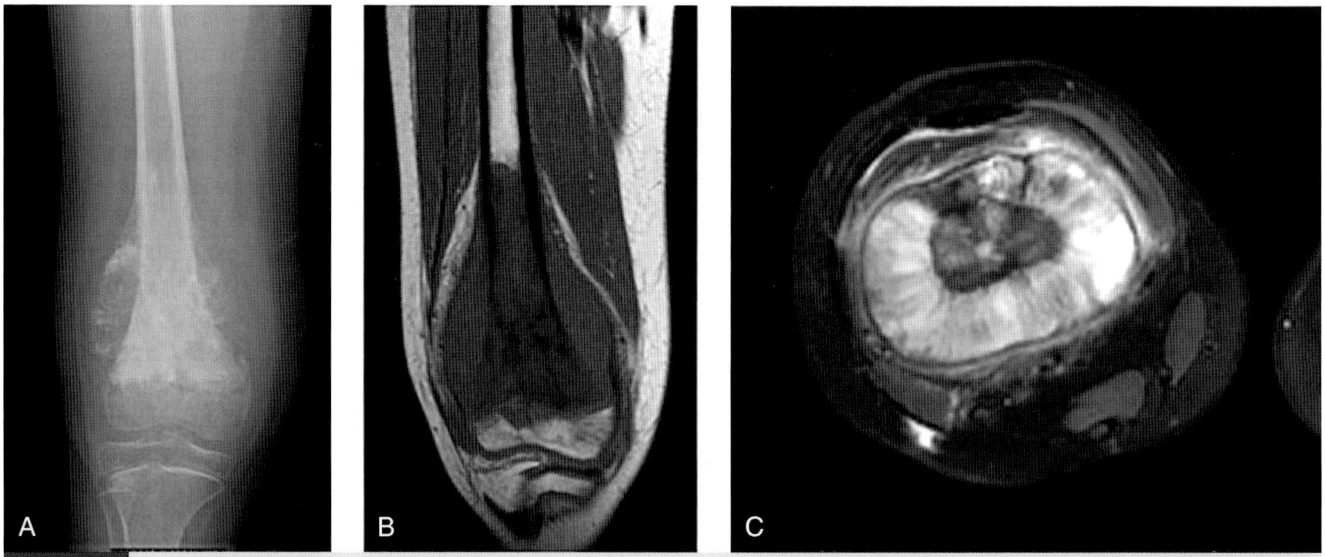

Figure 1 Images of osteosarcoma in a 9-year-old girl. **A,** AP radiograph of the distal right femur shows an obvious mixed lytic and blastic lesion in the metaphysis with a classic sunburst pattern of periosteal new bone formation in the soft tissue. **B,** T1-weighted coronal MRI shows the intraosseous and soft-tissue component. **C,** T2-weighted fat-suppressed axial MRI delineates the extensive soft-tissue involvement surrounding the distal femoral metaphysis.

sarcoma and osteosarcoma are the two most frequently encountered tumors in pediatric orthopaedics. Importantly, the genetic etiologies and landscapes of these tumors are very different.[14]

Osteosarcoma is the most common primary bone tumor that affects both children and young adults, with an incidence of 5 to 10 new cases per 1 million individuals each year (**Figure 1**). The overall survival rate of patients with this cancer is approximately 60%. In contrast to Ewing sarcoma, osteosarcoma tumors are genomically unstable and exhibit high rates of somatic mutations and rearrangements.[15] As such, the median somatic nonsilent mutational frequency has been estimated at 1.2 mutations per megabase.[12,15] Genes commonly mutated in osteosarcoma include the *TP53* gene as well as genes converging on the phosphatidylinositol 3-kinase/mammalian target of rapamycin (*PI3K/mTOR*) gene pathway.[15] Germline mutations in *TP53* are common in Li-Fraumeni syndrome,[16] a cancer predisposition condition in which multiple tumor types, including osteosarcoma, develop in affected individuals.[17] Unfortunately, despite substantial research, *TP53* has not been amenable to pharmacologic intervention.[18] Because the *PI3K/mTOR* gene pathway is amenable to pharmacologic intervention, future therapies might use drugs already in clinical use for other cancers.[19]

Ewing sarcoma is an aggressive primary bone (neuroectodermal) tumor that affects male children slightly more often than female children during adolescence or young adulthood, with an incidence of 3 new cases per 1 million individuals annually (**Figure 2**). Severe pain with or without an associated mass is the most common clinical symptom. In many patients, current therapy can be curative, although the prognosis for those with disseminated disease remains dismal. It has been known for more than 20 years that Ewing sarcoma is nearly always caused by a chimeric fusion between the EWS (Ewing sarcoma) and the ETS (E26 transformation-specific) family transcription factors,[20] with a paucity of additional somatic mutations detected in most tumors. However, somatic loss of the *STAG2*, *INK4A*, or *TP53* tumor suppressor genes is present in approximately 10% to 20% of tumors, where these molecular alterations have been associated with metastatic disease and a poor prognosis.[21,22]

Inherited genetic risk factors play a more important role than had previously been appreciated in Ewing sarcoma and may explain the low somatic mutational burden. A GWAS of 401 patients showed an association of Ewing sarcoma with high-risk common variants near the *TARDBP* and *EGR2* genes.[23] EGR2 is a zinc-finger transcription factor that promotes proliferation, differentiation, and survival. Relevant to Ewing sarcoma pathogenesis, the chimeric EWS-ETS fusion protein differentially binds and regulates its expression, depending on the presence or absence of the risk allele within its enhancer.[24]*EGR2* also is overexpressed in Ewing sarcoma, suggesting that pharmaceutical interventions aimed at reducing its expression may be a logical therapeutic option. Interestingly, the lower prevalence of this genetic risk variant in African-American populations is likely responsible for the ninefold lower incidence of Ewing

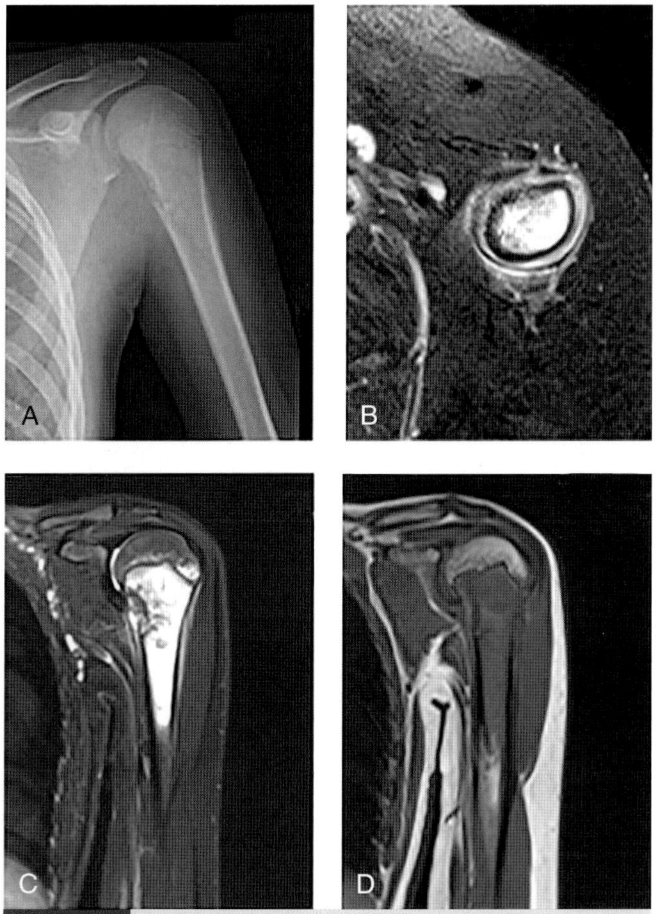

Figure 2 Images of Ewing sarcoma in an 11-year-old girl. **A,** AP radiograph of the left proximal humerus demonstrates medial lytic cortical destruction with a subtle permeative pattern of bone destruction throughout the metaphysis, along with a lateral periosteal reaction. **B,** T2-weighted fat-suppressed axial MRI shows minimal soft-tissue mass but the clear onion-skin pattern of a circumferential periosteal reaction. **C,** T1-weighted coronal MRI reveals distal intraosseous involvement of the shaft with proximal extension up to the physis. **D,** T2-weighted fat-suppressed coronal MRI shows the intraosseous involvement and periosteal reaction.

sarcoma in African Americans than in Caucasian Americans.[25] Overall, targeted therapies to correct these molecular defects, including cytosine arabinoside to suppress EWS-ETS expression, may yield new treatment strategies.

Somatic Mutations in Segmental Overgrowth Syndromes

A major shift in the understanding of sporadic overgrowth syndromes resulted from the discovery of a recurrent activating somatic mutation in Proteus syndrome.[26] The characteristic features of Proteus syndrome include overgrowth of skin, connective, fat, brain, and other tissues. Sequencing of paired samples taken from affected and unaffected tissues revealed somatic activating (gain-of-function) mutations in the growth-promoting serine/threonine kinase gene *AKT1*, which was only present in highly enriched affected tissue.[26] Interestingly, these *AKT1* mutations all occurred at the same nucleotide and resulted in a constitutively activated AKT1 kinase. In addition to *AKT1*, somatic mutations in the *PIK3CA* gene, now collectively referred to as *PIK3CA*-related overgrowth syndrome,[27] cause a wide spectrum of congenital abnormalities depending on the cell type containing the somatic mutations. Manifestations of these mutations include macrodactyly;[28] fibroadipose overgrowth;[29] muscle hemihypertrophy; congenital lipomatous overgrowth with vascular, epidermal, and skeletal anomalies (CLOVES) syndrome;[30] isolated brain malformations;[31] and other fibroadipose vascular anomalies[32] (**Figure 3**). Further genetic studies have revealed that additional mutations in genes that regulate the *PI3K/AKT/mTOR* gene pathway, including *PIK3R2*, *AKT3*, and *TOR*, are responsible for a wide spectrum of human segmental overgrowth syndromes.[33]

Genetic testing of genes that operate within the *PI3K/AKT/mTOR* gene pathway is warranted in clinically suspicious cases to guide tumor surveillance as well as personalize treatments using pharmacologic agents to inhibit these hyperactivated growth pathways. In many biopsy specimens, the percentage of cells harboring these somatic mutations may be quite small, arguing for the use of diagnostic testing with high-density sequence coverage. Although many of the genes implicated in overgrowth also have been demonstrated in sporadic cancers, the risk of true malignancy in affected tissues appears to be quite low.

Genetic Prediction of Comorbidities and Outcome in Clubfoot

Although the genetic basis for clubfoot in most patients remains unknown, evidence supports an important role for genes regulating early leg development. Disruption of genes in the *PITX1/TBX4/HOXC* gene pathway, by either point mutations or through microdeletions or microduplications,[34-37] is present in some families with autosomal dominant inherited clubfoot. Although clubfoot is the most common orthopaedic condition in these disorders, vertical talus is more common in families with *HOXC* gene cluster microdeletions.[38] Limb patterning defects, with small peroneus muscles and arteries supplying the lateral lower limb, appear to be present in patients with

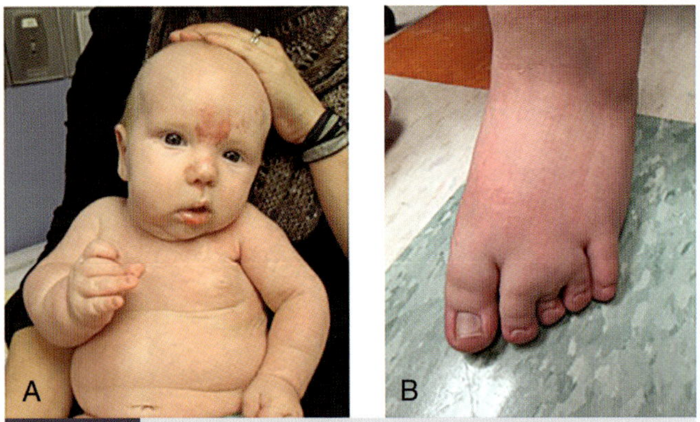

Figure 3 Clinical photographs of phenotypic manifestations of *PIK3CA*-related overgrowth syndrome. **A,** A male infant with facial asymmetry, midline facial capillary malformation, and hemimegalencephaly who has *PIK3CA* somatic mutation. **B,** A child with *PIK3CA* mutation showing two-three-four toe syndactyly.

mutations in the *PITX1/TBX4/HOXC* gene pathway, possibly contributing to the greater incidence of treatment resistance. Additional orthopaedic abnormalities, including hip dysplasia, polydactyly, and tibial hemimelia, are more common in these conditions. Although genetic testing is not yet recommended for all children with clubfoot because the yield of testing remains low, chromosomal microarray testing to identify microdeletions or microduplications may be helpful in familial cases or for children in whom additional congenital anomalies are present. Chromosomal microarray testing has the additional benefit of detecting large-scale chromosomal abnormalities, including trisomy and Klinefelter syndrome, which are both associated with an increased incidence of congenital foot contractures.[18,36]

Advances in the Genetic Basis of Adolescent Idiopathic Scoliosis

In addition to addressing the basic mechanisms of the pathogenesis of adolescent idiopathic scoliosis (AIS), genetic studies are now identifying the factors responsible for female sex bias and scoliosis curve progression. Although common genetic variants likely play only a minor role in overall AIS pathogenesis, multiple large-scale GWASs have strongly confirmed the importance of SNPs near *LBX1* (ladybird homeobox 1), a gene that is involved in muscle cell migration and cardiac and neural tube development.[39-41] AIS also is associated with an SNP near *GPR126* (G protein coupled receptor 126) that is essential for cardiac, neural, and ear development.[42] Interestingly, *GPR126* also regulates human height and binds to collagen, suggesting a possible role in mediating extracellular matrix stability.

In the first study to reveal an explanation for female sex bias in AIS, researchers reported an association of AIS with an SNP located in an enhancer near *PAX1* (paired box 1) that is present only in females.[43] *PAX1* is a transcription factor involved in spine development that has been implicated in congenital scoliosis in mice. Early-onset alopecia in males was previously associated with these risk alleles, suggesting the possibility that hormonal modulation of these regulatory sites contributes to both sexually dimorphic phenotypes. The paucity of males with scoliosis highlights the extent of the problem but also may hinder the identification of sex-specific risk factors because large numbers of male cases may be needed to definitively exclude an association. Notably, several GWASs used only females as cases, and, therefore, some of the previously reported loci may apply only to females.

The identification of genetic factors responsible for scoliosis curve progression is of major clinical importance because these markers could be used to prospectively design personalized treatment methods. Previous studies reported SNPs near calmodulin, estrogen receptors, tryptophan hydroxylase, insulin-like growth factor, neurotrophin 3, interleukin-17 receptor, melatonin receptor, and a group of SNPs that were predictive of scoliosis curve progression. However, a systematic review and a meta-analysis concluded a limited predictive value of these studies and a low level of evidence; none could be recommended for clinical use as a diagnostic criterion.[44] An association study using female patients with scoliosis curves greater than 40° demonstrated an association of AIS with SNPs around SOX9, a transcription factor involved in chondrogenesis, that had not previously been identified when individuals with lesser curves were included.[45] More recent studies, in which the protein coding region of the extracellular matrix genes *FBN1* (fibrillin 1) and *FBN2* (fibrillin 2) was sequenced in 852 AIS cases, demonstrated that rare variants in these genes were predictive of AIS curve progression.[46]

Mendelian forms of AIS are rare. Although large families have been described, few causative genes have been identified. Variants in *POC5*, a centriolar protein gene, and *CHD7*, a gene associated with CHARGE syndrome (coloboma of the eye, heart defects, atresia choanae, retarded growth and development, genital abnormalities, and ear abnormalities), may play a role in AIS pathogenesis in some families.[47,48] Because the genetic inheritance of AIS is complex, it is more likely that a polygenic burden of rare variants will contribute to disease susceptibility, which was recently shown for extracellular matrix genes as a whole.[49] Much larger studies are needed to confirm the genetic associations that have already been published and identify new disease and gene associations, particularly with rare variants that only recently have begun to be investigated in AIS. Eventually, if algorithms can be applied that take into account the role of both common and rare genetic variants, it is possible that better predictions of scoliosis risk and curve progression can be developed.

Summary

Technology is driving new disease gene discovery and genetic associations for pediatric orthopaedic disorders. These technologies have resulted in the identification of somatic mutations that may lead to cancer or segmental overgrowth syndromes. In the future, new pharmacogenetic data will be implemented in clinical practice to optimize efficacy and reduce the risk of adverse effects in selected populations.

Key Study Points

- Pharmacogenetic variants can identify individuals who are ultrarapid metabolizers of codeine and are at risk for adverse respiratory suppression and death.
- The genetic landscapes of Ewing sarcoma and osteosarcoma are very different; insights about these differences may lead to new therapeutic strategies.
- Segmental overgrowth syndromes are associated with somatic mutations that may increase cancer risk. Treatment with pharmacotherapeutic interventions may be possible.
- Rare genetic factors are predictive of comorbidities and treatment outcomes in some families with clubfoot.
- The genetic inheritance of AIS is complex, but factors responsible for female sex bias and scoliosis curve progression have recently been revealed.

Annotated References

1. Collins FS, Varmus H: A new initiative on precision medicine. *N Engl J Med* 2015;372(9):793-795.

   New research and clinical initiatives for developing personalized medicine in the United States are presented in this article.

2. Alkan C, Coe BP, Eichler EE: Genome structural variation discovery and genotyping. *Nat Rev Genet* 2011;12(5):363-376.

   Microarray methods for detecting structural variation and copy number variants have contributed to new understandings in inherited human diseases.

3. Manolio TA: Genomewide association studies and assessment of the risk of disease. *N Engl J Med* 2010;363(2):166-176.

4. Ronemus M, Iossifov I, Levy D, Wigler M: The role of de novo mutations in the genetics of autism spectrum disorders. *Nat Rev Genet* 2014;15(2):133-141.

   De novo mutations are responsible for many severe human developmental disorders, including autism. This study included 2,500 simplex autism families.

5. Shendure J, Akey JM: The origins, determinants, and consequences of human mutations. *Science* 2015;349(6255):1478-1483.

   This thorough review article presents an overview of human mutations and how they arise in the genome.

6. Green RC, Berg JS, Grody WW, et al; American College of Medical Genetics and Genomics: ACMG recommendations for reporting of incidental findings in clinical exome and genome sequencing. *Genet Med* 2013;15(7):565-574.

   The American College of Medical Genetics platform statement and guidelines regarding the return of incidental findings when patients undergo clinical exome or genome sequencing includes a list of 56 disease genes that are considered clinically actionable.

7. Biesecker LG, Spinner NB: A genomic view of mosaicism and human disease. *Nat Rev Genet* 2013;14(5):307-320.

   Mosaicism is reviewed as it relates to congenital birth defects and cancer.

8. Lee JW, Aminkeng F, Bhavsar AP, et al: The emerging era of pharmacogenomics: Current successes, future potential, and challenges. *Clin Genet* 2014;86(1):21-28.

   New applications of pharmacogenetics as they apply to the clinical care of patients are reviewed.

9. Madadi P, Amstutz U, Rieder M, et al; CPNDS Clinical Recommendations Group: Clinical practice guideline: CYP2D6 genotyping for safe and efficacious codeine therapy. *J Popul Ther Clin Pharmacol* 2013;20(3):e369-e396.

   The clinical practice guideline generated by the Canadian Pharmacogenetic Network for Drug Safety Clinical Recommendations Group addresses the utility of genotyping patients for the CYP2D6 enzyme before the initiation of codeine therapy and the management of patients with genotypic data.

10. Koren G, Cairns J, Chitayat D, Gaedigk A, Leeder SJ: Pharmacogenetics of morphine poisoning in a breastfed neonate of a codeine-prescribed mother. *Lancet* 2006;368(9536):704.

11. US Food and Drug Administration: Codeine Product Labeling Changes. Available at: http://www.fda.gov/Safety/

MedWatch/SafetyInformation/ucm356221.htm. Accessed May 26, 2016.

The FDA issued a policy statement after deaths were reported in patients taking appropriately prescribed codeine dosages.

12. Lawrence MS, Stojanov P, Polak P, et al: Mutational heterogeneity in cancer and the search for new cancer-associated genes. *Nature* 2013;499(7457):214-218.

Exome sequences from 3,083 tumor-normal pairs were analyzed and revealed wide differences in mutational processes between tumor types, resulting in substantial mutational heterogeneity in cancer.

13. Zhang J, Walsh MF, Wu G, et al: Germline mutations in predisposition genes in pediatric cancer. *N Engl J Med* 2015;373(24):2336-2346.

The sequencing and analysis of 565 cancer predisposition genes in 1,120 patients with cancer younger than 20 years showed a frequency of pathogenic or probably pathogenic germline mutations in 8.5% of the patients compared with 1.1% of the control group members. A family history of cancer was not predictive of germline mutations.

14. HaDuong JH, Martin AA, Skapek SX, Mascarenhas L: Sarcomas. *Pediatr Clin North Am* 2015;62(1):179-200.

This review article summarizes the epidemiology, molecular basis, and current treatment of human sarcomas, including osteosarcoma and Ewing sarcoma.

15. Perry JA, Kiezun A, Tonzi P, et al: Complementary genomic approaches highlight the PI3K/mTOR pathway as a common vulnerability in osteosarcoma. *Proc Natl Acad Sci USA* 2014;111(51):E5564-E5573.

Whole exome, whole genome, and RNA sequencing was performed on tumor and normal pairs. Only *TP53* was mutated frequently across all samples. Pathway analysis revealed convergence on the *PI3K/mTOR* pathway.

16. Srivastava S, Zou ZQ, Pirollo K, Blattner W, Chang EH: Germ-line transmission of a mutated p53 gene in a cancer-prone family with Li-Fraumeni syndrome. *Nature* 1990;348(6303):747-749.

17. Gorlick R: Current concepts on the molecular biology of osteosarcoma. *Cancer Treat Res* 2009;152:467-478.

18. Vogelstein B, Papadopoulos N, Velculescu VE, Zhou S, Diaz LA Jr, Kinzler KW: Cancer genome landscapes. *Science* 2013;339(6127):1546-1558.

This review article summarizes the genomic landscape of cancer and the definitions of driver and passenger mutations. It also describes 12 common growth-signaling pathways that are often mutated in cancer.

19. Yap TA, Bjerke L, Clarke PA, Workman P: Drugging PI3K in cancer: Refining targets and therapeutic strategies. *Curr Opin Pharmacol* 2015;23:98-107.

This review article describes the goals of targeting the *PI3K* gene pathway in cancer by describing the more than 30 small molecule *PI3K* inhibitors currently in clinical trials, including one already approved for the treatment of B cell malignancies.

20. Delattre O, Zucman J, Plougastel B, et al: Gene fusion with an ETS DNA-binding domain caused by chromosome translocation in human tumours. *Nature* 1992;359(6391):162-165.

21. Crompton BD, Stewart C, Taylor-Weiner A, et al: The genomic landscape of pediatric Ewing sarcoma. *Cancer Discov* 2014;4(11):1326-1341.

A large-scale sequencing study of 112 patients with Ewing sarcoma revealed few somatic mutations but found that the loss of *STAG2* expression was present in 15% of tumors and correlated with metastatic disease.

22. Tirode F, Surdez D, Ma X, et al; St. Jude Children's Research Hospital–Washington University Pediatric Cancer Genome Project and the International Cancer Genome Consortium: Genomic landscape of Ewing sarcoma defines an aggressive subtype with co-association of STAG2 and TP53 mutations. *Cancer Discov* 2014;4(11):1342-1353.

A collaborative whole genome sequencing study of 112 Ewing sarcoma samples and matched germline DNA revealed few single-nucleotide variants, indels, or copy number alterations. *STAG2* and *TP53* mutations were found in 7% to 17% of patients and were associated with poor outcomes.

23. Postel-Vinay S, Véron AS, Tirode F, et al: Common variants near TARDBP and EGR2 are associated with susceptibility to Ewing sarcoma. *Nat Genet* 2012;44(3):323-327.

A GWAS of Ewing sarcoma cases revealed an association with variants near TARDBP (Tat activating regulatory DNA-binding protein, TDP-43) and EGR2 (early growth response protein). The risk alleles were less common in African Americans, which possibly explains their lower incidence of Ewing sarcoma.

24. Grünewald TG, Bernard V, Gilardi-Hebenstreit P, et al: Chimeric EWSR1-FLI1 regulates the Ewing sarcoma susceptibility gene EGR2 via a GGAA microsatellite. *Nat Genet* 2015;47(9):1073-1078.

After the identification of common variants near *EGF2* associated with Ewing sarcoma, this study investigated the mechanism by which SNPs alter *EGF2*.

25. Jawad MU, Cheung MC, Min ES, Schneiderbauer MM, Koniaris LG, Scully SP: Ewing sarcoma demonstrates racial disparities in incidence-related and sex-related differences in outcome: An analysis of 1631 cases from the SEER database, 1973-2005. *Cancer* 2009;115(15):3526-3536.

26. Lindhurst MJ, Sapp JC, Teer JK, et al: A mosaic activating mutation in AKT1 associated with the Proteus syndrome. *N Engl J Med* 2011;365(7):611-619.

Exome sequencing of 158 affected and unaffected tissues from 29 patients with Proteus syndrome revealed somatic activating mutations at the same location (c.49G>A, p.Glu17Lys) in the oncogene *AKT1* in 25 patients.

27. Keppler-Noreuil KM, Sapp JC, Lindhurst MJ, et al: Clinical delineation and natural history of the PIK3CA-related overgrowth spectrum. *Am J Med Genet A* 2014;164A(7):1713-1733.

    This review summarizes the clinical variability and outcomes of patients with *PIK3CA* somatic mutations.

28. Rios JJ, Paria N, Burns DK, et al: Somatic gain-of-function mutations in PIK3CA in patients with macrodactyly. *Hum Mol Genet* 2013;22(3):444-451.

    Activating mutations in *PIK3CA* were found in patients with macrodactyly.

29. Lindhurst MJ, Parker VE, Payne F, et al: Mosaic overgrowth with fibroadipose hyperplasia is caused by somatic activating mutations in PIK3CA. *Nat Genet* 2012;44(8):928-933.

    Activating mutations in *PIK3CA* were identified in fibroadipose hyperplasia.

30. Kurek KC, Luks VL, Ayturk UM, et al: Somatic mosaic activating mutations in PIK3CA cause CLOVES syndrome. *Am J Hum Genet* 2012;90(6):1108-1115.

    Activating mutations in *PIK3CA* were identified as causative factors in CLOVES syndrome.

31. Poduri A, Evrony GD, Cai X, et al: Somatic activation of AKT3 causes hemispheric developmental brain malformations. *Neuron* 2012;74(1):41-48.

    Activating mutations in *AKT3* were identified as causative factors in hemimegalencephaly syndromes.

32. Alomari AI, Spencer SA, Arnold RW, et al: Fibro-adipose vascular anomaly: Clinical-radiologic-pathologic features of a newly delineated disorder of the extremity. *J Pediatr Orthop* 2014;34(1):109-117.

    The clinical and radiologic features of a series of 16 patients with fibroadipose vascular anomaly are presented. Level of evidence: III.

33. Lee JH, Huynh M, Silhavy JL, et al: De novo somatic mutations in components of the PI3K-AKT3-mTOR pathway cause hemimegalencephaly. *Nat Genet* 2012;44(8):941-945.

    Mutations in the *PI3K/AKT3/mTOR* pathway were identified in patients with similar hemimegalencephalic phenotypes.

34. Alvarado DM, Aferol H, McCall K, et al: Familial isolated clubfoot is associated with recurrent chromosome 17q23.1q23.2 microduplications containing TBX4. *Am J Hum Genet* 2010;87(1):154-160.

35. Alvarado DM, McCall K, Aferol H, et al: Pitx1 haploinsufficiency causes clubfoot in humans and a clubfoot-like phenotype in mice. *Hum Mol Genet* 2011;20(20):3943-3952.

    The PITX1 bicoid homeodomain transcription factor has been identified in a family with a spectrum of lower extremity abnormalities, including clubfoot, which is found in 1 in 1,000 live births.

36. Alvarado DM, Buchan JG, Frick SL, Herzenberg JE, Dobbs MB, Gurnett CA: Copy number analysis of 413 isolated talipes equinovarus patients suggests role for transcriptional regulators of early limb development. *Eur J Hum Genet* 2013;21(4):373-380.

    This study analyzed copy number variations in the etiology of isolated talipes equinovarus. The results do not support a major role for recurrent copy number variations, but they do suggest a role for genes involved in early embryonic patterning in some families.

37. Gurnett CA, Alaee F, Kruse LM, et al: Asymmetric lower-limb malformations in individuals with homeobox PITX1 gene mutation. *Am J Hum Genet* 2008;83(5):616-622.

38. Alvarado DM, McCall K, Hecht JT, Dobbs MB, Gurnett CA: Deletions of 5' HOXC genes are associated with lower extremity malformations, including clubfoot and vertical talus. *J Med Genet* 2016;53(4):250-255.

    Small microdeletions of the *HOXC* gene cluster were identified in three families with clubfoot or vertical talus, and point mutations in *HOXC12* segregate with familial clubfoot.

39. Takahashi Y, Kou I, Takahashi A, et al: A genome-wide association study identifies common variants near LBX1 associated with adolescent idiopathic scoliosis. *Nat Genet* 2011;43(12):1237-1240.

    A large GWAS of 1,376 Japanese girls with scoliosis revealed a substantial genome-wide association with common SNPs near *LBX1* that has since been widely replicated in additional populations.

40. Zhu Z, Tang NL, Xu L, et al: Genome-wide association study identifies new susceptibility loci for adolescent idiopathic scoliosis in Chinese girls. *Nat Commun* 2015;6:8355.

    A large GWAS of 4,317 AIS cases confirmed a strong association with common variants near *LBX1* and identified new loci near *PAX3* and *EPHA4*, *AJAP1*, and *BCL2*.

41. Londono D, Kou I, Johnson TA, et al; TSRHC IS Clinical Group; International Consortium for Scoliosis Genetics; Japanese Scoliosis Clinical Research Group: A meta-analysis identifies adolescent idiopathic scoliosis association with LBX1 locus in multiple ethnic groups. *J Med Genet* 2014;51(6):401-406.

    A meta-analysis across six Asian and three non-Asian cohorts confirmed the association of AIS with common polymorphisms around *LBX1*.

42. Kou I, Takahashi Y, Johnson TA, et al: Genetic variants in GPR126 are associated with adolescent idiopathic scoliosis. *Nat Genet* 2013;45(6):676-679.

    A stepwise association study of 1,819 cases revealed a strong association with *GPR126* that was replicated in Han Chinese and European-ancestry populations.

43. Sharma S, Londono D, Eckalbar WL, et al; TSRHC Scoliosis Clinical Group; Japan Scoliosis Clinical Research Group: A PAX1 enhancer locus is associated with susceptibility to idiopathic scoliosis in females. *Nat Commun* 2015;6:6452.

    A GWAS of 3,102 individuals revealed an association of idiopathic scoliosis to common variants near *PAX1*, a paired-box transcription factor involved in spine development that was present only in females, not males.

44. Noshchenko A, Hoffecker L, Lindley EM, et al: Predictors of spine deformity progression in adolescent idiopathic scoliosis: A systematic review with meta-analysis. *World J Orthop* 2015;6(7):537-558.

    A review of 25 published predictors of spine deformity, including clinical and genetic factors, revealed limited predictive value and a low level of evidence to support clinical use.

45. Miyake A, Kou I, Takahashi Y, et al: Identification of a susceptibility locus for severe adolescent idiopathic scoliosis on chromosome 17q24.3. *PLoS One* 2013;8(9):e72802.

    A large GWAS of more than 12,000 Japanese individuals revealed an association of severe AIS with a variant near the *SOX9* gene that was replicated in a Chinese cohort.

46. Buchan JG, Alvarado DM, Haller GE, et al: Rare variants in FBN1 and FBN2 are associated with severe adolescent idiopathic scoliosis. *Hum Mol Genet* 2014;23(19):5271-5282.

    An exome sequencing study revealed more fibrillin rare variants in patients with AIS compared with control subjects (7.6% versus 2.4%). These variants also were associated with tall stature and upregulation of the transforming growth factor-β pathway but not Marfan syndrome.

47. Patten SA, Margaritte-Jeannin P, Bernard JC, et al: Functional variants of POC5 identified in patients with idiopathic scoliosis. *J Clin Invest* 2015;125(3):1124-1128.

    Genetic linkage analysis and exome sequencing revealed a rare missense mutation in the centriolar protein gene *POC5* that segregated with scoliosis in several families, and overexpression *POC5* variants in zebrafish resulted in spine deformity.

48. Gao X, Gordon D, Zhang D, et al: CHD7 gene polymorphisms are associated with susceptibility to idiopathic scoliosis. *Am J Hum Genet* 2007;80(5):957-965.

49. Haller G, Alvarado D, Mccall K, et al: A polygenic burden of rare variants across extracellular matrix genes among individuals with adolescent idiopathic scoliosis. *Hum Mol Genet* 2016;25(1):202-209.

    An exome sequencing study revealed excess extracellular matrix gene variation in patients with AIS compared with control subjects. Although rare variants across multiple collagen genes were associated with AIS, the association was strongest with *COL11A2*.

Chapter 8

Skeletal Dysplasias

Jose A. Morcuende, MD, PhD

Abstract

Skeletal dysplasias are a group of more than 450 heterogeneous genetic disorders characterized by abnormal differentiation, development, growth, and maintenance of bone and cartilage. Albeit individually rare, collectively the incidence of these disorders is estimated to be approximately 1 per 5,000 live births, representing 5% of children born with a birth defect. An accurate diagnosis based on clinical and radiographic features is important to predict final height, allow specific genetic counseling, and permit the selection of the best treatment approaches to avoid potential complications. A multidisciplinary approach is highly recommended for the management of patients with skeletal dysplasia. It is helpful to be familiar with background information related to genetics; classifications; and key clinical characteristics, including the natural history and treatment options for some of the most common skeletal dysplasias seen in orthopaedics.

Keywords: classification; genetics; skeletal dysplasia

Introduction

The vertebrate skeleton is a fascinating and complex organ system; it is composed of 206 bones with many different shapes and sizes. Like every other organ system, the skeleton has specific developmental and functional characteristics that define its identity in biologic and pathologic terms. For normal skeletogenesis to take place, the coordination of temporal and spatial gene expression patterns is a crucial prerequisite. Any disturbances in these processes will lead to skeletal abnormalities.

It is helpful to be aware of the clinical characteristics and the genetic causes of musculoskeletal disorders so that appropriate referrals can be made for genetic counseling and to allow refinement of the prognosis and natural history for each patient. Given the large number of inherited musculoskeletal abnormalities and the power and speed of current genetic and developmental biologic information, only selected disorders are discussed in this chapter. Fundamental general concepts related to genetics; classifications; and key clinical characteristics, including natural history and treatment options, are reviewed.

The Genetic Basis and Classification of Musculoskeletal Disorders

Broadly defined, birth defects or congenital abnormalities occur in 6% of all live births, with 20% of infant deaths resulting from congenital anomalies. At present, the cause of approximately 50% of all birth defects is unknown. Chromosomal abnormalities account for 6% to 7% of birth defects, specific gene mutations account for 7% to 8% of birth defects, and environmental teratogens are responsible for 7% to 10% of birth defects. Combined genetic predisposition and environmental factors are responsible for the remaining 20% to 25% of congenital abnormalities.

Genetic disorders of the skeleton comprise a large group of clinically distinct and genetically heterogeneous conditions that now number 456 forms. Of these conditions, 316 are associated with one or more of 226 different genetic abnormalities. This increased expansion reflects the continued delineation of unique phenotypes that, in aggregate, represents approximately 5% of all children with birth defects. Although individually rare, the different forms result in a substantial number of individuals who are affected by musculoskeletal disorders, with substantial morbidity and mortality rates.

Clinical diversity often makes musculoskeletal disorders difficult to diagnose, and many attempts have been made to delineate single entities or groups of diseases to facilitate the diagnosis. The criteria used for their distinction have been based on a combination of clinical,

Dr. Morcuende or an immediate family member serves as an unpaid consultant to Clubfoot Solutions and serves as a board member, owner, officer, or committee member of the Orthopaedic Research and Education Foundation.

morphologic, radiographic, biochemical, and molecular characteristics.[1,2] The Nosology and Classification of Genetic Skeletal Disorders has been commonly used since its first publication in 1970; it was most recently revised in 2010.[3] However, it is becoming increasingly clear that several distinctive classifications are needed to reflect clinical signs and symptoms and molecular pathology. Several reviews of the rapidly changing molecular basis of skeletal dysplasias have been published focusing on a molecular-pathogenetic classification, including specific aspects such as transcriptional dysregulation, or a combination of molecular pathology and the developmental biology of the musculoskeletal system.[4-7] These new concepts directly link the clinical phenotype to the key cellular processes of skeletal biology and should assist in providing a framework accessible to clinicians as well as basic scientists for the future understanding of these disorders. It is likely that future insights will lead to reclassification.

Conceptually, it is useful to classify musculoskeletal disorders that are caused by gene mutations into groups broadly categorized by the function of the causative gene. Mutations in early patterning genes cause disorders called dysostoses that affect only specific skeletal elements, leaving the rest of the skeleton largely unaffected. In contrast, mutations in genes that are involved primarily in cell differentiation cause disorders called osteochondrodysplasias, which affect the development and growth of most skeletal elements in a generalized fashion (by affecting endochondral bone formation).

Skeletal dysplasias can be broadly classified into those caused by mutations in genes encoding one of the following types of proteins: structural proteins, proteins that regulate developmentally important signaling pathways, proteins that play a role in metabolic macromolecular processing, proteins implicated in neoplasia, and proteins that play a role in nerve or muscle function. In addition, many genes have important functions in both dysostoses and osteochondrodysplasias, so some inherited disorders can display features of both processes. Genes used during skeletal development may be important in other organs; when mutated, the resulting skeletal defects are part of a syndrome.

Numerous online services allow access to public information and services relevant to the genetics of musculoskeletal disorders. One database that contains a wealth of clinical and genetic data is the Online Mendelian Inheritance in Man.[8] It provides free text overviews of genetic disorders and gene loci, with the correspondent mouse correlates. In addition, the database is linked to a wealth of other genetic databases, allowing users to obtain information on gene structure, map location, function, phenotype, literature references, and other information.

Clinical Evaluation

With the increased availability of ultrasonography in prenatal screening, a diagnosis of skeletal dysplasias is being made in more fetuses.[9] When a skeletal dysplasia is suspected during ultrasonography, femoral length is the best biometric parameter. Further testing may be performed, if indicated, by chorionic villous sampling and karyotype/genetic mutation analysis.

Most skeletal dysplasias result in short stature, which is defined as a height more than two SDs less than the mean for the population at a given age. The resultant growth disproportion is commonly referred to as either short trunk or short limb. The short-limb types are further subdivided into categories based on the segment of the limb that is affected. Rhizomelic refers to shortening of the proximal part of a limb (humerus and femur); mesomelic, the middle segment (radius, ulna, tibia, and fibula); and acromelic, the distal segment (hands and feet).

In evaluating a patient with short stature or abnormal bone development, several aspects of the medical history and the physical examination should be investigated. An accurate history regarding the time of onset of short stature is essential before the physical examination commences. Among the 456 skeletal dysplasias identified to date, approximately 100 have prenatal onset, whereas others may be present only in newborns or children older than 2 years. Individuals with disproportionate short stature are likely affected by a skeletal dysplasia. Therefore, whenever an individual has evidence of short stature, it is essential to measure all body proportions.

Any history of heart disease, respiratory difficulty, immune deficiency, precocious puberty (that is, puberty that begins before age 8 years in girls and 9 years in boys), and malabsorption also should be obtained because these issues are associated with some skeletal disorders. Birth length, head circumference, and weight should be recorded, and any pertinent family history of short stature or dimorphism should be obtained. The height and weight percentiles should be determined by using standard charts. The physical examination should include a careful characterization of the patient's facial features, including the presence of cleft palate and abnormal teeth, the position of the ears, and any limb malformations. A thorough neurologic evaluation is necessary because of the frequent incidence of spinal compromise in many syndromes.

After the history and the physical examination, radiographs are obtained to identify the area of bone

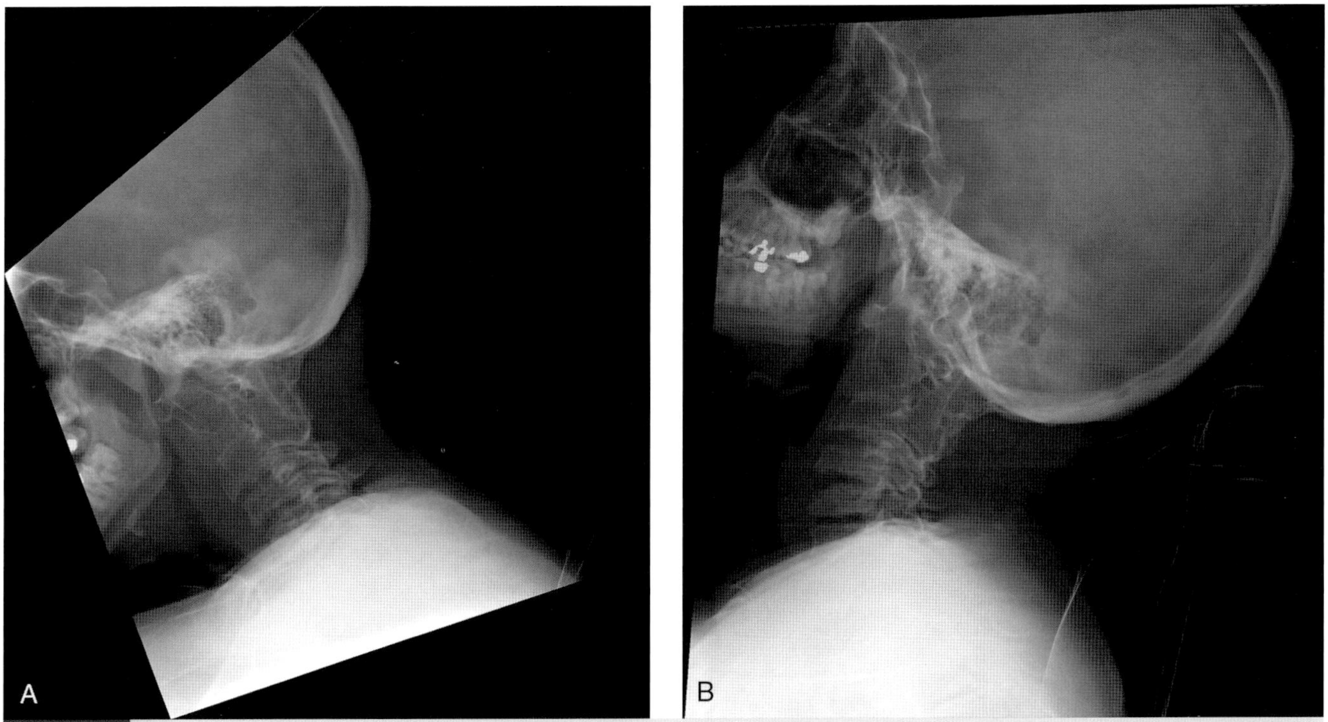

Figure 1 Flexion (**A**) extension (**B**) radiographic views of the cervical spine of a 17-year-old girl with spondyloepiphyseal dysplasia show multiple vertebral anomalies, including irregularities of the vertebral bodies and fusions.

involvement.[10] The so-called skeletal survey may vary from institution to institution, but it should include the following views: skull (AP and lateral), thoracolumbar spine (AP and lateral), chest, pelvis, one upper limb, one lower limb, and the left hand. Flexion-extension views of the cervical spine should be obtained if instability is suspected (**Figure 1**). In some instances, imaging of other family members suspected of having the same condition as the patient being examined may be helpful.

Laboratory tests may include calcium, phosphate, alkaline phosphatase, serum thyroxin, and protein levels to rule out metabolic disorders. If a progressive disorder is identified, urine should be checked for storage products. Referral to a pediatric geneticist often is helpful in determining a diagnosis in complex cases, providing genetic counseling to the family, and managing the many medical problems associated with musculoskeletal disorders.

Disorders Caused by Defects in Structural Proteins

A variety of proteins play important roles in the connective tissues, including the bones, articular cartilage, ligaments, and skin. Mutations in such genes disrupt the structural integrity of the connective tissues in which they are expressed. In most cases, the phenotype is absent or only minor manifestations are present at birth. The phenotype evolves with time because the abnormal structural components slowly fail or wear out as the individual grows. Deformity often recurs after surgery because the structural components are abnormal and will wear out again. If the structural abnormality involves cartilage, a growth abnormality may be caused by physeal mechanical failure or early degenerative disease of the joints resulting from articular cartilage failure. When a protein that is important for ligament or tendon strength is affected, joint subluxation is often present. Substantial heterogeneity may occur in the severity of the phenotype, depending on the exact way in which the mutation alters protein function. In patients with mild disease, life expectancy is normal; however, in patients with more severe disease, life expectancy may be shortened resulting from the secondary effects of structural defects on vital organs. These disorders tend to be inherited in an autosomal dominant manner.

Multiple Epiphyseal Dysplasia

Multiple epiphyseal dysplasia (MED) is one of the most widely known and commonly occurring skeletal dysplasias. It is most commonly inherited in an autosomal dominant fashion, although autosomal recessive forms also have been described. Its prevalence is estimated to be 1 in 10,000 individuals. The predominant feature of MED is the delayed and irregular ossification of numerous epiphyses. In most patients, pain and stiffness in the joints

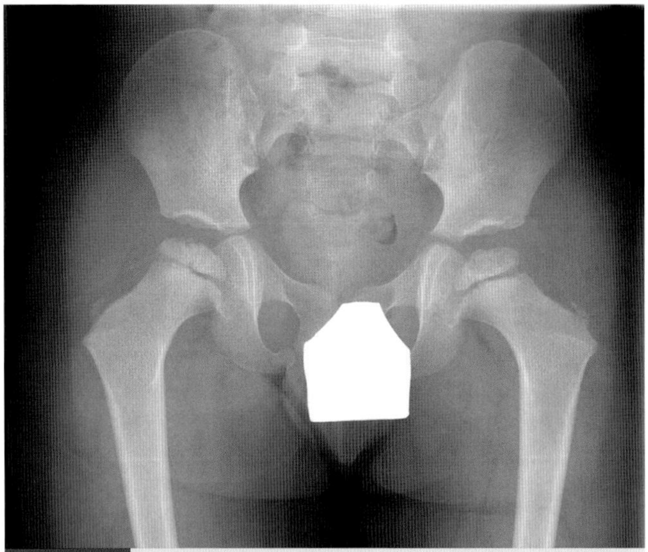

Figure 2 A 4-year-old boy underwent follow-up for a hip click detected when he was a newborn but had no current clinical symptoms. AP radiograph of the pelvis shows some flattening and ossification irregularities of the femoral heads, which are consistent with Meyer dysplasia.

is present, with the hips and knees being most commonly affected. In general, patients with MED have mild, short stature and early-onset osteoarthritis.

Historically, MED was described as occurring in two separate forms: Ribbing disease, with mild involvement, and Fairbank disease, a more severe type. However, with current genetic understanding, MED is now considered to represent a continuous spectrum from mild to severe, so these eponyms have been abandoned.

MED exhibits considerable genetic heterogeneity. To date, mutations have been reported in 40 patients or families with MED, and 15 of these are allelic with pseudoachondroplasia and result from mutations in the gene encoding cartilage oligomeric matrix protein (COMP). MED also can result from mutations in the genes encoding the α1, α2, and α3 chains of type IX collagen (*COL9A1*, *COL9A2*, *COL9A3*, respectively). Mutations in the gene encoding matrilin 3, a member of the matrilin family of extracellular oligomeric proteins, can cause a distinctive mild form of MED. It has been demonstrated that a form of recessively inherited MED, with a distinctive clinical presentation, including clubfoot and bilateral double-layered patellae, can result from mutations in gene *SLC26A2*. Therefore, MED is one of the more genetically heterogeneous of the bone dysplasias.[11]

In early adolescence, patients may report joint stiffness and contractures, lower extremity pain, angular deformities of the knees, gait disturbance, or short stature.[12] Depending on the severity of the epiphyseal dysplasia, symptoms may develop as early as age 4 or 5 years. It is common, however, for milder forms of the disorder to go unrecognized until young adulthood. Most patients have minimal short stature and are greater than the third percentile for standing height; so true dwarfism is not present. The face and spine are normal. Associated neurologic findings are nonexistent. Intelligence is not affected. The epiphyses of the upper extremities can be involved, but patients rarely report any important symptoms in this area. Mild limitation of motion in the elbow, wrist, and shoulder is found occasionally.

The principal finding on radiographs is a delay in the appearance of ossification centers. When the epiphyses do appear, they are fragmented, mottled, and flattened (**Figure 2**). The more fragmentation that is present in the capital femoral epiphysis, the earlier the onset of osteoarthritis. The proximal femur often is most affected, and its appearance may be easily confused with that of bilateral Legg-Calvé-Perthes disease. Several radiographic clues may be helpful in differentiating the two conditions. In Legg-Calvé-Perthes disease, usually one hip is involved before the other, so each hip is in a different stage of the disease. This characteristic is not the case in MED. In addition, acetabular changes are primary in MED and more pronounced. Metaphyseal cysts are seen in Legg-Calvé-Perthes disease but not in MED. Radiographs of the knees, ankles, shoulders, and wrists should be obtained in any child with a possible diagnosis of Legg-Calvé-Perthes disease to rule out MED.[13]

Coxa vara occurs in some patients. Radiographs of the knees often demonstrate flattening of the femoral condyles as well as genu valgum deformity. Osteochondritis dissecans may be superimposed. Lateral radiographs of the knees demonstrate a double-layered patella in some patients. When present, a double-layered patella is characteristic for MED. The ankles also are in valgus, mostly caused by deformity in the talus. Upper extremity involvement is less severe. The metacarpals and phalanges usually are short with irregular epiphyses. MED is distinguished from spondyloepiphyseal dysplasia by the absence of severe vertebral changes. Mild end plate irregularities may be present.

Hip pain or subluxation is a common reason that patients with MED seek orthopaedic care in adolescence. Containment surgery can be considered for those hips that show progressive subluxation. Although the principle of coverage is the same as that used in Legg-Calvé-Perthes disease, preexisting coxa vara often occurs in hips with MED, which contraindicates a proximal femoral varus osteotomy. In such instances, shelf acetabular augmentation can improve coverage of a misshapen femoral head.

If hinge abduction is present on arthrography, a valgus proximal femoral osteotomy may improve congruency and relieve pain. Osteotomies may be helpful in realigning angular deformities at the knees. For optimal surgical correction, the site of the deformity (the distal femur, the proximal tibia, or both) must be ascertained preoperatively. Degenerative joint disease is the most important problem, and it usually occurs in the second or third decade of life. If the femoral head is well formed at maturity, the onset of arthritis is delayed. The hip is the most common location of arthritis in this patient group and often leads to total joint arthroplasty.[14]

Pseudoachondroplasia

Pseudoachondroplasia is a form of short-limbed dwarfism that has a prevalence of approximately four per million. It is characterized by involvement of both the epiphyses and the metaphyses; individuals with pseudoachondroplasia have substantially short stature and a predisposition to premature osteoarthritis. The spine also is involved with this disorder.

Pseudoachondroplasia usually is transmitted as an autosomal dominant trait. The molecular genetics of pseudoachondroplasia have been extensively studied, and it now appears that this disease results almost exclusively from mutations in the gene encoding COMP. The *COMP* gene consists of 19 exons, and most mutations to date (95%) are clustered within exons 8 to 14, which encode the type III repeats. The fact that most of these mutations are in the conformationally sensitive type III repeats indicates that this region is critical for protein function. The remaining 5% of the mutations are in exons 16 and 18, which encode specific segments of the C-terminal globule.[11]

The cell-matrix pathology of pseudoachondroplasia resulting from COMP mutations has been well documented. Abnormal COMP is retained within the rough endoplasmic reticulum of cartilage, tendon, and ligament cells. This results in the secondary retention of type IX collagen, chondroitin sulfate proteoglycan 1 (aggrecan), and link protein. This retention of proteins leads to a reduction in the amount of these molecules available for interactions within the extracellular matrix of cartilage, resulting in cell death and the phenotypic picture of pseudoachondroplasia.[15-17] Additional studies are needed to delineate the mechanism leading to the excessive retention of proteins to develop treatment modalities.

Pseudoachondroplasia is a relatively straightforward disease for molecular diagnosis because it results almost exclusively from mutations along a very compact region in the *COMP* gene. Molecular diagnosis for pseudoachondroplasia is currently provided on a commercial basis and as part of the service provision of the European Skeletal Dysplasia Network for research and diagnosis.

Children with pseudoachondroplasia are normal at birth, and the condition is usually diagnosed at age 2 years after the onset of a waddling gait, when rhizomelic shortening becomes noticeable. Adult height ranges from 106 to 130 cm. Growth curve charts specific to pseudoachondroplasia are available. The clinical features are limited to the skeleton. The skull and facial features in pseudoachondroplasia are normal, which is helpful in differentiating it from achondroplasia, in which frontal bossing and midface hypoplasia are present. Abnormalities of the lower extremities are common and include genu valgum and varum deformities. Windswept deformity of the knees, in which genu valgum is present on one side and genu varum on the other, develops in some patients. The joints are extremely lax, especially in childhood and adolescence, with a predisposition to early osteoarthropathy. The large weight-bearing joints (hips and knees) are most often affected, and approximately one-third of patients need total hip replacement by their mid-30s. Scoliosis may occur in adolescence but generally is not severe. Cervical spine instability is seen in 10% to 20% of individuals. Development milestones and intelligence are normal, and premature mortality is not a reported problem.[18]

Typical radiographic changes include small, irregular epiphyseal and metaphyseal changes. Hand radiographs reveal delayed epiphyseal ossification, resulting in delayed bone age. In the long bones, these changes are seen as epiphyseal ossification delay. When the epiphyses do ossify, they appear irregular and fragmented. The hip and knee are most severely affected. In the pelvis, ossification of the capital femoral epiphysis is delayed, and when ossified, it is small and flattened. The femoral heads may resemble those seen in other spondyloepiphyseal dysplasias or bilateral Legg-Calvé-Perthes disease. Sclerosis and irregularity of the acetabular roof are commonly observed.[13] Subluxation of the hips often occurs, and degenerative arthritis develops in response to the incongruity. The vertebral changes in pseudoachondroplasia are characteristic and consist of anterior beaking in childhood that resolves in adolescence. The interpedicular distance in the lumbar spine is normal in pseudoachondroplasia, unlike achondroplasia. Odontoid hypoplasia may be present, resulting in atlantoaxial instability.

Patients with pseudoachondroplasia often have substantial angular deformities of the lower limbs that require corrective osteotomies. Careful preoperative assessment is necessary to properly realign the mechanical axis through the hip, knee, and ankle. For instance, in genu varum associated with achondroplasia, the deformity is present solely in the tibia; however, in pseudoachondroplasia, the deformity often is present in both the femur and the tibia, requiring osteotomies in both the distal femur and the proximal tibia. Care also must be taken in assessing the contribution of ligamentous laxity to the bowing deformity. After a corrective osteotomy, recurrence of the deformity with growth is common.

Premature osteoarthritis of the hip in early adulthood is a frequent problem in pseudoachondroplasia. Patients with symptomatic subluxation or incongruity may benefit from a realignment osteotomy of the proximal femur. Varus osteotomy of the proximal femur usually creates more incongruity. If hinge abduction is present, demonstrated by the femoral head levering out of the joint with abduction of the hip, a proximal femoral valgus osteotomy may improve joint congruity and abductor function. Before performing a proximal femoral valgus osteotomy, however, preoperative arthrography should be performed to demonstrate improved congruity with 15° to 20° of flexion and adduction of the femur. Abduction of the hip should demonstrate hinge abduction of the femoral head. Reconstructive pelvic osteotomies, such as a Salter osteotomy or the triple innominate osteotomy of Steel, are contraindicated in pseudoachondroplasia because concentric reduction is not present preoperatively, which is a prerequisite for these osteotomies. Salvage procedures such as shelf augmentation or the Chiari osteotomy can be done in select patients. As many as 50% of adult patients have undergone total hip arthroplasty.

Type II Collagenopathies

Type II collagenopathies include the lethal forms of achondrogenesis II and hypochondrogenesis (not discussed) and the congenital forms of spondyloepiphyseal dysplasia, Kniest syndrome, and Stickler syndrome.

Spondyloepiphyseal Dysplasia

Spondyloepiphyseal dysplasia not only affects the spine but also involves the epiphysis of the long bones. The congenital type is diagnosed at birth, and its mode of inheritance is autosomal dominant, whereas the late-onset type is X-linked or autosomal recessive. Most cases of congenital spondyloepiphyseal dysplasia are attributable to new mutations to the type II collagen gene (*COL2A1*), and the late-onset type is thought to involve the *SEDL* gene.[19,20]

Patients with the congenital form of the condition have pronounced coxa vara and short stature at birth. Hip flexion contracture and hyperlordosis of the lumbar spine also are present, along with a characteristic barrel chest. On radiographs, the femoral neck shows features that are reminiscent of pseudarthrosis, and the greater trochanter is displaced upward, whereas the femoral heads are normally centered (**Figure 3**). Platyspondyly and delayed epiphyseal ossification are present in both the congenital and late-onset forms. The cervical spine demonstrates a dysplastic dens with a risk for atlantoaxial instability. Kyphosis and scoliosis frequently develop. Possible associated abnormalities include cleft palate, hearing loss, myopia, cataracts, retinal detachment, and clubfeet. Early referrals to an ophthalmologist and an ear, nose, and throat specialist are important, with orthopaedic treatment directed toward early correction of the lower extremity and spinal deformities, especially coxa vara and atlantoaxial instability.[21,22]

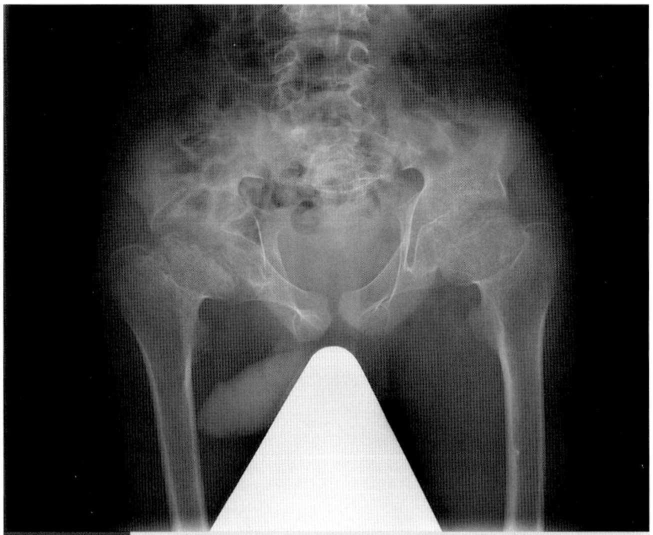

Figure 3 AP radiograph of the pelvis of a 16-year-old boy with spondyloepiphyseal dysplasia shows coxa magna with irregularities of femoral head ossification, femoral neck shortening, and overriding of the greater trochanters. Pelvic and acetabular development are abnormal and accommodate the femoral head deformities.

Kniest Syndrome

Kniest syndrome is a rare, autosomal dominant, skeletal dysplasia resulting from the deletion of several amino acids in the type II collagen gene (*COL2A1*). Children with Kniest syndrome have a normal trunk at birth but shortened extremities. Both the epiphysis and the metaphysis of the long bones are affected. Scoliosis and kyphosis often develop. The face is unusually flat with hypertelorism. Joint contractures in the knees and hips, dumbbell-shaped femurs, cleft palate, retinal detachment, otitis/hearing loss, and early osteoarthritis are present. Early referrals to an ophthalmologist and an ear, nose, and throat specialist are important, with orthopaedic treatment directed toward the correction of progressive lower extremity and spinal deformities.

Stickler Syndrome

Stickler syndrome, also known as arthro-ophthalmopathy, is genetically and phenotypically heterogeneous, with variations in both signs and symptoms and the age of onset. Most striking are ocular problems (myopia, retinal detachment, glaucoma, and blindness). In addition, patients have micrognathia, cleft palate, and hearing loss. Patients are of normal height and even show a marfanoid habitus, and mitral valve prolapse often is present. Joint involvement demonstrates some stiffness and pain with a radiographic flat epiphysis with remodeling defects and a relatively narrow diaphysis. Signs of early osteoarthritis are common in young adults. Similar to Kniest syndrome, early referrals to an ophthalmologist; an ear, nose, and throat specialist; and a pediatric cardiologist are important, with orthopaedic treatment directed toward correction of progressive lower extremity and spinal deformities.

Disorders Caused by Defects in Developmentally Important Signaling Pathways

Achondroplasia

Achondroplasia is the most common osteochondrodysplasia in humans and occurs in approximately 1 in 30,000 live births. It is inherited as an autosomal dominant trait, although it results from sporadic mutations in at least 80% of patients (with increased risk associated with paternal age). The mutation is always in the same location of the gene (a guanine to adenine change at nucleotide 1138, with the remainder of patients having a guanine to cytosine change at the same nucleotide) and results in uncontrolled activation of fibroblast growth factor receptor 3 (*FGFR3*), which leads to impaired growth in the proliferative zone of the physis. Intramembranous and periosteal ossification processes are normal. It was recently demonstrated that, as previously expected, *FGFR3* mutations in sporadic cases of achondroplasia occur exclusively on the parentally derived allele.

Because the *FGFR3* mutation in achondroplasia has been recognized, similar observations regarding the conserved nature of *FGFR3* mutations and the resulting phenotype have been made regarding hypochondroplasia, the lethal thanatophoric dysplasia, SADDAN (severe achondroplasia with developmental delay and acanthosis nigricans), and two craniosynostosis disorders: Muenke coronal craniosynostosis and Crouzon syndrome with acanthosis nigricans. More importantly, the relationships between mutations in the *FGFR3* gene and other *FGFR* genes, and the phenotypes that result from these mutations, have improved understanding of these disorders. It has been observed that a highly conserved relationship exists between mutations at a particular amino acid and the resulting phenotype.[23-26]

The skeletal manifestations of achondroplasia are related to a defect in endochondral bone formation.[27,28] The resulting growth disturbances are variable, with the proximal segments of limbs affected more often than the distal segments (rhizomelia) and relatively minor involvement of the growth of the spine. Achondroplasia is recognized at birth, and the appearance of a person with achondroplasia has numerous features that are uniform and predictable. Intelligence is normal, and life expectancy is not substantially diminished. The predicted adult height is 132 cm for men and 122 cm for women. Obesity is more common than in the general population. Developmental milestones are met later in children with achondroplasia than in children of average stature.

The cranium is enlarged, with frontal bossing, midface hypoplasia, flattening of the nasal bridge, and a prominent mandible. The foramen magnum is frequently narrowed, and it is associated with neurologic complications resulting from compression of the brain stem (quadriparesis, spasticity, sleep apnea, respiratory insufficiency, and sudden death). Spine length is in the lower range of normal, whereas the extremities are much shorter than normal, with the proximal segments—the humeri and the femora—the most foreshortened (rhizomelic) (**Figure 4**). Kyphosis of the thoracolumbar junction is present during infancy, but it usually improves with increasing age. Scoliosis is rare. Hyperlordosis of the lumbar spine increases with age, and a high incidence of symptomatic spinal stenosis (narrowing of the interpedicular distances with shortening of the pedicles) is present. Clinically, patients will have low back and leg pain, paresthesias, dysesthesias, weakness, and/or bowel and bladder incontinence.

Elbow extension is limited, and some patients may have asymptomatic radial head dislocations. Patients often will have a classic tridentate (three-pronged) hand, which is characterized by a persistent space between the long and ring fingers. The main functional limitations of the upper extremities are related to shortening of the humeri, which lead to difficulties in personal hygiene and dressing.

Radiographically, the pelvis is broad with a diminished vertical height. The iliac crest has a square appearance, and the superior acetabular roof is horizontal. The distal femoral metaphysis often flares out. Genu varum is very common, with ligamentous laxity and the fibula overgrowing the tibia. Internal tibial torsion is common with ankle varus.

Children with achondroplasia should be closely monitored in the first 2 years of life for signs of foramen magnum stenosis.[29] If the diagnosis is made and symptoms are persistent, decompression of the brain stem is indicated.[30] In some patients, associated hydrocephalus

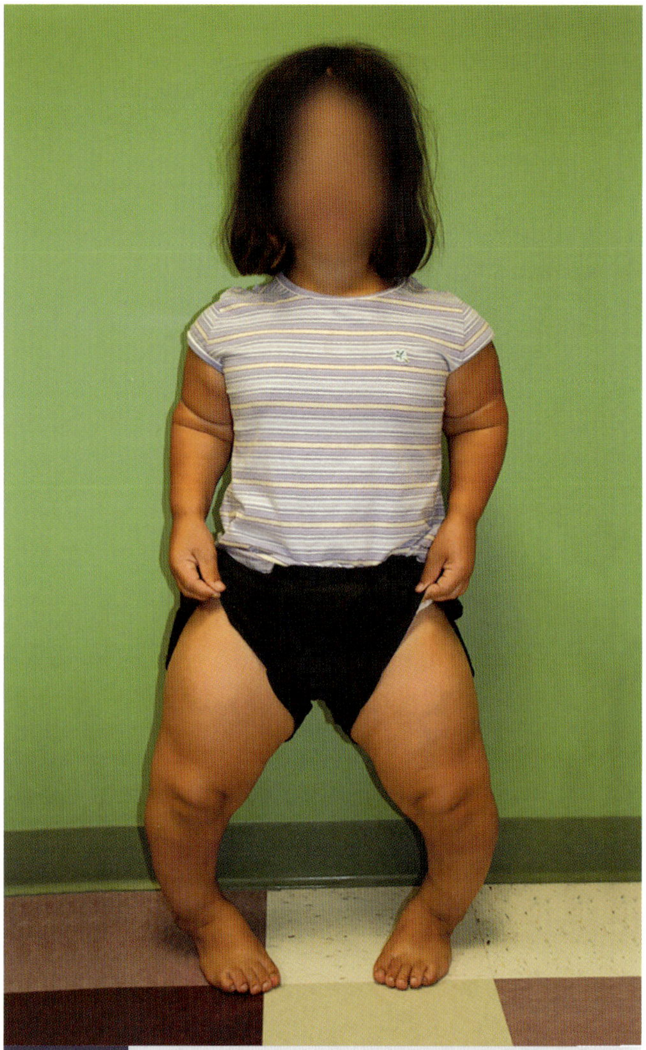

Figure 4 Clinical photograph of a 12-year-old girl with achondroplasia shows typical shorter-than-normal limbs, with the proximal segments—the humeri and the femora—the most foreshortened. (Reproduced from Baratela WAR, Mackenzie WG: Skeletal dysplasias, in Song KM, ed: *Orthopaedic Knowledge Update: Pediatrics 4*. Rosemont, IL, American Academy of Orthopaedic Surgeons, 2011, pp 71-82.)

will require shunting. Problems of the ear, nose, and throat are frequent but secondary to facial abnormalities. Recurrent otitis media may result in hearing loss, thus early hearing screening should be performed. Maxillary hypoplasia leads to dental crowding and malocclusion, which may require orthodontic treatment. Sleep apnea treatment, if necessary, begins with an adenotonsillectomy and may progress to include other procedures that are more complex.

The main orthopaedic problems include thoracolumbar kyphosis, spinal stenosis, shortening of the extremities, and angular deformities of the knees. Kyphosis is noncongenital and is centered in the thoracolumbar junction. Treatment may be indicated to prevent further development of the deformity and assist those in whom correction is not achieved with long-term bracing. In adulthood, surgical correction is performed if kyphosis contributes to symptomatic spinal stenosis.

Spinal stenosis is the most serious problem and usually develops in the third decade of life. Spinal decompression is indicated as soon as the diagnosis is made. Limb lengthening remains controversial but is gradually gaining greater acceptance. If the lower extremities are lengthened, the humeri also should be lengthened to facilitate personal care. The treatment of genu varum usually requires surgery because bracing is not effective. Fibular head epiphysiodesis, fibular shortening, and tibial osteotomies can be performed to correct the deformity but not before a child is at least age 4 years. Interestingly, severe degenerative arthritis is not common in adults with achondroplasia.

Hypochondroplasia

Hypochondroplasia manifestations are similar to but milder than those of achondroplasia. The gene mutation is in different locations compared with achondroplasia, thus more variability occurs in the phenotype.[31] Clinically, stunted growth first becomes apparent at approximately age 2 years; in some cases, it is not apparent until age 5 or 6 years. Children otherwise have a normal appearance apart from a disproportionately small stature, which is attributable solely to the shortening of the extremities plus small hands. Genu varum and flexion contractures of the knees and elbows develop over time, as well as lumbar hyperlordosis and mild stenosis. Radiographically, the long bones are broad and short, with the acetabular roof often more horizontal than normal and the sciatic notch slightly smaller. At the lumber level, some reduction in the interpedicular distance occurs. Patients with hypochondroplasia attain a height of 130 cm to 140 cm and have normal life expectancy. Orthopaedic treatment may be required for corrective osteotomies and symptomatic spinal stenosis.

Thanatophoric Dysplasia

Thanatophoric dysplasia is very severe and nearly always fatal before a patient reaches age 2 years. It is characterized by a severe disproportionate small stature with rhizomelic shortening, platyspondyly, a protuberant abdomen, and a small and narrow thoracic cavity that causes cardiorespiratory insufficiency. Children often die immediately after birth. Given its early lethality, pediatric orthopaedic surgeons are rarely confronted with this condition.

Camptomelic Dysplasia

The term camptomelic refers to bowing of the long bones, primarily the tibiae and femora, which appears to be caused by an abnormality in the formation of the cartilage anlagen during fetal development. Endochondral ossification is normal, but diaphyseal cylinderization is markedly abnormal. The first transcription factor discovered to cause a skeletal dysplasia was SOX9 in camptomelic dysplasia. The transcriptional targets of the *SOX9* gene include several cartilage matrix proteins, including types II and XI collagen and aggrecan. Hence, skeletal manifestations are, in part, caused by decreased expression of these molecules and explain some of the phenotypic overlap with some of the severe type II collagenopathies.

Camptomelic dysplasia is a dominantly inherited condition and a severe and rare form of short-limbed skeletal dysplasia that is sometimes fatal. Its primary characteristics are congenital bowing and angulation of long bones (camptomelia), primarily involving the tibiae and femora, and disproportionate short limb stature. Other characteristics include relative macrocephaly, a distinctive face (flattened face with a high forehead), a low nasal bridge, and a specific pattern of defective mineralization, including areas of the spine with progressive scoliosis that further compromise pulmonary function and lead to death if untreated. Hydromyelia and diastematomyelia have been reported, and neurologic complications and pseudarthrosis after spinal treatment are very common.[32,33] In addition, defective cartilage in the tracheal rings and the lower respiratory tract may cause respiratory failure. Other clinical features include a flattened head, cleft palate, micrognathia, defects of the heart and kidneys, and sex reversal (female with an XY karyotype).

Treatment is symptomatic and directed to the deformities. However, a high number of complications, such as pseudarthrosis and neurologic complications, occur with the XXX karyotype.

Cleidocranial Dysplasia

Although the name may suggest that only two bones are affected, cleidocranial dysplasia is a true dysplasia because numerous abnormalities are present in all parts of the skeleton, primarily those bones of membranous origin (primarily the clavicles, the cranium, and the pelvis). Cleidocranial dysplasia is an autosomal dominant condition, and the defect is in the *CBFA1* gene, which encodes for an osteoblast-specific transcription factor that is required for osteoblast differentiation.[34-36] Approximately two-thirds of the mutations are familial, and the remainder are new mutations.

Typically, the disorder is identified within the first 2 years of life. Classic features include widening of the cranium and dysplasia of the clavicles and pelvis. Patients have mild to moderate short stature and bossing in the frontal parietal and occipital regions. Maxillary micrognathia and common high palate and dental abnormalities also are present. The clavicles are partially or completely absent (10% of the time), which causes the shoulders to look droopy, the chest to be narrow, and the neck longer. The defect may be palpable. When it is bilateral, the classic diagnostic feature is that the child can touch his or her shoulders together. Brachial plexus irritation occurs in rare occasions. Pectus excavatum and sternal abnormalities also are common. Scoliosis and syringomyelia have been described, and MRI is recommended for patients with progressive scoliosis. The iliac wings appear small, and coxa vara may occur, causing limitation of abduction and a Trendelenburg gait. Widening of the symphysis pubis and coxa vara with short femoral necks is common, and 24% of patients have lumbar spondylolysis.[37]

Treatment of the clavicles is not necessary. However, if brachial plexus irritation, pain, and numbness occur, excision of the clavicular fragments can be performed to decompress the brachial plexus. Coxa vara is treated by corrective femoral osteotomies. Scoliosis should be treated in similar manner as idiopathic scoliosis.[38]

Nail-Patella Syndrome

The *LMX1B* gene is mutated in nail-patella syndrome, with the transcription factor involved in patterning the dorsoventral axis of the limbs and early morphogenesis of the glomerular basement membrane. This syndrome is inherited as an autosomal dominant trait, but marked intrafamilial and interfamilial variation occurs in the clinical features.[39,40] Its characteristics include dystrophy of the nails, an absent or hypoplastic patella, and iliac horns. Femoral condyle dysplasia and genu valgum are common. Varying degrees of cubitus valgus (hypoplasia of the lateral humerus) occur along with radial head posterior subluxation or dislocation. Other associated abnormalities include abnormal pigmentation of the iris in 50% of patients, with glaucoma and nephropathy leading to renal failure that develops in the third or fourth decade of life.

Cornelia de Lange Syndrome

Heterozygous mutations in *NIPBL* have been documented in 47% of unrelated individuals with Cornelia de Lange syndrome, with autosomal dominant inheritance in familial cases. *NIPBL* codes for a protein (delangin) that is important to chromosome function and DNA repair.[41] Orthopaedic manifestations show wide variability in severity, including short thumbs, clinodactyly of the small finger, flexion contractures of the elbow with radial head dislocations, and radial hemimelia with ray deficiencies. In the lower extremities, hip dysplasia, syndactyly of the second and third toes, and hallux valgus have been described. Patients also have short stature, microcephaly, mental retardation, cleft palate, and distinctive facial features (bushy eyebrows, a small nose, and full eyelashes). Congenital heart malformations are present in approximately 30% of patients.[42]

Disorders Caused by Defects in Metabolic Macromolecular Processing

Enzymes modify molecules or other proteins. They often modify substances for degradation and cause cell dysfunction when mutated because of an accumulation of these substances. Mutations in genes that encode for enzymes can have a wide variety of effects on cells, resulting in a broad range of abnormalities in cell function and a wide range of clinical findings. Many of these disorders result in the excess accumulation of proteins in cells. In these cases, the cells become larger than normal, which results in increased pressure in bones, causing osteonecrosis, and increased extradural material in the spine, potentially causing paralysis. Multiple systems are nearly always involved in these disorders. Medical treatments to replace the defective enzyme have been developed for many of these disorders, and such treatments often will arrest—but not reverse—the skeletal manifestations of the disorder. Early diagnosis and appropriate medical treatment are slowly decreasing the number of individuals who seek treatment for musculoskeletal problems. Most enzyme disorders are inherited in an autosomal recessive manner.

Mucopolysaccharidosis

Mucopolysaccharidosis (MPS) is a genetic disorder characterized by mucopolysaccharide excretion in urine. At least 13 types of MPS have been recognized, and each type produces a particular sugar in the urine because of a specific enzyme defect (**Table 1**). The incidence of MPS is approximately 1 in 20,000 live births. This disorders was among the first skeletal dysplasias to be described and the first to be understood at a biochemical level.[43,44]

All forms of MPS are autosomal recessive except for MPS type II, also known as Hunter syndrome, which is X-linked. The most common types of MPS are type I, also known as Hurler syndrome, and type IV, which is known as Morquio syndrome. A diagnosis of MPS can be made by urine screening using a toluidine blue-spot test. If the initial results are positive, specific blood testing is done to determine the associated sugar abnormality (**Table 1**).

Each type of MPS has a deficiency of a specific lysosomal enzyme that degrades the sulfated glycosamine glycans: heparan sulfate, dermatan sulfate, keratan sulfate, and chondroitin sulfate. The incomplete degradation product accumulates in the lysozymes themselves. The incomplete product accumulates in tissues such as the brain, the viscera, and the joints. This accumulation is responsible for the development of osteonecrosis, presumably because of too much material in the intramedullary space, and contributes to spinal cord compressive symptoms because of accumulation of material in the spinal canal.

This unremitting process leads to the clinical progression of the disorders. A child appears normal at birth, with the disorder biochemically detectable by age 6 to 12 months and clinically symptomatic by age 2 years. All these disorders lead to abnormally short stature. In some patients, severe mental retardation occurs (Hurler, Hunter, and Sanfilippo syndromes). Abnormalities of the skull (enlargement, with a thick calvarium) and facial features (coarse, gargoylism) along with deafness also are present. In some patients, hepatosplenomegaly and cardiovascular abnormalities are present. Radiographically, the clavicles are broad, and the scapulae are short and stubby. The vertebral bodies are ovoid, and scoliosis and kyphosis are frequent. Acetabular dysplasia and coxa valga are visible, and the iliac wings are flared.

The clinical course is variable, but, if untreated, most patients die in the first two decades of life. Treatment is evolving, and some of these disorders have been treated successfully with bone marrow transplantation. The preferred donor is a human leukocyte antigen identical sibling. After successful transplantation, accumulation of the mucopolysaccharide stops, with subsequent improvement in the coarse facial features, hepatosplenomegaly, and partially in hearing.[45-48] Research is currently underway in the field of gene therapy for some of these syndromes.

Orthopaedic treatment is directed to correcting musculoskeletal deformities that cause functional impairments. Hip flexion contractures and dysplasia often require surgical reconstruction, including reduction with femoral and pelvic osteotomies. Cervical instability may be present, and C1-C2 fusion and halo immobilization may be necessary. Kyphosis requires orthotic treatment or even surgical spine fusion. Genu valgus may be treated with corrective osteotomies.

MPS Type I

MPS type I is characterized by a deficiency of l-iduronidase, the enzyme that degrades dermatan sulfate and heparan sulfate. The Hurler and Scheie forms represent the severe and mild ends, respectively, of the clinical spectrum. Children with the Hurler form have progressive mental retardation, severe multiple skeletal deformities, and

Table 1

Mucopolysaccharidoses

Designation	Name	Enzyme Defect	Stored Substance	Inheritance Pattern
MPS I	Hurler/Scheie	α-L-iduronidase	HS + DS	Autosomal recessive
MPS II	Hunter	Iduronidase-2-sulfatase	HS + DS	X-linked recessive
MPS IIIA	Sanfilippo A	Heparan-sulfatase (sulfamidase)	HS	Autosomal recessive
MPS IIIB	Sanfilippo B	α-*N*-acetylglucosaminidase	HS	Autosomal recessive
MPS IIIC	Sanfilippo C	Acetyl-CoA: α-glucosaminidase-N-acetyltransferase	HS	Autosomal recessive
MPS IIID	Sanfilippo D	Glucosamine-6-sulfatase	HS	Autosomal recessive
MPS IVA	Morquio A	N-acetylgalactosamine-6-sulfatase	KS, CS	Autosomal recessive
MPS IVB	Morquio B	β-galactosidase	KS	Autosomal recessive
MPS IVC	Morquio C	Unknown	KS	Autosomal recessive
MPS V	Formerly Scheie disease, no longer used	NA	NA	NA
MPS VI	Maroteaux-Lamy	Arylsulfatase B, *N*-acetylgalactosamine-4-sulfatase	DS, CS	Autosomal recessive
MPS VII	Sly	β-glucuronidase	CS, HS, DS	Autosomal recessive
MPS VIII	DiFerrante	Glucosamine-6-sulfatase	CS, HS	Autosomal recessive

CS = chondroitin sulfate, DS = dermatan sulfate, HS = heparan sulfate, KS = keratan sulfate, MPS = mucopolysaccharidosis, NA = not applicable.

considerable organ and soft-tissue deformities and die before reaching age 10 years.[49] The Scheie form is characterized by stiffness of the joints and corneal clouding but no mental retardation; the diagnosis is usually made during the teen years, and patients have a normal life expectancy. Marrow transplantation is used in the treatment of the more severe forms. However, the results on bones are variable, with the development of typical skeletal phenotypic features in most of these children despite undergoing a successful bone marrow transplant. Some studies have cast doubt on the long-term effectiveness of marrow transplantation, but it provides short-term improvement, especially in the nonosseous manifestations. Musculoskeletal deformities that persist after marrow transplantation require treatment.[50]

Malalignment of the limbs can occur, and guided growth techniques, or osteotomies, may be necessary to treat genu valgum. Osteotomies may be associated with recurrence, and, as such, guided-growth approaches are an attractive alternative; however, comparative studies are lacking in the literature. Approximately 25% of patients have an abnormality of the upper cervical spine. The accumulation of degradation products in closed anatomic spaces, such as the carpal tunnel, causes triggering of the fingers and carpal tunnel syndrome.

MPS Types II and III

Patients with Hunter syndrome (MPS type II) and Sanfilippo syndrome (MPS type III) usually demonstrate milder skeletal manifestations.[51,52] Carpal tunnel syndrome is almost universal in Hunter syndrome, with ankle equinus contractures present in both types. Hip dysplasia is usually mild in these disorders and typically does not require surgical treatment. All patients with Sanfilippo syndrome have persistent neurocognitive decline, which is more variable in patients with Hunter syndrome.

MPS Type IV

Three types of Morquio syndrome, which are classified as subtypes of MPS type IV, have been identified. All are caused by enzyme defects involved in the degradation of keratan sulfate, and all patients with MPS type IV are normal at birth. For patients with the severe type (IVA), the diagnosis is made between 1 and 3 years of age; those with the mild type (IVC) are diagnosed as teenagers; and those with the intermediate form (type IVB) are diagnosed somewhere in the middle of this age range. Intelligence is normal in all patients with MPS type IV, and only rarely are facial features coarsened. All patients are short-trunked dwarfs with ligamentous laxity. The degree of genu valgus is substantial and aggravated by lax ligaments. Management of the knee proves difficult because of osseous malalignment and lax ligaments. Realignment osteotomies can restore plumb alignment, but recurrence is possible, and osteotomies may not control instability during ambulation. The prophylactic use of braces to prevent initial valgus or recurrent deformity after surgery has not been effective. Guided growth is an attractive alternative to osteotomies and avoids issues of recurrence; however, comparative studies are lacking. Arthritis develops early in the hips and knees. The hips show progressive acetabular dysplasia. Radiographs may show a small femoral ossific nucleus, but an MRI or an arthrogram will show a much larger cartilaginous femoral head. The femoral capital epiphyses are initially advanced for a patient's age, but for patients aged 4 to 9 years, the femoral heads grow smaller and then disappear. The pathophysiology of progressive hip disease is not completely understood, and no pharmacologic or surgical approach is currently available to improve the prognosis. Patients may require a total joint arthroplasty.

Odontoid hypoplasia or aplasia is common, with resultant C1-C2 instability. A soft-tissue mass in the spinal canal contributes to cord compression. The upper and lower extremities often are flaccid rather than spastic. Sudden death of patients with Morquio syndrome has been reported and is typically attributed to C1-C2 subluxation. C1-C2 fusion before the onset of symptoms is controversial but is promoted by some physicians, whereas others recommend surgical intervention for symptomatic patients. No comparative studies have evaluated the outcomes of the different management approaches. Elsewhere in the spine, the vertebrae show progressive platyspondylia with a thoracic kyphosis. Progressive deformity should be surgically stabilized. Despite these problems, many patients with Morquio syndrome live for decades. Cardiorespiratory disease is common, but problems in the upper cervical spine account for most disabilities.

Diastrophic Dysplasia

Diastrophic dysplasia is an autosomal recessive disorder that is characterized by rhizomelic dwarfism and is associated with multiple severe spinal deformities that can be life threatening.[53] It is the result of a sulfate transport protein defect (SLC26A2) that affects proteoglycan sulfation in cartilage. Interestingly, it is present in 1 in 70 Finnish citizens. The disorder is apparent at birth. Patients may have cleft palate, and cauliflower ears can develop from cystic swelling in the ear cartilage. The hands are short with characteristic hitchhiker thumbs. Joint contractures are common in the hips (which often can be dislocated on both sides) and knees, with genu valgus and dislocated patellae. Severe clubfeet often are present.

Cervical kyphosis occurs in up to 40% of the patients but resolves spontaneously in most children by age 6 years. Severe thoracic kyphosis (>60°) is usually associated with hypoplastic vertebrae and has a tendency to progress. In addition, spina bifida occulta has a high incidence rate (75%), and surgeons must be aware of the condition when planning surgical stabilization.[54-57]

Compressive wrapping is used with good results for cystic ear swelling. Progressive lower extremity deformities are difficult to treat and have a great tendency to recur. Hip dislocations are very difficult to reduce, and their reduction should be carefully discussed with the parents because the prognosis is poor even when the hips are centered. Treatment is indicated for progressive spinal deformity or cord compromise. However, severe complications can be expected, with multiple reports of quadriplegia and cardiopulmonary failure.

Disorders Caused by Defects in Tumor Suppressor Genes

Various cellular proteins are important in regulating cell reproduction or proliferation. A mutation that results in dysregulation of such pathways can cause overgrowth of a cell type or organ, and these pathways are frequently dysregulated in neoplasia. In many of these conditions, when a single copy (one of the two alleles) of a gene is mutated in the germline, the result is an overgrowth phenotype, but when the second copy (the other allele) becomes mutated in a somatic manner (in a certain cell type), the result is the development of a tumor. Because many of these disorders are usually caused by one copy of a defective gene, they are inherited in an autosomal dominant manner.

Hereditary Multiple Exostosis

Hereditary multiple exostosis (HME), or diaphyseal aclasia, is a highly penetrant, autosomal dominant trait characterized by slightly stunted growth of the long bones and multiple osteochondromas. Osteochondromas are cartilage-capped excrescences of bone that develop at the growth plate level during growth. These osteochondromas are indistinguishable morphologically from solitary cases. HME has an incidence of about 1 in 50,000 live births.[58] The median age at the time of diagnosis is approximately age 3 years. By the second decade of life, nearly all individuals who are affected will have exostoses; the penetrance of the disorder has been found to be 96% to 100%. Many patients with HME require resection of the lesions because of a mass effect or neurovascular impingement symptoms. Importantly, a malignant chondrosarcoma eventually develops in up to 3% of patients with HME.

During the past decade, advances in molecular biology and genetics have permitted a better understanding of the molecular factors underlying these lesions. Linkage analysis has located three etiologic genes for HME: *EXT1, EXT2,* and *EXT3*. Interestingly, mutations in any of these genes demonstrate very similar clinical manifestations.[59,60] These EXT loci have defined a new class of putative tumor suppressor genes, to which have been recently added three related genes: *EXTL1, EXTL2,* and *EXTL3*.

Because both HME and sporadic osteochondromas have been associated with a loss of heterozygosity at one or more of the EXT loci, a neoplastic model of pathogenesis has been suggested. The Knudson two-hit theory of carcinogenesis, derived from familial retinoblastoma, has been applied to HME. Both copies of the *EXT1* gene have been observed to be deleted, and gene losses and mutations have been observed in chondrosarcomas arising from osteochondromas. However, it is still unclear how *EXT1* and *EXT2* genes function as tumor suppressors.

Several hard, knobby lumps will be present near the joints. Numerous sites can be involved; typically five or six exostoses can be found in the upper and lower extremities.[61-66] The most common locations are the distal femur (70%), the proximal tibia (70%), the humerus (50%), and the proximal fibula (30%). Over time, there will be some shortening of the limbs in relation to the trunk, and there may be leg-length inequality. As the lesions enlarge, they may cause discomfort secondary to mechanical pressure to adjacent soft tissues and muscles. They rarely cause neurologic dysfunction. Often, patients report an undesirable cosmetic appearance. Valgus deformity of the knee and ankle are common, and osteochondromas of the proximal femur may lead to dysplasia of the hip, which may require corrective osteotomies. In adults, sarcomatous transformation will result in a painful and enlarging mass in an area of previous deformity.

The treatment of HME is surgical excision. However, not all the exostoses should be removed. Established indications for surgery include growth disturbances leading to angular deformities or hip dysplasia, functional limitation of joint range of motion, spinal cord compression with neurologic compromise, a painful mass and obvious cosmetic deformity, and rapid increase in the size of the lesion. Deformities in the forearm should be treated early to prevent further progression and reduce disability. Knee osteotomies are associated with a high incidence of peroneal nerve palsy.

Silver-Russell Syndrome

Patients with Silver-Russell syndrome have a low birth weight, an average head circumference, and a triangular shape to the face. Hemihypertrophy is present in 80% of the individuals who are affected. The management of leg-length equality can be difficult because individual growth curves may vary, not following normal predictive charts. Growth hormone has been administered in an attempt to improve stature; although the use of growth hormone will increase growth velocity, it is not yet known whether ultimate height is increased. Because Wilms tumor in an affected patient has been reported, some physicians recommend screening for Wilms tumor, as is done for other causes of hemihypertrophy.[67,68]

Proteus Syndrome

Proteus syndrome includes hemihypertrophy, macrodactyly, and partial gigantism of the hands or feet (or both), with a characteristic appearance to the plantar surface of the feet, often described as similar to the surface of the brain.[69] Existing symptoms worsen, and new symptoms appear over time. Unlike other overgrowth syndromes, an increased incidence of malignancy has not been reported in Proteus syndrome. Various cutaneous manifestations have been identified, including hemangiomas, pigmented nevi of various intensities, and subcutaneous lipomas. Varicosities are present, although true arteriovenous malformations are rare.

Skeletal deformities include focal and regional gigantism, scoliosis, and kyphosis. Rather large vertebral bodies, known as megaspondylodysplasia, are present. Angular malformations of the lower extremities, especially genu valgus, are common. Recurrences after surgical interventions are very common and are likely caused by an underlying growth advantage in affected tissues that cannot be corrected surgically. Thus, musculoskeletal deformities caused by Proteus syndrome can be very difficult to manage. Osteotomies can correct angular malformations, but the decision to undertake surgical correction must consider the possibility of a rapid recurrence of the deformity after corrective surgery. The use of growth modulation (for example, an eight-Plate [Orthofix]) to manage limb angular deformity is a rather promising approach, but data on the results of this approach are lacking. Nerve compression can be managed using decompression, but spinal cord compression is difficult, if not impossible, to successfully treat surgically because of vertebrae overgrowth. Scoliosis seems to be caused by overgrowth of one side of the spine. Functional ability depends on the severity of the limb deformity and the presence of intracranial abnormalities.

Summary

Skeletal dysplasias are a group of heterogeneous genetic disorders characterized by abnormal differentiation, development, growth, and maintenance of bone and cartilage. Given this heterogeneity, a multidisciplinary treatment approach is highly recommended for affected patients. Clinical and radiographic features can aid in making an accurate diagnosis. Knowledge of the diagnosis can assist in predicting the patient's final height and allows for specific genetic counseling and the selection of the best treatment for an individual patient.

Key Study Points

- Skeletal dysplasias represent a very heterogeneous group of disorders.
- An accurate diagnosis based on clinical, radiographic, and molecular criteria is important so that each patient can be provided with the best treatment options.
- A multidisciplinary approach in the management of these patients is highly recommended.

Annotated References

1. Carey JC, Viskochil DH: Status of the human malformation map: 2002. *Am J Med Genet* 2002;115(4):205-220.

2. Krakow D, Rimoin DL: The skeletal dysplasias. *Genet Med* 2010;12(6):327-341.

3. Warman ML, Cormier-Daire V, Hall C, et al: Nosology and classification of genetic skeletal disorders: 2010 revision. *Am J Med Genet A* 2011;155A(5):943-968.

   The authors present an overview of recognized diagnostic skeletal disorders and group them based on clinical and radiographic features and molecular pathogenesis. In this 2010 revision, 456 conditions were included and placed in 40 groups defined by molecular, biochemical, and/or radiographic criteria.

4. Kornak U, Mundlos S: Genetic disorders of the skeleton: A developmental approach. *Am J Hum Genet* 2003;73(3):447-474.

5. Hermanns P, Lee B: Transcriptional dysregulation in skeletal malformation syndromes. *Am J Med Genet* 2001;106(4):258-271.

6. Unger S: A genetic approach to the diagnosis of skeletal dysplasia. *Clin Orthop Relat Res* 2002;401:32-38.

7. Mortier GR: The diagnosis of skeletal dysplasias: A multidisciplinary approach. *Eur J Radiol* 2001;40(3):161-167.

8. U.S. National Library of Medicine, Online Mendelian Inheritance in Man (OMIM): Available at: http://www.ncbi.nlm.nih.gov/omim/. Accessed May 20, 2016.

   Online Mendelian Inheritance in Man is an authoritative compendium of human genes and genetic phenotypes that is freely available and updated daily.

9. Parilla BV, Leeth EA, Kambich MP, Chilis P, MacGregor SN: Antenatal detection of skeletal dysplasias. *J Ultrasound Med* 2003;22(3):255-258, quiz 259-261.

10. Alanay Y, Lachman RS: A review of the principles of radiological assessment of skeletal dysplasias. *J Clin Res Pediatr Endocrinol* 2011;3(4):163-178.

    An accurate diagnosis of a skeletal dysplasia is based on detailed evaluation of clinical and radiographic findings. This review outlines the diagnostic approach to patients with disproportionate short stature, with special emphasis on radiologic findings.

11. Briggs MD, Chapman KL: Pseudoachondroplasia and multiple epiphyseal dysplasia: Mutation review, molecular interactions, and genotype to phenotype correlations. *Hum Mutat* 2002;19(5):465-478.

12. Ingram RR: Early diagnosis of multiple epiphyseal dysplasia. *J Pediatr Orthop* 1992;12(2):241-244.

13. Crossan JF, Wynne-Davies R, Fulford GE: Bilateral failure of the capital femoral epiphysis: Bilateral Perthes disease, multiple epiphyseal dysplasia, pseudoachondroplasia, and spondyloepiphyseal dysplasia congenita and tarda. *J Pediatr Orthop* 1983;3(3):297-301.

14. Treble NJ, Jensen FO, Bankier A, Rogers JG, Cole WG: Development of the hip in multiple epiphyseal dysplasia: Natural history and susceptibility to premature osteoarthritis. *J Bone Joint Surg Br* 1990;72(6):1061-1064.

15. Acharya C, Yik JH, Kishore A, Van Dinh V, Di Cesare PE, Haudenschild DR: Cartilage oligomeric matrix protein and its binding partners in the cartilage extracellular matrix: Interaction, regulation and role in chondrogenesis. *Matrix Biol* 2014;37:102-111.

In this review, the authors compiled the interactions of COMP with other proteins in the cartilage extracellular matrix and summarized their importance in maintaining the structural integrity of cartilage and regulating cellular functions.

16. Posey KL, Alcorn JL, Hecht JT: Pseudoachondroplasia/COMP: Translating from the bench to the bedside. *Matrix Biol* 2014;37:167-173.

Pseudoachondroplasia is a skeletal dysplasia caused by mutations in the *COMP* gene. This review focus on the information learned from mutant *COMP* mouse model systems and discusses how it may translate to clinical therapies.

17. Cooper RR, Ponseti IV, Maynard JA: Pseudoachondroplastic dwarfism: A rough-surfaced endoplasmic reticulum storage disorder. *J Bone Joint Surg Am* 1973;55(3):475-484.

18. McKeand J, Rotta J, Hecht JT: Natural history study of pseudoachondroplasia. *Am J Med Genet* 1996;63(2):406-410.

19. Reardon W, Hall CM, Shaw DG, Kendall B, Hayward R, Winter RM: New autosomal dominant form of spondyloepiphyseal dysplasia presenting with atlanto-axial instability. *Am J Med Genet* 1994;52(4):432-437.

20. Zabel B, Hilbert K, Stöss H, Superti-Furga A, Spranger J, Winterpacht A: A specific collagen type II gene (COL2A1) mutation presenting as spondyloperipheral dysplasia. *Am J Med Genet* 1996;63(1):123-128.

21. Miyoshi K, Nakamura K, Haga N, Mikami Y: Surgical treatment for atlantoaxial subluxation with myelopathy in spondyloepiphyseal dysplasia congenita. *Spine (Phila Pa 1976)* 2004;29(212l):E488-E491.

22. Svensson O, Aaro S: Cervical instability in skeletal dysplasia: Report of 6 surgically fused cases. *Acta Orthop Scand* 1988;59(1):66-70.

23. Shiang R, Thompson LM, Zhu YZ, et al: Mutations in the transmembrane domain of FGFR3 cause the most common genetic form of dwarfism, achondroplasia. *Cell* 1994;78(2):335-342.

24. Horton WA: Fibroblast growth factor receptor 3 and the human chondrodysplasias. *Curr Opin Pediatr* 1997;9(4):437-442.

25. Yamanaka Y, Ueda K, Seino Y, Tanaka H: Molecular basis for the treatment of achondroplasia. *Horm Res* 2003;60(suppl 3):60-64.

26. Maynard JA, Ippolito EG, Ponseti IV, Mickelson MR: Histochemistry and ultrastructure of the growth plate in achondroplasia. *J Bone Joint Surg Am* 1981;63(6):969-979.

27. Ponseti IV: Skeletal growth in achondroplasia. *J Bone Joint Surg Am* 1970;52(4):701-716.

28. Hall JG: The natural history of achondroplasia. *Basic Life Sci* 1988;48:3-9.

29. Lutter LD, Longstein JE, Winter RB, Langer LO: Anatomy of the achondroplastic lumbar canal. *Clin Orthop Relat Res* 1977;126:139-142.

30. Baca KE, Abdullah MA, Ting BL, et al: Surgical decompression for lumbar stenosis in pediatric achondroplasia. *J Pediatr Orthop* 2010;30(5):449-454.

31. Rousseau F, Bonaventure J, Legeai-Mallet L, et al: Clinical and genetic heterogeneity of hypochondroplasia. *J Med Genet* 1996;33(9):749-752.

32. Coscia MF, Bassett GS, Bowen JR, Ogilvie JW, Winter RB, Simonton SC: Spinal abnormalities in camptomelic dysplasia. *J Pediatr Orthop* 1989;9(1):6-14.

33. Thomas S, Winter RB, Lonstein JE: The treatment of progressive kyphoscoliosis in camptomelic dysplasia. *Spine (Phila Pa 1976)* 1997;22(12):1330-1337.

34. Lee B, Thirunavukkarasu K, Zhou L, et al: Missense mutations abolishing DNA binding of the osteoblast-specific transcription factor OSF2/CBFA1 in cleidocranial dysplasia. *Nat Genet* 1997;16(3):307-310.

35. Mundlos S: Cleidocranial dysplasia: Clinical and molecular genetics. *J Med Genet* 1999;36(3):177-182.

36. Otto F, Kanegane H, Mundlos S: Mutations in the RUNX2 gene in patients with cleidocranial dysplasia. *Hum Mutat* 2002;19(3):209-216.

37. Cooper SC, Flaitz CM, Johnston DA, Lee B, Hecht JT: A natural history of cleidocranial dysplasia. *Am J Med Genet* 2001;104(1):1-6.

38. Richie MF, Johnston CE II: Management of developmental coxa vara in cleidocranial dysostosis. *Orthopedics* 1989;12(7):1001-1004.

39. Bongers EM, Gubler MC, Knoers NV: Nail-patella syndrome: Overview on clinical and molecular findings. *Pediatr Nephrol* 2002;17(9):703-712.

40. Beguiristáin JL, de Rada PD, Barriga A: Nail-patella syndrome: Long term evolution. *J Pediatr Orthop B* 2003;12(1):13-16.

41. Gillis LA, McCallum J, Kaur M, et al: NIPBL mutational analysis in 120 individuals with Cornelia de Lange syndrome and evaluation of genotype-phenotype correlations. *Am J Hum Genet* 2004;75(4):610-623.

2: Basic Science

42. Joubin J, Pettrone CF, Pettrone FA: Cornelia de Lange's syndrome: A review article (with emphasis on orthopedic significance). *Clin Orthop Relat Res* 1982;171:180-185.

43. Muenzer J: The mucopolysaccharidoses: A heterogeneous group of disorders with variable pediatric presentations. *J Pediatr* 2004;144(5 suppl):S27-S34.

44. Kircher S, Bajbouj M, Beck M: *Mucopolysaccharidoses: A Guide for Physicians and Parents*. Bremen, Germany, Uni-Med Verlag AG, 2007.

45. Sauer M, Grewal S, Peters C: Hematopoietic stem cell transplantation for mucopolysaccharidoses and leukodystrophies. *Klin Padiatr* 2004;216(3):163-168.

46. Wraith JE, Clarke LA, Beck M, et al: Enzyme replacement therapy for mucopolysaccharidosis I: A randomized, double-blinded, placebo-controlled, multinational study of recombinant human alpha-L-iduronidase (laronidase). *J Pediatr* 2004;144(5):581-588.

47. Muenzer J, Fisher A: Advances in the treatment of mucopolysaccharidosis type I. *N Engl J Med* 2004; 350(19):1932-1934.

48. Giugliani R, Federhen A, Rojas MV, et al: Mucopolysaccharidosis I, II, and VI: Brief review and guidelines for treatment. *Genet Mol Biol* 2010;33(4):589-604.

49. Taylor C, Brady P, O'Meara A, Moore D, Dowling F, Fogarty E: Mobility in Hurler syndrome. *J Pediatr Orthop* 2008;28(2):163-168.

50. Malm G, Gustafsson B, Berglund G, et al: Outcome in six children with mucopolysaccharidosis type IH, Hurler syndrome, after haematopoietic stem cell transplantation (HSCT). *Acta Paediatr* 2008;97(8):1108-1112.

51. White KK, Hale S, Goldberg MJ: Musculoskeletal health in Hunter disease (MPS II): ERT improves functional outcomes. *J Pediatr Rehabil Med* 2010;3(2):101-107.

52. White KK, Karol LA, White DR, Hale S: Musculoskeletal manifestations of Sanfilippo syndrome (mucopolysaccharidosis type III). *J Pediatr Orthop* 2011;31(5):594-598.

    The authors present the results of a retrospective case series of patients with MPS III from two institutions. Musculoskeletal findings, including scoliosis, carpal tunnel syndrome, trigger finger, and osteonecrosis of the hip, can cause severe discomfort in these patients. Level of evidence: IV.

53. Carten M, Gagne V: *Diastrophic Dysplasia*. Available at: http://www.pixelscapes.com/ddhelp/DD-booklet/. Accessed June 6, 2016.

    This website provides information on diastrophic dysplasia, with special emphasis on the cervical spine abnormalities that may have implications for anesthesia use.

54. Bethem D, Winter RB, Lutter L: Disorders of the spine in diastrophic dwarfism. *J Bone Joint Surg Am* 1980;62(4):529-536.

55. Poussa M, Merikanto J, Ryöppy S, Marttinen E, Kaitila I: The spine in diastrophic dysplasia. *Spine (Phila Pa 1976)* 1991;16(8):881-887.

56. Remes V, Marttinen E, Poussa M, Kaitila I, Peltonen J: Cervical kyphosis in diastrophic dysplasia. *Spine (Phila Pa 1976)* 1999;24(19):1990-1995.

57. Ryöppy S, Poussa M, Merikanto J, Marttinen E, Kaitila I: Foot deformities in diastrophic dysplasia: An analysis of 102 patients. *J Bone Joint Surg Br* 1992;74(3):441-444.

58. Black B, Dooley J, Pyper A, Reed M: Multiple hereditary exostoses: An epidemiologic study of an isolated community in Manitoba. *Clin Orthop Relat Res* 1993;287:212-217.

59. Hall CR, Cole WG, Haynes R, Hecht JT: Reevaluation of a genetic model for the development of exostosis in hereditary multiple exostosis. *Am J Med Genet* 2002;112(1):1-5.

60. Zak BM, Crawford BE, Esko JD: Hereditary multiple exostoses and heparan sulfate polymerization. *Biochim Biophys Acta* 2002;1573(3):346-355.

61. Peterson HA: Deformities and problems of the forearm in children with multiple hereditary osteochondromata. *J Pediatr Orthop* 1994;14(1):92-100.

62. Ballantyne JA, Simpson AH, Porter DE, Fraser M: Wrist and forearm dysfunction in hereditary multiple exostoses. *J Hand Surg [Br]* 2003;28(suppl 1):26.

63. Porter DE, Benson MK, Hosney GA: The hip in hereditary multiple exostoses. *J Bone Joint Surg Br* 2001;83(7):988-995.

64. Nawata K, Teshima R, Minamizaki T, Yamamoto K: Knee deformities in multiple hereditary exostoses: A longitudinal radiographic study. *Clin Orthop Relat Res* 1995;313:194-199.

65. Noonan KJ, Feinberg JR, Levenda A, Snead J, Wurtz LD: Natural history of multiple hereditary osteochondromatosis of the lower extremity and ankle. *J Pediatr Orthop* 2002;22(1):120-124.

66. Schmale GA, Conrad EU III, Raskind WH: The natural history of hereditary multiple exostoses. *J Bone Joint Surg Am* 1994;76(7):986-992.

67. Siklar Z, Berberoğlu M: Syndromic disorders with short stature. *J Clin Res Pediatr Endocrinol* 2014;6(1):1-8.

    The relatively more frequently seen syndromes associated with short stature (Noonan, Prader-Willi, Silver-Russell, and Aarskog-Scott syndromes) are discussed. These disorders are associated with a number of endocrinopathies, as well as with developmental, systemic, and behavioral issues. At present, growth hormone therapy is used in most syndromic disorders, although long-term studies evaluating this treatment are insufficient and some controversies exist regarding dosage, optimal age to begin therapy, and adverse effects. Before starting growth hormone treatment, patients with syndromic disorders should be extensively evaluated.

68. Azzi S, Abi Habib W, Netchine I: Beckwith-Wiedemann and Russell-Silver syndromes: From new molecular insights to the comprehension of imprinting regulation. *Curr Opin Endocrinol Diabetes Obes* 2014;21(1):30-38.

The authors discuss the recently identified molecular abnormalities at 11p15.5 involved in Silver-Russell and Beckwith-Wiedemann syndromes, which have led to the identification of cis-acting elements and transacting regulatory factors involved in the regulation of imprinting in this region. They also discuss the multilocus imprinting disorders identified in various human syndromes, their clinical outcomes, and their effect on commonly identified metabolic disorders.

69. Cohen MM Jr: Proteus syndrome review: Molecular, clinical, and pathologic features. *Clin Genet* 2014;85(2):111-119.

The author provides an overview of Proteus syndrome and addresses its diagnostic criteria, natural history, management, psychological issues, and differential diagnosis.

2: Basic Science

Chapter 9

Orthopaedic-Related Syndromes

Klane K. White, MD, MSc Benjamin A. Alman, MD

Abstract

Syndromes are characterized by a constellation of phenotypic findings that run together. Many syndromes are caused by genetic mutation; others may be caused by fetal environmental factors that alter cell behavior, often in a manner that mimics genetic mutation. An understanding of genetic etiology allows the classification of syndromes based on the function of the causative gene product: structural proteins, proteins that regulate developmentally important signaling pathways, proteins implicated in neoplasia, proteins that play a role in processing molecules such as enzymes, and proteins that play a role in nerve or muscle function. Each class of syndromes commonly shares similar clinical findings and responses to treatment. Advances in the understanding of the sequelae of the various genetic mutations also have identified novel possible treatments of some syndromes. Such therapies are being adopted in select patients. During the next decades, it is predicted that many such therapies will alter the orthopaedic manifestations of these conditions.

Keywords: development; dysplasia; overgrowth; syndrome

Introduction

The word "syndrome" is derived from the Greek "run together," and patients who are affected by musculoskeletal syndromes have a constellation of clinical findings that define each condition. Numerous syndromes affect the musculoskeletal system. As such, it is useful to group them into classes. As more is learned about the underlying genetic causes of syndromes, they can be categorized according to the function of the causative gene. The various conditions can be broadly classified into those caused by mutation in genes encoding one of the following types of proteins: structural proteins, proteins that regulate developmentally important signaling pathways, proteins implicated in neoplasia, proteins that play a role in processing molecules such as enzymes, and proteins that play a role in nerve or muscle function.[1-4] Syndromes within each broad group share similarities in the mode of inheritance and clinical behavior.

Dr. White or an immediate family member is a member of a speakers' bureau or has made paid presentations on behalf of BioMarin and Genzyme and serves as a board member, owner, officer, or committee member of the Pediatric Orthopaedic Society of North America. Dr. Alman or an immediate family member has stock or stock options held in ScarX Therapeutics and serves as a board member, owner, officer, or committee member of the Shriners Hospitals for Children Research Advisory Board.

Disorders Caused by Structural Genes

Connective tissues—bones, articular cartilage, ligaments, and skin—play an obvious, critical role in the skeleton. Structural proteins support these tissues, and mutations in genes that encode for these proteins disrupt the structural integrity of the tissues in which they are expressed. In these conditions, lethal structural defects may be present at birth, or minor manifestations in a phenotype may evolve with time. Because the structural components are abnormal, deformity often recurs after surgical correction. The phenotype of the condition depends on the tissues involved. When the mutation is in a protein expressed in cartilage, growth abnormality may be caused by physeal mechanical failure. When a protein in a ligament or a tendon is affected, joints may subluxate. There can be substantial heterogeneity in the severity of a phenotype, depending on the exact way in which the mutation alters protein function. Life expectancy is normal in patients with mild disease; however, in patients with severe disease, life expectancy may be shortened because of secondary effects on vital organs. These disorders, such as osteogenesis imperfecta, multiple epiphyseal dysplasia, and Marfan syndrome, tend to be inherited in an autosomal dominant manner.[1,5]

Disorders Caused by Tumor-Related Genes

Several proteins and cell signaling pathways regulate cell growth and death. Mutations in these genes can activate proteins that cause cells to proliferate or inactivate proteins that normally suppress cell growth. Conditions in this category can be autosomal dominant. However, some conditions are caused by mosaic somatic mutations, in which not all the cells in the body are mutated. In some instances, when a single copy (one of the two alleles) of a gene is mutated, the result is an overgrowth phenotype, whereas when the second copy (the other allele) becomes mutated in a somatic manner, the result is a tumor. Because these mutations cause tissue overgrowth, recurrence is frequent after surgery because the genetic defect that causes the overgrowth still is present.[2,6,7]

Neurofibromatosis

Neurofibromatosis is the most common single-gene disorder in humans, and neurofibromatosis type 1 is the type most frequently encountered by orthopaedic surgeons. The diagnosis is based on clinical findings, which are not usually apparent until later in life, often in the preteen years. At least two of following cardinal clinical findings are required to make the diagnosis[8]: at least six café au lait spots, larger than 5 mm in diameter in children and larger than 15 mm in diameter in adults; two neurofibromas or a single plexiform neurofibroma; freckling in the axillae or inguinal region; an optic glioma; at least two Lisch nodules (hamartoma of the iris); a distinctive osseous lesion such as vertebral scalloping or cortical thinning; and a first-degree relative with neurofibromatosis type 1.

Neurofibromatosis is caused by a mutation in the *NF1* gene. Its protein product, neurofibromin, acts as a tumor suppressor. Neurofibromin is expressed at higher levels in the neural crest during development, and these cells migrate to the common sites of abnormalities in the disorder. The mutation stimulates the conversion of Ras-GTP (guanosine-5'-triphosphate) to Ras-GDP (guanine diphosphate), activating Ras signaling, which is involved in the control of cell growth. Tumors that develop in affected individuals typically have only the mutated gene because the normal copy is lost. The gene defect also provides a clue to potential novel therapies because pharmacologic agents that block Ras signaling could be used to treat the disorder.[9] Farnesyl transferase inhibitors block the downstream effects of Ras signaling activation and thus have the potential to treat some of the neoplastic manifestations of neurofibromatosis type 1.[10] However, a recent randomized controlled trial suggested little benefit from this treatment.[11] Another approach is the use of statin inhibitors, which regulate Ras signaling by interfering with the membrane binding of Ras.[12,13] Clinical trials of these approaches are ongoing, but initial reports do not show a benefit in ameliorating cognitive deficits or behavioral problems.[11] Two recently reported approaches to treat the bone-specific phenotype target pyrophosphate, which accumulates at high levels in bone.[14,15] This could be corrected by using asfotase-α enzyme therapy.[14] Another approach is to target β-catenin signaling, which is hyperactive in osteogenesis in neurofibromatosis, preventing bone formation. Inhibiting its activity improves bone repair.[15] However, clinical studies are required to determine the efficacy of these approaches.

The orthopaedic manifestations of neurofibromatosis include scoliosis, overgrowth of the limbs, and pseudarthrosis of the tibia. Scoliosis is common, and curves can be dystrophic or idiopathic. Dystrophic scoliosis is associated with a short, sharp, single curve involving six or fewer vertebrae. It is associated with deformity of the ribs and vertebrae, with dural ectasia and rib penetration of the spinal canal. The onset is early in childhood, and it is relentlessly progressive. Curves in children younger than 7 years have almost a 70% chance of becoming dystrophic later in life. The most important risk factors for progression are an early age of onset; a high Cobb angle; and an apical vertebra that is severely rotated, scalloped bone (concave loss of bone) in the middle to lower thoracic area.[16] Dystrophic curves are refractive to brace treatment. Other spinal deformities such as kyphosis also can occur. In severe cases, the scoliosis has so much rotation that curve progression is more obvious on lateral rather than AP radiographs.[16] In those with severe angular kyphosis, a high risk of paraplegia is present.

Pseudarthrosis of bone can occur and most frequently affects the tibia. Tibial dysplasia with a characteristic anterolateral bow, which in infancy can progress to pseudarthrosis, is associated with neurofibromatosis type 1. The characteristic anterolateral bow that is obvious in infancy often progresses to fracture, with spontaneous union being rare.[17] Hamartoma of undifferentiated mesenchymal cells occurs at the pseudarthrosis site, which sometimes is associated with loss of the normal allele of the *NF1* gene.[18,19]

Pharmacologic approaches to pseudarthrosis in neurofibromatosis have been reported. A mouse model suggested the use of lovastatin, but human studies of this approach are needed.[13] Direct installation of bone morphogenetic protein to the pseudarthrosis site may help to achieve union, but variable results have been reported, and it is not known if the use of bone morphogenetic protein in patients with an inherited premalignant condition has long-term consequences.[20]

The incidence of malignancy in neurofibromatosis is reported to range from less than 1% to more than 20%. The most common tumor location is in the central nervous system, with lesions such as optic nerve glioma, acoustic neuroma, and astrocytoma. Malignant degeneration of a neurofibroma to a neurofibrosarcoma is a risk. This process can occur in a central or peripheral neurofibroma. It can be quite difficult to distinguish a malignant lesion from a benign lesion. CT scans show areas of low-enhancing density in neurofibrosarcomas,[21] but no studies have confirmed the sensitivity and specificity of this finding. Similar patterns also can be visualized using MRI. Routine surveillance for sarcomatous change is impossible because of the large number of neurofibromas. In children with a neurofibroma, the propensity exists for the development of other malignancies such as Wilms tumors or rhabdomyosarcomas.

Beckwith-Wiedemann Syndrome

Beckwith-Wiedemann syndrome is characterized by organomegaly, omphalocele, and a large tongue (that regresses in size as a child ages). It is linked to the insulin-like growth factor gene, with paternal genomic imprinting playing a role in inheritance.[22] Neonatal hypoglycemic episodes occur and may cause a cerebral palsy–like picture. The risk of tumor development is 10%, with Wilms tumor being the most common. Abdominal ultrasonographic imaging to screen for Wilms tumor is advocated at regular intervals until a child with Beckwith-Wiedemann syndrome reaches age 6 years.[23,24]

Silver-Russell Syndrome

Silver-Russell syndrome is associated with a triangular shape to the face, and hemihypertrophy is present in 80% of the individuals with the syndrome. Intrauterine growth retardation and a low birth weight often are hallmarks of the disorder. Approximately one-half of cases are caused by hypomethylation of the 11p.15.5 chromosome.[25] Managing limb-length equality can be difficult because individual growth curves may not follow normal predictive charts. Growth hormone has been administered in an attempt to improve stature; although the use of growth hormone will increase growth velocity, it is not yet known whether ultimate height is increased.[26,27] Some features of Silver-Russell syndrome also are associated with Wilms tumor,[28,29] leading some physicians to recommend screening for Wilms tumor in these patients as would be done for patients with other causes of hemihypertrophy.

Proteus Syndrome

A characteristic appearance on the plantar surface of the feet, which is similar to the surface of the brain, occurs in Proteus syndrome. Both hemihypertrophy and macrodactyly are present. A mosaic distribution of lesions, a progressive course, and sporadic occurrence are characteristics required to make the diagnosis. Symptoms worsen as time progresses, but unlike other overgrowth syndromes, an increased incidence of malignancy has not been reported. Hemangiomas, pigmented nevi, and subcutaneous lipomas are present in the skin. A somatic mosaic mutation (mutant only in involved cells) activating *AKT1* is associated with Proteus syndrome.[30]

Spinal deformity, including scoliosis, kyphosis, and large vertebral bodies, known as megaspondylodysplasia, can be present.[31] Angular malformations of the lower extremities, especially genu valgum, are common, along with regional gigantism. Recurrence after surgical intervention is very common[31] and likely is caused by an underlying growth advantage in affected tissues that cannot be corrected surgically. Osteotomies can correct angular malformations, but the decision to undertake surgical correction must consider the possibility of rapid recurrence of the deformity after corrective surgery. The use of growth modulation (for example, eight-Plate [Orthofix]) to manage limb angular deformity is a promising approach,[32] but published results are lacking. Nerve compression can be managed with decompression, but spinal cord compression is difficult, if not impossible, to successfully treat surgically because of vertebrae overgrowth.[33]

Disorders Caused by Developmentally Important Signaling Pathways

Gene expression and cell signaling pathways are regulated in a coordinated manner for cells to proliferate, move, and die, allowing an organism to pattern normally and develop into an adult. Mutations in the genes that regulate these processes will alter normal development, causing disturbances of growth or patterning.[4] Environmental events such as exposure to a teratogen also can dysregulate these same pathways, resulting in a similar phenotype. Because such problems generally cause shape changes in the skeleton, surgery to correct issues such as limb malalignment are usually successful. Manifestations frequently occur in other organ systems because the genes that play roles in skeletal development also play important roles in the development of other organs. These disorders are usually inherited in an autosomal dominant manner, although the inheritance pattern is variable. Many of these disorders are caused by mutations dysregulating the way growth plate chondrocytes function, and knowledge of the growth plate defect helps physicians understand the associated clinical manifestations.

Achondroplasia and Related Disorders

Achondroplasia, hypochondroplasia, and thanatophoric dysplasia are all caused by mutations activating the fibroblast growth factor receptor-3 (*FGFR-3*) gene. They have different levels of receptor activation and thus different levels of severity. Because fibroblast growth factor regulates growth plate chondrocyte proliferation, long-bone growth is inhibited in these conditions, with more involvement in bones with the most enchondral growth. This pathophysiology explains many of the clinical characteristics, with more involvement in longer bones (the femur and the humerus), the characteristic rhizomelia, and progressive spinal stenosis distally in the lumbar spine because larger vertebrae have more enchondral growth and are more affected. Recent studies have identified possible pharmacologic therapies that can correct the underlying cell defect, including statin treatment[34] and c-natriuretic protein.[35] Although both substances work in mice with *FGFR-3* mutations, neither approach is yet verified as efficacious in human patients.

Camptomelic Dysplasia

Camptomelic dysplasia is caused by a mutation in the *SOX9* gene, which regulates the differentiation of mesenchymal cells to chondrocytes. Although the enchondral process is normal, the number of cells undergoing this process is not, appearing to result in an abnormality in the formation of the cartilage anlagen during fetal development. For this reason, camptomelic dysplasia is a severe form of short-limbed dwarfism that it is sometimes fatal. The long bones, primarily the tibiae and the femora, are bowed. Defective tracheal and lower respiratory tract cartilage may cause respiratory failure in the neonatal period. Progressive spinal deformity (kyphosis and scoliosis), which further compromises pulmonary function, is common and leads to death if it is untreated. Hydromyelia and diastematomyelia have been reported, and neurologic complications and pseudarthrosis after spinal treatment are very common. Other clinical features include a flattened head, cleft palate, micrognathia, defects of the heart and kidneys, and sex reversal (a female with an XY karyotype). The *SOX9* gene is required for the development of male external genitalia.[36]

Cleidocranial Dysplasia

Cleidocranial dysplasia is caused by a mutation in *RUNX2*, a transcription factor that regulates the formation of osteoblasts directly from undifferentiated cells and the terminal differentiation of growth plate chondrocytes. Bones formed by intramembranous ossification (primarily the clavicles, the cranium, and the pelvis) are abnormal. It is inherited in an autosomal dominant manner. Clinically, the characteristic finding is hypoplasia or the absence of clavicles; when it is bilateral, a child can touch his or her shoulders together in front of the chest. Patients have mild short stature and large heads with petite faces. Coxa vara, if present, can be treated in the same manner as is done for idiopathic cases. Pectus excavatum and sternal abnormalities also are common.[37]

Disorders Caused by Multiple Genes and Chromosome Abnormalities

These conditions are not inherited, but instead are caused by a random event in the formation of the embryo. In many cases, missing segments or large duplications of chromosomes are incompatible with embryotic survival. Abnormalities occur in all cells in the body, and mental defects frequently are associated with abnormalities in the central nervous system.

Down Syndrome (Trisomy 21)

Down syndrome is the most frequent trisomy, and its incidence increases with maternal age. Most patients have three copies of chromosome 21, 4% have a translocation involving this chromosome, and 1% are mosaic (with some normal cells). Many features attributable to Down syndrome are found in a specific chromosomal region (D21S55), including hypotonia and joint hyperlaxity, with abnormalities in the upper cervical spine (atlantoaxial and occipitoatlantal). Patients have relatively short stature, a flat face, and varying degrees of mental retardation. Acetabular dysplasia or hip dislocations occur in 5% of patients aged 2 to 10 years, and slipped capital femoral epiphysis and osteonecrosis often are present.[38] Wide variability in acetabular version occurs, which must be taken into account to effectively reconstruct the hip.[39] Other common characteristics include short, broad hands; patellofemoral instability; flatfoot and hallux valgus; congenital heart defects; and thyroid dysfunction. Orthopaedic surgeons and pediatricians often are asked to evaluate children with Down syndrome to confirm their eligibility for participation in the Special Olympics. A broad variety of radiographic abnormities of the cervical spine are present, but radiographic findings often do not correlate with the symptoms. In addition, a high complication rate associated with cervical spine fusion occurs in Down syndrome. Thus, it is not clear how to best manage children who are asymptomatic but have radiographic abnormalities. Modern instrumentation techniques can decrease but not eliminate the associated complication rate. For children who want to participate in the Special Olympics and are asymptomatic but have radiographic findings, the most prudent approach is to have these children avoid tumbling activities.[40,41]

Turner Syndrome (X Chromosome)

Turner syndrome is caused by complete or partial absence of one of the X chromosomes, and it can occur only in women; a lack of this chromosome in males is incompatible with life. Clinical features include short stature; a wide, webbed neck; low-set ears and hairline; cubitus and genu valgum; swollen hands and feet; scoliosis; and a broad, flat chest shaped like a shield. Patients usually experience gonadal dysfunction, which results in absent or incomplete development at puberty, infertility, diabetes, increased weight, and osteoporosis. Additional observations include congenital heart disease; kidney abnormalities; and cognitive deficits, specifically in memory, visuospatial, and mathematical areas. Life expectancy is normal.[42]

Noonan Syndrome

Noonan syndrome often is confused with Turner syndrome because both share several clinical characteristics. Noonan syndrome equally affects both males and females. Ten types have now been identified; they have similar phenotypic features but different causative genes (**Table 1**). All but one form (type 2) is autosomal dominant.

The principal features of Noonan syndrome include congenital heart defects, short stature, cervical spine fusion, low set ears and hairline, scoliosis, pectus carinatum or excavatum, impaired blood clotting, and learning disabilities with hypotonia. Noonan syndrome is one of the common syndromes associated with congenital heart defects. Some patients have severe joint or muscle pain, often with no identifiable cause. Arnold-Chiari malformation (type I) has been noted in some patients.[43,44]

Table 1

Gene Mutations in Noonan Syndrome

Type	Mutated Gene
1	*PTPN11*
2	Not yet identified
3	*KRAS*
4	*SOS1*
5	*RAF1*
6	*NRAS*
7	*BRAF*
8	*RIT1*
9	*SOS2*
10	*LZTR1*

Prader-Willi Syndrome

Prader-Willi syndrome is caused by a partial deletion of the 15th chromosome involving a group of genes when the chromosome is inherited from the father. The distinction of chromosomes by paternal origin is the result of imprinting; thus, Prader-Willi has a sister syndrome called Angelman syndrome that affects maternally imprinted genes in the region (diagnosed by DNA-based methylation testing to detect the absence of the paternally contributed region). Prader-Willi syndrome is characterized by hypotonia, short stature (that responds to growth hormone therapy), and a failure to thrive in the early years, which is followed by an extreme and insatiable appetite often resulting in morbid obesity, hypogonadism, and mild mental retardation. Orthopaedic manifestations include scoliosis (affecting up to 90% of patients), small hands and feet, and joint hyperlaxity. Patients with Prader-Willi syndrome have complications from surgery secondary to an abnormal physiologic response to hypercapnia and hypoxia, obstructive sleep apnea, thick pulmonary secretions, obesity, prolonged exaggerated response to sedatives, and increased risk for aspiration. Growth hormone therapy is used in this disorder, which results in improvements in weight and behavior.[45] The effect of growth hormone therapy on skeletal deformity is unclear, but the results of a recent randomized controlled trial suggests that it does not negatively affect the sequelae of spinal deformity.[46]

Trichorhinophalangeal Syndromes

Two types of trichorhinophalangeal (TRP) syndromes have been identified. TRP types I and II are caused by either mutation or loss of the *TRSP1* gene. However, TRP type II has a larger loss of the chromosomal region, with loss of the adjacent *EXT-1* gene (responsible for hereditary multiple exostoses). This causes exostoses in TRP type II. Patients have a pear-shaped, bulbous nose; prominent ears; sparse hair; cone epiphyses; and short lateral metacarpals. They also have mild mental retardation. Skeletal manifestations are specific to the epiphyses. Hips mimic Legg-Calvé-Perthes disease in both radiographs and symptoms. The key distinguishing feature for TRP type II is the presence of multiple exostoses, especially involving the lower extremities.[47]

Disorders Caused by Protein Processing Genes (Enzymes)

Enzymes modify molecules or other proteins. The enzymes implicated in musculoskeletal pathology often modify substances for degradation. Thus, these conditions often are associated with cell dysfunction because of the accumulation of these substances. The excess accumulation of proteins in cells causes them to become larger than normal, and the increased space occupied by these large cells can mimic increased pressure in bones, causing osteonecrosis. They also can cause increased extradural material in the spine, potentially resulting in nerve compression symptoms. Accumulated cellular by-products can be biologically active, often resulting in bone and joint disease similar to that seen in autoimmune diseases. Multiple systems are nearly always involved in these disorders. Medical treatments to replace the defective enzyme have been developed for many of these disorders, and such treatments often will arrest but not reverse the skeletal manifestations of the disorder. Early diagnosis and appropriate medical treatment are slowly decreasing the number of individuals who have musculoskeletal problems. Most enzyme disorders are inherited in an autosomal recessive manner.

Summary

Various orthopaedic syndromes are caused by genetic mutations or fetal environmental factors that alter cell behavior, often in a manner that mimics genetic mutation. An understanding of genetic etiology allows the classification of syndromes based on the function of the causative gene product: structural proteins, proteins that regulate developmentally important signaling pathways, proteins implicated in neoplasia; proteins that play a role in processing molecules such as enzymes, and proteins that play a role in nerve or muscle function. Each class of syndromes shares common clinical findings and responses to treatment.

Key Study Points

- Knowledge about the genetic cause of a syndrome can explain the phenotype and predict treatment outcomes.
- Syndromes caused by mutations in genes encoding proteins that regulate cell growth can predispose individuals to cancers.
- Disorders caused by mutations in genes encoding for enzymes tend to be autosomal recessive, and enzyme replacement therapy typically arrests but does not fix skeletal deformity.
- Syndromes caused by large chromosomal abnormalities, such as a trisomy, are not inherited.
- Overgrowth conditions can be caused by mosaic (or somatic) mutations.

Annotated References

1. Alman BA: A classification for genetic disorders of interest to orthopaedists. *Clin Orthop Relat Res* 2002;401:17-26.

2. Alman BA: Skeletal dysplasias and the growth plate. *Clin Genet* 2008;73(1):24-30.

3. Alman BA: The role of hedgehog signalling in skeletal health and disease. *Nat Rev Rheumatol* 2015;11(9):552-560.

   The authors present a review of the role of developmentally important signaling pathways in bone growth and syndromes associated with deregulation of the hedgehog signaling cascade. Level of evidence: V.

4. Cohen MM Jr: The new bone biology: Pathologic, molecular, and clinical correlates. *Am J Med Genet A* 2006;140(23):2646-2706.

5. Armon K, Bale P: Identifying heritable connective tissue disorders in childhood. *Practitioner* 2012;256(1752):19-23.

   The authors present a review of the role of connective tissue disorders and mutations in causative genes. Level of evidence: V.

6. Schindeler A, Little DG: Recent insights into bone development, homeostasis, and repair in type 1 neurofibromatosis (NF1). *Bone* 2008;42(4):616-622.

7. Lublin M, Schwartzentruber DJ, Lukish J, Chester C, Biesecker LG, Newman KD: Principles for the surgical management of patients with Proteus syndrome and patients with overgrowth not meeting Proteus criteria. *J Pediatr Surg* 2002;37(7):1013-1020.

8. Ferner RE, Gutmann DH: Neurofibromatosis type 1 (NF1): Diagnosis and management. *Handb Clin Neurol* 2013;115:939-955.

   The authors present a review of the genetic and clinical presentation of neurofibromatosis type 1. Level of evidence: V.

9. Abramowicz A, Gos M: Neurofibromin in neurofibromatosis type 1: Mutations in NF1gene as a cause of disease. *Dev Period Med* 2014;18(3):297-306.

   The role of neurofibromin in cell signaling is discussed, with special attention to Ras/MAPK pathway regulation as well as organism development. Level of evidence: V.

10. Widemann BC, Salzer WL, Arceci RJ, et al: Phase I trial and pharmacokinetic study of the farnesyltransferase inhibitor tipifarnib in children with refractory solid tumors or neurofibromatosis type I and plexiform neurofibromas. *J Clin Oncol* 2006;24(3):507-516.

11. Widemann BC, Babovic-Vuksanovic D, Dombi E, et al: Phase II trial of pirfenidone in children and young adults with neurofibromatosis type 1 and

progressive plexiform neurofibromas. *Pediatr Blood Cancer* 2014;61(9):1598-1602.

Pirfenidone, an oral anti-inflammatory, antifibrotic agent was evaluated in an open-label, single-arm, phase II trial in children and young adults with inoperable plexiform neurofibromas. Pirfenidone was well tolerated, but did not demonstrate activity as defined in this trial. Level of evidence: IV.

12. Korf BR: Statins, bone, and neurofibromatosis type 1. *BMC Med* 2008;6:22.

13. Kolanczyk M, Kühnisch J, Kossler N, et al: Modelling neurofibromatosis type 1 tibial dysplasia and its treatment with lovastatin. *BMC Med* 2008;6:21.

14. de la Croix Ndong J, Makowski AJ, Uppuganti S, et al: Asfotase-α improves bone growth, mineralization and strength in mouse models of neurofibromatosis type-1. *Nat Med* 2014;20(8):904-910.

Neurofibromin is an essential regulator of bone mineralization. The authors suggest that altered pyrophosphate homeostasis contributes to skeletal dysplasias associated with neurofibromatosis type 1, and some skeletal conditions might be prevented pharmacologically. Level of evidence: V.

15. Ghadakzadeh S, Kannu P, Whetstone H, Howard A, Alman BA: β-Catenin modulation in neurofibromatosis type 1 bone repair: Therapeutic implications. *FASEB J* 2016; June 15 [Epub ahead of print].

Poor bone repair in neurofibromatosis is associated with hyperactivity of β-catenin. Inhibiting this pathway improves osteogenesis. A pharmacologic approach to inhibit β-catenin might be efficacious to improve fusion rates and success in treating pseudoarthrosis. Level of evidence: V.

16. Feldman DS, Jordan C, Fonseca L: Orthopaedic manifestations of neurofibromatosis type 1. *J Am Acad Orthop Surg* 2010;18(6):346-357.

17. Turra S, Santini S, Cagnoni G, Jacopetti T: Gigantism of the foot: Our experience in seven cases. *J Pediatr Orthop* 1998;18(3):337-345.

18. Cho TJ, Seo JB, Lee HR, Yoo WJ, Chung CY, Choi IH: Biologic characteristics of fibrous hamartoma from congenital pseudarthrosis of the tibia associated with neurofibromatosis type 1. *J Bone Joint Surg Am* 2008;90(12):2735-2744.

19. Stevenson DA, Zhou H, Ashrafi S, et al: Double inactivation of NF1 in tibial pseudarthrosis. *Am J Hum Genet* 2006;79(1):143-148.

20. Senta H, Park H, Bergeron E, et al: Cell responses to bone morphogenetic proteins and peptides derived from them: Biomedical applications and limitations. *Cytokine Growth Factor Rev* 2009;20(3):213-222.

21. Filippi G: The de Lange syndrome: Report of 15 cases. *Clin Genet* 1989;35(5):343-363.

22. Shah KJ: Beckwith-Wiedemann syndrome: Role of ultrasound in its management. *Clin Radiol* 1983;34(3):313-319.

23. Kuroiwa M, Sakamoto J, Shimada A, et al: Manifestation of alveolar rhabdomyosarcoma as primary cutaneous lesions in a neonate with Beckwith-Wiedemann syndrome. *J Pediatr Surg* 2009;44(3):e31-e35.

24. Mussa A, Di Candia S, Russo S, et al: Recommendations of the Scientific Committee of the Italian Beckwith-Wiedemann Syndrome Association on the diagnosis, management and follow-up of the syndrome. *Eur J Med Genet* 2016;59(1):52-64.

This article presents best practice guidelines and comprehensive recommendations on the complex management of patients with Beckwith-Wiedemann syndrome. Level of evidence: V.

25. Marczak-Hałupka A, Kalina MA, Tańska A, Chrzanowska KH: Silver-Russell syndrome: Part I. Clinical characteristics and genetic background. *Pediatr Endocrinol Diabetes Metab* 2015;20(3):101-106.

The genetic and clinical manifestations of Silver-Russell syndrome are reviewed in this article. Level of evidence: V.

26. Tsirikos AI, McMaster MJ: Goldenhar-associated conditions (hemifacial microsomia) and congenital deformities of the spine. *Spine (Phila Pa 1976)* 2006;31(13):E400-E407.

27. Ishida M: New developments in Silver-Russell syndrome and implications for clinical practice. *Epigenomics* 2016;8(4):563-580.

A comprehensive list of the molecular defects in Silver-Russell syndrome is reported to date, and the article highlights the importance of multiple loci/tissue testing and trio (both parents and proband) screening. The epigenetic and phenotypic overlaps with other imprinting disorders also are discussed. Level of evidence: V.

28. Incardona JP, Gaffield W, Kapur RP, Roelink H: The teratogenic Veratrum alkaloid cyclopamine inhibits sonic hedgehog signal transduction. *Development* 1998;125(18):3553-3562.

29. Palumbo O, Mattina T, Palumbo P, Carella M, Perrotta CS: A de novo 11p13 microduplication in a patient with some features invoking Silver-Russell syndrome. *Mol Syndromol* 2014;5(1):11-18.

This case report and review of the literature discussed the presentation and etiology of Silver-Russell syndrome. Level of evidence: IV.

30. Lindhurst MJ, Sapp JC, Teer JK, et al: A mosaic activating mutation in AKT1 associated with the Proteus syndrome. *N Engl J Med* 2011;365(7):611-619.

Exome sequencing in Proteus syndrome determined that this disorder is caused by a somatic activating mutation in *AKT1*, proving the hypothesis of somatic mosaicism and implicating activation of the PI3K (phosphatidylinositol 3-kinase)-AKT (also known as protein kinase B) pathway in the characteristic clinical findings of overgrowth and tumor susceptibility. Level of evidence: V.

31. Azouz EM, Costa T, Fitch N: Radiologic findings in the Proteus syndrome. *Pediatr Radiol* 1987;17(6):481-485.

32. Stevens PM, Klatt JB: Guided growth for pathological physes: Radiographic improvement during realignment. *J Pediatr Orthop* 2008;28(6):632-639.

33. Choi ML, Wey PD, Borah GL: Pediatric peripheral neuropathy in proteus syndrome. *Ann Plast Surg* 1998;40(5):528-532.

34. Yamashita A, Morioka M, Kishi H, et al: Statin treatment rescues FGFR3 skeletal dysplasia phenotypes. *Nature* 2014;513(7519):507-511.

    Statin treatment was evaluated in patient-specific, induced pluripotent stem cell models and a mouse model of *FGFR3* skeletal dysplasia. It was found that statins could correct the degraded cartilage in both chondrogenically differentiated thanatophoric dysplasia and achondroplasia-induced pluripotent stem cells. Treatment of the achondroplasia model mice with statins led to a substantial recovery of bone growth. Level of evidence: V.

35. Lorget F, Kaci N, Peng J, et al: Evaluation of the therapeutic potential of a CNP analog in a Fgfr3 mouse model recapitulating achondroplasia. *Am J Hum Genet* 2012;91(6):1108-1114.

    In this report on the pharmacologic activity of a 39 amino acid c-natriuretic protein analog in an *FGFR3* mutation mouse model, the authors observed an increase in axial and appendicular skeleton lengths and improvements in dwarfism-related clinical features, which included flattening of the skull, reduced crossbite, straightening of the tibias and femurs, and correction of the growth-plate defect. Level of evidence: V.

36. Jain V, Sen B: Camptomelic dysplasia. *J Pediatr Orthop B* 2014;23(5):485-488.

    This article is a case report and review of the literature on camptomelic dysplasia. Level of evidence: IV.

37. Vij R, Batra P, Vij H: Cleidocranial dysplasia: Complete clinical, radiological and histological profiles. *BMJ Case Rep* 2013;2013:pii.

    This article is a case report of cleidocranial dysplasia, with complete clinical, radiologic, histologic, and treatment profiles. Level of evidence: IV.

38. Talmac MA, Kadhim M, Rogers KJ, Holmes L Jr, Miller F: Legg-Calvé-Perthes disease in children with Down syndrome. *Acta Orthop Traumatol Turc* 2013;47(5):334-338.

    In a case series of children with trisomy 21 and Legg-Calvé-Perthes disease, the radiographic characteristics of Legg-Calvé-Perthes disease in patients with Down syndrome do not differ from those without it and should be followed accordingly. Level of evidence: V.

39. Abousamra O, Bayhan IA, Rogers KJ, Miller F: Hip instability in Down syndrome: A focus on acetabular retroversion. *J Pediatr Orthop* 2016;36(5):499-504.

    This report suggests that a wide range of acetabular anteversion measurements exist in children with Down syndrome. After detailed anatomic study of the hip, good results with a low complication rate can be expected in the intermediate term after hip reconstruction. Level of evidence: IV.

40. Caird MS, Wills BP, Dormans JP: Down syndrome in children: The role of the orthopaedic surgeon. *J Am Acad Orthop Surg* 2006;14(11):610-619.

41. McKay SD, Al-Omari A, Tomlinson LA, Dormans JP: Review of cervical spine anomalies in genetic syndromes. *Spine (Phila Pa 1976)* 2012;37(5):E269-E277.

42. Levitsky LL, Luria AH, Hayes FJ, Lin AE: Turner syndrome: Update on biology and management across the life span. *Curr Opin Endocrinol Diabetes Obes* 2015;22(1):65-72.

    This article reviews the pathophysiology, molecular biology, and management of Turner syndrome. Level of evidence: V.

43. Myers A, Bernstein JA, Brennan ML, et al: Perinatal features of the RASopathies: Noonan syndrome, cardiofaciocutaneous syndrome and Costello syndrome. *Am J Med Genet A* 2014;164A(11):2814-2821.

    This article reviews the pathophysiology, molecular biology, and management of Noonan syndrome, cardiofaciocutaneous syndrome, and Costello syndrome, with focus on the perinatal presentations. Level of evidence: V.

44. Tartaglia M, Zampino G, Gelb BD: Noonan syndrome: Clinical aspects and molecular pathogenesis. *Mol Syndromol* 2010;1(1):2-26.

45. Festen DA, de Lind van Wijngaarden R, van Eekelen M, et al: Randomized controlled GH trial: Effects on anthropometry, body composition and body proportions in a large group of children with Prader-Willi syndrome. *Clin Endocrinol (Oxf)* 2008;69(3):443-451.

46. de Lind van Wijngaarden RF, de Klerk LW, Festen DA, Duivenvoorden HJ, Otten BJ, Hokken-Koelega AC: Randomized controlled trial to investigate the effects of growth hormone treatment on scoliosis in children with Prader-Willi syndrome. *J Clin Endocrinol Metab* 2009;94(4):1274-1280.

47. Schinzel A, Riegel M, Baumer A, et al: Long-term follow-up of four patients with Langer-Giedion syndrome: Clinical course and complications. *Am J Med Genet A* 2013;161A(9):2216-2225.

    The authors review the clinical findings, natural history, and management of Langer-Giedion syndrome. Level of evidence: IV.

Chapter 10

Medical Therapy in Pediatric Orthopaedics

Andrew W. Howard, MD, MSc, FRCSC   Stephanie N. Moore, BS   Jonathan G. Schoenecker, MD, PhD

Abstract

The need for medical therapy in children with orthopaedic conditions is limited typically to analgesia, antibiotics, and medications that are designed to optimize bone integrity. It is helpful to have a broad overview of these therapies, including specific pathologic conditions in which these therapies are used, the mechanisms of action, and adverse side effects.

Keywords: analgesics; antibiotic; antibiotic resistance; bisphosphonate; diphosphonate; pain relief

Introduction

Pediatric orthopaedic surgeons treat a variety of conditions, including traumatic injuries, developmental and genetic skeletal manifestations, and musculoskeletal infections. Four overarching categories of therapeutics are commonly prescribed for this wide range of conditions: antibiotics targeting infection, analgesics targeting traumatic and postoperative pain, therapeutics targeting degenerative phenotypes, and therapies aimed at enhancing tissue regeneration. Although the treatment of traumatic injuries and musculoskeletal infections is common in orthopaedics as a whole, the pediatric orthopaedic specialty also regularly treats premature skeletal degeneration from pathologic causes (such as osteogenesis imperfecta, cerebral palsy, or Duchenne muscular dystrophy) and environmental causes (such as diet, obesity, and vitamin D deficiency). Numerous pharmacologic therapies are available for limiting skeletal degeneration, but no therapies have been approved by the FDA to improve musculoskeletal regeneration. As such, substantial activity is ongoing in both the development of novel therapeutics and the off-label use of currently approved therapeutics, although the latter must be prescribed with great caution. This chapter provides a broad overview of the common therapeutics used in pediatric orthopaedics to treat trauma-induced or postoperative pain, musculoskeletal degeneration, and infections.

Dr. Schoenecker or an immediate family member has received research or institutional support from Ionis pharmaceuticals. Neither of the following authors nor any immediate family member has received anything of value from or has stock or stock options held in a commercial company or institution related directly or indirectly to the subject of this chapter: Dr. Howard and Ms. Moore.

Analgesia

Principles of Acute Pain Relief

For the management of acute pain, the "ladder" concept espoused by the World Health Organization in 1986 (that was initially related to cancer pain) still applies.[1] This approach says that if pharmacologic agents are needed to manage pain, it is appropriate to start with simple analgesics (acetaminophen or ibuprofen) and progress to an opioid if pain is severe. The role of opioid use in chronic pain is being increasingly questioned because of its limited clinical effectiveness and the severe secondary problems for both patients and society associated with chronic opioid use.[2] The recent evidence regarding the pharmacologic management of acute pain in children's orthopaedics is discussed. Typically, acute pain includes pain from fractures and postoperative pain.

Pain Relief for Fractures

Multiple recent randomized controlled trials (RCTs) are available to guide the selection of analgesics to treat fracture pain in the emergency department. For nondisplaced fractures, all recent randomized trials indicate that ibuprofen is the preferred agent rather than morphine, codeine, acetaminophen, or codeine plus acetaminophen.[3-5] Ibuprofen provided equal or better analgesia compared with the other agents and had a better adverse event profile and better patient and parent satisfaction.

In displaced fractures requiring emergency department reduction, equal effectiveness was reported for fentanyl administered intranasally compared with intravenous morphine.[6,7] A Cochrane review confirmed this finding for nonfracture pain as well.[8]

Postoperative Pain Relief

The American Society of Anesthesiologists produces and updates practice guidelines that combine high-level scientific evidence with opinions from the society or experts when high-level evidence is lacking.[9] For pediatric postoperative pain, the guidelines emphasize multimodal approaches, a reduction of anxiety and emotional distress, and proactive and aggressive pain management based on the concern that pediatric postoperative pain has traditionally been undertreated.[9]

Combinations of nonopioid analgesics are the rational starting point for postoperative pain management. A meta-analysis of three RCTs involving 1,647 adult patients with wisdom tooth extraction (a common model for moderate pain) showed that a combination of ibuprofen and paracetamol was superior to either agent used alone.[10]

Postoperative pain that is more severe often is treated with an opioid in addition to simple analgesics. As with many common practices in medicine, the level of evidence supporting this practice is low. A 2014 Cochrane systematic review examined 10 RCTs that evaluated nalbuphine (an opioid) for postoperative pain management in children. Interestingly, five trials compared nalbuphine to a placebo, but nalbuphine was not superior to placebo or other comparator opioid medications based on the trials available.[11] The absence of evidence of effectiveness, however, should not be mistaken as evidence of no effectiveness. It would be difficult to design a proper placebo-controlled trial of opioid use for severe pain.

Patient-controlled analgesia is a means of administering a postoperative intravenous opioid with an automatic pump that responds to patient demand but limits total dosing. A 2015 Cochrane review of RCTs found that in adults, pain scores were better, opioid use was a little higher, and patient satisfaction was higher with patient-controlled analgesia compared with the conventional administration of opioid medications.[12] In pediatric patients, it is common to use a background infusion in addition to the on-demand analgesia; a recent systematic review found such infusions to be equally safe and effective.[13]

Adjunctive medications given intraoperatively can reduce postoperative pain and postoperative opioid requirements. In a systematic review of 11 RCTs involving 742 children, clonidine, an alpha-agonist, was found to be beneficial in reducing postoperative pain.[14] More recently, in a review of 14 RCTs involving 1,463 children, dexmedetomidine was shown to be effective in reducing postanesthesia care unit (PACU) pain scores and opioid use.[15] A second systematic review of 20 RCTs linked reduced PACU pain to a reduction in emergence agitation when dexmedetomidine was used as an adjunct to pediatric anesthesia.[16] Dexmedetomidine is a highly selective agonist of alpha-2 receptors that has a favorable profile in children regarding anxiolysis, analgesia, sympatholysis, and anesthetic-sparing effect with minimal respiratory depression.[17] Ketamine also can be used as an adjunct to general anesthesia; a systematic review of 35 pediatric RCTs showed that ketamine produced a reduction in PACU pain scores but did not have an opioid-sparing effect.[18]

Epidural, caudal, or regional anesthetics are commonly used to improve postoperative pain management and reduce opioid requirements in children's orthopaedics. According to a meta-analysis of four RCTs, epidural anesthesia was superior to patient-controlled morphine for pain relief after scoliosis surgery.[19] Evidence is less conclusive for other types of surgery. A comprehensive systematic review of regional blocks in pediatrics found six trials for an upper extremity, one trial for a hip, and five trials for a lower extremity and concluded that the literature supported the use of blocks, but the studies had low methodologic quality.[20]

Epidural, caudal, and regional blocks can be potentiated by adding agents to the local anesthetic. One meta-analysis compared neostigmine to clonidine and tramadol as adjuncts to a single-shot caudal anesthetic and found that neostigmine provided the greatest increase (8 hours) in the duration of effective analgesia.[21] A similar 8-hour increase in the duration of analgesia was noted in a more recent meta-analysis of six pediatric RCTs that evaluated dexmedetomidine as an adjunct to caudal anesthetic.[22]

A delay in the diagnosis of compartment syndrome is an ongoing concern with epidural or regional anesthesia. A recent review article evaluated all published cases (pediatric and adult) of compartment syndrome in the presence of regional anesthesia and concluded that the classic signs of compartment syndrome were present in 32 of 35 patients.[23] Although the authors determined that no conclusive evidence linked regional anesthesia to diagnostic delay, the important message is that a high index of clinical suspicion and ongoing assessment must apply. This observation is particularly true for children because invasive compartment pressure monitoring may not be indicated and may be less reliable.

Opioid Dependence and Withdrawal

Children can manifest withdrawal symptoms from the abrupt cessation of an opioid after as few as 5 to 7 days. Withdrawal symptoms can include anxiety, agitation, insomnia, and tremors and often are missed or misinterpreted in pediatric patients. Patients who have been in intensive care units for prolonged periods are most at risk because of both pain and procedural sedation. Current guidelines suggest that after 14 days or more of opioid use, children should be weaned with a gradually decreasing dose, and those who have been given an opioid for 7 to 14 days should be considered for weaning and monitored for withdrawal symptoms. Abrupt discontinuation of opioid use is generally well tolerated by children who have received such medication for less than 7 days.[24]

Osteoporosis

Calcium and Phosphate

Calcium and phosphorous, in the form of phosphate, are essential elements in many biologic processes. They are not only required for proper cellular function and signaling but also combine to make biologic crystals, most notably, hydroxyapatite, which is found in bone (**Figure 1**). Because of their essential nature, their anatomic distribution is tightly regulated, with 10,000 times more calcium and phosphate circulating in the extracellular space compared with the intracellular microenvironment. This ideal biologic gradient provides excess calcium and phosphate for cellular function; however, calcium and phosphate are at their saturation points when circulating in plasma (**Figure 2**). Although this is ideal for maintaining bone integrity, calcium and phosphate can aggregate in soft tissues, such as muscle, skin, and blood vessels. The fact that most soft tissues are free of calcium phosphate aggregates indicates that specialized biologic mechanisms are in place to prevent aberrant aggregation. Pyrophosphate directly inhibits calcium and phosphate aggregation, thus preventing in vivo mineralization. Circulating levels of pyrophosphate are maintained by pyrophosphate pumps, which, in turn, provide the frontline defense against soft-tissue calcification[25] (**Figure 2**). Thus, calcium, phosphate, and pyrophosphate homeostasis are critical for maintaining bone integrity and cellular function while also preventing soft-tissue calcification.

It follows that genetic mutations to elements of the pyrophosphate pump are considered the potential underlying cause of soft-tissue calcification disorders, such as pseudoxanthoma elasticum and generalized arterial calcification of infancy.[26] More commonly, pediatric orthopaedic surgeons are tasked with addressing deficiencies or disorders of calcium and/or phosphate that result in osteoporosis. Childhood osteoporosis is divided into primary and secondary causes. Osteogenesis imperfecta represents the prototypical primary osteoporosis of childhood. Secondary pediatric osteoporosis, incited by underlying diseases and/or their treatment, can be placed into two broad categories: glucocorticoid-treated diseases and disorders that compromise normal weight bearing and mobility.

First-line measures to optimize pediatric osteoporosis can be placed into three main categories: improve nutrition, increase physical activity, and treat the underlying condition and associated comorbidities.[27] The most well-described nutritional factors for pediatric bone health are vitamin D and calcium (**Figure 1**). However, several other nutrients also play a role in bone metabolism, including protein; potassium; magnesium; copper; iron; fluoride; zinc; and vitamin A, C, and K supplementation. Bisphosphonates, also known as diphosphonates, are synthetic analogues of pyrophosphate and are the most extensively published agents for treating childhood osteoporosis in the United States,[28] although their use remains off-label in many other countries.

Vitamin D

Vitamin D, a fat-soluble hormone that is synthesized and metabolized by all mammals, is a critical component of calcium homeostasis and, as a result, has a substantial effect on bone quality and mineralization (**Figure 1**). Vitamin D is first synthesized in the skin as a provitamin, 7-dehydrocholesterol, where subsequent exposure to sunlight converts 7-dehydrocholesterol to vitamin D_3 (cholecalciferol). Vitamin D also can be obtained from dietary supplementation, where it is absorbed from the small intestine and circulated in the blood. Whether from endogenous or dietary sources, all circulating vitamin D requires two successive modifications within the liver and kidneys to become the biologically active form, calcitriol [1,25$(OH)_2$D]. Although the primary function of vitamin D is regulation of calcium homeostasis, it is now well understood that vitamin D also plays important roles in multiple components of the musculoskeletal system. Specifically, vitamin D stimulates the intestinal absorption of calcium, which, in turn, indirectly promotes bone mineralization. Conversely, vitamin D also has been demonstrated to directly regulate the mobilization of calcium from bone back into circulation. In addition to effects on the skeletal system, vitamin D affects the function of skeletal muscle.[27,29,30]

Severe vitamin D deficiency causes rickets and/or hypocalcemia in infants and children. The clinical consequences of mild vitamin D deficiency are less well established. However, chronically low vitamin D levels are associated

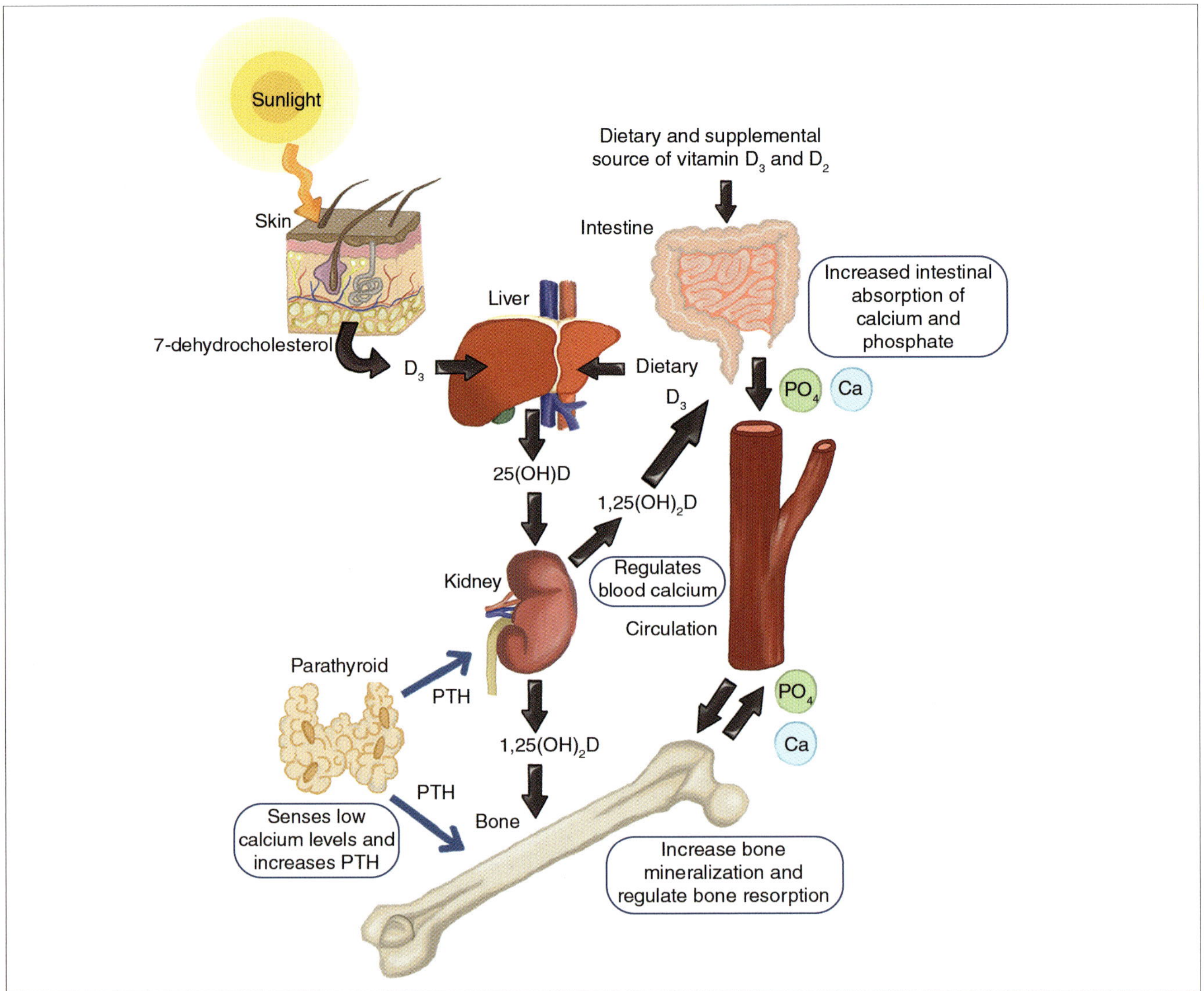

Figure 1 Illustration of calcium, phosphate, and vitamin D homeostasis. The classic pathway begins with either endogenous, dietary, or supplemental sources of vitamin D_3. Following metabolism by the liver to produce 25-hydroxyvitamin D [25(OH)D], the renal system converts 25(OH)D to the active form of vitamin D, calcitriol [$1,25(OH)_2D$], which circulates throughout the body in the picomolar range. $1,25(OH)_2D$ acts both on bone and the intestinal system to regulate circulating levels of calcium and phosphate. Because bone contains the body's primary reserve of calcium (Ca) and phosphate (PO_4), in the form of hydroxyapatite, resorption of bone via $1,25(OH)_2D$ signaling through osteoblasts and osteoclasts serves as a critical regulatory mechanism for circulating calcium and phosphate levels. In addition, $1,25(OH)_2D$ acts on the intestinal system to increase dietary absorption of calcium and phosphate by regulating both passive and active ion transport through the intestinal epithelium. Together, this system tightly regulates circulating calcium and phosphate levels, thereby allowing for proper intracellular signaling, muscle cell contraction, nerve cell activity, and bone and teeth health. D_2 = vitamin D_2 (ergocalciferol), D_3 = vitamin D_3 (cholecalciferol), PTH = pituitary hormone.

with the development of low bone mineral density and other measures of reduced bone health, even in the absence of rickets. Vitamin D deficiency is common in infants who are dark skinned and exclusively breast fed beyond ages 3 to 6 months.[27] More commonly, the pediatric orthopaedic surgeon should be aware of vitamin D deficiency when managing fracture repair, osteotomies, or fusion. These populations include children with chronic illnesses, on vegetarian or unusual diets, who are dark skinned, who use anticonvulsant or antiretroviral medications, or with malabsorptive conditions. Additional risk factors include residence at higher latitudes, the winter season, and other causes of low sun exposure.[27] Vitamin D deficiency in children in the United States and several other developed nations has been reported with increasing frequency since the mid-1980s.[29] According to large population-based studies, the overall prevalence of vitamin D deficiency or insufficiency in children in the United States is approximately 15%.[31]

Because of improved analytic methods for measuring vitamin D and more comprehensive data collection, low circulating levels of vitamin D and the reemergence of vitamin D–dependent rickets are common clinical findings. The level of calcifediol, also known as 25-hydroxyvitamin D [25(OH)D], is the best indicator of vitamin D status and stores because it is the main circulating form of vitamin D and has a half-life of 2 to 3 weeks. In contrast, $1,25(OH)_2D$ has a much shorter half-life (4 hours), circulates in much lower concentrations than 25(OH)D, and is susceptible to fluctuations induced by the pituitary hormone in response to subtle changes in calcium levels. The optimal serum 25(OH)D level remains controversial, and no clinical consensus exists for optimal vitamin D intake levels for children and infants. However, a minimum 25(OH)D level of 50 nmol/L (20 ng/mL) is recommended in youth through diet and/or supplementation. As such, the American Academy of Pediatrics recently recommended a vitamin D dietary allowance of 400 IU or 10 µg daily from the time of infancy through adolescence.[30] The initial basis for selecting this dose was from a well-established source of vitamin D supplementation, cod liver oil, in which 10 µg represents the amount of vitamin D found in 1 teaspoon, which had long been considered safe and effective at preventing rickets.[29] Beyond the time of adolescence and skeletal development, the recommendations for optimal vitamin D levels are less precise, resulting in reports that recommend daily vitamin D intake ranging from 200 to 4,000 IU per day. Therapeutic side effects and adverse consequences of vitamin D are rare and include toxicity associated with increased intestinal calcium and phosphate absorption; hypercalcemia and/or hyperphosphatemia; and suppression of the pituitary hormone, which results in renal pathology.

Calcium

Calcium is a key nutrient for adequate skeletal mineralization, with recommended intake amounts best achieved through a healthy diet. Pathologic calcium insufficiency is less common than vitamin D deficiency. Calcium supplementation in childhood was recently investigated by a meta-analysis, but it showed only a small effect on bone mineral density that is unlikely to alter fracture risk.[30] The Institute of Medicine recommends 700 mg/d for children aged 1 to 3 years, 1,000 mg/d for children aged 4 to 8 years, and 1,300 mg/d for children and adolescents aged 9 to 18 years.[30] Higher daily supplementation may be required for children with malabsorption or those taking medications that impair calcium retention or absorption (diuretics or glucocorticoid therapy).

Bisphosphonates

Bisphosphonates are a powerful family of pharmaceuticals that have been used by clinicians for more than 40 years to prevent osteoporosis.[28] These stable forms of pyrophosphate freely pass into cells and act as effective inhibitors of the HMG-CoA (3-hydroxy-3-methyl-glutaryl-coenzyme A) reductase pathway (**Figure 2**). In addition, bisphosphonates induce osteoclast apoptosis when they are metabolized into nonhydrolyzable adenosine triphosphate (ATP) analogues, which, following incorporation into replicating DNA, accumulate in cells and induce apoptosis (**Figure 2**). Bisphosphonates have pleiotropic effects on cellular function,[31] most notably attenuating osteoclast activity and reducing the ability to resorb bone. However, the industrial use of bisphosphonates to protect against aberrant mineralization predates their use to preserve bone by at least a century. Bisphosphonates were first used to soften public water supplies in the 1800s, thereby preventing the calcification of pipes. In addition, the first clinical studies regarding bisphosphonates and their uses in vivo in the 1960s also focused on their ability to prevent calcium and phosphate aggregation. Despite the well-documented antimineralization properties of bisphosphonates, their predominant clinical application has instead been concentrated on their antibone resorptive properties.

Most studies that describe the effects of bisphosphonate therapy in children are observational preadministration and postadministration reports; relatively few controlled studies of bisphosphonate therapy in children exist, and even fewer studies have been sufficiently powered to assess fracture outcomes. Bisphosphonate therapy is typically reserved for children with a history of low-trauma fractures; it also has limited potential for spontaneous (medication-unassisted) recovery caused by permanent or persistent osteoporosis risk factors. The most frequently prescribed bisphosphonate regimen is cyclic intravenous pamidronate (divided equally over 3 days and administered every 4 months).[28] With the resolution of risk factors during children's growth (for example, the cessation of secondary osteoporosis), discontinuation of therapy is usually considered after a child has been fracture free for at least 6 to 12 months and bone mineral density Z-scores are appropriate for the child's height.

The most frequent adverse side effects of bisphosphonate therapy, reported with both oral and intravenous treatment,[28] are collectively referred to as acute-phase reactions and include fever, malaise, back and bone pain,

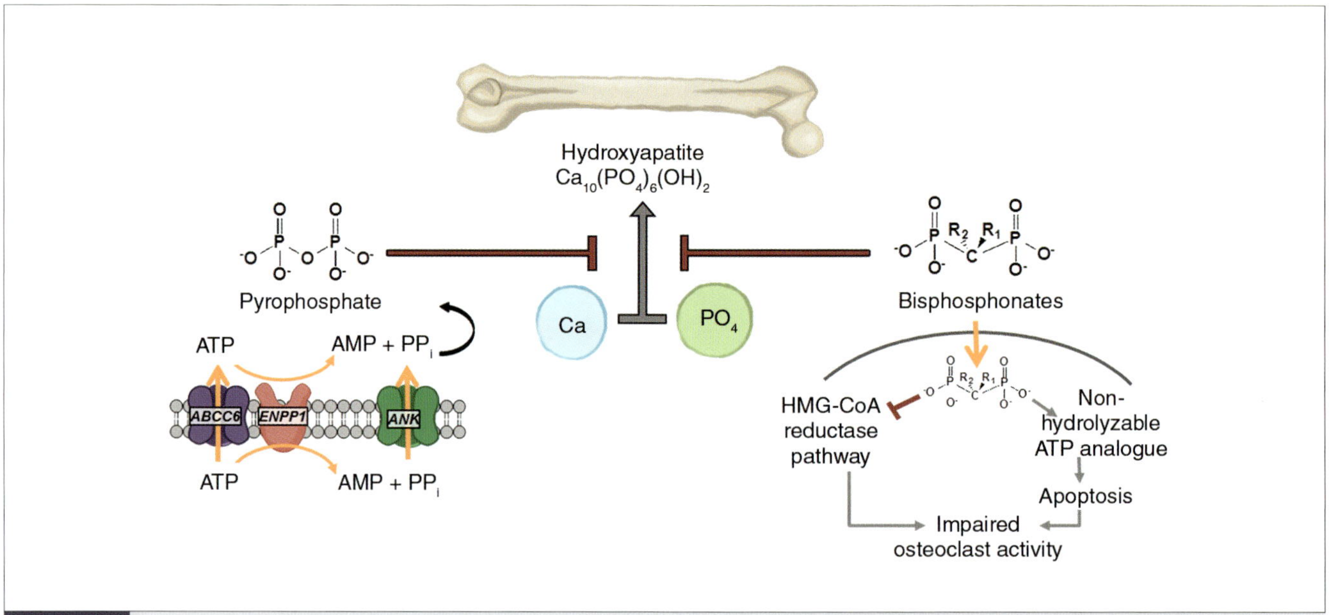

Figure 2 Illustration of pyrophosphate (PP_i) and bisphosphonate mechanisms of regulating mineralization. Pyrophosphate is a well-described antimineralization molecule that, as early as the 1930s, was shown to inhibit calcium (Ca) crystal buildup when used in small amounts as a water softener. Since that time, substantial research has been conducted to identify the biologic source and roles of pyrophosphate, such that pyrophosphate prevents calcification in soft tissues such as the skin, kidney, and smooth muscles while regulating bone mineralization. Pyrophosphate is regulated in circulation by a group of proteins found primarily within the liver and referred to as the pyrophosphate pump. Adenosine triphosphate (ATP)–binding cassette C subfamily, member 6 (ABCC6) exports ATP from inside the cell to the extracellular space where the enzyme ENPPI cleaves ATP to produce pyrophosphate and AMP (adenosine monophosphate). In addition to extracellular conversion, pyrophosphate also can be produced from ATP intracellularly and exported to the extracellular space by the transporter ANK (ANKH inorganic pyrophosphate transport regulator). Together, this system and enzymes that hydrolyze pyrophosphate to inorganic phosphate tightly regulate circulating pyrophosphate levels, which are critical for proper bone and teeth mineralization. Bisphosphonates are nonhydrolyzable analogues of pyrophosphate. As such, they possess the same antimineralization properties as pyrophosphate but cannot be removed from circulation by using hydrolyzing enzymes. Therefore, the half-lives of bisphosphonates are long, at times being present in the body for years after their initial administration. In addition to their antimineralization properties, bisphosphonates also impair osteoclast activity by inhibiting the HMG-CoA reductase pathway and/or becoming intercalated into DNA as an ATP analogue, thereby inducing cellular apoptosis. Because of their effects on osteoclast activity, the predominant clinical application of bisphosphonates has been concentrated on their antibone resorptive properties.

nausea, and vomiting. These reactions and are effectively managed with anti-inflammatory and antiemetic medications. The more serious acute side effects associated with bisphosphonate therapy in adults (such as osteonecrosis of the jaw and atypical subtrochanteric fractures, uveitis, and thrombocytopenia) are rare in children. Concerns about the effects of bisphosphonates on linear growth have ultimately been quelled by studies that confirm expected growth rates in children with bisphosphonate-treated osteogenesis imperfecta and osteoporosis; some studies have reported improved growth with long-term bisphosphonate therapy, which is likely attributable to the positive effect on vertebral height.[32]

Antibiotics

Antibiotic use is common in pediatric orthopaedic practice for two reasons: (1) the prevalence of spontaneous bone and joint infections among children, and (2) infection is a potentially severe and potentially preventable complication of elective orthopaedic surgery. The broad mechanisms of action are depicted in **Figure 3**.

The antibiotics in current use have actually changed the nature of the infections being treated. For example, methicillin-resistant *Staphylococcus aureus* (MRSA) is rapidly increasing in prevalence as a community-acquired pediatric musculoskeletal infection in many jurisdictions in the United States. MRSA infections can be more severe and difficult to treat than infections caused by methicillin-sensitive *Staphylococcus aureus* (MSSA). Careful, conscientious, and evidence-informed stewardship of antibiotic management is required of both individual clinicians and the medical community if orthopaedic surgeons are to maintain their ability to easily and effectively treat musculoskeletal infections.

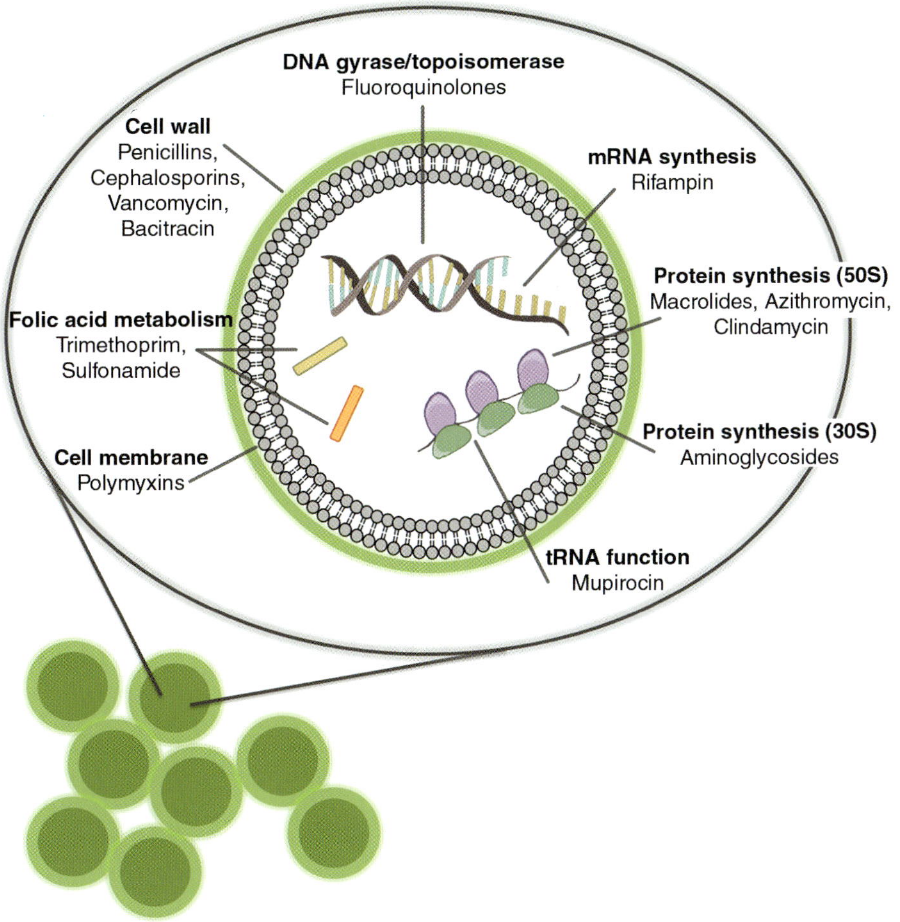

Figure 3 Illustration of the mechanism of action for common classes of antibiotics. Commonly prescribed antibiotics and their target(s) within the pathogen are depicted. Antibiotics are naturally occurring or chemically synthesized compounds that inhibit a wide range of critical bacterial functions. Specifically, antibiotics can impair cell wall and cell membrane structure, function, and synthesis; DNA replication and messenger RNA (mRNA) synthesis; protein production and folding; and cellular metabolism and folic acid synthesis of the pathogen. tRNA = transfer RNA.

Acute Hematogenous Osteomyelitis and Septic Arthritis

Local signs of inflammation and systemic signs of infection characterize hematogenous osteomyelitis; antibiotic treatment alone often is curative.[33] With septic arthritis, initial surgical drainage and irrigation of the joint are the mainstays of treatment, but antibiotic therapy is an important adjunct. In either case, the initial choice of antibiotic therapy is made based on the anatomic location (bone versus joint); the community prevalence of infectious agents; and the age, immunization status, and comorbidities of the patient.

For most children in most locations, *S aureus* is the most common cause of both osteomyelitis and septic arthritis.[33] The ongoing emergence of community-acquired MRSA is likely the most important determinant of the choice of empiric antibiotic coverage. Current recommendations are for a first-generation cephalosporin or antistaphylococcal penicillin if the community prevalence of MSSA is 90% or greater and for clindamycin or vancomycin if the community prevalence of MRSA is 10% or greater. The current prevalence of MRSA is higher than 10% in most states in the United States according to data from the Centers for Disease Control and Prevention.[34]

Recent trends are for a shorter course of intravenous therapy and a shorter total course of treatment of uncomplicated acute osteomyelitis treated within 4 days of symptom onset. A systematic review comparing intravenous dosing regimens of less than 1 week to more than 1 week showed no differences in response rates or complications, a result that has been shown in RCTs and multihospital cohort studies and is the subject of a current systematic review.[35-38] Recommendations for prolonged (6 weeks) intravenous treatment of patients with acute hematogenous osteomyelitis date back to a time when the condition had an appreciable mortality and long-term morbidity, but this is no longer the case in the United States and Europe.[33] Trends in the treatment of septic arthritis are similar—toward a brief course of intravenous antibiotics followed by oral administration—with RCT evidence supporting a shorter course of treatment.[36]

MRSA is not as easy to treat as typical hematogenous osteomyelitis, even if appropriate antibiotic coverage is selected. An initial case series of pediatric musculoskeletal MRSA infections published in 2009 described such infections as a "game changer" and reported that, of 27 children with MRSA musculoskeletal sepsis, 12 children required care in an intensive care unit. Of those 12 children, 5 children required inotrope support, and 4 children required extracorporeal membrane oxygenation in the presence of multisystem organ failure.[39] A later report contrasted MRSA with MSSA and described the pathogenic mechanisms involved, including Panton-Valentine leukocidin genes that produce powerful cytotoxins leading to increased tissue destruction and invasion.[40] MRSA remains associated with longer hospital stays, a higher chance of repeat surgery, and a higher chance of intensive care admission, although not to the extent described in the 2009 report. For patients with MRSA, the appropriate timing for changing from intravenous to oral antibiotic therapy is unknown, and the decision should be based on the clinical course in consultation with infectious disease specialists.

Chronic Osteomyelitis

Chronic osteomyelitis is rare in well-resourced countries but remains very common in less-resourced settings. An established sequestrum (devitalized bone separated from circulation) and an evolving involucrum (new periosteal bone created by a healing process) create an environment where surgical intervention is necessary to remove dead bone, and antibiotics may not be important to achieve healing—at least according to authors with experience in managing chronic osteomyelitis in less-resourced settings.[41] However, patients who are systemically ill with invasive infection should be treated with antibiotics, guided by the particular clinical presentation and the results of a blood culture.[41]

Surgical Prophylaxis

Strong evidence shows that prophylactic antibiotics are important in preventing surgical site infections,[42] although much of this evidence has been derived from adult populations undergoing total joint arthroplasty or spinal instrumentation procedures. A systematic review and meta-analysis found no benefit of additional antibiotics beyond a single preincision dose in closed fracture surgery.[43] Large, single-center retrospective studies have evaluated low-risk orthopaedic procedures in children (including percutaneous pinning of fractures, knee arthroscopy, implant removal, and the excision of benign bone tumors) and have found an equally low infection rate if antibiotic prophylaxis is used in low-risk settings.[44]

Antibiotic Resistance

Antibiotic resistance is an emerging public health crisis that has prompted the development of the National Action Plan for Combating Antibiotic-Resistant Bacteria.[45] According to this plan, the Centers for Disease Control and Prevention estimate that 2 million infections and 23,000 deaths annually occur because of resistant bacteria in the United States; more importantly, epidemiologic trends suggest that without good antibiotic stewardship, the drug resistance problem will continue to worsen. A return to a preantibiotic era where infections were frequently fatal is foreseen and must be avoided. Antibiotic stewardship means prescribing only for appropriate indications, whereas best estimates indicate that approximately 30% of outpatient antibiotic prescriptions in the United States are not clinically indicated.[46]

The widespread use of antibiotics creates selective pressure for the emergence of resistant organisms, a phenomenon predicted by Alexander Fleming in 1946 when he discovered penicillin.[47] Substantial evidence indicates that the clinical use of antibiotics in humans is responsible for much of the development of antibiotic resistance seen today. For example, the rate of prescribing antibiotics to outpatients varies more than threefold across European countries,[48] and a striking positive correlation exists between the volume of antibiotics consumed and the presence of antibiotic resistance across multiple classes of pathogenic bacteria.[48]

More than 15 classes of antibiotics are in current use, and bacterial resistance mechanisms exist for all these classes.[49] Antibiotics are naturally occurring compounds that inhibit a range of critical bacterial functions, including cell wall structure, function, and synthesis; protein production and folding; DNA synthesis and replication; RNA synthesis; and folic acid synthesis[49] (**Figure 3**). Bacteria acquire resistance either gradually by a stepwise process of mutation in relevant chromosomes or more rapidly through the sharing of genetic material by means of bacteriophages, plasmids, naked DNA, or transposons. Drug resistance can be transferred from one bacterium to another across taxonomic groups.[49] Membrane proteins that pump drugs from the bacterial cell can provide resistance to multiple classes of antibiotics simultaneously.[47]

Strategies to prevent and manage drug resistance include tracking the resistance frequency, reducing the prescription of antibiotics, isolating hospital patients with resistant infections, and developing new antibiotic agents.[49] Mathematical modeling supports the empiric observation that resistant organisms appear relatively quickly, but take a much longer time to disappear even if antibiotic use is restricted. However, empiric work from Finland has shown that a national program to restrict the outpatient use of macrolide antibiotics was successful in decreasing the frequency of erythromycin resistance among streptococcal infections.[50]

The development of new antibiotics has always been and will remain an important strategy in combatting resistance. A valid concern is that the pace of discovery and marketing of new antibiotic agents has slowed down.[51] Drug companies are said to have little incentive for the development of new antibiotics because a new antibiotic likely will be prescribed for only brief periods, for chronic use, and it eventually will become worthless when resistance develops. Regulatory agencies often restrict the use of new drugs, even if they are effective, to slow the development of resistance. In addition, the traditional source of antibiotic agents, soil organisms that can be cultured in the laboratory, has perhaps already yielded most of the useful agents possible.[51] Some of these marketplace and regulatory realities need to be considered and addressed by the medical community as part of its social responsibility and extended role in antibiotic stewardship.

A relatively new approach—culturing in soil—has opened up the possibility of discovering natural antibiotics among an estimated remaining 99% of soil organisms that cannot be cultured under traditional laboratory conditions.[52] The first of these new antibiotics, teixobactin, targets a bacterial cell wall lipid and shows high antibacterial activity and low toxicity to mammalian cells. Furthermore, its mechanism of action suggests that it evolved to minimize the development of antibiotic resistance. Other such natural compounds with similarly low susceptibility to resistance are likely present in nature. Thus, the development of new antibiotics and good stewardship of the use of current antibiotics should allow physicians to stay ahead in the antimicrobial arms race.

Summary

The overall treatment and care of pediatric orthopaedic patients is diverse. As such, a variety of pharmaceutical agents is used throughout treatment, including interventional, preoperative, and postoperative care. Common pharmacologic agents include analgesics, vitamin D supplementation, calcium supplementation, bisphosphonates, and antibiotics. Understanding their mechanisms of action, potential adverse side effects, and the pathologic conditions where the therapies are used will aid in providing the best care to pediatric patients.

Key Study Points

- A multimodal therapeutic approach to analgesic use in pediatric patients is paramount.
- Dependency and withdrawal after analgesic administration can occur rapidly in pediatric patients. Physicians should recognize and act on the signs of analgesic dependency and withdrawal.
- The regulation of vitamin D and calcium levels is critical to maintain pediatric bone health.
- Given limited controlled studies, bisphosphonates should be prescribed with caution.
- No FDA-approved therapies currently exist to improve bone regeneration. Off-label uses of therapies must be used with caution.
- Therapeutics and recommendations for the treatment of infection are consistently changing. Pediatric orthopaedic surgeons must stay up-to-date to provide the most informed care. Strategies for minimizing antibiotic resistance are critical in pediatric orthopaedics.

Annotated References

1. McGrath PA: Development of the World Health Organization guidelines on cancer pain relief and palliative care in children. *J Pain Symptom Manage* 1996;12(2):87-92.

2. Ballantyne JC, Kalso E, Stannard C: WHO analgesic ladder: A good concept gone astray. *BMJ* 2016;352:i20.

   This editorial addresses the World Health Organization's analgesic ladder for use in chronic pain. The authors state that although the ladder approach is a valuable tool for guiding the treatment of excruciating and short-lived pain, such an approach is not appropriate for highly complex chronic pain. Level of evidence: V.

3. Drendel AL, Gorelick MH, Weisman SJ, Lyon R, Brousseau DC, Kim MK: A randomized clinical trial of ibuprofen versus acetaminophen with codeine for acute pediatric arm fracture pain. *Ann Emerg Med* 2009;54(4):553-560.

4. Poonai N, Bhullar G, Lin K, et al: Oral administration of morphine versus ibuprofen to manage postfracture pain in children: A randomized trial. *CMAJ* 2014;186(18):1358-1363.

   No important differences in analgesic efficacy were found with the oral administration of morphine or ibuprofen for children with an uncomplicated extremity fracture. However, morphine was associated with a substantially greater number of adverse effects. Level of evidence: I.

5. Ali S, Klassen TP: Ibuprofen was more effective than codeine or acetaminophen for musculoskeletal pain in children. *Evid Based Med* 2007;12(5):144.

6. Borland M, Jacobs I, King B, O'Brien D: A randomized controlled trial comparing intranasal fentanyl to intravenous morphine for managing acute pain in children in the emergency department. *Ann Emerg Med* 2007;49(3):335-340.

7. Ali S, Klassen TP: Intranasal fentanyl and intravenous morphine did not differ for pain relief in children with closed long-bone fractures. *Evid Based Med* 2007;12(6):176.

8. Murphy A, O'Sullivan R, Wakai A, et al: Intranasal fentanyl for the management of acute pain in children. *Cochrane Database Syst Rev* 2014;10(10):CD009942.

   Intranasal fentanyl is an effective treatment of acute moderate to severe pain and appears to cause minimal distress in children. Based on current studies, it cannot be concluded if it is superior or equivalent to intramuscular or intravenous morphine. Level of evidence: II.

9. American Society of Anesthesiologists Task Force on Acute Pain Management: Practice guidelines for acute pain management in the perioperative setting: An updated report by the American Society of Anesthesiologists Task Force on Acute Pain Management. *Anesthesiology* 2012;116(2):248-273.

   Practice guidelines for acute pain management in a perioperative setting were reviewed based on new evidence from scientific literature and findings from surveys of experts. The new evidence did not necessitate a change in practice recommendations. Level of evidence: I.

10. Moore RA, Derry S, Aldington D, Wiffen PJ: Single dose oral analgesics for acute postoperative pain in adults: An overview of Cochrane reviews. *Cochrane Database Syst Rev* 2015;9:CD008659.

    Marked evidence demonstrates the efficacy of single-dose oral analgesics, in both fast-acting formulations and fixed-dose combinations. This review aimed to better inform the choices of both professionals and consumers. Level of evidence: II.

11. Schnabel A, Reichl SU, Zahn PK, Pogatzki-Zahn E: Nalbuphine for postoperative pain treatment in children. *Cochrane Database Syst Rev* 2014;7(7):CD009583.

    Because of insufficient evidence, this systematic review could not definitively show that the efficacy of nalbuphine was superior to a placebo or if nalbuphine treatment resulted in more or fewer adverse events compared with a placebo or other opioid administrations. Level of evidence: II.

12. McNicol ED, Ferguson MC, Hudcova J: Patient controlled opioid analgesia versus non-patient controlled opioid analgesia for postoperative pain. *Cochrane Database Syst Rev* 2015;6(6):CD003348.

    This study provided moderate quality to low quality evidence that patient-controlled analgesia is an effective substitute to non–patient-controlled systemic analgesia for postoperative pain relief. Level of evidence: II.

13. Hayes J, Dowling JJ, Peliowski A, Crawford MW, Johnston B: Patient-controlled analgesia plus background opioid infusion for postoperative pain in children: A systematic review and meta-analysis of randomized trials. *Anesth Analg* 2016; Apr 8 [Epub ahead of print].

    No substantial differences were found in patient pain scores 12 and 24 hours after surgery with the addition of an opioid background infusion to patient-controlled analgesia bolus doses of opioid. Further high-quality studies are required. Level of evidence: II.

14. Lambert P, Cyna AM, Knight N, Middleton P: Clonidine premedication for postoperative analgesia in children. *Cochrane Database Syst Rev* 2014;1(1):CD009633.

    Eleven relevant studies demonstrated that preadministration of clonidine at an adequate dosage of 4 µg/kg was likely to be beneficial for postoperative pain relief in children. Side effects were minimal, yet further research is necessary. Level of evidence: II.

15. Bellon M, Le Bot A, Michelet D, et al: Efficacy of intraoperative dexmedetomidine compared with placebo for postoperative pain management: A meta-analysis of published studies. *Pain Ther* 2016;5(1):63-80.

    A meta-analysis demonstrated that the intraoperative administration of a dexmedetomidine bolus (>0.5 µg/kg) in children reduces postoperative opioid consumption and pain in the PACU. Level of evidence: II.

16. Zhu M, Wang H, Zhu A, Niu K, Wang G: Meta-analysis of dexmedetomidine on emergence agitation and recovery profiles in children after sevoflurane anesthesia: Different administration and different dosage. *PLoS One* 2015;10(4):e0123728.

    Compared with fentanyl and midazolam, dexmedetomidine had no significant difference on the incidence of emergence agitation or postoperative pain in children after sevoflurane anesthesia. Level of evidence: III.

17. Mahmoud M, Mason KP: Dexmedetomidine: Review, update, and future considerations of paediatric perioperative and periprocedural applications and limitations. *Br J Anaesth* 2015;115(2):171-182.

    Because of many favorable therapeutic properties and limited adverse effects, the use of dexmedetomidine in pediatric populations has increased in recent years. This review focused on current pediatric perioperative and periprocedural applications, therapeutic limitations, and considerations for the future. Level of evidence: III.

18. Dahmani S, Michelet D, Abback PS, et al: Ketamine for perioperative pain management in children: A meta-analysis of published studies. *Paediatr Anaesth* 2011;21(6):636-652.

    The administration of ketamine was associated with decreased pain intensity during the PACU stay yet was unable to exhibit a postoperative opioid-sparing effect. Level of evidence: II.

19. Taenzer AH, Clark C: Efficacy of postoperative epidural analgesia in adolescent scoliosis surgery: A meta-analysis. *Paediatr Anaesth* 2010;20(2):135-143.

20. Suresh S, Schaldenbrand K, Wallis B, De Oliveira GS Jr: Regional anaesthesia to improve pain outcomes in paediatric surgical patients: A qualitative systematic review of randomized controlled trials. *Br J Anaesth* 2014;113(3):375-390.

    The objective of this review was to systematically evaluate the use of regional anesthesia techniques to minimize postoperative pain in pediatric patients. Only a limited number of regional anesthesia techniques were demonstrated to substantially improve postoperative pain. Level of evidence: II.

21. Engelman E, Marsala C: Bayesian enhanced meta-analysis of post-operative analgesic efficacy of additives for caudal analgesia in children. *Acta Anaesthesiol Scand* 2012;56(7):817-832.

    Compared with clonidine and tramadol, neostigmine provided the longest postoperative analgesia. Although the duration of analgesia is shorter and sedation is increased with clonidine, it may decrease the potential for postoperative nausea or vomiting. Level of evidence: II.

22. Tong Y, Ren H, Ding X, Jin S, Chen Z, Li Q: Analgesic effect and adverse events of dexmedetomidine as additive for pediatric caudal anesthesia: A meta-analysis. *Paediatr Anaesth* 2014;24(12):1224-1230.

    Dexmedetomidine, when used as an additive to local anesthetic, provides substantially longer postoperative analgesia with comparable adverse effects versus local anesthetic alone in pediatric patients undergoing orchidopexy or lower abdominal surgery. Level of evidence: II.

23. Mar GJ, Barrington MJ, McGuirk BR: Acute compartment syndrome of the lower limb and the effect of postoperative analgesia on diagnosis. *Br J Anaesth* 2009;102(1):3-11.

24. Galinkin J, Koh JL; Committee on Drugs; Section on Anesthesiology and Pain Medicine; American Academy of Pediatrics: Recognition and management of iatrogenically induced opioid dependence and withdrawal in children. *Pediatrics* 2014;133(1):152-155.

    The frequent dosing of an opioid can result in dependence in as few as 5 days. Currently, no recommendations are available for managing withdrawal in pediatric populations. This guideline aimed to summarize the existing literature and provide recommendations for treating pediatric populations. Level of evidence: III.

25. Dabisch-Ruthe M, Kuzaj P, Götting C, Knabbe C, Hendig D: Pyrophosphates as a major inhibitor of matrix calcification in pseudoxanthoma elasticum. *J Dermatol Sci* 2014;75(2):109-120.

    Pyrophosphate is a critical circulating compound that prevents matrix calcification in pseudoxanthoma elasticum. Therefore, supplementation of pyrophosphate analogues such as bisphosphonates may be therapeutically advantageous for treating pseudoxanthoma elasticum and related disorders. Level of evidence: II.

26. Uitto J, Jiang Q, Váradi A, Bercovitch LG, Terry SF: Pseudoxanthoma elasticum: Diagnostic features, classification, and treatment options. *Expert Opin Orphan Drugs* 2014;2(6):567-577.

    Alterations to diet can influence the severity of the mineralization phenotype found in mice with mutations in the *ABCC6* gene. Clinically, these observations suggest the use of dietary intervention and lifestyle modification in patients with pseudoxanthoma elasticum. Level of evidence: III.

27. Misra M, Pacaud D, Petryk A, Collett-Solberg PF, Kappy M; Drug and Therapeutics Committee of the Lawson Wilkins Pediatric Endocrine Society: Vitamin D deficiency in children and its management: Review of current knowledge and recommendations. *Pediatrics* 2008;122(2):398-417.

28. Russell RG: Bisphosphonates: The first 40 years. *Bone* 2011;49(1):2-19.

    This review discussed the history, molecular mechanisms, biologic effects, and development of different classes of bisphosphonates.

29. Weisberg P, Scanlon KS, Li R, Cogswell ME: Nutritional rickets among children in the United States: Review of cases reported between 1986 and 2003. *Am J Clin Nutr* 2004;80(6suppl):1697S-1705S.

30. Wagner CL, Greer FR; American Academy of Pediatrics Section on Breastfeeding; American Academy of Pediatrics Committee on Nutrition: Prevention of rickets and vitamin D deficiency in infants, children, and adolescents. *Pediatrics* 2008;122(5):1142-1152.

31. Ohba T, Cates JM, Cole HA, et al: Pleiotropic effects of bisphosphonates on osteosarcoma. *Bone* 2014;63:110-120.

    Bisphosphonates possess a diverse inhibitory effect on osteosarcoma by activating apoptosis and inhibiting cellular proliferation, inhibiting the expression of vascular endothelial growth factor A and vascular endothelial growth factor receptor 1 in osteosarcoma tumor cells, inhibiting tumor-induced angiogenesis, and directly inhibiting action on endothelial cells.

32. Thomas IH, DiMeglio LA: Advances in the classification and treatment of osteogenesis imperfecta. *Curr Osteoporos Rep* 2016;14(1):1-9.

Osteogenesis imperfecta, a rare collagen disorder characterized by an increased susceptibility to bony fractures, is now routinely treated with bisphosphonates. New therapies, such as anabolic agents, transforming growth factor-β antibodies, and other antiresorptive drugs, are currently under development. Level of evidence: III.

33. Peltola H, Pääkkönen M: Acute osteomyelitis in children. *N Engl J Med* 2014;370(4):352-360.

This article reviewed the epidemiology, diagnosis, and treatment of osteomyelitis in children.

34. Methicillin-resistant: *Staphylococcus aureus* (MRSA): MRSA tracking. Centers for Disease Control and Prevention. Available at: http://www.cdc.gov/mrsa/tracking/. Accessed June 27, 2016.

The number and kind of MRSA infections throughout the United States are tracked using the National Healthcare Safety Network and the Emerging Infections Program.

35. Le Saux N, Howard A, Barrowman NJ, Gaboury I, Sampson M, Moher D: Shorter courses of parenteral antibiotic therapy do not appear to influence response rates for children with acute hematogenous osteomyelitis: A systematic review. *BMC Infect Dis* 2002;2:16.

36. Peltola H, Pääkkönen M, Kallio P, Kallio MJ; Osteomyelitis-Septic Arthritis (OM-SA) Study Group: Prospective, randomized trial of 10 days versus 30 days of antimicrobial treatment, including a short-term course of parenteral therapy, for childhood septic arthritis. *Clin Infect Dis* 2009;48(9):1201-1210.

37. Zaoutis T, Localio AR, Leckerman K, Saddlemire S, Bertoch D, Keren R: Prolonged intravenous therapy versus early transition to oral antimicrobial therapy for acute osteomyelitis in children. *Pediatrics* 2009;123(2):636-642.

38. Grimbly C, Odenbach J, Vandermeer B, Forgie S, Curtis S: Parenteral and oral antibiotic duration for treatment of pediatric osteomyelitis: A systematic review protocol. *Syst Rev* 2013;2:92.

This systematic review updated the literature on best practices in treating pediatric osteomyelitis with either short- or long-term parenteral antibiotics. The effect of either treatment on clinical outcomes will be evaluated at the completion of the study. Level of evidence: II.

39. Vander Have KL, Karmazyn B, Verma M, et al: Community-associated methicillin-resistant Staphylococcus aureus in acute musculoskeletal infection in children: A game changer. *J Pediatr Orthop* 2009;29(8):927-931.

40. Sarkissian EJ, Gans I, Gunderson MA, Myers SH, Spiegel DA, Flynn JM: Community-acquired methicillin-resistant Staphylococcus aureus musculoskeletal infections: Emerging trends over the past decade. *J Pediatr Orthop* 2016;36(3):323-327.

At the Children's Hospital of Philadelphia, community-acquired pediatric MRSA musculoskeletal infections increased threefold, and the risk for complications during inpatient management were elevated. Regional epidemiologic trends will help facilitate timely and accurate clinical diagnosis and treatment. Level of evidence: II.

41. Jones HW, Beckles VL, Akinola B, Stevenson AJ, Harrison WJ: Chronic haematogenous osteomyelitis in children: An unsolved problem. *J Bone Joint Surg Br* 2011;93(8):1005-1010.

Chronic hematogenous osteomyelitis in pediatric populations remains a major cause of musculoskeletal morbidity. Following a review of the current literature, this review highlighted areas where research might improve treatment of this condition. Level of evidence: III.

42. Tsai DM, Caterson EJ: Current preventive measures for health-care associated surgical site infections: A review. *Patient Saf Surg* 2014;8(1):42.

Healthcare-associated infections impose a tremendous cost on the healthcare system annually and impose substantial patient morbidity and mortality. This review aimed to discuss the etiology of healthcare-associated infections and successful preventive measures used preoperatively, intraoperatively, and postoperatively. Level of evidence: III.

43. Slobogean GP, Kennedy SA, Davidson D, O'Brien PJ: Single- versus multiple-dose antibiotic prophylaxis in the surgical treatment of closed fractures: A meta-analysis. *J Orthop Trauma* 2008;22(4):264-269.

44. Formaini N, Jacob P, Willis L, Kean JR: Evaluating the use of preoperative antibiotics in pediatric orthopaedic surgery. *J Pediatr Orthop* 2012;32(7):737-740.

Prophylactic antibiotics may not be necessary for less invasive procedures when performed in a low-risk pediatric population because the incidence of infection did not substantially increase when antibiotics were not administered before surgery. Level of evidence: III.

45. White House: *National Action Plan for Combatting Antibiotic-Resistant Bacteria*. 2015. Available at: https://www.whitehouse.gov/sites/default/files/docs/national_action_plan_for_combating_antibotic-resistant_bacteria.pdf. Accessed June 20, 2016.

This plan to guide the United States in combating antibiotic-resistant bacteria was developed in response to an Executive Order issued by President Barack Obama in September 2014.

46. Fleming-Dutra KE, Hersh AL, Shapiro DJ, et al: Prevalence of inappropriate antibiotic prescriptions among US ambulatory care visits, 2010-2011. *JAMA* 2016;315(17):1864-1873.

In the United States between 2010 and 2011, of the 506 antibiotic prescriptions per 1,000 patients prescribed, only

353 prescriptions were likely appropriate, indicating a need for establishing a standard for outpatient antibiotic administration to better combat antibiotic-resistant bacteria. Level of evidence: II.

47. Alekshun MN, Levy SB: Molecular mechanisms of antibacterial multidrug resistance. *Cell* 2007;128(6):1037-1050.

48. Goossens H, Ferech M, Vander Stichele R, Elseviers M, Group EP; ESAC Project Group: Outpatient antibiotic use in Europe and association with resistance: A cross-national database study. *Lancet* 2005;365(9459):579-587.

49. Levy SB, Marshall B: Antibacterial resistance worldwide: Causes, challenges and responses. *Nat Med* 2004;10(12suppl):S122-S129.

50. Seppälä H, Klaukka T, Vuopio-Varkila J, et al; Finnish Study Group for Antimicrobial Resistance: The effect of changes in the consumption of macrolide antibiotics on erythromycin resistance in group A streptococci in Finland. *N Engl J Med* 1997;337(7):441-446.

51. Wright G: Antibiotics: An irresistible newcomer. *Nature* 2015;517(7535):442-444.

The author presented findings that suggest that a systematic search for gram-negative bacteria producing antibiotics that target gram-positive cell walls could identify other resistance-like antibiotics.

52. Ling LL, Schneider T, Peoples AJ, et al: A new antibiotic kills pathogens without detectable resistance. *Nature* 2015;517(7535):455-459.

Teixobactin, a new antibiotic discovered from a screen of uncultured bacteria, is able to inhibit cell wall synthesis and kill gram-positive bacteria. The method of cultivation suggests a new path toward the development of antibiotics that are able to avoid developing resistance.

Section 3

Neuromuscular, Metabolic, and Inflammatory Disorders

SECTION EDITOR:
Henry G. Chambers, MD

Chapter 11

Cerebral Palsy

Nirav K. Pandya, MD Scott P. Kaiser, MD

Abstract

Cerebral palsy is a nonprogressive disorder of movement, tone, and posture that is caused by injury to the immature brain in the prenatal, perinatal, or postnatal periods. The clinical manifestations of this disorder vary widely based on the location and degree of injury to the motor cortex. In addition, other areas of the brain may be affected, which leads to cognitive, speech, and sensory difficulties. Multiple advances have been made in the treatment of this disorder over the past several years.

Keywords: cerebral palsy; motor function; neuromuscular; spasticity; treatment

Introduction

Cerebral palsy (CP) is a nonprogressive disorder that affects movement, tone, and posture and is caused by injury to the immature brain. Brain injury occurs early in development, in the prenatal, perinatal, or postnatal periods. The location and degree of injury to the motor cortex affects the clinical manifestations of CP. Other areas of the brain also may be affected, leading to cognitive, speech, and sensory difficulties. Over the past several years, multiple advances have been made in the treatment of patients with CP.

Dr. Pandya or an immediate family member serves as a paid consultant to Histogenics and Orthopediatrics and serves as a board member, owner, officer, or committee member of the Pediatric Orthopaedic Society of North America. Neither Dr. Kaiser nor any immediate family member has received anything of value from or has stock or stock options held in a commercial company or institution related directly or indirectly to the subject of this chapter.

Epidemiology

CP is the most common neuromuscular disorder in children and currently has a prevalence ranging from 1.5 to 4 individuals per 1,000 live births.[1] Approximately 1 in 323 children is identified with cerebral palsy.[2] In particular, low birth weight (less than 1,500 g) drastically increases the risk of this condition.[3] Additional risk factors include premature birth (before 31 weeks) and multiple births (ie, twins or triplets).[4,5]

In addition to motor disease, nearly 50% of patients have concurrent epilepsy.[2] Other manifestations include cognitive impairment, sensory deficits, strabismus, gastrointestinal dysfunction, impaired oral motor function, decreased bone mass, spasticity, contractures, urinary incontinence, and emotional and behavioral problems. Functionally, approximately 60% of patients with CP are able to walk independently, approximately 10% use a mobility device, and approximately 30% have limited or no walking ability.[2]

Etiology

The etiology of CP in most patients is unknown. Although prematurity combined with very low birth weight is a risk factor, full-term birth is more common than premature birth in patients with CP. Prenatal, perinatal, and postnatal causes also should be considered. In the prenatal period, congenital brain defects, intrauterine infections, placental complications, Rh/ABO hemolytic disease, fetal anoxia, coagulopathies, and maternal disease (ie, seizure, hyperthyroidism, and chorioamnionitis) should be considered. Ischemic stroke is a major cause of CP in the perinatal period. Intracranial hemorrhage, hypoglycemia, trauma, hypoxic ischemic encephalopathy, infection, and hypothyroidism also are possible causes. A very small number of cases are caused by obstetric trauma. Possible postnatal causes of CP also include hypoxia, acidosis, bacterial meningitis, viral encephalitis, hyperbilirubinemia, traumatic brain injury, and toxin exposure. The common link, regardless of the specific etiology, is an insult to the developing motor system of the brain. This can include the motor cortex, but also includes the periventricular regions of the brain and, in those with associated dystonia, the basal ganglia.

Diagnosis

Prior to the initiation of treatment, an appropriate diagnosis should be made. Because of the varied manifestations of the disorder, making a diagnosis of CP can be challenging for the clinician. From a global standpoint, a patient with a developmental delay and/or persistence of primitive reflexes may have CP. Many patients do not achieve gross motor milestones such as head control by age 2 months, the ability to sit by age 6 months, or the ability to walk by age 14 months. On physical examination, patients may exhibit preferential use of limbs and abnormal tone. The differential diagnosis should include other metabolic or neurodegenerative disorders, particularly if the neurologic manifestations are progressive or there is a loss of previously acquired motor milestones.[6] Laboratory studies can be used to investigate genetic, metabolic, and endocrine disorders. Although MRI findings have been shown to be abnormal in 86% of patients with CP (patients with ataxia are more likely to have normal MRI findings), there is substantial heterogeneity in the clinical meaning of these imaging findings.[7] As a result, CP is usually diagnosed using clinical methods.

Classification

Accurate classification of CP also can be challenging because of its heterogeneous presentations. Geographic, physiologic, and functional classifications have been developed. The pattern of limb involvement is described by the geographic classification and is a reflection of the location of the insult to the motor cortex. Monoplegia (the involvement of one limb), hemiplegia (the involvement of both limbs on the same side), diplegia (greater involvement of both lower limbs than both upper limbs), and quadriplegia/tetraplegia (all four limbs equally involved) are common geographic terms used to describe CP. Poor reliability has been reported with this classification system.[8]

Even in instances in which the geographic classification accurately describes the pattern of limb involvement, the manner in which the involvement manifests can vary. The physiologic classification attempts to describe the nature of the involvement. In the most common form, spastic, patients exhibit an increase in muscle tone with rapid passive stretching. Joint contractures are frequently present in patients with spasticity.[2,9] Spasticity is a stretch reflex disorder that involves the pyramidal area of the brain. It is both velocity dependent (worse when the stretch is faster) and length dependent (worse when the muscle is shorter).

When CP involves the extrapyramidal areas of the brain, patients exhibit dyskinesia, which manifests as involuntary motor movements. Athetosis (purposeless movements with rare joint contractures), choreiform (continual purposeless movements), and dystonia (increased tone without spasticity, clonus, or hyperreflexia) may be present. Rigidity may be present in patients with severe involvement, but this manifestation is rare in children with CP. If the cerebellum is involved, patients may exhibit ataxia. This condition is less common and involves difficulty with coordinated movements and balance, particularly walking. In addition, some patients may be hypotonic and exhibit low muscle tone in the context of normal reflexes.

Not all patients can receive an accurate diagnosis using these specific physiologic definitions, because some patients may have a mixture of disease manifestations resulting from injury to multiple overlapping areas of the brain.[9]

From an orthopaedic standpoint, interventions are chosen to optimize function. Although terms such as household ambulator and community ambulator attempt to capture the functional ability of patients with CP, they do not recognize the unique functional needs of this patient population. The Gross Motor Function Classification System (GMFCS) describes the functional abilities of patients with developmental differences[10] (**Figure 1**). Different age-based criteria have been developed.[11] The GMFCS focuses on functional limitations for certain motor tasks such as walking and sitting as well as the need for assistive devices. This system has been shown to be reliable for classifying patients and helping to determine proper interventions.[11-13]

Goal Setting

The orthopaedic surgeon is one member of a multidisciplinary team of healthcare providers that should be involved in the management of patients with CP. The clinicians should be able to make a correct diagnosis; determine the etiology of the disease (if possible); identify the type, extent, and severity of the neuromuscular deficit; and address any associated conditions. Multiple aspects of the patient's condition should be addressed, including the interplay between pathophysiology, organ dysfunction, task performance, roles (responsibilities in society), and the various influences of each of these factors.[14] In combination with the family and other healthcare providers, goals need to be established that address independence,

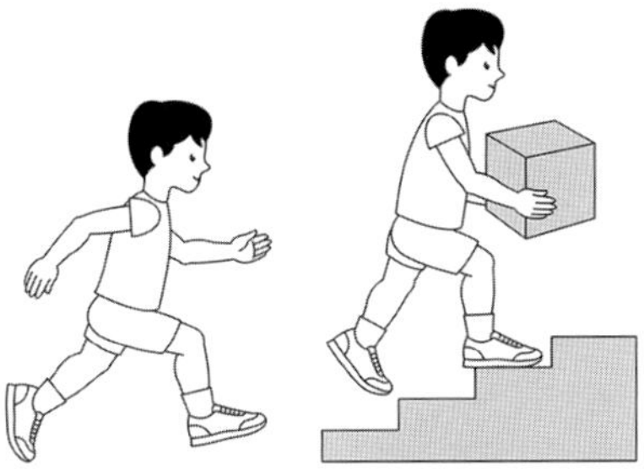

GMFCS Level I
Children walk at home, school, outdoors, and in the comunity. They can climb stairs without the use of a railing. Children perform gross motor skills such as running and jumping, but speed, balance, and coordination are limited.

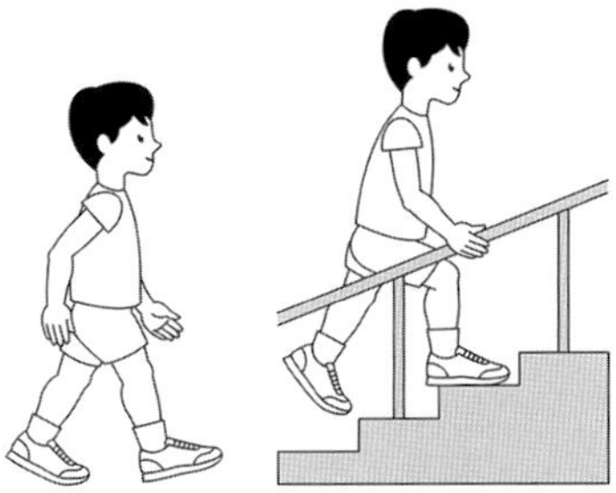

GMFCS Level II
Children walk in most settings and climb stairs holding onto a railing. They may experience difficulty walking long distances and balancing on uneven terrain, inclines, in crowded areas or confined spaces. Children may walk with physical assistance, a hand-held mobility device, or use wheeled mobility over long distances. Children have only minimal ability to perform gross motor skills such as running and jumping

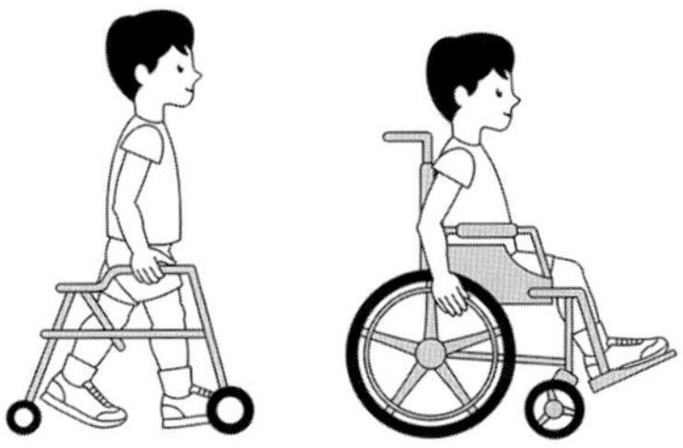

GMFCS Level III
Children walk using a hand-held mobility device in most indoor settings. They may climb stairs holding onto a railing with supervision or assistance. Children use wheeled mobility when traveling long distances and may self-propel for shorter distances.

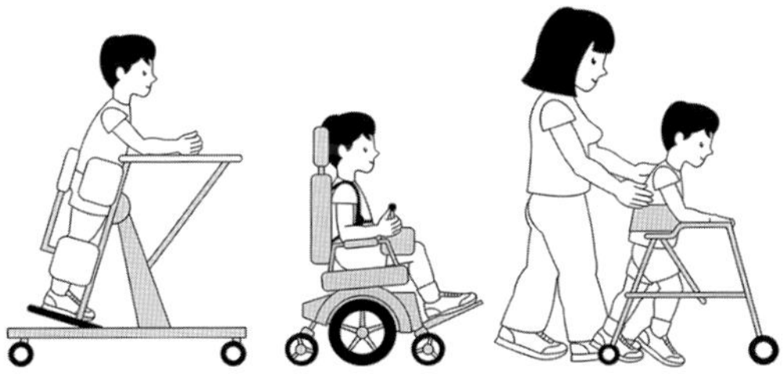

GMFCS Level IV
Children use methods of mobility that require physical assistance or powered mobility in most settings. They may walk for short distances at home with physical assistance or use powered mobility or a body support walker when positioned. At school, outdoors, and in the community, children are transported in a manual wheelchair or use powered mobility.

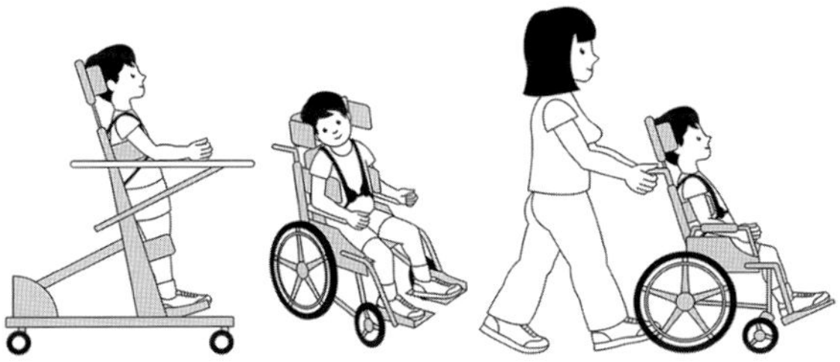

GMFCS Level V
Children are transported in a manual wheelchair in all settings. Children are limited in their ability to maintain antigravity head and trunk postures and control leg and arm movements.

Figure 1 Illustration of the Expanded and Revised Gross Motor Function Classification System (GMFCS) for children between the ages of 6 and 12 years. (Copyright Kerr Graham, Bill Reid, and Adrienne Harvey, The Royal Children's Hospital, Melbourne, Australia.)

working, communication, activities of daily living, mobility, and walking. It is important for clinicians to balance the perceived benefits of any intervention with the risks of disruption to education, social relationships, future employment, and independence. The clinicians and family should discuss treatments intended to correct the secondary issues resulting from the brain insult, not methods to reverse the brain injury.

Because goal setting for many caregivers focuses on the patient's ability to walk, clinicians should set realistic goals and discourage unrealistic expectations. Prognostic factors for poor ambulatory ability include the persistence of two or more primitive reflexes after age 1 year and the inability to sit independently by age 2 years.[15,16] It is critical to balance the patient's desire to walk with other desires such as the abilities to communicate and be mobile (not necessarily to achieve ambulation).

Nonorthopaedic Treatment

Multiple nonsurgical and surgical treatment modalities are at the disposal of the clinician. A recent systematic review found the following interventions effective in the treatment of patients with CP: botulinum toxin, diazepam/baclofen, and selective dorsal rhizotomy for reducing muscle spasticity; casting for improving and maintaining ankle range of motion; hip surveillance for maintaining hip joint integrity; various physical and occupational therapy programs for improving motor activity, self-care, and fitness; bisphosphonates (also known as diphosphonates) for treating low bone mineral density; pressure care for preventing ulcers; and anticonvulsant administration for managing seizures.[17]

Physical Therapy

Physical therapy is critical in the treatment of patients with CP, particularly before age 3 years and in postoperative periods. A recent study demonstrated a positive effect in older children with CP, but the largest effect was seen in younger patients and those with level II GMFCS.[18] However, the efficacy of physical therapy on the long-term function of patients with CP remains controversial. In a recent study that evaluated the effect of exercise on postural control in children with CP, the effectiveness of five interventions—gross motor task training, hippotherapy (horseback riding), treadmill training with no body-weight supported, trunk-targeted training, and reactive balance training—was supported by a moderate level of evidence.[19] Regardless of the type of physical therapy chosen, it is important that therapy programs do not place an undue burden on caregivers or unnecessarily disrupt the child's education.

Oral Medications

Oral medications such as baclofen and diazepam (gamma-aminobutyric acid receptor agonists) both act on spasticity by reducing muscle tone but also can cause sedation, balance and cognitive dysfunction, increased drooling, increased drug tolerance, and drug withdrawal symptoms because of their central mechanism of action. A recent systematic review demonstrated insufficient data to promote or refute oral baclofen for reducing spasticity or improving motor function in children with spastic CP.[20]

Botulinum Toxin

Botulinum toxin is derived from *Clostridium botulinum* and works at the neuromuscular junction by preventing the release of acetylcholine. Although there are several forms of botulinum toxin, only types A and B are available for use in the United States. Type A toxin, which has been available for the longest amount of time, lacks many of the systemic and regional anticholinergic effects of type B toxin and more data are available regarding its use in patients with CP. Although botulinum toxin has not been approved by the FDA for patients with CP, it has been used off-label for many years. Injections are performed in the affected muscles in the location where there is a preponderance of neuromuscular junctions. It is used to treat local and dynamic spasticity and can remain effective for 3 to 6 months. Botulinum toxin has been shown to be effective when combined with physiotherapy in the upper limbs and improves ease of care and comfort for nonambulatory children.[21,22]

Intrathecal Baclofen

Because of its local administration, intrathecal baclofen has a much lower risk of systemic side effects compared with oral baclofen. It is administered via a pump, which is implanted in the submuscular tissue of the anterior abdomen. The pump can be controlled by a clinician, who may vary the dosage based on the patient's clinical presentation. These pumps are generally used in nonambulatory patients with severe spasticity. A recent systematic review demonstrated a short-term benefit in the treatment of spasticity, with limited long-term data suggesting continued efficacy.[23] Complications with this treatment modality include infection, catheter problems, and pump malfunction. Because of limited battery life, these pumps should be reimplanted every 6 to 7 years. In addition, there is some concern that the incidence or progression of scoliosis is increased after pump insertion.

Selective Dorsal Rhizotomy

Selective dorsal rhizotomy is a procedure that decreases spasticity by selectively cutting the dorsal afferent nerve fibers from L1 to S1. The ideal patient for this procedure is generally ambulatory, has spastic diplegia, and is aged 3 to 8 years. A preoperative evaluation is needed to assess the patient's ambulatory ability and strength (which should be good, particularly in the trunk) as well as his or her motivation and cognitive ability to engage in intensive physical therapy. A multidisciplinary healthcare team is necessary to assess a patient's suitability for the procedure and ensure a good postoperative outcome. Although reported results have been mixed, a recent retrospective review demonstrated that the benefits of selective dorsal rhizotomy lasted throughout adolescence and early adulthood, particularly in patients with spastic diplegia at levels I through III GMFCS.[24] The benefits include improved muscle tone, gross motor function, and activities of daily living performance, and a decreased need for orthopaedic procedures and botulinum toxin injections.

Orthopaedic Treatment

Upper Extremity

Surgical treatment of upper extremity contractures in patients with CP focuses on promoting functional gains. For example, various treatments can be used to limit elbow postural flexion that occurs while running or performing activities, which is a common problem for these patients. Splinting and botulinum toxin injections can be used to prevent progressive and fixed contractures, including adduction at the shoulder, flexion at the elbow, pronation of the forearm, flexion of the wrist, adduction of the thumb into the palm, or flexion of the fingers. Surgery to achieve better cosmesis, such as repositioning the wrist, may alleviate anxiety about the social stigma of CP and may be considered for the cognitively aware patient.

The most common upper extremity contracture in CP results from spasticity and leads to imbalance in the forearm musculature. The deformity is a combination of forearm pronation, wrist flexion and adduction, with opposition of the thumb into the palm. Forearm pronation can be addressed with tenotomy or transfer of the pronator teres. Wrist flexion can be addressed with transfer of the flexor carpi ulnaris to the extensor carpi radialis brevis or common digital extensors, or a wrist fusion in the setting of fixed contracture. Thumb-in-palm deformity can be addressed with adductor pollicis release and extensor pollicis longus transfer from the third extensor compartment to the first extensor compartment. A prospective multicenter study at the Shriner's Hospital for Children network examined forearm surgery (including transfer of the flexor carpi ulnaris to the extensor carpi radialis brevis, pronator teres release, and extensor pollicis longus rerouting with adductor pollicis release) in children with CP and adequate selective control.[25] The authors reported that surgery achieved substantial sustained improvements compared with botulinum toxin injections and continued physical therapy.

A thorough patient assessment can help evaluate potential functional gains from surgery. When assessing the need for surgical intervention, specifically at the wrist, activity measurement tools can be helpful. Physical examination measurements such as range of motion have been shown to have poor correlation with measurements of activity. The Assisting Hand Assessment and the Shriners Hospital Upper Extremity Evaluation Dynamic Positional Analyses have been validated as activity limitation measurement tools.[26] Gripping ability may be improved by repositioning the wrist; however, adequate selective control of finger extension and flexion should exist. The grasp and release test can be performed to assess whether the patient can position his or her fingers with the wrist extended. Patients are given six objects to grasp, lift, and release to test their level of functioning, including lateral pinch and palmar grasp. Without adequate selective control, functional gains will not occur with surgical correction. When selective control is present, fusion of the wrist in the neutral position may enable grip, even in a child who could not grip before surgery. In patients without selective control or potential use of the hand, surgical release may be necessary to facilitate proper hygiene when nonsurgical management is unsuccessful.

Shoulder adduction and elbow contractures are often associated with more severe CP. Shoulder adduction can be improved with intramuscular lengthening of the pectoralis major. Elbow contractures can be improved with release of the lacertus fibrosus, lengthening of the biceps and brachialis tendons, and anterior capsule release. Postoperative extension casting with long-term intermittent splinting is needed to maintain the gains in range of motion made possible by these surgical procedures.

Spine

Indications for spine fusion in patients with CP are currently being debated. The risk-to-benefit ratio should be evaluated for each patient, especially those with level V GMFCS.[27] Neuromuscular scoliosis may be progressive after skeletal maturity. Bracing will not alter the course of the scoliosis but can potentially influence sitting balance. Spinal fusion is indicated when a curve is progressive and sitting balance is compromised. The goals of fusion are to establish a balanced spine and a level pelvis.

After a 2013 systematic review highlighted the paucity of evidence on surgical site infections in pediatric spine surgery,[28] more recent studies on spinal fusion have focused on identifying risk factors for complications.[29-34] A recent prospective cohort study reported a 39% rate of major perioperative complications after spine surgery in patients with CP. Surgical blood loss was the only important independent risk factor for major perioperative complications.[29] Blood loss in posterior spinal fusion is greater in patients with neuromuscular scoliosis resulting from CP than in patients with idiopathic scoliosis. Patients with active seizure disorders also have an increased risk of intraoperative complications. The presence of a gastrostomy or gastrojejunostomy tube is associated with an increased risk of perioperative complications, and patients with these devices are susceptible to and should be monitored for postoperative pancreatitis.[30] Patients with CP have an increased risk of infection after posterior spinal fusion compared with other patient populations. A recent multicenter prospective study of posterior spinal fusion in patients with CP reported a 6.4% infection rate and identified the presence of gastrostomy and gastrojejunostomy tubes, a higher preoperative serum white blood cell count, and longer surgical time as risk factors for infection.[31]

When perioperative complications and postoperative infection are successfully avoided, the results of spinal fusion in patients with CP can be positive, with good correction and improved sitting balance. Fixation to the pelvis is recommended; however, this can lead to complications associated with loss of fixation or skin complications associated with prominent implants.[32] The Luque-Galveston fixation technique and fixation with a unit rod are widely accepted procedures but are being replaced in many medical centers by third-generation hook and pedicle screw constructs.[33] A recent historical cohort study compared rigid constructs (with pedicle screws and iliac screw fixation with or without sacral screw fixation) with nonrigid constructs (with sublaminar wires). The study found lower pseudarthrosis rates with modern, rigid constructs.[34]

Neuromuscular scoliosis and neuromuscular hip dislocation are very common in children with CP, and both conditions increase in frequency and severity with increased GMFCS levels. Dislocation of a reduced hip is common after spinal fusion. If the dislocated hip is the down hip, it is more likely to become painful after dislocation.[35] Therefore, assessment of the hips before and after spinal fusion is crucial.

Hip

Treatment for neuromuscular hip subluxation can be divided into proactive and reactive strategies. Proactive strategies aim to slow the progression of subluxation and prevent dislocation. The goals are to prevent pain and progressive limitations in perineal care. A prevention strategy coupling radiographic surveillance with proactive surgical treatment can nearly eliminate hip dislocations in patients with CP. This was demonstrated by a prevention program undertaken in Sweden that eliminated hip dislocations in the CP population over a 20-year period.[36] Beginning at age 2 years, the hips of children with CP should be monitored with annual pelvic radiography up to age 5 years in ambulatory patients (levels I through III GMFCS) and up to skeletal maturity in nonambulatory patients (levels IV and V GMFCS). Monitoring may be discontinued at these end points if the hip is normal. If subluxation is present, the Reimer migration index is used to measure the progression of subluxation (**Figure 2**). When the Reimer migration index exceeds the 50% threshold, hip reconstruction is recommended.[37]

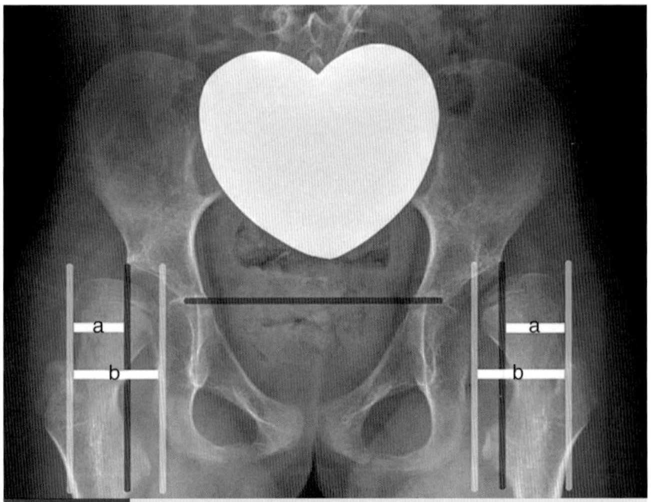

Figure 2 Pelvic radiograph shows parameters for measuring the Reimer migration index. The index equals a divided by b and is measured by drawing lines perpendicular to the axis of the triradiate cartilage at the lateral acetabular margins (black lines). Parallel lines are drawn at the lateral and medial margins of the proximal femoral physis (white lines). The Reimer migration index is the ratio of the width of the femoral head lateral to the acetabulum (a) divided by the total width of the femoral head (b).

Two osseous components, coxa valga and acetabular dysplasia, contribute to neuromuscular hip subluxation. In this condition, the femur is characterized by the persistence of immature hip morphology. At birth, coxa valga with increased anteversion is present in the proximal femur. A delay in walking prevents the normal pressure relationship between the femoral head and the acetabulum. Without early weight bearing, and in the setting of muscle spasticity (especially spasticity of the adductor and flexor muscles) and weakness of the hip extensor and abductor muscles, the neck-shaft angle and anteversion of the femur remain increased, and the triradiate cartilage is not stimulated to cover the femoral head with a deep acetabulum.

In the femur, coxa valga and excess anteversion can be treated with proximal varus derotation osteotomy. The goal is to maximize coverage of the femoral head at the time of surgery. The amount of varus depends on the child's preoperative ambulatory status and the potential for future ambulation. Hip coverage can be improved by increasing the degree of varus correction, but varus greater than 110° to 115° increases the risks of excessive shortening of the abductors and impairment of postoperative gait.

Acetabular dysplasia in CP is characterized by superior and posterior insufficiency. Therefore, incomplete osteotomies (eg, Pemberton, Dega, San Diego, and incomplete periacetabular osteotomies) are recommended over a complete innominate osteotomy (as described by Salter). The Pemberton and Dega osteotomies provide more anterior coverage and are not recommended for patients with levels IV and V GMFCS who have posterior acetabular insufficiency.

Maximizing coverage of the femoral head during hip reconstruction is important because the muscle imbalance that preceded the reconstruction will persist after the reconstruction. Unlike in developmental dysplasia of the hip, redirecting the femoral head toward the triradiate cartilage in neuromuscular hip subluxation does not reliably stimulate acetabular remodeling around the femoral head with continued growth. The risk of redislocation is proportional to potential growth remaining and disease severity. A retrospective study of 144 hips in 75 patients showed that progressive subluxation after hip reconstruction does not occur in levels II and III GMFCS hips but does occur in levels IV and V GMFCS hips.[38]

If a hip dislocates, the decision for hip reconstruction or salvage should take into consideration the patient's ambulatory status and level of pain, as well as the radiographic characteristics of the hip. A hip that remains subluxated will have progressive wear from the capsule and spastic abductor muscles. Because obvious wear can generate pain, reducing an arthritic femoral head into the acetabulum may be ill advised. In this case, salvage surgery is an option (**Figure 3**). Techniques include proximal femoral resection (Castle procedure) or proximal femoral valgus osteotomy with or without resection of the femoral head or neck.

The Castle procedure was originally described with a required period of 3 months of postoperative traction. A recent study reported improved success rates without postoperative traction.[39] A 2014 systematic review of salvage surgeries for painful dislocated hips in patients with CP found that each technique had approximately a 70% success rate. Complications included persistent pain, heterotopic ossification, and skin ulceration.[40]

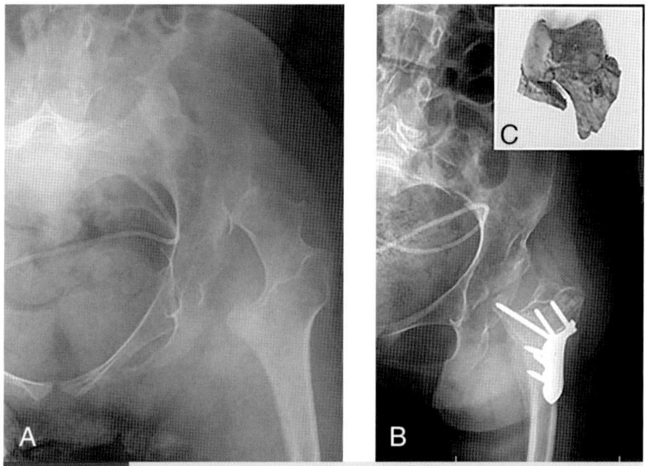

Figure 3 Radiographic images from a patient with cerebral palsy and level IV GMFCS who had severe groin pain in the left hip. **A,** AP pelvic radiograph shows a dislocated left hip, with extensive wear of the lateral femoral head. **B,** The patient was treated with salvage hip reconstruction. **C,** At the time of surgery, the resected femoral head showed severe wear laterally with destruction of the articular surface and exposed epiphyseal bone. After surgery, there was immediate improvement in pain; however, spasms continued for 8 months after surgery.

Lower Extremity Surgery in Ambulatory Children

The surgical treatment of gait abnormalities in children with CP involves addressing contractures that prevent joint range of motion at various levels (the hip, knee, and ankle), as well as realigning the rotation of the long bones. These procedures are done to improve kinetics and gait efficiency.

The decision for or against surgical treatment depends on the nature of the patient's disability and the potential for successful rehabilitation. Children with CP may have neurologic manifestations such as dystonia, ataxia, or choreoathetosis that limit gait and will not be improved by surgery. There may be an underlying weakness that prevents ambulation or behavioral or cognitive limitations that prevent participation in preoperative and/or postoperative therapy. These limitations can result in failed improvement in joint contractures or in malrotation. Inappropriate or excessive lengthening of tendons can decrease the patient's motor strength, and the surgeon should always consider the risk of an ambulatory child becoming nonambulatory after a major orthopaedic intervention.

Quantitative three-dimensional gait analysis provides substantial research benefits and serves as a clinical tool to analyze the relationship among forces (center of mass, ground reaction force, kinetics), joint motion (video-based kinematics), and muscle activity (electromyography) during each moment of the gait cycle. Quantitative data can be combined with observational and video-based gait analyses and physical examination findings to accurately diagnose gait pathology and develop a surgical plan. Because spasticity is eliminated by anesthesia, examination under anesthesia is the most useful method for determining the true mechanical limitations in range of motion. The limitations are caused by fixed contractures of muscle tendon units or capsular contractures at the joint. The decision for or against surgery should not be made until the examination under anesthesia has been completed so that the final decision can be made based on all available data.

The five priorities of gait have been described as follows: stability in stance phase, clearance in swing phase, appropriate pre-positioning before heel strike, adequate stride length, and conservation of energy.[41] Each priority builds on the preceding priorities. The goal of surgery in ambulatory patients with CP is to eliminate joint contractures and rotational abnormalities that affect gait biomechanics and impair function. Focusing on the priorities of gait allows the surgeon to define the impairment and determine the potential benefit of surgery. For example, the first priority of gait—stability in stance—is vital to gait. Without stability on the stance limb, gait is not possible. Ataxia will manifest as instability in the stance phase, and, subsequently, all other priorities of gait will be affected. Because orthopaedic surgery cannot change ataxia, surgery will fail to improve gait. However, if stability in stance is limited because of a fixed equinus contracture manifesting as a small base of contact, then stability may be improved with lengthening of the gastrocnemius-soleus complex. An equinus contracture also results in poor clearance, with the toe catching at the midswing phase, poor pre-positioning caused by limited dorsiflexion at terminal swing, decreased stride length caused by the inability to advance the center of mass over the talus during the stance phase, and poor conservation of energy caused by loss of the foot rockers. Orthopaedic surgery can reduce contractures (specifically, contractures at the hip, knee, and ankle) to increase stride length during the swing phase, decrease energy expenditure during the stance phase, and improve weight transition over the ankle during second rocker phase. Bony realignment, patellar tendon shortening, and tendon transfers can improve the biomechanics of gait to prevent collision of the knees during gait (scissoring) and improve the efficiency of existing strength to maximize ambulatory capacity.

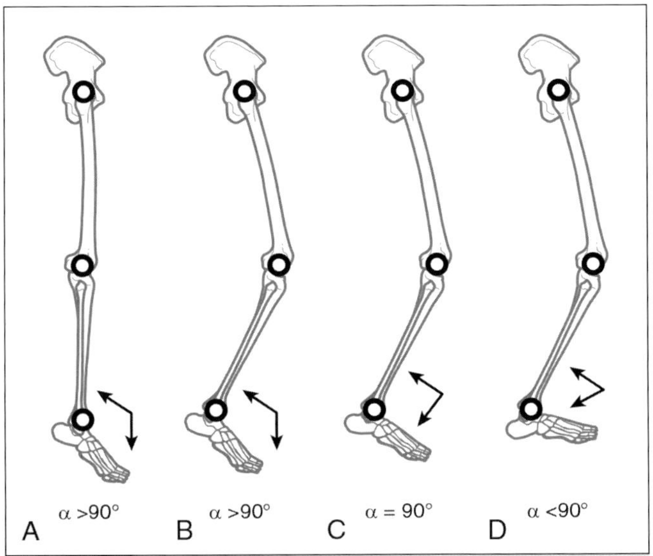

Figure 4 Illustrations of gait patterns seen in patients with spastic diplegia. Arrows show the alpha (α) angle. **A,** Group 1: true equinus is driven by a gastrocnemius contracture without flexion contracture at the knee or hip. **B,** Group 2: jump gait is characterized by an equinus contracture with compensatory knee and/or hip flexion contracture. **C,** Group 3: apparent equinus is similar to jump gait in appearance, but the toe walking is driven by a flexion contracture at the knee and/or hip, and there is no associated contracture of the gastrocnemius-soleus complex. **D,** Group 4: crouch gait is characterized by excessive ankle dorsiflexion and contractures at the knee and/or hip.

Fixed contractures can occur around any or all of the joints in the lower extremity. A patient's gait can be classified by the influence of contractures at each level (**Figure 4**).

True Equinus Gait

In true equinus gait, inadequate dorsiflexion through the ankle joint shifts first contact toward the forefoot. To maintain the center of mass, the knee, which does not have a fixed contracture, is kept bent through the midstance phase. When there is a fixed contracture of the gastrocnemius and/or soleus muscle, the patient will benefit from lengthening the gastrocnemius-soleus complex. This may be done through various gastrocnemius lengthening techniques such as the Vulpius, Strayer, and Baker techniques or Z-lengthening. A risk of overlengthening the gastrocnemius-soleus complex exists with any of these techniques and can lead to excessive dorsiflexion, weakness in plantar flexion, and iatrogenic progression into the crouch gait. A gastrocnemius recession procedure decreases the risk of overcorrection, compared with Achilles tendon lengthening, and does not weaken the gastrocnemius-soleus complex as much as Achilles tendon lengthening. Lengthening only the gastrocnemius fascia is preferable, if possible, to prevent weakness and maintain the plantar flexion–knee extension couple. Ankle dorsiflexors are weak in the setting of equinus. Lengthening of the gastrocnemius-soleus complex has the secondary benefit of improving active ankle dorsiflexion because it enables increased function of antagonist muscles and active ankle dorsiflexion during the swing phase, thereby improving clearance.[42] This benefit has been shown to be maintained at least 1 year after surgery.[43]

Jump Gait

When a fixed equinus at the ankle is coupled with a fixed flexion contracture at the knee and/or hip, the patient has jump gait. The ankle equinus and contractures at the knee and hip should be concurrently addressed. At the hip, psoas muscle lengthening should be performed at the pelvic brim as a fractional lengthening. If the psoas muscle is released from the lesser trochanter, the result will be weakened hip flexion, and ambulatory capacity will be affected. Gait analysis coupled with physical examination is important to accurately identify contractures because overlengthening can degrade gait. Recently proposed criteria for decision-making in proximal fractional psoas muscle lengthening highlights these risks. The criteria involve a complex decision algorithm that combines variables, including age, mass, speed, stride time, dimensionless stride time, the pelvis-hip deviation index, minimum swing phase pelvic rotation, and swing phase knee flexion range of motion. In children who met the criteria, 82% had good outcomes and, in those who did not meet the criteria, only 27% had good outcomes.[44]

Crouch Gait

Crouch gait is defined as increased hip and knee flexion with increased dorsiflexion of the ankle. Overlengthening the gastrocnemius-soleus complex is the most common cause of this gait deviation, but it also is seen in patients who are overweight or have severe pes valgus, which can mimic the effect of increased dorsiflexion of the ankle. Solid ankle-foot orthoses can be used to support the ankle and foot and attempt to prevent collapse of the foot into planovalgus; however, this is often unsuccessful. Ground reaction (or floor reaction) ankle-foot orthoses can be used to place an extension moment on the knee during the stance phase. Chronic knee flexion leads to traction injury of the knee extensor mechanism. This manifests as progressive elongation of the patellar tendon, and it often results in fragmentation of the distal patella. The quadriceps become inefficient and weak, and anterior knee pain ensues. Any single event multilevel surgery in this setting should address the extensor mechanism with a patellar tendon shortening or advancement.[45]

Rotational Abnormalities

Rotational abnormalities can manifest at the femur or tibia. This so-called lever arm syndrome is secondary to persistent femoral anteversion and internal tibial torsion, but external tibial torsion may develop in response to the increased femoral anteversion. Excessive femoral anteversion mimics the scissoring seen with true adduction contractures. There is also an apparent valgus leading to the knees colliding during gait. Children with excessive femoral anteversion coupled with excessive hip internal rotation benefit from proximal or distal femoral derotation osteotomy. However, femoral derotation osteotomy to correct excessive femoral anteversion in children with mild increases of hip internal rotation on examination can lead to overcorrection with an externally rotated foot-progression angle.[46] Long-standing proximal internal rotation may couple with secondary deformities in the lower limb segment such as tibial external rotation, distal tibial valgus, and foot planovalgus. The downstream effects of proximal derotation should be considered in surgical planning for each patient.

Foot and Ankle

The goal of foot and ankle surgery in an ambulatory patient with CP is restoration of a plantigrade, well-positioned foot to maximize gait efficiency. In a nonambulatory patient, the goal is to preserve adequate positioning of the foot to prevent or heal chronic skin breakdown and prevent osteomyelitis. Equinus usually is present and is a major factor in foot deformities in CP. It can be present in isolation or in conjunction with other deformities caused by muscle imbalance.

Contracture of the Achilles tendon combined with contractures of the anterior and/or posterior tibial tendons result in equinocavovarus foot deformity. Contracture of the Achilles tendon combined with collapse of the midfoot and/or contractures of the peroneal tendons lead to equinoplanovalgus foot deformity. Secondary deformities encountered include hallux valgus, toe flexion contractures, and distal tibial valgus. Successful surgical treatment requires identifying the contributing deforming forces and defining each as dynamic or fixed. Dynamic contractures can be corrected with manipulation and spasticity management such as botulinum toxin injections. They can be addressed with tendon lengthening, tendon transfer, and/or capsular release. Fixed contractures are not reducible, even in the absence of spasticity, and require bony realignment or fusion. It is often impossible to determine the true nature of the foot deformity until all spasticity is relieved with the patient under anesthesia. Recent evidence suggests that including foot reconstructions in single-event multilevel surgeries may increase the risks of long-term pain and complex regional pain syndrome.[47]

The loss of the medial arch and external rotation of the foot in equinoplanovalgus reduces the lever arm and results in weakness. Dorsiflexion through the midfoot can result in a crouch gait. Correcting the foot and restoring the lever arm can improve gait and increase extension at the knee.[48] Options for equinoplanovalgus deformity correction include lateral column lengthening (the modified Evans procedure) and calcaneo-cuboid-cuneiform osteotomies (medial slide calcaneal osteotomy, open wedge cuboid osteotomy, and closing wedge cuneiform osteotomy). In severe equinoplanovalgus deformity, lateral column lengthening may fail, which can lead to subluxation of the calcaneocuboid joint, unless it is augmented medially with a tibialis posterior reefing or talonavicular arthrodesis.[49] A recent study suggests greater correction can be obtained with calcaneo-cuboid-cuneiform osteotomies.[50]

In equinocavovarus deformity, differentiation of the deforming force between the tibialis anterior and tibialis posterior should guide the plan for correction. If the hindfoot is correctable into valgus, then isolated soft-tissue surgeries can be used to correct the deformity. A split transfer of the tibialis anterior tendon to the lateral cuneiform can maintain active dorsiflexion while reorienting the force vector out of varus. This tendon transfer is often coupled with lengthening of the tibialis posterior tendon and, occasionally, posteromedial capsular release. If the tibialis anterior tendon is weak, then a split tibialis posterior tendon transfer to the peroneus brevis should be used. If the hindfoot is not correctable into valgus, tendon transfer should be coupled with a calcaneal lateral closing wedge osteotomy or a slide osteotomy. The contribution of cavus and equinus to restriction of dorsiflexion also should be assessed. Cavus can be addressed with a plantar fascia release through either a plantar or a medial incision. Equinus can be addressed through Achilles tendon lengthening. If both are present, their correction should be staged because the surgeon cannot control the contributions of each procedure if done concurrently.

When deformities are too severe to correct through reconstruction, or when reconstruction fails, triple arthrodesis is an option. To address severe deformity, the addition of a lateral column lengthening to the triple arthrodesis has been described.[51] Although this results in good correction, it also results in a stiff foot that is at higher risk for skin breakdown. Reconstruction is preferred when indicated.

Summary

CP is a nonprogressive disorder of movement, tone, and posture caused by an injury to the brain during early development. Because CP manifests with great variability, the GMFCS classification helps to describe the functional ability of patients as they age. A multidisciplinary approach is necessary to optimize the patient's role in society. Nonsurgical treatment modalities such as botulinum toxin can aid in spasticity control and are a useful adjunct to physical and occupational therapy. Surgery can aid in improving function; however, before the decision for surgical intervention is made, it is important to identify the ambulatory potential and ability of a child and whether his or her contractures are dynamic (necessitating tendon transfer and/or lengthening) versus static or fixed (requiring bony surgery). Hip surveillance is important for all patients, and the high complication rate with spinal fusion should be noted. In the ambulatory patient, careful preoperative planning is necessary to identify gait abnormalities so that function can be improved and weakness prevented.

Key Study Points

- CP is a nonprogressive disorder of movement, tone, and posture caused by injury to the immature brain, which can occur in the prenatal, perinatal, or postnatal period.
- Orthopaedic surgery can address issues of anatomy (contractures and alignment). Limitations caused by spasticity might be addressed with nonsurgical treatment or selective dorsal rhizotomy. Functional limitation and need for self-care should be addressed.
- Dynamic contractures for which nonsurgical treatments have been unsuccessful can be addressed with tendon transfer and/or lengthening. Fixed contractures require joint release or bony surgery.
- Surgery to address lever arm dysfunction such as increased femoral anteversion, excessive internal or external tibial torsion, and pes valgus should be considered in ambulatory patients.
- Spinal fusion in children with CP has a high complication rate, and the risks of surgery may outweigh the benefits in some patients.
- Screening with pelvic radiography should be performed for all children with CP and neuromuscular hip subluxation until at least age 5 years. A Reimer migration index greater than 50% is an indication for hip reconstruction surgery.

Annotated References

1. Centers for Disease Control and Prevention: *Data and Statistics for Cerebral Palsy*. Available at http://www.cdc.gov/ncbddd/cp/data.html. Updated: May 2, 2016. Accessed December 14, 2015.

   This report provides an overview of the prevalence, characteristics, and risk factors for CP. Level of evidence: IV.

2. Christensen D, Van Naarden Braun K, Doernberg NS, et al: Prevalence of cerebral palsy, co-occurring autism spectrum disorders, and motor functioning: Autism and Developmental Disabilities Monitoring Network, USA, 2008. *Dev Med Child Neurol* 2014;56(1):59-65.

   A review of surveillance data for CP in the United States demonstrates that the prevalence has remained constant. Level of evidence: IV.

3. Winter S, Autry A, Boyle C, Yeargin-Allsopp M: Trends in the prevalence of cerebral palsy in a population-based study. *Pediatrics* 2002;110(6):1220-1225.

4. Pakula AT, Van Naarden Braun K, Yeargin-Allsopp M: Cerebral palsy: Classification and epidemiology, in Michaud LJ: *Cerebral Palsy*. Philadelphia, PA, WB Saunders, 2009, pp 425-452.

5. Bonellie SR, Currie D, Chalmers J: Comparison of risk factors for cerebral palsy in twins and singletons. *Dev Med Child Neurol* 2005;47(9):587-591.

6. Zarrinkalam R, Russo RN, Gibson CS, van Essen P, Peek AK, Haan EA: CP or not CP? A review of diagnoses in a cerebral palsy register. *Pediatr Neurol* 2010;42(3):177-180.

7. Reid SM, Dagia CD, Ditchfield MR, Carlin JB, Reddihough DS: Population-based studies of brain imaging patterns in cerebral palsy. *Dev Med Child Neurol* 2014;56(3):222-232.

   This meta-analysis examined cohort studies that evaluated imaging findings in patients with CP. A high rate of abnormalities was found in patients with the disease. Level of evidence: III.

8. Blair E, Stanley F: Interobserver agreement in the classification of cerebral palsy. *Dev Med Child Neurol* 1985;27(5):615-622.

9. Reid SM, Carlin JB, Reddihough DS: Distribution of motor types in cerebral palsy: How do registry data compare? *Dev Med Child Neurol* 2011;53(3):233-238.

   This retrospective review of the Victoria Australia Cerebral Palsy Register demonstrated considerable heterogeneity among the Victoria Register and other registers regarding motor classification, particularly mixed motor types. Level of evidence: IV.

10. Palisano R, Rosenbaum P, Walter S, Russell D, Wood E, Galuppi B: Development and reliability of a system to classify gross motor function in children with cerebral palsy. *Dev Med Child Neurol* 1997;39(4):214-223.

11. Palisano RJ, Rosenbaum P, Bartlett D, Livingston MH: Content validity of the expanded and revised Gross Motor Function Classification System. *Dev Med Child Neurol* 2008;50(10):744-750.

12. Shi W, Yang H, Li CY, et al: Expanded and revised gross motor function classification system: Study for Chinese school children with cerebral palsy. *Disabil Rehabil* 2014;36(5):403-408.

    The Chinese version of the Expanded and Revised GMFCS was given to various healthcare providers, teachers, and parents to classify 130 children. It was shown to be a valid measure of functional ability. Level of evidence: III.

13. Godwin EM, Spero CR, Nof L, Rosenthal RR, Echternach JL: The gross motor function classification system for cerebral palsy and single-event multilevel surgery: Is there a relationship between level of function and intervention over time? *J Pediatr Orthop* 2009;29(8):910-915.

14. National Center for Medical Rehabilitation Research: Report to the NACHHD Council. Washington, DC, US Department of Health and Human Services, 2006. Available at: https://www.nichd.nih.gov/publications/pubs/documents/ncmrr_report_online_2006_historical.pdf. Accessed December 14, 2015.

15. Sala DA, Grant AD: Prognosis for ambulation in cerebral palsy. *Dev Med Child Neurol* 1995;37(11):1020-1026.

16. Wu YW, Day SM, Strauss DJ, Shavelle RM: Prognosis for ambulation in cerebral palsy: A population-based study. *Pediatrics* 2004;114(5):1264-1271.

17. Novak I, McIntyre S, Morgan C, et al: A systematic review of interventions for children with cerebral palsy: State of the evidence. *Dev Med Child Neurol* 2013;55(10):885-910.

    This systematic review found several green-light interventions for children with CP, including physical therapy, botulinum toxin, hip surveillance, and selective dorsal rhizotomy. Level of evidence: II.

18. Chen YN, Liao SF, Su LF, Huang HY, Lin CC, Wei TS: The effect of long-term conventional physical therapy and independent predictive factors analysis in children with cerebral palsy. *Dev Neurorehabil* 2013;16(5):357-362.

    This retrospective review examined the long-term effects of physical therapy in patients with CP and found that physical therapy demonstrated long-term benefits, particularly in younger patients and those with level II GMFCS. Level of evidence: IV.

19. Dewar R, Love S, Johnston LM: Exercise interventions improve postural control in children with cerebral palsy: A systematic review. *Dev Med Child Neurol* 2015;57(6):504-520.

    A systematic review of exercise intervention studies demonstrated that gross motor task training, hippotherapy, treadmill training with no body weight support, trunk-targeted training, and reactive balance training are beneficial in children with CP. Level of evidence: III.

20. Navarrete-Opazo AA, Gonzalez W, Nahuelhual P: Effectiveness of oral baclofen in the treatment of spasticity in children and adolescents with cerebral palsy. *Arch Phys Med Rehabil* 2016;97(4):604-618.

    This systematic review identified six randomized controlled trials examining the use of oral baclofen in the treatment of spasticity in children with CP. The authors found conflicting evidence regarding reduction of muscle tone and improvements in motor function and level of activity. Level of evidence: III.

21. Ferrari A, Maoret AR, Muzzini S, et al: A randomized trial of upper limb botulinum toxin versus placebo injection, combined with physiotherapy, in children with hemiplegia. *Res Dev Disabil* 2014;35(10):2505-2513.

    This randomized controlled trial of botulinum toxin and physical therapy versus placebo injection and physical therapy in children with hemiplegia showed that botulinum toxin resulted in substantial improvement in function compared with placebo, particularly in children with disease involvement that was more severe. Level of evidence: I.

22. Copeland L, Edwards P, Thorley M, et al: Botulinum toxin A for nonambulatory children with cerebral palsy: A double blind randomized controlled trial. *J Pediatr* 2014;165(1):140-146.e4.

    The authors of this randomized controlled trial compared a sham procedure with botulinum toxin for nonambulatory patients with CP and found improved care and comfort of patients who had the botulinum toxin injections. Both groups received physical therapy. The Canadian Occupational Performance Measure was the primary end point. There was no increase in moderate and severe adverse events in the children who had botulinum injections compared with the control group. Level of evidence: I.

23. Hasnat MJ, Rice JE: Intrathecal baclofen for treating spasticity in children with cerebral palsy. *Cochrane Database Syst Rev* 2015;13(11):CD004552.

    This meta-analysis examined six studies that demonstrated the short-term benefit of intrathecal baclofen. The authors noted that long-term data were limited. Level of evidence: II.

24. Dudley RW, Parolin M, Gagnon B, et al: Long-term functional benefits of selective dorsal rhizotomy for spastic cerebral palsy. *J Neurosurg Pediatr* 2013;12(2):142-150.

    This retrospective study demonstrated the long-term benefits of selective dorsal rhizotomy. Level of evidence: IV.

25. Van Heest AE, Bagley A, Molitor F, James MA: Tendon transfer surgery in upper-extremity cerebral palsy is more effective than botulinum toxin injections or regular, ongoing therapy. *J Bone Joint Surg Am* 2015;97(7):529-536.

    The authors of this prospective study found tendon transfers (flexor carpi ulnaris to the extensor carpi radialis brevis, pronator teres release, and extensor pollicis longus rerouting with adductor pollicis release) were superior to botulinum toxin or physical therapy alone as measured by the Shriners Hospital Upper Extremity Evaluation Dynamic Positional Analyses activity measure and the Pediatrics Quality of Life tool. Level of evidence: II.

26. James MA, Bagley A, Vogler JB IV, Davids JR, Van Heest AE: Correlation between standard upper extremity impairment measures and activity-based function testing in upper extremity cerebral palsy. *J Pediatr Orthop* 2015.

    A study of 37 children with upper extremity CP found little correlation between impairment measures (range of motion and stereognosis) and newly validated activity measures (Assisting Hand Assessment, box and blocks test, and Shriners Hospitals Upper Extremity Evaluation Dynamic Positional Analyses). The authors concluded that range of motion may be a poor measure of function, and activity measures should be used in upper extremity surgical decision-making. Level of evidence: II.

27. Whitaker AT, Sharkey M, Diab M: Spinal fusion for scoliosis in patients with globally involved cerebral palsy: An ethical assessment. *J Bone Joint Surg Am* 2015;97(9):782-787.

    A systematic literature review of studies of spine fusion for neuromuscular scoliosis in patients with globally involved CP found little evidence to support that spine fusion leads to decreased morbidity or mortality or provides substantial benefits in terms of quality of life improvements. Level of evidence: III.

28. Glotzbecker MP, Riedel MD, Vitale MG, et al: What's the evidence? Systematic literature review of risk factors and preventive strategies for surgical site infection following pediatric spine surgery. *J Pediatr Orthop* 2013;33(5):479-487.

    A systematic review of 57 studies found that a diagnosis of CP, nonadherence to antibiotic administration regimens, and prominent implants were risk factors for surgical site infection. Level of evidence: III.

29. Samdani AF, Belin EJ, Bennett JT, et al: Major perioperative complications after spine surgery in patients with cerebral palsy: Assessment of risk factors. *Eur Spine J* 2016;25(3):795-800.

    The authors reported major perioperative complications in 39.4% of 127 patients with CP who underwent spine surgery. Although kyphosis, staged procedures, and lack of fibrinolytic use were substantially associated with an increased risk of complications in univariate analysis, only increased blood loss was an independent risk factor in multivariable analysis. Level of evidence: II.

30. Nishnianidze T, Bayhan IA, Abousamra O, et al: Factors predicting postoperative complications following spinal fusions in children with cerebral palsy scoliosis. *Eur Spine J* 2016;25(2):627-634.

    The authors of a retrospective study of 303 children found gastrostomy or gastrojejunostomy tube feeding was a risk factor for complications after spine surgery in CP patients. Level of evidence: III.

31. Sponseller PD, Jain A, Shah SA, et al: Deep wound infections after spinal fusion in children with cerebral palsy: A prospective cohort study. *Spine (Phila Pa 1976)* 2013;38(23):2023-2027.

    This prospective cohort study found that deep wound infection occurred in 6.4% of children with CP after spinal fusion. The presence of a gastrostomy/gastrojejunostomy tube was an important predictor of infection, and gram-negative organisms were the most common causative agents. Level of evidence: II.

32. Myung KS, Lee C, Skaggs DL: Early pelvic fixation failure in neuromuscular scoliosis. *J Pediatr Orthop* 2015;35(3):258-265.

    The authors of this retrospective review found that not placing bilateral pedicle screws at L5 and S1 in addition to two iliac screws was associated with a 35% early failure rate of pelvic fixation. Level of evidence: IV.

33. Piazzolla A, Solarino G, De Giorgi S, Mori CM, Moretti L, De Giorgi G: Cotrel-Dubousset instrumentation in neuromuscular scoliosis. *Eur Spine J* 2011;20(suppl 1):S75-S84.

    Cotrel-Dubousset instrumentation techniques were found to provide lasting correction of spinal deformity in patients with neuromuscular scoliosis. Lower complication rates were reported compared with second-generation instrumented spinal fusion. Level of evidence: IV.

34. Funk S, Lovejoy S, Mencio G, Martus J: Rigid instrumentation for neuromuscular scoliosis improves deformity correction without increasing complications. *Spine (Phila Pa 1976)* 2016;41(1):46-52.

    This retrospective study compared rigid and nonrigid constructs for neuromuscular scoliosis and found that rigid constructs improved deformity correction, had lower rates of pseudarthrosis, and decreased the need for anterior release. Level of evidence: III.

35. Crawford L, Herrera-Soto J, Ruder JA, Phillips J, Knapp R: The fate of the neuromuscular hip after spinal fusion. *J Pediatr Orthop* 2015.

    This retrospective study demonstrated a need for hip containment after posterior spinal fusion, whereas hips that were contained before posterior spinal fusion maintained their containment. Level of evidence: IV.

36. Hägglund G, Alriksson-Schmidt A, Lauge-Pedersen H, Rodby-Bousquet E, Wagner P, Westbom L: Prevention of dislocation of the hip in children with cerebral palsy: 20-year results of a population-based prevention programme. *Bone Joint J* 2014;96-B(11):1546-1552.

    The authors report on the 20-year results of a population-based hip surveillance prevention program in Sweden that demonstrated a significantly lower incidence of hip dislocation in CP patients. Level of evidence: IV.

37. Shore B, Spence D, Graham H: The role for hip surveillance in children with cerebral palsy. *Curr Rev Musculoskelet Med* 2012;5(2):126-134.

    The authors review the spectrum of treatments available for progressive hip displacement and examine the current literature on the success of hip surveillance in patients with CP. Level of evidence: V.

38. Bayusentono S, Choi Y, Chung CY, Kwon SS, Lee KM, Park MS: Recurrence of hip instability after reconstructive surgery in patients with cerebral palsy. *J Bone Joint Surg Am* 2014;96(18):1527-1534.

    This retrospective review demonstrated that patients with level IV or V GMFCS should be monitored for recurrence of hip instability. Level of evidence: III.

39. Dartnell J, Gough M, Paterson JM, Norman-Taylor F: Proximal femoral resection without post-operative traction for the painful dislocated hip in young patients with cerebral palsy: A review of 79 cases. *Bone Joint J* 2014;96-B(5):701-706.

    This retrospective review reports good outcomes for young patients with CP treated with proximal femoral resection without traction for painful dislocated hips. Level of evidence: IV.

40. Boldingh EJ, Bouwhuis CB, van der Heijden-Maessen HC, Bos CF, Lankhorst GJ: Palliative hip surgery in severe cerebral palsy: A systematic review. *J Pediatr Orthop B* 2014;23(1):86-92.

    This systematic review of techniques for palliative hip surgery in patients with severe CP did not show a preference for a particular technique, although the Castle resection arthroplasty technique had the best results and outcomes. Level of evidence: III.

41. Gage JR, DeLuca PA, Renshaw TS: Gait analysis: Principle and applications with emphasis on its use in cerebral palsy. *Instr Course Lect* 1996;45:491-507.

42. Davids JR, Rogozinski BM, Hardin JW, Davis RB: Ankle dorsiflexor function after plantar flexor surgery in children with cerebral palsy. *J Bone Joint Surg Am* 2011;93(23):e1381-e1387.

    In this retrospective cohort study, 53 children with CP underwent surgical lengthening of the gastrocnemius-soleus muscle group. Quantitative gait analysis was performed before and after surgery. The authors found that ankle dorsiflexion during the swing phase improved after patients underwent ankle plantar flexor lengthening surgery. Level of evidence: IV.

43. Dreher T, Buccoliero T, Wolf SI, et al: Long-term results after gastrocnemius-soleus intramuscular aponeurotic recession as a part of multilevel surgery in spastic diplegic cerebral palsy. *J Bone Joint Surg Am* 2012;94(7):627-637.

    The authors report on patients who underwent gastrocnemius-soleus complex intramuscular aponeurotic recession as a part of multilevel surgery for spastic diplegic CP. They found satisfactory correction of mild and moderate equinus deformity in the patients without relevant risk for overcorrection. Level of evidence: IV.

44. Schwartz MH, Rozumalski A, Truong W, Novacheck TF: Predicting the outcome of intramuscular psoas lengthening in children with cerebral palsy using preoperative gait data and the random forest algorithm. *Gait Posture* 2013;37(4):473-479.

This study demonstrated the use of preoperative gait analysis and the random forest algorithm to predict the rate of good hip outcomes in patients with diplegic CP who undergo surgery. Level of evidence: III.

45. Novacheck TF, Stout JL, Gage JR, Schwartz MH: Distal femoral extension osteotomy and patellar tendon advancement to treat persistent crouch gait in cerebral palsy: Surgical technique. *J Bone Joint Surg Am* 2009;91(suppl 2):271-286.

46. Schwartz MH, Rozumalski A, Novacheck TF: Femoral derotational osteotomy: Surgical indications and outcomes in children with cerebral palsy. *Gait Posture* 2014;39(2):778-783.

This study used the random forest algorithm to predict outcomes of femoral derotation osteotomy as part of single-event multilevel surgery in patients with CP. Level of evidence: IV.

47. Høiness PR, Capjon H, Lofterød B: Pain and rehabilitation problems after single-event multilevel surgery including bony foot surgery in cerebral palsy: A series of 7 children. *Acta Orthop* 2014;85(6):646-651.

The authors report on seven patients with CP who underwent single-event multilevel surgery, including foot reconstruction. Results were concerning, with five of the seven patients experiencing chronic regional pain syndrome, and two losing the ability to walk after surgery. Level of evidence: IV.

48. Kadhim M, Miller F: Crouch gait changes after planovalgus foot deformity correction in ambulatory children with cerebral palsy. *Gait Posture* 2014;39(2):793-798.

This retrospective case series of 34 feet in 21 children with crouch gait found improvement in knee extension after planovalgus foot deformity correction with either subtalar fusion or calcaneal lengthening. Level of evidence: IV.

49. Sung KH, Chung CY, Lee KM, Lee SY, Park MS: Calcaneal lengthening for planovalgus foot deformity in patients with cerebral palsy. *Clin Orthop Relat Res* 2013;471(5):1682-1690.

The authors report on 75 patients with CP treated with calcaneal lengthening for planovalgus foot deformity. Undercorrection of the deformity was found in patients with a preoperative anteroposterior talus/first metatarsal angle greater than 23°, a lateral talus-first metatarsal angle greater than 36°, and naviculocuneiform overlap greater than 72%. The authors recommend augmenting the lateral calcaneal osteotomy with medial stabilization procedures such as tibialis posterior tendon reefing and talonavicular arthrodesis. Level of evidence: IV.

50. Kim JR, Shin SJ, Wang SI, Kang SM: Comparison of lateral opening wedge calcaneal osteotomy and medial calcaneal sliding-opening wedge cuboid-closing wedge cuneiform osteotomy for correction of planovalgus foot deformity in children. *J Foot Ankle Surg* 2013;52(2):162-166.

This retrospective study of 38 patients compared calcaneal lengthening osteotomy versus triple calcaneo-cuboid-cuneiform osteotomies for the correction of planovalgus foot deformity in children. The clinical results were comparable, but in subgroup analysis the triple osteotomy was superior in treating severe planovalgus. Level of evidence: III.

51. Frost NL, Grassbaugh JA, Baird G, Caskey P: Triple arthrodesis with lateral column lengthening for the treatment of planovalgus deformity. *J Pediatr Orthop* 2011;31(7):773-782.

The authors report on 27 patients who underwent triple arthrodesis augmented by lateral calcaneal lengthening. Good clinical results were found in 86% of the patients who had no or minimal pain; however, the complication rate was 38%. Level of evidence IV.

Chapter 12

Myelomeningocele

Vineeta T. Swaroop, MD

Abstract

The orthopaedic care of patients with myelomeningocele has continued to evolve over the past 5 years. It is helpful to review the early outcomes of fetal surgery and issues affecting the function of patients with myelomeningocele.

Keywords: fetal surgery; myelomeningocele; neural tube defect; spina bifida

Introduction

Neural tube defects result from failure of the neural tube to close during embryogenesis. Although the incidence of these defects has declined in recent decades, it remains at 1 per 2,000 births in the United States.[1] Myelomeningocele, the most common neural tube defect, is a myelodysplasia of the neural elements that manifests in the vertebrae as a defect in the posterior elements. Dysplasia of the spinal cord and nerve roots leads to bowel, bladder, motor, and sensory paralysis below the level of the lesion. Patients may have concomitant lesions of the spinal cord, such as diastematomyelia or hydromyelia, or structural abnormalities of the brain, such as hydrocephalus or Arnold-Chiari malformation, which also can compromise neurologic function.

With advances in the management of several important complications, the survival rate into early adulthood for patients born with an open myelomeningocele has improved from 10% in the 1950s to 75% in the early 2000s.[2] Comprehensive treatment is necessary to prevent, monitor, and treat a variety of potential complications that can affect function, quality of life, and survival.

Dr. Swaroop or an immediate family member serves as a board member, owner, officer, or committee member of the Pediatric Orthopaedic Society of North America.

Treatment is best accomplished using a multidisciplinary team approach, including orthopaedic surgeons, neurosurgeons, urologists, rehabilitation specialists, physical and occupational therapists, and orthotists. Access to nutritionists, social workers, wound specialists, and psychologists also is helpful.

Both congenital and acquired orthopaedic deformities occur in patients with myelomeningocele. Congenital deformities include kyphosis, teratologic hip dislocation, clubfoot, and vertical talus. Acquired deformities are related to the level of involvement and are caused by muscle imbalance, paralysis, and decreased sensation in the lower extremities.[3]

Since the advent of computerized gait analysis (CGA) in the late 1980s, the orthopaedic care of myelomeningocele has changed substantially. The most important change has been a shift from the goal of radiographic improvement to a focus on functional improvement. The use of gait analysis as a preoperative diagnostic tool has provided a major step in establishing these changes. The main goal of orthopaedic care is to correct deformities that may prevent the patient from using an orthosis for ambulation. The negative effects of spasticity, poor balance, and tethered cord syndrome on ambulatory function are now better appreciated than in the past.[4] Functional outcome assessments, including gait analysis, oxygen consumption, and patient-based outcomes, provide better feedback for surgeons and families regarding which patients may achieve the most benefit from surgery.

Etiology

Myelomeningocele results from failure of fusion of the neural folds during the fourth week of embryogenesis. In contrast, conditions such as meningocele, lipomeningocele, and diastematomyelia arise from abnormalities during the canalization phase and are referred to as postneurulation defects.[5] The cause of these embryonic failures is suspected to be multifactorial in origin and includes genetic and environmental contributors. Folate deficiency is an important factor in the cause of neural tube defects, as evidenced by the 20% decline of anencephaly and 34% decline of myelomeningocele since folic acid fortification was added to the US food supply.[1] Other environmental factors examined for a potential role in neural tube defects include temperature; drug exposure; substance abuse; maternal infection; and other nutritional factors, including vitamin B_{12} and zinc deficiency.[6]

Genetic factors also play a role in the development of myelomeningocele. Some studies suggest a higher incidence of neural tube defects in siblings of affected children compared with the general population, with a positive family history reported in 6% to 14% of cases.[7,8] Association with single gene defects, increased recurrence risk among siblings, and higher frequency in twins also seem to indicate a genetic factor; however, the low frequency of families with a substantial number of neural tube defects makes research into genetic causation challenging. Animal studies have shown as many as 100 mutant genes that affect neurulation, and almost all have homologs in humans.[6] These candidate genes include those that are important in folic acid metabolism, glucose metabolism, retinoid metabolism, and apoptosis.[9] Future research directions such as genomewide association studies and whole genome sequencing may help to identify genes affecting the risk for human neural tube defects.

Outcomes of Fetal Surgery

Prenatal diagnosis of myelomeningocele has increased considerably since second trimester ultrasound evaluation has become routine. The current standard of neurosurgical care is closure of the defect within 48 to 72 hours of birth to prevent further deterioration. Prenatal surgery to perform intrauterine closure of the defect arose as an attempt to improve neurologic function based on the "two-hit" hypothesis. Under this hypothesis, the first hit is failure of neurulation in the embryonic period causing myelodysplasia, and the second hit is persistent exposure of neural tissue to the intrauterine environment, which leads to tissue damage and irreversible loss of neurologic function.[10] A recent study found elevated levels of phospholipase A_2, which is known to have neurotoxic properties, in the amniotic fluid of rats with myelomeningocele. This finding suggests that phospholipase A_2 may be a useful drug target to limit ongoing neurologic damage.[11]

The goal of fetal surgery for myelomeningocele is to prevent progressive neural tissue destruction and improve neurologic outcome at birth. In addition, in utero repair may stop leakage of cerebrospinal fluid, thus reducing hindbrain herniation and hydrocephalus. An endoscopic technique was first used to perform intrauterine repair in the mid 1990s, but was abandoned because of poor outcomes. The first open intrauterine surgeries were performed in the late 1990s, with encouraging outcomes of a decreased need for ventriculoperitoneal shunt (VPS) placement and reversion of brainstem herniation compared with postnatal surgery.[12] However, many complication were reported, including preterm labor, premature rupture of membranes, premature delivery, uterine dehiscence, and perinatal death. As a result of controversy over the benefits versus risks of intrauterine repair, a randomized controlled trial, Management of Myelomeningocele Study (MOMS), was conducted between 2003 and 2008 at three US medical centers. Although the intent of the study was to randomize 200 pregnant women to either intrauterine repair or postnatal surgery, the trial was stopped after 183 patients were treated because of the benefits of intrauterine surgery.

A report on the results of 158 of those patients showed rates of VPS placement of 40% in the group who received prenatal surgery compared with 82% in the group receiving postnatal surgery.[13] Prenatal surgery led to an improved composite score for mental development and motor function at 30 months, improved outcomes of hindbrain herniation by 12 months, and improved ambulation by 30 months. However, prenatal surgery was associated with an increased risk of preterm delivery and uterine dehiscence. After the trial, the participating medical centers published their post-MOMS experiences, reporting better outcomes, mainly in the rates of uterine dehiscence and premature rupture of membranes.[14]

Based on emerging outcomes data from prenatal surgery, there seems to be a positive effect on lower extremity function, although few studies have compared like groups undergoing prenatal or postnatal treatment. In 80 neonates treated with fetal repair, 55% were assigned a functional level of 1 or higher above their prenatal anatomic level.[14] Another report with no control group found motor function and ambulation ability that was better than expected based on the lesion level in patients who had fetal surgery.[15] The same group reported 10-year outcomes, which suggested improved long-term ambulatory status; 79% of the group were community ambulators and 9% were household ambulators.[16] Another study comparing six patients who underwent intrauterine repair to seven patients with postnatal repair found substantially greater improvement in functional level compared with anatomic level in the intrauterine repair cohort.[17]

Classification

Functional Classification

The classification of myelomeningocele is based on the neurologic level of the lesion. Four main groups were

Table 1

Functional Classification of Myelomeningocele

Group	Neurologic Level of Lesion	Prevalence	Functional Capacity	Ambulatory Capability	Functional Mobility Scale[a]
Thoracic/high lumbar	L1 or above	30%	No functional quadriceps (≤grade 2)	During childhood, require bracing to level of pelvis for ambulation (RGO, HKAFO)	1,1,1
Low lumbar	L3-L5	30%	Quadriceps, medial hamstring ≥grade 3 No functional activity (≤grade 2) of gluteus medius and maximus, gastrocnemius-soleus complex	Require AFOs for ambulation 80% to 95% of patients maintain community ambulation in adulthood	3,3,1
High sacral	S1-S3	30%	Quadriceps, gluteus medius ≥ grade 3 No functional activity (≤ grade 2) of gastrocnemius-soleus complex	Require AFOs for ambulation 94% to 100% of patients maintain community ambulation in adulthood	6,6,6
Low sacral	S3-S5	5% to 10%	Quadriceps, gluteus medius, gastrocnemius-soleus complex ≥grade 3	Ambulate without braces or support 94% to 100% of patients maintain community ambulation in adulthood	6,6,6

RGO = reciprocating gait orthosis, HKAFO = hip-knee-ankle-foot orthosis, AFO = ankle-foot orthosis

[a]The three numbers represent ratings for the level of function achieved at three separate distances, representing home, school, and community environments.

Reproduced with permission from: Swaroop VT, Dias L: Myelomeningocele, in Weinstein SL, Flynn JM, eds: *Lovell and Winter's Pediatric Orthopaedics*, ed 7. Philadelphia, PA, Lippincott Williams and Wilkins, 2014, pp 555-586.

identified based on the lesion level and associated functional capabilities (**Table 1**).

Functional Mobility Scale

The Functional Mobility Scale (FMS) was initially intended to describe functional mobility in children with cerebral palsy. Application of the FMS in the classification of populations with myelomeningocele reflects the increased focus on functional outcomes. The unique value of the FMS is that it allows quick, practical scoring of mobility over three distinct distances representing home (5 m), school (50 m), and community (500 m) (**Figure 1**). A score is assigned for each distance based on the assistive devices used, including crutches, a walker, or a wheelchair. The FMS provides an accurate clinical picture of a patient's functional status at a distinct point in time. A major advantage of the FMS is its ability to account separately for distances representing the home, the school, and the community, hence addressing the complexities of functional mobility in the real world.[5]

Prognosis for Ambulation

Among the many factors affecting the ambulatory potential of a patient with myelomeningocele, one of the most important is the neurologic level of involvement. Multiple studies have shown the critical role that neurologic level and resulting muscle group strength plays in achieving and maintaining ambulation. In particular, functional iliopsoas and quadriceps strength (grade 4 or 5) has shown a strong correlation with ambulatory ability.[18,19] Many other factors affect ambulation and, when present, can prevent a patient from reaching his or her expected potential based on muscle strength. These factors include poor balance; spasticity; the number of VPS placement revisions; the presence of a tethered cord; age; obesity; and musculoskeletal conditions,

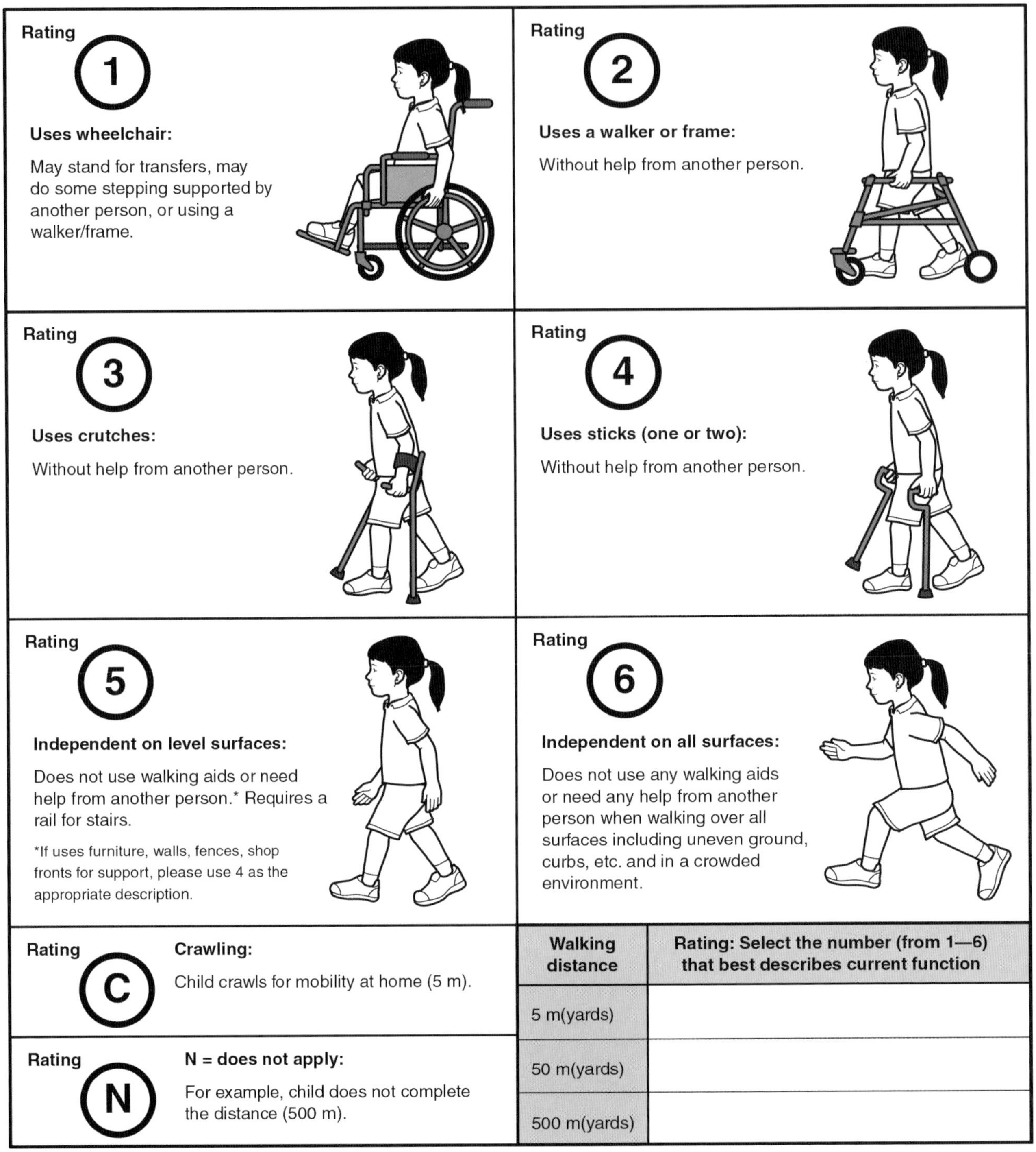

Figure 1 Illustration of the Functional Mobility Scale.

including hip contractures, scoliosis, and foot and ankle deformity.

The manual muscle test, which is performed by a physical therapist, helps to assign a functional level to patients with myelomeningocele (**Figure 2**). The results allow providers to counsel families from an early age regarding the expected potential for ambulation with or without assistive devices and orthoses. In general, patients with thoracic or high-lumbar (L1 or above) levels of neurologic involvement require a walker and a hip-spanning orthosis, such as a reciprocating gait orthosis or a hip-knee-ankle-foot orthosis (**Figure 3**), for short-distance ambulation during childhood. For these patients, achievement of independent sitting balance (a proxy for function of the central nervous system) is another predictor of potential for ambulation with orthoses. Most patients with high-level lesions require a wheelchair for mobility in adulthood because of the high energy cost of ambulation and the high incidence of scoliosis and hip and knee flexion contractures, which are prone to recurrence in adulthood despite aggressive treatment during childhood. Some controversy exists regarding whether patients in this group should be assisted to attain early ambulation. It was found that patients with high-level lesions who participated in a walking program early in life were more independent and better able to accomplish transfers later in life compared with those who did not achieve early walking.[20]

Patients with low lumbar lesions lack functional hip abductor strength and require crutches and ankle-foot orthoses (AFOs) for ambulation. Most patients in this group retain the ability for community ambulation in adulthood. Patients with high sacral lesions have functional activity of the quadriceps and gluteus medius but lack functional activity of the gastrocnemius-soleus complex; they usually can ambulate at the community level with AFOs and no assistive devices. The relatively rare patient with neurologic involvement at the low sacral level retains gastrocnemius-soleus complex function and can ambulate into adulthood without orthoses or assistive devices.

Issues Affecting Function

Bone Density and Fractures

Long-bone fractures occur in up to 40% of patients with myelomeningocele.[21,22] The increased risk for fracture is related to a variety of factors, including disuse osteoporosis, joint contractures, and postoperative immobilization, especially spica casting. A lesion at a higher level also has been shown to correspond to a higher incidence of fracture, with the risk of fracture six times greater with neurologic involvement at the thoracic level compared with the sacral level.[23] The correlation with the lesion level is thought to be caused by osteopenia related to mobility, and Z-scores have been shown to vary substantially based on neurologic level, with lower scores in patients who have a lesion at a higher level. Bone mineral density (BMD) is significantly related to ambulatory status, with lower BMD in both partial ambulators and nonambulators compared with full ambulators.[21] The bone health of partial ambulators and nonambulators should be monitored closely from an early age to identify patients who would benefit from a directed bone health program.

Hydrocephalus

Some degree of hydrocephalus will develop in many infants after closure of a spinal defect. The use of newer protocols may help to avoid VPS placement and its inherent long-term complications. Currently, approximately 50% of infants with myelomeningocele require a VPS.[24] Patients who do not require a VPS may have improved functional outcomes in terms of upper extremity function, trunk balance, and independent ambulation.[25] In addition, studies in adults have found a relationship between lifetime VPS revisions and increased mortality, achievement, IQ, memory, and quality of life.[24]

Obesity

Childhood and adolescent obesity is common in patients with myelomeningocele, affecting 40% of patients and likely resulting from a complex interaction of factors, including energy intake and the degree of motor impairment.[26] Studies have shown that many patients with myelomeningocele have a higher percentage of body fat compared with age-matched children with normal development.[27] Both neurologic level and ambulatory ability are associated with the percentage of body fat in a patient. In addition, a correlation has been shown between body fat and hydrocephalus, which suggests that the metabolic and nutritional maladaptation may be caused not only by inactivity but by the underlying condition itself.[28] Nutritional counseling and mobility programs should be initiated early to prevent the development of obesity.

Tethered Cord

Tethered cord syndrome occurs in 10% to 30% of patients with myelomeningocele. The most common clinical symptom is progressive scoliosis; other common symptoms are gait changes, loss of muscle strength, spasticity, back and leg pain, and bladder changes. If tethered cord is suspected, a VPS malfunction should be ruled out first. When the diagnosis of tethered cord is made, surgical untethering is indicated to prevent further deterioration. Improvements may be seen in pain, strength, gait, spasticity, bladder function, and other symptoms after surgical untethering.

Overview of Orthopaedic Treatment

The goal of orthopaedic care of patients with myelomeningocele is to prevent or correct deformities to maximize mobility, function, and independence. The role of the orthopaedic surgeon is to assist the patient and family

Myelomeningocele MMT/ROM
PATIENT: **DATE:**
DIAGNOSIS: Myelomeningocele **DOB:** **PHYSICIAN:**

RANGE OF MOTION °

HIP	RIGHT	LEFT
Flexion		
Abduction (hip extended)		
Adductor stretch reflex		
Abduction (hip flexed)		
Adduction		
Internal/external rotation		
Hip flexion contracture		
Ober test		

KNEE	RIGHT	LEFT
Flexion (prone)		
Flexion (supine)		
Extension		
Straight leg raise		
Popliteal angle (bilateral)		

ANKLE	RIGHT	LEFT
Dorsiflexion (knee flexed)		
Dorsiflexion (knee extended)		
Plantar flexor stretch (R1) (knee flexed/knee extended)		
Clonus (knee flexed/knee extended)		
Plantar flexion		
Thigh-foot angle		
Thigh foot angle range (ext/int)		
Forefoot abd/add		

Ligamentous Laxity	RIGHT	LEFT
Medial coll. (Knee Flexed)		
Medial coll. (knee extended)		
Lateral coll. (Knee Flexed)		
Lateral coll.(Knee extended)		

WEIGHT BEARING	RIGHT	LEFT
hindfoot valgus		
hindfoot varus		
correctable		
equinus		
correctable		
hallux valgus/varus		
rocker bottom midfoot		

MEASUREMENTS*	RIGHT	LEFT
leg length		
calf circumference		

*in centimeters

STRENGTH

		RIGHT		**LEFT**	
	COMMENTS:	CC	IP	CC	IP
Iliopsoas					
Sartorius					
Gluteus maximus					
Gluteus medius					
Tensor					
Adductors					
Medial hamstrings					
Lateral hamstrings					
Quadriceps					
Anterior tibialis					
Posterior tibialis					
Gastroc (hand test)					
Gastroc (standing)					
Soleus					
Peroneus longus					
Brevis					
Toe ext. longus					
Brevis					
Toe flex. Longus					
Brevis					
EHL					
EHB					
FHL					
FHB					
Lumbricales					

CC = cerebral control / IP = in pattern

		DEFINITION
X	Present	**Unable to be graded, but working**
5	Normal	**Complete range of motion against gravity with full resistance**
4	Good	**Complete range of motion against gravity with moderate resistance**
4-	Good Minus	**Complete range of motion against gravity with some resistance**
3+	Fair	**Complete range of motion against gravity with slight resistance**
3	Fair	**Complete range of motion against gravity**
3-	Fair Minus	**Incomplete (greater than 1/2 way) range of motion against gravity**
2+	Poor Plus	**Less than 1/2 way against gravity or full ROM with gravity eliminated plus slight resistance**
2	Poor	**Complete range of motion with gravity eliminated**
2-	Poor Minus	**Incomplete range of motion with gravity eliminated**
1	Trace	**Contraction is felt but there is no visible joint movement**
0	Zero	**No contraction is felt in the muscle**

rev. 2/03

Figure 2 A sample of a manual muscle test form. (Adapted with permission from Motion Analysis Center, Rehabilitation Institute of Chicago, Chicago, IL.)

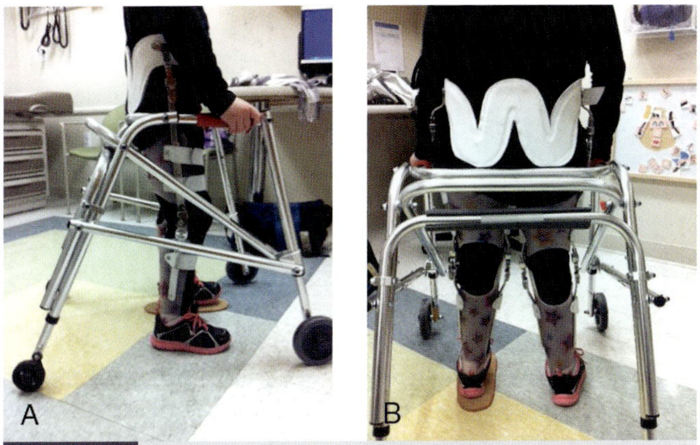

Figure 3 Lateral (**A**) and PA (**B**) views of a patient with a hip-knee-ankle-foot orthosis.

in developing realistic individualized goals based on the patient's functional neurosegmental level and provide the necessary care to meet established goals. To promote increased independence, care providers should emphasize intellectual and personality development through wheelchair mobility, wheelchair sports programs beginning in preschool, and educational mainstreaming.

At the time of the newborn examination of a patient with myelomeningocele, any associated conditions such as clubfoot or hip or knee contractures should be recognized and treated appropriately. A manual muscle test performed by a skilled physical therapist is done to evaluate the neurologic level of function for each limb. This should occur before closure of the spinal defect and should be repeated 10 to 14 days after closure and annually thereafter. A change in muscle strength on the manual muscle test may signal a tethered spinal cord.

Orthopaedic follow-up examinations should occur every 3 to 4 months during the first year of life, every 6 months until 12 years of age, and annually thereafter. Each visit should include assessment and monitoring of motor and sensory function, gait, spinal and lower extremity alignment, skin integrity, and orthoses use. The orthopaedic surgeon should remain vigilant for tethered cord syndrome and must monitor spinal balance and deformity and assist in monitoring the neurologic status of each patient.

Computerized Gait Analysis

CGA has been used in the evaluation of patients with myelomeningocele since the late 1980s. For patients with neurologic involvement at the low lumbar or sacral level, CGA has played a role in the identification of deformities affecting function such as hip and knee contractures, rotational deformities of the femur and tibia, and foot deformities. CGA also has a major influence on the selection of functional surgical procedures. For example, CGA has helped to identify the importance of hip abductor strength and its effect on gait. Knowing that hip abductor weakness causes excessive pelvic obliquity and rotation has led to the understanding that any surgery that affects pelvic motion will make gait more difficult. In addition, CGA has helped to identify negative effects on gait caused by surgical procedures that decrease the strength of the power generation muscles, iliopsoas, gluteus, and hamstrings. CGA also has been used to evaluate the relationship between energy consumption and gait, using oxygen cost to compare various orthoses and gait patterns.

Spinal Deformity

Spinal deformity in patients with myelomeningocele may occur as a congenital deformity resulting from a malformation such as hemivertebrae or unsegmented bar or may occur as an acquired developmental deformity related to the level of neurologic involvement.[5] The incidence of spinal deformity correlates with the neurologic level of involvement. The development of scoliosis in patients with involvement at the low lumbar or sacral levels should alert the care provider to the possibility of a tethered spinal cord because patients with neurologic involvement at these levels have a low incidence of scoliosis.

Scoliosis

Scoliosis is present in 60% to 90% of patients with myelomeningocele. Many factors, including functional level of involvement, ambulatory status, level of last intact laminar arch, hip displacement, and lower extremity spasticity, correlate with the development and progression of scoliosis. The goals for scoliosis treatment in patients with myelomeningocele are to prevent deformity progression, achieve solid fusion, maximize functional independence, increase sitting tolerance, and achieve a level pelvis with a balanced spine.[4]

Patients with a curve magnitude of less than 20° should be observed with serial radiographs. For patients with a curve magnitude greater than 20°, brace treatment may be considered; however, the general consensus is that brace treatment does not halt curve progression in this population. Rather, a brace may be used to support the trunk in a functional position and control the curve during growth in an attempt to delay surgical treatment. If a brace is prescribed, proper fitting and daily skin assessments are essential to avoid skin complications.

Surgical treatment is generally indicated for progressive curves greater than 50° that interfere with sitting balance. For each patient, the benefits of surgical treatment must be weighed against the increased risk of complications associated with scoliosis surgery in the myelomeningocele population. Complications include hardware problems in approximately 30% of the patients. These problems often lead to a loss of correction and pseudarthrosis in up to 75% of the patients, depending on the surgical technique (the highest rates are associated with isolated posterior fusion). Other common complications include infection and postoperative lower limb fractures. Neurologic complications occur infrequently but can be permanent.

Consideration should be given to the functional consequences of surgical treatment. Multiple studies have shown no substantial difference in the ability to perform activities of daily living after surgical intervention.[29,30] Comparisons of the long-term outcomes of scoliosis in patients with myelomeningocele who were treated surgically or nonsurgically showed that spinal fusion for scoliosis is effective in halting curve progression but has no clear effect on walking capability, motor level, sitting balance, or health-related quality of life.[31] Multiple authors have reported that ambulation may be more difficult after surgery.[29,30] However, it is possible that evolving surgical techniques, newer instrumentation, and improvements in postoperative management may eventually lead to improved functional outcomes for surgically treated patients.

For most patients, combined anterior and posterior instrumented arthrodesis is the treatment of choice to achieve fusion and provide the best long-term correction. The benefits of the combined approach include increased strength of the fusion mass from anterior interbody fusion and diskectomy to improve curve flexibility. The posterior-only approach has been associated with higher failure rates, hardware complications, and loss of correction. A select group of patients may benefit from the potential advantages of the anterior-only approach, which includes preservation of motion segments and maintenance of improved function. Patients who have a thoracolumbar curve of less than 75°, a compensatory curve of less than 40°, no increased kyphosis, and no syrinx are candidates for this approach.[32]

Pedicle screw instrumentation in patients with myelomeningocele allows for posterior segmental fixation, which is difficult to achieve with other forms of fixation that require intact laminae such as multihook systems or sublaminar wires. Pedicle screws allow for preservation of lumbar lordosis and motion in ambulatory patients. The limitations of this technique arise from the abnormal pedicles in patients with myelomeningocele, which are often small, dysplastic, and rotated or are small, tightly packed vertebrae in lordotic segments.[5]

Controversy exists as to whether it is necessary to extend posterior fusion to the pelvis to address associated pelvic obliquity. In general, the fusion should include all curves and should extend to the sacrum for nonambulators. Because preservation of pelvic motion is essential for function in ambulatory patients, lumbosacral arthrodesis should be avoided whenever possible.

Short-term results suggest that the vertical expandable prosthetic titanium rib (VEPTR; DePuy Synthes), a construct allowing for continued growth, is a reasonable alternative to fusion for skeletally immature patients. The VEPTR allows for correction and stabilization of spinal deformity while maintaining adequate respiratory function. The complication rate is similar to that of fusion techniques.[33]

Kyphosis

Rigid kyphotic deformities of the lumbar or thoracolumbar spine, which occur in 8% to 21% of patients with myelomeningocele, can lead to difficulty with sitting or lying supine and are prone to skin breakdown and the resulting risk of infection. Patients may have a large, rigid curve at birth; curve progression is related to the level of the neurologic lesion. Nonsurgical treatment with orthoses or modified seating systems has been largely ineffective. Surgical treatment is indicated to correct sitting posture, prevent skin breakdown, and prevent deformity progression.

Various surgical treatment options exist; however, surgery for rigid kyphosis is technically demanding and carries a high risk of associated complications, including skin issues, infection, and pseudarthrosis. Multiple studies have shown a high rate of revision surgery and lengthy hospital stays.[34,35] The standard surgical treatment is kyphectomy with osteotomy and resection of the vertebral bodies combined with cordotomy and segmental spinal instrumentation and fusion down to the pelvis (**Figure 4**). Despite the high complication rate, surgical treatment has been shown to achieve lasting correction, with improved seating balance and resolution of skin problems in most patients.

Growth-friendly techniques recently have been applied as an alternative to fusion after kyphectomy in patients with myelomeningocele to prevent further compromise of trunk height. Growth-friendly options include growing rods and the Luque trolley with Galveston instrumentation. Medium-term results suggest both options are reasonable alternatives to fusion to allow extra growth; however, the use of these techniques must be balanced against the risk of an increased number of surgeries.[36]

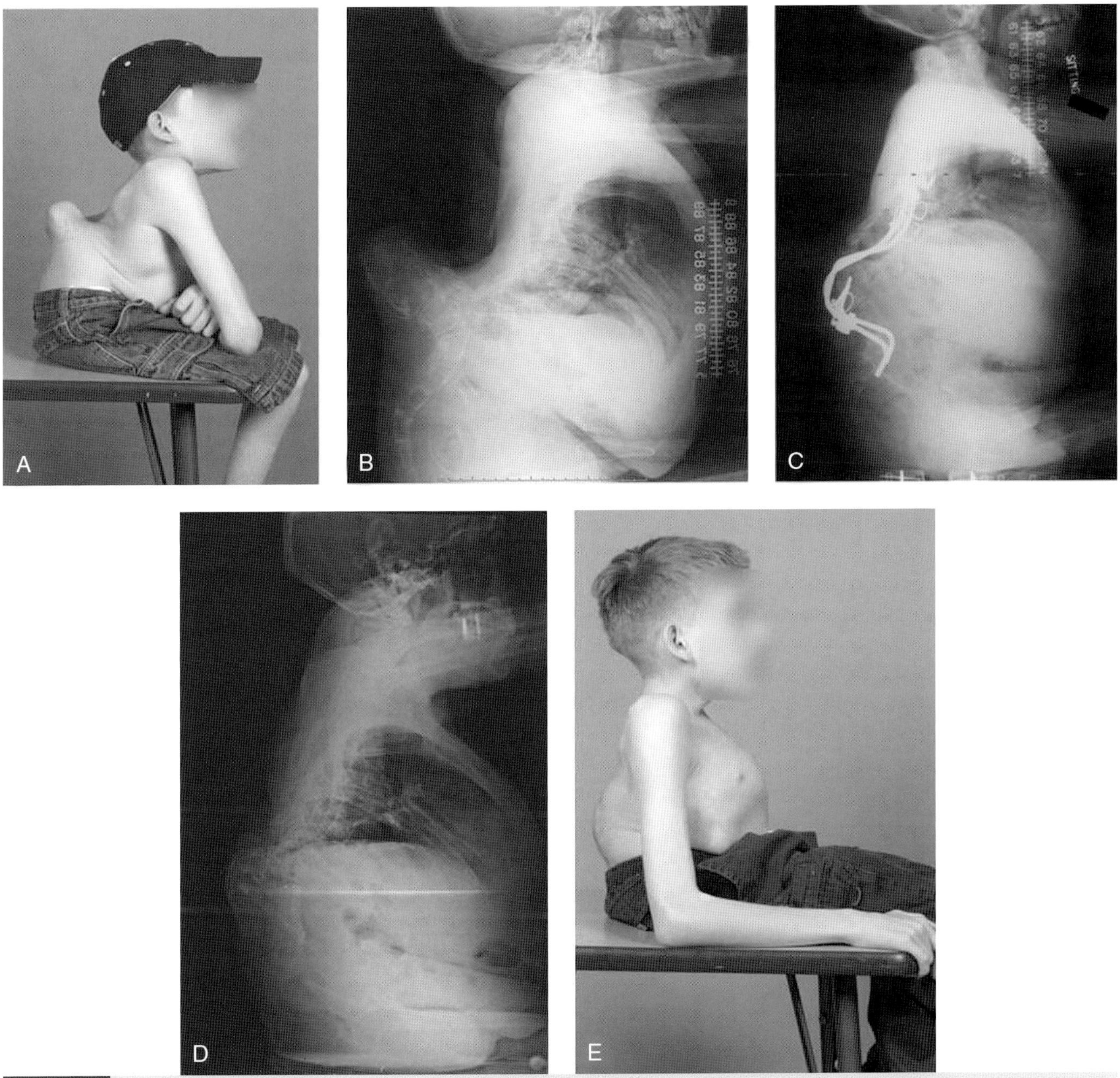

Figure 4 Images from a patient with thoracic-level myelomeningocele and a severe rigid kyphotic deformity. Preoperative lateral photograph (**A**) and lateral radiograph (**B**). **C,** Postoperative lateral radiograph after kyphectomy with segmental proximal fixation and distal sacral fixation. A deep infection developed and was treated with anterior fusion; a posterior infection was suppressed. Infection recurred after suppression therapy was discontinued, and implant removal was required. **D,** Final lateral radiograph shows solid anterior fusion. **E,** Photograph shows the final clinical appearance of the patient. (Reproduced with permission from: Garg S, Oetgen M, Rathjen K, et al: Kyphectomy improves sitting and skin problems in patients with myelomeningocele. *Clin Orthop Relat Res* 2011;469[5]:1279-1285.)

Hip Instability

Paralytic hip dislocation is a common and difficult problem in patients with myelomeningocele, and its management represents an example of a radical change in treatment strategy in recent years that has resulted from the increased emphasis on functional outcomes. CGA assessment of patients with neurologic involvement at a low lumbar level and a unilateral hip dislocation has shown that gait symmetry corresponds to the absence of hip contractures and is not related to hip dislocation.[37] An examination of functional results after surgical hip reduction showed no improvement in hip range of motion, ambulatory ability, decreased pain, or a decreased need for bracing. A review of the literature confirmed that current treatment goals should focus on maintaining hip range of motion, with contracture release as necessary. No role was identified for hip reduction in patients with low lumbar or higher functional levels of involvement.[38]

Optimal treatment remains controversial for the relatively rare patient who has sacral-level involvement, a dislocated hip, and the ability to walk without support. Without treatment, these patients may have a decline in gait function caused by limb-length discrepancy and increased lurch caused by the loss of a fulcrum resulting from the dislocated hip. These patients may benefit from surgical reduction to preserve independent gait function; however, surgical outcomes in this subgroup of patients are unknown and merit further study.[3]

Knee Deformity and Pain

Knee Flexion Contracture

Knee flexion contracture, which is common in patients with myelomeningocele, causes a crouch gait with high energy cost in ambulatory patients. Studies have shown that a fixed knee flexion contracture greater than 10° may lead to anterior knee pain, decreased endurance, difficulty with orthotic fitting, and a progressive crouch gait.[39,40] CGA is useful to quantify the amount of knee flexion during gait, which can be substantially greater than that seen during a static clinical examination. To preserve ambulatory potential, surgical treatment is indicated for knee flexion contracture greater than 20°.[41] Surgical options include anterior distal femoral epiphysiodesis, radical knee flexor release of the hamstrings and posterior capsule, or, for severe cases, distal femur supracondylar extension osteotomy. Epiphysiodesis has been shown to be safe and effective for knee flexion contracture in patients with myelomeningocele, with a rate of correction of approximately 1° per month. CGA has documented improvements in clinical knee flexion contracture, dynamic sagittal kinematics, and walking velocity after radical posterior knee capsulectomy.[41]

Knee Valgus Stress

Valgus knee deformity occurs frequently in patients with neurologic involvement at the low lumbar and sacral levels and can lead to instability, pain, and arthritis in adulthood. Knee pain plays an important role in a patient's decision not to walk. CGA has facilitated a better understanding of the multiple factors that can contribute to abnormal valgus stress. During the stance phase, the knee is subjected to forces of the upper body and ground reaction forces coming through the foot, which can lead to valgus positioning.[4] Contributing factors to knee valgus stress include rotational malalignment of the femur, femoral anteversion in association with excessive external tibial torsion, excessive trunk and pelvic motion, knee flexion contractures, and valgus foot deformities.

Although surgical correction of excessive rotational abnormalities leads to improvement in knee stress, it may not completely normalize the knee moment because of the many involved factors. Tibial derotation osteotomy can lead to improvement in knee pain and may prevent the onset of late degenerative changes,[42] but crutches still may be recommended to compensate for weak hip abductor muscles and protect the knees from excessive lateral sway. AFOs also should be used to increase stance-phase stability. If knee flexion contracture or hindfoot valgus is present, these conditions should be corrected surgically at the same time.[3] CGA has shown that patients with knee pain have increased knee flexion compared with patients who are asymptomatic; this suggests that increased knee flexion combined with inadequate control of hip transverse kinematics may lead to knee joint loading.[43]

Rotational Deformities

In patients with myelomeningocele, internal tibial torsion is typically a fixed deformity often associated with clubfoot. The etiology of external tibial torsion is unknown, but dynamic muscle imbalance may be a contributing factor.[44] Internal or external tibial torsion deformity should not be expected to resolve spontaneously without surgical correction. For ambulatory patients, rotational malalignment can substantially alter gait mechanics and velocity, affecting ambulatory efficiency. In an attempt to decrease risk of recurrence, surgical treatment is typically delayed until the age of 5 or 6 years. Prior to that time, AFOs with twister cables can be used to improve ambulatory function, although parents should be counseled not to expect the twister cables to correct the underlying bony torsion.

Surgical correction is recommended for deformity greater than 20° and leads to improved functional outcomes in terms of increased brace tolerance and gait parameters. When planning for correction of external tibial torsion, it is essential to assess for any concomitant hindfoot valgus, which should be addressed at the same time with a medial sliding osteotomy of the calcaneus to achieve a successful result.[3] Tibial derotation osteotomies in patients with myelomeningocele have traditionally been associated with a high rate of complications, including nonunion, delayed union, poor wound healing, and infection. However, the use of technique modifications, including drill corticotomy, rigid compression plating, and meticulous skin closure, have resulted in a substantial decrease in the complication rate.[44]

Foot Deformity

Foot deformity exists in almost all patients with myelomeningocele and can interfere with brace tolerance, which causes difficulties with ambulation. The goal of treatment is to preserve function and range of motion and avoid pressure sores by maintaining a plantigrade, flexible, and braceable foot.[45] Effort should be made to prevent rigid deformities by early intervention, with bracing or surgical treatment as needed. The principles of surgical treatment include use of tendon excisions rather than transfers or lengthenings to achieve a flail foot, which makes brace fitting easier. For fixed bony deformities, every effort should be made to preserve joint motion with extra-articular osteotomies. Arthrodesis should be avoided because the resulting stiffness combined with an insensate foot leads to a high risk of pressure sores. After surgical treatment, use of an AFO brace helps to maintain correction and prevent recurrence.

Clubfoot

Clubfoot is the most common foot deformity seen in patients with myelomeningocele (**Figure 5**) and is different from idiopathic clubfoot. In patients with myelomeningocele, clubfoot is a severely rigid deformity that is often recalcitrant to treatment and has a propensity for recurrence. The Ponseti method of manipulative treatment combined with Achilles tenotomy has been used to treat patients with myelomeningocele. Early study results show initial correction can be achieved in most patients; however, the recurrence rate is 60% to 70% with a high associated rate of complications, including skin breakdown and fractures.[46,47] No long-term follow-up reports are available at this time. Although the Ponseti method is useful as a noninvasive method to delay or avoid the need for extensive soft-tissue release, families should be educated about realistic expectations and prepared for the high risk of recurrence, the potential need for further treatment, and the risk of complications. Consideration should be given to performing an open excision of the Achilles tendon in the operating room, and a brace should be used on a full-time basis after casting to prevent recurrence.

Vertical Talus

Vertical talus is a rigid, rocker-bottom flatfoot deformity that occurs in 10% of patients with myelomeningocele. There is extreme, rigid plantar flexion of the talus with dorsolateral dislocation of the talonavicular joint, and the foot is not correctable by manipulation. Correction has traditionally been achieved with complete posteromedial, lateral, and dorsal release when the patient is between 10 and 12 months of age.[45] More recently, a minimally invasive treatment method has been reported consisting of serial manipulation and casting followed by open talonavicular pin fixation and Achilles tenotomy.[48] Initially described for isolated vertical talus, encouraging short-term results have now been reported for nonisolated cases as well, including patients with myelomeningocele[49] (**Figure 6**). Although long-term results and recurrence rates are not yet known, this method provides a noninvasive option for potentially avoiding the need for extensive soft-tissue release.

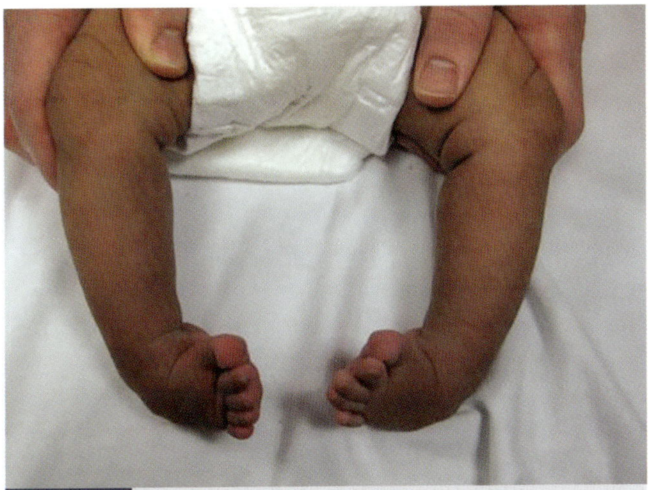

Figure 5 Clinical photograph of a child with bilateral severe, rigid clubfoot. Note the presence of deep medial and posterior creases.

Adult Care

With an increase in the number of patients surviving into adulthood, many patients with myelomeningocele now require transition to adult medical providers. This presents a challenge because adult providers may lack the expertise necessary to manage the issues unique to adult patients with myelomeningocele. Guiding principles for orthopaedic care include aggressive treatment of tethered cord syndrome, surgical correction of musculoskeletal deformities that have the potential to affect independence, and avoidance of arthrodesis of the foot.[50] Secondary conditions in adults such as obesity and urologic issues have a negative effect on autonomy, function, and the level of community participation. Lymphedema also is common in adult patients and can cause difficulties with brace fitting and lead to functional decline. Pressure sores are another major complication and occasionally require limb amputation.

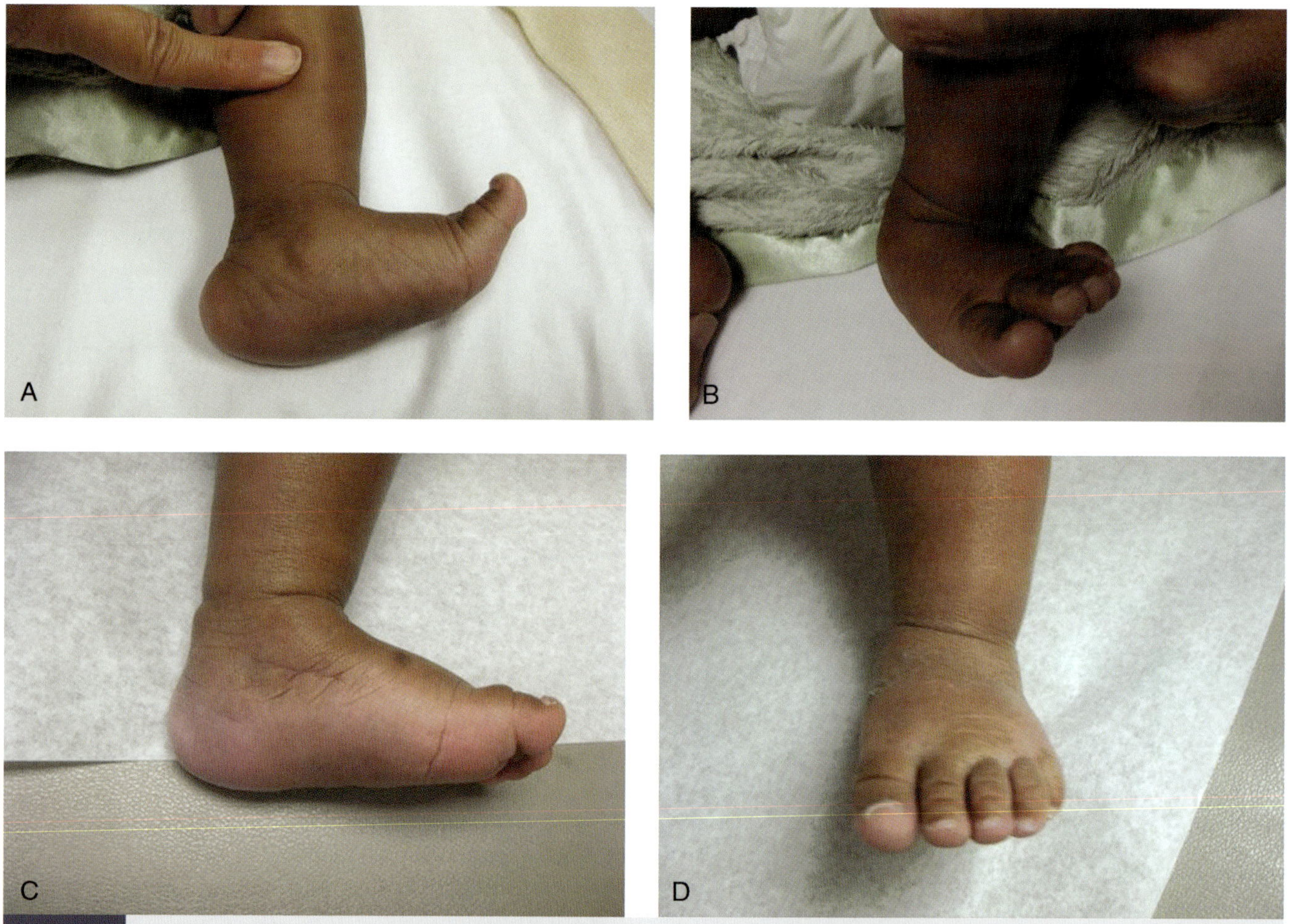

Figure 6 Lateral (**A**) and AP (**B**) clinical photographs of the foot of a child with rigid vertical talus. Lateral (**C**) and AP (**D**) clinical photographs of the foot after undergoing a minimally invasive method of treatment.

Multiple large cohort studies have reported on outcome and life satisfaction of adults with myelomeningocele. One study found myelomeningocele did not affect overall reported life satisfaction for adults.[51] Fifty-six percent of the patients completed a technical, associate, or college degree, and 47% were able to maintain employment. Twenty-eight percent had been married, and 18% had biological children. However, the presence of hydrocephalus substantially decreased the likelihood of these outcomes but did not contribute to decreased life satisfaction. Similarly, a 2011 study found adult patients who had never required a VPS placement had higher IQs.[52] All of the patients in that study with neurologic involvement at the thoracic or high lumbar level used wheelchairs; 78% of the patients with low lumbar-level involvement used a wheelchair on a part-time basis. All of the patients with neurologic involvement at the sacral level were ambulatory. In this cohort of patients, spinal fusions protected sitting balance, but hip surgery did not produce congruent hips and occasionally resulted in debilitating stiffness.

Summary

The orthopaedic care of patients with myelomeningocele continues to improve with increased attention to functional outcomes. Ideally, orthopaedic care should be administered as part of a multidisciplinary team approach to optimally manage the complex medical comorbidities of these patients. The goal of the orthopaedic surgeon is to minimize deformity, maximize function and mobility, and limit complications.

Key Study Points

- Fetal surgery for myelomeningocele, although associated with serious risks such as preterm delivery and uterine dehiscence, decreases the need for VPS placement and seems to improve lower extremity function in short-term follow-up studies.
- The most important factor influencing ambulatory potential in patients with myelomeningocele is the neurologic level of involvement.
- Many factors influence the functional level achieved by patients with myelomeningocele, including spasticity; tethered cord; obesity; neurosurgical complications; poor balance; and musculoskeletal conditions such as hip contractures, scoliosis, and foot deformity.

Annotated References

1. Shimoji K, Kimura T, Kondo A, Tange Y, Miyajima M, Arai H: Genetic studies of myelomeningocele. *Childs Nerv Syst* 2013;29(9):1417-1425.

   In a review of genetic studies of myelomeningocele, the genetic etiology of candidate genes related to the metabolic pathways of folate and glucose, animal models of neural tube defects, and recent studies of microRNA are described. Level of evidence: III.

2. Bowman RM, McLone DG, Grant JA, Tomita T, Ito JA: Spina bifida outcome: A 25-year prospective. *Pediatr Neurosurg* 2001;34(3):114-120.

3. Swaroop VT, Dias L: Orthopedic management of spina bifida: Part I. Hip, knee, and rotational deformities. *J Child Orthop* 2009;3(6):441-449.

4. Thomson JD, Segal LS: Orthopedic management of spina bifida. *Dev Disabil Res Rev* 2010;16(1):96-103.

5. Swaroop VT, Dias L: Myelomeningocele, in Weinstein SL, Flynn JM, eds: *Lovell and Winter's Pediatric Orthopaedics* ,ed 7. Philadelphia, PA, Lippincott Williams & Wilkins, 2014, pp 555-586.

6. Padmanabhan R: Etiology, pathogenesis and prevention of neural tube defects. *Congenit Anom (Kyoto)* 2006;46(2):55-67.

7. Doran PA, Guthkelch AN: Studies in spina bifida cystica: I. General survey and reassessment of the problem. *J Neurol Neurosurg Psychiatry* 1961;24:331-345.

8. Ingraham FD, Swam H: Spina bifida and cranium bifida: I. A survey of five hundred forty six cases. *N Engl J Med* 1943;228:559.

9. Au KS, Ashley-Koch A, Northrup H: Epidemiologic and genetic aspects of spina bifida and other neural tube defects. *Dev Disabil Res Rev* 2010;16(1):6-15.

10. Walsh DS, Adzick NS, Sutton LN, Johnson MP: The rationale for in utero repair of myelomeningocele. *Fetal Diagn Ther* 2001;16(5):312-322.

11. Agarwal R, Thornton ME, Fonteh AN, Harrington MG, Chmait RH, Grubbs BH: Amniotic fluid levels of phospholipase A2 in fetal rats with retinoic acid induced myelomeningocele: The potential "second hit" in neurologic damage. *J Matern Fetal Neonatal Med* 2015;1-6.

    Phospholipase A_2 activity was substantially increased in amniotic fluid of pregnant rats with myelomeningocele compared with controls and may contribute to ongoing neural injury. This pathway may be a useful drug target to limit ongoing damage and better preserve neurologic function. Level of evidence: II.

12. Tulipan N, Bruner JP, Hernanz-Schulman M, et al: Effect of intrauterine myelomeningocele repair on central nervous system structure and function. *Pediatr Neurosurg* 1999;31(4):183-188.

13. Adzick NS, Thom EA, Spong CY, et al; MOMS Investigators: A randomized trial of prenatal versus postnatal repair of myelomeningocele. *N Engl J Med* 2011;364(11):993-1004.

    A randomized trial of patients undergoing myelomeningocele repair prenatally compared with those treated with standard postnatal repair showed a decreased need for shunting and improved motor outcomes at 30 months in the patients treated prenatally; however, prenatal repair was associated with maternal and fetal risks. Level of evidence: I.

14. Moldenhauer JS, Soni S, Rintoul NE, et al: Fetal myelomeningocele repair: The post-MOMS experience at the Children's Hospital of Philadelphia. *Fetal Diagn Ther* 2015;37(3):235-240.

    A review of patients undergoing fetal myelomeningocele repair at a single institution showed a 6% perinatal demise. Fifty-five percent of the patients were assigned a functional level that was one (or more) better than the prenatal anatomic level. Level of evidence: III.

15. Danzer E, Gerdes M, Bebbington MW, et al: Lower extremity neuromotor function and short-term ambulatory potential following in utero myelomeningocele surgery. *Fetal Diagn Ther* 2009;25(1):47-53.

16. Danzer E, Thomas NH, Thomas A, et al: Long-term neurofunctional outcome, executive functioning, and behavioral adaptive skills following fetal myelomeningocele surgery. *Am J Obstet Gynecol* 2016;214(2):269.e1-269.e8.

    Results of fetal myelomeningocele repair at a median follow-up of 10 years showed that fetal surgery improves long-term ambulatory status. Spinal cord tethering is associated with functional loss. A more-than-expected number of children who had fetal repair were continent, but bowel and bladder control continue to be a challenging problem. Level of evidence: III.

17. Faria TC, Cavalheiro S, Hisaba WJ, et al: Improvement of motor function and decreased need for postnatal shunting in children who had undergone intrauterine myelomeningocele repair. *Arq Neuropsiquiatr* 2013;71(9A):604-608.

    A comparison of patients with myelomeningocele undergoing intrauterine repair to standard postnatal repair showed substantially improved function in the intrauterine repair group, with functional level higher than anatomic level by two or more spinal segments in all patients. Level of evidence: III.

18. Seitzberg A, Lind M, Biering-Sørensen F: Ambulation in adults with myelomeningocele. Is it possible to predict the level of ambulation in early life? *Childs Nerv Syst* 2008;24(2):231-237.

19. McDonald CM, Jaffe KM, Mosca VS, Shurtleff DB: Ambulatory outcome of children with myelomeningocele: Effect of lower-extremity muscle strength. *Dev Med Child Neurol* 1991;33(6):482-490.

20. Mazur JM, Shurtleff D, Menelaus M, Colliver J: Orthopaedic management of high-level spina bifida: Early walking compared with early use of a wheelchair. *J Bone Joint Surg Am* 1989;71(1):56-61.

21. Haas RE, Kecskemethy HH, Lopiccolo MA, Hossain J, Dy RT, Bachrach SJ: Lower extremity bone mineral density in children with congenital spinal dysfunction. *Dev Med Child Neurol* 2012;54(12):1133-1137.

    Dual-energy x-ray absorptiometry of the lateral distal femur was found to be a viable technique for assessing BMD in patients with myelomeningocele and was sensitive to differences in three categories of ambulation. Overall ambulatory status had more influence on BMD than neurologic level. Level of evidence: III.

22. Szalay EA, Cheema A: Children with spina bifida are at risk for low bone density. *Clin Orthop Relat Res* 2011;469(5):1253-1257.

    A retrospective review of patients with myelomeningocele showed that nonambulatory patients were more likely to have low BMD for age than unaffected individuals. Dual-energy x-ray absorptiometry of the lateral distal femur was useful in measuring BMD in this population. Level of evidence: IV.

23. Akbar M, Bresch B, Raiss P, et al: Fractures in myelomeningocele. *J Orthop Traumatol* 2010;11(3):175-182.

24. Bowman RM, McLone DG: Neurosurgical management of spina bifida: Research issues. *Dev Disabil Res Rev* 2010;16(1):82-87.

25. Battibugli S, Gryfakis N, Dias L, et al: Functional gait comparison between children with myelomeningocele: Shunt versus no shunt. *Dev Med Child Neurol* 2007;49(10):764-769.

26. Fiore P, Picco P, Castagnola E, et al: Nutritional survey of children and adolescents with myelomeningocele (MMC): Overweight associated with reduced energy intake. *Eur J Pediatr Surg* 1998;8(suppl 1):34-36.

27. Mueske NM, Ryan DD, Van Speybroeck AL, Chan LS, Wren TA: Fat distribution in children and adolescents with myelomeningocele. *Dev Med Child Neurol* 2015;57(3):273-278.

    The percentage of fat in patients with myelomeningocele compared with control subject was performed using dual-energy x-ray absorptiometry. The authors reported that the patients with myelomeningocele had higher than normal total body and leg fat, but only patients with higher-level lesions had increased trunk fat. Level of evidence: IV.

28. Mita K, Akataki K, Itoh K, Ono Y, Ishida N, Oki T: Assessment of obesity of children with spina bifida. *Dev Med Child Neurol* 1993;35(4):305-311.

29. Schoenmakers MA, Gulmans VA, Gooskens RH, Pruijs JE, Helders PJ: Spinal fusion in children with spina bifida: Influence on ambulation level and functional abilities. *Eur Spine J* 2005;14(4):415-422.

30. Mazur J, Menelaus MB, Dickens DR, Doig WG: Efficacy of surgical management for scoliosis in myelomeningocele: Correction of deformity and alteration of functional status. *J Pediatr Orthop* 1986;6(5):568-575.

31. Khoshbin A, Vivas L, Law PW, et al: The long-term outcome of patients treated operatively and non-operatively for scoliosis deformity secondary to spina bifida. *Bone Joint J* 2014;96-B(9):1244-1251.

    At an average follow-up of 14 years, this retrospective review of patients with myelomeningocele and scoliosis treated surgically or nonsurgically showed that both groups had statistically similar outcomes in walking capacity, neurologic motor level, sitting balance, and health-related quality-of-life outcomes. Level of evidence: III.

32. Sponseller PD, Young AT, Sarwark JF, Lim R: Anterior only fusion for scoliosis in patients with myelomeningocele. *Clin Orthop Relat Res* 1999;364:117-124.

33. Flynn JM, Ramirez N, Emans JB, Smith JT, Mulcahey MJ, Betz RR: Is the vertebral expandable prosthetic titanium rib a surgical alternative in patients with spina bifida? *Clin Orthop Relat Res* 2011;469(5):1291-1296.

    A review of skeletally immature, nonambulatory patients with myelodysplasia treated with VEPTR for scoliosis showed it is a reasonable option to correct spinal deformity, allow spinal growth, and maintain adequate respiratory function; the complication rate was similar to that of standard approaches. Level of evidence: IV.

34. Garg S, Oetgen M, Rathjen K, Richards BS: Kyphectomy improves sitting and skin problems in

patients with myelomeningocele. *Clin Orthop Relat Res* 2011;469(5):1279-1285.

The authors of this retrospective review of patients with thoracic-level myelomeningocele who were treated with kyphectomy and fusion found improved sitting balance and resolution of skin problems in 17 of 18 patients; however, a high complication rate and long hospital stays were reported. Level of evidence: IV.

35. Altiok H, Finlayson C, Hassani S, Sturm P: Kyphectomy in children with myelomeningocele. *Clin Orthop Relat Res* 2011;469(5):1272-1278.

This retrospective review of patients with myelomeningocele who were treated with kyphectomy and fusion showed that, although the procedure was technically demanding and had substantial risk, it allowed correction and maintenance of sagittal alignment. Level of evidence: IV.

36. Bas CE, Preminger J, Olgun ZD, Demirkiran G, Sponseller P, Yazici M; Growing Spine Study Group: Safety and efficacy of apical resection following growth-friendly instrumentation in myelomeningocele patients with gibbus: Growing rod versus Luque trolley. *J Pediatr Orthop* 2015;35(8):e98-e103.

A comparison of growth-friendly techniques for kyphosis management showed that both techniques were reasonable growth-preserving alternatives to fusion after kyphectomy; however, there are risks associated with an increased number of surgeries. Level of evidence: IV.

37. Gabrieli AP, Vankoski SJ, Dias LS, et al: Gait analysis in low lumbar myelomeningocele patients with unilateral hip dislocation or subluxation. *J Pediatr Orthop* 2003;23(3):330-334.

38. Swaroop VT, Dias LS: What is the optimal treatment for hip and spine in myelomeningocele? in Wright JG, ed: *Evidence-Based Orthopaedics* .Amsterdam, Netherlands, Elsevier Health Sciences, 2008, pp 273-277.

39. Spiro AS, Babin K, Lipovac S, et al: Anterior femoral epiphysiodesis for the treatment of fixed knee flexion deformity in spina bifida patients. *J Pediatr Orthop* 2010;30(8):858-862.

40. Dias LS: Surgical management of knee contractures in myelomeningocele. *J Pediatr Orthop* 1982;2(2):127-131.

41. Moen TC, Dias L, Swaroop VT, Gryfakis N, Kelp-Lenane C: Radical posterior capsulectomy improves sagittal knee motion in crouch gait. *Clin Orthop Relat Res* 2011;469(5):1286-1290.

This retrospective review used CGA to assess the outcomes of patients with low lumbar or high sacral involvement undergoing radical posterior capsulectomy for knee flexion contracture. Results showed improvement in clinical knee flexion contracture, dynamic sagittal kinematics, and walking velocity. Level of evidence: IV.

42. Dunteman RC, Vankoski SJ, Dias LS: Internal derotation osteotomy of the tibia: Pre- and postoperative gait analysis in persons with high sacral myelomeningocele. *J Pediatr Orthop* 2000;20(5):623-628.

43. Rao S, Dietz F, Yack HJ: Kinematics and kinetics during gait in symptomatic and asymptomatic limbs of children with myelomeningocele. *J Pediatr Orthop* 2012;32(1):106-112.

The authors used CGA to compare children with L3-L4 myelomeningocele involvement with age-matched control subjects. They found that the symptomatic limbs in patients with myelomeningocele had increased knee flexion and trended toward higher extension, adduction, and internal rotation moments. Level of evidence: IV.

44. Mednick RE, Eller EB, Swaroop VT, Dias L: Outcomes of tibial derotational osteotomies performed in patients with myelodysplasia. *J Pediatr Orthop* 2015;35(7):721-724.

In this retrospective review, the authors report on patient with myelodysplasia undergoing distal tibial derotational osteotomy. Results showed that it was a safe, effective method to treat tibial torsion, with an acceptable complication rate. Patients with lumbar-level involvement and initial internal torsion were at higher risk for rerotation. Level of evidence: IV.

45. Swaroop VT, Dias L: Orthopaedic management of spina bifida: Part II. Foot and ankle deformities. *J Child Orthop* 2011;5(6):403-414.

A review of diagnosis and management of foot deformities in patients with myelomeningocele is presented.

46. Dunkley M, Gelfer Y, Jackson D, et al: Mid-term results of a physiotherapist-led Ponseti service for the management of non-idiopathic and idiopathic clubfoot. *J Child Orthop* 2015;9(3):183-189.

A review of clubfeet treated with the Ponseti method by physiotherapists showed that this treatment was not as successful in nonidiopathic feet as it was in idiopathic feet. A 40% recurrence rate and the need for additional treatment were reported in the group with nonidiopathic clubfoot. Level of evidence: III.

47. Gerlach DJ, Gurnett CA, Limpaphayom N, et al: Early results of the Ponseti method for the treatment of clubfoot associated with myelomeningocele. *J Bone Joint Surg Am* 2009;91(6):1350-1359.

48. Dobbs MB, Purcell DB, Nunley R, Morcuende JA: Early results of a new method of treatment for idiopathic congenital vertical talus. Surgical technique. *J Bone Joint Surg Am* 2007;89(suppl 2 pt 1):111-121.

49. Chalayon O, Adams A, Dobbs MB: Minimally invasive approach for the treatment of non-isolated congenital vertical talus. *J Bone Joint Surg Am* 2012;94(11):e73.

This retrospective review of patients with nonisolated vertical talus treated with a minimally invasive method showed that initial correction was achieved in all patients; a 20% recurrence rate was reported. Level of evidence: IV.

50. Selber P, Dias L: Sacral-level myelomeningocele: Long-term outcome in adults. *J Pediatr Orthop* 1998;18(4):423-427.

51. Cope H, McMahon K, Heise E, et al: Outcome and life satisfaction of adults with myelomeningocele. *Disabil Health J* 2013;6(3):236-243.

A survey of adults with myelomeningocele showed a diverse range of outcomes in education, employment, relationships, and reproduction. Hydrocephalus was associated with difficulty attaining adult milestones but did not contribute to reduced life satisfaction. Level of evidence: IV.

52. Roach JW, Short BF, Saltzman HM: Adult consequences of spina bifida: A cohort study. *Clin Orthop Relat Res* 2011;469(5):1246-1252.

The authors of a retrospective review of adults with myelomeningocele reported a range of social and educational outcomes. All except one patient with neurologic involvement at the thoracic and high-lumbar level used wheelchairs, 78% of patients with low-lumbar involvement used a wheelchair part-time, and all patients with sacral-level involvement were ambulatory. Level of evidence: IV.

Chapter 13

Arthrogrypotic Syndromes

Kathryn S. Doughty, MD, MPH, MS Robert H. Cho, MD Christopher Stutz, MD

Abstract

Arthrogryposis refers to a constellation of syndromes characterized by multiple joint contractures. The treatment of any type of arthrogryposis can be challenging, but early intervention and proper nonsurgical and surgical management can achieve improvement in many patients. The goal for any treatment strategy is to maximize function with the minimal amount of hospitalization necessary to achieve that goal. Physical and occupational therapy and bracing can help improve function in many children so that surgical management can be mitigated or avoided. Surgical treatment should be reserved for enhancing function, not just correcting deformity.

Keywords: amyoplasia; arthrogryposis; arthrogryposis multiplex congenita; Bruck syndrome; contractures; distal arthrogryposis; Larsen syndrome; multiple pterygium syndrome

Introduction

Arthrogryposis multiplex congenita, which is also known as arthrogryposis, is an umbrella term rather than a diagnosis for a heterogeneous group of disorders characterized by multiple congenital joint contractures. Although the exact etiology is usually multifactorial (nerve, muscle, or connective tissue disorders; maternal disease; intrauterine constraint; and vascular compromise), the condition is associated with decreased fetal movement. The earlier the intrauterine insult resulting in fetal akinesis, the more severe the disease is at birth. Most deformities are nonprogressive and may improve over time with early treatment. Mental development is usually normal. The most common musculoskeletal deformities associated with arthrogryposis are clubfeet and hip dislocations. The incidence of arthrogryposis is approximately 1 per 3,000 live births.[1]

More than 300 different syndromes are associated with congenital contractures.[2] These conditions are associated with substantial morbidity and economic burden, so understanding the underlying etiology of a child's condition can aid in determining the prognosis and selecting the best treatment options. Approximately 50% of the conditions associated with arthrogryposis have an underlying genetic abnormality. Distal arthrogryposis is one of the most notable conditions because it can be inherited in an autosomal dominant manner.

Congenital contractures can be categorized as isolated or multiple[3] (**Figure 1**). In a child with multiple congenital contractures, it is necessary to determine if the neurologic examination has normal or abnormal findings. Amyoplasia and distal arthrogryposis are common types of arthrogryposis that are associated with normal neurologic development. A generalized connective tissue disorder and fetal crowding are less common causes of arthrogryposis that are associated with normal neurologic development. Conversely, an abnormal neurologic examination suggests that in utero movement was diminished as a result of central or peripheral nervous system disorders or intrinsic muscle disease.

Diagnosis

Prenatal ultrasounds may be able to document fetal movements and positions that suggest a typically developing fetus versus a fetus affected by multiple joint contractures. Genetic testing may be useful; however, only approximately 50% of arthrogrypotic conditions have an

Dr. Doughty or an immediate family member serves as a board member, owner, officer, or committee member of the American Academy for Cerebral Palsy and Developmental Medicine and the Pediatric Orthopaedic Society of North America. Dr. Cho or an immediate family member serves as a paid consultant to DePuy Spine, Medtronic Sofamor Danek, Nuvasive, and OrthoPediatrics. Neither Dr. Stutz nor any immediate family member has received anything of value from or has stock or stock options held in a commercial company or institution related directly or indirectly to the subject of this chapter.

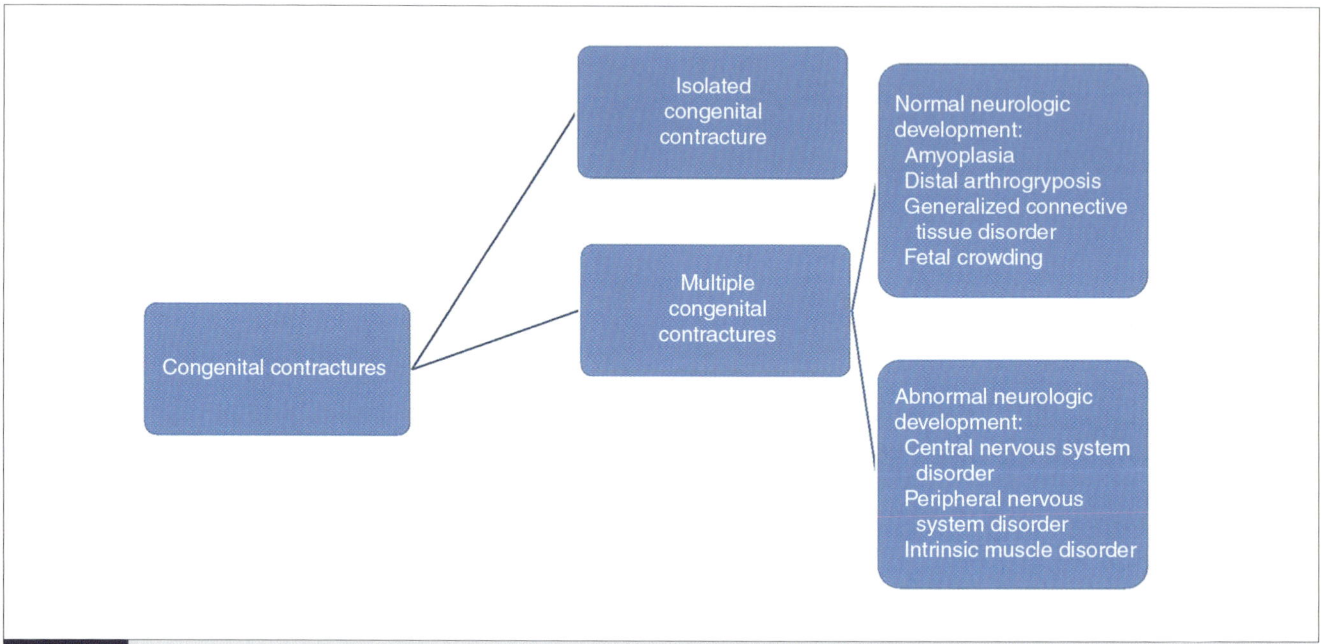

Figure 1 Congenital contractures can be divided into isolated or multiple contractures. Isolated congenital contractures affect only a single area of the body; the most common isolated contracture is congenital clubfoot. Amyoplasia falls under the category of multiple congenital contractures with normal neurologic development.

identifiable genetic abnormality. Genetic information can be helpful in counseling parents on the risks for future affected pregnancies. Arthrogryposis is not a hereditary condition, whereas distal arthrogryposis is often inherited in an autosomal dominant pattern (**Figure 2**).

Any child with multiple contractures should have a thorough initial history and physical examination, including a family history. Additional studies and consultations with specialists may be warranted if the condition affects the neurologic system or appears to be syndromic. A skeletal survey, including radiographs of the spine, shoulders, elbows, hips, knees, and feet, is usually obtained early in the examination process.

Depending on the results of the skeletal survey, a partial differential diagnosis may include spinal dysraphism, congenital muscular dystrophy, spinal muscular atrophy, structural brain anomalies, chromosomal abnormalities, thrombocytopenia with absent radius (TAR) syndrome, Möbius syndrome, Larsen syndrome, or Freeman-Sheldon syndrome.[4]

Types of Arthrogryposis

Amyoplasia

Amyoplasia is the classic form of arthrogryposis, comprising approximately one-third of all cases. The incidence of amyoplasia is approximately 1 per 10,000 live births.[5] It is not a hereditary condition. All four extremities are affected in approximately 60% of patients, only the lower extremities are affected in approximately 25% of patients, and only the upper extremities in approximately 15% of patients. Clinical features are often diagnostic, including a midline hemangioma on the forehead, although this usually disappears over time (**Figure 3**).

The lower extremities are usually held in a typical posture—flexed, abducted and externally rotated hips, rigid knees (flexed or extended), and clubfeet (**Figure 4**). A typical posture, which is described later in this chapter, also characterizes amyoplasia of the upper extremities. Amyoplasia literally means “without muscle,” so muscles are typically hypoplastic or absent; in fact, the skeletal muscle is replaced by dense fibrous tissue and fat. Joints lack flexion creases (**Figure 5**). Intelligence is normal, sensation is intact, and most affected children are able to function independently as adults.[6]

Distal Arthrogryposis

Distal arthrogryposis most notably affects the hands and feet, but it may also involve more proximal joints. Distal arthrogryposis is often inherited in an autosomal dominant manner. Clinical features are similar to, but less severe than, classic amyoplasia. The hands are usually held in a typical posture with flexed wrists and the thumb in the palm. The lower extremities may exhibit hip dislocations, clubfeet, or congenital vertical tali. Joints are notable for lack of flexion creases. These patients also

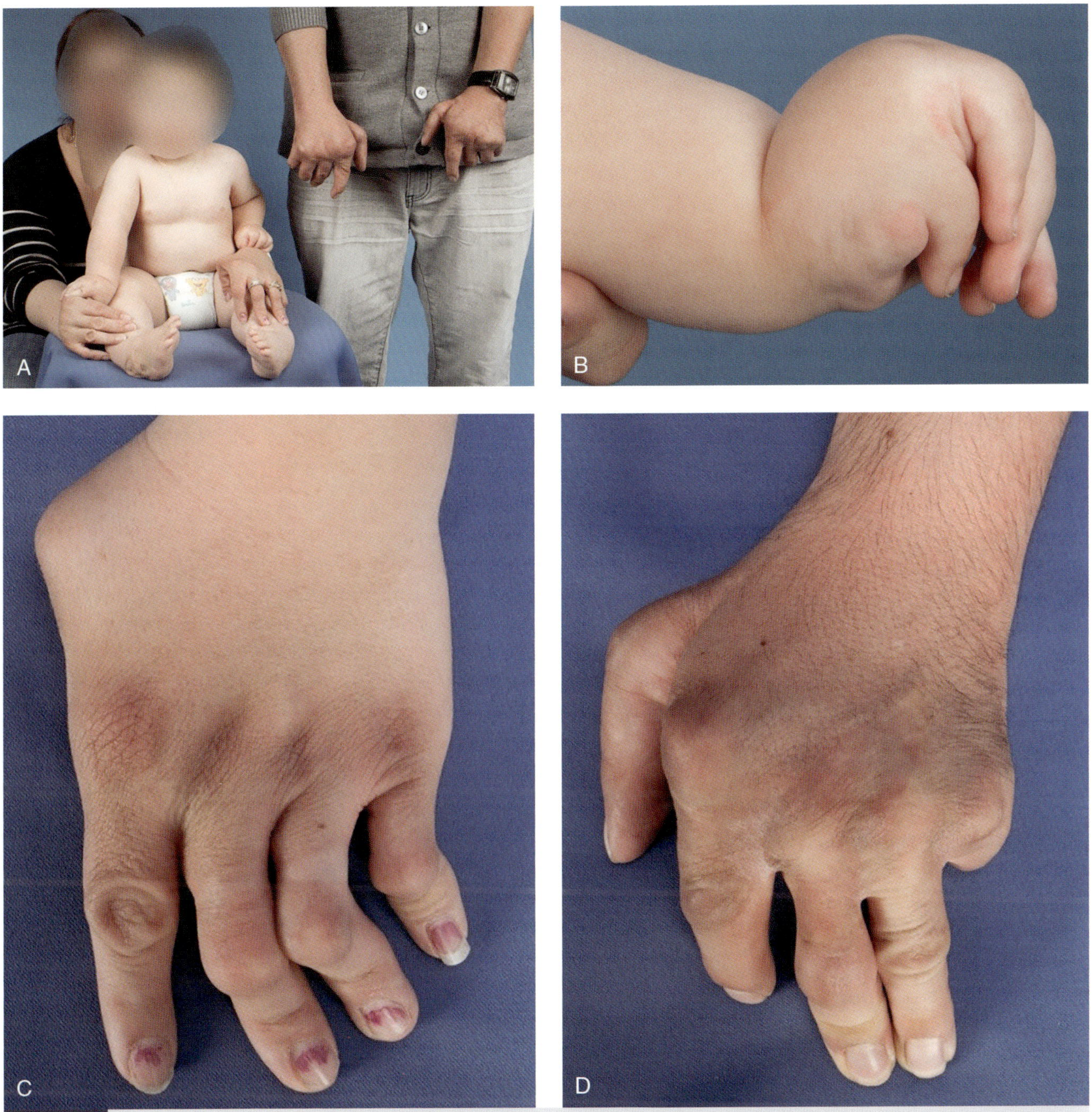

Figure 2 **A,** Photograph of a child with distal arthrogryposis with bilateral hand and foot deformities. His mother and uncle (pictured) also are affected, as is his maternal grandmother (not pictured). **B,** Photograph of the left hand of the child (**B**), the left hand of the child's mother (**C**), and the left hand of the child's uncle (**D**).

have normal intelligence, intact sensation, and most can function independently as adults.

Larsen Syndrome

Larsen syndrome, which was originally described in 1950, is a rare hereditary syndrome characterized by multiple joint dislocations from birth and characteristic facial features. Characteristics of the syndrome include a flattened dish-like face, bilateral dislocations of multiple joints, and equinovarus deformities of the feet.[7] Mutation occurs in the *FLNB* gene, which encodes for the protein filamin B and acts as a cytoskeletal binder to help chondrocytes differentiate and proliferate during development. The disease is characterized by a combination of laxity

3: Neuromuscular, Metabolic, and Inflammatory Disorders

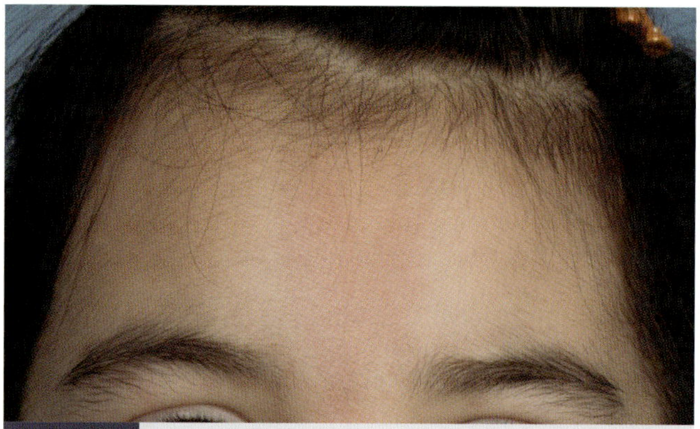

Figure 3 Photograph of a 4-year-old girl with a midline hemangioma, which is very common in patients with amyoplasia. Most hemangiomas disappear over time. Although this child's birthmark is vaguely visible, it becomes more prominent when the child is upset.

and dislocation in large joints that is present from birth (most commonly the cervical spine, hip, knee, and the radiocapitellar joints) and rigid talipes equinovarus deformities of the feet. The cervical spine and knee deformities are particularly challenging to manage, and the goals of treatment are stabilization and prevention of further deformity.[8,9] Unilateral hip dislocations are often treated surgically, but the treatment of bilateral hip dislocation is controversial and may be best left untreated.[10] Clubfoot deformities also are challenging to treat. Similar guidelines to the treatment of clubfeet for the other arthrogrypotic syndromes should be followed. Timing of treatment usually involves serial casting for clubfoot, followed by surgical stabilization of the cervical spine if necessary, and then treatment of knee or other joint dislocations.

Multiple Pterygium Syndromes

Multiple pterygium syndromes are a rare spectrum of disorders involving pterygia (skin webbing) of multiple joints, including the elbows and knees; congenital joint contractures; and facial anomalies. Multiple pterygium syndromes are further subcategorized into Escobar syndrome[11] (a milder disorder) and lethal multiple pterygium syndrome, which is often fatal in utero or shortly after birth. Most cases involve a mutation of the *CHRNG* gene, which encodes for the gamma subunit of the fetal acetylcholine receptor protein that allows for neuromuscular signaling. The lethal form involves complete absence of this subunit, whereas the Escobar form involves a decrease in the relative level of this protein. The fetal acetylcholine receptor gene is replaced in utero at approximately 33 weeks of gestation with an adult acetylcholine receptor gene; therefore, most patients with multiple pterygium

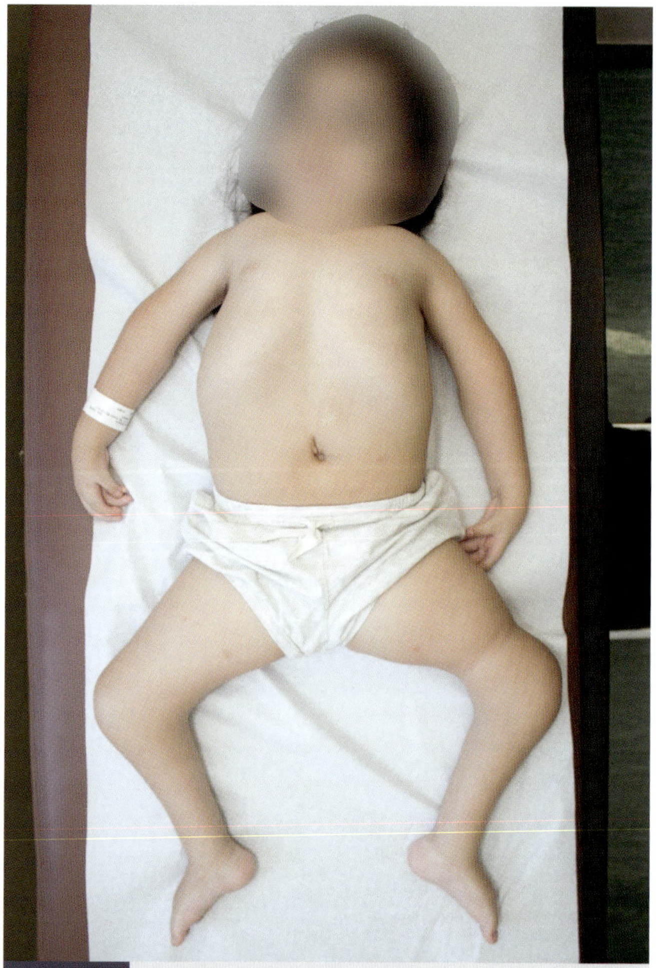

Figure 4 Clinical photograph of a child with amyoplasia shows the typical posture: narrow, sloping shoulders; rigid elbows (flexed or extended); flexed, abducted, externally rotated hips; and rigid knees (flexed or extended). This child also has evidence of an amniotic band around the left thigh. Her clubfeet have been surgically treated.

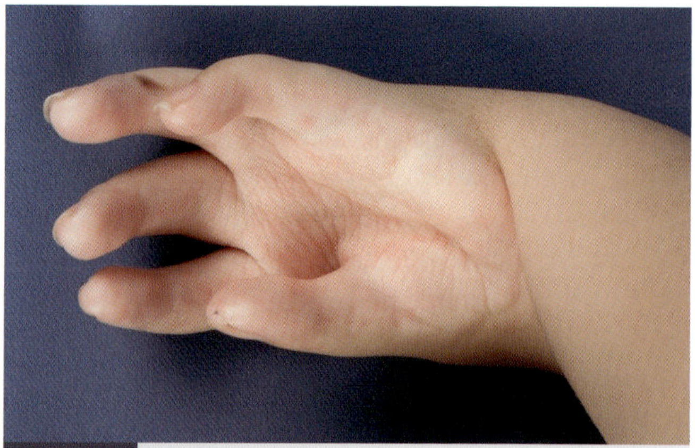

Figure 5 Clinical photograph shows the lack of flexion creases in the hand of a child with arthrogryposis.

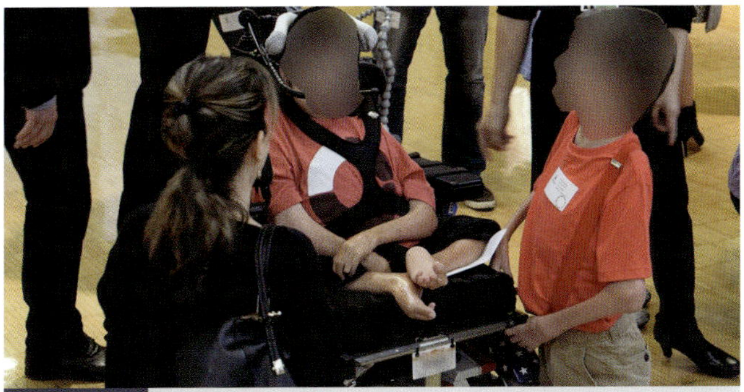

Figure 6 Photograph of a boy with Bruck syndrome participating in a publicity event for the hospital where he receives treatment. The patient controls his wheelchair with his lips.

syndrome have joint contractures without concomitant muscle weakness.

Bruck Syndrome

Bruck syndrome is an extremely rare syndrome, with approximately 20 patients with this condition reported in the medical literature. This syndrome is a combination of arthrogryposis and osteogenesis imperfecta. Two subtypes have been identified with different gene mutations but similar phenotypic presentations. This condition manifests in neonates with multiple joint contractures and pterygia; fractures are often seen in the postnatal period. Most patients are nonambulatory. Because Bruck syndrome is challenging to treat, realistic goals should be discussed with the patient and the family to achieve satisfactory outcomes (**Figure 6**).

General Management

Although each child with arthrogryposis is unique and requires a personalized treatment plan and goals, many management principles apply to most patients. Clinicians should aim to maximize function while minimizing repeated hospitalizations or medicalization of these children. An accurate diagnosis will help parents understand disease risks in future pregnancies. Some families may require counseling to deal with feelings of guilt (especially if the mother believes the condition is related to the size or shape of her uterus). Local and national arthrogryposis groups can provide valuable support to patients and their families.

Physical therapy and a stretching program done at home should be started as soon as possible. Stretching should be gentle and atraumatic. Stretching can be quite effective in reducing contractures, especially in children younger than 1 year.

Bracing may be necessary to provide joint stabilization, which can encourage the achievement of normal developmental milestones. Lightweight, nonarticulated ankle-foot and knee-ankle-foot orthoses are often most useful early in development. Bracing is also vital to maintaining any joint range of motion that was obtained through stretching or surgery. For patients with lower extremity or spinal arthrogryposis, adaptive equipment, such as walkers, scooters, and electric wheelchairs, is vital to encourage a child's sense of independence.

Surgical correction should be reserved for enhancing function, not merely correcting deformities. Surgical intervention should be delayed until the child is demonstrating some head and trunk control, which are indicators of the future ability to stand. The number of hospitalizations and periods of immobilization should be minimized to allow normal socialization and education. Procedures should be combined whenever possible so that only one recovery period is necessary. Hip extensor strength is mandatory for upright stance, so surgical correction of knee deformities may not be indicated if the child lacks the strength to stand.

Surgical intervention for the upper extremities should not be considered until the child demonstrates difficulty with activities of daily living; even then, the child's function may improve more with occupational therapy than with surgery.

The use of anesthesia in patients with arthrogrypotic conditions requires special considerations. Trismus, C-spine stiffness (or laxity in patients with Larsen syndrome), difficult intravenous access, gastroesophageal reflux disease, and postoperative airway obstruction are common in these patients. One type of pterygium syndrome is associated with malignant hyperthermia.[12]

Spine and Lower Extremity

Spine

Scoliosis in arthrogryposis has been reported to have an incidence of up to 70%.[13] Curvatures in these patients may be present at birth and often progress as the child grows. Most curve patterns involve thoracolumbar or lumbar curves with pelvic obliquity, but also can involve the thoracic spine. Most patients with arthrogryposis and scoliosis do not have congenital vertebral anomalies; however, congenital scoliosis with upper extremity arthrogryposis has been described in a small series of patients.[14] Although the use of a thoracolumbar orthosis in these patients is often unsuccessful, it may delay the need for surgical stabilization.

Medical literature provides little guidance for the treatment of children with arthrogryposis and scoliosis. One study found that nonsurgical management of curves may be effective for ambulatory patients who have less than 30° of curvature;[15] however, it is unclear how many of the curves would have progressed without brace treatment. Of the patients who required spinal fusion from the same study, 80% were nonambulatory and had involvement in all four limbs. Combined anterior and posterior fusion was recommended for this population, but this was prior to the widespread use of all-pedicle screw constructs and posteriorly-based osteotomies, which have much more corrective potential than older technologies.

Traditional spine-based growing rods or rib-based distraction using implants such as the Vertical Expandable Prosthetic Titanium Rib (VEPTR; DePuy Synthes) are viable alternatives to bracing in patients with progressive early-onset scoliosis. However, in a series of patients with arthrogryposis and early-onset scoliosis who were treated with VEPTR, a 60% incidence of proximal junctional kyphosis was reported. As with all growing spine implant systems, complications were frequent and at least one complication was seen in 40% of the patients.[16]

Newer growth modulation technologies, including the Magnetic Expansion Control (MAGEC; Ellipse Technology) device, are promising because they can be lengthened externally, which decreases the number of surgical procedures that the child must undergo. However, complications can occur. A recent study reported a 42% incidence rate of unplanned returns to the operating room in nonarthrogypotic patients treated with growing rod surgery.[17]

Hip Dislocation

The management of bilateral hip dislocations remains controversial because surgical intervention can cause hip stiffness and/or osteonecrosis. Closed reduction is rarely successful. Unilateral dislocation will result in a functional limb-length discrepancy. If surgery is elected, the hips should undergo reduction in infancy, and postoperative immobilization should be limited to 5 weeks to minimize the risk of postoperative stiffness. Although a risk of osteonecrosis exists with medial open reduction, the limited surgical dissection required with this approach compared with an anterior approach minimizes the risk of increasing inherent joint stiffness.[18] In the long term, a stiff hip may be more debilitating than a dislocated hip or a collapsed femoral head.

Hip External Rotation Contracture

External rotation contracture of the hip rarely requires surgical intervention and, in fact, surgical dissection around the hip should be avoided to minimize the risk of joint stiffness. If the external rotation of the limb is problematic (interfering with gait or wheelchair sitting), it can be addressed through distal femoral derotational osteotomies.

Knee Flexion Contracture

Early stretching may improve the arc of motion in a patient with knee flexion contracture. Casting or bracing should be used to maintain the range of motion. Older children who have not been successfully treated with casting or bracing may require hamstring lengthening, release of the gastrocnemius origin, posterior capsulectomy, and even femoral shortening via a popliteal fossa approach. The goal should be to correct the flexion deformity to approximately 15° to 20°, which can be accommodated in a postoperative knee-ankle-foot orthosis and is compatible with ambulation. Prolonged postoperative bracing is mandatory to prevent recurrent deformity.

Knee Extension Contracture

In a child younger than 1 year, the initial management of knee extension contractures should focus on gentle stretching. Casting, bracing, or a Pavlik harness can be used to maintain knee flexion throughout the process. If the knee is anteriorly dislocated, reduction may be obtained with serial casting or may require surgical quadriceps lengthening and/or femoral shortening. In children older than 1 year, management is more challenging. Quadriceps lengthening, anterior knee releases, or even flexion osteotomies may be required to improve the arc of motion.

Knee extension contractures often allow children to stand without the use of above-knee bracing; however, as the child grows, the contractures make sitting difficult in automobiles, at school, and in social settings such as movie theaters. When contemplating surgery for an older child with knee extension contractures, it is important to be aware that increasing the knee range of motion may inhibit the child's ability to stand without above-knee bracing. Knee disarticulation is one surgical option, especially when knee extension (or flexion) contractures are paired with irreparable foot deformities. If the child has good trunk musculature and hip extensor strength, knee disarticulations may allow increased mobility on the distal femoral condyles (**Figure** 7).

Talipes Equinovarus

Talipes equinovarus, which is more commonly known as clubfoot, is one of the most common arthrogrypotic musculoskeletal deformities. Early stretching, casting, percutaneous Achilles tenotomies, bracing, and repeat casting can achieve some correction, although this treatment course is not as successful as in children with idiopathic clubfeet.[19,20] Residual deformity can be corrected with limited posteromedial releases. Nighttime splinting is mandatory to prevent recurrence. Concomitant hip and knee deformities may preclude the use of traditional boots and bars for clubfoot treatment, so ankle-foot or knee-ankle-foot orthoses may be used. Talectomies may be an appropriate salvage procedure for older children who have substantial residual deformity. This procedure is often delayed until most of the foot growth is completed at approximately 10 years of age.[21]

Congenital Vertical Talus

Congenital vertical talus is the most severe form of pathologic flatfoot. This deformity is usually associated with other conditions such as spina bifida or arthrogrypotic syndromes. As in clubfoot, some correction may be obtained by serial casting; however, many patients with this type of stiff foot will require open reduction.

Upper Extremity

The findings associated with arthrogryposis in the upper extremity are largely dependent on the underlying cause, with the manifestations of amyoplasia being very different from those of distal arthrogryposis (Freeman-Sheldon or Sheldon-Hall syndromes). Despite the differences in phenotypic presentation, the treatment goals remain largely the same, with a focus on independent accomplishment of the activities of daily living and development of a functional capacity that allows the patient to become a productive member of society. The approach to accomplishing these goals differs based on the presenting limitations. Common objectives include positioning the limb for bimanual use and tabletop activities, facilitating self-care, permitting the use of assistive devices for locomotion if necessary, and enabling the patient to easily interact with communication devices.

Amyoplasia

The typical presentation of amyoplasia in the upper limb consists of a shoulder that is internally rotated and adducted, pronated forearms, flexed and ulnarly deviated wrists, stiff fingers, and clasped thumbs (**Figure 8**). In a patient with upper limb amyoplasia, treatment of the limb begins at an early age with occupational therapy. Stretching and splinting are the mainstays of early intervention. Elbow flexion is the most critical element in obtaining independence in activities of daily living. Stretching exercises to achieve passive elbow flexion past 90° are initiated as early as possible to allow for hand-to-mouth activity. The wrist is splinted to minimize flexion and ulnar deviation deformity that is often present. Passive stretching exercises are used to maximize finger and thumb range of motion. Despite the early initiation of stretching exercises and the diligence of caretakers and therapists, patients with upper limb amyoplasia often require surgery to optimize function. Surgical intervention most often focuses on passive positioning of the upper limb.

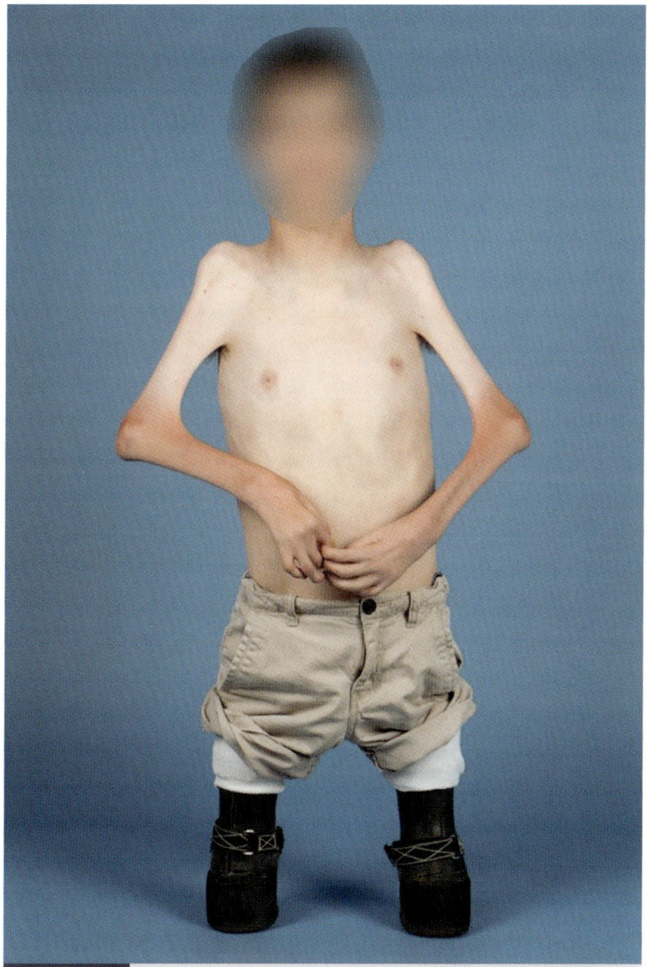

Figure 7 Knee disarticulations can allow ambulation in children with excellent trunk and hip extensor strength. Photograph of a child who had undergone multiple surgical procedures to treat rigid, painful knees and feet. After knee disarticulation he was fitted with prosthetic stubby feet, which improved his independence by allowing him to transfer from wheelchair to bed, walk in spaces his wheelchair would not fit, and sit more easily in an automobile and at a desk, and to skateboard. Rather than using full-height prostheses, the lower center of gravity of stubby feet helps prevent a head injury in the event of a fall; his upper extremity deformities will not allow him to break a fall.

Shoulder

An internal rotation deformity of the shoulder may require surgical intervention in more severe cases. An external

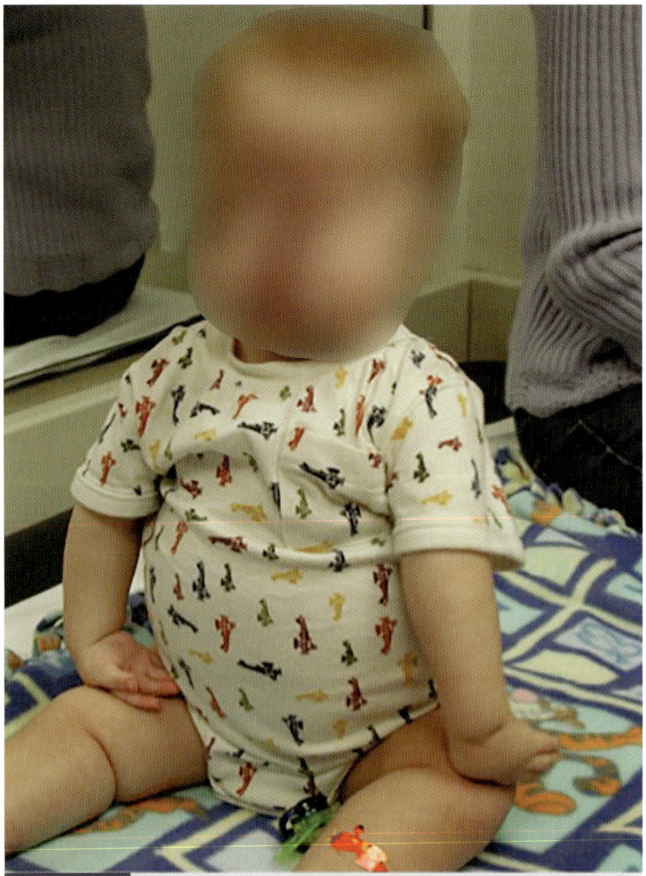

Figure 8 Clinical photograph of an infant with upper limb amyoplasia shows the typical appearance of adducted and internally rotated shoulders, extended elbows, flexed and ulnarly deviated wrists, stiff fingers, and clasped thumbs.

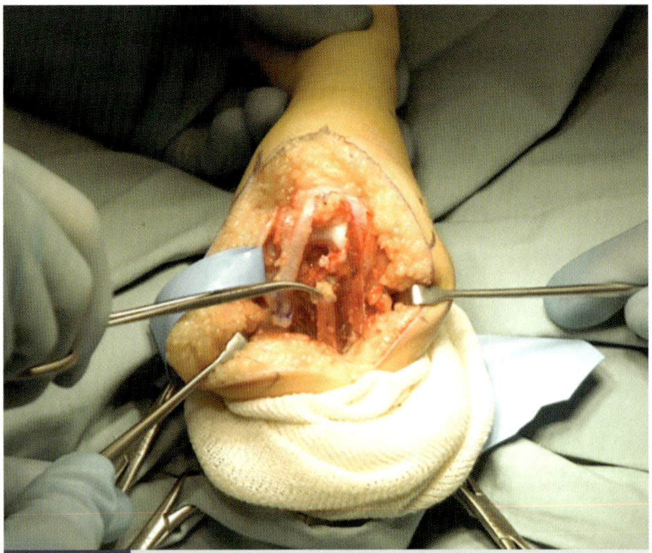

Figure 9 Intraoperative photograph shows surgical release of the elbow extension contracture performed through a posterior incision. The triceps tendon is lengthened using W-plasty with the medial and lateral limbs of the tendon remaining attached to the olecranon. Note the complete posterior capsulectomy and visualization of the trochlear cartilage. (Courtesy of Marybeth Ezaki, MD, Dallas, TX.)

rotation osteotomy of the humerus will provide an arm position that allows the forearm to clear the abdomen and will facilitate bimanual activities in a palm-facing-palm orientation.[22]

Elbow

Elbow extension contractures that fail to resolve sufficiently to allow for hand-to-mouth activities are treated with surgical release (**Figure 9**). The elbow is approached posteriorly using an extended incision. The ulnar nerve is identified, mobilized, and transposed anteriorly. The triceps tendon is lengthened using W-plasty or a similar technique, and the posterior capsule of the elbow is released. After passive elbow flexion greater than 90° is achieved, the triceps tendon is repaired in its lengthened position. The elbow is splinted at 90° postoperatively for 3 weeks and then placed in a removable splint to allow for mobilization and passive range-of-motion exercises. A subset of children with amyoplasia may be candidates for a muscle transfer to achieve active elbow flexion after the patient has recovered from the release surgery. Multiple procedures, including a triceps to biceps transfer, Steindler flexorplasty, bipolar pectoralis major or latissimus transfer, long head of triceps transfer, or a free functioning muscle transfer, have been described in an effort to achieve this goal.[23-28] Each technique possesses its own advantages and limitations, with the specific choice of procedure being tailored to the specific needs of the patient as well as the surgeon's preference. Regardless of the selected technique, these procedures are usually performed when the patient is older than 5 years to allow the child to participate in an intensive, active rehabilitation protocol that maximizes the chance for a favorable outcome.

Wrist

The flexed and ulnarly deviated position of the wrist in a patient with upper limb amyoplasia makes hand-to-mouth as well as bimanual activities more difficult. Surgical correction of the wrist is based on the severity of the deformity and the functional capacity of the muscles crossing the joint. Children who demonstrate active extension of the wrist to neutral often respond well to a volar wrist fascial release with or without wrist flexor lengthening and/or tenotomy. Centralization of the

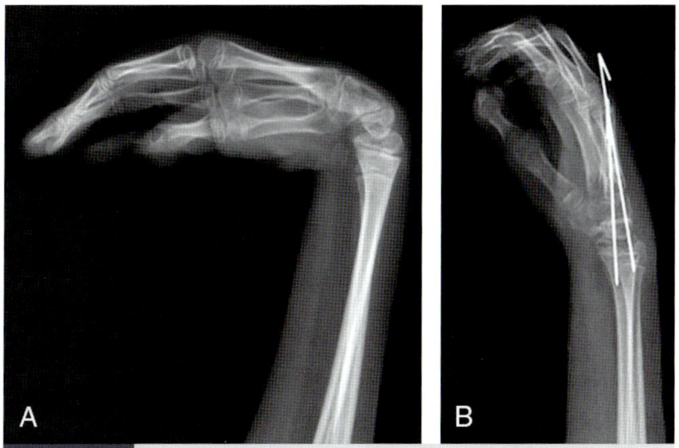

Figure 10 **A,** Preoperative lateral radiograph of the wrist of a child with amyoplasia shows the severe flexion deformity. **B,** Lateral radiograph after a dorsal carpal wedge osteotomy for correction of the flexion deformity.

extensor carpi ulnaris tendon to the anatomic insertion of the extensor carpi radialis brevis can strengthen the power of neutral extension while diminishing the forces of ulnar deviation. Children with a more severe wrist flexion contracture frequently require a bony procedure to attain neutral wrist extension. The procedure is commonly done using a dorsal carpal wedge osteotomy[29-31] (**Figure 10**). It takes advantage of the carpal coalitions often seen in the carpus of children with amyoplasia by obtaining extension and radial deviation through a biplanar wedge resection from the dorsum of the carpus.

Thumb and Fingers

A thumb-in-palm deformity is common in patients with amyoplasia and represents a complex contracture often involving multiple tissues, including skin, muscle, and occasionally, joint capsule. Surgical correction of the deformity often requires a formal volar thenar release as well as release of the adductor pollicis and first dorsal interossei muscles within the first web space. The skin contracture is commonly present in more than one plane, with shortages being present both within the first web space and over the volar aspect of the thumb metacarpophalangeal joint. Hence, a typical four-flap Z-plasty of the first web space skin is rarely sufficient for correction. Instead, a rotational flap from the radial aspect of the index finger is commonly used to bring needed additional tissue to both areas[32] (**Figure 11**). Occasionally, imbrication or advancement of the dorsal thumb extensor tendons (extensor pollicis longus and brevis) can be helpful in maintaining the thumb in a more extended position. These muscle-tendon units are variably present in the thumbs of children with amyoplasia.

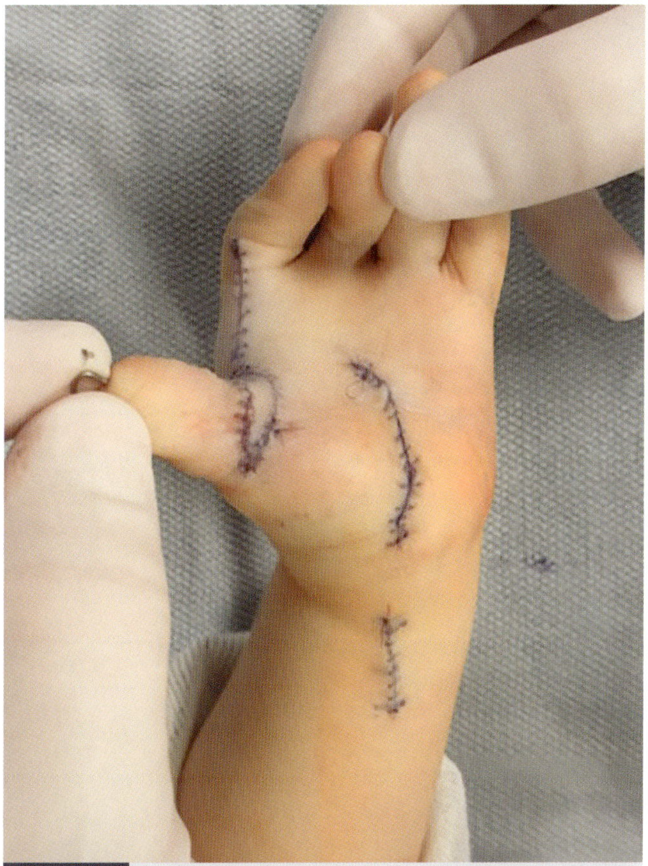

Figure 11 Photograph of the hand of a child with a thumb-in-palm deformity who underwent surgical treatment. An index finger rotational flap is used to release the skin contracture within the first web space as well as along the thenar eminence. The donor site is closed primarily.

The function of the fingers can range from a mild degree of stiffness to digits without flexion creases and little interphalangeal joint motion. Passive range-of-motion and stretching exercises can be helpful in the digits that possess some capacity for active digital flexion. In hands without active digital flexion, the fingers are often used as a single unit for gross grasping against an opposed thumb. At present, surgery plays an extremely limited role in obtaining improved digital function.

Distal Arthrogryposis

In distal arthrogryposis of the upper limb, the shoulders and elbows are largely spared of deformity and dysfunction, wrists are fixed in extension, fingers are flexed and ulnarly deviated, and a substantial thumb-in-palm deformity may exist (**Figure 12**). The first line of treatment is stretching and passive range-of-motion exercises with functional and corrective splinting as an adjunct.

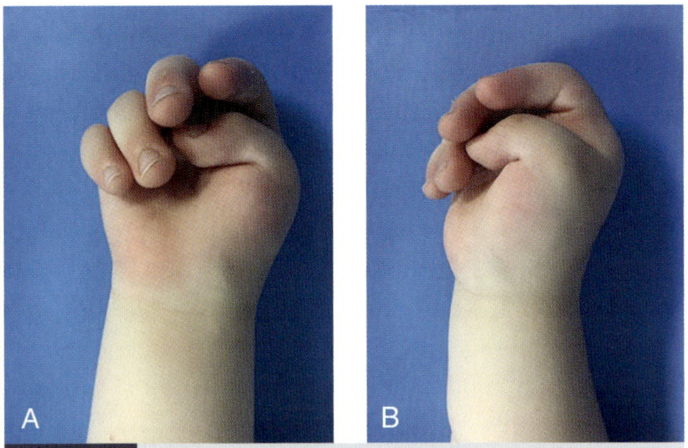

Figure 12 PA (**A**) and lateral (**B**) photographs show the typical presentation of the hand of a child with distal arthrogryposis. The wrist is positioned in extension, the fingers are flexed, and the thumb is clasped. (Courtesy of Scott Oishi, MD, Dallas, TX.)

Unfortunately, wrist and hand deformities are often recalcitrant to nonsurgical correction.[33]

Surgical correction of deformities associated with distal arthrogryposis has not proved particularly successful. A wrist extension contracture is rarely amenable to surgical correction. The abnormalities of the extensor mechanism (ranging from absent to extremely attenuated) also make it difficult to alleviate the flexion deformity of the digits. In rare instances, the extensor tendons are substantial enough that tenolysis and centralization of the tendon over the metacarpophalangeal joint can increase the extensor power and improve digital extension. The thumb-in-palm deformity in distal arthrogryposis is treated in a similar manner to the thumb deformity in amyoplasia. If the primary limitation is a camptodactyly deformity, improvement may be obtained with surgical release to increase proximal interphalangeal joint extension.

Summary

Arthrogryposis refers to a constellation of syndromes characterized by multiple joint contractures. Treatment of arthrogryposis of any type can be challenging, but improvement can be seen in many patients with early intervention and proper nonsurgical and surgical management. The goal for any treatment strategy should be to maximize function with the minimal amount of hospitalization necessary to achieve that goal. Physical and occupational therapy and bracing can help improve function in many children so that surgical management can be mitigated or avoided. Surgical treatment should be reserved for enhancing function, not just improving the appearance of the deformity.

Key Study Points

- Arthrogryposis is a constellation of different diseases with a similar phenotype of nonprogressive multiple joint stiffness and contractures.
- Treatment of patients with arthrogryposis focuses on improving a patient's function with as little hospitalization time as possible; physical and occupational therapy should be used to minimize or obviate the need for surgery.
- Surgical treatment should focus on improving function, not necessarily on correcting deformity.
- Both the surgical and nonsurgical management of upper extremity amyoplasia should focus on enhancing the patient's ability to complete hand-to-mouth activities.
- The creation or maintenance of an appropriate thumb-index web space is important for single-handed manipulation of objects.

Annotated References

1. Fahy MJ, Hall JG: A retrospective study of pregnancy complications among 828 cases of arthrogryposis. *Genet Couns* 1990;1(1):3-11.

2. Johns Hopkins University: OMIM. Online Mendelian inheritance in man. Available at: http://www.ncbi.nlm.nih.gov/sites/entrez?db=omim. Accessed January 17, 2016.

3. Bamshad M, Van Heest AE, Pleasure D: Arthrogryposis: A review and update. *J Bone Joint Surg Am* 2009;91(suppl 4):40-46.

4. Bernstein RM: Arthrogryposis and amyoplasia. *J Am Acad Orthop Surg* 2002;10(6):417-424.

5. Hall JG: Arthrogryposis multiplex congenita: Etiology, genetics, classification, diagnostic approach, and general aspects. *J Pediatr Orthop B* 1997;6(3):159-166.

6. Dubousset J, Guillaumat M: Long-term outcome for patients with arthrogryposis multiplex congenita. *J Child Orthop* 2015;9(6):449-458.

   Sixty-five patients with a history of arthrogryposis were followed into adulthood (age range, 22 to 65 years). Of those patients, 38 were married, and 34 of those patients had children, with only 4 of the children having arthrogryposis. Unassisted walking was achieved by 29 patients, whereas 18 patients required permanent wheelchair use, 9 patients used a wheelchair some of the time, and 8 patients used forearm crutches. Spine surgery was performed in 26 patients, with 14 patients requiring anterior/posterior procedures. Lower limb surgery was often repeated but almost always improved function and pain. Upper extremity involvement was determined to be the most debilitating issue and affected the patient much more than the inability to walk. The authors recommended closer attention to improvement of upper limb function during childhood. Level of evidence: IV.

7. Larsen LJ, Schottstaedt ER, Bost FC: Multiple congenital dislocations associated with characteristic facial abnormality. *J Pediatr* 1950;37(4):574-581.

8. Johnston CE II, Birch JG, Daniels JL: Cervical kyphosis in patients who have Larsen syndrome. *J Bone Joint Surg Am* 1996;78(4):538-545.

9. Munk S: Early operation of the dislocated knee in Larsen's syndrome: A report of 2 cases. *Acta Orthop Scand* 1988;59(5):582-584.

10. Laville JM, Lakermance P, Limouzy F: Larsen's syndrome: Review of the literature and analysis of thirty-eight cases. *J Pediatr Orthop* 1994;14(1):63-73.

11. Escobar V, Bixler D, Gleiser S, Weaver DD, Gibbs T: Multiple pterygium syndrome. *Am J Dis Child* 1978;132(6):609-611.

12. Oppitz F, Speulda E, Busley R (English translation): Anesthesia recommendations in patients suffering from arthrogryposis multiplex congenita. Last updated June 2011. Available at: https://www.orpha.net/data/patho/Pro/en/Arthrogryposis_EN.pdf. Accessed April 27, 2016.

The authors detail the main issues with providing anesthesia to patients with arthrogryposis multiplex congenita, including difficulty in establishing the airway, poor venous circulation, and intraoperative hyperthermia. Regional anesthesia is noted as a good option to minimize these issues for limb surgery. Regional anesthesia for spine surgery tends to be technically difficult to perform and does not provide adequate analgesia. Laryngeal mask airway works well for most patients, but there are case reports of complications related to its use. Blood loss and anticoagulation risks are not increased compared with similar surgeries in the general population.

13. Drummond DS, Mackenzie DA: Scoliosis in arthrogryposis multiplex congenita. *Spine (Phila Pa 1976)* 1978;3(2):146-151.

14. Fletcher ND, Rathjen KE, Bush P, Ezaki M: Asymmetrical arthrogryposis of the upper extremity associated with congenital spine anomalies. *J Pediatr Orthop* 2010;30(8):936-941.

15. Yingsakmongkol W, Kumar SJ: Scoliosis in arthrogryposis multiplex congenita: Results after nonsurgical and surgical treatment. *J Pediatr Orthop* 2000;20(5):656-661.

16. Astur N, Flynn JM, Flynn JM, et al: The efficacy of rib-based distraction with VEPTR in the treatment of early-onset scoliosis in patients with arthrogryposis. *J Pediatr Orthop* 2014;34(1):8-13.

Ten patients (7 female and 3 male) were evaluated retrospectively to see how well the VEPTR device performs in improving spinal deformity and maintaining correction with growth. The initial implantation of the VEPTR device decreased scoliosis from a mean of 67° to 43° (37% correction) and kyphosis from a mean of 65° to 48° (29% correction). At final follow-up, scoliosis measured 55° (17% correction) and kyphosis measured 62° (8% correction). Spinal growth increased by a mean of 4.2 cm (approximately 1 cm per year). A total of 62 procedures were performed, with 6 complications in four patients: 3 infections, 2 rib failures, and 1 implant failure. Level of evidence: IV.

17. Cheung KM: Complications of magnetically-controlled growing rod surgery: A prospective multicenter study with minimum 2 year follow-up. *Bone Joint J* 2014;96-B (suppl 15):10.Available at http://www.bjjprocs.boneandjoint.org.uk/content/96-B/SUPP_15/10. Accessed July 14, 2016.

In this multicenter study, the authors reported complications in 11 of 26 patients treated with a magnetically controlled rod device. Complications included five rod distraction failures, two broken rods, three failures of proximal implants, and one wound infection.

18. Gardner RO, Bradley CS, Howard A, Narayanan UG, Wedge JH, Kelley SP: The incidence of avascular necrosis and the radiographic outcome following medial open reduction in children with developmental dysplasia of the hip: A systematic review. *Bone Joint J* 2014;96-B(2):279-286.

Drawing on data from 14 studies that described 734 hips with developmental dysplasia (mean follow-up, 10.9 years; range, 2 to 28 years), the authors concluded that the rate of osteonecrosis increased with the length of follow-up to 24% at skeletal maturity. Type 2 osteonecrosis was the most predominant finding at the 5-year follow-up. A higher rate of osteonecrosis was identified when surgery was performed in children younger than 1 year and when hips were immobilized in 60° or more of abduction postoperatively. The presence of osteonecrosis resulted in a higher incidence of unsatisfactory outcomes.

19. Janicki JA, Narayanan UG, Harvey B, Roy A, Ramseier LE, Wright JG: Treatment of neuromuscular and syndrome-associated (nonidiopathic) clubfeet using the Ponseti method. *J Pediatr Orthop* 2009;29(4):393-397.

20. Matar HE, Beirne P, Garg N: The effectiveness of the Ponseti method for treating clubfoot associated with arthrogryposis: Up to 8 years follow-up. *J Child Orthop* 2016;10(1):15-18.

The Ponseti method was used to treat 17 clubfeet in 10 children with arthrogryposis. The authors reported initial correction in all of the children and satisfactory outcomes for two-thirds of the children at final follow-up.

21. Iskandar HN, Bishay SN, Sharaf-El-Deen HA, El-Sayed MM: Tarsal decancellation in the residual resistant arthrogrypotic clubfoot. *Ann R Coll Surg Engl* 2011;93(2):139-145.

Tarsal decancellation was performed in 12 children (15 feet) with residual arthrogrypotic clubfeet. All of the children had received past treatment with the Ponseti method. At a mean follow-up of 3.3 years, excellent results were reported in six feet, good results in six feet, and fair results in three feet.

22. Zlotolow DA, Kozin SH: Posterior elbow release and humeral osteotomy for patients with arthrogryposis. *J Hand Surg Am* 2012;37(5):1078-1082.

    Children with arthrogryposis often lack the ability to feed themselves, primarily because of their limited shoulder external rotation and elbow flexion. Patients who can achieve passive elbow flexion through a surgical release but who cannot externally rotate their shoulders are still unable to reach their mouths with their hands. Combining a posterior elbow capsular release with a simultaneous humeral osteotomy in these patients places the forearm and hand in a much better position for function with minimal additional surgical exposure.

23. Chomiak J, Dungl P, Včelák J: Reconstruction of elbow flexion in arthrogryposis multiplex congenita type I: Results of transfer of pectoralis major muscle with follow-up at skeletal maturity. *J Pediatr Orthop* 2014;34(8):799-807.

    The purpose of this study was to analyze the results of a pectoralis major transfer to restore active elbow flexion in patients with extension elbow contractures in arthrogryposis. A unipolar transfer technique was used for the pectoralis muscle transfer. The muscle transfer restored useful elbow flexion without flexion deformity if the passive flexion exceeded 90°. Level of evidence: II.

24. Gogola GR, Ezaki M, Oishi SN, Gharbaoui I, Bennett JB: Long head of the triceps muscle transfer for active elbow flexion in arthrogryposis. *Tech Hand Up Extrem Surg* 2010;14(2):121-124.

25. Goldfarb CA, Burke MS, Strecker WB, Manske PR: The Steindler flexorplasty for the arthrogrypotic elbow. *J Hand Surg Am* 2004;29(3):462-469.

26. Kay S, Pinder R, Wiper J, Hart A, Jones F, Yates A: Microvascular free functioning gracilis transfer with nerve transfer to establish elbow flexion. *J Plast Reconstr Aesthet Surg* 2010;63(7):1142-1149.

27. Stevanovic M, Sharpe F: Functional free muscle transfer for upper extremity reconstruction. *Plast Reconstr Surg* 2014;134(2):257e-274e.

    The authors present a review of their experiences in upper extremity reconstruction using functional free muscle transfer. The indications and techniques for functional free muscle transfer in the upper extremity are discussed, and surgical details for sites of reconstruction and the nuances of harvesting the main donor muscles are presented.

28. Van Heest A, Waters PM, Simmons BP: Surgical treatment of arthrogryposis of the elbow. *J Hand Surg Am* 1998;23(6):1063-1070.

29. Ezaki M, Carter PR: Carpal wedge osteotomy for the arthrogrypotic wrist. *Tech Hand Up Extrem Surg* 2004;8(4):224-228.

30. Foy CA, Mills J, Wheeler L, Ezaki M, Oishi SN: Long-term outcome following carpal wedge osteotomy in the arthrogrypotic patient. *J Bone Joint Surg Am* 2013;95(20):e150- e151.

    Wrist flexion and ulnar deviation deformity is common in children with amyoplasia congenita. Multiple surgical procedures have been reported to correct the deformity, enhance functional independence, and improve quality of life. Surgical correction of wrist flexion posture in children with amyoplasia congenita results in improvement that is sustained over time. Surveys and questionnaires completed by parents or guardians indicate satisfaction with the surgical results. Level of evidence: IV.

31. Van Heest AE, Rodriguez R: Dorsal carpal wedge osteotomy in the arthrogrypotic wrist. *J Hand Surg Am* 2013;38(2):265-270.

    The authors report on a study to assess the outcomes of patients who underwent dorsal carpal wedge osteotomy for the treatment of wrist flexion deformities causing functional limitations in patients with arthrogryposis. The excessively flexed wrist in children with arthrogryposis can safely and effectively be improved with this procedure, which, as reported by parents, facilitates independence in activities of daily living and school-related tasks. Greater recovery of wrist extension was found for patients older than 7 years at the time of surgery and for those treated with concomitant extensor carpi ulnaris transfer. Level of evidence: IV.

32. Ezaki M, Oishi SN: Index rotation flap for palmar thumb release in arthrogryposis. *Tech Hand Up Extrem Surg* 2010;14(1):38-40.

33. Smith DW, Drennan JC: Arthrogryposis wrist deformities: Results of infantile serial casting. *J Pediatr Orthop* 2002;22(1):44-47.

Chapter 14

Osteogenesis Imperfecta and Metabolic Bone Disease

Jared William Daniel, MD   Jennifer Harrington, MBBS, PhD   Andrew W. Howard, MD, MSc, FRCSC

Abstract

Osteogenesis imperfecta and metabolic bone diseases are seen with a variety of clinical presentations in pediatric orthopaedic clinics. Basic knowledge is essential for making a diagnosis and managing these conditions. Osteogenesis imperfecta is a group of inherited connective tissue conditions characterized by increased bone fragility and low bone mass. Medical and surgical management of this condition remains an integral part of successful treatment.

Despite many advancements in technology and understanding, rickets continue to affect many children throughout the world. Vitamin D deficiency continues to be the most common cause of calcipenic rickets in children. Prompt treatment is fundamental in the management of rickets and its orthopaedic manifestations. A better understanding of X-linked hypophosphatemia has allowed for improvements in medical and surgical management.

Secondary osteoporosis may be attributable to multiple etiologies; however, glucocorticoid-induced osteoporosis still affects children being treated for a variety of pediatric conditions.

Keywords: calcipenic rickets; glucocorticoid-induced osteoporosis; osteogenesis imperfecta; vitamin D deficiency; X-linked hypophosphatemia

None of the following authors or any immediate family member has received anything of value from or has stock or stock options held in a commercial company or institution related directly or indirectly to the subject of this chapter: Dr. Harrington, Dr. Howard, and Dr. Daniel.

Introduction

Fundamental knowledge about the underlying conditions and treatment options for osteogenesis imperfecta (OI) and metabolic bone diseases is essential for proper management. Advancements in technology and research have provided new treatments and a better understanding of these conditions.

Osteogenesis Imperfecta

OI is a broadly used term to describe a group of inherited connective tissue conditions characterized by increased bone fragility and low bone mass. The estimated prevalence of OI is 1 in 12,000 to 15,000 children.[1] OI has an expansive clinical phenotype, ranging from perinatal lethality to mild forms without fractures. This condition has substantially heterogeneity, even within affected family members. Patients may have substantial skeletal deformities in long bones, or simple fragility fractures. Scoliosis and joint laxity are orthopaedic conditions seen in patients with OI. Other clinical extraskeletal manifestations include hearing loss, dental abnormalities, blue-gray sclera, hypercalciuria, aortic root dilatation, neurologic conditions (macroencephaly, hydrocephalus, and basilar invagination), and skin hyperlaxity.

Classification

Published in 1979, the Sillence classification described four types of OI: type I, mild nondeforming OI; type II, perinatal lethal OI; type III, severely progressing and deforming OI; and type IV, moderately deforming OI. The most common mutations involve the two genes (*COL1A1* and *COL1A2*) that encode the alpha chains of type I collagen. With the increased awareness of the genetic complexity and phenotypic heterogeneity of OI, alternative classification schemes such as deforming and nondeforming OI (**Figure 1**) have been proposed. In a practical and functional manner, these schemes help to

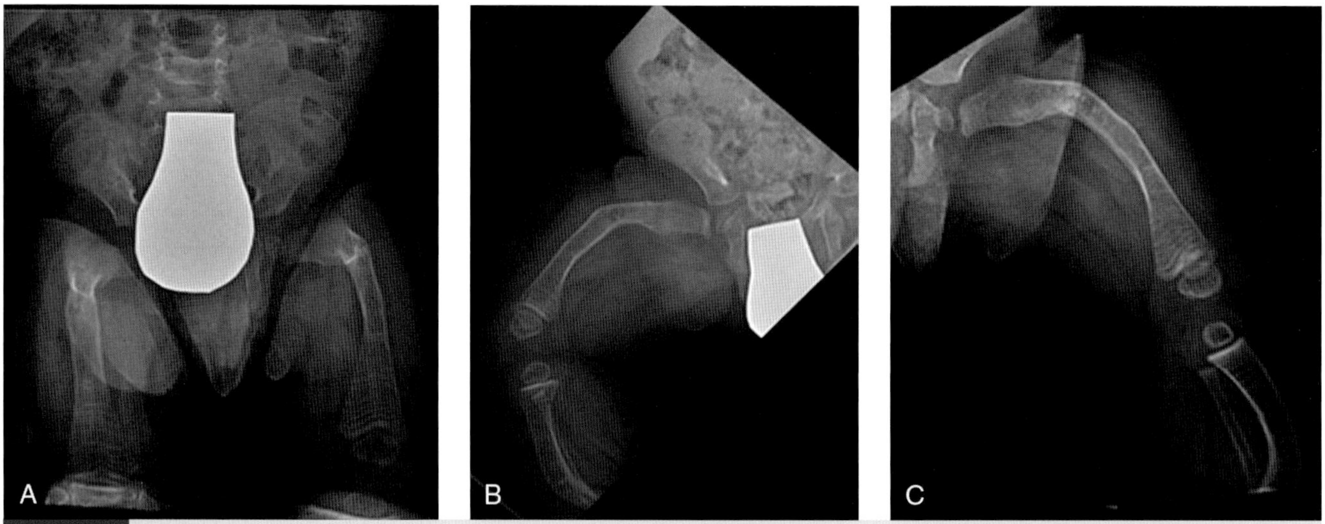

Figure 1 AP (**A**) and lateral (**B** and **C**) radiographs from a 20-month-old boy with osteogenesis imperfecta and recurrent femoral fractures.

encompass the ever-expanding list of new genetic mutations leading to OI (**Table 1**).

Characteristics of OI

Making a diagnosis of OI typically is done based on family history and associated radiographic and clinical features. Radiographic features include generalized osteopenia and gracile long bones with evidence of bowing. Vertebral fractures are common, with a 71% prevalence rate in patients with type I OI.[1,2] Spiral and transverse fractures are the most frequently seen fractures in long bones. Avulsion-type fractures such as olecranon and patellar fractures are particularly characteristic of OI and occur as a result of the decreased tensile strength of the bone.[1,2] The underlying genetic mutation is more frequently being identified because of the increased ability to test multiple OI-related genes at one time using techniques such as exome sequencing.

In infants, it is essential to differentiate OI from other fracture etiologies, particularly nonaccidental injury. Other causes of fracture in older children include idiopathic juvenile osteoporosis and secondary causes of osteoporosis such as glucocorticoid-induced osteoporosis, hormone deficiency, acute lymphoblastic leukemia, and immobilization.

Low bone mass is a characteristic clinical feature of children with OI.[3] Patients tend to have low bone mineral density (BMD), leading to decreased bone size, decreased volumetric BMD, or both.[4,5] With decreased bone mass, OI is typically associated with an increased risk of fracture. Newer research is exploring fracture prediction

Table 1

Alternative Classification Scheme for Osteogenesis Imperfecta

Phenotype	Gene Involved	Inheritance Pattern
Nondeforming	*COL1A1*	AD
	COL1A2	AD
	CRTAP	AR
	PPIB	AR
	SP7	AR
	PLS3	XL
Progressively deforming	*COL1A1*	AD
	COL1A2	AD
	CRTAP	AR
	LEPRE1	AR
	PPIB	AR
	BMP1	AR
	FKBP10	AR
	PLOD2	AR
	SERPINF1	AR
	SERPINH1	AR
	TMEM38B	AR
	WNT1	AR
	CREB3L1	AR
	SPARC	AR
Osteogenesis imperfecta with calcification of interosseous membranes	*IFITM5*	AD

AD = autosomal dominant; AR = autosomal recessive; XL = X-linked based on mechanical models. Applied finite element models have been used to predict fractures in patients with OI.[3,6] These finite element models are continuing to be modified to improve geometric biofidelity and update mechanical property data through advanced meshing techniques. Finite element modeling has been used to estimate the effects of teriparatide treatment on vertebral strength in adults with OI. A finite element model has been used to assess fracture risk at the tibia in children with OI using simulated loading experienced during two-legged hopping, lateral loading, and torsional loading.[3,7] Future finite element modeling may provide quantification of fracture risk in OI and identify activities that pose the greatest risk of fracture. By understanding the fracture risk of each patient with OI, education and counseling can be maximized. However, given the combination of reduced bone mass and decreased bone quality, bone and/or spinal deformity can occur and further contribute to the risk of fracture.

Treatment and Symptom Management

The goals of treatment of OI are to maximize a patient's mobility and ability to accomplish the activities of daily living. Treatment also should focus on decreasing bone pain and bone fragility, and correcting deformity. Management typically is multidisciplinary and includes rehabilitation and medical, pharmacologic, and surgical interventions.

Patients with OI usually are seen by an orthopaedic surgeon because of a fracture. It is important to understand that fracture healing time in children with OI is normal, even with bisphosphonate (also known as diphosphonate) treatment.[8] The goals of orthopaedic treatment of OI fractures are to stabilize or protect the whole bone and avoid excessive mobilization. Prolonged immobilization will lead to weak, stiff muscles and secondary disuse osteopenia, which leads to more fractures in this population. Fractures affecting infants are typically treated with the simplest form of immobilization that provides comfort to the limb; 2 to 3 weeks of immobilization is usually required. Toddlers and older children undergo treatment based on the fracture pattern and the amount of deformity present. Treatment with plates should be avoided because of the high risk of subsequent peri-implant fractures. However, transverse fractures of the olecranon or patella (caused by tensile failure) are best treated with tension-band wiring and early motion (**Figure 2**).

Because of the association of OI with potential deformities of the femur and tibia, orthopaedic surgeons must have a full understanding of prior fractures and fixation methods spanning the entire bone length. Deformities can be in a single plane or multiple planes and can be acute or chronic. Preoperative planning is essential to assist with deformity correction. Newer technology allows for full computerized preoperative deformity correction. With the advancement in intramedullary instrumentation, OI long bone deformities can be treated with osteotomies and intramedullary fixation, which maintains straight mechanical alignment and supports the whole bone, allowing for early mobilization, weight bearing, and strengthening.[1] Growing rods provide the mechanical advantages of a rigid nail but reduce the number of revision surgeries needed because of ongoing growth.[1,9]

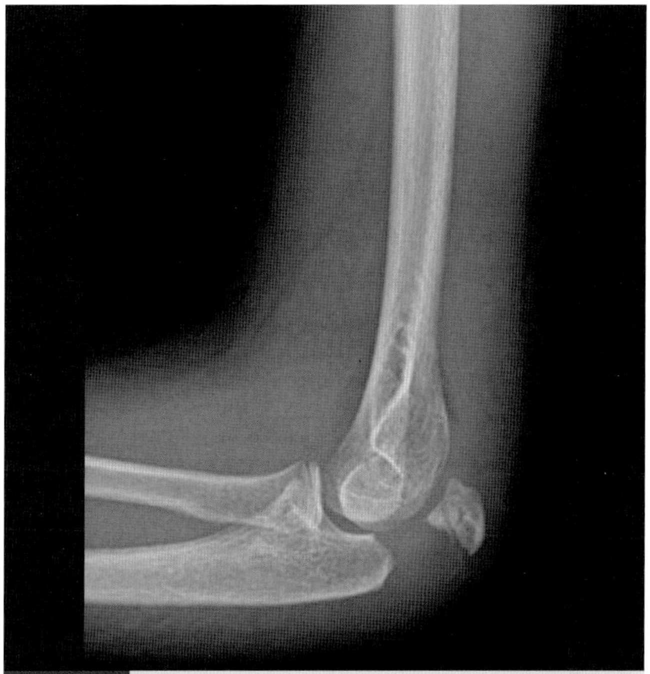

Figure 2 Lateral radiograph shows an avulsion fracture of the olecranon in a patient with osteogenesis imperfecta.

Children with severe OI often have scoliosis and/or kyphosis. The incidence of scoliosis in OI is between 39% and 80%[10] (**Figure 3**). Up to 60% of patients with OI also have substantial chest wall deformities. Pulmonary compromise is the leading cause of death in adults with OI. Thoracic scoliosis of more than 60° in patients with OI has severe adverse effects on pulmonary function.[10] The use of spinal fusion with instrumentation has been reported in selected patients, but it has a high complication rate and is not universally recommended.[1,11] A 2014 study described the surgical technique of using cement augmentation to improve pedicle screw instrumentation and pull-out strength in osteoporotic patients with OI; however, this was a small case series with limited follow-up.[12] In the past 5 years, there have been few advancements in the surgical treatment of spinal deformities in patients with OI.

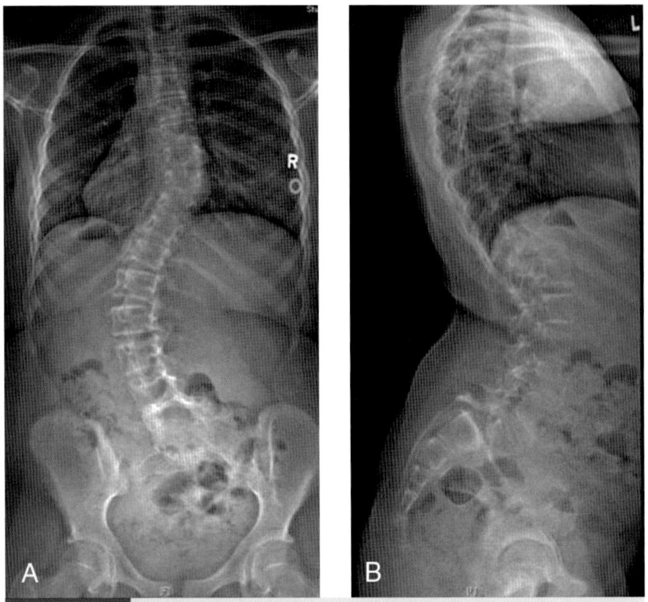

Figure 3 PA (**A**) and lateral (**B**) radiographs of the spine a 13-year-old girl with osteogenesis imperfecta, scoliosis, and spondylolisthesis.

Pediatric patients with OI also have a higher incidence of spondylolysis and spondylolisthesis compared with the normal pediatric population. The authors of a 2011 study retrospectively evaluated radiographs of 110 pediatric patients with OI and concluded that the overall incidence of spondylolysis was 8.2%, with an overall incidence of spondylolisthesis of 10.9%.[13] In contrast, in a normal patient cohort, the incidence of spondylolysis was reported to be 2.6% to 4.0%, with the incidence of spondylolisthesis reported at 4.2%. These findings suggest that it is important to monitor children early in their clinical care to properly manage back pain symptoms.

Physical therapy is important to improve motor skills and maximize the effects of weight-bearing exercises to prevent fracture or facilitate rehabilitation after a fracture. Hydrotherapy can be an important modality to allow for gradual return to weight bearing. Patients with upper limb deformities also may benefit from an occupational therapy evaluation to promote self-care and activities of daily living.

Pharmacologic treatment remains an important aspect in the clinical management of OI. Children should be assessed to ensure sufficient dietary calcium and 25-hydroxyvitamin D intake. The decision to initiate pharmacologic intervention depends on the clinical severity of the disease, not the BMD or collagen mutation. Bisphosphonate therapy continues to remain the mainstay of medical treatment for OI and has been shown in observational studies to decrease bone pain, enhance well-being, improve muscle strength and mobility, improve vertebral shape, and decrease fracture rates. Both controlled and observational trials have demonstrated that bisphosphonate therapy substantially increases BMD, with most of the clinical gain occurring within the first 2 to 4 years.[1,4] However, two meta-analyses showed that bisphosphonate therapy increased BMD in patients with OI but did not show definitive evidence of fracture reduction.[14,15]

Recent literature has described a change in the mechanism and location of femoral fractures in patients with OI receiving bisphosphonate therapies.[16,17] The atypical fractures of the femur consist of proximal third femoral fractures involving the subtrochanteric region and more transverse fracture patterns resulting from low-energy injuries. These fractures contrast with the more typically seen high-energy, spiral, middiaphyseal fracture patterns.[16,17] A similar atypical fracture pattern has been described in adults undergoing bisphosphonate therapy for osteoporosis. The exact mechanism causing the change in the trend of fracture patterns despite prior intramedullary fixation is unclear, but it may be related to the effects of bisphosphonate on bone remodeling and bone stress relationships involving the proximal femur.

Bisphosphonate treatment can be associated with flu-like symptoms in up to 85% of children after the first dose and also can lead to transient hypocalcemia.[18] The use of bisphosphonates also has been linked to a decrease in bone remodeling and delayed healing of osteotomy sites after intramedullary nailing. Osteonecrosis of the jaw is a described adverse reaction in adults, but it has not been reported in pediatric patients with OI.

Other pharmacologic treatments currently are under trial for the medical management of OI. Teriparatide, an anabolic agent that stimulates bone formation, is being evaluated for the management of adults with OI. Growth hormone has been trialed in patients with OI for its anabolic effects on bone through the stimulation of osteoblasts, collagen synthesis, and bone growth. The current literature is insufficient to support the use of growth hormone as a standard treatment of OI. Denosumab, a monoclonal antibody to receptor activator of nuclear factor-$\kappa\beta$ ligand, decreases bone resorption, increases bone density, and reduces fracture rates in postmenopausal women. In a study of four children with OI type VI, denosumab treatment resulted in an increase in BMD, mobility, and improved vertebral shape.[19] Follow-ups on larger studies of denosumab use in children with other genetic forms of OI are ongoing. Future therapies include antisclerostin antibodies, transforming growth factor-β antagonism, and gene- and cell-based therapies. More research is needed, however, before transitioning to new treatment options.

Table 2

Factors Affecting Bone Mass

Nonmodifiable	Genetics Sex Ethnicity
Modifiable	Nutrition (calcium, vitamin D, sodium, protein) Exercise and lifestyle Body weight and composition Hormonal status Medication taken

Metabolic Bone Disease

Metabolic bone disease describes a diverse set of conditions that can affect bone health and pediatric growth. Good nutritional status is essential for normal bone growth in pediatric patients. Bone mass can be affected by multiple factors, both modifiable and nonmodifiable[20] (Table 2).

Despite medical and nutritional advancements, rickets still exists in various parts of the world. Rickets can be classified into two types: calcipenic and phosphopenic rickets. Secondary causes of osteoporosis are becoming more prevalent and should be considered in the management of pediatric orthopaedic conditions.

Calcipenic Rickets

Vitamin D deficiency is the most common cause of calcipenic rickets in children and osteomalacia in both children and adults. Rickets is characterized by a failure or delay in endochondral ossification at the growth plate (zone of provisional calcification) of long bones, which can lead to deformities in ambulatory children. Osteomalacia is characterized by defective mineralization of osteoid on the trabecular and cortical surfaces of bone and is associated with widened osteoid seams and the presence of Looser transformation zones. Both conditions can lead to bone pain and muscle weakness in the limbs. Vitamin D deficiency also has been linked to an increased risk of other diseases, including osteoporosis, cardiovascular disease, diabetes, some cancers, and infectious diseases.[21-24]

Vitamin D deficiency continues to be the most common nutritional deficiency worldwide, with children and adults at equal risk. Vitamin D deficiency is defined by the Institute of Medicine as a 25-hydroxyvitamin D level of less than 20 ng/mL (50 nmol/L), whereas vitamin D insufficiency is defined as a 25-hydroxyvitamin D level of 21 to 29 ng/mL (51 to70 nmol/L). The introduction of food fortification programs and improvements in air quality has substantially reduced the prevalence of rickets in developed countries. However, in the United States, more than 50% of Hispanic and African-American adolescents in Boston[25] and 48% of white preadolescent girls in Maine had levels below 20 ng/mL.[26] The overall prevalence of rickets has been reported to be up to 70% in developing counties.[27]

Many risk factors predispose the pediatric population to rickets and vitamin D deficiency. Risk factors include poor nutritional intake, premature birth, dark skin, living in areas of limited sun exposure (>37.5° latitude), obesity, taking medications that affect the concentration of vitamin D, and diseases causing nutritional malabsorption (for example, celiac disease and cystic fibrosis). In 2010, the Institute of Medicine published recommendations for administration of vitamin D to healthy children and healthy children at risk for vitamin D deficiency.[28,29] If a pediatric patient has rickets associated with a vitamin D deficiency, the American Academy of Pediatrics recommends an initial 2- to 3-month regimen of high-dose vitamin D therapy of 1,000 international units (IU) daily in neonates, 1,000 to 5,000 IU daily in infants 1 to 12 months old, and 5,000 IU daily in patients older than 12 months.[30] After appropriate levels are obtained, treatment can be adjusted to a maintenance dose of 400 IU of vitamin D daily, depending on the patient's age and risk factors. If a pediatric patient is determined to be at risk for vitamin D deficiency, a maintenance dose (800 IU/day) should be considered. An alternative treatment regimen is providing 50,000 IU of vitamin D_2 once per week for 6 weeks, then transitioning to a maintenance dose of 600 to 1,000 IU daily.[28,29] Supplementation with calcium in conjunction with vitamin D is important for the successful treatment of rickets; the calcium dosage is based on the patient's age.[20]

Phosphopenic Rickets

Phosphopenic rickets most commonly occurs because of excess urinary phosphate losses, resulting from either genetic mutations leading to isolated phosphaturia or from generalized renal tubular dysfunction such as occurs in Fanconi syndrome. X-linked hypophosphatemic rickets is the most common form of inheritable rickets, with an incidence of 1 in 20,000 live births.[31] X-linked hypophosphatemia is inherited in an X-linked dominant fashion, with prominent bowing of the legs, short stature, and medial tibial torsion seen in early childhood. Disease progression may result in progressive bone deformity, dental abscesses, enthesopathy, arthritis, and severe osteomalacia. X-linked hypophosphatemia is caused by mutations in the phosphate-regulating endopeptidase homolog X-linked (*PHEX*) gene, which are expressed in osteocytes. Mutations of the gene result in an increase in fibroblast growth factor-23 (FGF-23), which leads to phosphaturia.

Medical Management

Early recognition of X-linked hypophosphatemia is essential for appropriate treatment. Early intervention with medical management improves clinical outcomes but does not completely heal the mineralization defect.[32] The current mainstay of treatment is based on phosphate and 1,25-hydroxyvitamin D supplementation. Medical management should begin at the time of the diagnosis in childhood and continue through adolescence until growth has ceased; however, many patients continue to require treatment in adulthood. Medical management with supplementation of phosphate and vitamin D has been shown to alleviate bowing, improve attained height, and reduce the need for corrective surgery.[31-35] Recommended treatment is the administration of a 20- to 30-ng/kg dose of calcitriol (split among two to three daily doses), along with 20 to 40 mg/kg of elemental phosphorus (split among three to five daily doses).[34] Multiple daily doses are vital to maintain steady serum levels of phosphorus and reduce adverse gastrointestinal side effects. In a developing child, medical therapy should be closely monitored with laboratory values, renal ultrasound, and radiography.

Newer treatment strategies are being developed to target the deficiencies of the *PHEX* gene or the aberrations in FGF-23. A recent randomized clinical trial studied the safety, tolerability, pharmacokinetics, pharmacodynamics, and immunogenicity of an anti-FGF-23 antibody versus placebo in 38 adult patients with X-linked hypophosphatemia.[36] The authors reported that the anti-FGF-23 antibody increased the maximum renal tubular threshold for phosphate reabsorption, serum inorganic phosphate, and serum 1,25-dihydroxyvitamin D and had a favorable safety profile. Currently, a randomized study is evaluating the effectiveness of an anti-FGF-23 antibody in prepubescent children.

Surgical Treatment

Although nonsurgical management is the mainstay of X-linked hypophosphatemia treatment, bone deformities can occur that necessitate surgical intervention. The natural history of bony deformity in X-linked hypophosphatemia makes appropriate treatment in young children challenging because it is unclear when surgical deformity correction is needed. One study reported that deformities of less than 15° frequently correct spontaneously when there is good metabolic control; however, no subsequent study has confirmed these finding.[37] Despite surgical intervention and proper medical management, the rate of deformity recurrence is as high as 90%.[38]

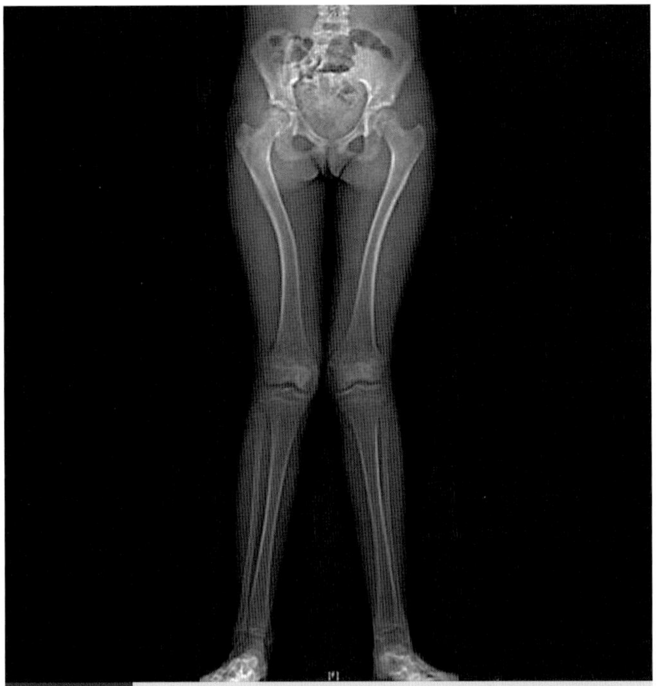

Figure 4 Long-leg standing AP radiograph from a 12-year-old girl with X-linked hypophosphatemic rickets with a multiapical femoral deformity.

Decisions about surgical care involve anticipating the effects of growth. The understanding of multiapical deformity and preoperative planning has been key to the proper treatment of the deformities associated with X-linked hypophosphatemia (**Figure 4**).

Guided growth techniques can provide substantial correction of angular deformities with low complication rates and a limited burden of care, whereas complex deformities with multiple apices require multiple levels of correction to achieve an anatomic result. In adults, simultaneous correction of multiple deformities has been advocated with fixator-assisted nailing. Because deformity in children can recur because of growth, it is necessary to plan care based on an analysis of the complete deformity. The timing of surgery, the wisdom of staged correction, and the burden of care also should be considered.

Surgery may be indicated for children with progressive bony deformities that result in substantial gait disturbances, activity limitations, and pain. Various treatment techniques can be used or combined to correct bony deformities, including acute correction and fixation of osteotomies with Kirschner wires, plates, external fixators, and intramedullary nails. Gradual correction of deformities also has been described using an Ilizarov external fixator or a Taylor Spatial Frame (Smith & Nephew). A 2015 review described bone lengthening with corrective osteotomy in a select number of patients who also had been treated with deformity correction. The authors reported that more major complications, including recurrent deformity and refracture, occurred in patients treated with bone lengthening with corrective osteotomy than in patients treated only with deformity correction.[32]

Another important advancement has been a return to low-energy, percutaneous, tissue-sparing osteotomies.[32] Because of the concern about recurrent deformity or refracture, intramedullary nailing has been recommended in conjunction with treatment or after treatment with an external fixator because it minimizes the risk of recurrence and refracture.

The use of a minimally invasive technique for guided growth for the treatment of bone deformity in patients younger than 10 years with X-linked hypophosphatemia has been described.[39,40] This technique corrects the mechanical axis to allow for more normal growth and functioning of the physis and avoids major osteotomy, which could result in early recurrence of a deformity (**Figure 5**). It was found that staples had a higher migration rate and resulted in rebound deformity, but tension-band plates had no hardware migration. Gradual deformity correction maintains alignment, minimizes secondary bony deformity, and avoids the need for future osteotomies for angular correction.

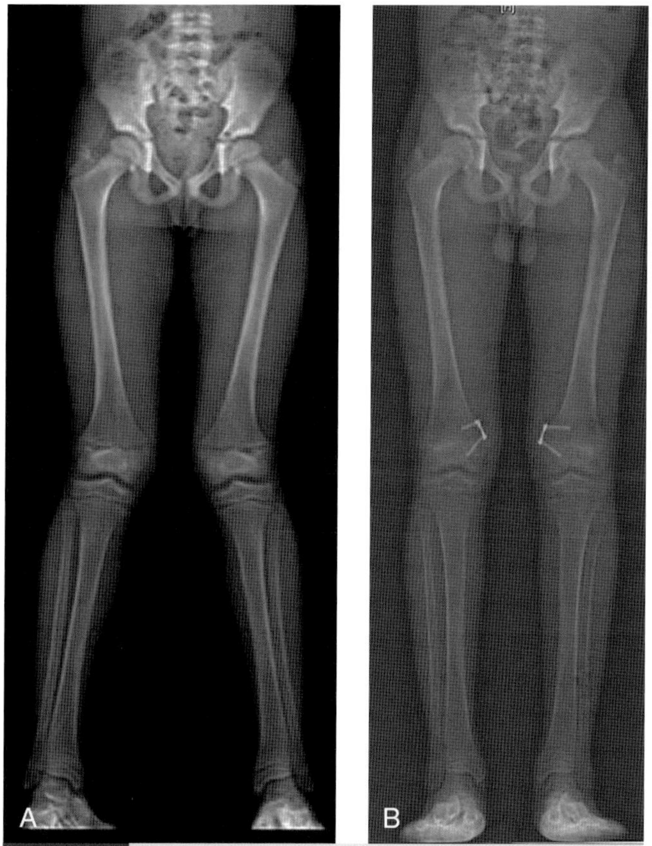

Figure 5 **A,** Long-leg standing AP radiograph of a 13-year-old boy with X-linked hypophosphatemia with a genu valgus deformity. **B,** Long-leg AP radiograph after the patient was managed with a guided growth system for 2 years.

Secondary Causes of Osteoporosis

Osteoporosis is defined as a skeletal disorder characterized by compromised bone strength, which predisposes an individual to an increased risk of fracture. Osteoporosis in children can have many primary and secondary etiologies (**Table 3**). This section focuses on the recent literature regarding glucocorticoid-induced osteoporosis.

Glucocorticoid-induced osteoporosis is the most common form of secondary osteoporosis. Systemic glucocorticoid therapy is associated with an initial increase in bone resorption (especially trabecular bone resorption), which is more pronounced in the first months of therapy. This is followed by decreased bone formation arising from the decreased activity of osteoblasts. A 10% to 20% loss of trabecular bone occurs in the first 6 months of glucocorticoid therapy, followed by a 2% per-year loss in subsequent years.[41] In addition, a 2% to 3% loss of cortical bone occurs in the first year; thereafter, a slow and continuous loss is maintained.[42] The architectural deterioration of bone related to systemic glucocorticoid therapy leads to increased fracture risk.

The risk of chronic glucocorticoid therapy is well established in adults. Several medications are available for the prevention and treatment of glucocorticoid-induced osteoporosis in adults. However, no evidence-based guideline exists for managing children who require long-term oral glucocorticoid therapy. Glucocorticoid use in growing children may decrease peak bone mass accrual and increase lifelong fracture risk, but the underlying disease process requiring glucocorticoid therapy may also have an adverse effect on the growing skeleton. A recent systematic review compared reported bone health outcomes in children treated with systemic glucocorticoid therapy with those of control subjects.[43] Children treated with systemic glucocorticoids had lower spine BMD and high rates of vertebral fractures compared with age- and sex-matched healthy control subjects.[43] However, given the paucity of long-term safety and efficacy data regarding the optimal medical treatment of children with glucocorticoid-induced osteoporosis, the use of bisphosphonate

Table 3

Primary and Secondary Etiologies for Osteoporosis in Children

Etiology	
Primary	Structural gene abnormalities (eg, osteogenesis imperfecta, Marfan syndrome, Ehlers-Danlos syndrome, Bruck syndrome, homocystinuria) Osteoporosis pseudoglioma Idiopathic juvenile osteoporosis
Secondary	Neuromuscular (eg, Duchenne muscular dystrophy, cerebral palsy, myelomeningocele) Endocrine (eg, growth hormone deficiency, hyperthyroidism) Infiltrative conditions (eg, leukemia, thalassemia) Chronic inflammatory conditions (eg, juvenile idiopathic arthritis, inflammatory bowel disease) Nutritional and vitamin deficiencies (eg, celiac disease, anorexia nervosa) Drug-related (eg, glucocorticoid, anticonvulsant, methotrexate, cyclosporine)

therapy should be limited in duration and administered only to children with substantial bone fragility.

Osteonecrosis is a devastating consequence of the medical management of several pediatric conditions. Glucocorticoid use is a well-known risk factor for osteonecrosis and there appears to be a dose-related correlation. In a 2014 review of the rate of osteonecrosis in children after chemotherapy and high-dose steroid treatment for hematologic malignancy (acute lymphoblastic leukemia, acute myeloid leukemia, or non-Hodgkin lymphoma), the authors reported that osteonecrosis developed in 7.6% of the patients.[44] It was concluded that osteonecrosis mainly affects the weight-bearing epiphyses, and the risk of osteonecrosis increases with age and higher doses of steroids (mean cumulative dose, 5,967 mg). Early screening for osteonecrosis was recommended in high-risk patients. Dexamethasone is associated with a higher risk of osteonecrosis compared with prednisolone and a higher risk of fractures compared with prednisone.[45,46]

Summary

Bone health is an important aspect of musculoskeletal care. Pediatric patients typically are seen by an orthopaedic surgeon for fracture care; however, it is important to understand the biology of other commonly occurring bone conditions. Future research will continue to provide insight for the nonsurgical and surgical treatment of patients with OI and metabolic bone diseases.

Key Study Points

- OI describes a group of inherited connective tissue conditions characterized by increased bone fragility and low bone mass. A multidisciplinary team should be involved in management.
- The goals of treatment of OI are to maximize a patient's mobility (decreasing bone pain and preventing or correcting deformity) and ability to accomplish the activities of daily living.
- Rickets can be classified into calcipenic and phosphopenic rickets. Rickets caused by vitamin D deficiency is the most common form of calcipenic rickets worldwide. Medical management of patients with rickets is essential.
- X-linked hypophosphatemia is the most common form of inheritable rickets. Mutations of the *PHEX* gene result in an increase in fibroblast growth factor-23 (FGF-23), which leads to phosphaturia. Surgical treatment may be required for correcting angular deformities caused by the condition.
- Glucocorticoid-induced osteoporosis is the most common form of secondary osteoporosis. Systemic glucocorticoid therapy is associated with an initial increase in bone resorption (especially trabecular bone resorption), which is more pronounced in the first months of therapy, then followed by decreased bone formation arising from the decreased activity of osteoblasts.

Annotated References

1. Harrington J, Sochett E, Howard A: Update on the evaluation and treatment of osteogenesis imperfecta. *Pediatr Clin North Am* 2014;61(6):1243-1257.

   The authors present a review of OI genetics and diagnosis and treatment strategies.

2. Ben Amor IM, Roughley P, Glorieux FH, Rauch F: Skeletal clinical characteristics of osteogenesis imperfecta caused by haploinsufficiency mutations in COL1A1. *J Bone Miner Res* 2013;28(9):2001-2007.

   The authors describe the clinical skeletal manifestations of mild OI caused by mutations in *COL1A1*. Spinal deformity and spinal compression fractures were commonly associated with *COL1A1* mutations.

3. Shaker JL, Albert C, Fritz J, Harris G: Recent developments in osteogenesis imperfecta. *F1000Res* 2015;4(F1000 Faculty Rev):681.

   This review article discusses recent updates on genetics factors related to OI and management of the condition.

4. Rauch F, Plotkin H, Zeitlin L, Glorieux FH: Bone mass, size, and density in children and adolescents with osteogenesis imperfecta: Effect of intravenous pamidronate therapy. *J Bone Miner Res* 2003;18(4):610-614.

5. Rauch F, Tutlewski B, Schönau E: The bone behind a low areal bone mineral density: Peripheral quantitative computed tomographic analysis in a woman with osteogenesis imperfecta. *J Musculoskelet Neuronal Interact* 2002;2(4):306-308.

6. Fritz JM, Guan Y, Wang M, Smith PA, Harris GF: Muscle force sensitivity of a finite element fracture risk assessment model in osteogenesis imperfecta: Biomed 2009. *Biomed Sci Instrum* 2009;45:316-321.

7. Caouette C, Rauch F, Villemure I, et al: Biomechanical analysis of fracture risk associated with tibia deformity in children with osteogenesis imperfecta: A finite element analysis. *J Musculoskelet Neuronal Interact* 2014;14(2):205-212.

   The authors describe the development of a finite element model to predict the risk of tibial fracture associated with tibia deformity in OI patients. Through their model, objective criteria were determined to assess the necessity of surgical intervention.

8. Pizones J, Plotkin H, Parra-Garcia JI, et al: Bone healing in children with osteogenesis imperfecta treated with bisphosphonates. *J Pediatr Orthop* 2005;25(3):332-335.

9. Fassier F, Glorieux FH: Surgical management of osteogenesis imperfecta, in Duparc J, ed: *Surgical Techniques in Orthopaedics and Traumatology* .Paris, France, Elsevier SAS, 2003, pp 1-8.

10. Widmann RF, Bitan FD, Laplaza FJ, Burke SW, DiMaio MF, Schneider R: Spinal deformity, pulmonary compromise, and quality of life in osteogenesis imperfecta. *Spine (Phila Pa 1976)* 1999;24(16):1673-1678.

11. Topouchian V, Finidori G, Glorion C, Padovani JP, Pouliquen JC: Posterior spinal fusion for kypho-scoliosis associated with osteogenesis imperfecta: Long-term results [French]. *Rev Chir Orthop Reparatrice Appar Mot* 2004;90(6):525-532.

12. Yilmaz G, Hwang S, Oto M, et al: Surgical treatment of scoliosis in osteogenesis imperfecta with cement-augmented pedicle screw instrumentation. *J Spinal Disord Tech* 2014;27(3):174-180.

    This retrospective review of 10 consecutive patients with OI who were treated with all-pedicle screw instrumentation (7 with cement-augmented pedicle screws) found that pedicle screw instrumentation in OI scoliosis was safe and effective, and cement augmentation improved pedicle screw pull-out strength. Level of evidence: IV.

13. Hatz D, Esposito PW, Schroeder B, Burke B, Lutz R, Hasley BP: The incidence of spondylolysis and spondylolisthesis in children with osteogenesis imperfecta. *J Pediatr Orthop* 2011;31(6):655-660.

    The authors present a retrospective radiographic review of patient treated in an OI clinic to assess the incidence of spondylolysis and spondylolisthesis. Radiographic morphology was evaluated to identify abnormalities or dysplasia. Level of evidence: IV.

14. Phillipi CA, Remmington T, Steiner RD: Bisphosphonate therapy for osteogenesis imperfecta. *Cochrane Database Syst Rev* 2008;4:CD005088.

15. Hald JD, Evangelou E, Langdahl BL, Ralston SH: Bisphosphonates for the prevention of fractures in osteogenesis imperfecta: Meta-analysis of placebo-controlled trials. *J Bone Miner Res* 2015;30(5):929-933.

    This meta-analysis of placebo-controlled trials evaluating the effectiveness of fracture prevention in patients with OI concluded that the effect of bisphosphonates on fracture prevention was inconclusive. Recommended further investigation. Level of evidence: I.

16. Nicolaou N, Agrawal Y, Padman M, Fernandes JA, Bell MJ: Changing pattern of femoral fractures in osteogenesis imperfecta with prolonged use of bisphosphonates. *J Child Orthop* 2012;6(1):21-27.

    This retrospective review compared the location of femoral fractures in patients with OI who were treated with bisphosphonates over a 2-year period with the femoral fracture location in a historical control group who did not receive bisphosphonate treatment. The bisphosphonate group had more subtrochanteric fractures compared with the control group and fracture patterns similar to those seen in adult patients with osteoporosis who were treated with bisphosphonates. Level of evidence: IV.

17. Hegazy A, Kenawey M, Sochett E, Tile L, Cheung AM, Howard AW: Unusual femur stress fractures in children with osteogenesis imperfecta and intramedullary rods on long-term intravenous pamidronate therapy. *J Pediatr Orthop* 2015.

The authors present a retrospective review of six children with OI in whom unusual stress femoral fractures developed after treatment with cyclic bisphosphonates. Level of evidence: IV.

18. Munns CF, Rajab MH, Hong J, et al: Acute phase response and mineral status following low dose intravenous zoledronic acid in children. *Bone* 2007;41(3):366-370.

19. Hoyer-Kuhn H, Netzer C, Koerber F, Schoenau E, Semler O: Two years' experience with denosumab for children with osteogenesis imperfecta type VI. *Orphanet J Rare Dis* 2014;9:145.

Treatment with denosumab was evaluated for children with OI type VI. After 2 years of treatment, the authors reported an increase in BMD, normalization of vertebral shape, increased mobility, and a reduced fracture rate. Level of evidence: IV.

20. Golden NH, Abrams SA; Committee on Nutrition: Optimizing bone health in children and adolescents. *Pediatrics* 2014;134(4):e1229-e1243.

The authors provide a clinical report on improving the understanding of bone health in children and adolescents. The report provides recommendation on screening, testing, and managing vitamin D deficiency, and describes the role of pediatricians in optimizing bone health.

21. Scientific Advisory Committee on Nutrition: *Update on Vitamin D* .London, England, The Stationery Office, 2007.

22. Bischoff-Ferrari HA, Giovannucci E, Willett WC, Dietrich T, Dawson-Hughes B: Estimation of optimal serum concentrations of 25-hydroxyvitamin D for multiple health outcomes. *Am J Clin Nutr* 2006;84(1):18-28.

23. Lips P: Vitamin D deficiency and secondary hyperparathyroidism in the elderly: Consequences for bone loss and fractures and therapeutic implications. *Endocr Rev* 2001;22(4):477-501.

24. Liu PT, Stenger S, Li H, et al: Toll-like receptor triggering of a vitamin D-mediated human antimicrobial response. *Science* 2006;311(5768):1770-1773.

25. Gordon CM, DePeter KC, Feldman HA, Grace E, Emans SJ: Prevalence of vitamin D deficiency among healthy adolescents. *Arch Pediatr Adolesc Med* 2004;158(6):531-537.

26. Sullivan SS, Rosen CJ, Halteman WA, Chen TC, Holick MF: Adolescent girls in Maine are at risk for vitamin D insufficiency. *J Am Diet Assoc* 2005;105(6):971-974.

27. Prentice A: Vitamin D deficiency: A global perspective. *Nutr Rev* 2008;66(10suppl 2):S153-S164.

28. Holick MF, Binkley NC, Bischoff-Ferrari HA, et al; Endocrine Society: Evaluation, treatment, and prevention of vitamin D deficiency: An Endocrine Society clinical practice guideline. *J Clin Endocrinol Metab* 2011;96(7):1911-1930.

The authors describe the clinical practice guidelines compiled by the Endocrine Society for the evaluation, treatment, and prevention of vitamin D deficiency.

29. Institute of Medicine of the National Academies: *Dietary Reference Intake for Calcium and Vitamin D.* Report Brief, November 2010. Available at: http://iom.edu/~/media/Files/Report%20Files/2010/Dietary-Reference-Intakes-for-Calcium-and-Vitamin-D/Vitamin%20D%20and%20Calcium%202010%20Report%20Brief.pdf. Accessed May 4, 2016.

30. Misra M, Pacaud D, Petryk A, Collett-Solberg PF, Kappy M; Drug and Therapeutics Committee of the Lawson Wilkins Pediatric Endocrine Society: Vitamin D deficiency in children and its management: Review of current knowledge and recommendations. *Pediatrics* 2008;122(2):398-417.

31. Petersen DJ, Boniface AM, Schranck FW, Rupich RC, Whyte MP: X-linked hypophosphatemic rickets: A study (with literature review) of linear growth response to calcitriol and phosphate therapy. *J Bone Miner Res* 1992;7(6):583-597.

32. Sharkey MS, Grunseich K, Carpenter TO: Contemporary medical and surgical management of X-linked hypophosphatemic rickets. *J Am Acad Orthop Surg* 2015;23(7):433-442.

This review article details the recent medical and surgical management of X-linked hypophosphatemic rickets.

33. Carpenter TO: New perspectives on the biology and treatment of X-linked hypophosphatemic rickets. *Pediatr Clin North Am* 1997;44(2):443-466.

34. Carpenter TO, Imel EA, Holm IA, Jan de Beur SM, Insogna KL: A clinician's guide to X-linked hypophosphatemia. *J Bone Miner Res* 2011;26(7):1381-1388.

Clinicians present recommendations for the diagnosis and management of X-linked hypophosphatemic rickets, arising from the Advance in Rare Bone Diseases Scientific Conference.

35. Tsuru N, Chan JC, Chinchilli VM: Renal hypophosphatemic rickets: Growth and mineral metabolism after treatment with calcitriol (1,25-dihydroxyvitamin D3) and phosphate supplementation. *Am J Dis Child* 1987;141(1):108-110.

36. Carpenter TO, Imel EA, Ruppe MD, et al: Randomized trial of the anti-FGF23 antibody KRN23 in X-linked hypophosphatemia. *J Clin Invest* 2014;124(4):1587-1597.

The results of a randomized clinical trial comparing anti-FGF-23 antibody with placebo for the medical management of X-linked hypophosphatemia are discussed.

The trial found that anti-FGF-23 antibody had positive effects and a favorable safety profile. Level of evidence: I.

37. Rubinovitch M, Said SE, Glorieux FH, Cruess RL, Rogala E: Principles and results of corrective lower limb osteotomies for patients with vitamin D-resistant hypophosphatemic rickets. *Clin Orthop Relat Res* 1988;237:264-270.

38. Petje G, Meizer R, Radler C, Aigner N, Grill F: Deformity correction in children with hereditary hypophosphatemic rickets. *Clin Orthop Relat Res* 2008;466(12):3078-3085.

39. Novais E, Stevens PM: Hypophosphatemic rickets: The role of hemiepiphysiodesis. *J Pediatr Orthop* 2006;26(2):238-244.

40. Stevens PM, Klatt JB: Guided growth for pathological physes: Radiographic improvement during realignment. *J Pediatr Orthop* 2008;28(6):632-639.

41. Pereira RM, Carvalho JF, Paula AP, et al; Committee for Osteoporosis and Bone Metabolic Disorders of the Brazilian Society of Rheumatology; Brazilian Medical Association; Brazilian Association of Physical Medicine and Rehabilitation: Guidelines for the prevention and treatment of glucocorticoid-induced osteoporosis. *Rev Bras Reumatol* 2012;52(4):580-593.

    A bibliographic review of scientific articles to establish guidelines for the prevention and treatment of glucocorticoid-induced osteoporosis is presented. Level of evidence: II.

42. van Staa TP, Leufkens HG, Cooper C: The epidemiology of corticosteroid-induced osteoporosis: A meta-analysis. *Osteoporos Int* 2002;13(10):777-787.

43. Hansen KE, Kleker B, Safdar N, Bartels CM: A systematic review and meta-analysis of glucocorticoid-induced osteoporosis in children. *Semin Arthritis Rheum* 2014;44(1):47-54.

    A systematic review and meta-analysis of existing literature was done to determine the effects of systemic glucocorticoid therapy on BMD and fracture risk in children. Sixteen studies were identified. Data showed lower spine BMD compared with healthy children. Level of evidence: II.

44. Salem KH, Brockert AK, Mertens R, Drescher W: Avascular necrosis after chemotherapy for haematological malignancy in childhood. *Bone Joint J* 2013;95-B(12):1708-1713.

    In this review of 105 children with hematologic malignancy who were managed with chemotherapy, osteonecrosis developed in 8 children. All of the children with osteonecrosis received treatment with steroids. The study concluded that the risk of osteonecrosis increases with age and higher doses of steroids. Level of evidence: IV.

45. Vora A: Management of osteonecrosis in children and young adults with acute lymphoblastic leukaemia. *Br J Haematol* 2011;155(5):549-560.

    A review of treatment strategies for the management of osteonecrosis in children and young adults with acute lymphoblastic leukemia is presented. The author provides information on the pathogenesis of the osteonecrosis, clinical features, natural history, and management.

46. Rayar MS, Nayiager T, Webber CE, Barr RD, Athale UH: Predictors of bony morbidity in children with acute lymphoblastic leukemia. *Pediatr Blood Cancer* 2012;59(1):77-82.

    The authors of this review article attempt to determine predictors of bony morbidity based on a single cancer center's protocol for the treatment of acute lymphoblastic leukemia. Level of evidence: IV.

Chapter 15

Progressive Neuromuscular Diseases in Childhood and Adolescence

Michael D. Sussman, MD

Abstract

A variety of diseases exist that cause muscle weakness and tend to be progressive during childhood. These include muscular dystrophies (specifically, Duchenne muscular dystrophy), spinal muscular atrophy, congenital myotonic dystrophy, and Charcot-Marie-Tooth disease. All these conditions are hereditary and have a genetic basis; in many cases, the responsible genes have been identified. It is helpful to be aware of the pathophysiology, clinical course, and orthopaedic treatment interventions for these diseases.

Keywords: Charcot-Marie-Tooth disease; congenital myotonic dystrophy; Duchenne muscular dystrophy; spinal muscular atrophy

Introduction

This chapter discusses the most commonly seen progressive neuromuscular diseases in children. These are diseases of the motor unit, which is defined as the combination of the motor neuron in the anterior horn of the spinal cord, its nerve connecting through the neuromuscular junction to the muscle, and the muscle itself. Duchenne muscular dystrophy (DMD) is the most prevalent of the many childhood-onset diseases of muscle that cause progressive weakness; however, there are other muscular dystrophies and myopathies with onset in childhood. A muscular dystrophy is characterized by a progressive loss of muscle cells and increasing weakness over time, whereas a myopathy will affect the function of a muscle fiber causing weakness, but tends to be nonprogressive. Congenital myotonic dystrophy is the second most prevalent muscle disease in pediatric patients. Other muscle diseases exist that do not manifest until later in life. These include limb-girdle muscular dystrophy, which is a group of muscular dystrophies, most of which manifest in adulthood, although some appear during childhood.

Spinal muscular atrophy (SMA) is caused by progressive loss of the motor neurons in the anterior horn of the spinal cord, which results in progressive paralysis. In many patients, this leads to early death from respiratory failure. There is no sensory involvement.

A variety of neuropathies (hereditary sensory motor neuropathies) exist that affect the axon between the motor neuron and neuromuscular junction. The most prevalent of these are the group of heritable conditions known as Charcot-Marie-Tooth (CMT) disease; however, other neuropathies can affect both motor and sensory nerves and may be hereditary (such as distal SMA, which may be better referred to as hereditary motor neuropathy and is distinguished from CMT by the lack of sensory involvement) or acquired (such as the inflammatory polyneuropathies).

These progressive neuromuscular diseases share certain characteristics, including a hereditary, a congenital, and a genetic basis. In many of these conditions, the specific gene abnormality has been identified. This allows for a precise diagnosis and treatment interventions specific to the particular gene defect causing the condition. Progressive neuromuscular diseases may be inherited in an autosomal dominant, an autosomal recessive, or an X-linked manner. If they are inherited in an autosomal dominant manner, a family history of the disease may exist, whereas this is less likely in an X-linked condition, and unlikely in an autosomal recessive condition unless there is consanguinity with a common ancestor. Most

Dr. Sussman or an immediate family member has stock or stock options held in Ionis Pharmaceuticals and CASI Pharmaceutical and has participated as a member of the medical advisory board of Sarepta Therapeutics and Marathon Pharmaceuticals.

of these conditions tend to get worse over time. Some neuromuscular diseases may manifest early in life, but others may not manifest until the second decade of life or even later. The conditions all cause weakness, but not spasticity. The weakness is not homogeneous and, in general, conditions affecting the muscle tend to manifest more in proximal muscles, whereas those affecting the neuron or axon manifest initially in the distal muscles. Asymmetric muscle weakness can lead to equinus, equinovarus, or cavovarus deformities of the foot. Conditions causing more proximal weakness and truncal weakness may predispose an affected individual to hip dislocation and scoliosis.

In many neuromuscular diseases, multiple organ systems may be involved. The treatment team may include an orthopaedic surgeon, a neurologist, a geneticist, a gastroenterologist, a nutritionist, and a developmental pediatrician, as indicated by organ system involvement. If cardiac and pulmonary dysfunction are involved, these possibly life-threatening conditions will require consultation with a pulmonologist and cardiologist and may require priority treatment.

Duchenne Muscular Dystrophy

DMD is a disease of muscle in which the muscle progressively deteriorates over time and is replaced by fibroadipose tissue. This results in a loss of functional fibers, weakness, scarring, and relative rigidity of the muscles. The incidence of DMD is 1 in 3,500 male births, and it is estimated that there are 15,000 affected males in the United States. Progressive weakness develops, and patients lose the ability to walk by age 8 to 12 years; death usually occurs by age 20 years due to respiratory failure. Although there is no cure for DMD, administration of high-dose corticosteroid markedly ameliorates the degenerative process, leading to a longer life and avoidance of scoliosis. Respiratory and cardiac medications also are critical. Currently, new molecular and genetically based treatment approaches are being investigated and hold great promise.

Pathophysiology and Genetics

DMD is caused by the absence of the muscle protein dystrophin, which constitutes only a small portion of the total muscle proteins. Dystrophin plays a critical role in the physical and biomechanical stabilization of the myofiber membrane and also provides an attachment site for enzymes (such as nitrous oxide synthetase) that help support muscle function. Several dystrophin-associated proteins that link the actin-myosin network to the extracellular matrix are not incorporated into the muscle when dystrophin is absent in DMD. Primary abnormalities in specific dystrophin-associated proteins are the cause of many of the limb-girdle dystrophies, which only occasionally manifest in the pediatric age group and are not discussed in this chapter.

The absence of dystrophin is secondary to a mutation in the gene for dystrophin, which is located on the X chromosome. A variety of gene abnormalities can result in the lack of dystrophin production. The most common abnormality (65% of patients) is the deletion of a segment of the gene that interrupts the normal triplet sequence of the DNA, which constitutes the reading frame, so that when the gene is spliced back together, all of the triplet sequences downstream from the deletion are nonsense. This results in the production of an incomplete protein, which is degraded, and no functional dystrophin is produced.

In 15% of the patients, there is a single nucleotide mutation known as a premature stop codon, which causes the ribosome to stop transcribing the gene. Any protein that is made up to this point is degraded, so that no dystrophin is produced. A variety of other gene abnormalities, including splice-site mutations and duplications, are responsible for the remainder of the genetic errors. It is important to ascertain the specific gene mutation because there are new treatments being developed that are specific to the type of genetic abnormality present. A test to determine the gene mutation is available at a reasonable cost.

In a similar but milder condition known as Becker muscular dystrophy, a gene segment deletion also exists in most patients, but the deletion does not interrupt the reading frame, and a smaller than normal dystrophin is produced in less than normal quantities.

Because the gene for dystrophin is located on the X chromosome, DMD and Becker muscular dystrophy are inherited in an X-linked fashion. This means that carrier mothers are clinically unaffected, 50% of their daughters will be carriers, and 50% of their sons will be affected with the disease. Because of a variety of factors, even though this is an X-linked recessive trait, some of the mothers who are carriers will also manifest mild signs of muscle disease, including cardiomyopathy. Given this X-linked inheritance pattern, if the mother had no brothers who were affected and no one in the lineage was previously affected to her knowledge, the gene could still be carried through several generations of females before manifesting in an affected male offspring. This explains why DMD may be a completely unexpected disease. In some instances, there may be a new mutation; this most frequently arises in the germline of the affected patient's maternal grandfather. Although most affected patients are male, DMD may rarely fully manifest in females for a variety of underlying genetic reasons.

Table 1

Duchenne Muscular Dystrophy: Clinical Symptoms and Historical Findings

Male sex (boy)
Ambulation begins later than 16 to 18 months of age
Difficulty in keeping up with peers
Inability to run normally (excessive use of arms)
Ability to jump and hop is unlikely
Unable to climb stairs reciprocally
Positive finding for Gowers maneuver
Cognitive delay
Easily fatigued
Calf enlargement
Positive family history for Duchenne muscular dystrophy or Becker muscular dystrophy

Genetic Modifiers of DMD

It recently has been determined that the DMD disease process may be modified on the basis of the presence of other inherited gene mutations unrelated to the dystrophin gene. For example, a mutation in the *LTBP4* gene can modify the disease process to produce a milder form of the disease. Patients with this mutation are able to ambulate for 1.8 years longer than those who do not have the mutation, although this effect has been seen only in Caucasian boys. This effect may be the result of a reduction in transforming growth factor-β signaling. In contrast, a mutation in the gene for osteopontin (*SPP1*) results in more severe disease progression, with the anticipated age of ambulation cessation occurring at a mean of 1 year earlier than the generally expected age. The *SPP1* gene encodes an inflammatory cytokine and seems to affect the response to corticosteroids, thus making corticosteroid treatment less effective. In patients with this gene mutation, those who were identified as Hispanic or South Asian lost ambulation 2.7 and 2 years earlier than Caucasian boys, respectively.[1] Tests for these mutations are not yet clinically available, but knowledge of the mutations will be important in clinical medication trials. An excessive number of mutations in a group can modify the disease process and could skew the results, especially in studies with a small number of patients.

In a 2015 study, a naturally occurring mutation in the *Jagged1* gene, which results in an overexpression of a protein that stimulates muscle regeneration, was found in a population of golden retrievers with a Duchenne-like muscular dystrophy. The presence of this gene completely reversed the dystrophic process, and dogs with this mutation developed normally despite the absence of dystophin.[2]

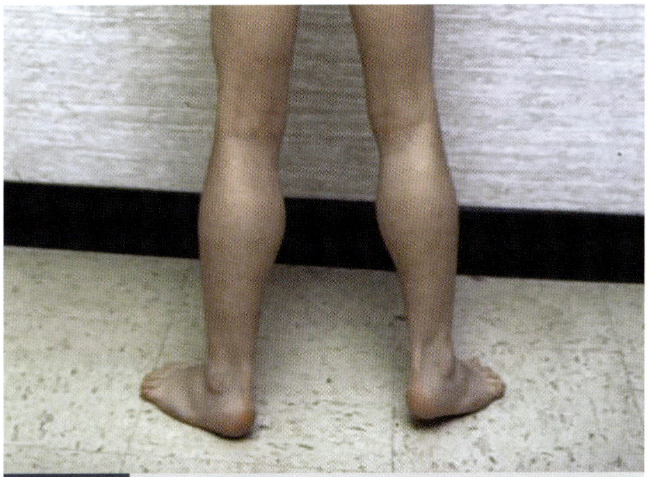

Figure 1 Clinical photograph shows calf enlargement in a boy with DMD.

Diagnosis

A diagnosis of DMD, which is often missed initially, should be suspected in boys who have delayed motor development. It is recommended that any boy who is not walking independently by 16 to 18 months of age (without other reasons for this motor delay) should be evaluated for DMD (**Table 1**). Affected patients do not run in a completely normal manner and always have difficulty ascending and descending stairs, usually using a handrail and ascending and descending one step at a time rather than reciprocally. Patients with DMD are rarely able to hop on one leg or jump. One of the first obvious changes seen in many but not all patients is calf enlargement,[3] which is specific for DMD and Becker muscular dystrophy and is not seen in any other neuromuscular diseases (**Figure 1**).

The Gowers maneuver is a particularly useful clinical finding. Although it occurs in patients with significant weakness of the pelvic girdle musculature from other causes, it is seen in all patients with DMD. The Gowers maneuver describes the method used by a patient to rise from the floor. First, the child will transition from a sitting position on the floor into the prone position on his hands and knees, as if he were intending to crawl. After assuming this crawling position, the child will then extend his knees into the "bear position." The trunk is then brought upright by hip extension, and the child put his hands on his thighs to assist in the process of getting the trunk in the upright position (**Figure 2**).

As determined by a study from the United Kingdom, the average age at diagnosis is 5.2 years and the delay from the time a patient was first seen by an orthopaedic

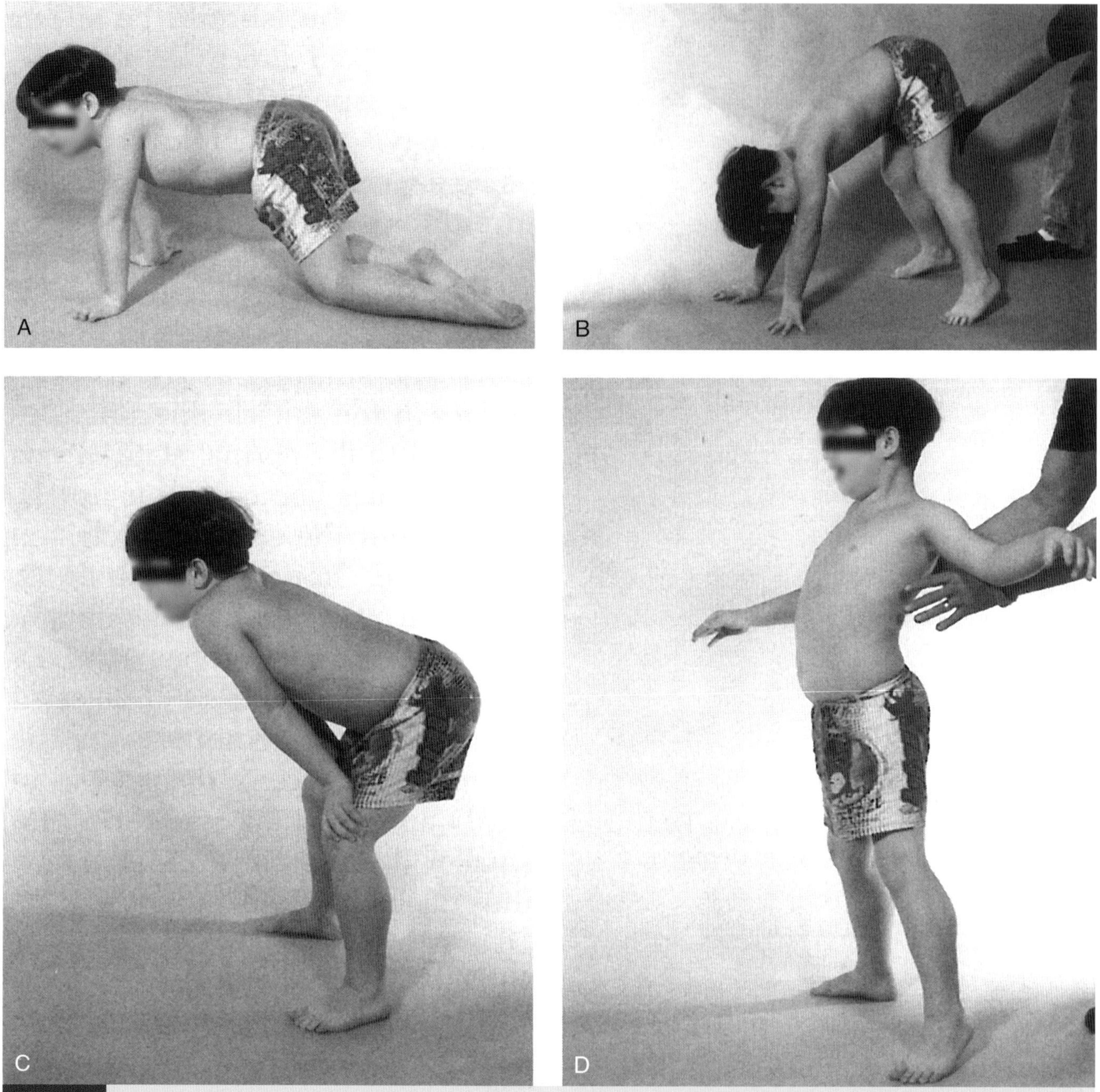

Figure 2 Clinical photographs of a child with Duchenne muscular dystrophy demonstrating the Gowers maneuver. **A,** The child moves from sitting on the floor to the prone position on all four limbs. **B,** The child extends his knees and assumes the "bear" position with all four limbs extended. **C,** The trunk is brought to the upright position using hands and arms on the upper thighs. **D,** The child achieves the upright position. (Reproduced from Sussman M: Duchenne muscular dystrophy. *J Am Acad Orthop Surg* 2002;10[2]:138-151.)

consultant and subsequently referred for DMD testing was 2 years.[4] The delay did not improve over a 10-year period despite a regional educational campaign.

If DMD is suspected, the first diagnostic step is to test for the serum creatinine kinase level, which can be ascertained with a relatively inexpensive blood test. The normal level is up to 200 international units (IU)/L; affected patients have levels that are usually greater than 10,000 to 15,000 IU/L. Milder elevations of the serum creatinine kinase level can occur after strenuous activity or bruising, but also are seen in other types of muscle disease such as limb-girdle muscular dystrophy. A diagnosis of DMD is made in some young patients when liver function studies are performed for unrelated reasons and their creatinine kinase level is found to be massively elevated.

If the serum creatinine kinase level is greater than 1,000 IU/L, a blood sample or cheek swab should be obtained to test for the dystrophin gene. This test is readily available, costs less than $500, is very specific and reliable, provides a definitive diagnosis, and will confirm the diagnosis and define the exact type of abnormality present in the gene in approximately 95% of boys with DMD. Although a muscle biopsy was frequently performed in the past, biopsy is now rarely indicated and should be performed only in those few patients with an elevated serum creatinine kinase level and clinical findings consistent with DMD, but who have negative genetic test results. Muscle biopsy also may be infrequently required to confirm other muscle diseases that cannot be diagnosed based on clinical findings and genetic tests. Although liver enzymes such as alanine transaminase and aspartate transaminase are typically elevated in patients with DMD and Becker muscular dystrophy, these findings do not indicate liver disease, and liver biopsy is not indicated.

Newborn screening for DMD can be done by measuring the serum creatinine kinase level on a neonatal blood spot examination. Because there is a transient elevation of the serum creatinine kinase level immediately following birth, the recommended threshold for further evaluation for DMD is a neonatal level greater than 1,000 IU/L. Early diagnosis is important so that the family can be provided with appropriate genetic counseling to allow for future pregnancy planning. Because a diagnosis of DMD is often not made until age 5 years, the affected mother may have other affected boys before she is recognized as a carrier. For known maternal carriers, in vitro fertilization allows preimplantation selection whereby only disease-free embryos are implanted. Prenatal diagnosis of DMD is also possible via amniocentesis or chorionic villus sampling. In addition, early diagnosis also is important because most new treatments will likely be most effective if started early in life when muscle damage is minimal.

Natural History

In affected patients, muscle weakness is difficult to appreciate in infancy, but it becomes more apparent with growth. Walking is usually delayed until after 16 months of age. When patients begin to walk, the gait is relatively widely based, and increased lumbar lordosis is present. As time progresses, the gait becomes increasingly abnormal.[5] There is improvement in walking speed over the first 5 years, as assessed by the 6-minute timed walk test, until the disease process overwhelms the developmental process between the ages of 5 and 7 years. As patients age, gait progressively deteriorates. Three-dimensional gait analysis shows that the knee flexion that occurs immediately after weight acceptance is usually lost sometime between the ages of 6 and 8 years. This means that when the stance phase is initiated, the knee is in full extension and remains in full extension throughout the entire stance phase. Before age 6 years, loss of hip extensor moments and power during the early stance phase occurs.[6] Tightness usually develops in the triceps surae beginning at age 4 to 5 years, and limitation of passive dorsiflexion can be found on physical examination. Loss of dorsiflexion occurs during the stance phase, and there is early rise of the heel from the floor in the late stance phase. As the Achilles tendon contracture progresses, patients will remain on their toes during all of the stance phase. This toe walking helps maintain knee extension as the ground reaction force from the plantar flexed foot forces the knee into extension. Between the ages of 8 and 10 years, gait becomes substantially more labored, with a wider stance base, greater lumbar lordosis, and increased fatigability. Affected patients who receive no treatment will generally stop walking sometime between the age of 8 and 12 years of age. The ability to ambulate after the age of 12 years is rare.

At approximately the time the ability to ambulate is lost, scoliosis can be clinically and radiologically demonstrated. Curves usually have their apex in the thoracolumbar region and will affect more than 90% of patients with DMD. Curves do not respond to brace treatment or adaptive seating, and they continue to progress to a severe magnitude, which interferes with comfort and function during the patients' teenage years.

An associated decline in pulmonary function begins in the teenage years; however, it appears that the scoliosis is not a major contributor to this decline. The major cause of respiratory decline is weakening of the muscles that support respiration, including the intercostal muscles and the diaphragm. A 2013 study found that stabilization of the scoliosis did not change the rate of respiratory decline based on a comparison with a contemporaneous group who did not undergo surgical correction.[7] Forced vital capacity (FVC) should be measured on a regular basis, which can be done accurately in a clinic by a skilled therapist using a handheld spirometer. If FVC substantially declines, a CoughAssist device (Philips Respironics) should be provided for daily use. Patients who have sleeping difficulty should have polysomnography and may benefit from bilevel positive airway pressure ventilation during sleep. The usual cause of death in boys with DMD is respiratory failure, which may be chronic, but also may occur in association with an acquired respiratory infection that has progressed to pneumonia. Death usually occurs by age 20 years, but a patient's lifespan may be extended by artificial ventilation.

Cardiac function progressively deteriorates because of associated cardiomyopathy. Beginning in the second decade of life, ejection fraction monitoring should be followed by echocardiography, because treatment with angiotensin converting enzyme inhibitors and beta blockers will help preserve cardiac function.[8]

Orthopaedic and Rehabilitation Treatment

At approximately age 5 or 6 years when tightness of the Achilles tendon develops as evidenced by limitations in passive dorsiflexion, an ankle-foot orthosis (AFO) used at nighttime, which has been custom molded in a neutral position, is recommended to help prevent progression of the Achilles tightness. However, AFOs should not be used during the daytime because they make ambulation more difficult. Even in the absence of contractures, patients will begin walking on their toes, which is an adaptation (known as the plantar flexion–knee extension couple) that creates a moment to help support the knee in extension. The hip extensors weaken early, before changes in hip motion can be appreciated. Because patients with DMD are unable to propel their center of mass forward using their weak hip extensor muscles, the triceps surae are used to compensate by helping to propel the center of mass forward during the stance phase of gait.[6]

In 20% of patients, the Achilles contracture is progressive and patients walk completely on their toes with no heel contact. When the contracture reaches approximately 30° or more of fixed equinus, walking becomes unstable. If the patient is a strong ambulator, has full knee extension against gravity, and the ability to handle some resistance with knee extension (grade 4), a careful Achilles tendon lengthening using an open sliding technique to avoid inadvertent complete tenotomy may be undertaken. Short leg casts are placed, and standing and walking are initiated on the first postoperative day. Short leg casts are continued for 4 weeks, and a custom-molded posterior leaf spring AFO is then placed to provide support in the stance phase of gait and control footdrop in swing. After this procedure, some patients will choose to use their AFOs for ambulation; however, the AFOs can be used only at night to prevent contracture recurrence if the patient can achieve stability during ambulation without AFOs.

As the disease progresses, contractures develop in most patients because of prolonged sitting and muscle imbalance. Tightness in the hip flexors and the tensor fasciae lata develops in all patients and results in abduction contractures, which contribute to the adoption of a widely based gait. Knee flexion contractures also may develop and can progress to 80° to 90° in some patients. If knee flexion contracture develops while the patient is still ambulating, the weak quadriceps will be unable to support knee extension and this may lead to the inability to continue ambulation. In the past, prophylactic multilevel tendon releases in the lower extremity were performed by some surgeons, but this technique is no longer generally recommended. The data supporting this approach are relatively weak. When walking ceases, full-time AFO use is still recommended to slow progression of the equinovarus deformity, which will inevitably occur. If severe equinovarus develops, it is rarely uncomfortable and does not require treatment unless the patient desires more stylish shoe wear. In those instances, simple tenotomies of the Achilles tendon can be performed, and, if substantial varus exists, tenotomies of the posterior tibial, flexor hallucis longus, and flexor digitorum longus tendons just above the ankle can be added. After surgery, short leg casts are placed, kept in place for 3 to 4 weeks, and then followed by the continuous use of a well-molded AFO that secures the foot in the corrected position. Releasing hip flexors and abductors and hamstrings in nonambulatory patients with DMD is not performed because correction is minimal after such surgery. Stretching has been advocated to control hip and knee flexion contractures, but no evidence exists that this offers any benefits, and stretching may cause discomfort. Night extension orthoses for the knees are not recommended because their efficacy is unproven, they can be uncomfortable, and they may interfere with sleep. Knee flexion contracture can approach 90°, but rarely exceed 90°, and it does not interfere with sitting but will make positioning for sleep difficult. In some patients with lower extremity contractures, moving or even touching the legs causes extreme discomfort.

Occupational and Physical Therapy

During the first decade of life, regular physical or occupational therapy is not usually necessary, although a therapist may provide the patient's school with recommendations regarding activities to be performed within the daily school setting. Although stretching exercises are frequently advocated and prescribed, there is no evidence for their efficacy, and they may place an additional burden on patients and their families. Adaptive recreation may be beneficial, and adaptation of a school's physical education program is important because patients with DMD will not be able to perform at the level of their peers. An independent education program should be instituted.

Experimental studies in animals have shown that eccentric muscle activity hastens muscle deterioration in DMD (but not necessarily other neuromuscular diseases);[9] therefore, activities that have a large eccentric component, such as weight lifting or walking on soft sand, should be avoided. When walking becomes difficult, patients will require powered devices for mobility. In patients with good upper limb function, a powered scooter may be an appropriate device, particularly for patients taking corticosteroids who can expect a reasonably long period of upper limb function. In those with poor upper limb function, a powered wheelchair with a variety of components, such as the tilt-in-space function (to allow differential pressure relief) and an elevating seat (to bring the patient to the level of his peers) should be prescribed. When upper limb function becomes compromised, occupational therapy can help the patient to master the use of adaptive equipment. A computer or tablet with voice-recognition software may be particularly helpful for completing schoolwork.

When ambulation ceases, a pneumatic standing device can provide good support for the trunk and lower extremities to allow standing for up to 30 minutes. Ultimately, standing in this device will become impractical because of the progression of hip, knee, and ankle contractures. In the past, knee-ankle-foot orthoses (KAFOs) were recommended to help prolong ambulatory ability, but it is now apparent that these devices are quite cumbersome, do not allow functional walking, and interfere with toileting. KAFOs are no longer recommended.

In addition to motor delays, cognitive impairment is common in DMD, with patients having an IQ of approximately 90. Because a large component of this impairment occurs in the area of expressive language, processing of information may be relatively better than its translation into expressive speech. Some patients may be severely cognitively impaired, but others may be very intelligent. Cognitive differences should be considered when establishing an independent education program.

With age and as muscle weakness increases, the patient may be unable to change positions while sleeping. Caregivers may need to turn the patient in bed. Enuresis is common in patients taking corticosteroids and more prevalent in those taking prednisone than in those taking deflazacort.[10]

Spinal Deformity

Progressive scoliosis develops in 90% of untreated patients and has its onset at approximately 10 to 12 years of age. In the 10% of patients in whom scoliosis does not develop, total thoracolumbar lordosis seems to prevent scoliosis. This is a naturally occurring phenomenon. Although a variety of seating and bracing techniques have been tried to induce this lordotic pattern, they have not been successful. No orthotic devices or seating adaptations have proven to be beneficial in controlling scoliosis in patients with DMD. After a curve reaches 20° to 30°, it is always continually and relentlessly progressive. Spinal instrumentation and fusion from the upper thoracic spine to L5 or the sacrum is recommended as soon as curves reach this magnitude. Performing the surgery at this stage of the disease is advantageous because patients have better pulmonary function and are likely to have an easier recovery.

The preferred treatment for scoliosis is posterior segmental instrumentation with sublaminar wires and pedicle screws for distal fixation at the lower lumbar spine or the upper sacrum or an all-pedicle screw construct. Anterior spinal surgery is contraindicated. Extending the fusion to the sacrum may not be necessary if pelvic obliquity is mild. All patients being considered for spinal fusion should have a thorough preoperative evaluation, including pulmonary and cardiac assessments. At least the first postoperative night should be spent in an intensive care unit for respiratory care; however, in most instances, extubation is possible on the first postoperative night and return to a standard nursing care environment can occur thereafter. A total intravenous anesthetic technique should be used in all patients with DMD to avoid anesthesia-induced rhabdomyolysis.

Although correction and stabilization of scoliosis is essential to maintain comfort and function in patients with spinal deformity, spinal stabilization may decrease but not eliminate the progressive decline in pulmonary function. A 2011 study reported a loss of pulmonary function in the immediate postoperative period, followed by a rate of decline similar to the preoperative trajectory;[11] however, other authors have reported that spinal fusion reduces the rate of pulmonary decline.[12] With careful perioperative management, patients with severe curves and pulmonary compromise can undergo successful surgical correction. A Japanese group reported that, in 14 patients with DMD and severe scoliosis (mean curve, 98°) and poor pulmonary function (mean FVC, 22%), FVC improved to 26% after a 6-week pulmonary training program before surgery.[13] Following surgery, all the patients were extubated on the same day and had no decline in pulmonary function at 6 weeks postoperatively but had the expected level of pulmonary decline 2 years after surgery. A Cochrane collaboration report on scoliosis surgery for patients with DMD concluded that because no randomized trials were available to evaluate the effectiveness of scoliosis surgery, no conclusion was possible regarding the efficacy of surgery.[14] However, in a published clinical care guideline, the group strongly recommended that spinal fusion be provided for patients with DMD and progressive curves.[15] In a review of 58 patients with progressive neuromuscular scoliosis, 27 of whom had DMD, a Korean group reported substantial improvements in sitting balance, body pain, and social functioning after spinal fusion, although parents did not report improvement in quality of life.[16] In contrast, some patients experience greater difficulty with self-feeding after spinal stabilization because they can no longer bend their trunk forward to meet their hand. Patients should be informed of this possible side effect before surgery.

Bone Health

Dual-energy x-ray absorptiometry has shown that osteopenia is associated with DMD and occurs early in life. Because patients with DMD are prone to long-bone fractures, aggressive treatment is needed to prevent periods of nonambulation, which lead to a more marked progression of weakness. Depending on the degree of weakness, patients may lose the ability to ambulate after a lower limb fracture. Upper limb fractures can cause balance problems and impair ambulatory ability, so physiotherapy to maintain ambulation may be useful. Fixation methods for lower limb fractures should allow minimal interruption of ambulation. In one large study of 143 patients with DMD, the fracture rate for long bones in patients treated with corticosteroids was 2.6 times greater than in patients who did not receive steroid treatment. In addition, vertebral compression fractures occurred in 32% of the patients treated with steroids, but none of the untreated patients. However, this difference may have been influenced by the fact that most of the patients who had not received steroid treatment had undergone thoracolumbar spinal fusion for scoliosis.[17]

In poor ambulators and nonambulators, casts may be used to treat lower limb fractures. Nonambulatory patients commonly sustain distal femoral fractures in the metaphyseal area in falls during wheelchair transfers. These fractures can be treated with long leg casts. Although, healing is usually rapid, flexion at the fracture site should be avoided because it can limit the patient's ability to stand for transfers. Fat embolism, although unusual, may occur even in minimally displaced femoral fractures and should be suspected if there is hypoxia and tachycardia after fracture of a long bone. The role of bisphosphonates (also known as diphosphonates) or other medications that may improve bone density has not been established in this patient group, although there is some interest in this among pediatric endocrinologists.

Anesthesia-Induced Rhabdomyolysis

Anesthesia-induced rhabdomyolysis is an unusual and frequently fatal reaction to general anesthetic. Triggering agents such as succinylcholine and halogenated hydrocarbon anesthetic gases have been implicated and neither should be used in patients with DMD. A total intravenous technique is recommended for any patient with DMD undergoing a surgical procedure, including spinal fusion. Anesthesia-induced rhabdomyolysis differs from malignant hyperthermia and, although it is not absolutely known, probably does not respond to intravenous dantrolene. In a typical scenario, as the patient is emerging from anesthesia, cardiac arrhythmia and tachycardia occur, followed by cardiac collapse associated with ventricular fibrillation. Most cases are associated with hyperkalemia. Rescue treatment should include rapid reduction of elevated potassium levels, usually by the administration of insulin, glucose, and bicarbonate, and the use of hyperventilation therapy. Younger patients seem most susceptible to anesthesia-induced rhabdomyolysis.[18] Families should be counseled that children with DMD should not be surgically treated outside of major hospitals where anesthesiologists are aware of anesthesia-induced rhabdomyolysis and have the resources to provide a rapid response.

Medical Treatment

The natural history of DMD (and presumably Becker muscular dystrophy) is dramatically altered by the daily administration of pharmacologic doses of corticosteroid. This treatment has become standard practice and is endorsed by the American Academy of Neurology and is included in care guidelines developed under the guidance of the US Centers for Disease Control.[15,19] (These guidelines are currently in the process of being updated.) Medications used are corticosteroids, either prednisone at 0.75 mg/kg daily or deflazacort at 0.9 mg/kg daily, up to a maximum of 35 mg per day. Therapy is usually initiated between the ages of 5 and 8 years, although some centers are initiating therapy at even younger ages. However, earlier initiation of steroid therapy may result in more severe growth retardation and other adverse side effects. Deflazacort, a derivative of prednisolone, has been shown to be associated with less weight gain than prednisone and is alleged by some clinicians to be associated with fewer behavioral problems. Deflazacort is available in Europe but not in North America, and it is not approved by the FDA.

Initial studies of corticosteroid use in patients with DMD published in the early 1990s showed improvement in muscle strength with the initiation of corticosteroid treatment, which was followed by a dramatic deviation from the anticipated loss of muscle strength, as determined by the combined muscle scores over succeeding years. Some functional tests also were shown to be much more stable. A 2015 Canadian study using deflazacort reported dramatic improvements in a variety of functional tests,

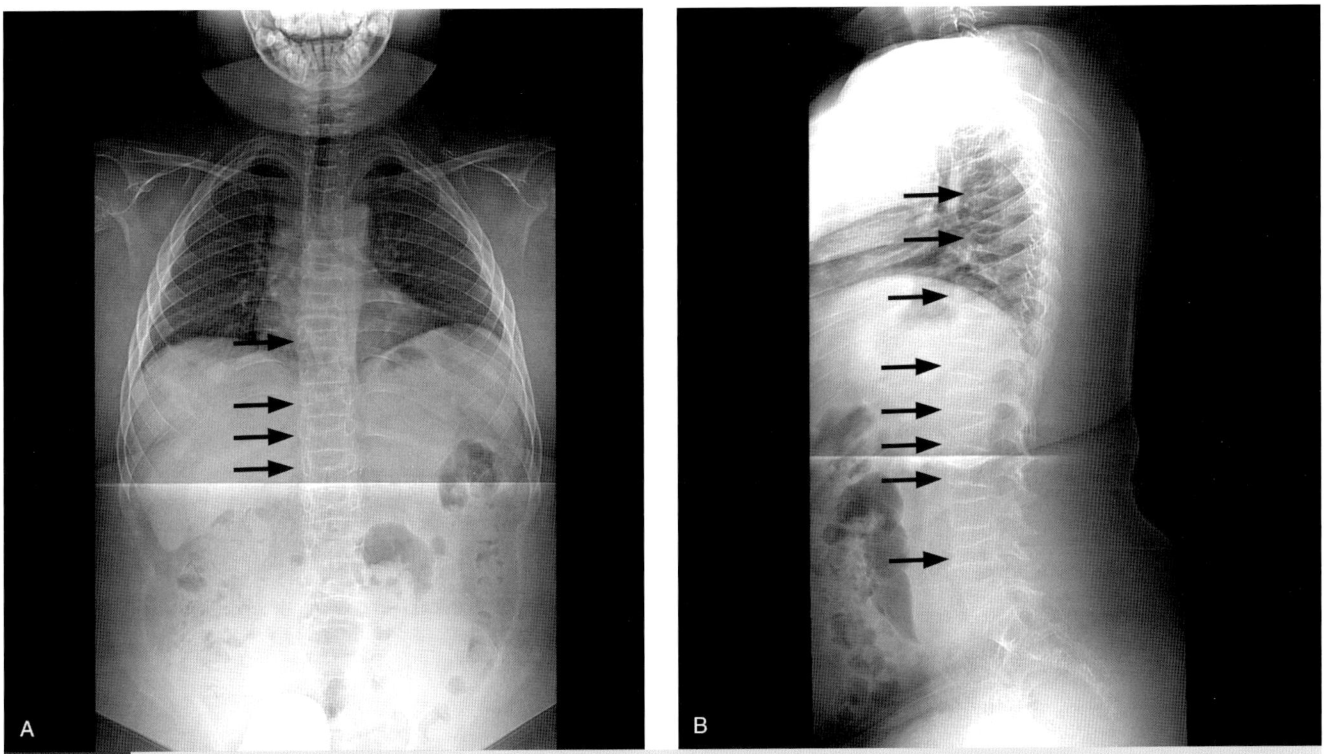

Figure 3 AP (**A**) and lateral (**B**) standing spinal radiographs of a 10-year-old boy with Duchenne muscular dystrophy who reported back pain. Multiple vertebral compression fractures can be seen (arrows). (Copyright Shriners Hospitals for Children, Portland, OR.)

including walking (at least 2 additional years longer than the expected ambulatory period), pulmonary function (at age 18 years, 80% in the group treated with deflazacort versus 33% in the group not treated with corticosteroid), longer maintenance of self-feeding, a decreased need for assisted ventilation during the daytime and nighttime, and longer survival into the fourth decade.[20] In addition, cardiac function deteriorated much less rapidly in patients taking corticosteroid therapy. A very dramatic effect of corticosteroid use is a decreased incidence in the need for spinal surgery. A 2013 Canadian study reported that 90% of untreated patients required surgery for scoliosis compared with 20% of those treated with deflazacort.[21]

Patients who do not undergo spinal fusion and who do not have scoliosis usually have a total thoracolumbar kyphosis, which, in conjunction with osteopenia, results in a high incidence of vertebral compression fractures (frequently at the thoracolumbar junction) (**Figure 3**). These fractures may be painful but are not associated with neurologic damage. In patients with substantial pain, the administration of oral bisphosphonate (off-label use of alendronate at 5 mg/day) has led to a rapid resolution of pain. This improvement occurs too rapidly to be the result of a change in bone density and may occur because of decreased bone turnover. The exact duration of bisphosphate treatment is unclear. Although it is unknown whether spinal bone density improves, femoral bone density does not improve. In a 2012 study, seven boys with DMD who had painful vertebral compression fractures were treated with intravenous pamidronate or zoledronic acid infusions.[22] Pain improved in four of the patients and completely resolved in the other three patients. The vertebral height of the affected vertebrae either remained the same or improved and lumbar spine dual-energy x-ray absorptiometry Z-scores improved, although new compression fractures occurred. Further studies are needed in this area.

Unfortunately, long-term corticosteroid use has adverse side effects[10] (**Table 2**). Corticosteroid should be continued for the patient's lifetime, even after ambulation ceases, to help preserve pulmonary, cardiac, and upper extremity functions.

Novel New Therapies Undergoing Clinical Trials

An exciting development in the treatment of DMD is the potential availability of a variety of innovative therapies that may arrest or slow disease progression with fewer side effects than corticosteroids. Some of these treatments are based on a specific gene abnormality and are applicable only to patients with that specific abnormality.

Table 2

Adverse Side Effects of Corticosteroid Use

Moon facies, as seen in Cushing syndrome, may occur.
Puberty may be delayed into late teens, including delayed development of facial and body hair.
Potential height may be lost (as much as 10 to 12 inches if medication is started at age 7).
Cataracts may develop, although treatment is rarely needed.
Substantial weight gain may occur (less weight gain with deflazacort than prednisone).
Behavioral problems may occur, including aggressive behavior toward classmates and siblings. Overt behavior problem may be less frequent with deflazacort use compared with prednisone. Depression is more prevalent with deflazacort.
Osteopenia may worsen, although this has not been definitively proven.
Vertebral compression fractures may occur when the spine is not fused because of scoliosis.
There is an increased risk of long-bone fractures.

The first broad group of potential new treatments is gene-based therapy. Antisense oligonucleotides are compounds that attach to the pre-mRNA of dystrophin and mask the deletion that interrupts the reading frame and thereby establish a normal reading frame to allow production of a truncated dystrophin. This abnormal dystrophin is produced in smaller quantities, similar to the dystrophin in patients with Becker muscular dystrophy. Because antisense oligonucleotides are specific for each deletion, these compounds are being developed for several of the most common deletions in DMD. These therapies are not intended to cure the disease, but to alleviate it and convert a Duchenne phenotype to a milder Becker phenotype. Currently, two different compounds are in phase 3 trials. Both compounds block the expression of exon 51 and allow resplicing of the pre-RNA and resumption of synthesis of a smaller dystrophin. Approximately 15% of patients with DMD have deletions that are amenable to the partial correction provided by this first antisense oligonucleotide; however, 80% of patients with deletions (who account for 65% of all patients with DMD) have deletions that are likely to be amenable to this exon-skipping approach. Clinical trials are underway for these agents.[3] Each additional exon-skipping agent will require its own clinical trial. Although data are still being analyzed, it is likely that the earlier these medications are started, the greater will be the benefits. Unfortunately, the initial trials have shown only minimal benefit, with only 1% to 2% dystrophin synthesis and small functional gains. These results may be due to the fact that treatment was not initiated until the patients were age 6 years of age or older, at which time substantial muscle damage had already occurred.

In the future, it is possible that the use of CRISPR/Cas9 technology for editing DNA may supersede the antisense oligonucleotide approach by editing the abnormal gene to yield a normal, functional dystrophin gene. This targeted genome editing technology is in the laboratory stage where it has shown success in mice with both deletions and premature termination codons.[23] Satellite cells, from which the muscle originates, also could be removed from the patient, have the normal gene inserted in vitro, and then be injected back into the patient. This approach also should immortalize the correction.

Another treatment approach is applicable to approximately 15% of DMD patients in whom the defect is the result of a single nucleotide change in the DNA, which results in an abnormal premature termination codon that stops synthesis of pre-RNA dystrophin. This partially synthesized chain is degraded, and no dystrophin is produced. There is normally a stop codon at the end of each protein sequence, but not within the protein sequence where synthesis of dystrophin is prevented. Several compounds have been developed that allow "reading through" of this stop codon, so that a minimally different dystrophin is produced. Ataluren is currently in clinical trial with 288 patients; treated patients have shown a modest benefit in their 6-minute timed walk tests compared with control subjects. This medication has been approved in some European countries but is not approved by the FDA. With a cost of approximately $400,000 to $700,000 US dollars per year, the British National Health Service has decided that the clinical benefit of the drug does not merit the cost and will not pay for the drug for patients in the United Kingdom. It should be noted that advocacy groups for patients with DMD are actively lobbying for a change in this decision.

Other Innovative Nonspecific Therapies

Other therapies may be applicable to all patients with DMD, regardless of the genetic defect. These include inhibition of myostatin, which is a normal circulating protein that inhibits muscle growth and regeneration. Myostatin is suppressed during fetal development but is expressed after birth. Inhibition of the circulating myostatin protein by antimyostatin antibodies should reduce the effect of circulating myostatin, thereby increasing muscle regeneration. A drug containing antimyostatin antibodies delayed the clinical muscle deterioration in DMD animal models and is currently in clinical trials. Facilitating a greater degree of muscle regeneration may enhance the action of other genetically based therapies because the regenerated muscle produced by those therapies is likely to be produced with genetically modified dystrophin.

CAT-1004 (Catabasis), an anti-inflammatory drug, also has been tested in animal models. This drug is alleged to have the positive anti-inflammatory effects of corticosteroid without the major adverse side effects. A clinical trial is beginning in multiple centers.

The upregulation of utrophin, a muscle protein similar to dystrophin and possibly able to substitute for dystrophin in patients with DMD, is being studied in ongoing clinical trials. A high concentration of utrophin is found in eye muscles, which are unaffected in patients with DMD. The upregulation of utrophin has produced beneficial effects in animal models.

Tadalafil is a drug that stimulates the synthesis of nitric oxide and may help increase muscle blood flow, reduce ischemia, and, in turn, diminish the muscle damage seen in DMD. A clinical trial was underway to establish the role of this treatment program in DMD, but it recently has been suspended for lack of a clinically meaningful effect.

Idebenone, a formulation of coenzyme Q, was tested in a prospective, double blind, randomized trial of 64 boys with DMD. Pulmonary function was measured to assess outcomes. In the group treated with idebenone, there was substantially less decline in pulmonary function, but no other functional measures were used.[24]

As these clinical trials are completed and analyzed, it may become clear that patients may benefit from a cocktail of several of these medications, which may have complementary effects. Treating physicians should be aware of these trials so that families who want to participate can be informed and counseled.

Spinal Muscular Atrophy

SMA is an inherited autosomal recessive disease in which there is progressive loss of the motor neurons (anterior horn cells) of the spinal cord. The loss of motor neurons results in progressive weakness and, ultimately, paralysis of the limbs and trunk and the bulbar enervated muscles (with the exception of the extraocular muscles). SMA is the most common genetic disease that causes childhood mortality. The incidence of SMA ranges from 4 per 100,000 individuals in England to 10 per 100,000 individuals in the United States and Germany. The carrier state of SMA ranges from 1 in 50 to 1 in 90 individuals, depending on the country being studied.[25] Affected patients have normal intelligence.

SMA is divided into three major subtypes (**Table 3**). The first type, known as SMA type 1 or Werdnig-Hoffman disease, has very early onset, with weakness seen at birth or before age 6 months in a child who seemed to be developing normally. These children will begin to develop skills such as rolling over but never achieve independent sitting. Acquired skills begin to be lost. Sucking ability may be deficient from birth, and feeding impairment is a predominant feature of SMA type 1. Weakness, including weakness of the muscles that support respiratory function, rapidly progresses. Death by the age of 2 years occurs in 70% of patients because of pulmonary insufficiency. Tongue fasciculations are frequently seen, which represent spontaneous activity of "sick" motor

Table 3

Characteristics of the Types of Spinal Muscular Atrophy

Type 1: Werdnig-Hoffman
Onset: 0 to 6 months of age
Absent deep tendon reflexes
Tongue fasciculations
Highest attainable function: Never able to sit independently
Life expectancy: <2 years
Death caused by pulmonary insufficiency; with newer molecular treatments, function may be preserved and lifespan increased. However, scoliosis and dislocated hips will likely develop, similar to type 2 disease.
Type 2: Intermediate (most commonly seen by orthopaedic surgeons)
Onset: 6+ months of age, with loss of previously acquired skills
Absent deep tendon reflexes
Tongue fasciculations
Highest attainable function: Sits unassisted, but no independent standing
Life expectancy: 15+ years
Death caused by pulmonary insufficiency
Scoliosis: almost universal
Dislocated hips: almost universal
Type 3: Kugelberg-Welander
Onset: After age 10 months; may not appear until teenage years
Highest attainable function: Walking more than 25 meters unassisted
Life expectancy: 25 years to normal
Scoliosis: possible
Dislocated hips: uncommon, but possible

neurons. In a natural history study, the median age at death or of respirator use greater than 16 hours per day, was 13.5 months.[26] If patients are provided with artificial ventilation via a tracheostomy, they may survive for many decades. However, full-time care will be needed because the patient will be totally paralyzed, with the exception of the eye musculature. If patients survive with full-time assisted ventilation, severe scoliosis and dislocated hips will develop in all of these patients.

SMA type 2 has an onset between 6 months and 3 years of age. Progression is less rapid than in SMA type 1, and survival is variable depending on the severity of involvement, with life expectancy between 15 and 30 years. These patients have similar orthopaedic problems as those with SMA type 1, including dislocated hips and scoliosis in all patients, usually during the first decade of life. Tongue fasciculation is seen, as is a fine tremor in the fingers. Patients with more severe disease will have marked drooping of the ribs, which results in a pear-shaped chest. Most patients breathe primarily with their diaphragm, so abdominal expansion is observed on inspiration. Scoliosis also begins in the first decade of life and frequently in the first several years of life. If untreated, scoliosis will progress to severe degrees. During the first or second decade of life, a decline in pulmonary function will require varying degrees of respiratory support; pulmonary medicine is a critical need. Feeding difficulties develop in many patients, and they may have difficulty maintaining adequate caloric intake and will require a gastrostomy tube to maintain nutrition and prevent aspiration.

SMA type 3, also known as Kugelberg-Welander syndrome, has a later onset (usually after 2 years of age), and progression is slower than in patients with SMA type 2. These patients will achieve independent standing and walking, although they may lose the ability to walk by the end of the first decade or early into the second decade of life. In patients who lose the ability to walk before skeletal maturity, scoliosis may occur and will require treatment. In addition, hip dislocation also may occur, but may not occur until the second decade of life. Hip pain is seen in some patients, particularly if hip dislocation occurs in the teen years. In patients with SMA type 3, respiratory function declines slowly and may not manifest as a problem until the second decade of life or later. Many patients have a relatively normal life span, but will become substantially disabled as adults.

Type 4 SMA (adult-onset) also exists, but it is not seen in the pediatric population.

Genetic Basis

SMA is caused by a deficiency in the SMN (survival motor neuron) protein that results from an abnormality in the *SMN1* gene (located on chromosome 5), which is responsible for producing this protein. Each parent has one mutated and nonfunctional allele of the *SMN1* gene. There are no clinical abnormalities associated with this heterozygous state; however, each child who is born to a set of parents who are carriers has a 25% chance of receiving two nonfunctional alleles and will be affected. Children with SMA have no functional SMN protein produced by the *SMN1* gene; however, a second gene, also located on chromosome 5, produces 10% to 15% of the normal amount of complete SMN protein. This *SMN2* gene has an alteration in a single base pair in exon 7, so an incomplete, nonfunctional, degraded SMN protein is produced. However, the *SMN2* gene also produces approximately 10% of the normal quantity of full-length and fully functional SMN protein. Therefore, the number of *SMN2* genes, which is variable, determines how much fully functional SMN protein is produced. The severity of the disease is determined by the number of *SMN2* genes in the patient. If there are no functional *SMN2* genes, the condition is lethal. With one or two functional *SMN2* genes present, the child will have the more severe SMA1 phenotype. However, children with four or five copies of the *SMN2* gene have a much milder form of the disease, probably SMA type 3. Although the number of gene copies of *SMN2* can be determined by genetic testing, and is relatively predictive of the type of SMA, the classification of SMA is determined not by genotyping but by assessing the child's clinical condition. The SMN protein is apparently involved in messenger and ribosomal RNA transcription and processing, and it is reduced from 5% up to 95% in patients with SMA. The defect manifests mainly in anterior horn cells, but subtle abnormalities may be present in other somatic cells.

In autosomal recessive conditions such as SMA, there is usually no family history of the disorder unless the parents share a common ancestor. In populations where consanguinity is relatively high, such as Saudi Arabia, the prevalence of SMA also will be high if there is an abnormal gene in the lineage.[27] If a common ancestor carried one copy of the abnormal gene, the chance of offspring in subsequent generations also carrying this gene will be high. If two carriers have a common ancestor from whom they both inherited the carrier state, there is a 25% chance that their child will have SMA.

Diagnosis

A diagnosis of SMA should be suspected if an infant has obvious weakness, sucking problems, and difficulty breathing at birth or if the child starts to lose acquired motor skills at any time during growth and development. Children may begin to crawl, sit, and even walk and then lose those abilities. The limbs become atrophic and, unlike DMD, calf hypertrophy is not seen.

If SMA is suspected, the child is usually referred to a child neurologist. The clinical examination will reveal weakness and the absence of deep tendon reflexes, tongue fasciculations, and finger tremors at rest, particularly in younger children. In the past, electromyography was used to provide diagnostic information, and spontaneous potentials known as fibrillation potentials and giant potentials were noted. Electromyography is no longer used as a diagnostic test in children with suspected SMA; genetic testing for the *SMN* gene deletion, which is positive in 98% of patients, is now favored. Muscle biopsy also is no longer indicated. Newborn screening is not currently performed; however, this test is likely to be added to the newborn screening panel because there now appears to be an effective treatment, which provides maximum benefit before the loss of a large percentage of anterior horn cells. If the family has one affected child, chorionic villus sampling or amniocentesis can be done in utero to detect SMA in the developing embryo. Preimplantation testing and selection of eggs fertilized in vitro also can be done, although this procedure may not be covered by insurance providers.

Orthopaedic Issues

In all patients with SMA type 1, most patients with SMA type 2, and some patients with SMA type 3, bilateral hip subluxation, which progresses to dislocation, will occur. However, hip dislocation is rarely symptomatic and no preventive interventions such as abduction bracing or surgical correction are indicated. Surgical procedures to prevent or correct the progressive dislocation usually are unsuccessful. Unlike patients who have cerebral palsy with muscle spasticity that pulls the femoral head against the pelvis, the muscles are flaccid and pain is not problematic in patients with SMA. As subluxation progresses, there is associated acetabular dysplasia. During a transitory period, a positive Barlow sign may be present and it will be possible to feel the hip going in and out of the acetabulum. This is not painful for the patient, and instability will disappear over time as the hip becomes completely dislocated. Dislocations are most frequently bilateral. In instances in which only one hip becomes dislocated, pelvic obliquity is not problematic, and, although some abduction may be lost, this is not a clinical problem.

Contractures at the hip (flexion and abduction), knee (flexion), and the foot and ankle (equinovarus) will develop in nonambulatory patients but usually do not develop in patients who are still walking. Contractures may interfere with the child's ability to stand in a standing frame. Surgical treatment of contractures is not usually indicated in children with SMA unless the contractures interfere with function. In patients with unilateral hip abduction contractures, standing is difficult. Release of the anterior part of the gluteus medius and tensor fasciae femoris from the pelvis along with sectioning of the proximal fascia lata (Ober-Yount procedure) will allow contracture relief and make standing much easier. In a child with severe hip flexion contracture that affects the ability to stand, anterior hip release may be performed to allow continued standing; tenotomies of the anterior gluteus medius, the tensor fascia femoris, the sartorius, and the direct head of the rectus femoris may be included in the surgery. Hamstring lengthening is not usually successful. An alternative approach for knee flexion deformity is an anterior distal femoral hemiepiphysiodesis, although this should be done before the deformity becomes severe, because a maximum of only 20° to 30° of correction is possible with this procedure. The development of equinovarus in a child who can stand is uncommon, particularly if prophylactic treatment with an AFO has been instituted; however, if equinovarus occurs, it can be treated with tenotomies. Tendon transfer does not seem to improve function in this patient population.

Scoliosis will develop in essentially all patients with SMA type 1 and SMA type 2 and many patients with SMA type 3, especially those who manifest substantial weakness before the early teenage years. Curves may develop before 2 years of age in SMA type 1 and SMA type 2 patients with more severe involvement. Although there have been no controlled studies in the use of spinal orthotics to slow curve progression, a progressive curve can be stabilized for a short period of time with a well-molded custom thoracolumbosacral orthosis (TLSO). This orthosis also provides sitting stability and increases comfort. The TLSO must be custom molded and provide an extremely large abdominal opening because these patients are abdominal breathers. The abdominal hole should not be covered with fabric, and the abdomen should protrude substantially through the opening. Consultation with the orthotist who is fabricating the TLSO is recommended because the belly hole must extend laterally at least to the anterior axillary line (**Figure 4**). The TLSO may compromise the patient's ability to eat, even with a large belly hole, and may need to be loosened during feedings. In general, the TLSO should be worn whenever the patient is sitting; however, the wearing schedule should be adjusted based on the patient's tolerance for the device, and wearing time can be gradually increased. If there is concern about the effect of the TLSO on respiration, vital capacity can be assessed in and out of the orthosis by a therapist with a handheld spirometer.

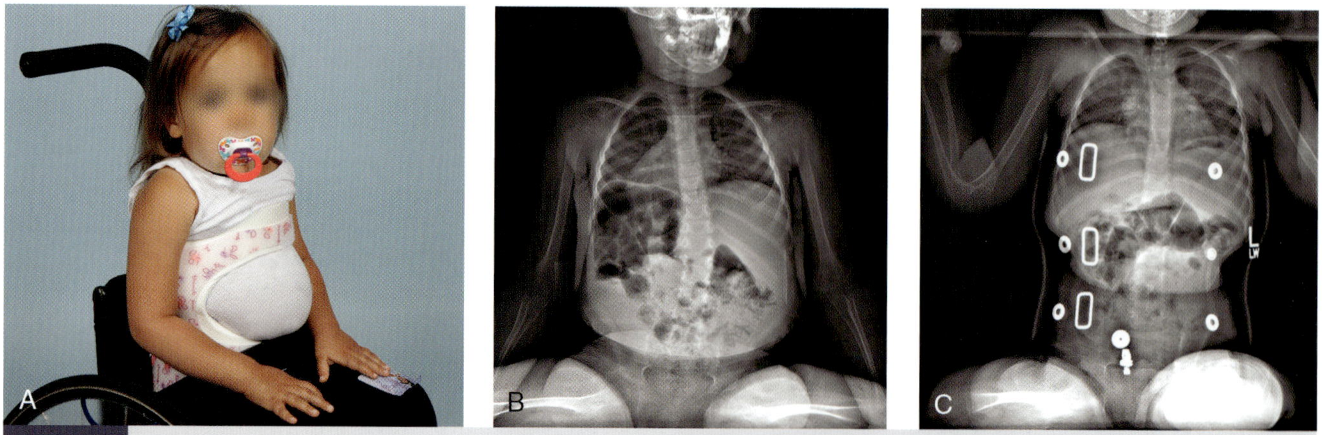

Figure 4 **A,** Photograph of a 2-year-old girl with spinal muscular atrophy wearing a thoracolumbosacral orthosis. The abdomen should be allowed to protrude through abdominal opening in the orthosis to reduce abdominal compression. **B,** Radiograph of the girl's spine prior to bracing shows a Cobb angle of 30°. **C,** Radiograph after 6 months of brace treatment shows no curvature. (Copyright Shriners Hospitals for Children, Portland, OR.)

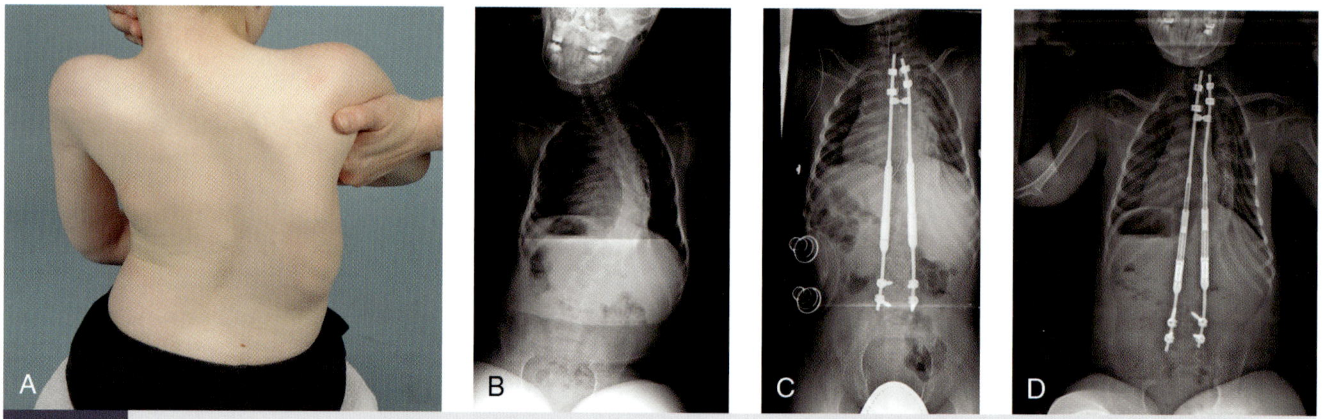

Figure 5 Images of a patient with spinal muscular atrophy and scoliosis. **A,** Clinical photograph of the child's spine before surgery. **B,** Preoperative radiograph shows a 70° Cobb angle. **C,** Radiograph immediately after the surgical insertion of a MAGEC rod shows a Cobb angle of 43°. **D,** Radiograph at the 18-month follow-up shows a Cobb angle of 40°. (Courtesy of Charles R. D'Amato, MD, Portland, OR and copyright Shriners Hospitals for Children, Portland, OR.)

Surgical treatment of a spinal deformity is indicated when the curves can no longer be controlled by the TLSO and exceed 50°. Because patients may be osteopenic and have very small bones, the size of instrumentation is a consideration. In the past, growing rods and the Vertical Expandable Prosthetic Titanium Rib (VEPTR; DePuy Synthes) have been used, but the MAGEC system (Ellipse Technologies), which can be extended without the need for subsequent surgeries, is currently preferred. The MAGEC rods are extended in an outpatient clinic by placing an external controller over the rod; incremental extension is produced through a magnetic signal (**Figure 5**).

Physical and Occupational Therapy and Adaptive Equipment

As the disease progresses, there is a concomitant process of normal growth and development and organization of motor skills as the child ages, which is modified by progressive muscle weakness. Because these two processes occur simultaneously, the progression of the disease will eventually overcome the developmental acquisition of motor skills, and function will begin to decline. Children who are more severely affected may have difficulty sitting and maintaining head support, so having an appropriate adaptive seat with a headrest is beneficial for environment interaction and feeding. Although a seating device will not prevent scoliosis, lateral pad stabilizers help keep the trunk and head centered and allow for better function. A powered wheelchair should be provided for nonambulatory children by the age of 2 years to allow independent mobility. As children age, special controls may be needed for their wheelchairs, depending on the child's level of weakness. Wheelchairs should be equipped with a tilt-in-space function and an attachment for a tablet or computer for schoolwork and/or communication.

For patients who are unable to stand independently, standing devices that control the lower extremities and trunk may provide supported standing. Standing has psychological and physical benefits, particularly in younger children with SMA who have reasonable trunk control. Many standing devices are not easily adaptable to small-size children and will not be able to support the lower extremities. A one-piece custom-molded KAFO with no knee articulation may make it easier for a patient to be placed in the standing position. If reasonable knee stability can be obtained without a KAFO, a custom-molded rigid AFO will also facilitate the ability to stand. Regardless of the child's ambulatory status, as soon as Achilles tightness (<10° of dorsiflexion) begins to develop, custom AFOs should be provided and used full time to slow the progression of equinovarus deformity.

Strength training may be useful in patients with SMA, and resistance strength training has been shown to improve strength and motor function in children with SMA type 2 and SMA type 3.[28] As in other pediatric disabling conditions, adaptive recreation is very important to the well-being of affected children because most of these patients do not have recreational and social outlets. Some patients with SMA seem to enjoy swimming because it allows movement and limb use.

Other Systemic Problems

Cardiac problems are not associated with SMA, and patients have normal intelligence. Eating becomes difficult because of chewing and swallowing problems. In patients with advanced disease, maintaining an adequate caloric intake may be problematic, so a gastrostomy may be necessary. However, it can be difficult to ascertain if patients are actually undernourished. The standard body mass index is not relevant in these patients because of diminished muscle mass and the high percentage of adipose tissue in the limbs.

Occasionally, patients may experience a metabolic crisis with tachycardia and hypotension after a mild systemic illness or if they become dehydrated. If the patient has metabolic acidosis and hypoglycemia, a rapid intervention with rehydration and correction of hypoglycemia and acidosis should be done in a hospital to allow careful monitoring. As this problem is prone to recurrence, arrangements should be made to allow rapid hospitalization when early symptoms occur. It has been suggested that the reduced muscle mass in these patients may be a contributing factor.[25] Gastrostomy may be indicated to prevent dehydration and allow rapid home hydration when indicated.

Pulmonary function is a major issue as muscle weakness progresses. Patients should be followed by a pediatric pulmonary specialist on a regular basis, including sleep studies when indicated. Bilevel positive airway pressure support during sleep will eventually be indicated. When pulmonary function begins to decline, patients should be provided with a CoughAssist device, which should be used on a regular basis (and even more often at the first sign of a respiratory infection). As respiratory function declines, assisted ventilation via a face mask may be required for portions of the day as well as at night, and this will eventually lead to full-time assisted ventilation. In late stages of the disease, a tracheostomy for full-time ventilator support may be chosen by the patient and family, although this is a difficult decision because the patient at this point is very disabled and requires full-time care.

Medical Treatment

As in DMD, exciting and innovative developments are occurring in the field of medical therapy for SMA. One therapy uses an antisense oligonucleotide that eliminates the abnormal sequence that causes skipping of exon 7 in the *SMN2* gene, thereby allowing the *SMN2* gene to synthesize a full-length SMN protein. In recent clinical trials of infants with SMA type 1 younger than 1 year treated with this therapy, maintenance of motor function and development of motor milestones have been achieved. Based on the natural history of the disease, untreated patients would be expected to deteriorate quite rapidly. Multiple studies of this therapy are ongoing, including a study of presymptomatic infants with genetically confirmed SMA. Intrathecal injection of the medication with the antisense oligonucleotide attached to a ligand allows it to be taken into the anterior horn cell. Increased circulating levels of SMN protein have been reported in this trial.

A second treatment approach inserts a full-length *SMN1* gene using a nontoxic adeno-associated viral vector. This treatment is administered intravenously on only one occasion and does not require intrathecal injection. Infants treated within a short time of disease onset have shown almost complete resolution of weakness and reestablishment of close to normal development.[29] In the small series of children who have been treated, it has been noted that the earlier treatment is instituted after a diagnosis of SMA, the more effective the therapy has been. These developments are very exciting and, if proven effective, will likely lead to newborn genetic screening for SMA so that treatment can be started early, before neurons are lost.

Positive results also have been reported in animal studies using the enzyme CRISPR-Cas9, which can alter the DNA of experimental animals who manifest the genetic

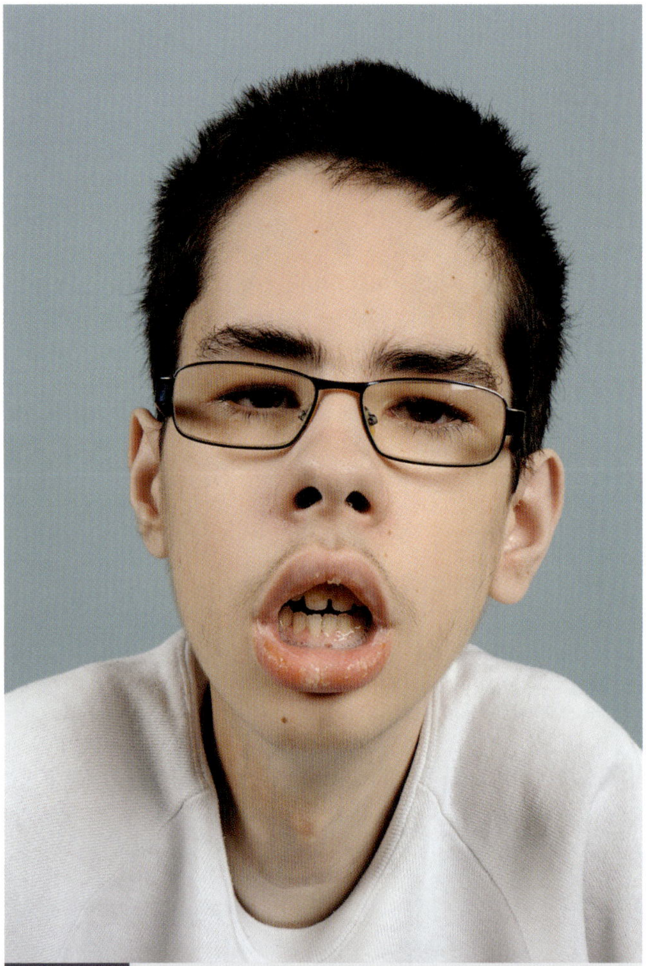

Figure 6 Clinical photograph of a patient with congenital myotonic dystrophy shows the typical facial appearance with a head that is elongated and narrowed in the coronal plane and a tented upper lip. (Copyright Shriners Hospitals for Children, Portland, OR.)

defect of SMA. The earlier after birth the therapy is initiated, the more likely is a positive response. In one study, mice with a severe form of SMA who were expected to die within 2 weeks have survived for more than 1 year and have exhibited few deficits.

An entirely different treatment approach, which does not address gene function, is the administration of a compound known as olesoxime. This compound is alleged to have neuroprotective properties that improve mitochondrial function. In a clinical trial, which is now in phase 3, there are indications that olesoxime slows the deterioration of muscle function. The compound has not yet been approved by the FDA. No peer-reviewed publications are currently available concerning any of these treatments.[30]

Congenital Myotonic Dystrophy

Myotonic dystrophy is a muscle disease that causes weakness, primarily distally, and is associated with myotonia, which is the inability of muscles to relax after a strong contraction (particularly in the hands). The milder adult-onset form of this disease is the most prevalent progressive neuromuscular disease in adults. A severe form of the disease, known as congenital myotonic dystrophy, has an incidence of 2 individuals per 100,000 live births. Newborn infants exhibit weakness, which may be profound; however, improvement occurs in the first year of life but is followed by a slow loss of strength during the teenage years. Congenital myotonic dystrophy is also characterized by cognitive impairment, potentially lethal cardiac issues, and a very typical facial appearance (**Figure 6**).

Congenital myotonic dystrophy is classified as type I or type II based on the underlying genetic defect. Because type I myotonic dystrophy accounts for 95% of the patients with the disease, this chapter will focus on type I disease.

Genetics

Congenital myotonic dystrophy is inherited in an autosomal dominant fashion and has some interesting genetic characteristics. When the male parent is affected, the child usually has the same degree of disease severity as the father. However, when the mother is affected, even with mild unrecognized disease, the child may be severely affected and require immediate, full-time ventilator support. The disease is caused by an expansion of a CTG trinucleotide sequence on chromosome 9 near the *MPK* gene, and the severity of disease is proportional to the number of trinucleotide repeat sequences, which increase during oogenesis but not spermatogenesis.

The classification is based on the clinical picture, and the limits are approximate. This trinucleotide insertion results in the synthesis of an elongated and toxic messenger RNA that accumulates in the cells. The normal *MPK* gene alters the function of RNA-binding proteins. Other adjacent genes also may be affected, which explains the early onset of cataracts seen in this disease.[31]

Natural History and Orthopaedic Treatment

Newborns with congenital myotonic dystrophy may have profound weakness and require intubation and full-time ventilator support to survive. However, during the first few months of life, infants gain strength and are usually able to be weaned from the ventilator by the time they are a few weeks to a few months old. Over the next few years, generalized muscle strength increases, and most affected children become strong enough to stand and walk by age 5 years (at the latest) if foot deformities are not present. Some children are strong enough to stand but are unable to stand independently because of contracture of the Achilles tendon or fully developed talipes equinovarus. These deformities should be surgically corrected to achieve a plantigrade foot to facilitate standing and walking. After surgery, patients should begin standing in short leg casts on the first postoperative day. This cast treatment is continued for 4 weeks, then followed by the use of a custom-molded AFO, which will be needed for standing and walking. If a patient develops sufficient strength and balance, the AFOs may be discontinued; however, the AFO should be worn at nighttime to prevent contracture recurrence.

In a study of 30 children and adolescents with congenital myotonic dystrophy treated at the Muscular Dystrophy Association Clinic at the Shriners Hospital for Children (Portland, Oregon), the mean age of ambulation was 30 months and the latest age was 5 years, with the exception of 1 of the 30 patients who was unable to walk.[32] Seventy percent of the patients (22 of 30) required orthopaedic surgery during the study period. Ten patients had one surgical procedure, eight patients had two surgical procedures, and four patients had three or more surgical procedures. These procedures involved the lower extremities and spine; no upper extremity surgery was indicated. None of the patients had hip subluxation, dislocation, or fixed adduction; however, two patients had unilateral abduction contractures that interfered with standing and walking. These patients had a good response to abductor release consisting of an Ober-Yount bipolar release of the tensor fascia femoris, wherein the anterior portion of the gluteus medius and the tensor fascia femoris were released and stripped from the iliac crest. In addition, tenotomy of the proximal iliotibial band in the upper thigh just below the insertion of the tensor fascia femoris muscle was performed. One patient had knee flexion contracture, which was treated by distal femoral extension osteotomy. Five patients had congenital clubfoot, and all of these patients underwent surgery before referral to the clinic. None of the patients were treated with the Ponseti method; however, this would be the currently preferred method. Five patients had Achilles tendon lengthening only. Most of these patients were unable to stand independently or walk before the lengthening procedure, but rapidly gained ambulation skills after the procedure. Other surgeries included rotational osteotomies of the tibia or femur, subtalar arthrodesis for severe planovalgus deformity, and correction of miscellaneous toe deformities.

Spinal deformities, including midthoracic to upper thoracic kyphosis and scoliosis, occurred in approximately 30% of patients and frequently were seen in the first decade of life.[32] Spinal bracing was attempted in most of the patients, but it is not clear that bracing was helpful, although it may have slowed curve progression. Surgical correction was done in three patients in this series and can be done safely and successfully. The guidelines for kyphosis surgery have not been well established. Some patients seem to tolerate the kyphosis well during childhood and adolescence, but stand with excessive cervical lordosis to maintain an upright head.[32] A more recent study reported similar findings.[33]

Gross motor skills and strength continue to improve over the first decade of life. However, toward the end of the second decade of life, hand weakness and myotonia begin to develop.

Other Systemic Issues

Cognitive delay occurs in most patients and generally parallels the severity of the motor impairment, which is secondary to the severity of the genetic defect. Patients also have a typical myopathic facial appearance, with the head elongated and narrowed in the coronal plane and a tented upper lip (**Figure 6**). Because the facial appearance is so characteristic of the disease, a diagnosis can be strongly suspected based only on facial appearance. The speech of these patients also has a very nasal character.

Even with mild involvement, patients have a high sensitivity to opiates and may experience excessive and prolonged sedation, including profound respiratory depression, after administration. Opiates should be avoided or used sparingly. If administered, close monitoring of the patient is required. In some patients with mild degrees of involvement, a diagnosis of congenital myotonic dystrophy is made only after a surgical procedure in which opiates are administered. These patients may require full-time ventilator assistance for several days.

Cardiac involvement includes arrhythmia or conduction disturbances, which can progress to ventricular fibrillation that leads to sudden death in a substantial number of affected individuals. Cardiac problems usually are seen beginning in the third decade of life and thereafter. Arrhythmia can be assessed with 24-hour Holter monitoring. Simple electrocardiography and echo examinations are insufficient for assessing arrhythmia. Cardiac arrhythmia also may occur in parents with milder degrees of involvement, so parents should be counseled to have their cardiac status assessed on a regular basis. If evidence of rhythm problems is found, insertion of a demand pacemaker reduces the risk of sudden cardiac death. Hypertrophic cardiomyopathy also may be a problem.[34]

Feeding may be a problem, particularly in infants, who may require a gastrostomy; however, most patients acquire the ability to eat and graduate to oral feeding. Constipation remains a lifetime problem because of bowel dysmotility. Other systemic problems include cataracts, premature male-pattern baldness, insulin resistance, hypersomnolence, and sterility in males.[35]

In a study of 150 parents of children with congenital myotonic dystrophy who were surveyed regarding the biggest issues for their children, the most frequently reported symptomatic themes were issues of communication (82%) and problems with the hands and fingers (80%). Other important issues involved fatigue (77%), cardiac disorders (24%), and anesthesia-associated problems (24%).[36]

Medical Treatment

Because congenital myotonic dystrophy is caused by an elongated trinucleotide segment known as DMPK, it potentially should be amenable to treatment with antisense oligonucleotides such as those being investigated in patients with DMD and SMA. Current clinical trials are underway for a drug called Ionis-dmpk.2.5$_{Rx}$ (Ionis Pharmaceuticals). The drug is injected subcutaneously on a weekly basis, and results are reported to be encouraging, although no specific data have yet been published.

Charcot-Marie-Tooth Disease

CMT is a group of more than 40 hereditary motor-sensory neuropathies, which are distinguished by different underlying gene defects and clinical manifestations. As in most neuropathies, there is initial distal weakness, which manifests as foot deformity caused by muscle imbalance and weakness and often contracture of the hands. In addition, an increased incidence of both scoliosis and hip dysplasia has been associated with CMT. Except in patients with unusually severe involvement, independent ambulation continues into adulthood; however, treatment may be needed to prevent the development of severe foot deformities that could affect the ability to ambulate. Deep tendon reflexes are frequently diminished or absent. Patients also may have sensory deficits, including a proprioceptive deficit leading to a positive Romberg test. Some patients may experience dysesthesia, particularly in the feet, and this condition may be exacerbated after foot surgery. Other abnormalities, such as optic atrophy and hearing loss, may accompany the primary condition and may help distinguish the specific genetic subtype.

Classification and Diagnosis

CMT is separated into four broad groups on the basis of motor nerve electrodiagnostic studies, inheritance pattern, and the specific genetic mutation.[37] In general, the diagnostic strategy should be to classify the condition based on the inheritance pattern and electrodiagnostic studies and then focus in on the specific genetic mutations for testing. Panels to identify the gene abnormality are being developed for multiple categories of CMT and will aid in making a diagnosis. However, genetic testing may be expensive and not covered by insurance providers. Nerve biopsy is not indicated for diagnosing this condition. Identification of the specific type of CMT disease is important for determining a prognosis, potential interventions, associated problems, and accurate genetic counseling. Identification of the specific gene abnormality will become essential when gene-based therapies are developed.

CMT type 1 disease is comprised of five subtypes (1A through 1E), all of which are autosomal dominant and characterized by decreased motor and sensory nerve conduction velocity (>50 m/s). The basis of the disease in CMT type 1 is demyelination of nerve axons. Large myelinated sensory nerves are also affected, which may explain the symptoms of pain and dysesthesia in some patients. Seventy percent of all patients with CMT disease have CMT type 1 disease, and 70% of those patients have type 1A.

CMT type 2 disease is autosomal dominant and includes 18 subtypes. CMT type 2 is distinguished by normal or slightly slowed motor nerve conduction velocity and a substantial decrease in the amplitude of the compound motor action potential. This type of CMT disease is caused by neuronal/axonal abnormalities.

CMT type X is the X-linked form of the disease, and CMT type X1 accounts for 10% of the overall cases of CMT. In this form, which is also called intermediate-type CMT, there is mild slowing of the motor nerve conduction.

CMT type 4 includes 11 autosomal recessive forms, some of which are associated with severe generalized involvement that results in loss of ambulation in the first or second decade of life.

Orthopaedic Treatment

CMT type 1A is the type of CMT disease most frequently seen by pediatric orthopaedic surgeons because the onset of foot deformity usually occurs in the early to middle part of the second decade of life. CMT type 1A accounts for approximately 50% of all patients with the diagnosis of CMT disease. The genetic defect in this type of CMT is a complete duplication of *PMP* gene on chromosome 22; an accurate genetic test is available. Because it has not been demonstrated that genetic confirmation will influence treatment, genetic testing is usually not covered by insurance providers. Some variability exists in the expressivity and severity of progression even within families, presumably resulting from the modification of the basic abnormality by other genes. Hand weakness, which begins with an intrinsic minus pattern, may occur, but it usually is not clinically important until the third decade of life. An occupational therapist may provide adaptive devices, such as pencil grips, special utensils, and computer devices to facilitate schoolwork. Voice-recognition software for dictation also may be indicated for some patients with more severe hand involvement.

The major musculoskeletal deformity associated with CMT type 1A in the teenage years is foot deformity. In the first decade of life patients may have flexible, flat feet. Subsequently, cavus posturing of the foot develops and progresses to a cavovarus deformity. Manual muscle testing demonstrates weakness of eversion as the first finding, which may precede the development of the cavovarus deformity.

Cavus deformity can be radiographically measured on standing lateral radiographs of the feet by measuring the Meary angle, which is the angle between the longitudinal axis of the talus and the first metatarsal. This measurement may be difficult to obtain in some patients because the first metatarsal may be difficult to distinguish, but generally it is the shortest and broadest of the metatarsals. In milder deformities, the Meary angle is probably reasonably accurate, but in feet with more severe deformity a great deal of variation in measurements of the Meary angle may occur depending on whether the x-ray beam is aligned perpendicular to the midfoot or perpendicular to the hindfoot. In some instance, two lateral views (one aligned to the midfoot and one aligned to the hindfoot) should be obtained to allow better assessment of the deformity. The calcaneal pitch also is increased in patients with CMT type 1A. Although the foot clinically appears to be in equinus, radiographs will demonstrate that the foot is not in equinus. The appearance of equinus when looking at the foot is actually a manifestation of the cavus deformity, with flexion of the midfoot on the hindfoot with associated dorsiflexion of the calcaneus, which is seen radiographically as increase calcaneal pitch. The Achilles tendon is actually elongated, so it is important not to confuse this cavus with equinus, because lengthening of the Achilles tendon will potentially aggravate the deformity and weaken the triceps surae.[38] As the disease progresses, hindfoot varus increases, and clinical evidence of excessive weight bearing can be seen on the lateral side of the midfoot and forefoot. Callosities develop at the head of the first metatarsal and the base of the fifth metatarsal, with a prominence at the base of the fifth metatarsal. The tripod position of the foot can be appreciated clinically with callus under the first and fifth metatarsal heads.

Although the deformities are initially dynamic and relatively flexible, over time they become relatively fixed and not passively correctable. Flexibility can be assessed by evaluating subtalar motion with the patient prone and the hip and the knee flexed to 90° so that the hindfoot varus can be observed. In addition, the Coleman block test can be performed with the patient standing on a block, such as the type used to clinically assess limb-length discrepancy. The patient stands on a block that is placed under the heel and second through fifth rays, leaving the first metatarsal head "floating" off the block. If the foot is still flexible, the heel, which was previously in varus, will come to neutral or even slight valgus.

Studies of foot pressure (pedobarographs) using a dynamic foot pressure measurement system are helpful in monitoring the progression of the foot deformity and will show increasing pressure at the fifth metatarsal head and base as the disease progresses. Manual muscle testing will show weak peroneal muscles, whereas the posterior tibial, toe flexors, extensors, and anterior tibial tendons maintain good strength. Although the literature has suggested that the tibialis anterior muscle is weak, this assumption may be incorrect, because testing for active dorsiflexion often indicates a strong anterior tibial tendon by palpation during active dorsiflexion. As a manifestation of this weakness, and probably in an effort to overcome the equinus positioning of the forefoot, the toe extensors are often overactive during gait, causing the toes to dorsiflex during swing phase to assist in foot clearance. This has the effect of tightening the plantar fascia, which is contiguous with the fascia of the toes, and this tightness further increases the cavus deformity. Toe dorsiflexion during initiation of the swing phase is an early sign of CMT disease.

Treatment

When the Meary angle is greater than 20° and the clinical examination and foot pressure show palpable plantar fascia tightness and cavus, a plantar fascia release, with stripping of the plantar muscles from the calcaneus (Steindler stripping), can be performed. This is done through an incision on the plantar-medial aspect of the foot at the proximal end of the arch. The skin and fibrofatty tissue are incised down to the fascia, which is then exposed by sweeping attached tissue off the thick fascia with a Cobb elevator; the plantar fascia is then completely incised from lateral to medial. The short plantar muscles are then teased off the calcaneus with the Cobb elevator, taking care to stay superficial to the deep fascia to avoid injury to the lateral plantar branch of the posterior tibial nerve. Postoperatively, the patient is allowed full weight bearing in a walking cast for 3 weeks; this is followed by nightly wear of AFOs. The AFO should be molded with the foot at 90° of dorsiflexion; amounts greater than 90° should not be attempted because this could lead

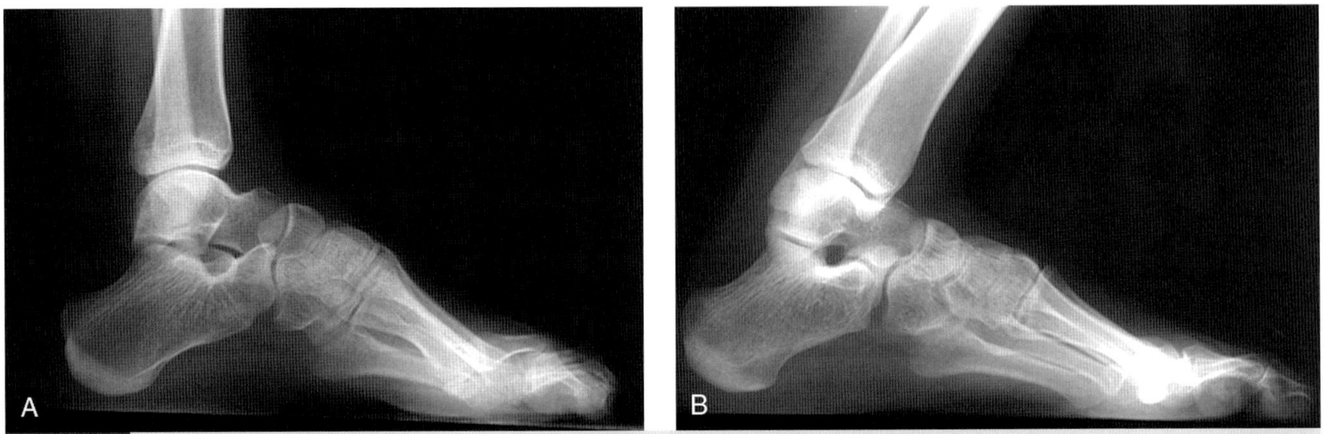

Figure 7 Lateral radiographs of the foot of a patient with type 1 Charcot-Marie-Tooth disease prior to surgery (**A**) and after a plantar fasciotomy, demonstrating a reduction in the Meary angle (**B**). (Copyright Shriners Hospitals for Children, Portland, OR.)

to discomfort and rejection of the AFO. This approach appears to reduce cavus and slow the progression of the deformity (**Figure 7**).

The deformity, however, will ultimately recur and progress. When this occurs and the heel is clearly in varus but is still passively correctable to or past neutral, a number of procedures are used for rebalancing the muscles. Some surgeons prefer to perform the following procedures at a single setting, followed by 6 weeks in a non–weight-bearing short leg cast, and then followed by use of a posterior leaf spring AFO. (1) The tibialis anterior tendon is transferred to the lateral cuneiform. The tendon is released from its insertion on the navicular, preserving as much length as possible; brought up to the extensor retinaculum, which may be released 1 to 2 cm; then tunneled subcutaneously to its new location on the lateral cuneiform; and then fixed into the bone with moderate tension using an interference screw. (2) The toe extensors II through V are transferred as a bundle to the lateral cuneiform using an interference screw for tendon fixation. (3) The tibialis posterior tendon is transferred through the interosseous membrane to the lateral cuneiform using an interference screw for tendon fixation.[39] Once the posterior tibial tendon is detached, the increased mobility of the foot out of varus can be appreciated. If a large amount of varus is present, the tendon will not be long enough to attach into the bone. In these instances, 2 to 3 cm of length can be added by creating a distally based flap of tendon and taking half of the tendon and folding it down. If the tendon is taken off the navicular at the level of the bone, the distal end of the tendon will have a fibrocartilaginous structure; therefore, a distally placed flap of half of the tendon will tend not to separate from the body of the tendon. A suture placed through both sides of the tendon flap will help reinforce and secure it. (4) In addition, a Jones transfer of the extensor hallucis longus to the first metatarsal neck through a drill hole in the metatarsal neck is performed and the tendon is sewn back onto itself.[40] (5) If a Jones transfer is performed, the interphalangeal joint of the great toe should be fused because when the long toe extensor is removed from its insertion on the distal phalanx and transferred to the metatarsal neck, the interphalangeal joint of the great toe will go into flexion. However, in a skeletally immature patient, the surgeon may not want to fuse the interphalangeal joint and instead can perform a tenodesis of the stump of the extensor hallucis longus to the extensor hallucis brevis.[41] (6) If the heel remains in varus after these procedures are performed, a medial slide of the calcaneal tuberosity with screw fixation can be added.[41] (7) If residual cavus exists, a dorsal closing wedge osteotomy of the first metatarsal also can be performed.[40] (8) Transfer of the peroneus longus into the peroneus brevis can be performed to remove the deforming force on the first ray to reduce cavus and supplement the weak eversion strength[40] (**Figure 8**). (9) Plantar fascia release also should be included as part of these reconstruction procedures if it has not been done previously.

The extensor digitorum communis and posterior tibial and anterior tibial transfers should all be inserted into the lateral cuneiform because of its central location in the foot. If the transfer were to be attached into the cuboid, too great of a pronating force may be exerted, and a pronated flatfoot will occur over time. After the surgery, an AFO should be molded and a short leg, non–weight-bearing cast should be worn for 6 weeks. After healing and cast removal, patients should be fitted with a posterior leaf spring AFO. This type of AFO will stabilize the foot and allow some dorsiflexion during the second rocker phase of stance gait. As the disease progresses,

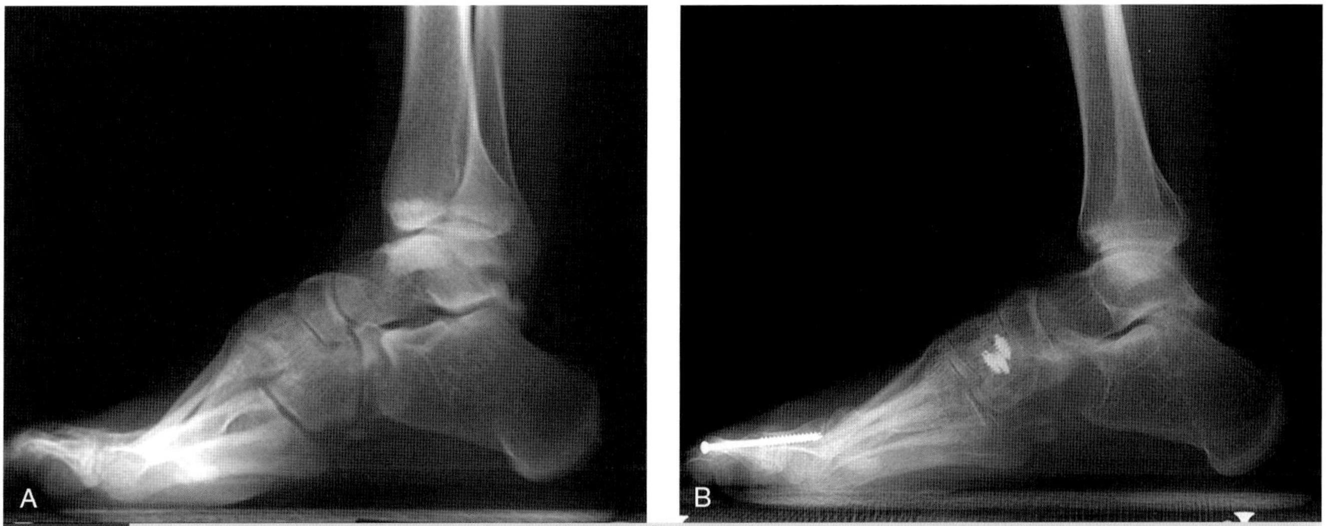

Figure 8 Lateral radiographs of the foot of a 17.5-year-old patient with type 1 Charcot-Marie-Tooth disease prior to surgery (**A**) and after multiple tendon transfers (**B**) as described in this chapter. (Copyright Shriners Hospitals for Children, Portland, OR.)

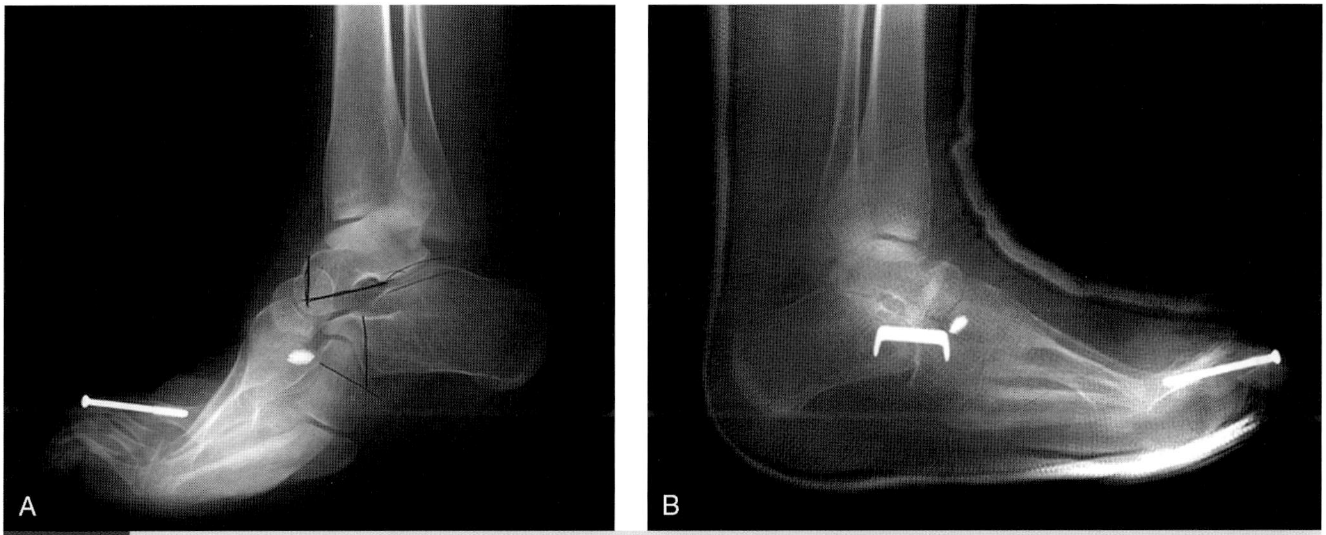

Figure 9 **A,** Lateral radiograph of the foot of a patient with Charcot-Marie-Tooth disease with incomplete correction after tendon transfers. **B,** Lateral radiograph of the foot after a Lambrinudi triple arthrodesis. (Copyright Shriners Hospitals for Children, Portland, OR.)

the transfers will weaken, and the patient will require an AFO to control footdrop and medial-lateral instability; however, deformity should not recur because the transfers were placed centrally (so as the foot weakens there is no muscle imbalance).

In almost all patients with CMT type 1A, the Achilles tendon should not be lengthened, because it is elongated rather than shortened, and lengthening will cause weakness and increase the calcaneal pitch. In rare instances of true equinus, in which equinus of the hindfoot can be radiographically documented, the Achilles tendon should be lengthened.

If the foot deformity is rigid and not passively correctable after release of the posterior tibial tendon, the transfers will be unable to correct the deformity and a Lambrinudi-type triple arthrodesis will be needed to achieve a plantigrade foot (**Figure 9**).

Because patients with CMT have protective sensation, pressure sores rarely develop, but a thick callus may develop over pressure points. A molded sole insert can be used to redistribute pressure more evenly. If the foot is plantigrade, most patients will continue to ambulate well into middle age. After middle age, more generalized weakness may develop and the need for assisted mobility will progress. In patients with proprioceptive deficits, an AFO will provide stability.

Although CMT type 2 disease is heterogeneous, general cavovarus does not develop and hand weakness is more prominent. Frequently, patients will have generalized weakness of all the muscles controlling the foot and ankle, resulting in a flail but plantigrade foot or flatfoot. These patients will benefit from a posterior leaf spring AFO to control footdrop in swing and provide stability in stance. Some subtypes of CMT type 2 disease are associated with severe proprioceptive sensory loss. Affected patients may lose the ability to walk in their second decade of life, but the use of an AFO may be helpful.

Scoliosis in CMT Disease

Scoliosis may occur in many types of CMT disease. In a study of 298 patients with CMT disease, scoliosis was radiographically identified in 45 patients.[42] In this study, CMT type 1 was the most prevalent type of disease. In the patients with scoliosis, 18 were females and 27 were males, which is a reversal of the sex ratio seen in idiopathic scoliosis in which more females than males are affected. Twenty-nine of 47 curves were thoracic and 50% of those were left thoracic curves, which also is unusual. Forty-nine percent of the curvatures were associated with increased kyphosis. During the term of the study, curve progression occurred in 70% of the patients. Bracing was attempted in 16 patients, but appeared to be successful in only 3 patients. In this group of patients, 14 had posterior spinal instrumentation and fusion without complications. Although intraoperative somatosensory-evoked potential monitoring was attempted in 12 patients, adequate signals were obtained only in 3 patients. Although the age of scoliosis onset was not defined, it is clear that all patients with CMT should have a yearly clinical assessment for scoliosis until skeletal maturity, and radiographic studies should be obtained when indicated. Scoliosis is particularly common in patients with CMT type 4C.[37]

Hip Dysplasia in CMT Disease

Patients with CMT disease are predisposed to the development of acetabular dysplasia with hip subluxation at a much higher rate than the unaffected population. This may lead to degenerative arthritis in adulthood. Dysplasia tends to be severe, with coxa valga and acetabular dysplasia associated with increased acetabular anteversion, which leads to decreased acetabular containment (**Figure 10**). In a study of 74 patients with CMT, hip radiographs showed hip dysplasia in 6 patients (8%).[43] The age of onset of the dysplasia is unclear. Hip dysplasia during childhood and adolescence is generally asymptomatic. Because symptoms do not manifest until degenerative arthritis develops later in life, AP pelvic radiographs for surveillance should be obtained for all patients with CMT. Radiographs should be obtained at the time of the CMT diagnosis and every several years thereafter until skeletal maturity. When acetabular dysplasia is severe, surgical correction is needed. Surgical correction of the acetabulum and the proximal femur may be required. Good coverage was reported in a group of patients treated with Bernese periacetabular osteotomy.[44]

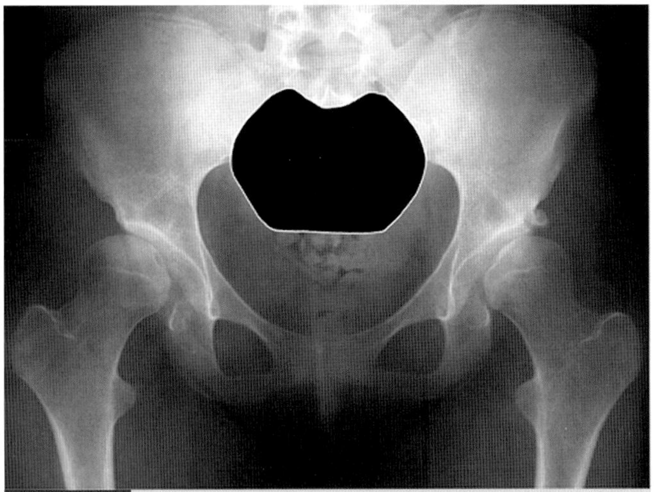

Figure 10 Radiograph of the pelvis of a 13-year-old girl with type 1A Charcot-Marie-Tooth disease shows bilateral hip dysplasia. (Copyright Shriners Hospitals for Children, Portland, OR.)

Summary

Children affected by any of the progressive neuromuscular diseases of childhood and adolescence will benefit from care by an orthopaedic surgeon as part of the multidisciplinary team. A predictable set of orthopaedic deformities is associated with each of the neuromuscular diseases. The treatment of these conditions, which all have a genetic basis, is advancing rapidly. It is hoped that new treatments will ameliorate or eliminate the deterioration associated with these diseases in the future.

Key Study Points

- Orthopaedic surgeons should be part of the multidisciplinary clinic team involved in the care of patients with progressive neuromuscular disorders. They can help to control deformities (primarily in the lower extremities and spine) with bracing and surgery, when indicated.
- Most of the neuromuscular diseases of childhood associated with weakness are the result of genetic mutations; however, in some instances, the disease may not manifest until later in life. The genetic mutations allows for precise diagnosis by genetically based studies using blood or cheek swabs through DNA analysis.
- The orthopaedic surgeon should be aware of the early clinical signs of DMD to make an early diagnosis, which will allow proper genetic counselling for the family. In addition, this will allow early institution of pharmacologic treatment as newer treatments become available.
- In patients with DMD, progressive weakness, functional loss, and deformity can be delayed, and the need for scoliosis surgery can be dramatically reduced, by the pharmacologic daily administration of corticosteroid.
- New treatments for DMD, SMA, and congenital myotonic dystrophy are being developed based on the specific genetic defect. These treatments are promising, and some are currently in clinical trials.

Annotated References

1. Bello L, Kesari A, Gordish-Dressman H, et al; Cooperative International Neuromuscular Research Group Investigators: Genetic modifiers of ambulation in the Cooperative International Neuromuscular Research Group Duchenne Natural History Study. *Ann Neurol* 2015;77(4):684-696.

   This important study demonstrated the modification of the clinical course of patients with DMD who possess mutations in two other genes—*LTBT4* (which makes the disease milder) and *SPP1* (which makes the disease more severe). In addition, the authors reported resistance to corticosteroid therapy in Hispanic and South Asian patients. Level of evidence: III.

2. Vieira NM, Elvers I, Alexander MS, et al: Jagged 1 rescues the Duchenne muscular dystrophy phenotype. *Cell* 2015;163(5):1204-1213.

   The authors describe the naturally occurring mutations in a cohort of golden retriever dogs carrying the gene for DMD in whom the expected clinical deterioration of the disease was not manifested. The dogs possessed a mutation in the *Jagged1* gene. Level of evidence: III.

3. Aartsma-Rus A, Fokkema I, Verschuuren J, et al: Theoretic applicability of antisense-mediated exon skipping for Duchenne muscular dystrophy mutations. *Hum Mutat* 2009;30(3):293-299.

4. Marshall PD, Galasko CS: No improvement in delay in diagnosis of Duchenne muscular dystrophy. *Lancet* 1995;345(8949):590-591.

5. Posselt H: The Duchenne timeline. Available at: https://www.youtube.com/watch?v=KA8W5UfE4ts&feature=youtu.be. Posted May 2010. Accessed May 9, 2016.

6. Heberer K, Fowler E, Staudt L, et al: Hip kinetics during gait are clinically meaningful outcomes in young boys with Duchenne muscular dystrophy. *Gait Posture* 2016;48:159-164.

   Gait laboratory study demonstrated the early loss of hip extensor moment and power, which was normalized after administration of corticosteroid. Level of evidence: I.

7. Alexander WM, Smith M, Freeman BJ, Sutherland LM, Kennedy JD, Cundy PJ: The effect of posterior spinal fusion on respiratory function in Duchenne muscular dystrophy. *Eur Spine J* 2013;22(2):411-416.

   The authors report that stabilization of the scoliosis in patients with DMD did not change the rate of respiratory decline based on a comparison with a contemporaneous group who did not undergo surgical correction.

8. Duboc D, Meune C, Pierre B, et al: Perindopril preventive treatment on mortality in Duchenne muscular dystrophy: 10 years' follow-up. *Am Heart J* 2007;154(3):596-602.

9. Proske U, Morgan DL: Muscle damage from eccentric exercise: Mechanism, mechanical signs, adaptation and clinical applications. *J Physiol* 2001;537(Pt 2):333-345.

10. Sienko S, Buckon C, Fowler E, et al: Prednisone and deflazacort in Duchenne muscular dystrophy: Do they play a different role in child behavior and perceived quality of life? PLOS Currents Muscular Dystrophy. Available at: http://currents.plos.org/md/article/prednisone-and-deflazacort-in-duchenne-muscular-dystrophy-do-they-play-a-different-role-in-child-behavior-and-perceived-quality-of-life/. Accessed June 19, 2016.

    An assessment using standardized behavior measures of boys with DMD and their families showed an increase in aggressive behavior in patients taking prednisone and an increase in depression in those taking deflazacort. Level of evidence: I.

11. Roberto R, Fritz A, Hagar Y, et al: The natural history of cardiac and pulmonary function decline in patients with Duchenne muscular dystrophy. *Spine (Phila Pa 1976)* 2011;36(15):E1009-E1017.

The authors report on cardiac and pulmonary functional decline in a group of patients with DMD. Level of evidence: III.

12. Chua K, Tan CY, Chen Z, et al: Long-term follow-up of pulmonary function and scoliosis in patients with Duchenne's muscular dystrophy and spinal muscular atrophy. *J Pediatr Orthop* 2016;36(1):63-69.

    The authors reported a substantial decline in the loss of pulmonary function in patients with DMD and in those with SMA after spinal fusion.

13. Takaso M, Nakazawa T, Imura T, et al: Surgical management of severe scoliosis with high risk pulmonary dysfunction in Duchenne muscular dystrophy: Patient function, quality of life and satisfaction. *Int Orthop* 2010;34(5):695-702.

14. Cheuk DK, Wong V, Wraige E, Baxter P, Cole A: Surgery for scoliosis in Duchenne muscular dystrophy. *Cochrane Database Syst Rev* 2015;10:CD005375.

    The authors of this systematic review of scoliosis surgery in patients with DMD were unable to reach a conclusion because of the absence of level I studies.

15. Bushby K, Finkel R, Birnkrant DJ, et al; DMD Care Considerations Working Group: Diagnosis and management of Duchenne muscular dystrophy: Part 2. Implementation of multidisciplinary care. *Lancet Neurol* 2010;9(2):177-189.

16. Suk KS, Baek JH, Park JO, et al: Postoperative quality of life in patients with progressive neuromuscular scoliosis and their parents. *Spine J* 2015;15(3):446-453.

    A questionnaire was used to assess the quality of life of patients with progressive neuromuscular disease after scoliosis surgery. The authors concluded that there was a substantial benefit after surgery. Level of evidence: III.

17. King WM, Ruttencutter R, Nagaraja HN, et al: Orthopedic outcomes of long-term daily corticosteroid treatment in Duchenne muscular dystrophy. *Neurology* 2007;68(19):1607-1613.

18. Hayes J, Veyckemans F, Bissonnette B: Duchenne muscular dystrophy: An old anesthesia problem revisited. *Paediatr Anaesth* 2008;18(2):100-106.

19. Bushby K, Finkel R, Birnkrant DJ, et al; DMD Care Considerations Working Group: Diagnosis and management of Duchenne muscular dystrophy: Part 1. Diagnosis, and pharmacological and psychosocial management. *Lancet Neurol* 2010;9(1):77-93.

20. Bello L, Gordish-Dressman H, Morgenroth LP, et al; CINRG Investigators: Prednisone/prednisolone and deflazacort regimens in the CINRG Duchenne Natural History Study. *Neurology* 2015;85(12):1048-1055.

    This randomized controlled trial of prednisone/prednisolone and deflazacort showed that deflazacort had greater efficacy in maintaining function in patients with DMD. Level of evidence: I.

21. Lebel DE, Corston JA, McAdam LC, Biggar WD, Alman BA: Glucocorticoid treatment for the prevention of scoliosis in children with Duchenne muscular dystrophy: Long-term follow-up. *J Bone Joint Surg Am* 2013;95(12):1057-1061.

    A review of the incidence of scoliosis in patients with DMD treated with deflazacort from a single center showed a dramatic reduction in the development of scoliosis in boys taking deflazacort compared with those not taking a corticosteroid. Level of evidence: III.

22. Sbrocchi AM, Rauch F, Jacob P, et al: The use of intravenous bisphosphonate therapy to treat vertebral fractures due to osteoporosis among boys with Duchenne muscular dystrophy. *Osteoporos Int* 2012;23(11):2703-2711.

    The authors review the clinical response of boys with DMD and vertebral compression fractures to bisphosphonate therapy for treatment of painful vertebral compression fractures. Level of evidence: IV.

23. Ousterout DG, Kabadi AM, Thakore PI, Majoros WH, Reddy TE, Gersbach CA: Multiplex CRISPR/Cas9-based genome editing for correction of dystrophin mutations that cause Duchenne muscular dystrophy. *Nat Commun* 2015;6:6244.

    The authors discuss an experimental study of the use of the CRISPR/Cas 9 approach to correction of the dystrophin defect in an animal model of DMD.

24. Buyse GM, Voit T, Schara U, et al; DELOS Study Group: Efficacy of idebenone on respiratory function in patients with Duchenne muscular dystrophy not using glucocorticoids (DELOS): A double-blind randomised placebo-controlled phase 3 trial. *Lancet* 2015;385(9979):1748-1757.

    This study compared the effect of idebenone versus a placebo on respiratory function in patients with DMD. The authors reported that idebenone reduced the loss of respiratory function. Level of evidence: I.

25. Prior TW, Russman BS: Spinal muscular atrophy, in Pagon RA, Adam MP, Ardinger HH, et al, eds: *Gene Reviews*. Seattle, WA, 1993.

26. Finkel RS, McDermott MP, Kaufmann P, et al: Observational study of spinal muscular atrophy type I and implications for clinical trials. *Neurology* 2014;83(9):810-817.

    The authors provide a careful assessment of clinical deterioration in patients with SMA type 1. Level of evidence: IV.

27. Al-Jumah M, Majumdar R, Al-Rajeh S, et al: Molecular analysis of the spinal muscular atrophy and neuronal apoptosis inhibitory protein genes in Saudi patients with spinal muscular atrophy. *Saudi Med J* 2003;24(10):1052-1054.

28. Lewelt A, Krosschell KJ, Stoddard GJ, et al: Resistance strength training exercise in children with spinal muscular atrophy. *Muscle Nerve* 2015;52(4):559-567.

The authors report on the response of patients with SMA to resistance strength training. Trends in improved motor function and strength were seen. Level of evidence: I.

29. Mendell JR: Gene therapy studies show promise for pediatric patients with fatal disorders, in Redefining Pediatric Health Care: Nationwide Children's Hospital 2013-2014 Annual Report, 2015, p. 26. Available at: http://www.nationwidechildrens.org/annual-report/neurology-neurosurgery.html. Accessed May 16, 2016.

    The author briefly describes the dramatic response of infants with SMA type 1 to viral transfer of *SMN1* gene.

30. Wertz MH, Sahin M: Developing therapies for spinal muscular atrophy. *Ann N Y Acad Sci* 2016;1366(1):5-19.

    Reviews of various genetically based approaches to treat patients with SMA are presented.

31. Ho G, Cardamone M, Farrar M: Congenital and childhood myotonic dystrophy: Current aspects of disease and future directions. *World J Clin Pediatr* 2015;4(4):66-80.

    The authors provide a thorough review of all aspects of congenital myotonic dystrophy.

32. Canavese F, Sussman MD: Orthopaedic manifestations of congenital myotonic dystrophy during childhood and adolescence. *J Pediatr Orthop* 2009;29(2):208-213.

33. Schilling L, Forst R, Forst J, Fujak A: Orthopaedic disorders in myotonic dystrophy type 1: Descriptive clinical study of 21 patients. *BMC Musculoskelet Disord* 2013;14:338.

    The authors review musculoskeletal disorders in patients with congenital myotonic dystrophy from a single clinic. Level of evidence: IV.

34. Lau JK, Sy RW, Corbett A, Kritharides L: Myotonic dystrophy and the heart: A systematic review of evaluation and management. *Int J Cardiol* 2015;184:600-608.

    A review of generally accepted approaches to the evaluation and management of cardiac problems in patients with myotonic dystrophy is presented.

35. Campbell C: Congenital myotonic dystrophy. *J Neurol Neurophysiol* 2012. Available at: http://www.omicsonline.org/congenital-myotonic-dystrophy-2155-9562.S7-001.pdf. Accessed June 17, 2016.

    The author presents a comprehensive review of congenital myotonic dystrophy, including genetics, natural history, and clinical management.

36. Johnson NE, Ekstrom AB, Campbell C, et al: Parent-reported multi-national study of the impact of congenital and childhood onset myotonic dystrophy. *Dev Med Child Neurol* 2015.

    The authors report on the overall effect of congenital myotonic dystrophy on children and their families. Level of evidence: IV.

37. Harel T, Lupski JR: Charcot-Marie-Tooth disease and pathways to molecular based therapies. *Clin Genet* 2014;86(5):422-431.

    A thorough and clear review of all of the subtypes of CMT is presented.

38. Aktas S, Sussman MD: The radiological analysis of pes cavus deformity in Charcot Marie Tooth disease. *J Pediatr Orthop B* 2000;9(2):137-140.

39. Williams PF: Restoration of muscle balance of the foot by transfer of the tibialis posterior. *J Bone Joint Surg Br* 1976;58(2):217-219.

40. Ward CM, Dolan LA, Bennett DL, Morcuende JA, Cooper RR: Long-term results of reconstruction for treatment of a flexible cavovarus foot in Charcot-Marie-Tooth disease. *J Bone Joint Surg Am* 2008;90(12):2631-2642.

41. Hansen ST Jr: *Functional Reconstruction of the Foot and Ankle*. Philadelphia, PA, Lippincott Williams and Wilkins, 2000.

42. Karol LA, Elerson E: Scoliosis in patients with Charcot-Marie-Tooth disease. *J Bone Joint Surg Am* 2007;89(7):1504-1510.

43. Walker JL, Nelson KR, Heavilon JA, et al: Hip abnormalities in children with Charcot-Marie-Tooth disease. *J Pediatr Orthop* 1994;14(1):54-59.

44. Novais EN, Kim YJ, Carry PM, Millis MB: Periacetabular osteotomy redirects the acetabulum and improves pain in Charcot-Marie-Tooth hip dysplasia with higher complications compared with developmental dysplasia of the hip. *J Pediatr Orthop* 2015.

    The outcomes of patients with hip dysplasia caused by CMT disease and treated with Bernese osteotomy with and without femoral osteotomy are discussed. Level of evidence: IV.

Chapter 16

Arthritis

Robert Sheets, MD Johanna Chang, MD Suhas Radhakrishna, MD

Abstract

Arthritis in children encompasses a wide variety of diseases. Reactive arthritis can include arthritis that lasts less than 6 weeks and includes transient arthritis, poststreptococcal arthritis, and Lyme disease arthritis. Chronic arthritis includes various subtypes of juvenile idiopathic arthritis and the arthritis that can be associated with a wide variety of vasculitic diseases. In addition, chronic recurrent multifocal osteomyelitis can mimic bacterial osteomyelitis and a bone tumor. Consultation with a pediatric rheumatologist early in a child's disease course can be helpful in making a diagnosis.

Keywords: chronic recurrent multifocal osteomyelitis (CRMO); enthesitis-related arthritis; juvenile arthritis; Lyme disease arthritis; poststreptococcal arthritis; psoriatic arthritis; reactive arthritis; transient synovitis

Introduction

An orthopaedic surgeon often is the first specialist consulted to evaluate a child with persistent but nontraumatic joint pain. Although many such children will have benign conditions, it is essential to consider juvenile arthritis and other systemic rheumatic diseases that occur along with arthritis in the differential diagnosis.

It is important to be familiar with juvenile arthritis and its subtypes, including details about how these disorders are treated. Information about reactive arthritis, which includes transient synovitis; poststreptococcal arthritis; Lyme disease arthritis; chronic recurrent multifocal osteomyelitis (CRMO); and the arthritis that accompanies granulomatosis with polyangiitis, Kawasaki disease, Henoch-Schönlein purpura, sarcoidosis, and Behçet syndrome, is presented. Key points are the emphasis on a broad differential diagnosis of joint pain and swelling along with an understanding of how these diseases can mimic septic arthritis, osteomyelitis, and benign and malignant diseases of both blood and bone.

None of the following authors or any immediate family member has received anything of value from or has stock or stock options held in a commercial company or institution related directly or indirectly to the subject of this chapter: Dr. Sheets, Dr. Chang, and Dr. Radhakrishna.

Juvenile Arthritis

Juvenile arthritis is a diagnosis of exclusion based on the patient's history, physical examination, and supportive laboratory and imaging results. An understanding of the subtypes of juvenile arthritis enables timely referral to a pediatric rheumatologist for definitive evaluation and early treatment. The classification nomenclature for the subtypes of juvenile arthritis is based on specific patterns of joint involvement, laboratory prognostic markers, and systemic features such as the presence of a psoriatic rash or inflammatory bowel disease.[1] Fortunately, with the advent of early treatment strategies using targeted biologic medications, long-term outcomes have improved greatly, and the need for surgical intervention is far less than in previous generations.[2]

Immune-mediated arthritis is defined by the presence of chronic synovial inflammation in the absence of another etiology, such as infection. Immune-mediated arthritis is clinically manifested by swelling, mild warmth, pain, and decreased range of movement. Joint swelling must be continuously present for a minimum of 6 weeks in the same joint. Synovitis of shorter duration is considered viral or postinfectious (reactive) until the 6-week threshold is reached. Erythema is unusual and suggests infection or malignancy. The degree of pain can vary; most patients have more stiffness than pain. Joint pain alone—in the absence of other inflammatory signs—is defined as arthralgia, not arthritis. Imaging, such as ultrasound or MRI, may be required to demonstrate synovitis in equivocal cases.[3,4]

Because pathognomonic laboratory tests or clinical findings do not exist for juvenile arthritis, it is imperative to exclude all other etiologies before establishing the diagnosis. Joint swelling has a broad differential diagnosis, including injury, infection, malignancy, a foreign body, hemophilia, and rare entities such as pigmented villonodular synovitis. Pathologies in close proximity to the joint space, such as osteomyelitis, bone lesions, hemangiomas, and arteriovenous malformations, may be mistaken for joint swelling. Joint pain without swelling has a more extensive differential diagnosis, including other entities such as benign limb pain of childhood, known colloquially as "growing pains"; benign joint hypermobility; pes planus; osteochondroses; amplified pain syndrome; and genetic disorders of both connective tissue and metabolism.

History

Several historical clues point toward arthritis. The gel phenomenon of morning and cold-induced stiffness is typical. Synovial fluid becomes more viscous with rest and cold and more fluid with movement and warmth. Parents often will notice a limp present in the morning when their child first arises or after naps. Conversely, a noninflammatory etiology is characterized by intermittent pain with activity and is primarily present in the evening and relieved by rest. Red flag symptoms prompting a broad workup for malignancy or infection include awakening from sleep because of pain, weight loss, fever, and pain disproportionate to any clinical findings.

Physical Examination

The physical examination should entail a brief but comprehensive assessment of range of motion, swelling, pain with motion, and tenderness in all joints. Special attention should be given to the neck's range of motion, the temporomandibular joint (assessed by opening the mouth), and the proximal interphalangeal (PIP) joints. Asking a patient to flex the PIP joints while keeping the metacarpophalangeal joints in extension (allowing the fingertips to touch the palm) is a quick assessment of PIP joint range of motion. Sometimes indirect observation is most helpful. Observation of gait as well as a child's movement on the examination table and in the room is essential. Younger children may be assessed through play or reaching for toys. Children may have had long-standing arthritis, which could be missed without a thorough examination.

Laboratory Tests

Laboratory tests cannot be used to diagnose or rule out arthritis. They are used mainly as supportive data and to exclude other etiologies. Inflammatory markers may be normal, especially in arthritis affecting only a few joints. Highly elevated inflammatory markers with minimal arthritis suggest another etiology. Rheumatoid factor (RF) and antinuclear antibody screening tests are not helpful because these substances are present in only a minority of patients with juvenile arthritis and have low specificity. These tests may be obtained in patients with known arthritis, and the RF may be helpful in polyarticular disease because a high titer suggests a poor prognosis. Antinuclear antibodies can be helpful in screening for systemic lupus erythematosus. An antistreptolysin O titer (blood test) may be useful for screening for poststreptococcal disease. Human leukocyte antigen B27 may be helpful in defining spondyloarthritis. The history and physical examination, rather than laboratory tests, are the main criteria for making a diagnosis of juvenile arthritis.[5,6]

Imaging

Imaging helps establish the presence of synovitis. At the time of the initial clinical visit, radiographs often lack the sensitivity to detect a joint effusion, but they can be helpful in excluding other etiologies. Radiographs in early arthritis typically show only periarticular osteopenia. In advanced arthritis, radiographs can delineate the extent of joint space narrowing, advancement of bone age, erosions, subluxation, and ankylosis (fusion).

MRI is the preferred imaging modality for defining synovitis, with intravenous contrast used to demonstrate synovial hyperemia. Noncontrast MRI with a high T2 signal still can be diagnostic.[3,4] Early arthritis is characterized on MRI by joint effusion, synovial proliferation, and enhancement; later disease is characterized by cartilage thinning and joint erosions (**Figure 1**).

Ultrasonography is emerging as an excellent modality for joint assessment.[3,4] Imaging also is used to monitor radiographic disease progression across time, which may occur even in clinically quiet disease.

Epidemiology

The incidence of juvenile arthritis is approximately 5 to 10 per 100,000 children. In general, it is more common in Caucasian children than in ethnic minorities, and it is seen in girls more often than in boys.[7] The etiology is multifactorial, with genetic contributions from immune genes, particularly in antigen presentation and cytokine pathways, and still undefined environmental and hormonal influences.

Treatment

The prompt diagnosis of juvenile arthritis enables the pediatric rheumatologist to institute aggressive therapy aimed at achieving early clinical remission. Long-term outcomes are greatly improved by using anti-tumor necrosis factor (anti-TNF) and other biologic medications.[2] However, if arthritis remains active, long-term sequelae include joint contracture, muscular atrophy, bone overgrowth, limb-length discrepancy, subluxation, micrognathia, short stature, and loss of function. Both physical and occupational therapy are vital adjunctive services in the management of these complications. Orthopaedic reconstructive surgery is warranted in patients with advanced arthritis if medical therapy has been unsuccessful. Such procedures include total joint arthroplasty, synovectomy, arthrodesis, and soft-tissue release.

Subtypes of Juvenile Arthritis

The nomenclature for juvenile arthritis continues to evolve. The 1977 American College of Rheumatology criteria defined three forms of juvenile rheumatoid arthritis: systemic, polyarticular, and pauciarticular. The classification used most commonly today is the 2001 International League of Associations for Rheumatology criteria,[1] which has seven subtypes of juvenile idiopathic arthritis (JIA), including oligoarticular JIA, polyarticular JIA (RF positive or negative), psoriatic arthritis, enthesitis-related arthritis, systemic juvenile idiopathic arthritis (sJIA), and undifferentiated arthritis. All subtypes are characterized by the presence of arthritis in one or more joints of at least 6 weeks' duration in a child younger than 16 years in the absence of another etiology. The exception is sJIA, which is diagnosed based on fever, rashes, and a marked systemic inflammatory response rather than the duration or pattern of arthritis.

Oligoarticular JIA is typically diagnosed in toddlers, who have fewer than five involved joints during the first 6 months after diagnosis. These children are generally afebrile, well appearing, and have large lower limb joint effusions of insidious onset. Distinctive features of other subtypes will develop in many children as they age. Uveitis, or ocular inflammation, is clinically silent and may lead to irreversible vision loss in up to 30% of these children, necessitating close monitoring by an ophthalmologist. However, oligoarticular JIA can occur in older children. The maximum age of definition of onset of JIA is 16 years.

Psoriatic arthritis can appear either oligoarticularly or polyarticularly and with or without psoriasis. However, a substantial family history of psoriasis exists in the families of children in whom psoriatic arthritis eventually develops. Blepharitis and nail pits as well as changes of the nails (that is, onycholysis) are common findings with psoriatic arthritis.[8]

Two categories for polyarticular JIA have been defined based on the involvement of five or more joints and the presence or absence of RF. The joint pattern is typically symmetric, often involving small joints, such as the metacarpophalangeal and PIP joints, the cervical spine, and the temporomandibular joint. RF-negative polyarticular JIA is typical in preschool children, whereas RF-positive polyarticular JIA more often is seen in adolescents. A positive RF indicates a higher likelihood of erosive arthritis. Cyclic citrullinated peptide antibodies are likely to replace RF because these are more specific for arthritis. Adolescents with arthritis should be evaluated for other systemic diseases, such as systemic lupus erythematosus.

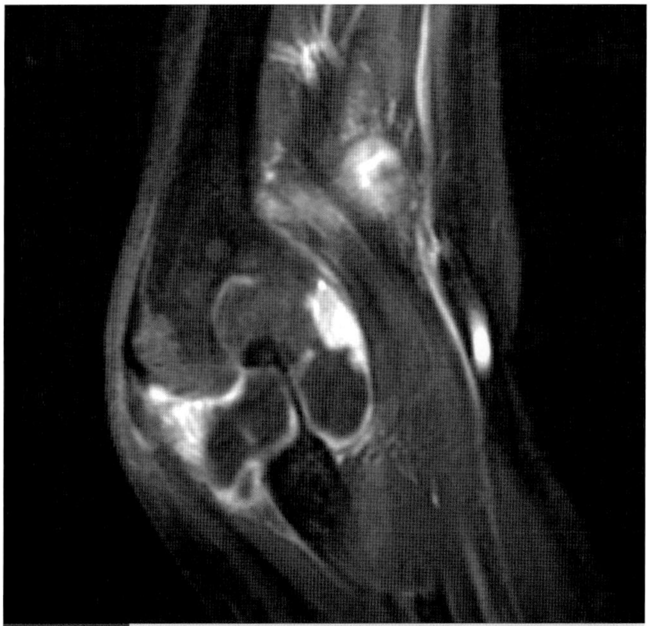

Figure 1 MRI shows oligoarticular juvenile idiopathic arthritis of the right elbow.

Although the term spondyloarthropathy was not defined in the juvenile arthritis criteria, it still is used clinically to refer to a constellation of disease manifestations that tend to be associated with arthritis involving the sacroiliac joints and the vertebrae. These manifestations include inflammatory bowel disease, acute symptomatic anterior uveitis, psoriasis, and enthesitis (inflammation at the insertion point of tendons). In the International League of Associations for Rheumatology criteria, juvenile psoriatic arthritis and enthesitis-related arthritis are separate entities.

Undifferentiated arthritis encompasses arthritis that has overlapping criteria or is not well defined in other criteria, such as arthritis associated with inflammatory bowel disease and juvenile ankylosing spondylitis. In the International League of Associations for Rheumatology criteria, enthesitis-related arthritis is the preferred designation for patients who previously may have been deemed to have juvenile spondyloarthritis and who now have enthesitis. This designation draws attention to the fact that the earliest manifestation for many children is enthesitis, particularly of the Achilles insertion point on the calcaneus. Enthesitis-related arthritis should be considered in children with Sever disease that is not responding to nonsurgical therapy. Most children with juvenile ankylosing spondylitis have enthesitis and thus are classified as having enthesitis-related arthritis. In the International League of Associations for Rheumatology criteria, psoriatic arthritis is distinguished from enthesitis-related arthritis based on a family history of psoriasis, dactylitis, or nail pitting.[9] Given the hereditary pattern of psoriasis and inflammatory bowel disease, knowledge of the family history is important when evaluating a child with arthritis.

Although sJIA is a subtype of JIA, its clinical and immunologic features suggest that it may, in fact, be part of a different disease spectrum. Many rheumatologists consider sJIA part of the autoinflammatory disorders that include familial Mediterranean fever and cryopyrin-associated periodic syndromes.[10,11]

Unlike other forms of JIA, patients with sJIA typically have a high fever accompanied by rash, with laboratory testing showing elevated inflammatory markers. Diagnosis requires the presence of arthritis for a minimum of 2 weeks and quotidian fevers for at least 3 days accompanied by at least one of the following: an evanescent, nonfixed, erythematous rash; generalized lymphadenopathy; hepatomegaly or splenomegaly; or serositis.[12] Although patients with sJIA often have symmetric, polyarticular arthritis, some children may not exhibit arthritis until later in the disease course.

The incidence of sJIA is 4% to 17% in patients with JIA and accounts for 5% to 10% of cases in the United States and Europe.[11] Although no peak onset has been established, children aged 1 to 5 years are the most frequently affected. Males and females are affected equally. Forty percent of patients with sJIA have a monophasic disease course characterized by variable disease severity and duration, and 50% of patients have disease that is refractory to treatment, with persistent inflammation and arthritis. The remaining 10% of patients have a polycyclic course with episodes of inflammation alternating with disease remission. A life-threatening complication known as macrophage activation syndrome, also known as secondary hemophagocytic lymphohistiocytosis, develops in approximately 10% of children with sJIA. Possible triggers for macrophage activation syndrome include viral illness and the addition of or a change in medication. Clinically, patients appear severely ill and have a persistent fever accompanied by rash, hepatosplenomegaly, lymphadenopathy, liver failure, and neurologic changes. Laboratory testing shows disproportionately low acute phase reactants, cytopenia, elevated ferritin (≥500 μg/L), coagulopathy, elevated liver enzymes, hypofibrinogenemia, and hypertriglyceridemia. A bone marrow biopsy can show phagocytosis of other hematopoietic cells by macrophages or histiocytes.[12,13]

The overall prognosis depends on the disease type and response to drug therapy, although sJIA often is considered the most severe of all JIA subtypes and has a reported disease-related mortality rate ranging from 0.5% to 1%.[11] Treatment-related adverse effects account for a substantial part of disease morbidity. Chronic steroid use results in Cushing syndrome, decreased bone health, and increased risk of infection.

Therapeutic Management of JIA

The main objectives for the treatment of JIA are pain relief, disease control, and the prevention of damage and disability. Because a standardized approach to the treatment of the various subtypes of juvenile arthritis is lacking, rheumatologists are working to establish evidence-based guidelines for the medical management of JIA. The Childhood Arthritis and Rheumatology Research Alliance recently published consensus treatment plans for new-onset polyarticular JIA and sJIA.[13,14] The medications described in these consensus treatment plans as well as other medications used in the treatment of JIA are discussed in this section.

NSAIDs, such as ibuprofen and naproxen, are arguably considered first-line therapy, but the development of more effective medications has limited the use of NSAID monotherapy to no more than 2 months in patients who have persistently active arthritis.[15] Aspirin is generally not used. The average time to symptomatic improvement from an NSAID is 1 month; however, 25% of children do not demonstrate clinical improvement until 8 to 12 weeks have passed. NSAIDs are well tolerated, with the most common adverse effects being abdominal pain and anorexia. Patients experiencing substantial gastritis can benefit from using antacids, histamine-2 blockers, or proton pump inhibitors or from switching to a cyclooxygenase-2 inhibitor. A complete blood count, liver enzyme levels, and serum creatinine levels should be checked before or soon after the initiation of routine NSAID use, with repeat laboratory testing every 6 months for long-term daily use.[15]

Intra-articular steroid injections provide quick symptomatic relief while waiting for systemic medications to take effect and can be done with or without additional therapy in patients, especially those with monoarticular or oligoarticular arthritis. However, one study described weak evidence for decreased clinical symptoms of arthritis in patients who had received intra-articular steroid injections in a lower limb.[16] Although intra-articular steroid injections are rarely curative, rapid pain relief can encourage normal activity and prevent the formation of joint contractures.[12,17] Triamcinolone hexacetonide has been shown to be more effective than triamcinolone acetonide and is the recommended glucocorticoid for use in joint injections. Clinical improvement for at least 4 months is expected, and intra-articular steroid injections can be repeated as needed.[15]

Disease-modifying antirheumatic drugs (DMARDs), a large category that includes methotrexate (MTX), sulfasalazine, leflunomide, azathioprine, cyclosporine, and hydroxychloroquine, are steroid-sparing medications that have been shown to reduce joint damage. These medications are immunosuppressants. MTX, a folic acid analog and inhibitor of enzymes in the folate pathway that leads to anti-inflammatory effects, is the most commonly prescribed DMARD for JIA. MTX can be given either orally or subcutaneously; some studies have shown increased bioavailability of the subcutaneous pathway compared with oral MTX at higher doses. MTX is felt to be an efficacious and safe medication that has been used effectively since the beginning of the practice of pediatric rheumatology.[18] Concomitant use of daily folic acid helps decrease the frequency and severity of MTX adverse effects, including oral ulcers, decreased appetite, and nausea. A complete blood count with differential, hepatic enzyme levels, and serum creatinine level is recommended to be checked before initiation, approximately 1 month after initiation, and then every 3 to 4 months in patients with stable doses and normal prior laboratory results.[15]

Sulfasalazine is another DMARD that previously was used frequently to treat JIA. It is an analogue of 5-aminosalicylic acid linked to sulfapyridine and is both antibacterial and anti-inflammatory. However, current guidelines support its use in only enthesitis-related arthritis, not in other JIA subtypes.[15] Sulfasalazine may trigger macrophage activation syndrome in patients with sJIA and has been shown to cause increased toxicity in adult-onset Still disease.[2,18]

Leflunomide inhibits pyrimidine synthesis and may have similar effects as MTX. It often is used as an alternative medication for patients who cannot tolerate MTX. Cyclosporine is more frequently used in patients with sJIA and features of macrophage activation syndrome.

The main risk associated with using DMARDs is the increased risk of infection. In addition, patients treated with DMARDs should have various laboratory tests checked at monthly intervals. Many DMARDs, including MTX, leflunomide, and sulfasalazine, have bone marrow–suppressing effects. These medications also may have gastrointestinal adverse effects. In particular, sulfasalazine has been reported to have complications that are more serious, such as Stevens-Johnson syndrome.[19]

If substantial synovitis or other signs of active disease persist despite the addition of nonbiologic DMARDs, many rheumatologists consider additional treatment with biologic agents. This relatively new category of medications includes TNF inhibitors, interleukin (IL)-1 inhibitors, tocilizumab, abatacept, rituximab, ustekinumab, and tofacitinib. Only a few of these medications are approved by the FDA for the treatment of JIA, but many are used off-label in patients with refractory JIA.

The TNF cytokine has been implicated in the inflammatory cascade leading to the development of JIA. The three most commonly used anti-TNF medications for JIA treatment are etanercept (a fusion protein consisting of the extracellular domain of the p75 TNF receptor linked to the Fc region of human immunoglobulin-1), adalimumab (a humanized monoclonal antibody to TNF), and infliximab (a chimeric mouse/human monoclonal antibody to TNF). The FDA approved etanercept for the treatment of polyarticular JIA in May 1999 and adalimumab for the treatment of polyarticular JIA in February 2008. Etanercept is administered as a once- or twice-weekly subcutaneous injection, whereas adalimumab is administered every 1 to 2 weeks. Infliximab is administered intravenously on a monthly basis. Anti-TNF medications are usually combined with MTX or other nonbiologic medications when tolerated. One study showed that children treated with etanercept plus MTX had improved treatment responses compared with etanercept alone, without an increase in adverse events.[2] Because the use of TNF-α inhibitors is associated with reactivated tuberculosis, a negative purified protein derivative skin test should be demonstrated in patients who will be treated with TNF-α inhibitors before starting anti-TNF therapy, and then repeated annually. A complete blood count, hepatic enzyme levels, and serum creatinine level should be obtained before initiating therapy and then repeated every 3 to 6 months.[15]

In 2009, the FDA required that a boxed warning be added to all anti-TNF therapies, highlighting the increased risk of cancer in children receiving these drugs to treat JIA. However, subsequent studies, including several randomized controlled studies, have not demonstrated any important safety concerns of these medications or any other biologic medication. Although some studies showed an increased risk of lymphoma or other malignancy in children treated with anti-TNF therapies, other studies have shown an increased baseline incidence of malignancy in children with JIA.[19] Again, most complications arising from anti-TNF therapies are caused by increased infectious risks, although studies have claimed that the risk is not greater when using anti-TNF therapy compared with use of MTX alone.[19]

IL-1 is an inflammatory cytokine most notably implicated in autoinflammatory syndromes and sJIA. The three commercially available IL-1 antagonists used in the treatment of sJIA are administered subcutaneously and include anakinra (IL-1 receptor antagonist), rilonacept (soluble fusion protein of human immunoglobulin-1 linked to the IL-1 receptor), and canakinumab (monoclonal antibody to IL-1β). All three medications are recommended for the treatment of sJIA in the consensus treatment plans from the Childhood Arthritis and Rheumatology Research Alliance; anakinra monotherapy can be considered an initial treatment in patients with sJIA who have physical findings that raise concern for active disease.[20] The FDA approved canakinumab for the treatment of sJIA in May 2013.

Tocilizumab is a monoclonal antibody to the IL-6 receptor and the only biologic agent that is FDA approved for use in both sJIA and polyarticular JIA. IL-6 is a proinflammatory cytokine. Tocilizumab is available as both an infusion and a subcutaneous injection.

Abatacept is a soluble fusion protein that consists of cytotoxic T cell lymphocyte antigen-4 fused with the Fc region of human immunoglobulin and blocks signal transduction between T cells and antigen-presenting cells. It is an infused medication administered on a monthly basis and was FDA approved for the treatment of polyarticular JIA in April 2008. However, it also is considered effective maintenance therapy in patients with sJIA who do not have physical findings concerning for active disease.[20]

Rituximab is a chimeric monoclonal antibody to the CD20 receptor that is present only on B cells. The FDA has approved rituximab combined with MTX in adults with rheumatoid arthritis who have not had adequate response with anti-TNF therapies. Studies in adults with rheumatoid arthritis suggest that the presence of an RF may lead to better response with rituximab therapy,[21] but these studies have not been performed in children. It seems to have some effectiveness in patients with various JIA subtypes, although studies are limited.

The number of biologic medications being developed for the treatment of inflammatory arthritis continues to grow, although studies for safety and efficacy in JIA have not yet been published. Ustekinumab, a human monoclonal antibody targeting the p40 subunit of IL-12/23, was FDA approved for the treatment of psoriatic arthritis in September 2013 but has not yet been studied in juvenile psoriatic arthritis. However, a randomized phase III trial of ustekinumab in adolescents with plaque psoriasis showed substantially improved signs and symptoms of psoriasis without any unexpected adverse events.[22] Tofacitinib is a Janus-kinase inhibitor that is approved by the FDA for the treatment of adults with rheumatoid arthritis but also seems to be efficacious in psoriasis and inflammatory bowel disease. Unlike other biologic medications, tofacitinib is administered orally. A randomized withdrawal, double-blind, placebo-controlled study of this medication in patients with JIA is expected to take place late in 2016.

The last category of medications used in the treatment of JIA is corticosteroids. Although systemic steroids work quickly to decrease inflammation, they have a limited role in the treatment of JIA. Steroids have never been proved to be disease modifying and have serious toxic adverse effects with long-term use. Low doses (5-15 mg/d) are helpful in cases of severe arthritis in patients with polyarticular JIA and enthesitis-related arthritis. In sJIA and patients with severe uveitis, moderate to high doses (>1 mg/kg/d) are used to control underlying inflammation. The toxicities of steroids include immunosuppression, hypertension, diabetes, cataracts, osteoporosis, osteonecrosis, obesity, and many others.[12,17] In the modern practice of rheumatology, steroids are mainly used as a bridging therapy until the effects of the more slowly acting DMARDs or biologic medications take place.

Reactive Arthritis

In pediatric rheumatology, specialists usually use the term reactive arthritis to describe a transient arthritis of any joint lasting less than 6 weeks, thus differentiating this diagnosis from JIA. In adults, the term is usually used in reference to transient arthritis that is linked to spondyloarthritis.

Transient Synovitis

The term transient synovitis often is applied to arthritis of the hip that follows a recent viral upper respiratory tract infection or viral intestinal disease. However, transient synovitis can involve other joints, usually a large joint and often only a single joint. The symptoms are usually acute, and a fever may be present. Inflammatory markers also may be elevated.[23] The major differential diagnosis is septic arthritis, but JIA also can appear in this fashion. Frequently, transient arthritis will respond within 1 or 2 days to an NSAID, such as naproxen. Most patients improve within days rather than weeks, so it becomes a diagnosis of exclusion. The workup consists of a complete blood count, the erythrocyte sedimentation rate, and the C-reactive protein level; joint aspiration is considered to rule out infection. Initial treatment with antibiotics may be warranted based on the erythrocyte sedimentation rate, C-reactive protein level, and joint aspiration.[24,25]

Table 1

Jones Criteria for the Diagnosis of Acute Rheumatic Fever[a]

Major Criteria	Minor Criteria
Carditis	Fever
Arthritis	Arthralgia
Erythema marginatum	Elevated erythrocyte sedimentation rate or C-reactive protein level
Subcutaneous nodules	Prolonged PR interval or other heart block
Sydenham chorea	

[a]To make a diagnosis of rheumatic fever, two major and one minor criteria or one major and two minor criteria must be present, along with evidence of a recent streptococcal infection as evidenced by a positive throat culture or increasing or elevated streptococcal antibody titers.

Table 2

CDC Criteria for Lyme Disease

Positive ELISA or immunofluorescence assay test

If symptoms present for <30 days: positive Western blot IgM with 2 of 3 bands positive, or Western blot IgG with ≥5 of 10 bands positive

If symptoms present for >30 days: Western blot with ≥5 of 10 bands positive

CDC = Centers for Disease Control and Prevention, ELISA = enzyme-linked immunosorbent assay, IgG = immunoglobulin G, IgM = immunoglobulin M.

Poststreptococcal Arthritis

The primary difference between transient synovitis, which is considered a postviral disease, and poststreptococcal arthritis is simply the documentation of a recent strep infection. However, this determination is not always simple because symptoms of a prior sore throat may be lacking. A prior sore throat and a positive culture for strep usually have an onset of arthritis in 1 to 2 weeks. However, titers for antistreptolysin O and anti–DNAase-B should be done to confirm that the culture was not a false-positive or an indicator of a streptococcal carrier. The interpretation of streptococcal antibody titers also can be difficult and is, at best, 90% sensitive. The course of poststreptococcal arthritis is more variable than transient synovitis. The streptococcal infection should be treated, and NSAIDs may be needed for a longer term course.[26] A streptococcal infection also needs to be distinguished from rheumatic fever, which often is manifested by migratory, very painful arthritis of large joints, and the Jones criteria would need to be fulfilled[27] (**Table 1**).

Lyme Disease Arthritis

In many but not all parts of the United States, Lyme disease arthritis has been well documented.[28] The diagnosis must be suspected clinically by a careful history and fulfillment of the diagnostic criteria from the Centers for Disease Control and Prevention[29] (**Table 2**). Lyme disease arthritis often occurs in the knee and initially may be indistinguishable from other forms of reactive arthritis or juvenile arthritis and may be self-limited or persistent. A history of exposure in an endemic area, a tick bite, flu-like symptoms, and an erythema chronicum migrans rash make the diagnosis much more likely, but one or more of these elements may not be present.[30-34] Misdiagnosis is a common problem if the serology criteria are not applied appropriately.

Chronic Recurrent Multifocal Osteomyelitis

The presentation of CRMO, although a rare disease, is extremely important to the orthopaedic surgeon. CRMO can include osteomyelitis that mimics bacterial osteomyelitis with bony changes and periosteal elevation, osteitis of a long bone, osteolytic lesion of a bone, or a mixed picture of any of these with arthritis.[33,34] The pathophysiology of CRMO is considered immune mediated.[35,36]

Radiographic evidence can be very helpful, and some features suggest the diagnosis early in the course. Plain radiographs, bone scans, and MRI have all been used, but MRI seems to be particularly helpful.[37-40] Persistence of a bony lesion, negative bone cultures, a negative bone biopsy for malignancy or other bone tumor, and a lack of response to antibiotics are all useful in developing a suspicion of CRMO. In addition to mimicking infection, the lesions also can have the characteristics of a bone tumor.[41] Recurrence of what seems to be osteomyelitis in the same or, more importantly, in a new area is highly suspicious for CRMO (**Figures 2, 3, and 4**). Laboratory testing shows persistent elevation of inflammatory markers if the patient is symptomatic, but these markers may resolve completely if the CRMO remits.

The treatment of CRMO is complicated, and a highly variable response can be seen. Medications may include NSAIDs, MTX, or a biologic medication.[42]

Arthritis in Other Systemic Rheumatic Diseases

Arthritis can occur in children with more complex rheumatic disease, such as systemic lupus erythematosus, juvenile dermatomyositis, sarcoidosis, and in some of the vasculitic diseases, including granulomatosis with polyangiitis, Henoch-Schönlein purpura, Kawasaki disease,

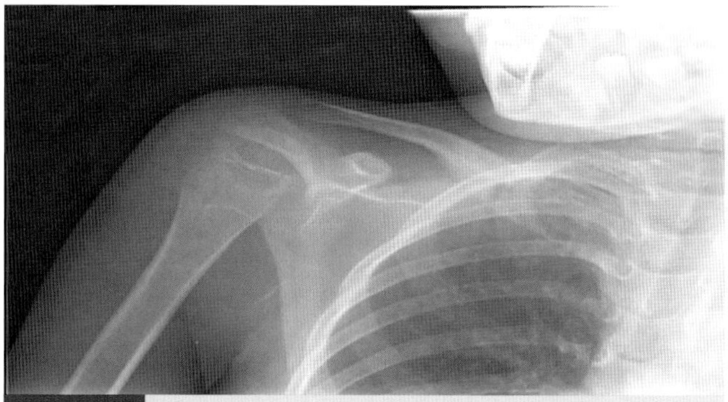

Figure 2 AP radiograph shows chronic recurrent multifocal osteomyelitis in the right clavicle.

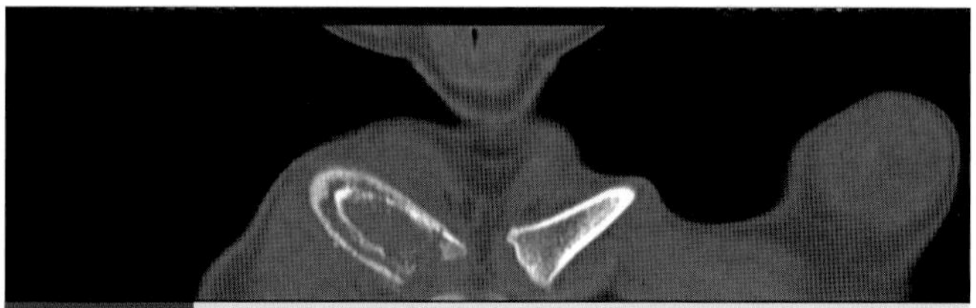

Figure 3 CT scan shows chronic recurrent multifocal osteomyelitis in the right clavicle.

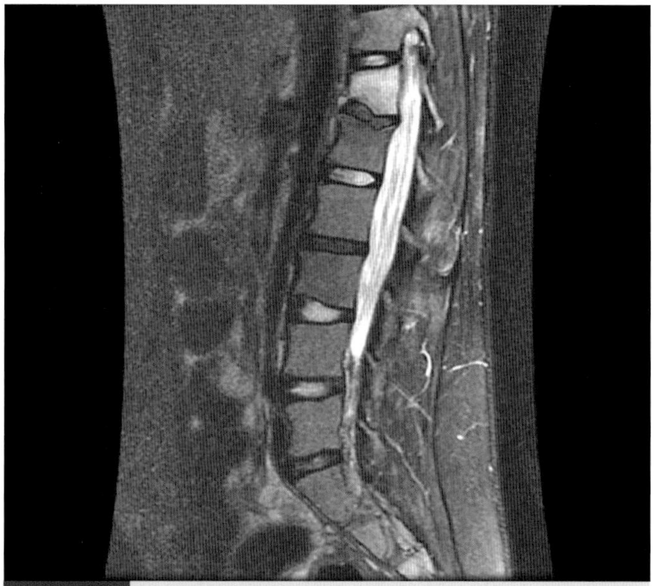

Figure 4 MRI shows chronic recurrent multifocal osteomyelitis in the spine.

eosinophilia with polyangiitis, and polyarteritis nodosa. The history and physical examination are usually able to differentiate these diseases from an orthopaedic etiology toward a rheumatic etiology.

Systemic lupus erythematosus is diagnosed in a preteen or teenage patient and includes one or more of the following symptoms: fever, fatigue, hair loss, the Raynaud phenomenon, a malar rash, weight loss, pericarditis, pneumonitis, and a pleural effusion.[43,44]

Juvenile dermatomyositis often occurs as proximal muscle weakness and frequently will have a characteristic rash on the face, extensor elbows, and knee, as well as the dorsum of the hands with lesions that are called Gottron papules. Patients frequently also have changes of the nail fold capillary bed that are visible with a magnifier.[45]

The characteristics of Kawasaki disease typically are a high daily fever with injected sclera; a red tongue; dry, red, vertically fissured lips; polymorphous dermatitis of the body; and lymphadenopathy. Patients are usually very irritable and have a marked increase in inflammatory markers as well as in alanine aminotransferase and γ-glutamyltransferase. Most importantly, coronary artery disease may develop in patients.[46]

Henoch-Schönlein purpura usually starts with a petechial or palpable purpuric rash of the distal lower legs that usually spreads to involve most of both legs and the buttocks. The arthritis can follow the onset of the rash within several days, occur at the same time as the purpura, or precede any other symptoms. Abdominal pain that may be severe frequently develops. The arthritis is usually a large-joint arthritis of the ankles and/or knees.[47]

Granulomatosis with polyangiitis (formerly known as Wegener granulomatosis) may include arthritis but usually includes other symptoms, notably significant pneumonitis, sinusitis, or nephritis. Many patients will have a positive antineutrophil cytoplasmic antibody test.[48]

In younger children, sarcoidosis usually manifests as multiple, very swollen joints and may include dermatitis and uveitis. In older children, pulmonary involvement is a more common indication.[49] Behçet syndrome can occur with arthritis, but it usually occurs with recurrent aphthous ulcers, dermatitis, fever, or intestinal symptoms.

Summary

Arthritis in children encompasses a wide variety of diseases ranging from brief forms of reactive arthritis to various forms of juvenile arthritis. Symptoms and clues to the diagnosis vary with the disease subtype. The patient's history and physical examination are still the most important components of the diagnosis; however, laboratory and imaging studies can be helpful in differentiating these disorders from other orthopaedic conditions. Because the treatment of arthritis has changed dramatically in the past 15 years, making a correct diagnosis is very important. Involvement of a pediatric rheumatologist early in the course of a child's disease can help in determining an accurate diagnosis and selecting the proper treatment.

Key Study Points

- Postviral reactive arthritis is fairly common in children and can be difficult to differentiate from orthopaedic disorders and chronic rheumatic diseases.
- Chronic forms of juvenile arthritis can present with either systemic features or one or more joints that are typically associated with morning stiffness and pain.
- MRI, with and without contrast, can be helpful in differentiating orthopaedic disorders from various forms of childhood arthritis.

Annotated References

1. Petty RE, Southwood TR, Manners P, et al: International League of Associations for Rheumatology classification of juvenile idiopathic arthritis: Second revision, Edmonton, 2001. *J Rheumatol* 2004;31(2):390-392.

2. Stoll ML, Cron RQ: Treatment of juvenile idiopathic arthritis: A revolution in care. *Pediatr Rheumatol Online J* 2014;12:13.

   This article provides an excellent review about treatment that has changed the course of JIA. Level of evidence: V.

3. Lanni S, Martini A, Malattia C: Heading toward a modern imaging approach in juvenile idiopathic arthritis. *Curr Rheumatol Rep* 2014;16(5):416.

   The imaging modalities for JIA are discussed in this article. Level of evidence: V.

4. Restrepo R, Lee EY, Babyn PS: Juvenile idiopathic arthritis: Current practical imaging assessment with emphasis on magnetic resonance imaging. *Radiol Clin North Am* 2013;51(4):703-719.

   This article analyzes the value of MRI in some patients with JIA. Level of evidence: V.

5. Saikia B, Rawat A, Vignesh P: Autoantibodies and their judicious use in pediatric rheumatology practice. *Indian J Pediatr* 2016;83(1):53-62.

   The latest guidelines for the use of laboratory tests in pediatric patients with arthritis are presented. Level of evidence: V.

6. Spencer CH, Patwardhan A: Pediatric rheumatology for the primary care clinicians: Recognizing patterns of disease. *Curr Probl Pediatr Adolesc Health Care* 2015;45(7):185-206.

   Guidelines for the approach to pediatric joint disease based on the pattern of symptoms and joint findings are presented. Level of evidence: V.

7. Krause ML, Crowson CS, Michet CJ, Mason T, Muskardin TW, Matteson EL: Juvenile idiopathic arthritis in Olmsted County, Minnesota, 1960-2013. *Arthritis Rheumatol* 2016;68(1):247-254.

   This article discusses epidemiology data for JIA in one county in Minnesota.

8. Stoll ML, Nigrovic PA, Gotte AC, Punaro M: Clinical comparison of early-onset psoriatic and non-psoriatic oligoarticular juvenile idiopathic arthritis. *Clin Exp Rheumatol* 2011;29(3):582-588.

   This helpful review of oligoarticular JIA underscores the importance of psoriatic arthritis in the differential diagnosis of JIA. Level of evidence: II.

9. Ramanathan A, Srinivasalu H, Colbert RA: Update on juvenile spondyloarthritis. *Rheum Dis Clin North Am* 2013;39(4):767-788.

   This article is a good review of the differentiation of spondyloarthritis in pediatrics compared with other forms of juvenile arthritis. Level of evidence: V.

10. Nirmala N, Grom A, Gram H: Biomarkers in systemic juvenile idiopathic arthritis: A comparison with biomarkers in cryopyrin-associated periodic syndromes. *Curr Opin Rheumatol* 2014;26(5):543-552.

    This article is a good discussion of the laboratory tests that are helpful for children who are febrile (feverish) and have arthritis. Level of evidence: II.

11. Bruck N, Schnabel A, Hedrich CM: Current understanding of the pathophysiology of systemic juvenile idiopathic arthritis (sJIA) and target-directed therapeutic approaches. *Clin Immunol* 2015;159(1):72-83.

    This article is a good review of sJIA as well as the change in medical approaches to the disease based on the newer understanding of sJIA pathophysiology. Level of evidence: V.

12. Cassidy J, Petty R: *Textbook of Pediatric Rheumatology Expert Consult,* ed 6. London, UK, Elsevier Health Sciences, 2010, pp 236-248.

13. Ringold S, Weiss PF, Colbert RA, et al: Childhood Arthritis and Rheumatology Research Alliance consensus treatment plans for new-onset polyarticular juvenile idiopathic arthritis. *Arthritis Care Res (Hoboken)* 2014;66(7):1063-1072 .

    The treatment guidelines for patients with polyarticular JIA were developed by a consensus of pediatric rheumatologists. Level of evidence: V.

14. DeWitt EM, Kimura Y, Beukelman T, et al: Consensus treatment plans for new-onset systemic juvenile idiopathic arthritis. *Arthritis Care Res (Hoboken)* 2012;64(7):1001-1010.

    Guidelines for the treatment of sJIA, which were established by a consensus of pediatric rheumatologists, are presented. Level of evidence: V.

15. Beukelman T, Patkar NM, Saag KG, et al: 2011 American College of Rheumatology recommendations for the treatment of juvenile idiopathic arthritis: Initiation and safety monitoring of therapeutic agents for the treatment of arthritis and systemic features. *Arthritis Care Res (Hoboken)* 2011;63(4):465-482.

Additional guidelines for using medications and monitoring any adverse effects from the medications as established by the American College of Rheumatology are presented. Level of evidence: V.

16. Jennings H, Hennessy K, Hendry GJ: The clinical effectiveness of intra-articular corticosteroids for arthritis of the lower limb in juvenile idiopathic arthritis: A systematic review. *Pediatr Rheumatol Online J* 2014;12:23.

This article emphasizes the value of a steroid joint injection in the management of patients with JIA. Level of evidence: V.

17. Szer I: *Arthritis in Children and Adolescents: Juvenile Idiopathic Arthritis*. Oxford, England, Oxford University Press, 2006.

18. Coulson EJ, Hanson HJ, Foster HE: What does an adult rheumatologist need to know about juvenile idiopathic arthritis? *Rheumatology (Oxford)* 2014;53(12):2155-2166.

Guidelines for adult rheumatologists about the care of patients with JIA are presented. Level of evidence: V.

19. Kessler EA, Becker ML: Therapeutic advancements in juvenile idiopathic arthritis. *Best Pract Res Clin Rheumatol* 2014;28(2):293-313.

Detailed information about changes in the therapy of JIA is presented in this article. Level of evidence: V.

20. Ringold S, Weiss PF, Beukelman T, et al: 2013 update of the 2011 American College of Rheumatology recommendations for the treatment of juvenile idiopathic arthritis: Recommendations for the medical therapy of children with systemic juvenile idiopathic arthritis and tuberculosis screening among children receiving biologic medications. *Arthritis Rheum* 2013;65(10):2499-2512.

Guidelines for the use of biologic medications in the treatment of JIA and the screening needed for tuberculosis are presented. Level of evidence: V.

21. Chatzidionysiou K, Lie E, Nasonov E, et al: Highest clinical effectiveness of rituximab in autoantibody-positive patients with rheumatoid arthritis and in those for whom no more than one previous TNF antagonist has failed: Pooled data from 10 European registries. *Ann Rheum Dis* 2011;70(9):1575-1580.

Specific information is presented about the use of rituximab for JIA that fails to respond to treatment that is more conventional. Level of evidence: I.

22. Landells I, Marano C, Hsu MC, et al: Ustekinumab in adolescent patients age 12 to 17 years with moderate-to-severe plaque psoriasis: Results of the randomized phase 3 CADMUS study. *J Am Acad Dermatol* 2015;73(4):594-603.

Newer understandings of the pathophysiology and treatment options emerging for psoriatic arthritis are presented. Level of evidence: I.

23. Nouri A, Walmsley D, Pruszczynski B, Synder M: Transient synovitis of the hip: A comprehensive review. *J Pediatr Orthop B* 2014;23(1):32-36.

This article is a good discussion about the diagnosis and management of transient synovitis of the hip. Level of evidence: V.

24. Liberman B, Herman A, Schindler A, Sherr-Lurie N, Ganel A, Givon U: The value of hip aspiration in pediatric transient synovitis. *J Pediatr Orthop* 2013;33(2):124-127.

This article discusses and analyzes hip aspiration in differentiating transient synovitis from septic hip arthritis. Level of evidence: V.

25. Taekema HC, Landham PR, Maconochie I: Towards evidence based medicine for paediatricians: Distinguishing between transient synovitis and septic arthritis in the limping child. How useful are clinical prediction tools? *Arch Dis Child* 2009;94(2):167-168.

26. Shulman ST, Ayoub EM: Poststreptococcal reactive arthritis. *Curr Opin Rheumatol* 2002;14(5):562-565.

27. van der Helm-van Mil AH: Acute rheumatic fever and poststreptococcal reactive arthritis reconsidered. *Curr Opin Rheumatol* 2010;22(4):437-442.

28. Mead PS: Epidemiology of Lyme disease. *Infect Dis Clin North Am* 2015;29(2):187-210.

The distribution of cases of Lyme disease in North America and Europe is presented. Level of evidence: II.

29. Sood SK: Lyme disease in children. *Infect Dis Clin North Am* 2015;29(2):281-294.

This article is an excellent and thorough discussion of Lyme disease, including criteria and treatment. Level of evidence: V.

30. Oliveira CR, Shapiro ED: Update on persistent symptoms associated with Lyme disease. *Curr Opin Pediatr* 2015;27(1):100-104.

A longer term course for the treatment of Lyme disease arthritis is presented in this article. Level of evidence: IV.

31. Esposito S, Bosis S, Sabatini C, Tagliaferri L, Principi N: Borrelia burgdorferi infection and Lyme disease in children. *Int J Infect Dis* 2013;17(3):e153-e158.

This article is a good review of Lyme disease. Level of evidence: V.

32. O'Connell S: Lyme borreliosis: Current issues in diagnosis and management. *Curr Opin Infect Dis* 2010;23(3):231-235.

33. Walsh P, Manners PJ, Vercoe J, Burgner D, Murray KJ: Chronic recurrent multifocal osteomyelitis in children: Nine years' experience at a statewide tertiary paediatric rheumatology referral centre. *Rheumatology (Oxford)* 2015;54(9):1688-1691.

This article is an excellent but brief review of CRMO.

34. Wipff J, Costantino F, Lemelle I, et al: A large national cohort of French patients with chronic recurrent multifocal osteitis. *Arthritis Rheumatol* 2015;67(4):1128-1137.

This article presents an extensive review of CRMO. Level of evidence: V.

35. Scianaro R, Insalaco A, Bracci Laudiero L, et al: Deregulation of the IL-1β axis in chronic recurrent multifocal osteomyelitis. *Pediatr Rheumatol Online J* 2014;12:30.

The theory of the pathophysiology of CRMO is discussed in this article. Level of evidence: V.

36. Ferguson PJ, Sandu M: Current understanding of the pathogenesis and management of chronic recurrent multifocal osteomyelitis. *Curr Rheumatol Rep* 2012;14(2):130-141.

Information on the pathophysiology and treatment of CRMO is presented. Level of evidence: V.

37. von Kalle T, Heim N, Hospach T, Langendörfer M, Winkler P, Stuber T: Typical patterns of bone involvement in whole-body MRI of patients with chronic recurrent multifocal osteomyelitis (CRMO). *Rofo* 2013;185(7):655-661.

This article is a helpful discussion and study of the use of MRI in the diagnosis of CRMO based on the distribution of lesions. It also includes additional discussion on the pathophysiology and treatment of CRMO. Level of evidence: II.

38. Falip C, Alison M, Boutry N, et al: Chronic recurrent multifocal osteomyelitis (CRMO): A longitudinal case series review. *Pediatr Radiol* 2013;43(3):355-375.

A clinical review of the course of treatment of CRMO is presented in this article. Level of evidence: II.

39. Guérin-Pfyffer S, Guillaume-Czitrom S, Tammam S, Koné-Paut I: Evaluation of chronic recurrent multifocal osteitis in children by whole-body magnetic resonance imaging. *Joint Bone Spine* 2012;79(6):616-620.

The value of MRI in the diagnosis of CRMO is presented in this article. Level of evidence: II.

40. Fritz J, Tzaribachev N, Thomas C, et al: Magnetic resonance imaging-guided osseous biopsy in children with chronic recurrent multifocal osteomyelitis. *Cardiovasc Intervent Radiol* 2012;35(1):146-153.

This article presents helpful guidelines for using MRI for diagnosis and biopsy of CRMO lesions. Level of evidence: II.

41. Jibri Z, Sah M, Mansour R: Chronic recurrent multifocal osteomyelitis mimicking osteoid osteoma. *JBR-BTR* 2012;95(4):263-266.

A case report of osteoid osteoma that mimicked CRMO is discussed.

42. Eleftheriou D, Gerschman T, Sebire N, Woo P, Pilkington CA, Brogan PA: Biologic therapy in refractory chronic non-bacterial osteomyelitis of childhood. *Rheumatology (Oxford)* 2010;49(8):1505-1512.

43. Santiago MB, Galvão V: Jaccoud arthropathy in systemic lupus erythematosus: Analysis of clinical characteristics and review of the literature. *Medicine (Baltimore)* 2008;87(1):37-44.

44. Tucker LB: Making the diagnosis of systemic lupus erythematosus in children and adolescents. *Lupus* 2007;16(8):546-549.

45. Quartier P, Gherardi RK: Juvenile dermatomyositis. *Handb Clin Neurol* 2013;113:1457-1463.

This article presents a general review of juvenile dermatomyositis in children, including rheumatic symptoms. Level of evidence: V.

46. Gong GW, McCrindle BW, Ching JC, Yeung RS: Arthritis presenting during the acute phase of Kawasaki disease. *J Pediatr* 2006;148(6):800-805.

47. Yang YH, Yu HH, Chiang BL: The diagnosis and classification of Henoch-Schönlein purpura: An updated review. *Autoimmun Rev* 2014;13(4-5):355-358.

Henoch-Schönlein purpura is reviewed in this article, including some emphasis on the arthritic involvement of the disease. Level of evidence: V.

48. Twilt M, Benseler S, Cabral D: Granulomatosis with polyangiitis in childhood. *Curr Rheumatol Rep* 2012;14(2):107-115.

Granulomatosis with polyangiitis, formerly known as Wegener granulomatosis, is reviewed in this article. Level of evidence: V.

49. Wouters CH, Maes A, Foley KP, Bertin J, Rose CD: Blau syndrome: The prototypic auto-inflammatory granulomatous disease. *Pediatr Rheumatol Online J* 2014;12:33.

This article discusses sarcoid presentation in younger children that can occur with substantial arthritis. Level of evidence: IV.

Section 4

Upper Extremity

SECTION EDITOR:

Charles A. Goldfarb, MD

Chapter 17

Congenital Upper Limb Differences

Lindley B. Wall, MD   Charles A. Goldfarb, MD

Abstract

Congenital upper limb anomalies are uncommon. Advancements in the treatment of these conditions has progressed slowly using information gained from retrospective analyses and reports of evolving surgical techniques. To provide better patient care, it is helpful to be familiar with knowledge gained from the most recent studies concerning congenital upper limb differences.

Keywords: congenital; limb development; upper extremity; upper limb

Introduction

The upper limbs develop within the first 2 months of gestation. The upper limb buds begin to emerge at 4 weeks of gestation and achieve final formation at approximately 8 weeks. As the fetus continues to grow, the hands double in size by the time of birth, and the hands again double in size from birth to age 2 years and then again from age 2 years to skeletal maturity. The upper limbs develop by a complex interaction of multiple factors along three axes: proximal-distal, anterior-posterior (radioulnar), and dorsal-ventral. Proximal-distal development results from signaling between the apical ectodermal ridge and the underlying mesoderm, primarily through the secretion of fibroblast growth factors. Anterior-posterior development, which results in differentiation between the radial and ulnar aspects of the upper limb, is guided by the release of Sonic Hedgehog morphogen from the zone of polarizing activity located on the posterior aspect of the limb. Dorsal-ventral differentiation occurs through signaling of WNT-7a, which acts to create dorsal structures such as nails.[1]

A better understanding of developmental biology has influenced the classification of congenital upper limb anomalies. Originally, the Swanson classification used purely phenotypic descriptions to classify congenital anomalies.[2] Recently, the Oberg, Manske, and Tonkin (OMT) scheme has been used to reclassify congenital upper limb anomalies using current knowledge of limb development.[3] In 2014, a modified OMT classification system was accepted by the International Federation of Societies for Surgery of the Hand (IFSSH).

Using the OMT classification system, recent studies have reported both the prevalence and the epidemiology of congenital upper limb anomalies. Two studies from Scandinavia reported an incidence ranging from 5.25 to 21.5 per 10,000 live births;[4,5] the difference between the studies was based on inclusion criteria. Failure of differentiation was the most common pattern, followed by duplication and failure of formation. Radial ray deficiencies were the most common anomaly identified in the Finnish study.[5] A US study reported limb malformations as the most common type of anomaly, specifically those affecting the hand plate, with radial polydactyly being the most frequently reported.[6] Continued research efforts will likely contribute to a better understanding of upper limb discrepancies and a more accurate determination of their prevalence.

Malformations

Entire Limb

Transverse Deficiency

A transverse deficiency most commonly relates to a diagnosis of symbrachydactyly. The proposed etiology for symbrachydactyly is a prenatal vascular insult.[7] An insufficient vascular supply to the progress zone of the growing

Dr. Goldfarb or an immediate family member serves as a paid consultant to or is an employee of Arthrex and serves as a board member, owner, officer, or committee member of the American Academy of Orthopaedic Surgeons and the American Society for Surgery of the Hand. Neither Dr. Wall nor any immediate family member has received anything of value from or has stock or stock options held in a commercial company or institution related directly or indirectly to the subject of this chapter.

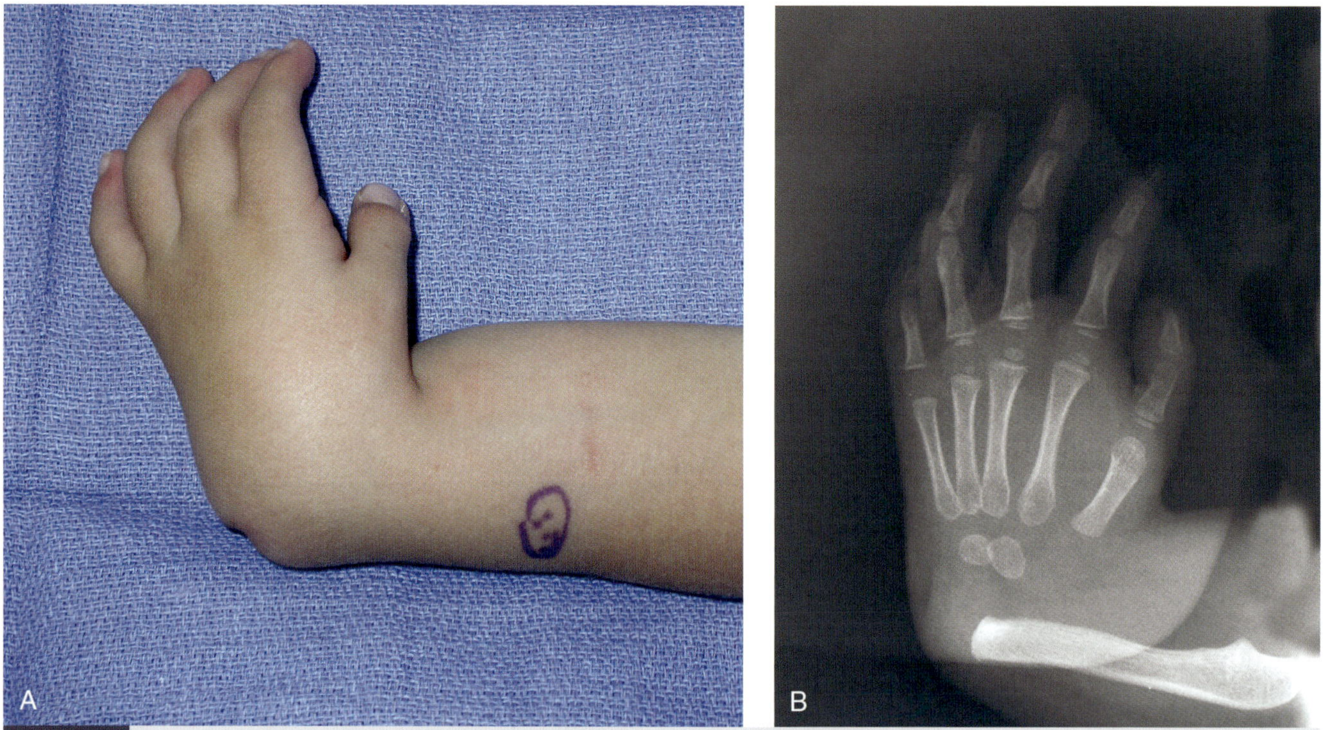

Figure 1 Clinical (**A**) and radiographic (**B**) images of a radial longitudinal deficiency.

limb results in a truncated limb. This mesodermal insult results in a truncated limb, with the presence of small nubbins of ectodermal origin (including nails and small tufts of bone). The proximal third of the forearm is the most common level of deficiency. The level of truncation varies and may occur through the elbow, in the forearm below the elbow, or at the wrist.

Historically, treatment of children with this deficiency included prosthetic fitting at approximately 6 months of age or when the child had achieved sitting balance. However, because prosthetic limbs are heavy and can interfere with sensory input, the philosophy concerning the fitting of an upper limb prosthesis has changed. Currently, it has been shown that upper limb prostheses do not improve function or quality of life, although they may be useful for specific tasks or functions.[8] Therefore, upper limb prosthetic fitting should not be universally performed, but should be provided when requested by the patient or family.

Radial Longitudinal Deficiency

A radial longitudinal deficiency (RLD) results from a failure of formation of the radial aspect of the forearm and hand. Historically, classification systems concentrated on the presence and length of the radius, whereas newer classification modifications include the carpus and proximal limb.[9,10] An RLD is often associated with other medical conditions and syndromes such as thrombocytopenia absent radius syndrome, Holt-Oram syndrome, Fanconi anemia, and vertebral-anal-cardiac-tracheal-esophageal-renal-limb (VACTERL) association.

Pediatric orthopaedic surgeons and hand surgeons are in a critical position to evaluate children with RLD for associated medical conditions because they may be the first physicians to examine these patients. Spinal radiographs, cardiac and renal ultrasound studies, and a complete blood count with differential are recommended for children with RLD. Smaller children with atypical facial features should be evaluated for Fanconi anemia, and a chromosomal challenge test should be obtained.

RLD of the forearm results in hypoplasia or aplasia of the radius. This anomaly results in a short forearm and radial deviation of the wrist (**Figure 1**). In a young child, radial deviation is initially treated with stretching and splinting. As the child ages, severe deformities can be surgically treated to improve the position of the hand in relation to the forearm. Classically, these children were treated with an acute centralization of the wrist, which involved an extensive soft-tissue release and placement of the hand on top of the distal ulna with pin fixation. Radialization is a variation of centralization in which tendons are transferred to the ulnar wrist at the time of wrist centralization.[11] More than 20 years of long-term follow-up of patients treated with centralization/radialization compared with those who were managed nonsurgically showed that the surgically treated patients had better cosmetic outcomes along with improved finger and wrist motion, grip strength, and increased ease in performing functional daily activities.[12]

More recently, the use of soft-tissue distraction followed by a staged centralization procedure has been described.[13-16] During centralization, the surgeon must take care to prevent injury to the distal ulna physis to prevent additional shortening of an already short forearm.

An alternative approach uses a volar bilobed flap with soft-tissue release to maintain motion of the wrist and decrease radial deviation.[17] If necessary, this procedure is followed by a free vascularized metatarsophalangeal joint transfer to stabilize the radial aspect of the wrist.[18] Currently, the optimal treatment of radial deviation of the wrist in patients with RLD is debatable.

Ulnar Longitudinal Deficiency

Ulnar longitudinal deficiency (ULD) results from failure of formation of the ulnar aspect of the forearm and hand. Unlike RLD, ULD is not associated with internal organ anomalies, but it can be associated with fibular hemimelia. ULD also can extend proximally and affect the elbow, including radiohumeral synostosis. Classically, children with ULD are described as having a hand that looks backward; however, these children typically have high functional ability. The performance of daily tasks may become more challenging with growth because children may no longer be able to reach their hands to their month. If necessary, an osteotomy of the synostosis and repositioning of the limb may improve function. Alternatively, surgery may focus primarily on the hand as described later in this chapter.

Madelung Deformity

Madelung deformity is a condition involving abnormal growth of the distal radial physis. The condition can be idiopathic or can result from an autosomal dominant trait with variable penetrance. When associated with Léri-Weill dyschondrosteosis, a form of dwarfism, it is associated with a *SHOX* gene (short stature homeobox gene) deficiency.[19] Clinically and radiographically, the wrist has classic ulnar and dorsal curvatures. There is limited growth at the volar ulnar aspect of the distal radial physis, which results in an increase in radial tilt, ulnar translation of the carpus, triangulation of the carpus, and a prominent dorsal distal ulna[20] (**Figure 2**). Typically, there is a thick volar ligament (Vickers ligament) that tethers the lunate to the distal radial metaphysis and is believed to contribute to the deformity. The severity of Madelung deformity varies. In some patients, the entire length of the radius is affected in addition to the wrist.[21]

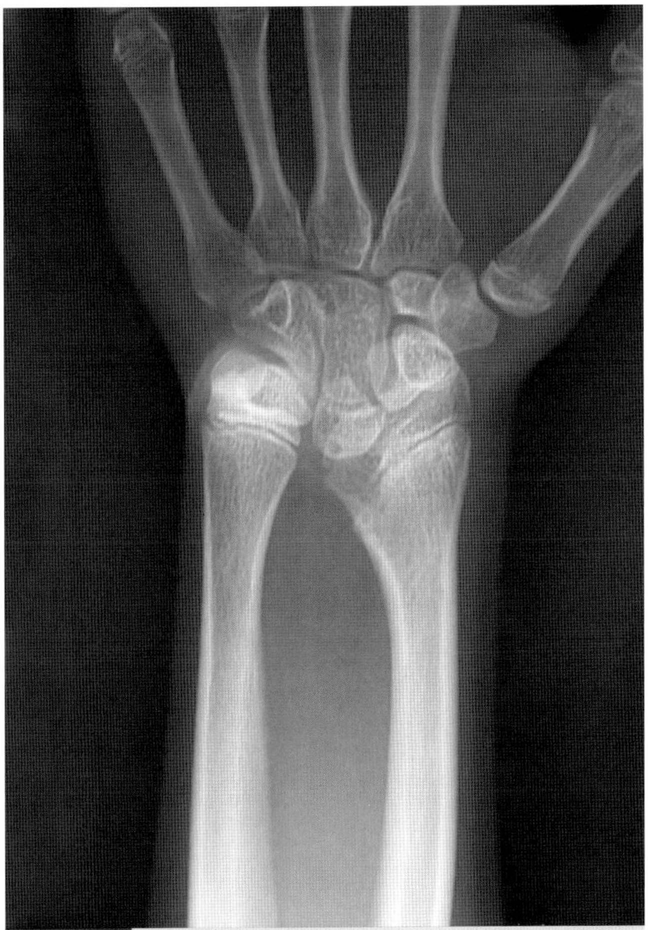

Figure 2 AP radiograph shows typical appearance of a Madelung deformity, with increased radial tilt, ulnar translation of the carpus, and triangulation of the carpus.

Madelung deformity typically presents in adolescence and is characterized by the classic wrist deformity, limited wrist motion, and wrist pain. Treatment of the deformity may subsequently improve range of motion and reduce pain. The recommended treatment includes excision of the Vickers ligament and a dome osteotomy of the distal radius, which corrects the distal radial deformity in multiple planes.[22] Results of this treatment at an average 11-year follow-up showed maintenance of motion and deformity correction. Patients with more severe deformities had worse functional and radiographic outcomes.[23] In young patients without pain, who have mild deformity and growth remaining, ligament release may be considered to potentially alter and limit the development of wrist deformity, maintain motion, and limit future pain.

Hand Plate Only

Symbrachydactyly

Symbrachydactyly affecting the hand plate can have a range of presentations from shortened digits to absent digits.[24] Short-finger symbrachydactyly varies in severity and may occur with or without syndactyly. Although patients with symbrachydactyly often do not need treatment, deepening of the web spaces may be considered. Short-finger symbrachydactyly is most commonly associated with Poland syndrome, with hypoplasia of the ipsilateral chest wall muscles and thorax.

Cleft-type symbrachydactyly, historically known as atypical cleft hand, is characterized by an ulnar-sided digit and a thumb; nubbins may be present within the u-shaped cleft. The severity of the thumb involvement is predictive of the child's ability to use the hand. If the thumb can be opposed to the ulnar-sided digit, function can be excellent. If the thumb is positioned in the plane of the hand, side-to-side pinch is used and function is more limited. The thumb position and function can be improved with a rotational osteotomy.

Monodactylous symbrachydactyly is the presence of a single digit on the radial side. Although most children with this type of symbrachydactyly have good hand function, some patients will benefit from the creation or lengthening of an ulnar-sided digit to provide a post for thumb pinch.[25-27] Peromelic symbrachydactyly is a hand without digits and with varying levels of deficiency (metacarpal, carpal, or through the radiocarpal joint).

Overall, the goals of symbrachydactyly treatment are to improve a child's functional ability and optimize his or her independence and hand use. Frequently, these children have good functional abilities because symbrachydactyly is a unilateral condition.

Radial Longitudinal Deficiency

RLD affecting the hand plate results in carpal hypoplasia and/or thumb hypoplasia or aplasia. Children with RLD should be medically evaluated as previously detailed. Typically, carpal anomalies do not require treatment. Thumb involvement in RLD ranges from a small thumb to complete thumb aplasia as classified by the Blauth classification system.[28] Manske et al[29] modified the Blauth classification based on the stability of the thumb carpometacarpal joint. This modification has implications with regard to the treatment of hypoplastic thumbs.

Blauth type I thumbs are small but have well developed structures and do not need treatment. Type II thumbs have hypoplastic intrinsic thenar muscles and thumb metacarpophalangeal (MCP) joint laxity and often are improved by either a Huber or flexor digitorum superficialis (FDS) opponensplasty. The Huber opponensplasty is a rotational flap of the adductor digiti minimi muscle to the radial side of the thumb. This flap must often be supplemented by capsular imbrication of the ulnar side of the MCP joint to manage instability. The FDS opponensplasty uses the FDS tendon from the ring finger, transferring it across the palm to the thumb MCP joint; the extra tendon length is used to reconstruct the ulnar collateral ligament. Similar reconstruction is applied to type IIIA hypoplastic thumbs. Type III thumbs also demonstrate hypoplasia of the thumb extrinsic muscles, which may need to be treated with tendon transfers. In the Western world, thumbs classified as Blauth types IIIB, IV, or V are treated with index finger pollicization. The hypoplastic thumb is removed (types IIIB and IV) and the index finger is shortened through the metacarpal and repositioned 90° to 110° from the middle finger and abducted out of the plane of the hand.[30]

Ulnar Longitudinal Deficiency

ULD of the hand includes hypoplasia or absence of the ulnar-sided structures. There are two commonly used classification systems for ULD of the hand. ULD of the hand was originally classified according to the number of absent digits.[31] Alternatively, Cole and Manske[32] classified ULD based on the degree of narrowing of the first web space, which directly correlates with functional use of the hand. Treatment of the ulnar-deficient hand includes deepening of a narrowed first web space and rotational osteotomy of the thumb to improve pinch and grasp as indicated.

Radial Polydactyly

Radial polydactyly or preaxial polydactyly is the presence of an additional thumb. The classification of thumb polydactyly is based on the level of duplication, starting with the distal phalanx and extending to the metacarpal level.[33] A Flatt type IV thumb, with duplication at the level of the MCP joint, is the most common type (**Figure 3**).

Patients with thumb polydactyly often have acceptable function, but the additional thumb is aesthetically abnormal. Reconstruction procedures depend on the level of duplication but generally consist of removal of the more hypoplastic thumb, which is typically the more radial thumb, and reconstruction of the remaining thumb to provide a straight, stable, functional thumb. In selected types, including Flatt types I and II, reconstruction includes either excision of the small thumb and stabilization of the remaining thumb or surgical combination of the thumbs, which is technically more challenging.[34-36] To achieve a stable thumb in Flatt type IV thumbs, the radial collateral ligament of the MCP joint is re-created with a periosteal sleeve from the excised radial thumb.

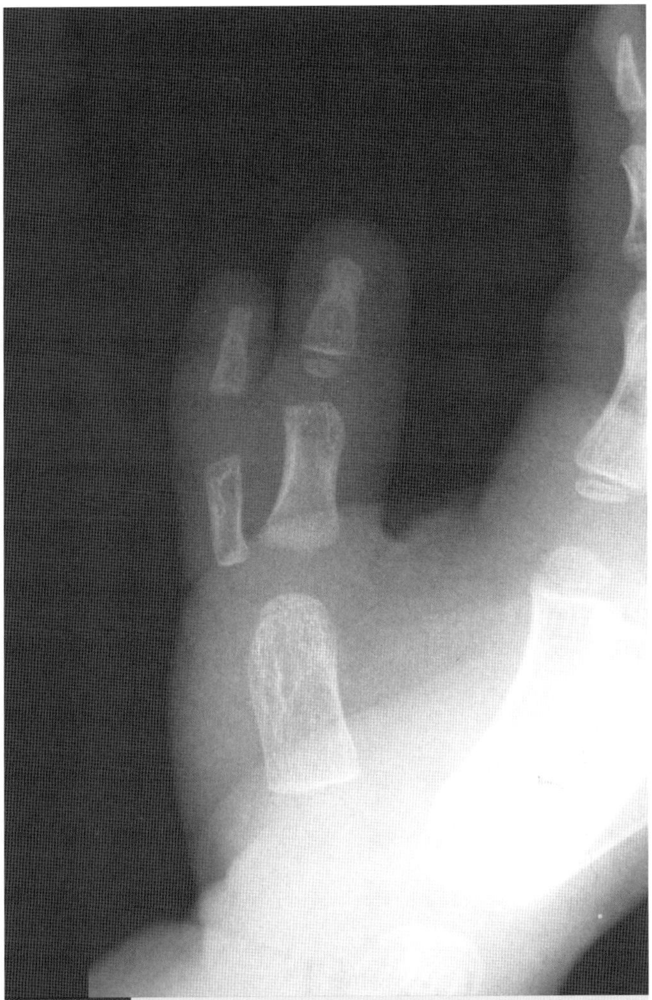

Figure 3 Radiograph shows a Flatt type IV radial polydactyly with duplication at the level of the proximal phalanx.

Residual deformity is treated with an osteotomy to correct angulation. Eccentric insertion of the flexor and/or the extensor tendons that create an abnormal line of pull can contribute to angulation. For correction, the tendons can be elevated and reinserted to direct the tendon force more centrally.

Clinical outcomes assessments report that remaining thumb angulation and reduced nail width is associated with decreased patient satisfaction.[37] Recently, long-term follow-up results from polydactyly reconstructions have been reported.[38] At an average follow-up of more than 10 years, a revision rate of 19% was reported. Arthrodeses for joint instability and pain was associated with 50% of the revision surgeries. Flatt type III and IV thumbs had weaker pinch than the contralateral side. All of the patients were satisfied with their surgical outcomes.

Ulnar Polydactyly

Ulnar polydactyly (postaxial polydactyly) is duplication of the small finger. This is one of the most common congenital anomalies and is predominantly seen in individuals of African descent. The level of duplication ranges from a small tag-like digit (type B) to a complete duplication of the small finger ray (type A), as classified by Temtamy and McKusick.[39] The type B fingers are often tied off in the nursery and are never evaluated by a surgeon.

Type A polydactyly has recently been further classified according to the level of duplication.[40] An associated syndrome or additional congenital anomaly was reported in 24% of the individuals evaluated; however, there is no standard recommendation for syndromic workup in these patients. Type A polydactyly is equally seen in Caucasian patients and those of African descent in contrast to type B polydactyly, which is more commonly seen in patients of African descent.

Reconstruction of ulnar polydactyly is a more straightforward procedure than radial polydactyly reconstruction. Type B digits can be tied off with suture or clipped at the base of the stalk. If the base is greater than 1 cm in width, surgical excision is the most reliable treatment. Type A digits are removed surgically, and the ulnar collateral ligament of the small finger MCP joint may be reconstructed with a periosteal flap from the excised digit. Stability is less of a concern with the small finger than with the thumb.

Syndactyly

Syndactyly results from incomplete recession of the interdigital skin during limb development—a failure of apoptosis. Syndactyly is classified by the extent of involvement and presence of an osseous connection. Syndactyly that extends the entire length of the digits is called complete syndactyly, whereas lesser involvement is termed partial or incomplete syndactyly. Cutaneous syndactyly describes digits that are connected simply by skin. In contrast, a complex syndactyly consists of a bony bridge between the two digits, typically seen at the distal phalanges. When syndactyly is associated with a syndrome, it is classified as complicated. Bilateral involvement is often observed. Involvement of the third web, between the long and ring fingers, is the most common presentation. When ulnar-sided syndactyly involving the small and ring finger is present, the possible association with oculodentodigital dysplasia syndrome should be evaluated[41] (**Figure 4**). In addition to hand involvement, oculodentodigital dysplasia syndrome, which is an autosomal dominant condition, includes dental and urologic abnormalities as well as neurologic problems such as paraparesis and cognitive difficulties. Patients with oculodentodigital dysplasia

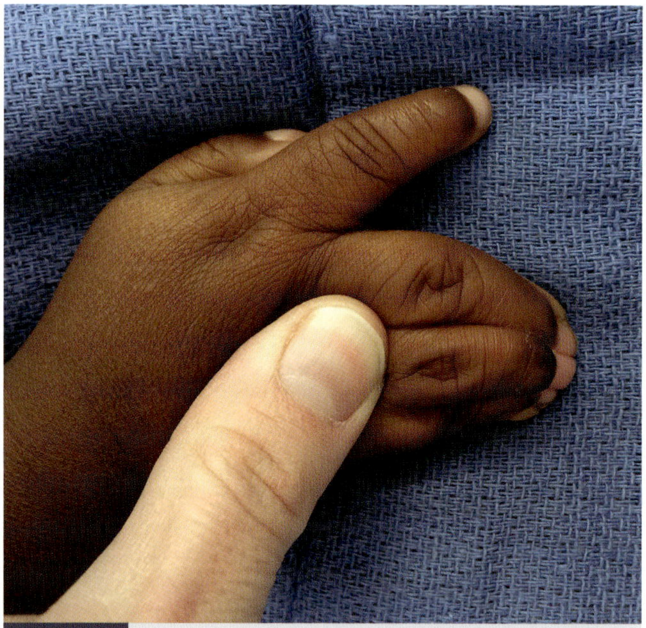

Figure 4 Clinical image of the hand of a child with oculodentodigital dysplasia. Note the ulnar-sided syndactyly.

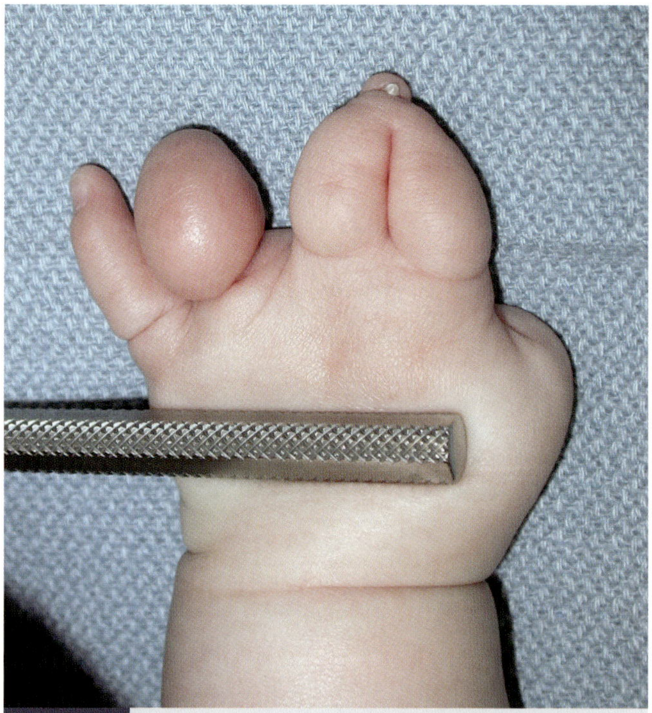

Figure 5 Clinical image of the hand of an infant with amniotic band syndrome. Note the constrictive band around the ring finger with distal amputation and acrosyndactyly between the index and middle digits.

syndrome should be referred to appropriate subspecialists to identify and treat the associated conditions in a timely manner.

Syndactyly reconstruction of central web spaces is recommended for children at 18 months to 2 years of age.[42,43] If there is syndactyly involving the border digits, earlier reconstruction, before 1 year of age, is advised to prevent contractures or deviation of the tethered digits.

Numerous techniques for syndactyly reconstruction have been described, with the general groups including reconstruction with or without skin grafting.[44-47] Techniques that do not use skin grafts require less surgical time and have no donor-site morbidity. Skin grafts can also have a less than optimal aesthetic appearance because of darkening over time and the potential for hair growth if skin is harvested from the groin. The advantages of skin grafting include decreasing the dorsal scar, providing complete wound coverage, and minimizing creep. If skin grafting is used, it can be harvested from the antecubital fossa or wrist flexion crease. Recently, the use of synthetic matrix has been reported in place of skin grafts for open areas after reconstruction.[48] This technique minimizes surgical time, morbidity, and scarring. Outcome evidence is limited as this time.

Deformations

Amniotic Band Syndrome

Amniotic band syndrome (ABS) is a condition characterized by circumferential bands around the limbs, acrosyndactyly, and amputated digits (**Figure 5**). The etiology of ABS is still unknown, but there are two prevailing theories: intrinsic and extrinsic.[49] The intrinsic theory hypothesizes that there is a genetic etiology for the bands. The common association of ABS with cleft palate supports this theory. In contrast, the extrinsic theory states that bands of amnion form and then wrap around the limbs and digits. This theory is supported by the presence of bands seen at birth and fused distal segments of digits with developed web spaces (acrosyndactyly).

Reconstruction of hands affected by ABS include release of the fused digits with skin grafting as needed and release of bands. Band reconstruction is performed by full-thickness band excision and repair with Z-plasty to break up the resulting scar.

Osteochondromatosis

Osteochondromatosis or multiple hereditary exostosis is a condition affecting the entire skeletal system and is frequently seen by pediatric orthopaedic surgeons. The condition results from mutations in the exostosin (*EXT*) genes (specifically *EXT1* or *EXT2* genes) and is autosomal dominant. Benign bony growths occur as the child grows, primarily at the ends of long bones or on flat bones, such as the scapula. The exostoses appear in childhood and then stop growing after the individual reaches skeletal maturity. If the exostoses continue to grow after skeletal maturity, evaluation for malignant transformation is needed.

With increasing size, the exostoses can cause pain or limb deformity, irritate adjacent structures, or limit joint motion. In any of these instances, surgery is indicated. Within the upper limbs, forearm exostoses can alter the growth and relationship of the radius and the ulna. Notably, distal ulnar exostoses can tether the distal radius and, over time, lead to radial head dislocation.[50] In addition, it has been shown that both decreased ulnar length and radial head dislocation are risk factors for limited forearm motion.[51]

Varied surgical approaches are available to treat forearm exostoses, with the goals of maintenance of forearm rotation and avoidance of radial head dislocation. One approach is the excision of exostoses and lengthening or corrective osteotomy of the radius or ulna. Alternatively, the radius and ulna can be untethered to allow continued but independent growth. The best timing for surgical treatment is currently unknown. Children can be monitored with serial radiographic studies; however, some investigators have found that simple excision of the exostoses is the optimal treatment of forearm exostoses.[52]

Summary

Congenital upper limb anomalies are uncommon. Efforts continue to determine the actual prevalence and global effects of these conditions. The functional and cosmetic implications of each anomaly are unique, and surgical intervention is dependent on the needs of the child and his or her family. Unfortunately, most research concerning surgical treatment is currently limited to small retrospective studies. There is a need for large, multicenter, prospective studies to advance the care of patients with congenital upper limb anomalies.

Key Study Points

- The OMT classification has been accepted for classifying congenital upper limb anomalies and is based on the developmental biology of the upper limb.
- Unilateral anomalies are often well tolerated; the child is able to compensate with the well-developed limb for function.
- An orthopaedic surgeon may be the first physician to identify a specific congenital anomaly in a child and therefore must be aware of associated conditions and syndromes and recommend appropriate testing or referral.

Annotated References

1. Sammer DM, Chung KC: Congenital hand differences: Embryology and classification. *Hand Clin* 2009;25(2):151-156.

2. Swanson AB: A classification for congenital limb malformations. *J Hand Surg Am* 1976;1(1):8-22.

3. Tonkin MA, Tolerton SK, Quick TJ, et al: Classification of congenital anomalies of the hand and upper limb: Development and assessment of a new system. *J Hand Surg Am* 2013;38(9):1845-1853 .

   The authors present and validate a new classification system of upper limb anomalies using the current knowledge of embryogenesis.

4. Ekblom AG, Laurell T, Arner M: Epidemiology of congenital upper limb anomalies in Stockholm, Sweden, 1997 to 2007: Application of the Oberg, Manske, and Tonkin classification. *J Hand Surg Am* 2014;39(2):237-248.

   This study was the first to apply the OMT classification to a specific population to determine feasibility and accuracy. The upper limb anomalies of all individuals born in Stockholm County between 1997 and 2007 were classified. Malformations were the most common anomaly, followed by deformations and dysplasias. Level of evidence: III.

5. Koskimies E, Lindfors N, Gissler M, Peltonen J, Nietosvaara Y: Congenital upper limb deficiencies and associated malformations in Finland: A population-based study. *J Hand Surg Am* 2011;36(6):1058-1065.

   This Finnish population study identified the incidence of congenital upper limb anomalies to be 5.25 in 10,000 live births. The classification system of the International Federation of Societies for Surgery of the Hand was used. Radial deficiencies were found to be the most common anomaly.

6. Goldfarb CA, Wall LB, Bohn DC, Moen P, Van Heest AE: Epidemiology of congenital upper limb anomalies in a Midwest United States population: An assessment using

the Oberg, Manske, and Tonkin classification. *J Hand Surg Am* 2015;40(1):127-32.e1-2.

Malformations were reported to be the most common congenital anomaly in this study, with 62% involving only the hand plate, and radial polydactyly being the most common hand anomaly. Level of evidence: III.

7. Bavinck JN, Weaver DD: Subclavian artery supply disruption sequence: Hypothesis of a vascular etiology for Poland, Klippel-Feil, and Möbius anomalies. *Am J Med Genet* 1986;23(4):903-918.

8. James MA, Bagley AM, Brasington K, Lutz C, McConnell S, Molitor F: Impact of prostheses on function and quality of life for children with unilateral congenital below-the-elbow deficiency. *J Bone Joint Surg Am* 2006;88(11):2356-2365.

9. James MA, Green HD, McCarroll HR Jr, Manske PR: The association of radial deficiency with thumb hypoplasia. *J Bone Joint Surg Am* 2004;86(10):2196-2205.

10. Goldfarb CA, Manske PR, Busa R, Mills J, Carter P, Ezaki M: Upper-extremity phocomelia reexamined: A longitudinal dysplasia. *J Bone Joint Surg Am* 2005;87(12):2639-2648.

11. Buck-Gramcko D: Radialization as a new treatment for radial club hand. *J Hand Surg Am* 1985;10(6 pt 2):964-968.

12. Kotwal PP, Varshney MK, Soral A: Comparison of surgical treatment and nonoperative management for radial longitudinal deficiency. *J Hand Surg Eur Vol* 2012;37(2):161-169.

At 20-years' follow-up, individuals treated with centralization or radialization were found to have better subjective and objective outcomes than nonsurgical control patients.

13. Damore E, Kozin SH, Thoder JJ, Porter S: The recurrence of deformity after surgical centralization for radial clubhand. *J Hand Surg Am* 2000;25(4):745-751.

14. Goldfarb CA, Murtha YM, Gordon JE, Manske PR: Soft-tissue distraction with a ring external fixator before centralization for radial longitudinal deficiency. *J Hand Surg Am* 2006;31(6):952-959.

15. Sabharwal S, Finuoli AL, Ghobadi F: Pre-centralization soft tissue distraction for Bayne type IV congenital radial deficiency in children. *J Pediatr Orthop* 2005;25(3):377-381.

16. Taghinia AH, Al-Sheikh AA, Upton J: Preoperative soft-tissue distraction for radial longitudinal deficiency: An analysis of indications and outcomes. *Plast Reconstr Surg* 2007;120(5):1305-1312, discussion 1313-1314.

17. Vuillermin C, Wall L, Mills J, et al: Soft tissue release and bilobed flap for severe radial longitudinal deficiency. *J Hand Surg Am* 2015;40(5):894-899.

RLD treated with soft-tissue release and a bilobed flap maintain wrist motion and achieve satisfying results in both function and appearance. Level of evidence: IV.

18. de Jong JP, Moran SL, Vilkki SK: Changing paradigms in the treatment of radial club hand: Microvascular joint transfer for correction of radial deviation and preservation of long-term growth. *Clin Orthop Surg* 2012;4(1):36-44.

The technique for using second metatarsophalangeal joint transfer for the treatment of RLD is described. The results in 24 cases are presented, with deformity correction reported in all of the patients, a 54% complication rate, and minimal donor-site morbidity.

19. Leri-Weill dyschondrosteosis. *Online Mendelian Inheritance in Man*. Available at: http://omim.org/entry/127300?search=leri-weill%20dyschondrosteosis&highlight=leriweill%20weill%20leri%20dyschondrosteosi. Accessed January 12, 2016.

Léri-Weill dyschondrosteosis is described along with clinical features, inheritance characteristics, molecular genetics, and diagnostic implications.

20. McCarroll HR Jr, James MA, Newmeyer WL III, Molitor F, Manske PR: Madelung's deformity: Quantitative assessment of x-ray deformity. *J Hand Surg Am* 2005;30(6):1211-1220.

21. Zebala LP, Manske PR, Goldfarb CA: Madelung's deformity: A spectrum of presentation. *J Hand Surg Am* 2007;32(9):1393-1401.

22. Harley BJ, Brown C, Cummings K, Carter PR, Ezaki M: Volar ligament release and distal radius dome osteotomy for correction of Madelung's deformity. *J Hand Surg Am* 2006;31(9):1499-1506.

23. Steinman S, Oishi S, Mills J, Bush P, Wheeler L, Ezaki M: Volar ligament release and distal radial dome osteotomy for the correction of Madelung deformity: Long-term follow-up. *J Bone Joint Surg Am* 2013;95(13):1198-1204.

At an average 25-years follow-up, volar ligament release and dome osteotomy for Madelung deformity provided a lasting correction with good to excellent functional outcomes. Patients with more severe disease or whole-bone involvement had less positive outcomes. Level of evidence: IV.

24. Ogino T, Minami A, Kato H: Clinical features and roentgenograms of symbrachydactyly. *J Hand Surg Br* 1989;14(3):303-306.

25. Dhalla R, Strecker W, Manske PR: A comparison of two techniques for digital distraction lengthening in skeletally immature patients. *J Hand Surg Am* 2001;26(4):603-610.

26. Goldberg NH, Watson HK: Composite toe (phalanx and epiphysis) transfers in the reconstruction of the aphalangic hand. *J Hand Surg Am* 1982;7(5):454-459.

27. Kay SP, Wiberg M: Toe to hand transfer in children: Part 1. Technical aspects. *J Hand Surg Br* 1996;21(6):723-734.

28. Blauth W: Der hypoplastische Daumen. *Arch Orthop Unfallchir* 1967;62:224-246.

29. Manske PR, McCarroll HR Jr, James M: Type III-A hypoplastic thumb. *J Hand Surg Am* 1995;20(2):246-253.

30. Manske PR: Index pollicization for thumb deficiency. *Tech Hand Up Extrem Surg* 2010;14(1):22-32.

31. Ogino T, Kato H: Clinical and experimental studies on ulnar ray deficiency. *Handchir Mikrochir Plast Chir* 1988;20(6):330-337.

32. Cole RJ, Manske PR: Classification of ulnar deficiency according to the thumb and first web. *J Hand Surg Am* 1997;22(3):479-488.

33. Wassel HD: The results of surgery for polydactyly of the thumb: A review. *Clin Orthop Relat Res* 1969;64:175-193.

34. Tonkin MA, Bulstrode NW: The Bilhaut-Cloquet procedure for Wassel types III, IV and VII thumb duplication. *J Hand Surg Eur Vol* 2007;32(6):684-693.

35. Baek GH, Gong HS, Chung MS, Oh JH, Lee YH, Lee SK: Modified Bilhaut-Cloquet procedure for Wassel type-II and III polydactyly of the thumb: Surgical technique. *J Bone Joint Surg Am* 2008;90(suppl 2 pt 1):74-86.

36. Baek GH, Gong HS, Chung MS, Oh JH, Lee YH, Lee SK: Modified Bilhaut-Cloquet procedure for Wassel type-II and III polydactyly of the thumb. *J Bone Joint Surg Am* 2007;89(3):534-541.

37. Goldfarb CA, Patterson JM, Maender A, Manske PR: Thumb size and appearance following reconstruction of radial polydactyly. *J Hand Surg Am* 2008;33(8):1348-1353.

38. Stutz C, Mills J, Wheeler L, Ezaki M, Oishi S: Long-term outcomes following radial polydactyly reconstruction. *J Hand Surg Am* 2014;39(8):1549-1552.

At more than 10 years follow-up, a revision rate of 19% was identified after radial polydactyly reconstruction. Patients with Flatt types III and IV had weaker pinch than the unaffected sides. All patients were satisfied with the surgical outcomes. Level of evidence: IV.

39. Temtamy S, McKusick VA: Synopsis of hand malformations with particular emphasis on genetic factors. *Birth Defects Orig Artic Ser* 1969;3:125-184.

40. Pritsch T, Ezaki M, Mills J, Oishi SN: Type A ulnar polydactyly of the hand: A classification system and clinical series. *J Hand Surg Am* 2013;38(3):453-458.

Type A polydactyly ranges in level of development, from metacarpal duplication to distal phalanx duplication. The authors of this study found that duplication at the metacarpal level was the most common type, with bilateral hand polydactyly involvement in 69% of patients. Associated syndromes or a congenital anomaly was reported in 24% of the patients. Level of evidence: IV.

41. Jones C, Baldrighi C, Mills J, Bush P, Ezaki M, Oishi S: Oculodentodigital dysplasia: Ulnar-sided syndactyly and its associated disorders. *J Hand Surg Am* 2011;36(11):1816-1821.

Oculodentodigital dysplasia is an autosomal dominant condition characterized by specific facial features, eye conditions, dental disorders, and ulnar-sided syndactyly. In addition, a 29% incidence of neurologic abnormalities were identified in this population. Level of evidence: IV.

42. Hutchinson DT, Frenzen SW: Digital syndactyly release. *Tech Hand Up Extrem Surg* 2010;14(1):33-37.

43. Dao KD, Shin AY, Billings A, Oberg KC, Wood VE: Surgical treatment of congenital syndactyly of the hand. *J Am Acad Orthop Surg* 2004;12(1):39-48.

44. Aydin A, Ozden BC: Dorsal metacarpal island flap in syndactyly treatment. *Ann Plast Surg* 2004;52(1):43-48.

45. Wafa AM: Hourglass dorsal metacarpal island flap: A new design for syndactylized web reconstruction. *J Hand Surg Am* 2008;33(6):905-908.

46. Greuse M, Coessens BC: Congenital syndactyly: Defatting facilitates closure without skin graft. *J Hand Surg Am* 2001;26(4):589-594.

47. Withey SJ, Kangesu T, Carver N, Sommerlad BC: The open finger technique for the release of syndactyly. *J Hand Surg Br* 2001;26(1):4-7.

48. Landi A, Garagnani L, Leti Acciaro A, Lando M, Ozben H, Gagliano MC: Hyaluronic acid scaffold for skin defects in congenital syndactyly release surgery: A novel technique based on the regenerative model. *J Hand Surg Eur Vol* 2014;39(9):994-1000.

At 24 months after surgery, 22 patients treated with graftless syndactyly reconstruction using hyaluronic acid scaffold had satisfactory outcomes, normal skin pigmentation, and minimal web creep. This approach presents a promising alternative to skin grafting for reconstruction.

49. Goldfarb CA, Sathienkijkanchai A, Robin NH: Amniotic constriction band: A multidisciplinary assessment of etiology and clinical presentation. *J Bone Joint Surg Am* 2009;91(suppl 4):68-75.

50. Gottschalk HP, Kanauchi Y, Bednar MS, Light TR: Effect of osteochondroma location on forearm deformity in patients with multiple hereditary osteochondromatosis. *J Hand Surg Am* 2012;37(11):2286-2293.

This retrospective study showed that patients with multiple hereditary osteochondromatosis had a 35% rate of radial head dislocation when there was a solitary distal ulnar osteochondroma. Level of evidence: IV.

51. Clement ND, Porter DE: Forearm deformity in patients with hereditary multiple exostoses: Factors associated with range of motion and radial head dislocation. *J Bone Joint Surg Am* 2013;95(17):1586-1592.

In a study of 212 forearms, the authors found that radial head dislocation and proportional ulnar length were independent risk factors for limited forearm motion in patients with multiple hereditary exostoses. Level of evidence: III.

52. Akita S, Murase T, Yonenobu K, Shimada K, Masada K, Yoshikawa H: Long-term results of surgery for forearm deformities in patients with multiple cartilaginous exostoses. *J Bone Joint Surg Am* 2007;89(9):1993-1999.

Chapter 18

Birth Brachial Plexus Palsy

Ann E. Van Heest, MD   Michael D. Partington, MD

Abstract

During the birthing process, injuries can occur to the brachial plexus that affect both motor and sensory functions of the upper limb. These injuries can be classified based on the anatomic characterization of the neurologic deficit. The patient evaluation primarily relies on serial physical examinations to track neurologic recovery, which is commonly documented using validated assessment tools such as the Active Movement Scale. Ancillary evaluations, including nerve conduction velocity studies, electromyography, MRI, CT, and ultrasonography, may be needed to further assess the extent of the neurologic injury and the prognosis for recovery. Neurosurgical treatment options include primary nerve surgery and/or nerve transfers. The shoulder is the most common site of chronic sequelae, including internal rotation contractures and the possible development of glenohumeral dysplasia.

Keywords: brachial plexus palsy; glenohumeral dysplasia; Narakas classification; primary nerve surgery

Introduction

Birth brachial plexus palsy (BBPP) is a neurologic injury occurring during the birthing process that results in paralysis and/or paresis and loss of sensation in the affected limb. BBPP occurs in approximately 0.4% to 2.6% of infants per 1,000 live births in the United States.[1] Risk factors for this neurologic injury include babies of abnormally large size (macrosomia); previous deliveries resulting in BBPP; prolonged labor, with vacuum or forceps delivery assistance; shoulder dystocia; and multiparous deliveries.[2] Although delivery via cesarean section does not eliminate the possibility of BBPP, the likelihood declines to 0.02% compared with 0.2% for a vaginal delivery.[1]

Approximately 75% of infants with BBPP will recover, leaving up to 25% of children with long-term deficits.[3] The reported degrees of clinical recovery may vary based on the time of treatment referral, the type of injury pattern, and subsequent treatment.

Evaluation

Classification

The original Seddon and Sunderland descriptions of nerve injuries are commonly used to classify peripheral nerve injuries in patients with BBPP.[4] Seddon described patterns of peripheral nerve injury as neurapraxia, axonotmesis, and neurotmesis. Sunderland expanded this classification to include neurapraxia (degree I), axonotmesis (degrees II and III), neuroma in continuity (degree IV), and neurotmesis (degree V). The Seddon and Sunderland classifications evaluate postganglionic peripheral nerve injuries and aid in predicting the prognosis for neurologic recovery and the need for surgical intervention[4] (**Table 1**).

An avulsion injury is another type of injury occurring specifically as part of BBPP. This preganglionic injury occurs at the spinal cord origin of the nerve roots. Avulsion injuries have the worst prognosis because spontaneous recovery is not possible, and such injuries cannot be surgically repaired. BBPP can include different types of preganglionic or postganglionic injury for each of the involved nerve roots, trunks, or divisions.

The Narakas classification is the most commonly used classification system for BBPP.[5] Narakas[6] subdivided these injuries based on the extent of plexus involvement, with type I involving the typical upper trunk (C5 and C6), type II including C5 and C6 with the addition of C7, type III

Dr. Van Heest or an immediate family member serves as a board member, owner, officer, or committee member of the Ruth Jackson Orthopaedic Society, the American Board of Orthopaedic Surgery, the American Society for Surgery of the Hand, and the American Orthopaedic Association. Neither Dr. Partington nor any immediate family member has received anything of value from or has stock or stock options held in a commercial company or institution related directly or indirectly to the subject of this chapter.

Table 1

Seddon and Sunderland Classification of Nerve Injury

Degree of Injury	Recovery	Rate of Recovery	Surgical Management
I, Neurapraxia	Complete	Up to 12 weeks	None
II, Axonotmesis	Complete	1 inch per month	None
III, Axonotmesis	Partial	1 inch per month	None or neurolysis
IV, Neuroma in continuity	None	None	Nerve repair, graft, or transfer
V, Neurotmesis	None	None	Nerve repair, graft, or transfer

being a pan-plexus injury, and type IV being a pan-plexus injury with associated Horner syndrome. Differentiating these types of injuries in a newborn is based on physical examination findings. The Narakas classification provides prognostic information that can help guide treatment. Patients with Narakas types I and II nerve injuries have substantially higher rates of recovery than those with Narakas types III or IV nerve injuries.[3,7] In the past, terminology has included terms such as Erb palsy; however, it is now preferable to describe the anatomic lesion (for example, upper trunk BBPP or pan-plexus BBPP).

Patient Evaluation

Making a diagnosis of BBPP requires a careful patient history, physical examination, and often radiographic studies. No other specific diagnostic testing is required if the history and physical examination are consistent with the characteristic features of BBPP. Most commonly, BBPP is diagnosed at the time of delivery. Most children with BBPP are large for their gestational age and are delivered after prolonged labor, often requiring the use of vacuum or forceps assistance. A known shoulder dystocia is common. After birth, abnormal movement of one upper limb is frequently noted. The muscle tone in the affected arm is usually flaccid or limp.

A radiograph may be taken to assess for fracture; radiography is mandated if the limb is painful with palpation. Initial management includes fracture management if a fracture is present; in these situations, it is difficult to discern whether the loss of normal movement of the arm is associated with pain from the fracture or concomitant BBPP. If loss of normal arm movement persists after the fracture heals, the diagnosis of BBPP is made.

The type of Narakas nerve injury is determined based on the physical examination of the newborn using active range of motion of the shoulder, elbow, forearm, wrist, and hand. All patients with Narakas type III or IV nerve injuries are referred directly to a center dedicated to treatment of BBPP. For patients with signs of recovery from Narakas type I or II nerve injuries, referral often is made at 2 to 4 weeks after birth if recovery is not complete. Some BBPPs are transient, and resolution is seen by the first checkup; these patients do not require referral. In infants who recover antigravity upper muscle strength in the first 2 months of life, a full and complete neurologic recovery can be expected.[8]

Each infant is examined for passive range of motion, active range of motion, and strength testing. Determining the presence or absence of Horner syndrome is important because signs of this syndrome are associated with a worse prognosis.[5,7] Horner syndrome is characterized by miosis (constricted pupils), partial ptosis (drooping eyelids), and anhidrosis (loss of hemifacial sweating).

Particular attention is given to assessing passive range of motion of the shoulder into external rotation with the arm at the side because loss of shoulder external rotation is associated with shoulder subluxation or dislocation.[9] It also is necessary to assess the infant's ability to bring his or her hand to his or her mouth against gravity (commonly called the cookie test) because absence of this ability has been used as an indication for surgical intervention.[10] In children with a pan-plexus injury, including Horner syndrome, phrenic nerve function is carefully assessed. Involvement can be assessed with ultrasound or chest radiographs and is important if general anesthesia is planned.[11]

Serial examinations of infants with BBPP allow tracking of neurologic recovery and determination of the need for surgery. For infants at a center dedicated to the treatment of BBPP, the Active Movement Scale (AMS) is the most commonly used and validated physical examination tool for tracking neurologic recovery.[9] The AMS gives an objective and validated measure to assess nerve deficits and subsequent recovery. Strength is graded on a 0 to 7 scale, with grades 0 to 4 as active movement with gravity eliminated and grades 5 to 7 as active movement against gravity; each level requires a demonstration of motion at the previous level.[5,9] The presence of any contracture is recorded, monitored, and treated with physical therapy interventions. For infants with a loss of shoulder external rotation, further evaluation with radiographic imaging or ultrasound is indicated.

Evaluation Methods

A recent meta-analysis of 307 articles examining BBPP found that the four most commonly used modalities for the diagnostic assessment of BBPP are electromyographic evaluations (standard and intraoperative), MRI, CT, and radiography.[5] The five most common methods for physically assessing the extent of BBPP are measurements of active and passive range of motion, the Mallet scale, the AMS, the Medical Research Council scale for muscle strength,[12] and the Narakas Motor Scale.[5] Only the AMS, the Mallet scale, and the Narakas Motor Scale have been validated in the BBPP population. In addition, performance-based functional outcome measures, such as the Assisting Hand Assessment, have been standardized and validated (per reports) within the BBPP population.[13]

Treatment

Early Therapy

Therapy starts immediately at the time of diagnosis, usually at birth, unless a concomitant fracture is present. If fracture is excluded and BBPP is diagnosed, initial management includes a supervised home therapy program to maintain passive range of motion. During the period of infancy, neurologic return is potentially occurring. Because the infant is not able to actively carry out certain movements because of paresis or paralysis, the caregiver must perform those movements for the infant to prevent contracture and promote awareness for neurologic return. Therapists monitor motor recovery and age-appropriate functional use of the limb. Cortical recognition and awareness of the affected limb is promoted using methods such as sensory stimulation. When neurologic return is imbalanced across a joint, the risk of contracture exists. This is particularly true in the shoulder. Because of the risk of internal rotation contracture, scapular stabilization and passive glenohumeral mobilization are frequently necessary. Instruction in performing a home therapy program and supervised professional monitoring are recommended.

Botulinum Toxin Injections: Techniques and Outcomes

Botulinum toxin injections have been described for use in BBPP for children with dynamic imbalance across a joint caused by disparate levels of neurologic return. The two most common case scenarios in BBPP are (1) neurologic return to the triceps that overpowers poor neurologic return to the biceps and (2) neurologic return to the shoulder internal rotator muscles that overpowers weak neurologic return to the shoulder external rotator muscles. For both of these clinical scenarios, botulinum toxin has been described for injection into the overpowering muscle (for example, the elbow extensor muscle or the shoulder internal rotator muscle) to facilitate functional use of the weak antagonist muscle. In a report of 1-month and 1-year results after the injection of botulinum toxin into the shoulder internal rotator muscles in 19 children with shoulder imbalance and into the elbow extensor muscles in 8 children with elbow imbalance, the results showed initial improvement in AMS scores in those with shoulder imbalance at 1 month; however, this improvement was not sustained at 1 year. The AMS scores of patients with elbow imbalance improved slightly at 1 month, and even greater improvement was found at 1 year because of the ongoing return of biceps neurologic function.[14] The use of botulinum toxin injections may be a temporizing measure only, but they are a treatment option in select children with BBPP with shoulder or elbow muscle imbalance.[14]

Primary Nerve Surgery: Technique and Outcomes

Most patients with BBPP recover spontaneously; however, for those who do not recover or those who have an incomplete recovery, surgical intervention is warranted. The indications for surgery are varied, but in infants with Narakas types III and IV pan-plexus injuries, the consensus is that surgery is indicated at 3 months of age. The rationale for surgery is that studies have consistently shown that all these children will have profound neurologic deficits without intervention.[8-10] Early surgical intervention in pan-plexus lesions may help minimize motor end plate loss and provide sufficient time for the return of neurologic function to the forearm and the hand. The three preferred options for primary nerve surgery in a patient with a pan-plexus lesion are plexus exploration with neurolysis, neuroma excision with sural nerve grafting, and outside-the-plexus reconstruction with nerve transfer procedures. Nerve procedures include transferring the terminal motor branches of the spinal accessory nerve to the suprascapular nerve or transferring the thoracic intercostal nerves to the musculocutaneous nerve for preganglionic avulsions.[2,8,9,15,16] Neurolysis alone has been shown to be ineffective in patients with pan-plexus injuries.[17]

The indications for and timing of treatment for infants with Narakas types I and II injuries are more controversial. Historically, it had been recommended that the absence of return of biceps function by 3 months of age was an indication for microsurgical intervention.[18] More recently, a failure to demonstrate elbow flexion as evaluated by the cookie test at 6 months of age has been advocated as an indication for microsurgical intervention.[8,9] However, a recent, large meta-analysis reported that delaying surgery (even beyond 6 months of age) for this patient group may yield better outcomes.[19] Currently, the inability to bring the hand to the mouth against gravity by 6 months of age is an accepted indication for surgical intervention.[2,11]

The preferred primary nerve surgery for patients with Narakas types I and II also is controversial. Although plexus exploration and neurolysis with excision of a nonconducting neuroma and nerve grafting are commonly used,[2,11] neurolysis alone for conducting neuromas in the upper trunk also has been described.[15,17,20]

Nerve Transfers: Techniques and Outcomes

Recent innovations in the treatment of infants with BBPP have included the increased use of nerve transfers, which also is known as secondary nerve surgery. Although the results of nerve transfer procedures have been increasingly reported in the adult population, such procedures in the treatment of infants remains unclear. A 2015 report by the International Federation of Societies for Surgery of the Hand stated that no existing evidence is available for using nerve transfers for primary nerve surgery in patients with BBPP. However, nerve transfers have been reported to be effective in infants with BBPP in specific clinical circumstances, including late presentation, isolated deficits, failed primary reconstruction, and the presence of multiple nerve root avulsions.[16] Two nerve transfer procedures for secondary nerve reconstruction to provide elbow flexion (the Oberlin procedure) and shoulder abduction (the Leechavengvongs procedure) have garnered notable attention.

Transfer of the ulnar and/or median nerve fascicles to the musculocutaneous nerve to provide elbow flexion is commonly termed the Oberlin procedure. Because this procedure has been used primarily in adult brachial plexus injuries, reports regarding results in children with BBPP are limited. A 2012 study reported on 17 infants treated with an Oberlin transfer at an average age of 12 months for absent elbow flexion caused by nerve root avulsion or failed primary nerve reconstruction.[21] At a mean follow-up of 31 months, the authors reported good to excellent results, with 3 patients achieving a modified British Medical Research Council scale grade of 2, 3 patients achieving a grade of 3, and 11 patients achieving a grade of 4. A 2014 study reported on 31 infants with BBPP treated with an Oberlin nerve transfer at 8 months of age.[22] At a mean follow-up of 35 months, 27 of the patients had an AMS score of 6 or 7, which is considered functional use of the elbow. In this study, four patients did not regain functional use of the elbow (final AMS score of less than 5). In these two reports, one patient had a transient anterior interosseous nerve deficit; no other donor deficit was noted.[16,21-26]

The Leechavengvongs procedure is one in which one branch of the radial nerve to the triceps muscle is transferred to the axillary nerve (deltoid muscle).[25] When combined with other shoulder stabilization procedures, improved shoulder function can be achieved with no weakness in elbow extension.[24]

Shoulder Techniques and Outcomes

A residual shoulder deficit is the most common chronic sequelae of BBPP. The authors of a 2014 study reviewed 69 children (median age, 14 years) to determine outcomes of BBPP. Reduced shoulder external rotation was found to be the most common deficit.[27] Early identification and treatment of glenohumeral dysplasia is a key factor in preventing chronic shoulder deficits.

The shoulder joint is particularly at risk for poor neurologic return, functional weakness, and skeletal deformity because of several neurologic factors. The upper trunk is most at risk for injury during the birthing process. In infants with Narakas type I injuries, the suprascapular nerve is at the greatest risk for injury because it is the first branch off the upper trunk, and it is tethered in its distal course into the suprascapular notch, which subjects it to the greatest stretch during shoulder dystocia during delivery. Across the shoulder joint, the internal rotator muscles (subscapularis, pectoralis major, latissimus dorsi, and teres major) often have excellent neurologic return and good functional strength in an isolated upper truck lesion. In contrast, the shoulder external rotator muscles (supraspinatus, infraspinatus, and teres minor) often have poor neurologic return and limited functional strength because of substantial injury to the suprascapular nerve and the axillary nerve in an upper trunk lesion. The strong internal rotators overpower the weak external rotators, leading to a power imbalance. A long-standing power imbalance between the two muscle groups can lead to internal rotation shoulder contractures and, eventually, shoulder subluxation and dislocation with the secondary skeletal changes of glenohumeral dysplasia.

During the past 10 years, ultrasound has been used extensively at most BBPP centers to diagnose glenohumeral subluxation or dislocation in infants during their first 12 months of life, before ossification of the humeral head. Ultrasound has been used in the diagnosis of hip dysplasia for decades, but its use in the shoulder for the diagnosis and treatment of glenohumeral dysplasia has more recently been described and validated, with comparison to the contralateral side to verify normal values based on patient age.[28] The most common sonographic measurements

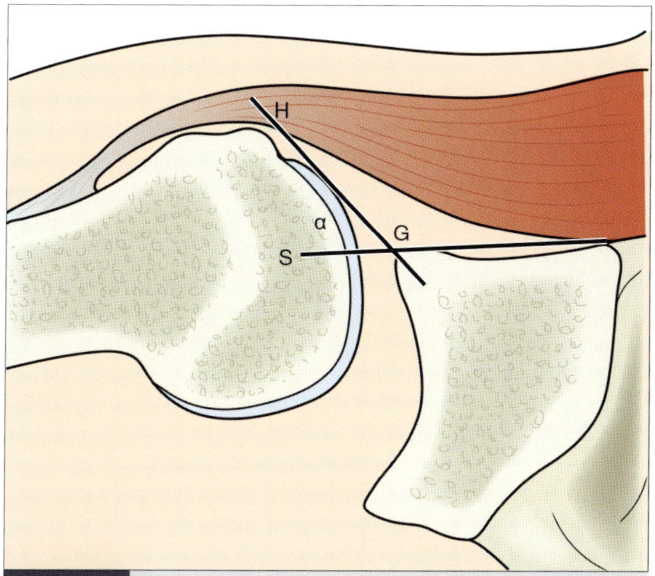

Figure 1 Illustration shows the method for calculating the α angle. The posterior osseous lip of the glenoid is identified (point G). A reference line (S) is drawn along the posterior scapular margin through point G. A tangential reference line (H) is drawn from the humeral head through point G.

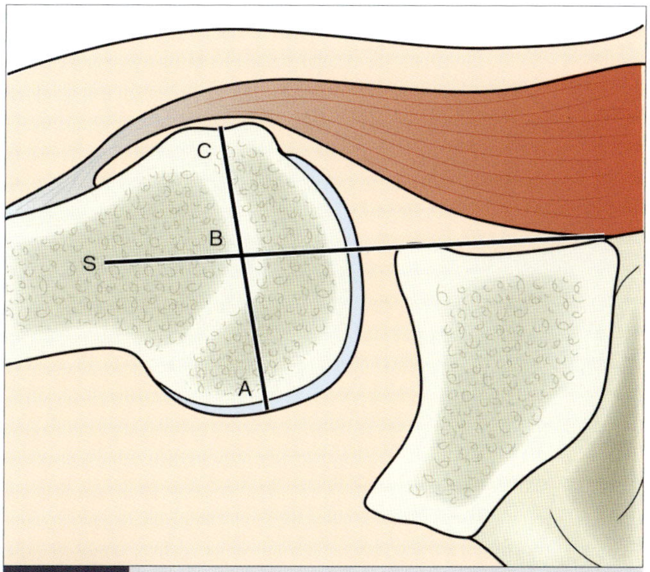

Figure 2 Illustration demonstrating the elements needed to calculate the percentage of humeral head displacement. A reference line (S) is drawn along the posterior scapular margin through the posterior osseous lip of the glenoid. Line AC is drawn at the greatest diameter of the humeral head. Point B is the intersection of line AC and line S. The humeral head displacement equals BC divided by AC multiplied by 100.

for assessing glenohumeral development are the alpha (α) angle and the percentage of humeral head dysplasia. Ultrasound can be performed in patients as young as 6 weeks. Normal values for the α angle are 30° or less, with the percentage of humeral head dysplasia less than 10% different from the contralateral (normal) side. The α angle is formed by the posterior scapular margin and a line tangent to the humeral head passing through the posterior osseous lip of the glenoid (**Figure 1**).

The second measurement is the percentage of humeral head displacement that is posterior to the posterior scapular margin. This measurement is determined from the ratio of the distance from the posterior scapular line to the posterior margin of the humeral head divided by the greatest diameter of the humeral head and then multiplied by 100 (**Figure 2**).

Shoulder Management

In a newborn, it is imperative to begin passive range of motion for all joints that are affected by a neurologic injury. In the shoulder, loss of shoulder external rotation is an indication that shoulder internal rotation contracture is developing, and the child is at risk for shoulder subluxation or dislocation. Prior to ossification, ultrasound can be used to diagnose subluxation or dislocation (**Figure 3**). MRI is an alternative advanced imaging option, but it requires general anesthesia for patients in this age group.

The treatment of shoulder dysplasia depends on the age at presentation. In children younger than 1 year, closed reduction with cast placement and botulinum toxin injection into the shoulder internal rotator muscles has been described. Surgery is indicated for children older than 1 year, those with persistent subluxation despite attempts at closed reduction, and when neurologic function of the shoulder external rotator muscles fails to return. A tendon transfer of the latissimus dorsi and the teres major is most commonly performed. Concomitant open or arthroscopic anterior release or open reduction with posterior capsulorrhaphy may be considered. Controversy exists in the literature regarding the timing and indications for these procedures.[2] In children younger than 18 months, remodeling of the glenohumeral joint after extra-articular procedures has been reported.[29] In children older than 7 years with a fixed glenohumeral dysplasia, treatment with derotation osteotomy of the proximal humerus may be considered[2] (**Figure 4**).

Summary

The ultimate goal of patient care during the birthing process is to prevent all birth injuries. The appropriate

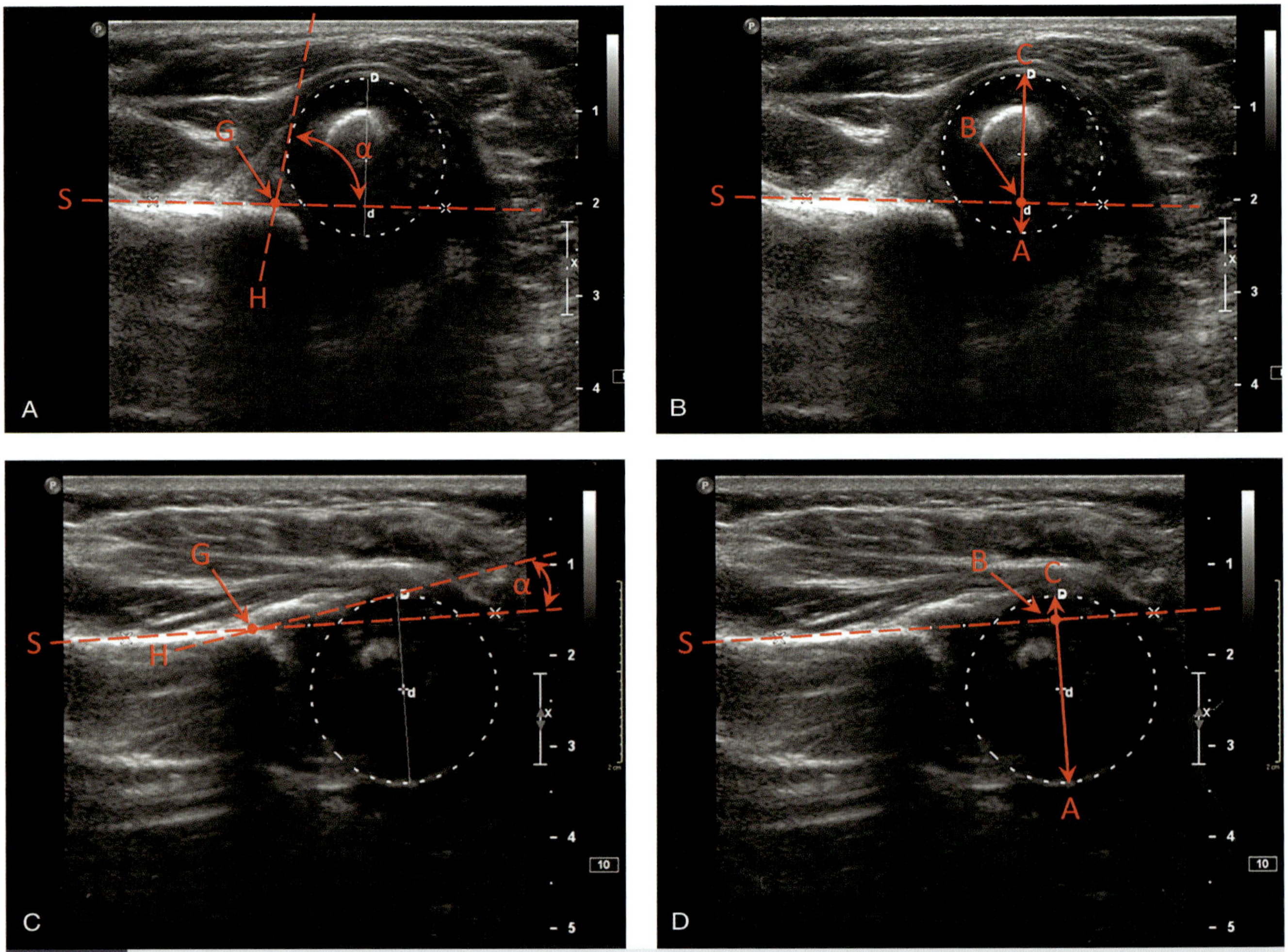

Figure 3 Ultrasound images of the shoulder of a 6-month-old infant who had loss of passive shoulder external rotation. Superimposed lines allow calculation of the α angle (see Figure 1) and the percentage of humeral head coverage (see Figure 2). **A,** Preoperative image shows a dislocated right shoulder in neutral position with a preoperative α angle of 81°. **B,** The preoperative humeral head coverage was calculated to be 19%. **C,** The patient was treated with a closed reduction while under general anesthesia. A shoulder spica cast was applied, and botulinum toxin was injected into the shoulder internal rotator muscles. Ultrasound image after treatment shows the reduced right shoulder in the neutral position with a postoperative α angle of 14°. **D,** Postoperative image shows humeral head coverage of 87%.

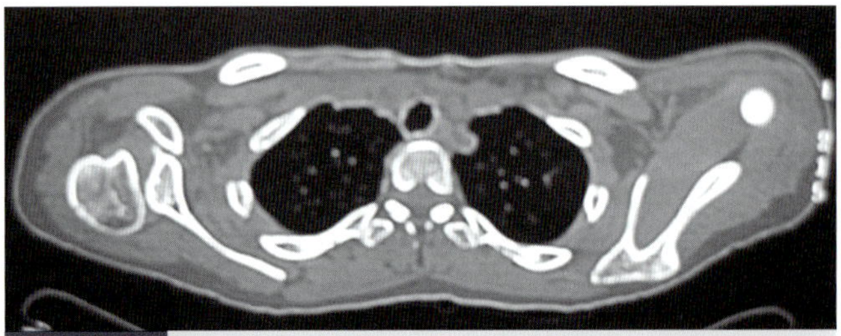

Figure 4 CT of the left shoulder of a 16-year-old patient with fixed glenohumeral dysplasia shows a flattened humeral head, retroversion of the glenoid, and posterior subluxation of the humeral head.

management of second-stage delivery, the appropriate use of forceps or vacuum suction, work on evidence-based guidelines for preventing shoulder dystocia in the delivery of large infants, and guidelines for proceeding to cesarean section may help decrease the number of infants with BBPP.

Although most infants with BBPP recover, approximately 25% of children have long-term deficits. Early therapy is important in the treatment of these patients and often leads to favorable outcomes. In those patients who do not have neurologic recovery or have only an incomplete recovery, surgical intervention is warranted.

Key Study Points

- During the birthing process, shoulder dystocia most commonly leads to injury of the upper trunk of the brachial plexus (C5-C6), which is a Narakas type I injury. The next most common injury occurs in the upper and middle trunk of the brachial plexus (C5 through C7), which is a Narakas type II injury.
- If a patient with a Narakas type I or II injury does not show sufficient neurologic return by 6 months of age (allowing the child to bring his or her hand to the mouth), surgical exploration with neurolysis or nerve resection and grafting is indicated.
- If a pan-plexus injury exists with no neurologic return by 3 months of age, brachial plexus exploration with nerve grafting is indicated, provided nerve root avulsions are not present.
- Nerve root avulsions are not surgically repairable and require alternative strategies such as nerve transfer to provide neurologic return.

Annotated References

1. Foad SL, Mehlman CT, Ying J: The epidemiology of neonatal brachial plexus palsy in the United States. *J Bone Joint Surg Am* 2008;90(6):1258-1264.

2. Hale HB, Bae DS, Waters PM: Current concepts in the management of brachial plexus birth palsy. *J Hand Surg Am* 2010;35(2):322-331.

3. Andersen J, Watt J, Olson J, Van Aerde J: Perinatal brachial plexus palsy. *Paediatr Child Health* 2006;11(2):93-100.

4. Sunderland S: *Nerves and Nerve Injuries* ,ed 2. London, England, Churchill Livingstone, 1978.

5. Chang KW, Justice D, Chung KC, Yang LJ: A systematic review of evaluation methods for neonatal brachial plexus palsy: A review. *J Neurosurg Pediatr* 2013;12(4):395-405.

   In a review of 307 articles on neonatal brachial plexus palsy, 126 clinical evaluation methods were identified, of which only five are specifically validated for this population. These methods include the AMS, the Toronto Scale Score, the Mallet Scale, the Assisting Hand Assessment, and the Pediatric Outcomes Data Collection Instrument. Level of evidence: II.

6. Narakas AO: Injuries of the brachial plexus and neighboring peripheral nerves in vertebral fractures and other trauma of the cervical spine [German]. *Orthopade* 1987;16(1):81-86.

7. Foad SL, Mehlman CT, Foad MB, Lippert WC: Prognosis following neonatal brachial plexus palsy: An evidence-based review. *J Child Orthop* 2009;3(6):459-463.

8. Waters PM: Comparison of the natural history, the outcome of microsurgical repair, and the outcome of operative reconstruction in brachial plexus birth palsy. *J Bone Joint Surg Am* 1999;81(5):649-659.

9. Clarke HM, Curtis CG: An approach to obstetrical brachial plexus injuries. *Hand Clin* 1995;11(4):563-580, discussion 580-581.

10. Michelow BJ, Clarke HM, Curtis CG, Zuker RM, Seifu Y, Andrews DF: The natural history of obstetrical brachial plexus palsy. *Plast Reconstr Surg* 1994;93(4):675-680, discussion 681.

11. Al-Qattan MM, Clarke HM, Curtis CG: The prognostic value of concurrent phrenic nerve palsy in newborn children with Erb's palsy. *J Hand Surg Br* 1998;23(2):225.

12. Frese E, Brown M, Norton BJ: Clinical reliability of manual muscle testing: Middle trapezius and gluteus medius muscles. *Phys Ther* 1987;67(7):1072-1076.

13. Holmefur M, Krumlinde-Sundholm L, Eliasson AC: Interrater and intrarater reliability of the Assisting Hand Assessment. *Am J Occup Ther* 2007;61(1):79-84.

14. Arad E, Stephens D, Curtis CG, Clarke HM: Botulinum toxin for the treatment of motor imbalance in obstetrical brachial plexus palsy. *Plast Reconstr Surg* 2013;131(6):1307-1315.

    The authors retrospectively reviewed 27 patients with BBPP treated with botulinum toxin injection for muscle imbalance. Outcomes were measured by comparing the change in AMS scores from preinjection scores to scores at 1 month and 1 year after injection. Botulinum toxin injections for shoulder movement imbalance produce improvement in external rotation that is not sufficiently sustained over time to be of clinical benefit; however, injections for elbow movement imbalance produce a sustained and clinically useful improvement. Level of evidence: IV.

15. Lin JC, Schwentker-Colizza A, Curtis CG, Clarke HM: Final results of grafting versus neurolysis in obstetrical brachial plexus palsy. *Plast Reconstr Surg* 2009;123(3):939-948.

16. Tse R, Kozin SH, Malessy MJ, Clarke HM: International Federation of Societies for Surgery of the Hand committee report: The role of nerve transfers in the treatment of neonatal brachial plexus palsy. *J Hand Surg Am* 2015;40(6):1246-1259.

    The International Federation of Societies for Surgery of the Hand reported that, although the role of nerve transfers for primary nerve reconstruction remains to be defined, nerve transfers have been found to be effective and useful in specific clinical circumstances, including late presentations, isolated deficits, failed primary reconstructions, and multiple nerve root avulsions. Level of evidence: V.

17. Clarke HM, Al-Qattan MM, Curtis CG, Zuker RM: Obstetrical brachial plexus palsy: Results following neurolysis of conducting neuromas-in-continuity. *Plast Reconstr Surg* 1996;97(5):974-982, discussion 983-984.

18. Gilbert A, Tassin JL: Surgical repair of the brachial plexus in obstetric paralysis [French]. *Chirurgie* 1984;110(1):70-75.

19. Ali ZS, Bakar D, Li YR, et al: Utility of delayed surgical repair of neonatal brachial plexus palsy. *J Neurosurg Pediatr* 2014;13(4):462-470.

    In a large meta-analysis of clinical series used to develop decision analysis, it was found that decision for surgery at 12 months versus no surgery or surgery at 3 or 6 months was strongly associated with differences in outcomes in patients with BBPP. Later surgery is associated with better outcomes. Level of evidence: IV.

20. Andrisevic E, Taniguchi M, Partington MD, Agel J, Van Heest AE: Neurolysis alone as the treatment for neuroma-in-continuity with more than 50% conduction in infants with upper trunk brachial plexus birth palsy. *J Neurosurg Pediatr* 2014;13(2):229-237.

    In a series of 17 patients with upper trunk injuries, neurolysis was effective in improving motor outcome at 1 year. More than 50% of the patients had improvements in shoulder flexion, shoulder abduction, and elbow flexion. Another one-third of the patients experienced improved shoulder external rotation. Level of evidence: IV.

21. Siqueira MG, Socolovsky M, Heise CO, Martins RS, Di Masi G: Efficacy and safety of Oberlin's procedure in the treatment of brachial plexus birth palsy. *Neurosurgery* 2012;71(6):1156-1160, discussion 1161.

    A series of 17 patients with BBPP underwent Oberlin nerve transfers (ulnar nerve to musculocutaneous nerve) after surgical confirmation of a nerve root avulsion, a failed primary repair procedure, or a late referral. A good to excellent biceps score was reported in more than 82% of the patients, with no new hand deficits. Level of evidence: IV.

22. Little KJ, Zlotolow DA, Soldado F, Cornwall R, Kozin SH: Early functional recovery of elbow flexion and supination following median and/or ulnar nerve fascicle transfer in upper neonatal brachial plexus palsy. *J Bone Joint Surg Am* 2014;96(3):215-221.

    The authors retrospectively reviewed 31 patients at three institutions who had undergone ulnar and/or median nerve fascicle transfer to the biceps and/or brachialis branches of the musculocutaneous nerve after BBPP. Twenty-seven of the 31 patients (87%) achieved functional elbow flexion (AMS $\geq$ 6), and 24 of the 31 patients (77%) had full recovery of elbow flexion against gravity (AMS = 7). Level of evidence: IV.

23. Al-Qattan MM, Al-Kharfy TM: Median nerve to biceps nerve transfer to restore elbow flexion in obstetric brachial plexus palsy. *Biomed Res Int* 2014;2014:854084.

    The authors reported on 10 children with BBPP who were treated with partial median nerve transfer to the musculocutaneous nerve. All the patients were 13 to 19 months of age with poor or no recovery of elbow flexion. After the nerve transfer, nine children recovered elbow flexion (AMS score of 6 or 7). The remaining child did not recover elbow flexion. Level of evidence: IV.

24. Leechavengvongs S, Witoonchart K, Uerpairojkit C, Thuvasethakul P, Malungpaishrope K: Combined nerve transfers for C5 and C6 brachial plexus avulsion injury. *J Hand Surg Am* 2006;31(2):183-189.

25. Leechavengvongs S, Witoonchart K, Uerpairojkit C, Thuvasethakul P: Nerve transfer to deltoid muscle using the nerve to the long head of the triceps, part II: A report of 7 cases. *J Hand Surg Am* 2003;28(4):633-638.

26. Oberlin C, Béal D, Leechavengvongs S, Salon A, Dauge MC, Sarcy JJ: Nerve transfer to biceps muscle using a part of ulnar nerve for C5-C6 avulsion of the brachial plexus: Anatomical study and report of four cases. *J Hand Surg Am* 1994;19(2):232-237.

27. Hulleberg G, Elvrum AK, Brandal M, Vik T: Outcome in adolescence of brachial plexus birth palsy: 69 individuals re-examined after 10-20 years. *Acta Orthop* 2014;85(6):633-640.

    In a cohort of 69 children with BBPP who were seen at a mean follow-up age of 14 years, 17 had a permanent lesion but were mainly independent in activities of daily living. Shoulder external rotation was the most common deficit. Level of evidence: IV.

28. Vathana T, Rust S, Mills J, et al: Intraobserver and interobserver reliability of two ultrasound measures of humeral head position in infants with neonatal brachial plexus palsy. *J Bone Joint Surg Am* 2007;89(8):1710-1715.

29. Van Heest A, Glisson C, Ma H: Glenohumeral dysplasia changes after tendon transfer surgery in children with birth brachial plexus injuries. *J Pediatr Orthop* 2010;30(4):371-378.

Chapter 19

Congenital Transverse Deficiency of the Upper Limb

Apurva S. Shah, MD, MBA   Stephanie Thibaudeau, MD

Abstract

Transverse deficiency is a rare congenital anomaly that is typically sporadic and unilateral. This deficiency reflects the failure of embryonic limb development in the proximodistal axis and results in the absence of the distal limb but with proximal structures essentially spared. The treatment of a patient with a transverse deficiency involves function optimization as well as patient and family education to improve the child's quality of life.

Keywords: congenital hand; prosthesis; transverse deficiency

Introduction

A transverse deficiency is a rare congenital anomaly that occurs in approximately 1 in 12,300 live births.[1] The most common form is a congenital proximal forearm (below-elbow) amputation that is typically sporadic and unilateral (70% to 96% of all instances) and rarely associated with other congenital anomalies.[1,2]

Incidence and Embryology

Transverse deficiency reflects the failure of embryonic limb development in the proximodistal axis and results in the absence of the distal limb but with proximal structures essentially spared (**Figure 1**). The limb bud appears during the fourth week of gestation, with growth and development occurring in three planes: proximodistal, ventrodorsal, and anterior-posterior (radioulnar). The apical ectodermal ridge (AER), a rim of epithelial cells at the distal extent of the limb bud, has been shown to be critical for outgrowth of the limb. AER function is mediated through fibroblast growth factor signaling to the underlying mesenchymal cells, thus preventing cell death and maintaining mesenchymal cell proliferation.[3,4] In animal models, injury to the AER results in transverse deficiency.[5] Traditionally, the area of proliferating mesenchymal cells underlying the AER was characterized by the progress zone model, where the fate of these pluripotent cells depended on their time of exit from the influence of the AER, with later exit giving rise to more distal elements. Some authors have recently questioned the time-dependent nature of this model and rather propose the prespecified model,[3,4,6,7] in which all the precursor cells are present early in the limb bud, with cells contributing to the proximal limb elements proliferating earlier than cells contributing to distal elements (**Figure 2**).

In most patients, transverse deficiency is unilateral and affects the upper limb two to three times more commonly than the lower limb.[8,9] One study noted that 93% of patients with a transverse deficiency have soft-tissue nubbins, skin invaginations, or hypoplasia of the proximal radius and ulna on the residual limb.[10] These findings support the concept that transverse deficiency and symbrachydactyly represent a continuum of a single disease process.[10]

The exact mechanism or teratogens through which transverse deficiency occurs are unknown, although an impediment in the vascular supply of the limb during development is thought to contribute to the pathophysiology. This theory arose from associating symbrachydactyly with Poland syndrome, which, along with the Klippel-Feil and Möbius syndromes, is grouped under the subclavian disruption sequence hypothesis.[11] Approximately 40% of patients with Poland syndrome, which is an absence of the pectoralis major muscle, also have

Dr. Shah or an immediate family member serves as a board member, owner, officer, or committee member of the Pediatric Orthopaedic Society of North America and the American Society for Surgery of the Hand. Neither Dr. Thibaudeau nor any immediate family member has received anything of value from or has stock or stock options held in a commercial company or institution related directly or indirectly to the subject of this chapter.

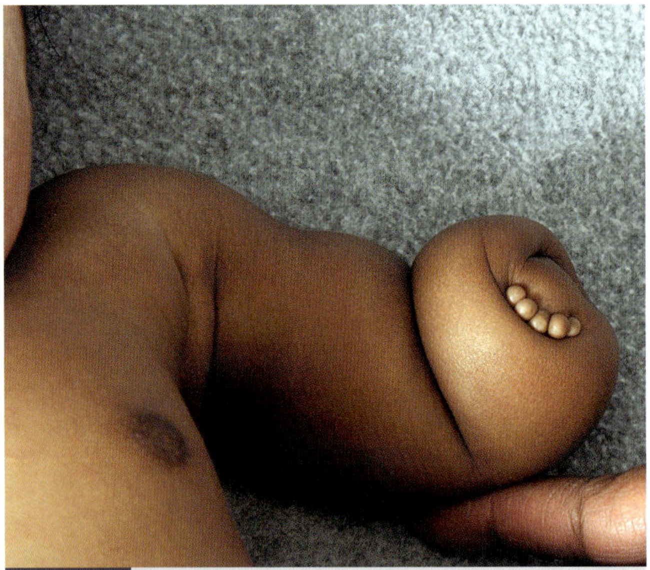

Figure 1 Photograph of the limb of a child with transverse deficiency of the upper limb. (Courtesy of Charles Goldfarb, MD, St. Louis, MO.)

symbrachydactyly.[12] Adams-Oliver syndrome often occurs in conjunction with aplasia cutis congenita and may indicate a vascular pathway as an etiology of transverse deficiency.[13] Maternal misoprostol ingestion also has been associated with transverse deficiency (odds ratio of 11.9).[14]

The pathophysiology and characteristics of transverse deficiency are important to recognize to differentiate transverse deficiency from other congenital limb anomalies that also may appear to have a transverse loss. The differential diagnoses include amniotic band syndrome (1 in 16,100 live births), longitudinal deficiency (1 in 3,700 live births), and hypodactyly/undergrowth (1 in 8,400 live births).[1] Longitudinal deficiencies affect anteroposterior growth, resulting in the absence of radial or ulnar structures. In contrast, in transverse deficiency or symbrachydactyly, where the ectodermal elements (nails, distal phalanges) are preserved, hypodactyly results in the loss of all ectodermal elements.[15] Amniotic band syndrome can be differentiated by other associated features, such as multiple limb involvement, cleft lip, lymphedema, acrosyndactyly, and lower limb constriction bands or amputations.[16]

Evaluation: Upper Limb Function and Quality of Life

In congenital hand deficiencies, clinicians often disproportionately focus on physical domains, such as body structure and function, because they are more tangible and easier to measure objectively compared with psychosocial issues. To integrate the psychosocial effects of health status on an individual, the World Health Organization created the International Classification of Functioning, Disability, and Health (WHO-ICF), which describes a health state by four domains: body structure, body function, environmental factors, and activity and participation.[17] Ideally, patient-reported outcome measures (PROMs) should address all WHO-ICF domains. A recent comprehensive review of the literature evaluated whether PROMs used to evaluate the treatment of congenital hand deficiency captured WHO-ICF domains.[18] PROMs covered a mean of 1.3 WHO-ICF domains when evaluating the treatment of congenital hand deficiency. The Prosthetic Upper Limb Functional Index was the only PROM in the review that was specifically validated for children with transverse deficiencies. Further development of PROMs that specifically address congenital hand deficiency and its subclassifications is required.

Importantly, patients' and parents' perception of the disability may be discordant, reflecting the importance of collecting information from both patients and parents.[19] A group of 439 children and adolescents with congenital below-elbow transverse deficiency and their parents were administered the Pediatric Outcomes Data Collection Instrument (PODCI) and the Pediatric Quality of Life Inventory (PedsQL).[20] High social functioning and upper limb function were reported within the normal range by both children and their parents. However, the children reported better upper limb function on the PODCI and better social functioning on the PedsQL compared with the reports of their parents. However, the parents overestimated the scores for comfort in the pain-comfort domain of the PODCI.[20] As the child ages, clinicians may need to pay particular attention to physical domains, such as bodily pain and comfort, because these have been correlated with lower health-related quality of life (HRQoL) scores in adults.[21] It is hypothesized that chronic compensatory behaviors and prosthetic use can lead to increased strain and pain that are eventually manifested as decreased HRQoL scores.[21] However, early psychosocial support and a multidisciplinary team approach in treating children with complex limb deformities may facilitate acceptance and improved self-esteem.[22]

Treatment and Upper Limb Prostheses

The treatment of patients with transverse deficiency involves function optimization as well as patient and family education to improve the child's quality of life. Surgery is infrequently needed. Historically, many healthcare

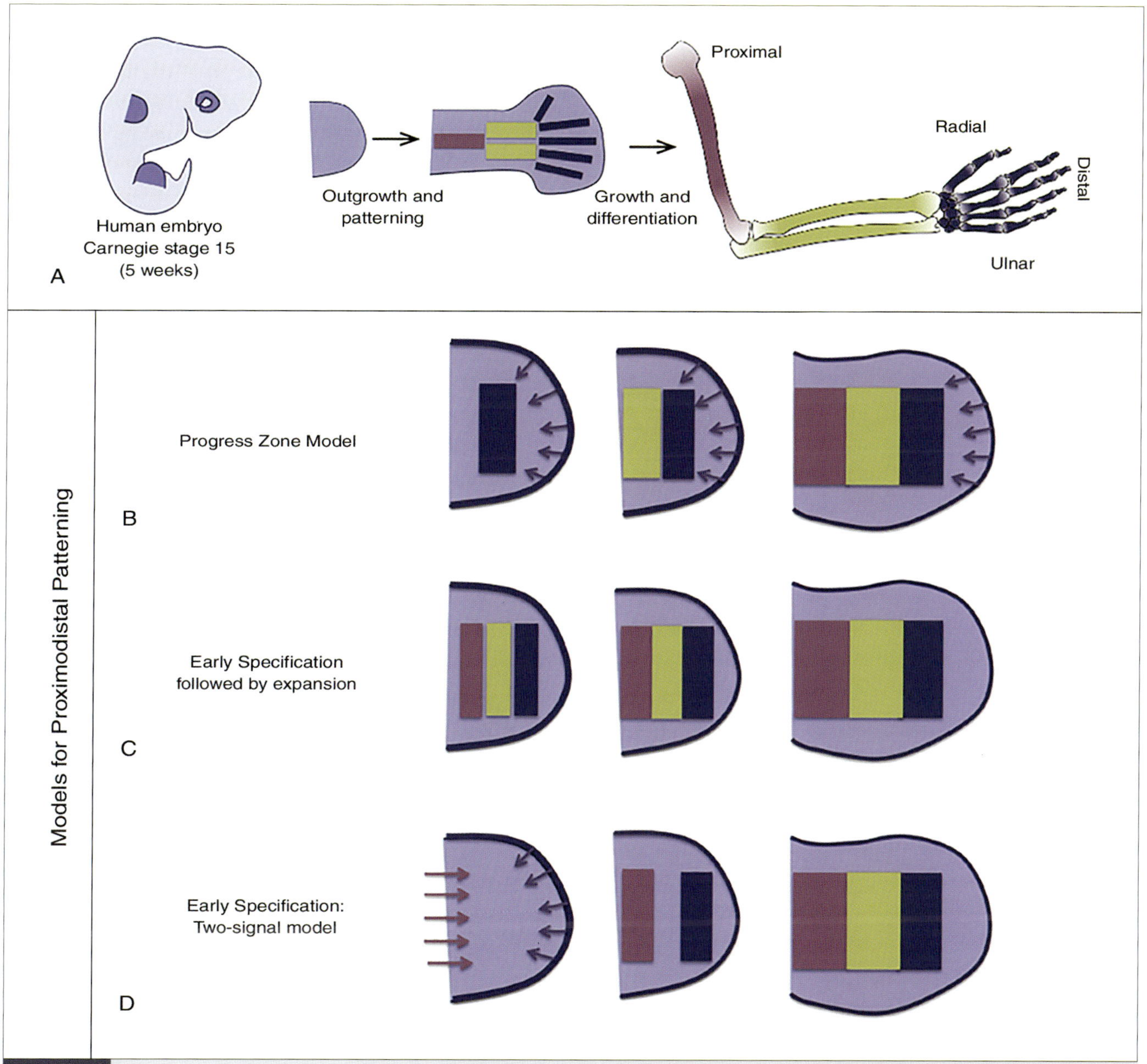

Figure 2 Illustration of embryology of proximodistal limb development. **A,** The limb bud emerges as a bud of mesenchymal cells encased in an ectodermal hull. Patterning (indicated by the color coding) is needed to establish the different proximodistal compartments of the limb. Three models (**B** through **D**) have been proposed to describe how this patterning arises. The validity of the progress zone model has recently been questioned. (Reproduced with permission from Vogeli KM, Mariani FV, Lightdale N: Updated embryology of the upper limb. *J Hand Surg Am* 2014;39[4]:811-812.)

professionals thought that the function of a child with transverse deficiency would improve by using an upper limb prosthesis. Traditionally, a passive prosthesis was fitted at 6 months of age, approximately when a child begins to sit independently and perform basic bimanual tasks at the midline. As time progresses, with increasing strength and functional demands, the passive prosthesis is replaced with an active prosthesis, often between the ages of 2 and 5 years. However, prosthesis rejection rates have been reported to range from 10% to 49%, and the optimal timing and use of prostheses in children with congenital transverse deficiency is controversial.[23-27] In a large cohort study of 256 patients, 49% of the patients were noncompliant in prosthesis use.[25] Fitting a child prior to 3 years of age improved long-term compliance, although there was no difference in compliance if a child was fitted prior to 1 year of age. Prosthetic fitting before 1 year of age may inhibit neurosensory input during the learning of bimanual activities and may delay the achievement of developmental milestones such as crawling.

Upper limb prostheses can be divided into passive and active groups, with the active group further subdivided into body-powered or myoelectric prostheses. A body-powered prosthesis is controlled through residual shoulder muscles that mechanically transmit movement through a harness to a voluntary opening or voluntary closing terminal device. A myoelectric prosthesis is electrically powered through electromyographic (EMG) signals of one or two groups of residual muscles. A group of 34 children from the Shriners Hospital for Children in Minnesota was given multiple prosthetic choices; these children most often selected a simple cosmetic passive hand (passive prosthesis) and a body-powered prosthesis with a voluntary closing terminal device. A myoelectric prosthesis was preferred in fewer than 15% of the children.[28] Another study found higher success rates with active prostheses if application of the active terminal device was accompanied with an intensive training program that involved short-term hospitalization.[25] Offering a variety of different prosthetic options appears to improve long-term prosthetic use.[25,28,29]

A multicenter study across Shriners Hospitals in North America explored the reasons for prosthetic rejection by children with unilateral congenital transverse forearm total deficiency.[24] The two most common reasons for discontinuing the use of prosthesis were lack of functional gain (53%) and lack of comfort (49%). Overall, the literature seems to indicate that traditional prosthetic wear in children with transverse deficiency does not translate into improved functionality or improvement in HRQoL scores.[30]

A multidisciplinary approach, with surgeons, therapists, and prosthetists working with the family and patient throughout growth, might provide patients with transverse deficiencies with the tools and prosthetic flexibility required for optimal use and cosmesis. Cost, limited funding, and the need for frequent prosthetic adjustments in a growing child can further contribute to prosthetic rejection rates.[29] A body-powered prosthesis for a below-elbow amputation ranges from $4,000 to $8,000, whereas a myoelectric prosthesis ranges between $25,000 and $50,000.[31] The process of three-dimensional printing of upper-limb prostheses may soon become streamlined. Increased access to advanced computer imaging, the decreased cost of three-dimensional printed prostheses, and the ability to allow remote fitting of a prosthesis may allow more children access to prosthetic devices.[32,33] In a case study for an adult patient with a transradial amputation, the cost of a three-dimensional printed myoelectric prosthesis was $300.[33] Nonprofit organizations, such as Enabling the Future, which provides free three-dimensional printed upper limb prostheses for children in need, may further help the medical community improve and tailor prostheses for the specific needs of children.[34]

Loss of sensory feedback from prosthetic wear is arguably the primary reason for limited functional gains and low compliance. Technologic advances in prosthetics, such as targeted muscle reinnervation and sensory biofeedback through neural interfaces, may overcome these obstacles. Targeted muscle reinnervation consists of transferring nerves from the nonfunctional limb segment to the chest wall or upper arm musculature (pectoralis major) to provide additional EMG output signals, thus refining the control and complexity of prosthetic actions.[35] Targeted sensory nerve transfers provide reinnervated areas on the chest wall that represent the amputated hand.[36] Sensory input through direct peripheral nerve interfaces (that is, intraneural electrodes) and regenerative peripheral nerve interfaces (muscle neurotized through a sensory nerve fascicle) are under investigation and have a promising future for real-time sensory feedback, obviating the need for visual cues.[37] Brain-machine interfaces are another novel method to control a prosthesis through electroencephalography and bypass the peripheral nervous system. The development of hybrid brain-machine interfaces with multiple inputs, including electroencephalography, EMG, and electrooculography, will improve the ability of patients to perform functional tasks through brain control.[38]

Further treatment options may arise from the microsurgical reconstruction of transverse deficiencies. The success of a pediatric hand transplant in the United States for a young child already receiving immunosuppression therapy for a kidney transplant and with below-elbow amputations secondary to sepsis, may open the door for future applications of vascularized composite allotransplantation.[39] Careful candidate selection cannot be overemphasized because vascularized composite allotransplantation requires lifelong immunosuppression therapy; its side effects have important ethical implications and potentially serious health repercussions in pediatric patients. Future advances in immunosuppression therapy and regeneration may broaden the indications for vascularized composite allotransplantation.[40]

Organ regeneration may present additional opportunities in the distant future. Organ regeneration requires three steps: (1) the formation of all cell types comprising the organ, (2) tissue organization, and (3) the creation of a three-dimensional morphology of the organ.[41] Major strides in molecular biology and genetics have helped in the better understanding of limb regeneration in vertebrate models, such as the zebra fish and the axolotl.[41,42] Amputation of the limb is followed by epithelization from cells at the circumference of the stump. These epithelial cells then proliferate to form the apical epithelial cap. The blastemal cells, which are undifferentiated mesenchymal cells, proliferate under the apical epithelial cap and contribute to limb regeneration. Most interestingly, these cells maintain positional memory of their proximodistal location and thus allow for maintenance of the three-dimensional morphology of the regenerating limb.[41] Maintenance of the apical epithelial cap and blastemal cell formation is dependent on peripheral nerve innervation.[43] Further characterization of these events, in particular the ability of blastemal cells to maintain positional memory, may allow researchers to develop blastemal cells for mammalian embryos and eventually limb regeneration.

Summary

Congenital transverse deficiency results from the failure of embryonic limb development in the proximodistal axis. Injury, whether mechanical or vascular, to the AER in utero is thought to result in transverse deficiency. Because of shared clinical features, transverse deficiency appears to represent the proximal continuum of symbrachydactyly. The use of prosthetics in patients with transverse deficiency remains controversial, but providing patients and families with multiple options appears to maximize adoption rates for prosthesis use. Technologic advances in engineering and computing have allowed for technologic advances in prostheses, including targeted muscle reinnervation and three-dimensional printed prostheses. Future advances in molecular biology and genetics may allow for limb regeneration and/or immune tolerance for vascularized composite allotransplantation.

Key Study Points

- Congenital transverse deficiency results from the failure of embryonic upper limb development in the proximodistal axis.
- Patients with transverse deficiency and their parents report social functioning and upper limb function within normal ranges.
- Pediatric prosthesis rejection ranges from 10% to 49%. Two main reasons for prosthetic discontinuation are a lack of functional gains and discomfort.

Annotated References

1. Koskimies E, Lindfors N, Gissler M, Peltonen J, Nietosvaara Y: Congenital upper limb deficiencies and associated malformations in Finland: A population-based study. *J Hand Surg Am* 2011;36(6):1058-1065.

   The incidence of upper limb deficiencies, as classified by the International Federation of Societies for Surgery of the Hand in Finland, was analyzed with data from the 1993 to 2005 Finnish Register of Congenital Malformations. The incidence of transverse arrest was 0.81 per 10,000 live births.

2. Jain SK: A study of 200 cases of congenital limb deficiencies. *Prosthet Orthot Int* 1994;18(3):174-179.

3. Dudley AT, Ros MA, Tabin CJ: A re-examination of proximodistal patterning during vertebrate limb development. *Nature* 2002;418(6897):539-544.

4. Sun X, Mariani FV, Martin GR: Functions of FGF signalling from the apical ectodermal ridge in limb development. *Nature* 2002;418(6897):501-508.

5. Oberg KC, Feenstra JM, Manske PR, Tonkin MA: Developmental biology and classification of congenital anomalies of the hand and upper extremity. *J Hand Surg Am* 2010;35(12):2066-2076.

6. Duboule D: Making progress with limb models. *Nature* 2002;418(6897):492-493.

7. Saunders JW Jr: Is the progress zone model a victim of progress? *Cell* 2002;110(5):541-543.

8. Gold NB, Westgate MN, Holmes LB: Anatomic and etiological classification of congenital limb deficiencies. *Am J Med Genet A* 2011;155A(6):1225-1235.

   The incidence of limb deficiencies was tabulated from the hospital-based Active Malformations Surveillance Program at Brigham and Women's Hospital in Boston (from 1972 to 1974 and 1979 to 2000). Infants who were affected were classified based on the anatomy and apparent cause of their deficiencies.

9. Ephraim PL, Dillingham TR, Sector M, Pezzin LE, Mackenzie EJ: Epidemiology of limb loss and congenital limb deficiency: A review of the literature. *Arch Phys Med Rehabil* 2003;84(5):747-761.

10. Kallemeier PM, Manske PR, Davis B, Goldfarb CA: An assessment of the relationship between congenital transverse deficiency of the forearm and symbrachydactyly. *J Hand Surg Am* 2007;32(9):1408-1412.

11. Bavinck JN, Weaver DD: Subclavian artery supply disruption sequence: Hypothesis of a vascular etiology for Poland, Klippel-Feil, and Möbius anomalies. *Am J Med Genet* 1986;23(4):903-918.

12. Woodside JC, Light TR: Symbrachydactyly: Diagnosis, function, and treatment. *J Hand Surg Am* 2016;41(1):135-143.

This article reviews the various clinical presentations of symbrachydactyly and its treatment.

13. Snape KM, Ruddy D, Zenker M, et al: The spectra of clinical phenotypes in aplasia cutis congenita and terminal transverse limb defects. *Am J Med Genet A* 2009;149A(8):1860-1881.

14. da Silva Dal Pizzol T, Knop FP, Mengue SS: Prenatal exposure to misoprostol and congenital anomalies: Systematic review and meta-analysis. *Reprod Toxicol* 2006;22(4):666-671.

15. Knight JB, Pritsch T, Ezaki M, Oishi SN: Unilateral congenital terminal finger absences: A condition that differs from symbrachydactyly. *J Hand Surg Am* 2012;37(1):124-129.

The authors present a retrospective review of 19 patients with unilateral congenital anomalies consisting of either absent or short bulbous fingers that lack terminal ectodermal elements, which is consistent with hypodactyly, a clinical entity distinct from symbrachydactyly or amniotic band syndrome. Level of evidence: IV.

16. Ogino T: Clinical features and teratogenic mechanisms of congenital absence of digits. *Dev Growth Differ* 2007;49(6):523-531.

17. World Health Organization: *Towards a Common Language for Functioning, Disability and Health: ICF. The International Classification of Functioning, Disability and Health.* Available at: http://www.who.int/classifications/icf/icfbeginnersguide.pdf?ua=1. Accessed March 31, 2016.

18. Adkinson JM, Bickham RS, Chung KC, Waljee JF: Do patient- and parent-reported outcomes measures for children with congenital hand differences capture WHO-ICF domains? *Clin Orthop Relat Res* 2015;473(11):3549-3563.

This review of the literature validated whether PROMs for evaluating surgery for children with congenital hand deficiency captured WHO-ICF domains. Level of evidence: III.

19. Ardon MS, Selles RW, Roebroeck ME, Hovius SE, Stam HJ, Janssen WG: Poor agreement on health-related quality of life between children with congenital hand differences and their parents. *Arch Phys Med Rehabil* 2012;93(4):641-646.

In a survey of 115 children with congenital hand deficiency and 106 of their parents regarding health-related quality of life as assessed by the PedsQL, the children scored the same as their parents (on a group level). However, the authors suggested caution when using parental responses in place of an affected child's response because high variation on scoring on an individual level was evident, with children reporting both higher and lower scores than their parent proxy. Level of evidence: III.

20. Sheffler LC, Hanley C, Bagley A, Molitor F, James MA: Comparison of self-reports and parent proxy-reports of function and quality of life of children with below-the-elbow deficiency. *J Bone Joint Surg Am* 2009;91(12):2852-2859.

21. Johansen H, Østlie K, Andersen LØ, Rand-Hendriksen S: Health-related quality of life in adults with congenital unilateral upper limb deficiency in Norway: A cross-sectional study. *Disabil Rehabil* 2016;1-10.

The authors report on the outcomes of 131 children, 116 with congenital deficiencies, who were fitted with upper limb prostheses at the Ontario Crippled Children's Centre between 1965 and 1975. The level of deficiency was a key factor in long-term compliance, with longer forearms having decreased compliance. Fifty percent of the children older than 2 years who were fitted with prostheses abandoned them. Level of evidence: III.

22. Andersson GB, Gillberg C, Fernell E, Johansson M, Nachemson A: Children with surgically corrected hand deformities and upper limb deficiencies: Self-concept and psychological well-being. *J Hand Surg Eur Vol* 2011;36(9):795-801.

Ninety-two patients with congenital hand deformities, which were subdivided into mild versus complex hand deformities, were administered the Piers-Harris Children's Self-Concept Scale to assess their well-being and self-esteem. When compared with a cohort of children with no hand deformities, the overall results of the groups with hand deformities did not differ. Compared with the group with complex hand deformities, the group with the mild deformities scored lower on seven items of the scale, reflecting lower self-esteem. Level of evidence: III.

23. Scotland TR, Galway HR: A long-term review of children with congenital and acquired upper limb deficiency. *J Bone Joint Surg Br* 1983;65(3):346-349.

24. Wagner LV, Bagley AM, James MA: Reasons for prosthetic rejection by children with unilateral congenital transverse forearm total deficiency. *J Prosthet Orthot* 2007;19(2):51-54.

25. Davids JR, Wagner LV, Meyer LC, Blackhurst DW: Prosthetic management of children with unilateral congenital below-elbow deficiency. *J Bone Joint Surg Am* 2006;88(6):1294-1300.

26. Postema K, van der Donk V, van Limbeek J, Rijken RA, Poelma MJ: Prosthesis rejection in children with a unilateral congenital arm defect. *Clin Rehabil* 1999;13(3):243-249.

27. Glynn MK, Galway HR, Hunter G, Sauter WF: Management of the upper-limb-deficient child with a powered prosthetic device. *Clin Orthop Relat Res* 1986;209:202-205.

28. Crandall RC, Tomhave W: Pediatric unilateral below-elbow amputees: Retrospective analysis of 34 patients given multiple prosthetic options. *J Pediatr Orthop* 2002;22(3):380-383.

29. Krebs DE, Edelstein JE, Thornby MA: Prosthetic management of children with limb deficiencies. *Phys Ther* 1991;71(12):920-934.

30. James MA, Bagley AM, Brasington K, Lutz C, McConnell S, Molitor F: Impact of prostheses on function and quality of life for children with unilateral congenital below-the-elbow deficiency. *J Bone Joint Surg Am* 2006;88(11):2356-2365.

31. Resnik L, Meucci MR, Lieberman-Klinger S, et al: Advanced upper limb prosthetic devices: Implications for upper limb prosthetic rehabilitation. *Arch Phys Med Rehabil* 2012;93(4):710-717.

    The authors review challenges in the implementation and use of advanced upper limb prosthetic technology in adults.

32. Zuniga J, Katsavelis D, Peck J, et al: Cyborg beast: A low-cost 3d-printed prosthetic hand for children with upper-limb differences. *BMC Res Notes* 2015;8:10.

    In this case report, two children fitted with three-dimensional printed prosthetic hands using virtual long-distance fitting are compared with nine children with a similar prosthesis prepared and fitted in a laboratory environment. No differences in outcomes occurred between the two fitting techniques, and three-dimensional techniques may represent a future low-cost option. Level of evidence: IV.

33. Gretsch KF, Lather HD, Peddada KV, Deeken CR, Wall LB, Goldfarb CA: Development of novel 3D-printed robotic prosthetic for transradial amputees. *Prosthet Orthot Int* 2015.

    This article is a case report of a three-dimensional printed prosthesis for a transradial amputee. Level of evidence: IV.

34. E-Nable Community: Enabling the Future. Available at: http://enablingthefuture.org/about/. Accessed November 2, 2015.

    A nonprofit organization provides three-dimensional printed prostheses to children with congenital hand deficiencies.

35. Kuiken TA, Li G, Lock BA, et al: Targeted muscle reinnervation for real-time myoelectric control of multifunction artificial arms. *JAMA* 2009;301(6):619-628.

36. Kuiken TA, Marasco PD, Lock BA, Harden RN, Dewald JP: Redirection of cutaneous sensation from the hand to the chest skin of human amputees with targeted reinnervation. *Proc Natl Acad Sci U S A* 2007;104(50):20061-20066.

37. Nghiem BT, Sando IC, Gillespie RB, et al: Providing a sense of touch to prosthetic hands. *Plast Reconstr Surg* 2015;135(6):1652-1663.

    This article reviews the latest technology in sensory feedback and the future of peripheral nerve interfaces for prosthetic hands.

38. McMullen DP, Hotson G, Katyal KD, et al: Demonstration of a semi-autonomous hybrid brain-machine interface using human intracranial EEG, eye tracking, and computer vision to control a robotic upper limb prosthetic. *IEEE Trans Neural Syst Rehabil Eng* 2014;22(4):784-796.

    This case report of two patients evaluates a pilot model of the Hybrid Augmented Reality Multimodal Operation Neural Integration Environment system, a brain-machine interface to control an advanced prosthesis using electroencephalography, eye tracking, and computer vision control. Level of evidence: IV.

39. Scudder L, Levin LS: *World's First Pediatric Bilateral Hand Transplant*. 2015. Available at: http://www.medscape.com/viewarticle/848727. Accessed November 2, 2015.

    An interview description of the first pediatric bilateral upper limb vascularized allotransplant is presented.

40. Leonard DA, Kurtz JM, Cetrulo CL Jr: Achieving immune tolerance in hand and face transplantation: A realistic prospect? *Immunotherapy* 2014;6(5):499-502.

    This article is a brief review of the advances of immune tolerance for vascularized composite allotransplantation.

41. Tamura K, Ohgo S, Yokoyama H: Limb blastema cell: A stem cell for morphological regeneration. *Dev Growth Differ* 2010;52(1):89-99.

42. Monaghan JR, Maden M: Cellular plasticity during vertebrate appendage regeneration. *Curr Top Microbiol Immunol* 2013;367:53-74.

    The authors review the developmental biology and the molecular basis for appendage regeneration in vertebrate models.

43. Stocum DL: The role of peripheral nerves in urodele limb regeneration. *Eur J Neurosci* 2011;34(6):908-916.

    The author reviews developments in molecular biology that suggest that nerve axons in the apical epithelial cap are essential for its maintenance and blastema formation through expression of anterior gradient protein.

Section 5

Lower Extremity

SECTION EDITOR:
Vishwas R. Talwalkar, MD

Chapter 20

Developmental Dysplasia of the Hip

Pablo Castañeda, MD

Abstract

Early diagnosis is of paramount importance in attempts to favorably alter the natural history of developmental dysplasia of the hip. This condition can be identified in most patients on the basis of a careful physical examination, although ultrasonography allows better detection of subtleties not appreciated by means of physical examination or plain radiography.

Evaluating children with risk factors for developmental dysplasia of the hip is important; however, in most instances the condition occurs in girls who have no other risk factors. Prenatal and postnatal environmental factors, such as maternal nutrition and swaddling, may have a role in preventing dysplasia. Early treatment of an unstable hip with a Pavlik harness or a similarly effective orthosis is generally effective, safe, and strongly advised, especially for lower grades of dislocation. Follow-up is recommended until 5 years of age for hips successfully treated for dysplasia and until skeletal maturity for hips that were dislocated and successfully treated.

Keywords: developmental dysplasia of the hip (DDH); diagnosis; treatment

Introduction

Developmental dysplasia of the hip (DDH) is one of the most common abnormal conditions present at birth, affecting up to 15% of infants based on ultrasonography findings.[1] However, most mild cases may resolve spontaneously. DDH is a spectrum of disease affecting the femoral head, the acetabulum, or both, and ranges from frank dislocation in infants to mild acetabular dysplasia in adults. Instability of the hip that can be identified by clinical examination occurs in approximately 1 in 1,000 newborns;[2] however, the precise prevalence is difficult to determine and may be as high as 1 in 50 newborns.[3] Approximately 5 in 1,000 newborns are ultimately treated for neonatal hip dysplasia.[4]

Although dysplasia is probably the most common etiology of hip osteoarthritis, less than 10% of young adults requiring arthroplasty had hip instability at birth.[5] The overall prevalence of hip dysplasia in the adult population is unknown, because advanced deterioration of the hip joint may obscure the underlying diagnosis,[6] but it has been shown that a high proportion of cases of osteoarthritis of the hip can be attributed to some form of dysplasia.[5,6] Defining dysplasia can be difficult, and radiographic measurements such as the center-edge angle are not uniformly associated with osteoarthritis in all populations.[7] Subluxation has been proven to be a more reliable predictor of early arthritis than a center-edge angle of less than 20°.[8,9]

Outcomes are directly related to the severity of the condition and the patient's age at the time of initial treatment. The best results and long-term outcomes occur in patients who are treated successfully with nonsurgical methods during the neonatal period.[10]

Etiology

Because a single cause of DDH is unlikely, it is considered a condition with multiple causes.[11] Although there is a proven genetic predisposition for DDH, environmental, hormonal, and biomechanical influences can increase the risk for the condition.[12] Genetic causes may not be modifiable, but environmental factors should be addressed if possible.

The incidence of DDH is variable between ethnic and cultural groups, and some specific populations have a very high risk.[13] It is well known that DDH is much more common in females, with a reported relative incidence of up to 10:1.[11]

Dr. Castañeda or an immediate family member serves as an unpaid consultant to Orthopediatrics and serves as a board member, owner, officer, or committee member of the Sociedad Mexicana de Ortopedia Pediátrica and the Sociedad de Especialistas en Cirugía Ortopédica del Centro Médico ABC.

Certain mechanical and obstetric factors are known to increase the risk for DDH, such as being a firstborn child, a breech presentation, or oligohydramnios.[14] The left hip is involved with a greater frequency than the right hip. Positioning after birth, such as tightly swaddling the infant with hips and knees in extension, also can influence the development of DDH.[15] Other causes, including environmental and nutritional factors, have been implicated, but further research is necessary.[16,17]

Pathologic Anatomy

Three major pathoanatomic factors in DDH—capsular laxity, acetabular dysplasia, and femoral anteversion—tend to be present in varying degrees in most patients.[18] Progressive changes of varying severities (mild instability to subluxation to frank dislocation) occur in all tissues as the femoral head displaces. The labrum becomes deformed as greater pressure is applied by the femoral head; when the head dislocates, a pseudoacetabulum is formed superior to the true acetabulum. The acetabulum is filled with fibroadipose tissue known as pulvinar, which fills the void left by the femoral head. The joint capsule becomes constricted, and the transverse acetabular ligament is pulled laterally, obstructing the inferior acetabulum. The ligamentum teres is stretched and hypertrophic and, with the hip in extension, the iliopsoas tendon constricts the capsule. Some morphologic changes are not present at birth but develop with varying degrees of severity[19] (**Figure 1**).

Strategies for reducing the incidence of DDH have focused on postnatal positioning that avoids knee and hip extension. It has been reported that late-presenting dislocations can be almost eliminated and the need for surgery substantially decreased with the routine use of a bulky diaper in newborns.[20]

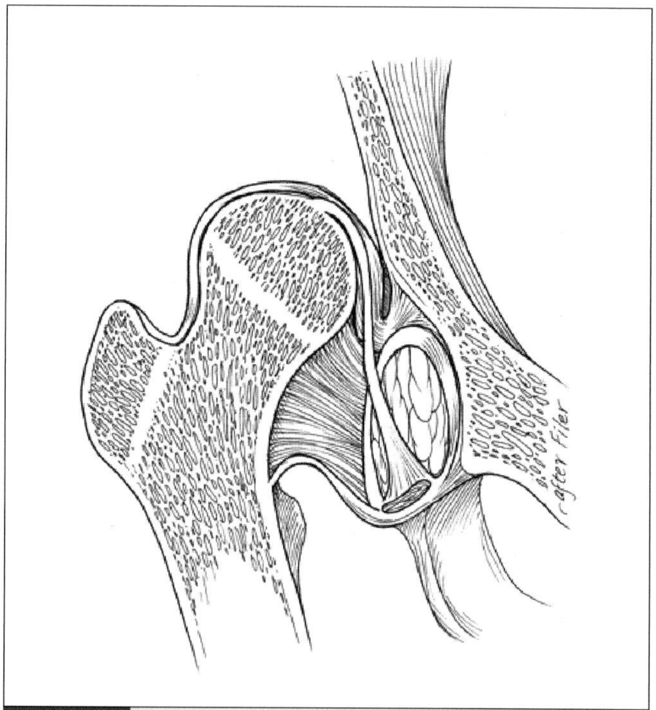

Figure 1 Illustration shows pathoanatomy of developmental dysplasia of the hip, including femoral anteversion, acetabular insufficiency, and capsular laxity, which are always present in varying degrees. Hypertrophy of the ligamentum teres, the transverse ligament, and an hourglass constriction of the capsule are present. In a dislocated hip, the so-called pulvinar tissue fills the empty acetabulum. (Reproduced from Guille JT, Pizzutillo PD, MacEwen G, Dean G: Developmental dysplasia of the hip from birth to six months. *J Am Acad Orthop Surg* 2000;8[4]:232-242.)

Screening

Universal screening for DDH has not been implemented because of a lack of evidence that it prevents adverse outcomes.[21] However, primary care physicians should continue to follow the clinical practice guidelines outlined by the American Academy of Pediatrics[21] and ultrasonography should be considered as an adjunct when there is high risk or examination findings are equivocal (**Figure 2**). Several studies have determined that routine neonatal examination combined with selective screening with ultrasonography is the optimal method for early detection and, without treatment, DDH can lead to early-onset osteoarthritis.[22-24]

In the first months of life, infants may exhibit limited hip abduction, an apparent limb-length discrepancy (the Galeazzi sign), and the classic signs of hip instability described by the Barlow maneuver (hip in place at rest but dislocatable with stress) and Ortolani maneuver (hip dislocated at rest but reducible with manipulation). However, newer imaging techniques have shown that physical examination alone may not be sufficient to detect pure dysplasia and milder forms of instability.[25] Imaging examinations generally include ultrasonography and radiography.

Imaging

Ultrasonography

Ultrasonography is the imaging modality of choice for DDH during an infant's first 6 months of life because it is capable of defining the nonosseous components of the hip. In addition, it is a dynamic test that allows the observation of changes in hip position with movement and can be performed while the child is in an orthosis.[26]

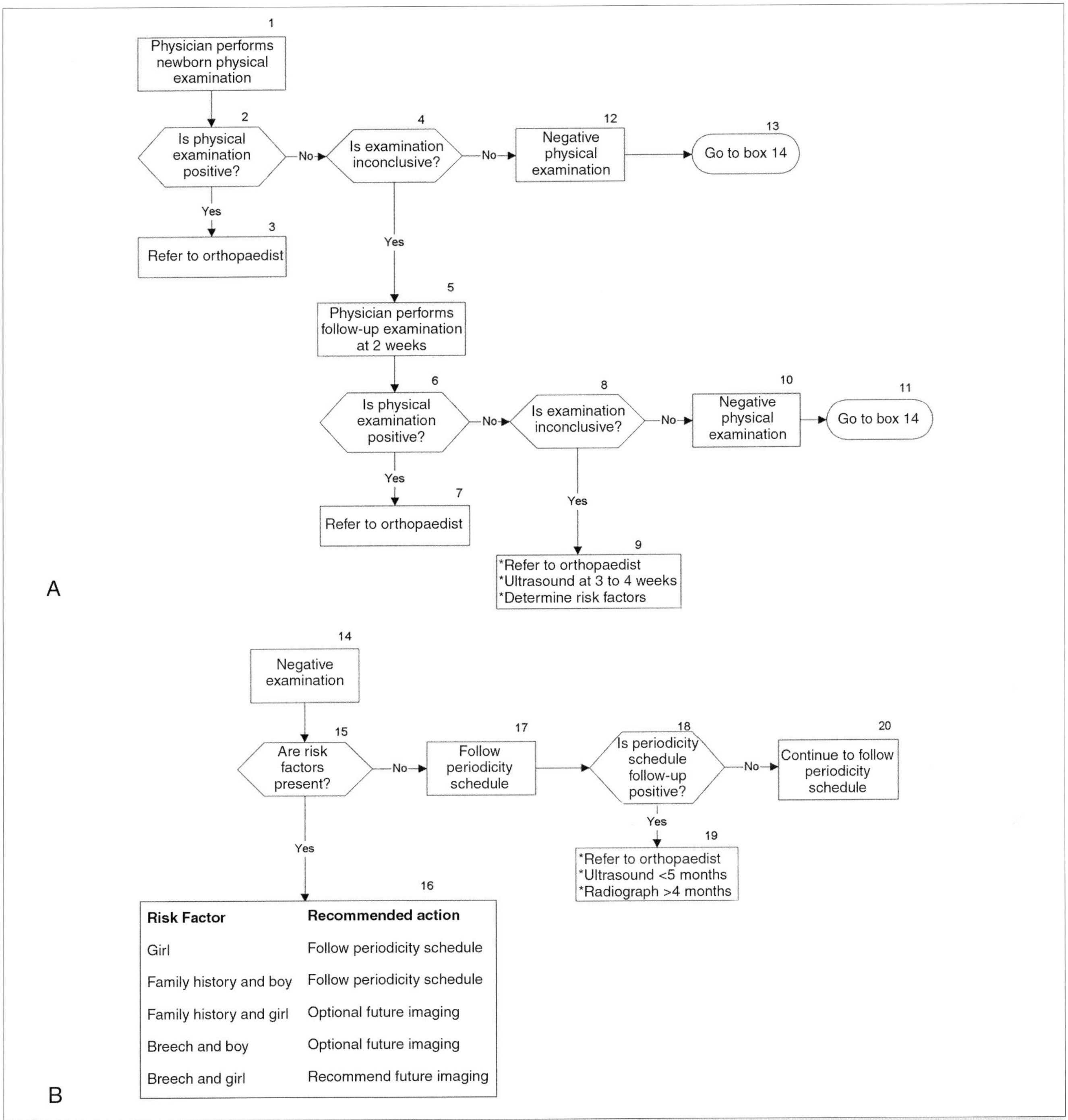

Figure 2 Clinical algorithm for screening for developmental dysplasia of the hip. (Reproduced with permission from Clinical Practice Guideline: Early detection of developmental dysplasia of the hip. Committee on Quality Improvement, Subcommittee on Developmental Dysplasia of the Hip: American Academy of Pediatrics. *Pediatrics* 2000; 105[4 pt 1]:896-905.)

Most clinicians currently use the Dynamic Standard Minimum Examination, which combines a morphologic approach using the measurement of specific parameters on a coronal ultrasonographic image, and a dynamic component, which assesses the hip in positions produced by physical maneuvers[26,27] (**Figure 3**). Measurements are made on a coronal view in the midacetabulum; a quality image should show the lateral wall of the ilium as horizontal and flat (**Figure 4**). Three lines are constructed: a baseline is drawn parallel to the ossified lateral wall of the

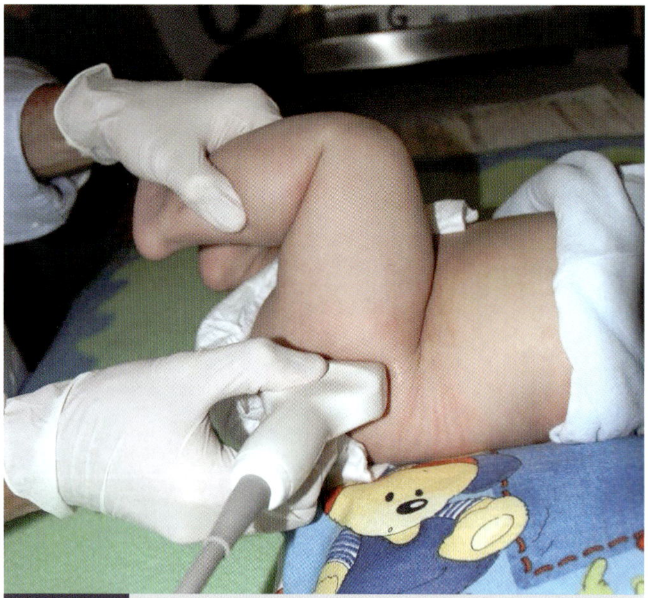

Figure 3 Clinical photograph shows placement of the clinician's hands and the transducer to obtain a coronal ultrasonographic view of an infant's hip. Note that the transducer is perpendicular to the femoral axis.

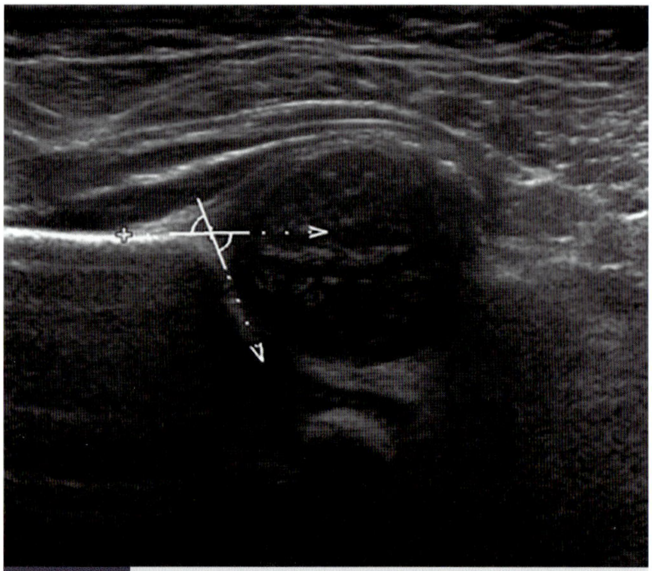

Figure 4 Coronal ultrasonogram of an infant's hip shows the ilium on left and the femoral head, which is the hypoechoic circle in the middle. The lines indicate measurement of the α-angle.

ilium; a second line (termed the bony roof line) is drawn from the inferior edge of the osseous acetabulum (the inferior iliac margin) at the roof of the triradiate cartilage to the most lateral point on the ilium; and a third line (termed the cartilage roof line) is drawn along the roof of the cartilaginous acetabulum from the intersection of the first two lines to the center of the labrum. Two angles are created. The α-angle is formed by the intersection of the baseline and the bony roof line; its lower limit of normal is approximately 60°. This angle reflects osseous coverage of the femoral head by the acetabulum. An α-angle less than 60° reflects acetabular dysplasia of progressively increasing severity. The β-angle is formed by the intersection of the baseline and the cartilage roof line and reflects cartilaginous coverage of the femoral head. A β-angle greater than 55° represents an increasing degree of subluxation or dislocation[26] (**Figure 5**).

The dynamic component of hip ultrasonography is a visual representation of the maneuvers done on clinical examination. An image is obtained with the hip flexed to 90° as posterior stress is applied to the knee with the palm of the hand, reproducing the Barlow provocative test; any resultant subluxation is then noted (**Figure 6**). During the first 4 weeks of life, the femoral head may be reduced in the acetabulum at rest, but up to 4 mm of displacement (physiologic laxity) may be seen under stress. In infants older than 4 weeks, more than 2 mm of subluxation of the femoral head on the transverse view or less than 50%

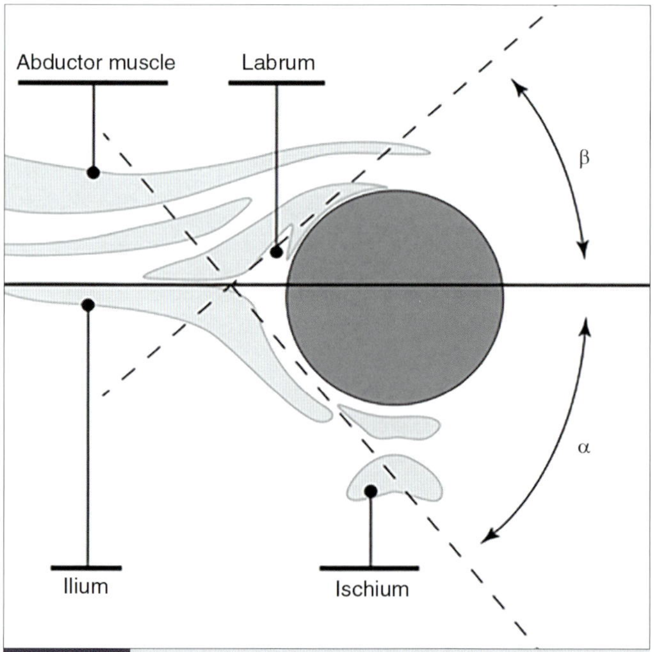

Figure 5 Illustration shows the parameters used with measurements on a coronal ultrasonogram to determine the α-angle and the β-angle.

coverage of the femoral head on the longitudinal view is considered abnormal[26] (**Figure 7**).

It has been recognized that universal screening of newborns for DDH has the risks of overdiagnosis and unnecessary treatment. It is now recommended that ultrasonography be performed between 2 and 6 weeks after birth on any newborn with a questionable physical examination finding and that ultrasonography be performed between 6 and 8 weeks after birth on any newborn with a risk factor but no abnormal physical examination findings.[25]

Radiography

As the ossification center grows and matures, it increases in size until it becomes large enough to obscure the echoes from the inferior iliac margin at the medial part of the acetabulum, making ultrasonography less valuable by 4 to 6 months of age; at this time, radiography becomes increasingly reliable for making a diagnosis of DDH.

When the hip is dislocated or subluxated, the femoral head is displaced laterally and proximally. Based on the Tönnis system, this displacement can be classified according to the level of the ossific nucleus relative to the lateral margin of the acetabulum (**Figure 8**). Lesser Tönnis grades of dysplasia correlate with an improved prognosis for satisfactory long-term outcomes. Each increase in the Tönnis grade at the time of diagnosis doubles the likelihood of failure of nonsurgical treatment.[28,29]

A useful radiographic measurement in children younger than 8 years is the acetabular index.[29] It is a measure of the inclination of the ossified acetabulum as determined by the angle formed between a horizontal line and a line drawn from the iliac margin at the upper edge of the triradiate cartilage to the most lateral edge of the ossified acetabulum (**Figure 9**). The acetabular index progressively decreases with age but will remain abnormally high in a dysplastic hip. The range for normal acetabular indices has been defined by Tönnis[29] (**Figure 10**).

Although there is no single accepted definition of radiographic dysplasia in adolescents or adults, there are a number of possible measurements that can aid in assessing this condition. Increased acetabular inclination can be

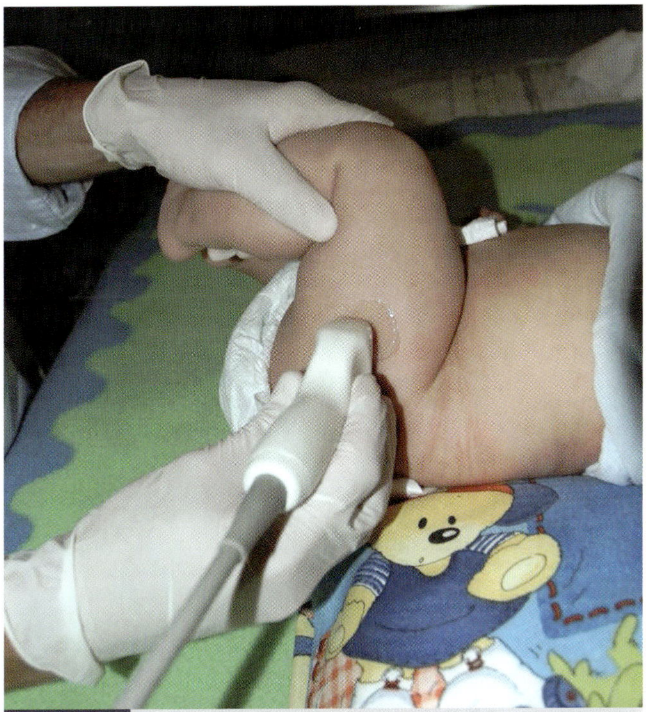

Figure 6 Clinical photograph shows placement of the clinician's hands and the transducer to obtain a transverse ultrasonographic view of an infant's hip. Note that the transducer is parallel to the femoral axis.

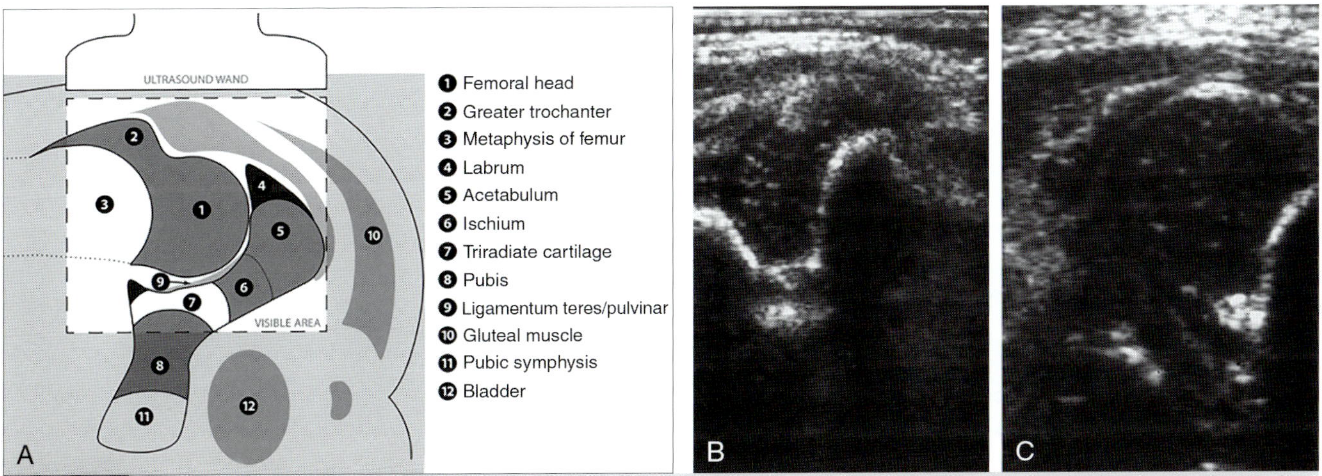

Figure 7 **A,** Diagram describes the anatomy seen on a longitudinal ultrasonogram of an infant's hip. Ultrasonograms of an unstable hip demonstrate that the distance from the femoral head to the acetabulum (**B**) increases (**C**) when posterior stress is applied.

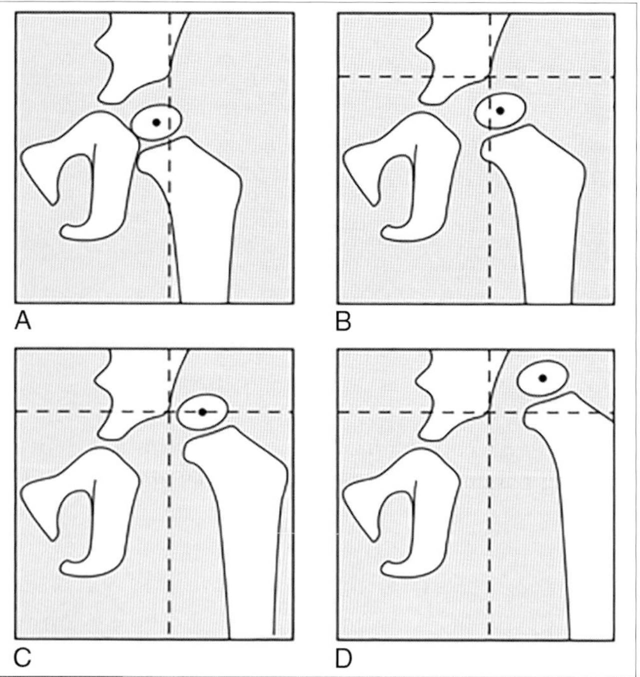

Figure 8 Illustrations of grade I (**A**), grade II (**B**), grade III (**C**), and grade IV (**D**) of the Tönnis classification of developmental dysplasia of the hip, in which femoral head displacement is determined based on the level of the ossific nucleus relative to the lateral margin of the acetabulum.

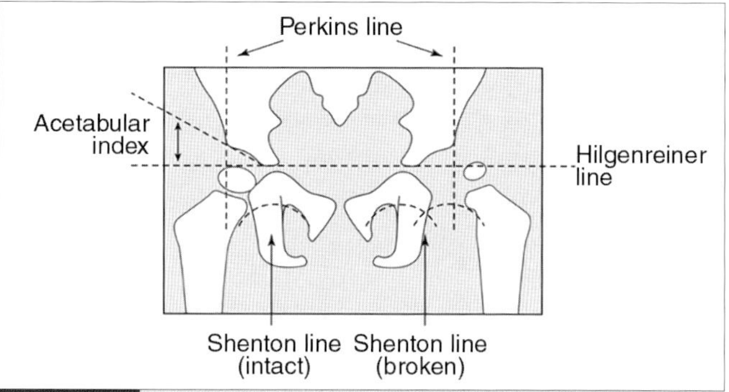

Figure 9 Illustration shows basic radiographic parameters used in determining the acetabular index.

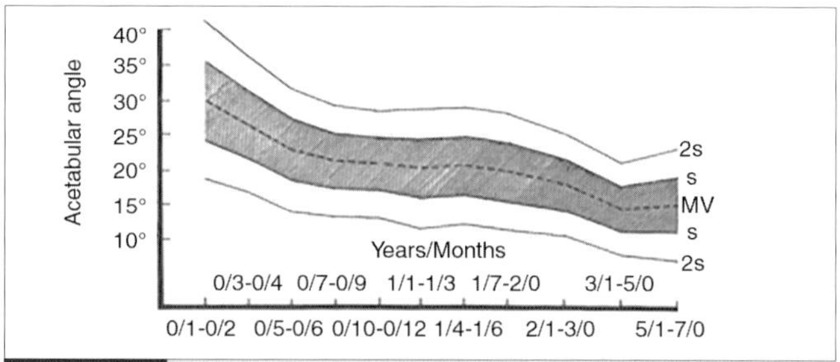

Figure 10 Nomogram developed by Tönnis shows means and SDs for the acetabular index based on the patient's age. (Reproduced with permission from Tonnis D: Normal values of the hip joint for the evaluation of X-rays in children and adults. *Clin Orthop Relat Res* 1976;119:39-47.)

defined as a high Tönnis angle. This angle is measured by drawing three lines on an AP pelvic radiograph: a horizontal line connecting the base of the acetabular teardrops (line 1); a horizontal line parallel to line 1 (line 2), running through the most inferior point of the sclerotic acetabular sourcil (point 1); and a line (line 3) extending from point 1 to a point at the lateral margin of the acetabular sourcil (the sclerotic weight-bearing portion of the acetabulum). The Tönnis angle is formed by the intersection of lines 2 and 3, and it should be no greater than 10°.

Other quantitative indicators of instability are the lateral and anterior center-edge angles, both useful measures of acetabular coverage of the femoral head. The lateral center-edge angle, also known as the center-edge angle of Wiberg, is determined from an AP pelvic radiograph and is used to assess the superolateral coverage of the femoral head. It is calculated by measuring the angle between a line through the center of the femoral head that is perpendicular to the transverse axis of the pelvis and a line through the center of the femoral head that passes through the most superolateral point of the sclerotic weight-bearing zone of the acetabulum. A value less than 25° may indicate inadequate coverage of the femoral head, and values less than 20° have been associated with early-onset osteoarthritis of the hip.[8] The anterior center-edge angle, also known as the angle of Lequesne, is similar, except it is measured on a false profile radiographic view, thus representing the degree of anterior coverage of the femoral head.

Infants Younger Than 6 Months

Treatment

Treatment is indicated at the time a dislocation is noted or when sonographic instability or dysplasia persist beyond 6 weeks of age. Clinical instability, which is determined by the presence of a positive Barlow sign, should be treated if it persists beyond the second week of extrauterine life. Before this time, it may be acceptable to wait, because some hips resolve spontaneously. However, if the instability is present after the second extrauterine week, it is generally agreed that most hips should receive treatment because spontaneous resolution is unlikely. The definition of instability or dysplasia is not universal.[3] Instability is considered to be present when the femoral head displaces more than 4 mm from the acetabulum in an infant older than 6 weeks. Dysplasia is considered to be present when the bony coverage of the femoral head is less than 50% or the α-angle is less than 50°. Because these values decrease with increasing age, more than 2 mm of displacement is considered abnormal in a child older than 3 months, and the mean α-angle also should be substantially higher than 60° in a child older than 3 months.[26,27]

Of the multiple devices available for treatment of DDH, the most commonly used in North America is the Pavlik harness, which is most successful when applied before the age of 4 months. However, good results have been reported in older children with lower grades of dysplasia.[30,31]

The method developed by Pavlik consists of obtaining dynamic abduction while allowing the child to move freely within the confines of the harness, which consists of a chest strap that provides sites of attachment for two lower extremity straps. These straps prevent hip extension and allow dynamic abduction while avoiding adduction and maintaining flexion, generally between 90° and 110°. Avoiding forced abduction results in a decreased risk for the development of osteonecrosis. The harness is worn full time for the treatment of instability; bathing privileges can be allowed after the hip is stable. Typically, follow-up and adjustments are done on a weekly basis, with testing for stability performed by ultrasonographic evaluation.[32-34] In almost 98% of patients, reduction is achieved within the first 3 weeks in the harness.[32] Prolonged treatment of a hip that does not reduce with the Pavlik harness within 3 to 4 weeks is not recommended because of potential damage to the posterior wall of the acetabulum, which leads to worsening dysplasia and instability.[32-35] The harness should be worn until the hip is normal and stable within the acetabulum and has bony coverage of at least 50% and an α-angle of at least 60°.[33]

Complications

Complications, which can include transient femoral nerve palsy caused by hyperflexion of the hips and osteonecrosis caused by excessive abduction, are rare and usually originate in physician or parental misunderstanding regarding proper application of the harness. A report of 30 cases of femoral nerve palsy identified an incidence of 2.5%.[34] Femoral nerve palsy is more likely to occur in larger infants with more severe dislocations. Most nerve palsies occur in the first week after application of the harness, and recovery typically occurs with harness removal. Osteonecrosis of the femoral epiphysis has been reported in the normal and abnormal hips of infants treated with a Pavlik harness.[35] A 28% rate of osteonecrosis was reported for hospitalized infants who were managed with prolonged forced abduction. Current methods that avoid excessive abduction have reported osteonecrosis rates of less than 10%. A more recent study, which used ultrasonography to monitor reduction, reported osteonecrosis in less than 2% of patients.[36]

Outcomes

The success rates with the Pavlik method is varied and dependent on the severity of the dysplasia and the definition of success. Success rates of 100% have been reported in studies that generally include lower grades of hip dysplasia, whereas lower success rates (65% to 90%) have been reported in hips that are dislocated but are reducible at the start of treatment.[36,37] The success rate decreases substantially with higher grades of dislocation and increasing patient age. Few children older than 3 months with high-grade dislocations are successfully treated with the Pavlik harness.[37] If reduction is not obtained within 3 to 4 weeks but the hip can be reduced by manipulation, rigid abduction bracing can be of value; however, success is not uniform and fixed dislocations are unlikely to respond to rigid abduction bracing after unsuccessful Pavlik harness treatment.[38,39]

Based on long-term studies, follow-up until skeletal maturity is currently recommended for all patients with DDH.[40] It has been shown that additional surgery may be required in approximately 15% of patients treated with a Pavlik harness.[38,39]

Radiographic signs of improvement include a decreasing acetabular index, the development of a smooth horizontal sourcil (dense bone on the weight-bearing surface of the acetabulum), and the development of a narrow U-shaped teardrop bone lateral to the ilioischial line. Mild residual dysplasia may be improved by abduction splinting during sleep;[39] however, the patient should be monitored for signs of poor development, which can lead to the need for secondary surgery. These signs include an acetabular index greater than 35° more than 2 years after initial treatment ended, an acetabular index higher than 2 SDs from the mean after the age of 5 years, or no improvement over a substantial period of time.[37,39] MRI also has been used to predict the presence of residual dysplasia[41,42] (**Figure 11**)

Older Children

Treatment

The treatment of DDH becomes increasingly challenging as a child ages. The ideal treatment obtains a timely, stable reduction while minimizing the need for further surgery and the risk for development of complications such as redislocation or osteonecrosis. After the age of approximately 4 to 6 months or when orthotic treatment has failed, other treatments should be considered.

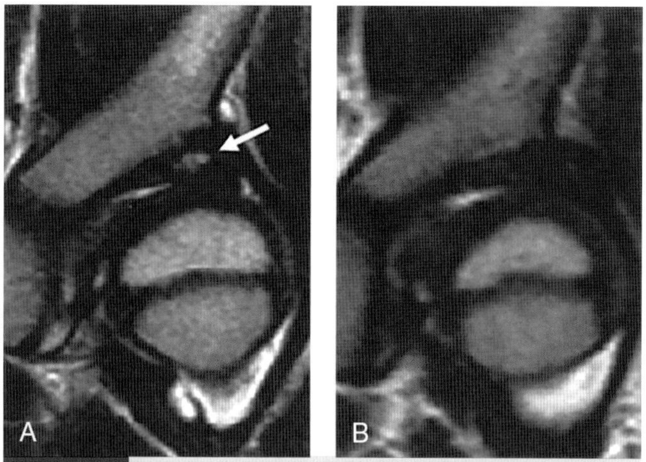

Figure 11 MRIs of the hips of infants with a positive high-signal intensity area (**A**) and negative high-signal intensity area (**B**). A high-signal intensity area correlates with an increased likelihood of residual dysplasia after a closed reduction. (Reproduced with permission from Wakabayashi K, Wada I, Horiuchi O, Mizutani J, Tsuchiya D, Otsuka T: MRI findings in residual hip dysplasia. *J Pediatr Orthop* 2011;31[4]: 381-387.)

Closed reduction is indicated for two groups of children: (1) those with a dislocated hip in which orthotic treatment has failed and (2) those with a late presenting dislocated hip for whom primary Pavlik harness treatment is not suitable. These children generally range from 4 to 12 months of age. Imaging should be obtained to determine the severity of the dislocation and rule out the presence of a so-called teratologic hip (a hip that has been dislocated since a very early time in embryonic development), which is not amenable to closed reduction. Teratologic dislocations tend to show very marked and advanced changes in the hip joint and can be associated with various conditions, including arthrogryposis multiplex congenita, lumbosacral agenesis, chromosomal abnormalities, diastrophic dwarfism, and Larsen syndrome. Teratologic hips can be difficult to distinguish radiographically; however, these hips tend to have certain characteristics such as the absence of a sulcus. A sulcus is typically seen on the lateral border of the acetabulum and is caused by the mechanical effect of the femoral head "sliding" out of the acetabulum; however, in teratologic dislocations this phenomenon is not seen because the femoral head has never been in the acetabulum. The ilium also tends to be smaller, and the degree of dysplasia tends to be greater than in typical dysplasia. A teratologic hip is best managed with open reduction at a minimum age of 8 to 9 months. Relative contraindications for closed reduction are the existence of an important medical problem or evidence of a failure to thrive. Treatment can be delayed until the child's medical condition has improved.

Although a discussion of the closed reduction technique is beyond the scope of this chapter, it is important to understand that the hip should be held in a stable position without forced abduction, and advanced imaging should be obtained within 24 hours to confirm maintenance of hip reduction. MRI is the modality of choice because of the lack of radiation and greater ability to visualize the cartilaginous femoral head and other soft tissues. Gadolinium can be added to the study to evaluate perfusion of the femoral head after the reduction, although the relationship of perfusion to the possible development of osteonecrosis is unclear.[43] CT can be of use, but the amount of radiation is substantial. A cast change can be performed if the hip is not reduced, but the goal is maintenance of the human position of at least 90° of flexion and the least amount of necessary abduction to retain a stable hip while avoiding the risk of osteonecrosis. Bracing after casting has not been shown to have a substantial effect on the development of the acetabulum when a quality stable reduction has been obtained.

Open reduction can be considered if closed reduction is unobtainable or would require excessive force.[18] In general, the indications for an open reduction and innominate osteotomy are a developmental hip dislocation in a child older than 18 months.[6] Femoral shortening may be added after 3 years of age to reduce the tension across the hip joint after reduction; however, it should be considered whenever the soft-tissue tension across the reduction appears excessive. Although controversial, the upper age limit for a safe reduction to improve on the natural history of a dislocated hip is generally considered to be approximately 8 years. Incongruity and stiffness are contraindications for surgery. In the setting of neuromuscular disease, the pathology is likely to differ because posterior acetabular dysplasia is more common than the typical anterolateral dysplasia seen in patients with DDH.[7]

In children younger than 18 months, substantial remodeling of the acetabulum can occur after a closed or open reduction without bony surgery. Pelvic osteotomies are rarely required in these younger children. In addition, the bone in the pelvis of children younger than 18 months is too soft to allow optimal correction or maintain correction with an innominate osteotomy. After 18 months of age, acetabular remodeling is much less assured. Because the primary bony defect is on the acetabular side of the joint, performing an innominate osteotomy at the time of open reduction adds little morbidity to the procedure. For these reasons, a pelvic osteotomy often is recommended in the treatment of DDH in children older than 18 months.[5]

An innominate osteotomy reliably obtains 15° of anterior and 25° of lateral coverage if performed properly. Technical errors such as pulling up on the proximal iliac fragment, allowing the posterior aspect of the osteotomy to open, or allowing the distal fragment to fall posteriorly will not allow anterolateral rotation of the acetabular fragment in the correct plane.[6,18]

From the age of 18 months to 3 years, a femoral osteotomy is not usually required. In most patients, stability of the hip can be ensured with open reduction, capsulorrhaphy, and an innominate osteotomy. Small amounts of femoral deformity such as anteversion will correct spontaneously with stable reduction and the resumption of normal muscle tension across the joint. In addition, the capsulorrhaphy is designed to add some internal rotation to the femoral position at the end of the procedure to account for anteversion. In some patients between the ages of 18 months and 3 years, excessive femoral anteversion of greater than 60° exists. A derotational femoral osteotomy can be added to the reconstruction in these patients because, even after pelvic osteotomy, there may be persistent instability and a failure to direct the femoral head toward the center of the acetabulum. The decision is based on the following three factors: (1) the severity of dysplasia on a preoperative radiograph, (2) the assessment of femoral anteversion on fluoroscopic screening of the hip at the start of the procedure, and (3) the direct visualization of the femoral anteversion after open reduction. At least 20° of anteversion must remain after derotation to prevent the possibility of posterior dislocation. After a child is older than 3 years, a femoral shortening osteotomy is generally required to assist gentle reduction and prevent osteonecrosis, although excessive shortening may lead to a loss of tension and redislocation. Judicious derotation and varus may be added at the discretion of the operating surgeon, although varus is rarely needed.

In patients with severe acetabular dysplasia in which instability persists after open reduction, capsulorrhaphy, innominate osteotomy, femoral osteotomy, and the resolution of all technical issues, the use of a transarticular fixation pin has been shown to be safe and effective.[44] The pin is removed through a window in the spica cast after 4 weeks. The hip should never be left subluxated at the conclusion of the primary procedure because redislocation will invariably occur, and any revision will be considered salvage surgery.

Complications and Revision Procedures

The two most serious and common complications in the surgical management of DDH are osteonecrosis and redislocation. Osteonecrosis is an iatrogenic complication because it does not occur as part of the natural history of DDH,[8] but it can occur even when treatment is performed by an experienced orthopaedic surgeon. Redislocation usually results from a technical failure on the part of the operating surgeon. The most common cause of redislocation is failure to identify the true acetabulum. This failure may occur because established dislocations often have a well-formed pseudoacetabulum located superolateral to the true acetabulum.

The first attempt at surgical reduction of a dislocated hip has the best chance for achieving a satisfactory result. Secondary procedures on a redislocated hip are technically challenging and the results are far less ensured than those of a primary open reduction; therefore, revision procedures are considered salvage procedures.

The treatment of redislocation varies depending on when it is identified; in the immediate postoperative period, the issue is likely a technical surgical failure. All steps in the surgical procedure should be reviewed to identify the primary problem. CT can help identify structural problems such as inadequate correction by pelvic osteotomy or excessive derotation of the femur. Revision surgery is appropriate in these cases to correct problems, and the addition of a transfixion pin should be considered. A less-than-satisfactory result can be expected if hip subluxation is present in the immediate postoperative period because the hip will not stabilize spontaneously.

If redislocation is identified at a later stage (for example, after removal of the hip spica cast), early revision surgery is not recommended because the hip will be stiff and osteopenic. These factors make surgery far more challenging, and the risk of further complications, including pathologic fracture, are more likely. A prerequisite for any osteotomy is an adequate range of motion in the adjacent joints. In this situation, a delay in open reduction revision is indicated after a rehabilitation period of approximately 3 months with weight bearing as tolerated to allow range of motion of the hip to return and promote strengthening of bone stock. During this time, the technical reasons for dislocation should be assessed, essential imaging such as CT should be obtained, and the revision should be planned.

Osteonecrosis, even in its mildest form, can affect the long-term function of a hip and has been reported to occur in up to 43% of hips after open reduction. Osteonecrosis may be compatible with satisfactory function until the teenage years, at which point the hip may become symptomatic with stiffness, pain, and degenerative changes. It has been reported that the rate of osteonecrosis can be reduced to as little as 6% in hips with congenital dislocation and subluxation treated with innominate osteotomy.[18] Technical factors, such as avoiding excessive tension across the hip joint, damage to the circulation to the femoral head, and excessive abduction in the spica cast, clearly have a role in reducing the rate of osteonecrosis.[18]

Long-term results for patients with late-presenting developmental dislocation have shown good outcomes, with approximately one-third of patients undergoing open reduction and innominate osteotomy requiring a hip replacement at a mean of 43 years after initial treatment. Successful primary surgery correlates with better long-term outcomes.[45] Risk factors for poor outcomes include bilateral surgery (a 2.9 times greater risk of needing a subsequent hip replacement than those who initially underwent unilateral surgery) and the need for revision surgery.[45]

Excellent and reproducible results have been reported in patients with adolescent dysplasia using variations on the periacetabular osteotomy method developed by Ganz.[46] Studies have demonstrated the durability of different types of periacetabular osteotomies at long-term follow-up, although poorer results were seen in patients with worsening degrees of osteoarthritis as demonstrated on imaging studies, specifically delayed gadolinium enhanced MRI.[47,48] Having adequate cartilage to preserve is a prerequisite for any joint preservation procedure.

Summary

Early diagnosis is an important factor in altering the natural history of DDH. A diagnosis of DDH usually can be made on the basis of careful physical examination, although ultrasonography allows improved detection of subtleties not appreciated by means of physical examination or plain radiography. Although the evaluation of children with risk factors for DDH is important, most dysplasia occurs in girls who have no other risk factors. Prenatal and postnatal environmental factors may have a role in the prevention of DDH.

Early treatment of an unstable hip with a Pavlik harness or similarly effective orthosis is recommended, especially for patients with lower grades of dislocation. Follow-up is recommended until 5 years of age for hips successfully treated for dysplasia and until skeletal maturity for hips that were dislocated and successfully treated. Adolescent hip dysplasia has been successfully treated with various types of periacetabular osteotomy procedures with excellent long-term results when adequate cartilage was present.

Key Study Points

- Hip dysplasia is one of the most prevalent conditions seen in musculoskeletal pathology.
- Early detection of DDH is paramount for good results.
- Nonsurgical treatment in infants has provided excellent results.
- Follow-up until skeletal maturity is warranted because the rates of adolescent and adult dysplasia have been underestimated in the past.
- Adolescent hip dysplasia can be treated with periacetabular osteotomy if adequate cartilage is present.

Annotated References

1. Rosendahl K, Markestad T, Lie RT: Developmental dysplasia of the hip: Prevalence based on ultrasound diagnosis. *Pediatr Radiol* 1996;26(9):635-639.

2. Boeree NR, Clarke NM: Ultrasound imaging and secondary screening for congenital dislocation of the hip. *J Bone Joint Surg Br* 1994;76(4):525-533.

3. Roposch A, Liu LQ, Protopapa E: Variations in the use of diagnostic criteria for developmental dysplasia of the hip. *Clin Orthop Relat Res* 2013;471(6):1946-1954.

   This article highlights the difficulties in terminology regarding DDH. The authors concluded that the consistency of diagnostic criteria for DDH is poor and considerable variation exists in the application of diagnostic criteria. These inconsistencies may explain the differing prevalence estimates and management standards for DDH.

4. Bialik V, Bialik GM, Blazer S, Sujov P, Wiener F, Berant M: Developmental dysplasia of the hip: A new approach to incidence. *Pediatrics* 1999;103(1):93-99.

5. Engesaeter IØ, Lie SA, Lehmann TG, Furnes O, Vollset SE, Engesaeter LB: Neonatal hip instability and risk of total hip replacement in young adulthood: Follow-up of 2,218,596 newborns from the Medical Birth Registry of Norway in the Norwegian Arthroplasty Register. *Acta Orthop* 2008;79(3):321-326.

6. Hoaglund FT, Steinbach LS: Primary osteoarthritis of the hip: Etiology and epidemiology. *J Am Acad Orthop Surg* 2001;9(5):320-327.

7. Dudda M, Kim Y-J, Zhang Y, et al: Morphologic differences between the hips of Chinese women and white women: Could they account for the ethnic difference in the prevalence of hip osteoarthritis? *Arthritis Rheum* 2011;63(10):2992-2999.

The authors highlight the differences in the incidence of DDH among different ethnic groups and discuss a genetic basis for the condition.

8. Cooperman DR, Wallensten R, Stulberg SD: Acetabular dysplasia in the adult. *Clin Orthop Relat Res* 1983;175:79-85.

9. Morvan J, Bouttier R, Mazieres B, et al; KHOALA Cohort Study Group: Relationship between hip dysplasia, pain, and osteoarthritis in a cohort of patients with hip symptoms. *J Rheumatol* 2013;40(9):1583-1589.

   This study presents further proof that one of the most common morphologic alterations leading to early degenerative arthritis is acetabular dysplasia determined by a high angle of acetabular inclination.

10. Albinana J, Dolan LA, Spratt KF, Morcuende J, Meyer MD, Weinstein SL: Acetabular dysplasia after treatment for developmental dysplasia of the hip: Implications for secondary procedures. *J Bone Joint Surg Br* 2004;86(6):876-886.

11. Carter CO, Wilkinson JA: Genetic and environmental factors in the etiology of congenital dislocation of the hip. *Clin Orthop Relat Res* 1964;33:119-128.

12. Shi D, Dai J, Ikegawa S, Jiang Q: Genetic study on developmental dysplasia of the hip. *Eur J Clin Invest* 2012;42(10):1121-1125.

    The authors examine the gap between a genetic basis for DDH and molecular mechanisms involved in the condition.

13. Wynne-Davies R: A family study of neonatal and late-diagnosis congenital dislocation of the hip. *J Med Genet* 1970;7(4):315-333.

14. Paton RW, Hinduja K, Thomas CD: The significance of at-risk factors in ultrasound surveillance of developmental dysplasia of the hip: A ten-year prospective study. *J Bone Joint Surg Br* 2005;87(9):1264-1266.

15. Mahan ST, Kasser JR: Does swaddling influence developmental dysplasia of the hip? *Pediatrics* 2008;121(1):177-178.

16. Nagamine S, Sonohata M, Kitajima M, et al: Seasonal trends in the incidence of hip osteoarthritis in Japanese patients. *Open Orthop J* 2011;5:134-137.

    The authors found that the prevalence of hip osteoarthritis was substantially higher in patients born in winter. The seasonal trend in hip osteoarthritis might be caused by the prevalence of congenital dislocation of the hip in children born in winter. The multifactorial nature of DDH is supported.

17. Fries CL, Remedios AM: The pathogenesis and diagnosis of canine hip dysplasia: A review. *Can Vet J* 1995;36(8):494-502.

18. Salter RB: Role of innominate osteotomy in the treatment of congenital dislocation and subluxation of the hip in the older child. *J Bone Joint Surg Am* 1966;48(7):1413-1439.

19. Li LY, Zhang LJ, Li QW, Zhao Q, Jia JY, Huang T: Development of the osseous and cartilaginous acetabular index in normal children and those with developmental dysplasia of the hip: A cross-sectional study using MRI. *J Bone Joint Surg Br* 2012;94(12):1625-1631.

    This study reported on the difference in measuring the bony and cartilaginous aspects of the acetabulum and found that the normal cartilaginous acetabular index is fully formed at birth and is maintained constantly throughout childhood.

20. Klisić P, Zivanović V, Brdar R: Effects of triple prevention of CDH, stimulated by distribution of "baby packages." *J Pediatr Orthop* 1988;8(1):9-11.

21. Clinical practice guideline: Early detection of developmental dysplasia of the hip. Committee on Quality Improvement, Subcommittee on Developmental Dysplasia of the Hip: American Academy of Pediatrics. *Pediatrics* 2000;105(4 pt 1):896-905.

22. Mahan ST, Katz JN, Kim YJ: To screen or not to screen? A decision analysis of the utility of screening for developmental dysplasia of the hip. *J Bone Joint Surg Am* 2009;91(7):1705-1719.

23. Shorter D, Hong T, Osborn DA: Cochrane Review: Screening programmes for developmental dysplasia of the hip in newborn infants. *Evid Based Child Health* 2013;8(1):11-54.

    This systematic Cochrane review found insufficient evidence to provide clear practice recommendations on screening programs for DDH. The authors concluded that universal ultrasonography screening results in a substantial increase in treatment compared with the use of targeted ultrasonography or clinical examination alone; however, neither of the ultrasonography strategies have been proven to improve clinical outcomes, including the late diagnosis of DDH and surgical outcomes.

24. Sink EL, Ricciardi BF, Torre KD, Price CT: Selective ultrasound screening is inadequate to identify patients who present with symptomatic adult acetabular dysplasia. *J Child Orthop* 2014;8(6):451-455.

    This study showed that most patients with symptomatic acetabular dysplasia at skeletal maturity would not have met current recommendations for selective ultrasonography screening in the United States had they been born during the current period. This finding highlights the need for a better screening strategy.

25. Clarke NM, Castaneda P: Strategies to improve nonoperative childhood management. *Orthop Clin North Am* 2012;43(3):281-289.

    This review paper highlights the need for better detection strategies and improved treatment modalities and evaluation for DDH.

26. Graf R: Fundamentals of sonographic diagnosis of infant hip dysplasia. *J Pediatr Orthop* 1984;4(6):735-740.

27. Clarke NM, Harcke HT, McHugh P, Lee MS, Borns PF, MacEwen GD: Real-time ultrasound in the diagnosis of congenital dislocation and dysplasia of the hip. *J Bone Joint Surg Br* 1985;67(3):406-412.

28. Rosen A, Gamble JG, Vallier H, Bloch D, Smith L, Rinsky LA: Analysis of radiographic measurements as prognostic indicators of treatment success in patients with developmental dysplasia of the hip. *J Pediatr Orthop B* 1999;8(2):118-121.

29. Tönnis D: Normal values of the hip joint for the evaluation of X-rays in children and adults. *Clin Orthop Relat Res* 1976;119:39-47.

30. Wilkinson AG, Sherlock DA, Murray GD: The efficacy of the Pavlik harness, the Craig splint and the von Rosen splint in the management of neonatal dysplasia of the hip: A comparative study. *J Bone Joint Surg Br* 2002;84(5):716-719.

31. van de Sande MA, Melisie F: Successful Pavlik treatment in late-diagnosed developmental dysplasia of the hip. *Int Orthop* 2012;36(8):1661-1668.

    With proper use of the Pavlik harness and supervised treatment, successful outcomes can be obtained in older children with DDH who are traditionally difficult to treat. However, in this study, the mean age of patients was 27 weeks, which could be considered a young population.

32. Malkawi H: Sonographic monitoring of the treatment of developmental disturbances of the hip by the Pavlik harness. *J Pediatr Orthop B* 1998;7(2):144-149.

33. Job-Deslandre C: Pathologie de la hanche chez l'enfant, Diagnosis of hip pain in childhood. *Rev Rhum* 2009;76:361-366.

34. Murnaghan ML, Browne RH, Sucato DJ, Birch J: Femoral nerve palsy in Pavlik harness treatment for developmental dysplasia of the hip. *J Bone Joint Surg Am* 2011;93(5):493-499.

    This is one of only a few studies with a detailed description of the complications of Pavlik harness treatment. The authors concluded that femoral nerve palsy, which is strongly predictive of unsuccessful treatment, is an uncommon, yet clinically important, complication of Pavlik harness treatment.

35. Pap K, Kiss S, Shisha T, Marton-Szücs G, Szöke G: The incidence of avascular necrosis of the healthy, contralateral femoral head at the end of the use of Pavlik harness in unilateral hip dysplasia. *Int Orthop* 2006;30(5):348-351.

36. Swaroop VT, Mubarak SJ: Difficult-to-treat Ortolani-positive hip: Improved success with new treatment protocol. *J Pediatr Orthop* 2009;29(3):224-230.

37. Atalar H, Sayli U, Yavuz OY, Uraş I, Dogruel H: Indicators of successful use of the Pavlik harness in infants with developmental dysplasia of the hip. *Int Orthop* 2007;31(2):145-150.

38. Ibrahim DA, Skaggs DL, Choi PD: Abduction bracing after Pavlik harness failure: An effective alternative to closed reduction and spica casting? *J Pediatr Orthop* 2013;33(5):536-539.

    This study with a limited number of patients reported no benefits from prolonged abduction bracing after failed treatment with a Pavlik harness. Level of evidence: IV.

39. Gans I, Flynn JM, Sankar WN: Abduction bracing for residual acetabular dysplasia in infantile DDH. *J Pediatr Orthop* 2013;33(7):714-718.

    In patients with residual dysplasia after a successful hip reduction, substantial improvement in the acetabular index was reported in patients who used an abduction brace. Level of evidence: III.

40. Modaressi K, Erschbamer M, Exner GU: Dysplasia of the hip in adolescent patients successfully treated for developmental dysplasia of the hip. *J Child Orthop* 2011;5(4):261-266.

    The authors highlight the need for follow-up at least until skeletal maturity in patients treated for DDH in infancy because not all hips deemed normal in infancy will have normal morphology in adolescence. Level of evidence: IV.

41. Wakabayashi K, Wada I, Horiuchi O, Mizutani J, Tsuchiya D, Otsuka T: MRI findings in residual hip dysplasia. *J Pediatr Orthop* 2011;31(4):381-387.

    A prognostic sign for poor acetabular development is a high intensity MRI signal within the labrum of a dysplastic hip. This finding could justify intervention at an earlier age than traditionally recommended.

42. Douira-Khomsi W, Smida M, Louati H, et al: Magnetic resonance evaluation of acetabular residual dysplasia in developmental dysplasia of the hip: A preliminary study of 27 patients. *J Pediatr Orthop* 2010;30(1):37-43.

43. Tiderius C, Jaramillo D, Connolly S, et al: Post-closed reduction perfusion magnetic resonance imaging as a predictor of avascular necrosis in developmental hip dysplasia: A preliminary report. *J Pediatr Orthop* 2009;29(1):14-20.

44. Castañeda P, Tejerina P, Nualart L, Cassis N: The safety and efficacy of a transarticular pin for maintaining reduction in patients with developmental dislocation of the hip undergoing an open reduction. *J Pediatr Orthop* 2015;35(4):358-362.

    This retrospective review of patients undergoing open reduction showed that using a transarticular pin to temporarily stabilize the joint was not associated with a higher complication rate and was associated with a very low rate of redislocation.

45. Thomas SR, Wedge JH, Salter RB: Outcome at forty-five years after open reduction and innominate osteotomy for late-presenting developmental dislocation of the hip. *J Bone Joint Surg Am* 2007;89(11):2341-2350.

46. Matheney T, Kim YJ, Zurakowski D, Matero C, Millis M: Intermediate to long-term results following the Bernese periacetabular osteotomy and predictors of clinical outcome. *J Bone Joint Surg Am* 2009;91(9):2113-2123.

47. Wells J, Millis M, Kim YJ, Bulat E, Miller P, Matheney T: Survivorship of the Bernese periacetabular osteotomy: What factors are associated with long-term failure? *Clin Orthop Relat Res* 2016; May 12 [Epub ahead of print].

This study demonstrates that Bernese periacetabular osteotomy is a reasonable treatment option that provides good long-term results for symptomatic hip dysplasia. Risk factors for poor results include an age older than 25 years, severe symptoms, and a loss of joint space. Level of evidence: III.

48. Yasunaga Y, Ochi M, Yamasaki T, Shoji T, Izumi S: Rotational acetabular osteotomy for pre- and early osteoarthritis secondary to dysplasia provides durable results at 20 years. *Clin Orthop Relat Res* 2016; April 27 [Epub ahead of print].

The authors reported excellent long-term results in patients with hip dysplasia and pre- or early-stage osteoarthritis after treatment with a rotational acetabular osteotomy, even in patients who were considered to be of advanced age in other large cohort studies. Level of evidence: IV.

Chapter 21

Slipped Capital Femoral Epiphysis and Femoroacetabular Impingement

Rachel Mednick Thompson, MD   David A. Podeszwa, MD

Abstract

Slipped capital femoral epiphysis (SCFE) is one of the most common and most challenging hip disorders affecting adolescents. Although the etiology is unknown, obesity may be a modifiable risk factor for SCFE. In situ pinning remains the preferred treatment for stable and unstable SCFE. However, even with relatively minimal displacement, the residual deformity has been shown to lead to a high rate of subsequent disability. Open reduction and fixation of unstable SCFE using the modified Dunn procedure can restore normal hip motion with very low rates of associated osteonecrosis when highly trained surgeons administer treatment.

A diagnosis of femoroacetabular impingement also is common in adolescents and young adults who have hip pain with an unclear etiology. This disorder has a likely association with high-level athletic participation and cam lesions in males. Femoroacetabular impingement can be treated through either open or arthroscopic approaches, with excellent clinical outcomes and return to sports.

Keywords: FAI; femoroacetabular impingement; SCFE; slipped capital femoral epiphysis; surgical hip dislocation

---

Dr. Podeszwa or an immediate family member serves as a board member, owner, officer, or committee member of the Pediatric Orthopaedic Society of North America and the American Academy of Orthopaedic Surgeons. Neither Dr. Thompson nor any immediate family member has received anything of value from or has stock or stock options held in a commercial company or institution related directly or indirectly to the subject of this chapter.

Introduction

Slipped capital femoral epiphysis (SCFE) is one of the most common hip disorders affecting adolescents, and although it is ubiquitous, treatment remains a challenge. Epiphysiolysis and the subsequent displacement of the proximal femoral epiphysis relative to the metaphysis result in a three-dimensional deformity that most commonly involves varus, extension, and external rotation. Even when relatively minimal displacement is present, the residual deformity has been shown to lead to a high rate of subsequent disability. Although a proportion of femoroacetabular impingement (FAI) results from SCFE, FAI is a distinct clinical entity whose etiology varies. Ultimately, the surgical treatment of SCFE-related deformity and FAI is complementary and is be reviewed jointly in this chapter.

Slipped Capital Femoral Epiphysis

Epidemiology

The incidence of SCFE is somewhat regional, ranging from 0.2 per 100,000 children in eastern Japan to 17.15 children in the northeastern United States,[1] with an overall US incidence of approximately 10.8 per 100,000 children. The increasing incidence in certain regions correlates with the rise in obesity. Children who are obese have an earlier onset of SCFE than children who are not obese, and the age at initial presentation has decreased substantially in the past 20 years because obesity has become increasingly more common in younger children. The mean age at presentation is 12 years in boys and 11.2 years in girls. SCFE affects boys more often than girls.

The incidence of SCFE varies not only by region but also with race and ethnicity. However, numerous epidemiologic studies contradict one another in regard to the influence of race, and the reported variability may actually be reflective of differences between typical body mass indices (BMI) in certain ethnic and racial groups.[1]

Etiology

The underlying causality in SCFE has not been definitively established and is likely multifactorial. No established genetic predilection for SCFE exists, regardless of the marked variability between different races and regions.

More than 50% of children with SCFE are classified as being in greater than the 95th percentile for weight, and the average BMI in children with SCFE is 25 to 30 kg/m^2 (>85th percentile).[1] Morphologic changes in the proximal femoral physis associated with obesity may biomechanically predispose children who are obese to SCFE. Increased femoral retroversion, which is common in these children, results in elevated physeal shear stress, which is then compounded by the shear stress associated with elevated proximal femoral physeal inclination seen in children with SCFE. Acetabular depth also may play a role, particularly in unstable SCFE.[2]

A recent review of 173 patients who were treated for SCFE demonstrated that those with posttreatment obesity had an odds ratio of 3.5 for the development of a contralateral slip.[3] Conversely, weight loss after SCFE treatment is protective against the development of a contralateral slip. Thus, obesity may be a modifiable risk factor for SCFE.

Classification

SCFE can be classified based on the duration of symptoms, the degree of radiographic displacement, or the patient's ability for mobilization. Perhaps the most clinically relevant classification is that of functional stability,[4] in which a slip is defined as stable if a patient is able to bear weight with or without crutches. Unstable SCFEs are classically associated with much higher rates of osteonecrosis compared with stable slips (4.7% to 58% versus zero to 1.4%, respectively). However, two high-volume centers recently reported poor sensitivity (39%) and moderate specificity (76%) of the functional stability classification scheme compared with an intraoperative evaluation of physeal stability.[5] Because this classification scheme largely drives treatment decisions, a more comprehensive scheme that better reflects stability status and the risk of osteonecrosis is needed.

Treatment

Stable SCFE

The goals of initial surgical management for all slips are the prevention of further slips and the avoidance of osteonecrosis. A systematic review of the literature confirmed that a single central screw placed in situ is the best method of treatment and has the lowest incidence of associated complications in stable slips.[6]

Previous cadaver, animal, and biomechanical studies have demonstrated the importance of placing the screw perpendicular to the physis, with at least four threads crossing the physis, while avoiding placing the screw head medial to the intertrochanteric line. However, the ability to judge the depth of the screw with fluoroscopy can be limited. The distance between the tip of the screw to the subchondral bone has been shown to be, on average, 2.1 mm closer on a CT scan than the distance seen on an AP radiographic view, with a smaller discrepancy between the lateral radiographic view and the CT scan.[7]

Unstable SCFE

A systematic literature review suggests that urgent reduction with internal fixation and a decompressive arthrotomy results in the lowest risk of osteonecrosis (excluding those treated with surgical dislocation).[6] In situ pinning remains the preferred treatment for internal fixation, with the treating surgeon determining the need to add a decompressive arthrotomy. In addition, biomechanical studies have shown that a two-screw construct provides greater stability than one screw for unstable slips.[8]

There has been great enthusiasm for open reduction and fixation of unstable SCFE using the modified Dunn procedure.[9] Anatomic reduction with resultant restoration of normal hip motion is a preferred outcome, but it is a technically demanding procedure. Early reports suggested very low rates of associated osteonecrosis when highly trained surgeons performed the procedure; however, the actual rate of osteonecrosis may be substantially higher when the procedure is attempted in lower-volume centers. A multicenter prospective series of 27 unstable slips with an average 22-month follow-up revealed that, although near-anatomic correction can be achieved with this approach (average slip angle = 6°), the rate of osteonecrosis remains high (26%).[10] This series also reported a 15% rate of broken hardware that required revision fixation. In those patients in whom osteonecrosis did not develop, excellent clinical outcomes were reported at nearly 2 years postoperatively. All outcomes scores were substantially lower in the patients with osteonecrosis.

Two recent prospective European series reflected similar radiographic and clinical outcomes with lower associated rates of osteonecrosis.[11,12]

Contralateral Prophylactic Pinning

A contralateral slip will subsequently develop in 15% to 24% of patients with SCFE.[2,13,14] The relatively high risk of a contralateral slip has prompted many surgeons to recommend prophylactic pinning in all children presenting with unilateral SCFE; however, the possible consequences of this additional procedure must be considered. With a minimum follow-up of 12 months after prophylactic pinning, a multicenter retrospective case series reported a 2% risk of osteonecrosis, a 2% risk of peri-implant fracture, and a 3% risk of symptomatic hardware.[15] A subsequent contralateral slip was prevented in the 99 patients in the study.

A review of 260 patients initially treated for a unilateral SCFE who were followed to skeletal maturity or until the development of a contralateral slip demonstrated that demographic factors were not predictive of a contralateral slip, but the modified Oxford bone score provides probability data for predicting a contralateral slip.[14] The positive predictive value for a modified Oxford bone score between 16 and 18 is 96%, and the negative predictive value is 92%. Excellent intraobserver reliability and very good interobserver reliability also were reported for the modified Oxford bone score.[16]

Reconstruction of Residual Deformity

Even with relatively minimal displacement, the residual deformity after in situ fixation of SCFE results in an increased risk of osteoarthritis. A series of 92 hips treated with in situ fixation had an average α angle of 72.7°, which is a radiographic finding associated with symptomatic FAI.[17] In addition, a linear relationship existed between the degree of deformity and subsequent degenerative changes.

Historically, osteotomy at the intertrochanteric level has been the preferred procedure for moderate or severe slips because it provides adequate deformity correction with a low risk of osteonecrosis. A review of 32 symptomatic patients treated with a flexion osteotomy templated from preoperative CT scans showed excellent clinical outcomes. Hip flexion was greater than 90° in more than 90% of the patients, and the anterior impingement sign had resolved in 75% of the patients at the most recent follow-up.[18] A similar review of eight patients treated with an Imhäuser osteotomy demonstrated substantial improvement in postoperative hip range of motion, the gait deviation index, Pediatric Outcomes Data Collection Instrument scores, and radiographic measures of FAI.[19] The addition of a concomitant proximal femoral osteochondroplasty (open or arthroscopic) may offer improved outcomes without a substantial increase in associated complications; however, larger studies with longer follow-up are still needed[20,21] (**Figure 1**).

A more powerful deformity correction can be achieved with subcapital osteotomy performed through a surgical hip dislocation approach. This technically demanding procedure may substantially improve hip function, but it is associated with a high complication rate (25%).[22]

Outcomes

Osteonecrosis is one of the most concerning outcomes associated with the treatment of SCFE. A systematic literature review of unstable SCFE showed an overall osteonecrosis rate of 21%.[23] A 2013 literature review (excluding surgical hip dislocation) reported an overall osteonecrosis rate of 23.9%. No correlation was found between the osteonecrosis rate and the method of fixation, the use of capsulotomy, or attempted reduction.[24] When comparing the treatment of surgical hip dislocation by using a modified Dunn procedure with in situ pinning in 88 patients with unstable SCFE, the results showed a 43% rate of osteonecrosis with in situ pinning and a 29% rate with a modified Dunn procedure.[25] For patients with stable SCFE, no instances of osteonecrosis occurred with in situ pinning, but the modified Dunn procedure had a 20% rate of osteonecrosis.

The preferred treatment for SCFE is still considered to be in situ screw fixation. However, recent midterm and long-term clinical studies have reported that in situ screw fixation leads to high rates of residual deformity and moderate rates of associated pain and osteoarthritis. A review of 176 hips treated with in situ fixation resulted in an 89.5% fixation survival rate (no corrective osteotomy or conversion to arthroplasty) at 10 years.[26] In 105 patients not treated with additional reconstruction surgery and who were available for evaluation with outcome measures, 33% of the patients reported pain (more than 3 on a 10-point visual analog scale) at an average of 23 years after initial treatment. Similar 20-year outcomes were reported from a tertiary care center in Mexico. Of 121 patients, 96 had clinical (positive impingement sign) and radiographic (α angle > 55°) evidence of impingement, and all patients had radiographic evidence of osteoarthritis.[27] Of the patients with FAI, the mean Harris hip score was 75.4, which was substantially lower than the mean Harris hip score of patients without FAI (89.3). Similarly, at an average follow-up of 37 years, patients with SCFE had higher α angles compared with age- and sex-matched control subjects. Higher α angles correlated with worse outcomes, as quantified by the Harris hip score.[28]

Femoroacetabular Impingement

Epidemiology

FAI is a clinical diagnosis supported by radiographic findings of proximal femoral or acetabular dysmorphology (decreased femoral head-neck offset and/or increased acetabular coverage or depth). This condition typically manifests as anterior hip and/or groin pain with flexion-related activities. Radiographic findings in the absence of symptoms are common. A review of 473 CT scans showed

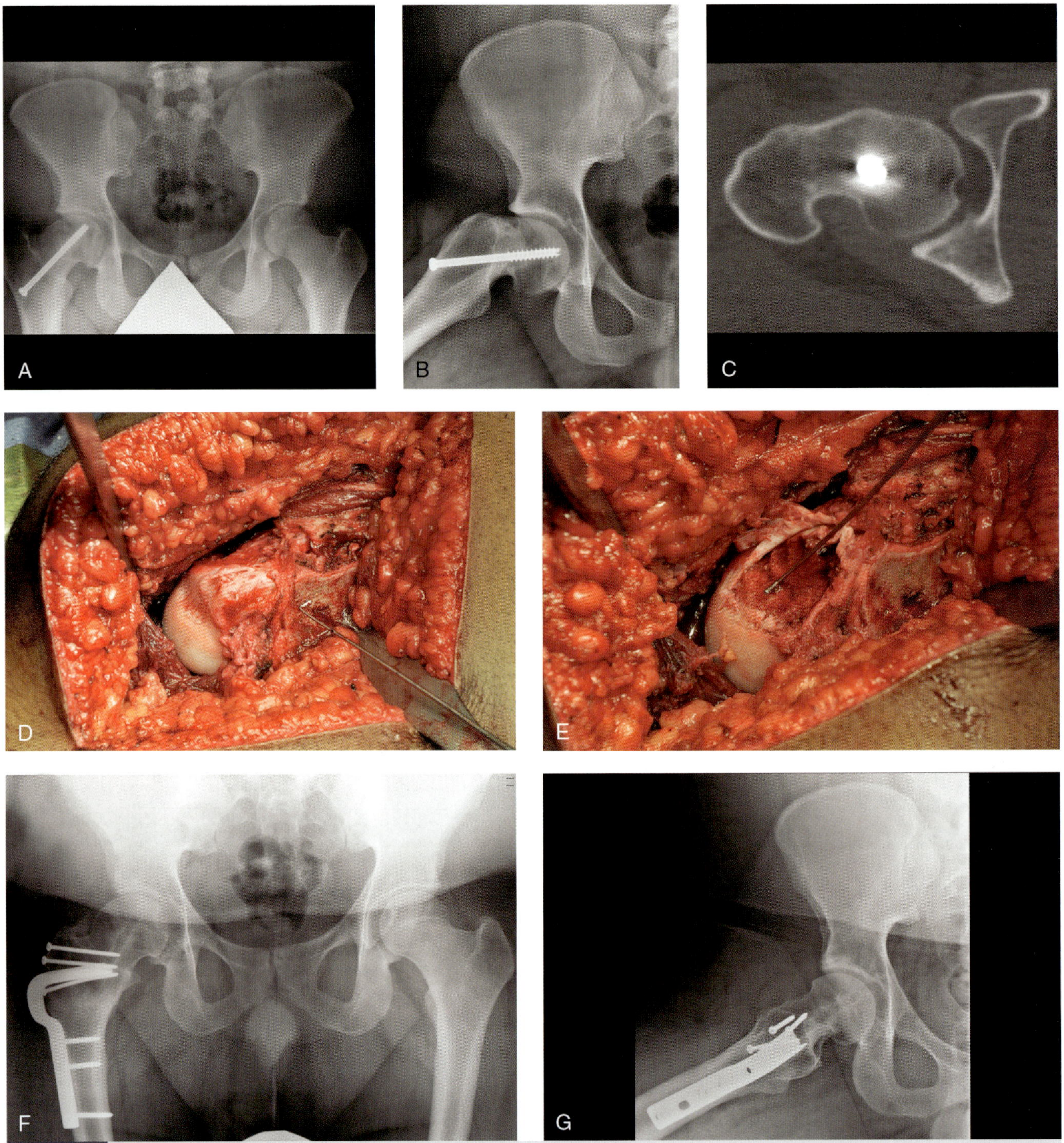

Figure 1 Standing AP pelvic (**A**) and lateral (**B**) radiographs of the right hip of a symptomatic 17-year-old adolescent boy with severe deformity secondary to a slipped capital femoral epiphysis. **C,** Axial CT scan demonstrates severe posterior displacement of the femoral epiphysis and metaphyseal prominence. Typical intraoperative photographs of a femoral head-neck junction before (**D**) and after (**E**) resection of the metaphyseal prominence. Standing AP pelvic (**F**) and lateral (**G**) radiographs of the right hip 2 years postoperatively show correction of the trochanteric height and the head-neck offset.

that 40% of asymptomatic hips had radiographic findings associated with FAI,[29] with these findings more common in men than in women. Similar findings were reported in a review of hip CT scans in otherwise healthy asymptomatic adolescents. The study demonstrated a 16.8% rate of cam deformity in asymptomatic adolescents (defined as an α angle ≥ 55°), a 32.4% rate of pincer deformity (defined as a lateral center edge angle ≥ 40°), and a 6.1% rate of mixed-type deformity.[30] Cam morphology was substantially more common in males, and pincer deformities were equally distributed among males and females.

A high prevalence of radiographic findings is consistent with FAI, but poor correlation exists between radiographic FAI and degenerative radiographic changes. The authors of a 2011 study evaluated 96 asymptomatic hips with radiographic findings consistent with FAI. The patients had been treated with arthroplasty of the contralateral hip. Because 82.3% of the patients had remained free of radiographic arthritic changes at a mean follow-up of 18.5 years, the authors recommend against treatment of asymptomatic radiographic FAI.[31]

A multicenter prospective study of patients undergoing surgical treatment of symptomatic FAI reported that 55% of the patients were female, 88% were Caucasian, the average age was 28.4 years, and the average BMI was 25.1.[32] Cam-type FAI was most common (47.6%), followed by mixed-type (44.5%) and pincer-type (7.9%).

Etiology

Pincer-type deformities are generally believed to be idiopathic morphologic differences in acetabular ossification, but cam lesions may result from multiple etiologies, including SCFE, Legg-Calvé-Perthes disease, infection, trauma, or increased repetitive loading. However, most lesions do not have a direct cause and are deemed idiopathic.

In males, a likely association exists between participation in high-level athletic activities and the presence of cam lesions. In a case-control study that compared 72 hips in elite-level basketball players with 76 hips in age-matched control subjects, the athletes had a tenfold increased likelihood of having a cam lesion, which was defined as an α angle greater than 55° measured on MRI. Although there was a definitive propensity toward an increased α angle in athletes at all ages, the differences were magnified after physeal closure.[33] It was hypothesized that the repetitive stress of loading coupled with the directional change of loading through the proximal femur may alter growth patterns, resulting in a cam deformity at skeletal maturity.

Assessment

In a patient with signs and symptoms of FAI, radiographic examination will likely confirm the diagnosis. The initial imaging should include a standing AP pelvic radiograph and a lateral projection of the affected hip. A recent retrospective review comparing lateral radiographs with radial MRIs in 60 patients who received a clinical diagnosis of FAI reported sensitivity for cam deformity of 96.4% with the 45° Dunn view compared with 70.6% for the cross-table lateral view. The specificity for cam deformity was 90% and 100%, respectively.[34] Dunn lateral views were recommended over cross-table lateral views for FAI evaluation. The Dunn lateral view also has a relatively low effective radiation dose compared with cross-table lateral and single frog-lateral views, and the need for repeated exposure is lowest with a Dunn lateral radiograph.[35]

Treatment

Using the surgical hip dislocation approach for the treatment of symptomatic FAI enables all osseous and soft-tissue abnormalities to be addressed as needed. Arthroscopic management of FAI, despite some limitations in treating all potential intra-articular pathology, has become increasingly more popular. A matched cohort of 60 consecutive patients treated surgically for FAI by either surgical hip dislocation or arthroscopy reported similar improvement in all radiographic measures of FAI except the AP α angle, which was treated more effectively with surgical hip dislocation.[36] The study authors recommended surgical hip dislocation for treating patients with superolateral or posterosuperior loss of femoral offset because an arthroscopic approach is limited in its ability to fully access and address cam-type deformities in these anatomic regions.

A similar retrospective review of patients treated for cam- or mixed-type FAI found statistically comparable improvement in radiographic parameters with open or arthroscopic treatment.[37] However, the authors reported a 2.2% rate of nonunion of the greater trochanter in the cohort treated with surgical hip dislocation. In addition, the need for arthroscopic lysis of adhesions was substantially higher in the surgical hip dislocation cohort than in the arthroscopically treated cohort (12% versus 6.1%, respectively).[37]

An alternative approach uses a modified Smith-Peterson interval in a mini-open approach. A prospective case series reviewed 49 hips at an average follow-up of 22 months. Substantial improvements in the Harris hip score, the Western Ontario and McMaster Universities Index (WOMAC), and the Medical Outcomes Study 36-Item Short Form measures were reported, with return to preinjury activity levels. Of note, a 20% rate of meralgia paresthetica was reported in this cohort.[38]

A similar minimally invasive approach used an anterolateral approach in 118 hips. At a mean follow-up of 26 months, similar improvements in functional outcomes were reported as assessed by the Harris hip score, WOMAC, and the Nonarthritic Hip score.[39] However, a 6.8% revision rate, a 3.5% rate of conversion to total hip arthroplasty (THA), and a 15% rate of increased Tönnis stage within 1 year were reported.[39] Long-term comparative studies are required to further evaluate the efficacy of minimally invasive approaches and define their role in treating FAI compared with surgical hip dislocation and arthroscopic approaches.

Outcomes

General

Surgical hip dislocation is a powerful tool for correcting cam- and pincer-type deformities. A review of 75 patients (minimum 5-year follow-ups) showed a 91% hip preservation survival rate (no conversion to THA, progression of osteoarthritis, or a Meryl d'Aubigné-Postel score <15).[40] Excessive acetabular rim trimming, preoperative arthritic changes, older age at surgery, and increased weight were predictive of failure. At the 10-year follow-up of this cohort, the hip preservation survival rate was 80%.[41]

Initial outcomes after arthroscopic treatment have been encouraging. A review of the outcomes of 243 patients who underwent arthroscopic surgery for FAI showed substantial improvement in all patient-reported outcome measures (as assessed by the modified Harris hip score, the Hip Outcome Score, and the International Hip Outcome Tool), with most of the patients improving at least by the minimal clinically important difference.[42] A similar review of 201 patients with a minimum 36-month follow-up reported a mean improvement in the Nonarthritic Hip score from 56.1 to 78.2 ($P < 0.001$), a mean visual analog pain scale improvement from 6.8 to 2.7 ($P < 0.001$), and a 5.7% conversion rate to THA.[43]

Regardless of the treatment method, whether open or arthroscopic, the failure of hip preservation surgery is most commonly associated with residual intra-articular impingement (74.8% of all revision cases) followed by extra-articular impingement (9.5% of cases). The rate of revision surgery was comparable in patients who were initially treated by arthroscopy or surgical hip dislocation (7.01% versus 7.25%, respectively), and most revisions could be accomplished arthroscopically.[44]

Adolescent Population

Because FAI is increasingly being recognized as a cause of disability that leads to degenerative arthritic changes, surgical treatment is more often being considered for adolescents with FAI. A review of 27 hips treated for symptomatic FAI in patients 19 years or younger (minimum 1-year follow-up) reported substantial improvement in self-reported functional outcomes, and all the patients reported improvement in their postoperative levels of athletic competition.[45] Similarly, a prospective cohort of 60 patients aged 11 to 16 years who underwent arthroscopic surgery for symptomatic FAI reported encouraging midterm results. At a minimum follow-up of 36 months, the modified Harris hip score increased from 57 to 91; however, there was a 13% rate of secondary surgery for lysis of adhesions and a subsequent decrease in functional scores.[46]

At 1 year after treatment with surgical hip dislocation, adolescent athletes with a University of California at Los Angeles (UCLA) physical activity score of 6+ appeared able to maintain preoperative functional activity levels.[47] Surgical hip dislocation resulted in substantial improvement in pain, with an average WOMAC-pain subscale improvement of 1.5 ($P = 0.002$). Of the 29 athletes included in the cohort study, 23 (79%) maintained or improved their activity level after surgical hip dislocation for FAI at 1 year postoperatively. Of the six athletes whose UCLA physical activity scores decreased postoperatively, only three had significant decreases.

Summary

Both SCFE and FAI remain difficult entities to treat. Although recently reported radiographic and clinical results of newer surgical approaches are encouraging, the inexperienced practitioner should approach these patients with caution and should recognize the risks and nuances associated with the more advanced surgical treatment of these conditions.

Key Study Points

- The modified Dunn osteotomy is a powerful tool for the treatment of unstable SCFE, but the learning curve is steep. The procedure should be reserved for surgeons with specific training in this approach.
- Prophylactic contralateral in situ pinning is not without risks and should be reserved for patients with substantial risks for a contralateral slip based on the modified Oxford bone score or those with an underlying endocrinopathy.
- FAI is a clinical diagnosis. A high prevalence of radiographic findings is consistent with FAI, but poor correlation exists between the radiographic findings and ultimate degenerative radiographic changes. Therefore, treatment should be reserved for patients with symptomatic FAI.

Annotated References

1. Loder RT, Skopelja EN: The epidemiology and demographics of slipped capital femoral epiphysis. *ISRN Orthop* 2011;2011:486512.

   This extensive literature review reports geographic and racial variability in the incidence of SCFE, highlighting the association between BMI and SCFE.

2. Podeszwa DA, Gurd D, Riccio A, De La Rocha A, Sucato DJ: Increased acetabular depth may influence physeal stability in slipped capital femoral epiphysis. *Clin Orthop Relat Res* 2013;471(7):2151-2155.

   A review of 232 patients with unilateral SCFE showed that the presence of increased acetabular depth was associated with unstable SCFE. Level of evidence: II.

3. Nasreddine AY, Heyworth BE, Zurakowski D, Kocher MS: A reduction in body mass index lowers risk for bilateral slipped capital femoral epiphysis. *Clin Orthop Relat Res* 2013;471(7):2137-2144.

   After treatment for obesity, the odds ratio for the development of a contralateral slip was 3.5. Weight loss was protective against the development of a contralateral slip. Level of evidence: III.

4. Loder RT, Richards BS, Shapiro PS, Reznick LR, Aronson DD: Acute slipped capital femoral epiphysis: The importance of physeal stability. *J Bone Joint Surg Am* 1993;75(8):1134-1140.

5. Ziebarth K, Domayer S, Slongo T, Kim YJ, Ganz R: Clinical stability of slipped capital femoral epiphysis does not correlate with intraoperative stability. *Clin Orthop Relat Res* 2012;470(8):2274-2279.

   The authors report on 82 patients who underwent open treatment of SCFE. The Loder stability classification had poor sensitivity (39%) and moderate specificity (76%) for intraoperative physeal stability. Level of evidence: III.

6. Loder RT, Dietz FR: What is the best evidence for the treatment of slipped capital femoral epiphysis? *J Pediatr Orthop* 2012;32(suppl 2):S158-S165.

   A systematic review of the literature found that the best treatment for stable SCFE is in situ single-screw fixation, whereas the best recommended treatment for unstable SCFE, excluding surgical dislocation, is urgent reduction, capsular decompression, and internal fixation. Level of evidence: IV.

7. Senthi S, Blyth P, Metcalfe R, Stott NS: Screw placement after pinning of slipped capital femoral epiphysis: A postoperative CT scan study. *J Pediatr Orthop* 2011;31(4):388-392.

   AP and lateral fluoroscopic views underestimate, on average, the tip-subchondral bone distance by 2.1 mm.

8. Kishan S, Upasani V, Mahar A, et al: Biomechanical stability of single-screw versus two-screw fixation of an unstable slipped capital femoral epiphysis model: Effect of screw position in the femoral neck. *J Pediatr Orthop* 2006;26(5):601-605.

9. Leunig M, Slongo T, Kleinschmidt M, Ganz R: Subcapital correction osteotomy in slipped capital femoral epiphysis by means of surgical hip dislocation. *Oper Orthop Traumatol* 2007;19(4):389-410.

10. Sankar WN, Vanderhave KL, Matheney T, Herrera-Soto JA, Karlen JW: The modified Dunn procedure for unstable slipped capital femoral epiphysis: A multicenter perspective. *J Bone Joint Surg Am* 2013;95(7):585-591.

    At an average follow-up of 22 months, a multicenter prospective case series of 27 unstable SCFEs treated with surgical hip dislocation and a Dunn osteotomy found that, although near-anatomic correction may be achieved (average slip angle of 6°), the rate of osteonecrosis remains high (26%).

11. Huber H, Dora C, Ramseier LE, Buck F, Dierauer S: Adolescent slipped capital femoral epiphysis treated by a modified Dunn osteotomy with surgical hip dislocation. *J Bone Joint Surg Br* 2011;93(6):833-838.

    A prospective case series of 30 consecutive hips treated with surgical hip dislocation and a modified Dunn osteotomy had an average final slip angle of 5.2°, an average Harris hip score of 97.8, flexion of 90° or more, and mean internal rotation of 33.3° in all patients except one patient with osteonecrosis.

12. Madan SS, Cooper AP, Davies AG, Fernandes JA: The treatment of severe slipped capital femoral epiphysis via the Ganz surgical dislocation and anatomical reduction: A prospective study. *Bone Joint J* 2013;95-B(3):424-429.

    At an average follow-up of 38.6 months, a case series reviewing the treatment of severe SCFE with Ganz surgical dislocation and anatomic reduction reported an average final slip angle of 7.5°, a mean modified Harris hip score of 89.1, an average Nonarthritic Hip score of 91.3, and 4 of 28 patients (14.3%) with osteonecrosis.

13. Baghdadi YM, Larson AN, Sierra RJ, Peterson HA, Stans AA: The fate of hips that are not prophylactically pinned after unilateral slipped capital femoral epiphysis. *Clin Orthop Relat Res* 2013;471(7):2124-2131.

    A review of 133 patients with a minimum follow-up 2 years after treatment of unilateral SCFE found a 15% risk for contralateral slip development. Overall health scores were lower than for age-matched control subjects. Level of evidence: III.

14. Popejoy D, Emara K, Birch J: Prediction of contralateral slipped capital femoral epiphysis using the modified Oxford bone age score. *J Pediatr Orthop* 2012;32(3):290-294.

    Demographic factors were not predictive of a contralateral slip in patients with SCFE, but the modified Oxford bone

5: Lower Extremity

score provides reliable probability data for predicting a contralateral slip. Level of evidence: IV.

15. Sankar WN, Novais EN, Lee C, Al-Omari AA, Choi PD, Shore BJ: What are the risks of prophylactic pinning to prevent contralateral slipped capital femoral epiphysis? *Clin Orthop Relat Res* 2013;471(7):2118-2123.

    This multicenter retrospective case series of 99 patients with prophylactic contralateral pinning revealed a 2% risk of osteonecrosis, a 2% risk of peri-implant fracture, and a 3% risk of symptomatic hardware. None of these risks was directly linked to specific implant positioning. Level of evidence: IV.

16. Zide JR, Popejoy D, Birch JG: Revised modified Oxford bone score: A simpler system for prediction of contralateral involvement in slipped capital femoral epiphysis. *J Pediatr Orthop* 2011;31(2):159-164.

    Excellent intraobserver reliability and very good interobserver reliability were reported for the modified Oxford bone score. Level of evidence: II.

17. Kamegaya M, Saisu T, Nakamura J, Murakami R, Segawa Y, Wakou M: Drehmann sign and femoro-acetabular impingement in SCFE. *J Pediatr Orthop* 2011;31(8):853-857.

    In 92 hips treated with in situ fixation, the average α angle was 72.7°, which was associated with an increased risk of obligate external rotation.

18. Saisu T, Kamegaya M, Segawa Y, Kakizaki J, Takahashi K: Postoperative improvement of femoroacetabular impingement after intertrochanteric flexion osteotomy for SCFE. *Clin Orthop Relat Res* 2013;471(7):2183-2191.

    A review of 32 symptomatic patients treated with flexion osteotomy templated from preoperative CT scans resulted in hip flexion greater than 90° in more than 90% of the patients, and 75% of the patients did not have the anterior impingement sign at the latest follow-up. Level of evidence: IV.

19. Caskey PM, McMulkin ML, Gordon AB, Posner MA, Baird GO, Tompkins BJ: Gait outcomes of patients with severe slipped capital femoral epiphysis after treatment by flexion-rotation osteotomy. *J Pediatr Orthop* 2014;34(7):668-673.

    Imhäuser osteotomies for SCFE deformity substantially improved the gait deviation index, Pediatric Outcomes Data Collection Instrument scores, and radiographic measures. Level of evidence: IV.

20. Bali NS, Harrison JO, Bache CE: A modified Imhäuser osteotomy: An assessment of the addition of an open femoral neck osteoplasty. *Bone Joint J* 2014;96-B(8):1119-1123.

    Combining a femoral neck osteochondroplasty with an Imhäuser osteotomy does not result in increased complication risks and trends toward higher postoperative Nonarthritic Hip scores.

21. Chen A, Youderian A, Watkins S, Gourineni P: Arthroscopic femoral neck osteoplasty in slipped capital femoral epiphysis. *Arthroscopy* 2014;30(10):1229-1234.

    Arthroscopic osteoplasty for residual symptomatic SCFE deformity resulted in reduction in α angles and resolution of obligate external rotation in 32 of 34 patients. Level of evidence: IV.

22. Anderson LA, Gililland JM, Pelt CE, Peters CL: Subcapital correction osteotomy for malunited slipped capital femoral epiphysis. *J Pediatr Orthop* 2013;33(4):345-352.

    Subcapital correction osteotomy for residual SCFE deformity in 12 hips resulted in substantial improvement in the α angle and the Harris hip scores but was associated with a complication rate of 25%. Level of evidence: IV.

23. Loder RT: What is the cause of avascular necrosis in unstable slipped capital femoral epiphysis and what can be done to lower the rate? *J Pediatr Orthop* 2013;33(suppl 1):S88-S91.

    A review of the literature of unstable SCFE reveals an overall osteonecrosis rate of 21%.

24. Zaltz I, Baca G, Clohisy JC: Unstable SCFE: Review of treatment modalities and prevalence of osteonecrosis. *Clin Orthop Relat Res* 2013;471(7):2192-2198.

    A literature review (excluding surgical hip dislocation) found an overall osteonecrosis rate of 23.9%. No correlation existed between the rate of osteonecrosis and the method of fixation, the use of capsulotomy, or attempted reduction.

25. Souder CD, Bomar JD, Wenger DR: The role of capital realignment versus in situ stabilization for the treatment of slipped capital femoral epiphysis. *J Pediatr Orthop* 2014;34(8):791-798.

    A review comparing the modified Dunn procedure with in situ pinning found a 43% rate of osteonecrosis with in situ pinning and a 29% rate of osteonecrosis with the modified Dunn procedure in patients with unstable SCFE compared with no cases of osteonecrosis with in situ pinning and a 20% rate of osteonecrosis with the modified Dunn procedure in those with stable SCFE. Level of evidence: III.

26. Larson AN, Sierra RJ, Yu EM, Trousdale RT, Stans AA: Outcomes of slipped capital femoral epiphysis treated with in situ pinning. *J Pediatr Orthop* 2012;32(2):125-130.

    The authors report that 176 hips treated with in situ fixation resulted in an 89.5% survival rate (no corrective osteotomy or arthroplasty required) at 10 years; however, 33% of the patients reported substantial pain at an average of 23 years after initial treatment. Level of evidence: IV.

27. Castañeda P, Ponce C, Villareal G, Vidal C: The natural history of osteoarthritis after a slipped capital femoral epiphysis/the pistol grip deformity. *J Pediatr Orthop* 2013;33(suppl 1):S76-S82.

    Of 121 patients reviewed, 96 had clinical (positive impingement sign) and radiographic (α angle > 55°) evidence of impingement. All patients had radiographic evidence of osteoarthritis at 20 years after in situ pinning.

28. Wensaas A, Gunderson RB, Svenningsen S, Terjesen T: Femoroacetabular impingement after slipped upper femoral epiphysis: The radiological diagnosis and clinical outcome at long-term follow-up. *J Bone Joint Surg Br* 2012;94(11):1487-1493.

    At a mean follow-up of 37 years, patients with SCFE had higher α angles compared with age- and sex-matched control subjects. The higher α angles correlated with worse outcomes.

29. Kim J, Choi JA, Lee E, Lee KR: Prevalence of imaging features on CT thought to be associated with femoroacetabular impingement: A retrospective analysis of 473 asymptomatic adult hip joints. *AJR Am J Roentgenol* 2015;205(1):W100-W105.

    A review of 473 CT scans showed that 40% of asymptomatic hips have radiographic evidence of FAI. Radiographic abnormalities were more commonly seen in men.

30. Li Y, Helvie P, Mead M, Gagnier J, Hammer MR, Jong N: Prevalence of femoroacetabular impingement morphology in asymptomatic adolescents. *J Pediatr Orthop* 2015; Jul 9 [Epub ahead of print].

    A review of hip CT scans in healthy, asymptomatic adolescents found a 16.8% rate of cam deformity, a 32.4% rate of pincer deformity, and a 6.1% rate of mixed-type deformity. Level of evidence: III.

31. Hartofilakidis G, Bardakos NV, Babis GC, Georgiades G: An examination of the association between different morphotypes of femoroacetabular impingement in asymptomatic subjects and the development of osteoarthritis of the hip. *J Bone Joint Surg Br* 2011;93(5):580-586.

    The authors report on 96 patients with asymptomatic hips and radiographic findings consistent with FAI who were followed for a mean of 18.5 years. Results showed that 82.3% of the patients remained free of radiographic arthritic changes.

32. Clohisy JC, Baca G, Beaulé PE, et al; ANCHOR Study Group: Descriptive epidemiology of femoroacetabular impingement: A North American cohort of patients undergoing surgery. *Am J Sports Med* 2013;41(6):1348-1356.

    In a multicenter cohort of patients undergoing surgical treatment of symptomatic FAI, 55% were female, 88% were Caucasian, the average age was 28.4 years, and the average BMI was 25.1.

33. Siebenrock KA, Ferner F, Noble PC, Santore RF, Werlen S, Mamisch TC: The cam-type deformity of the proximal femur arises in childhood in response to vigorous sporting activity. *Clin Orthop Relat Res* 2011;469(11):3229-3240.

    In a case-control study comparing 72 hips in elite-level basketball players with 76 hips in age-matched control subjects, the athletes had a tenfold increased likelihood of having a cam lesion, defined as an α angle greater than 55° as measured on MRI. Level of evidence: II.

34. Domayer SE, Ziebarth K, Chan J, Bixby S, Mamisch TC, Kim YJ: Femoroacetabular cam-type impingement: Diagnostic sensitivity and specificity of radiographic views compared to radial MRI. *Eur J Radiol* 2011;80(3):805-810.

    A review comparing lateral radiographs to radial MRIs reported a sensitivity for cam deformity of 96.4% with the 45° Dunn view compared with 70.6% with the cross-table lateral view.

35. Young M, Dempsey M, Rocha DL, Podeszwa DA: The cross-table lateral radiograph results in a significantly increased effective radiation dose compared with the Dunn and single frog lateral radiographs. *J Pediatr Orthop* 2015;35(2):157-161.

    Cross-table lateral radiographs resulted in the highest effective radiation dose, followed by Dunn and single frog-lateral radiographs, with the need for repeat exposure lowest with the Dunn lateral views. Level of evidence: II.

36. Bedi A, Zaltz I, De La Torre K, Kelly BT: Radiographic comparison of surgical hip dislocation and hip arthroscopy for treatment of cam deformity in femoroacetabular impingement. *Am J Sports Med* 2011;39(suppl):20S-28S.

    A matched cohort of 60 patients treated for FAI by either surgical hip dislocation or arthroscopy reported similar improvement in all radiographic measures except the AP α angle, which was addressed more effectively with open treatment. Level of evidence: III.

37. Büchler L, Neumann M, Schwab JM, Iselin L, Tannast M, Beck M: Arthroscopic versus open cam resection in the treatment of femoroacetabular impingement. *Arthroscopy* 2013;29(4):653-660.

    A retrospective review of patients treated for cam- or mixed-type FAI found statistically comparable improvement in radiographic parameters with open or arthroscopic treatment, along with a 2.2% rate of greater trochanteric nonunion in the cohort treated with surgical hip dislocation. Level of evidence: III.

38. Cohen SB, Huang R, Ciccotti MG, Dodson CC, Parvizi J: Treatment of femoroacetabular impingement in athletes using a mini-direct anterior approach. *Am J Sports Med* 2012;40(7):1620-1627.

    The authors evaluated 49 hips treated for FAI through a mini-open anterior approach. At an average follow-up of 22 months, substantial improvement occurred in the Harris hip scores (24 points) and in the WOMAC and the Medical Outcomes Study 36-Item Short Form measures, along with minimal changes in preinjury to postoperative activity scores. Level of evidence: IV.

39. Chiron P, Espié A, Reina N, Cavaignac E, Molinier F, Laffosse JM: Surgery for femoroacetabular impingement using a minimally invasive anterolateral approach: Analysis of 118 cases at 2.2-year follow-up. *Orthop Traumatol Surg Res* 2012;98(1):30-38.

    The authors report on 118 hips with FAI treated with a mini-open anterolateral approach (mean follow-up = 26 months). Substantial improvement was found in the

5: Lower Extremity

Nonarthritic Hip scores, the Harris hip scores, and the WOMAC scores. The revision rate was 6.8%, with 3.5% of the hips revised with arthroplasty. Fifteen percent of the cases progressed by one Tönnis stage. Level of evidence: III.

40. Steppacher SD, Huemmer C, Schwab JM, Tannast M, Siebenrock KA: Surgical hip dislocation for treatment of femoroacetabular impingement: Factors predicting 5-year survivorship. *Clin Orthop Relat Res* 2014;472(1):337-348.

    A review of 75 patients with a minimum 5-year follow-up showed a 91% hip survival rate following surgical hip dislocation and associated procedures for FAI.

41. Steppacher SD, Anwander H, Zurmühle CA, Tannast M, Siebenrock KA: Eighty percent of patients with surgical hip dislocation for femoroacetabular impingement have a good clinical result without osteoarthritis progression at 10 years. *Clin Orthop Relat Res* 2015;473(4):1333-1341.

    A review of 72 patients with a minimum 10-year follow-up reported an 80% hip survival rate after surgical hip dislocation and associated procedures for FAI.

42. Fabricant PD, Fields KG, Taylor SA, Magennis E, Bedi A, Kelly BT: The effect of femoral and acetabular version on clinical outcomes after arthroscopic femoroacetabular impingement surgery. *J Bone Joint Surg Am* 2015;97(7):537-543.

    A review of 243 patients who underwent arthroscopic surgery for FAI reported substantial improvement in all patient-reported outcome measures.

43. Palmer DH, Ganesh V, Comfort T, Tatman P: Midterm outcomes in patients with cam femoroacetabular impingement treated arthroscopically. *Arthroscopy* 2012;28(11):1671-1681.

    At a minimum follow-up of 36 months, patients treated arthroscopically for FAI reported substantial improvement in Nonarthritic Hip scores and visual analog pain scores; however, the conversion rate to THA was 5.7%. Level of evidence: IV.

44. Ricciardi BF, Fields K, Kelly BT, Ranawat AS, Coleman SH, Sink EL: Causes and risk factors for revision hip preservation surgery. *Am J Sports Med* 2014;42(11):2627-2633.

    The failure of surgical management is most commonly associated with residual intra-articular impingement (74.8% of all revision cases) followed by extra-articular impingement (9.5%). The rate of revision surgery is comparable between those treated with arthroscopy and surgical hip dislocation (7.01% versus 7.25%, respectively). Level of evidence: III.

45. Fabricant PD, Heyworth BE, Kelly BT: Hip arthroscopy improves symptoms associated with FAI in selected adolescent athletes. *Clin Orthop Relat Res* 2012;470(1):261-269.

    A review of 27 hips treated for symptomatic FAI in patients 19 years or younger with a minimum 1-year follow-up showed improvement in the average modified Harris hip score of 21 points. All patients reported improvement in their postoperative levels of athletic competition.

46. Philippon MJ, Ejnisman L, Ellis HB, Briggs KK: Outcomes 2 to 5 years following hip arthroscopy for femoroacetabular impingement in the patient aged 11 to 16 years. *Arthroscopy* 2012;28(9):1255-1261.

    The authors report on 60 patients aged 11 to 16 years (minimum follow-up of 36 months) treated with arthroscopic surgery for symptomatic FAI. The mean modified Harris hip score increased from 57 to 91. Level of evidence: IV.

47. Novais EN, Heyworth BE, Stamoulis C, Sullivan K, Millis MB, Kim YJ: Open surgical treatment of femoroacetabular impingement in adolescent athletes: Preliminary report on improvement of physical activity level. *J Pediatr Orthop* 2014;34(3):287-294.

    Adolescents with a UCLA physical activity score of 6+ undergoing surgical hip dislocation for symptomatic FAI reported a substantial improvement in pain, with 79% maintaining or improving their levels of athletic competition at 1 year after surgery.

Chapter 22

Legg-Calvé-Perthes Disease

Holly B. Leshikar, MD, MPH Jonathan G. Schoenecker, MD, PhD

Abstract

Legg-Calvé-Perthes disease is a disruption of the normal physiology of the capital femoral epiphysis, physis, and metaphysis. Although its exact pathophysiology remains uncertain, strong associations between the development of this condition in late childhood and an ischemic etiology have been demonstrated. The unique vascularity of the pediatric hip likely plays a role in the development of the condition. The goals of treatment in Legg-Calvé-Perthes disease are focused on maintaining containment and motion of the femoral head within the acetabulum as the disease progresses through the characteristic stages, with the femoral head initially more susceptible to deformation until blood flow returns. Outcomes vary, with some patients having no subsequent difficulty with the affected hips whereas other patients ultimately require total hip arthroplasty because of early degenerative changes.

Keywords: femoroacetabular impingement; Legg-Calvé-Perthes disease; osteonecrosis; physeal bar

Introduction

Legg-Calvé-Perthes disease (LCPD) is an ailment of skeletal immaturity that manifests as idiopathic necrosis of the proximal femoral epiphysis, physis, and, in severe cases, the metaphysis. The segregation of the epiphyseal vasculature from the metaphyseal vasculature of the proximal femur during development and the relatively feeble epiphyseal vasculature make the epiphysis uniquely susceptible to osteonecrosis. The disease follows a protracted course, which is readily observed by plain radiography, and is characterized by sclerosis, fragmentation, reossification, and remodeling. The predominant feature of sclerosis is avascular necrotic bone. The fragmentation stage of LCPD features bone resorption and metaplastic development of a neocartilage anlage, which promotes subsequent revascularization and ossification.

The overwhelmingly benign course of the disease in children younger than 6 years suggests that the age of the patient is the single most important factor in disease severity. In older children, disease severity is initially correlated with the extent of proximal femoral involvement, but the outcome is ultimately associated with the resultant geometry and condition of the articular cartilage of the hip. Loss of containment and the development of a physeal bar contribute to poor hip geometry. Femoroacetabular impingement, subluxation, and the extent of revascularization of the epiphysis are among the factors that influence the health of the articular cartilage. Therefore, the optimal treatment is to minimize geometric deformity of the proximal femur and acetabulum, promote complete revascularization, and avoid the development of a physeal bar. Because no current therapies exist that alter the extent of revascularization of the epiphysis or physeal bar development, containment is the only factor associated with outcome that is treatable. Initially, containment is treated by any combination of range-of-motion therapy, bracing, activity modification, and anti-inflammatory drugs. Surgical management may be considered if containment cannot be maintained. Proposed surgical containment methods range from adductor tenotomy and casting to femoral and pelvic osteotomies. Better outcomes are achieved if containment occurs early in the disease process. Late LCPD deformity, especially in the setting of a physeal bar, characteristically includes coxa magna, a short femoral neck, and a high-riding greater trochanter with variable acetabular dysplasia. These deformities can cause impingement between the anterior head-neck junction and the anterior aspect of the acetabular rim and external impingement of the

Dr. Schoenecker or an immediate family member has received research or institutional support from Ionis Pharmaceuticals. Neither Dr. Leshikar nor any immediate family member has received anything of value from or has stock or stock options held in a commercial company or institution related directly or indirectly to the subject of this chapter.

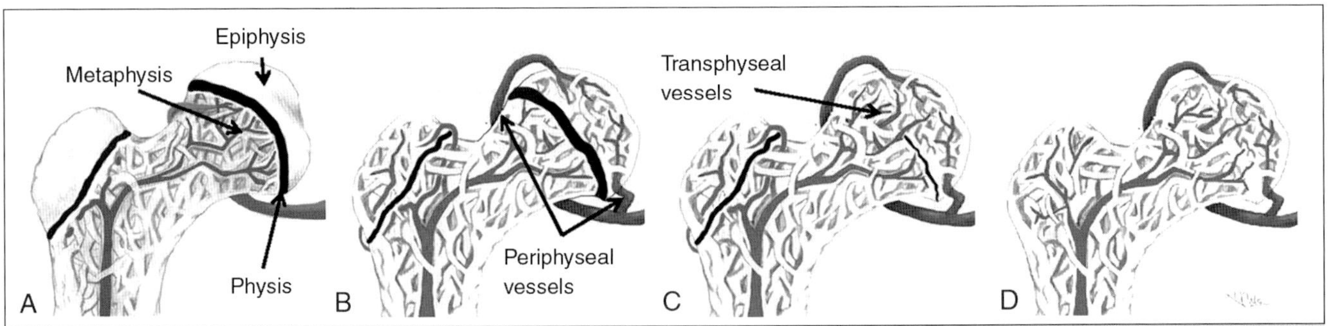

Figure 1 Illustrations show the development of the proximal femur in humans. **A,** Initially, the proximal femoral epiphysis in humans consists of avascular cartilage. **B,** At approximately 6 months of age, a secondary ossification center develops as a result of a vascular system that does not cross the physis (arrows indicate periphyseal vessels). At skeletal maturity (**C**), transphyseal vessels (indicated by the arrow shown crossing the physis) develop that result in physeal closure (**D**).

posterosuperior greater trochanter and ischium. In severe LCPD, propagated acetabular dysplasia also may include paradoxic joint instability transposed on femoroacetabular impingement. These geometric deformities instigate degradation of the chondrolabral junction and articular cartilage. The goal of addressing these late deformities is to achieve impingement-free and stable, normal hip range of motion in an effort to delay the development of osteoarthritis.

Epidemiology

LCPD is a unique process of osteonecrosis of the proximal femur that typically involves the capital epiphysis and physis and, variably, the metaphysis. LCPD occurs in skeletally immature patients, with the typical onset occurring from 4 to 8 years of age. The incidence tends to increase with closer proximity to Northern Europe and is highest in Caucasians, although it ranges widely from 0.4 to 29.0 children per 100,000.[1] Children with LCPD have a short stature. Most epidemiologic studies show delay in bone maturation of more than 1 year, suggesting that the disease is likely more systemic and not limited to the proximal femur.[2] Affected patients are disproportionately male by a 4:1 ratio.[1,3] A large case series reported no important difference in the age of presentation between female and male patients.[4] Because the natural history differs substantially, it is important to highlight the distinction between LCPD and that of osteonecrosis of the femur, which occurs in older children, adolescents, and adults.

Pathophysiology

The work of Trueta in 1957 demonstrated that the epiphyseal vascularity is segregated from the metaphysis in the growing skeleton by the avascular physis.[5] At skeletal maturity, resorption of the physis allows blood vessels from the metaphysis to form anastomoses with those of the epiphysis. With a less redundant vasculature, the capital femoral epiphysis in children is a watershed area of bone and is susceptible to pathologies different from those of adults (**Figure 1**). This unique aspect of the vascular anatomy, the relatively feeble epiphyseal vasculature, and the timing of the onset of LCPD suggest that the condition is caused, at least in part, by insufficient vascularity at a particular point in skeletal development when the epiphysis is most susceptible to osteonecrosis. This theory of an insufficient blood supply to the proximal femoral epiphysis is reinforced by the universal involvement of the anterior aspect of the femoral head, which is most susceptible because of its vascular supply.

A sudden or catastrophic loss of perfusion to the femoral head seems a less likely cause given the rare history of injury in patients with LCPD and the insidious onset of symptoms.[6] Instead, a vascular mechanism is supported, but the exact underlying pathology remains unknown. In a study that examined the brachial arteries of children, those with LCPD tended to have smaller caliber arteries and impaired arterial function compared with their healthy counterparts.[3] This microvascular dysfunction, which is known to play a role in cardiovascular disease, may help explain the increased prevalence of ischemic heart disease and hypertension in young adults with a prior diagnosis of LCPD.[7] Environmental risk factors for vascular dysfunction, such as exposure to tobacco smoke, also have been associated with higher rates of LCPD.[8-10] These findings suggest an underlying vascular mechanism.

A thrombotic etiology also has been proposed. In a large case-control study of 169 patients with LCPD and 474 control subjects, a higher incidence of factor V Leiden mutation, protein S deficiency, elevated factor VIII, and prothrombin G20210A mutations were found in the children with LCPD.[11] Leptin, which is an angiogenic factor and positive vascular endothelial growth factor regulator known to affect bone metabolism, has been considered as a factor in the pathogenesis of the disease.[12,13] A case-control study reported that leptin resistance was elevated in children with LCPD compared with control subjects. The authors hypothesized that the increased leptin resistance may contribute to the pathology of the disease.[12-14] The authors of a recent study suggested that elevated interleukin-6 levels, which were found to be high in patients with LCPD during the initial and fragmentation phases of the disease, may result in a portion of the osteoclastic activity.[15] The prolonged injury to the physis and epiphysis that occurs in LCPD may act as a potent instigator that induces an acute phase response. It is premature to assign causation of the disease course to these mediators (even when elevated) because they may represent only the downstream outcomes of the course of the condition.

Natural History

The initial radiographic observations of LCPD progression described by Waldenström have continued to frame the stages of the disease process (**Figure 2**). An inciting event occurs during stage I with observable sclerosis followed by subsequent fragmentation of the epiphysis in stage II and reossification in stage III. Remodeling may occur in stage IV. Disease severity is initially correlated with the extent of proximal femoral involvement during stage II. The predominant feature of sclerosis is osteonecrosis. Unlike adult forms of osteonecrosis, the fragmentation stage features bone resorption and metaplastic development of a neocartilage anlage (**Figure 3**). Especially if uncontained, the deforming forces act on the soft cartilage that predominates this stage of the disease, which leads to the resultant change in geometry of the femoral head (**Figure 4**).

By undergoing metaplastic change, the resultant cartilaginous anlage has the biologic capacity to initiate endochondral vascularization and ossification (stage III). This important feature of LCPD is the principal factor that differentiates it from less efficient and often futile revascularization and ossification through the process of creeping substitution, which is observed in osteonecrosis without metaplasia and is seen in older children and adults. Thus, the pediatric hip has a substantially greater potential for revascularization of avascular areas, which effectively resets the hip back to a stage in development at which the epiphysis was largely a cartilaginous anlage, before ossification. Reossification (stage III) is directed by revascularization of the capital epiphysis, and the method by which this occurs and whether it is complete directs the disease severity.

The following three main outcomes exist regarding revascularization: (1) revascularization without consequence, (2) revascularization with consequence, and (3) incomplete revascularization. Anatomically, restoration of the blood flow to the epiphysis may occur through creation of periphyseal vessels, which spare the physis, maintain segregation of the metaphyseal and epiphyseal blood flow, and lead to the maintenance of the characteristic proximal femoral geometry. Alternatively, injury to the physis during the first two stages of the disease can promote channels of vascularity through the physis, leading to premature ossification across the physis and physeal bar formation.[16,17] With a healthy physis and periphyseal revascularization, the hip may remodel (stage IV) in the plane of motion, which results in a hip with relatively little deficiency in motion. Alternatively, revascularization via physeal bar formation impedes the ability of the hip to remodel and may instead propagate further geometric changes in the proximal femur. The role of physeal bar formation in the overall deformity has been described and suggests a poorer outcome with characteristic residual post-LCPD deformities, including femoral head widening (coxa magna) and flattening (coxa plana), a shortened neck (coxa breva), and relative overgrowth of the greater trochanter.

The outcome is ultimately associated with the resultant geometry of the femoral head and the condition of the articular cartilage of the hip[18,19] (**Figure 5**). Although healing occurs in many patients with little or no permanent change in the morphology of the femoral head and acetabulum, long-term studies have shown that a substantial change develops in approximately 50% of patients, which leads to premature degenerative joint disease and disability.[20,21] Factors that are known to negatively influence the resultant hip geometry are a loss of containment and the development of a physeal bar. Factors that are known to negatively influence the health of the articular cartilage are femoroacetabular impingement and/or subluxation and the extent of revascularization of the epiphysis.

Classification and Imaging

Classification systems are based on the radiographic course of the femoral head in LCPD. As previously discussed, Waldenström divided the disease course into four stages based on radiographic characteristics. Other classifications include the Catterall, Salter-Thompson, and Herring lateral pillar systems. The lateral pillar classification was suggested by Herring and associates in 1992 and then

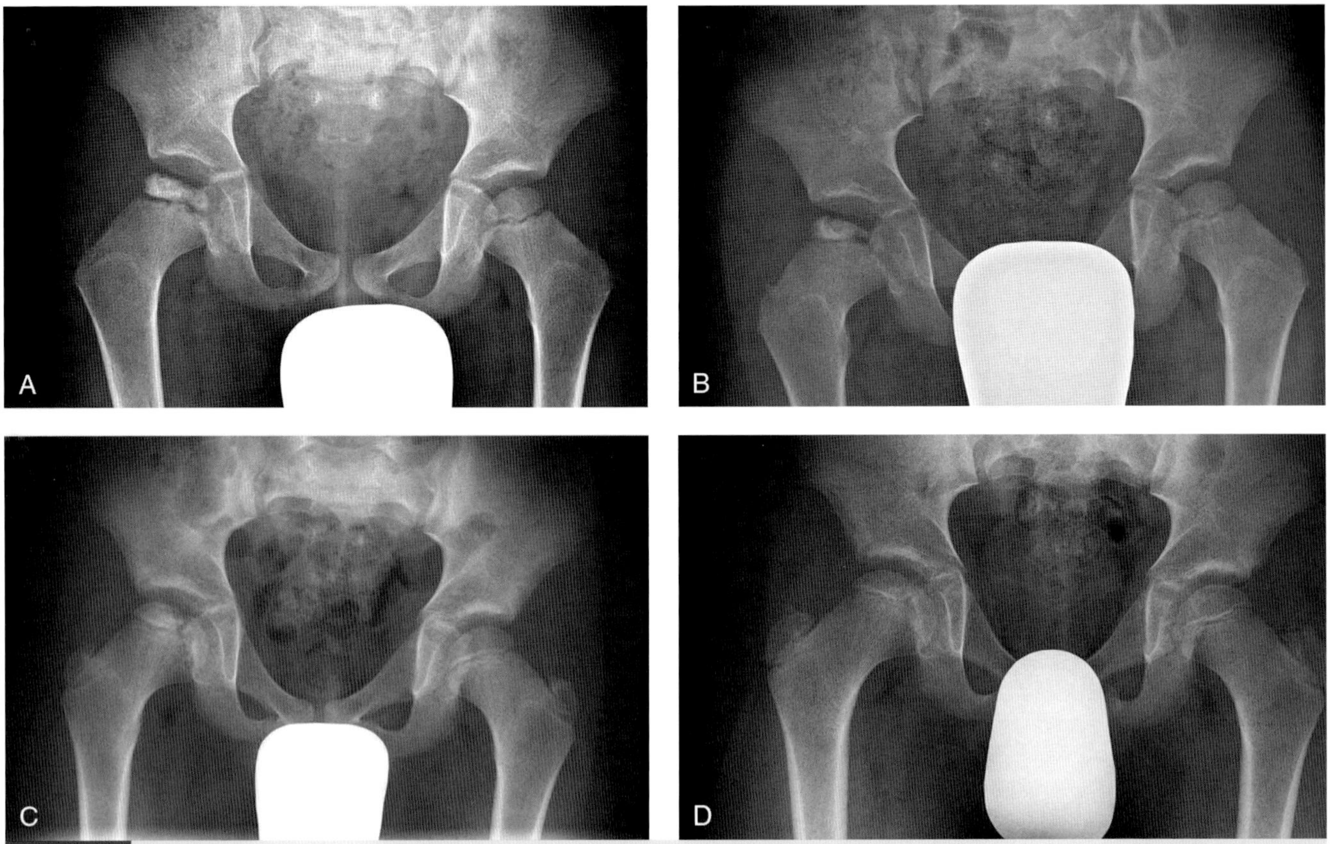

Figure 2 AP radiographs show the four stages of Legg-Calvé-Perthes disease described by Waldenström. **A,** Sclerosis. **B,** Fragmentation. **C,** Reossification. **D,** Remodeling.

modified in 2004. It is based on the height of the lateral epiphysis and the extent of the collapse in the fragmentation stage[22] (**Figure 6**). Many studies have shown the excellent interobserver and intraobserver reliability of this classification system.[23] Although widely used, it should be applied cautiously in the early fragmentation stage because progression to a group other than the previously assigned group can occur in up to 75% of hips initially classified as Herring lateral pillar group A. Twenty-one percent to 33% of hips are ultimately assigned a more severe group later in the fragmentation stage.[24,25]

The most widely used system for outcome measurements in LCPD is the Stulberg classification, which categorizes the mature hip into one of five classes. The Stulberg system is based on the shape of the femoral head and its congruency and has been shown to predict degeneration.[26] The reproducibility of this classification was improved by pooling class I and II hips and class III and IV hips.[27]

Visual assessment of the degree of femoral head deformity in LCPD is unreliable, and most authors have advocated for a more objective classification.[28] A new classification has been developed that relies on digitalized imaging to determine the sphericity deviation score, extent of enlargement, and composite femoral congruity arc of the femoral head in final outcome classifications.[29] Intraobserver and interobserver reliability were found to be good to excellent for all measures, and good correlation with the Stulberg classification also was reported.

The role of advanced imaging in classifying and predicting outcomes in LCPD remains unclear. Recently, there has been substantial interest in the use of early diffusion MRI for making a prognosis. In a 2014 study, 31 hips were imaged and classified using the Herring lateral pillar system. A diffusion MRI was obtained when the patient was first treated and again when the fragmentation stage was reached.[30] The apparent diffusion coefficient (ADC) of the metaphysis correlated with the Herring lateral pillar classification as early as the condensation (sclerotic) phase, but more studies to elucidate its role in prognosis beyond plain radiography remain unsupported. Interestingly, the authors of a 2011 study suggested that diffusion MRI may play a role later in the disease process to illustrate a pattern of reperfusion during the reossification stage.[31] In their study, substantial differences in metaphyseal diffusion ratios between hips

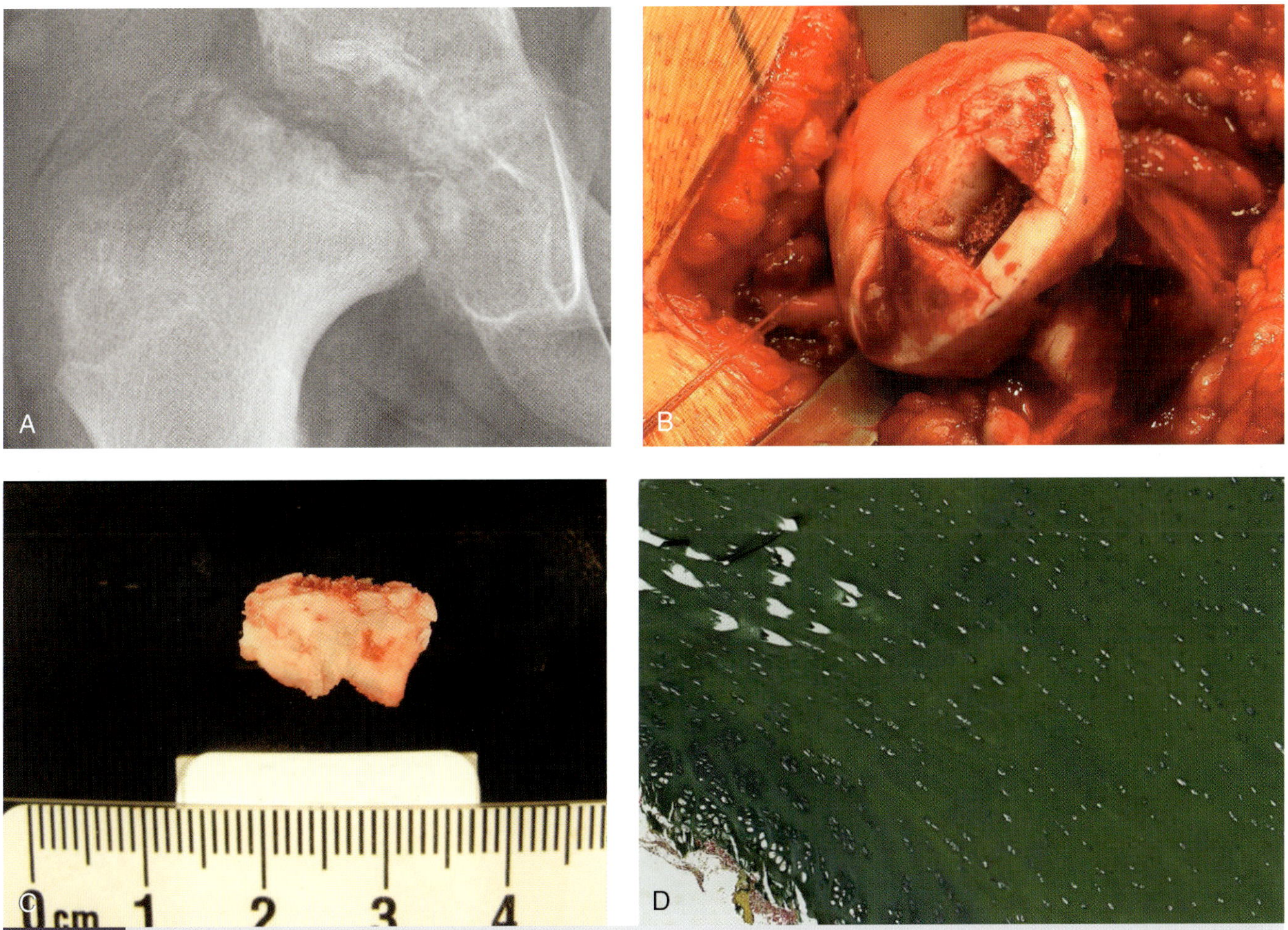

Figure 3 **A,** Radiograph of the femur in a patient with stage II Legg-Calvé-Perthes disease. **B,** Femoral head during surgical hip dislocation for containment. **C,** Photograph of a specimen removed during femoral head reshaping. **D,** Histologic analysis of the specimen found cartilage instead of necrotic bone.

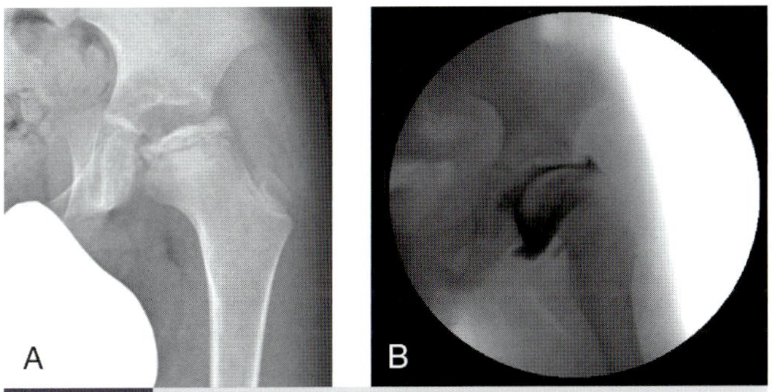

Figure 4 **A,** Radiograph of the femoral head in an 8-year-old boy with stage II Legg-Calvé-Perthes disease. **B,** Arthrogram demonstrating the cartilage anlage.

were reported, with the hips having the higher ratios being statistically more likely to have transphyseal reperfusion and focal physeal irregularity. This finding was suggestive of physeal bar formation and worse outcomes.

Residual deformity, including the femoroacetabular impingement, can occur and is best characterized on axial imaging or dynamically by arthrography.

Clinical Presentation

A typical child with LCPD will have a limp. In the early stages of the disease, the limp may or may not be associated with pain in the hip, and radiographs may appear normal. As the process progresses into the fragmentation stage, pain usually localizes to the hip but may be referred to the thigh, knee, or groin as a reduction in abduction and internal rotation occurs. LCPD has a variable course from the initial presentation to the final revascularization and healing of the femoral epiphysis, with the disease process lasting between 2 and 5 years. The inflammatory stage of fragmentation is characterized by a decrease in motion but an improvement in pain. During the reossification stage, there is little pain,

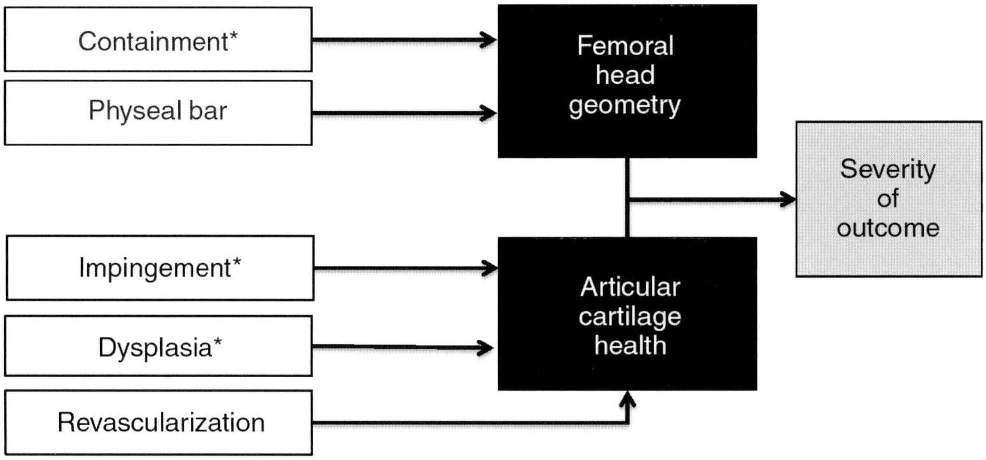

Figure 5 Algorithm of factors that contribute to the severity of the outcome in Legg-Calvé-Perthes disease. Outcome is associated with the resultant geometry of the femoral head and the health of the articular cartilage at the end of the disease process. The asterisks indicate factors that currently can be treated.

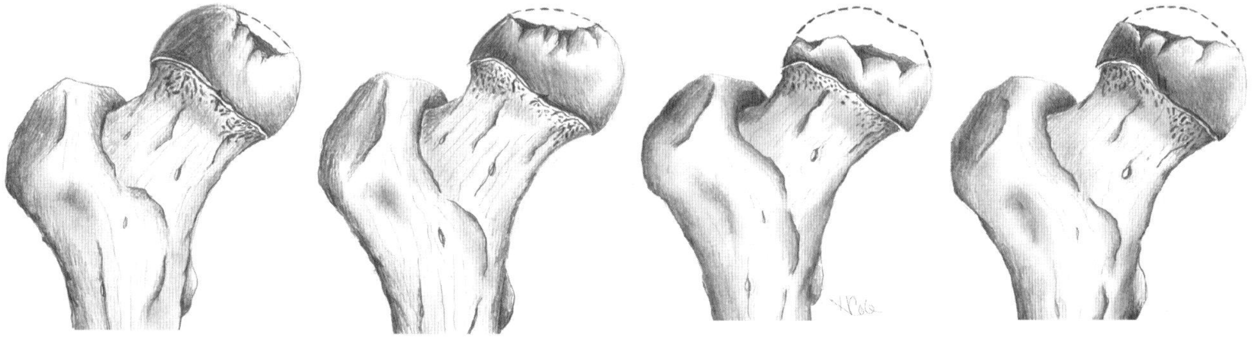

Figure 6 Illustrations of the Herring lateral pillar classification of Legg-Calvé-Perthes disease. The lateral one-third of the epiphysis, usually located lateral to the central sequestrum, is compared with the contralateral hip and measured for grading during the fragmentation stage. The epiphysis is considered group A if the height is equal to the contralateral epiphysis, group B if there is partial collapse but the height is greater than 50% of the contralateral epiphysis, and group C if there is greater collapse and the height is less than 50% of the contralateral epiphysis. A fourth type, called B/C, is a borderline group that was included to categorize hips with a thin or poorly ossified lateral pillar and loss of exactly 50% of the original height of the lateral pillar.

but improvement in motion depends on the residual deformity.

Musculoskeletal infections, including proximal femoral osteomyelitis, septic arthritis, and pyomyositis should be ruled out by clinical examination, imaging, and laboratory analysis. Slipped capital femoral epiphysis may also be included in the differential diagnosis in older children. Bilaterality suggests the possibility of epiphyseal dysplasia, sickle cell disease, or other conditions with greater systemic manifestations such as Meyer dysplasia, Gaucher disease, or hypothyroidism. It is important to recognize that LCPD may involve bilateral disease, but different stages of the disease are likely to be seen in each hip.

Treatment and Outcomes

The goal of treatment in LCPD is to minimize geometric deformity and maintain congruency of the hip as revascularization occurs and the hip progresses through the stages of this condition. The biologic plasticity suggested by Salter[32] creates a condition of malleable cartilage. It follows that the shape of the cartilaginous epiphysis governs the shape of the ossified femoral head at the completion of the disease course. Therefore, containment of the femoral head within the acetabulum is most important during the early disease stages (I and II) when the femoral head is most susceptible to deforming forces. Although no current treatments exist that can influence the rate of revascularization or prevent physeal bar formation, methods are available to maintain containment. At each stage of the disease, treatment should be directed by the underlying occurring physiology.

The hip is painful early in the disease process. The loss of vascularity to the epiphysis is accompanied by synovitis of the joint.[8] Limited range of motion is often a clinical sign of pain, which is caused by irritability of the hip more than deformity or subluxation of the joint. Treatment is aimed at minimizing pain by the administration of anti-inflammatory medications, activity restrictions, and periods of non–weight-bearing. The range of motion directs therapy. If the child's motion is excellent, there is no need for further treatment other than observation. When range of motion cannot be maintained or dramatically diminishes, dynamic observation with arthrography and clinical examination under anesthesia can be helpful in defining the problem and assessing congruity.

When lateral subluxation is present but joint congruity has been maintained, multiple treatment strategies have been suggested; these strategies range from bracing to osteotomies of both the femur and the acetabulum. These treatments help to contain the hip and prevent subluxation, which may prevent further deformity by promoting congruity.

Bracing

A 2013 study suggested that a well-developed approach that uses soft-tissue releases (adductor tenotomy to achieve abduction), Petrie casting (to achieve containment), and an A-frame orthosis (to maintain containment) can achieve excellent outcomes. These outcomes can be achieved even in children with Herring lateral pillar B or B/C hips and are equivalent to outcomes reported after osteotomy containment techniques.[33] This technique avoids osteotomies, which may lead to abnormal force distribution across the epiphyseal cartilage and possibly further flattening of the femoral head. The unsuccessful maintenance of femoral head containment with nonsurgical management may be an indication for surgical intervention.

Femoral or Acetabular Osteotomy

A prospective multicenter study of LCPD treatment, which included patients older than 6 years of age, reported good radiographic results (Stulberg class I or II) in 61% of hips treated surgically with femoral or acetabular osteotomy and in 46% of hips treated nonsurgically.[34] In patients with onset of LCPD after 8 years of age who had Herring lateral pillar B and B/C hips, a higher rate of good results was reported with surgical treatment than with nonsurgical management. However, Herring lateral pillar C hips frequently had poor radiographic results, and outcomes were similar in the surgically and nonsurgically treated groups. This highlights the challenge of obtaining optimal containment in patients with extensive lateral ischemic changes. A review of the results of femoral osteotomy from the study resulted in a recommendation that caution be exercised in creating more than 15° of varus correction of the proximal femur, which often fails to remodel.[35]

Various acetabular osteotomies to achieve containment also have been reported. A shelf osteotomy was described for treatment in the early stages of LCPD; however, it did not show clear superiority over femoral or nonosteotomy techniques in terms of radiographic markers of containment or the final Stulberg classification.[16]

Although early surgery has not been definitively shown to prevent deformity in all patients, it is logical that containment of the femoral head within the acetabulum is most important during the early disease stages when the femoral head is most susceptible to deforming forces. Other procedures such as arthrodiastasis also have been used to contain the hip while preventing weight bearing through the soft epiphysis; however, this procedure is used less frequently because there is insufficient evidence to support or refute its efficacy as a treatment method. Drilling of the epiphysis in early stages to stimulate vascular ingrowth has been advocated by some surgeons, but the potential to create a physeal bar with revascularization from the metaphysis to the epiphysis suggests that this treatment should be studied further before being widely accepted.

In a child younger than 6 years with little or no involvement of the lateral epiphysis, the prognosis and outcome tends to be favorable regardless of the chosen treatment. The consensus among authors is for nonosteotomy treatment protocols, with emphasis on range of motion and symptom management.

When deformity occurs quickly in stages 1 and 2, femoral head extrusion may occur where the anterolateral portion of the femoral head is unable to roll under the acetabulum with abduction. This creates impingement of the lateral portion of the femoral head with the lateral acetabulum, resulting in pain and loss of motion. This phenomenon has been termed hinge abduction and is best demonstrated with arthrography. With this dynamic deformity, containment of the hip may not be achieved through abduction alone. Studies suggest that there is little advantage to treatment to contain the femoral head when hinge abduction exists; therefore, many surgeons prefer a salvage procedure to improve a mechanically disadvantaged situation.[21] The goal of a valgus osteotomy is to reorient the medial femoral head superiorly so that it becomes load bearing. Although a full arc of motion is not restored, the more congruent medial head is able to roll under the acetabulum without hinging.

The authors of a 2013 study reported on 25 patients (18 Herring lateral pillar C and 7 lateral pillar B hips) in the late fragmentation stage or early reossification stage with hinge abduction who were treated with valgus femoral osteotomy (VFO).[36] At a mean follow-up of 6.3 years (range, 3.1 to 11.2 years), the mean Iowa hip score improved from 71 to 90. Some authors advise that VFO should be performed when reossification has occurred so that further deformity will not develop in the reoriented head.[37]

On the acetabular side, hinge abduction has been addressed with a Chiari or shelf osteotomy, with the goal of alleviating impingement by extending the effective edge of the acetabulum over the extruded portion of the femoral head. In a study of 27 consecutively treated hips with hinge abduction, which was demonstrated by arthrography, substantial improvements in pain scores and abduction were reported after shelf osteotomy (even in Catterall III and IV grade hips at the time of surgery).[38,39]

Residual Deformity at Skeletal Maturity

At skeletal maturity, the incongruent hip with substantial residual deformity represents a complex treatment challenge. The constellation of acetabular and femoral deformities cause pain and functional deficits and eventually progress to osteoarthritis. Long-term outcomes reported in a 2013 study suggested that impingement plays an important role in the frequency of pain and is associated with lower hip scores in mature patients with LCPD.[21] Joint preservation surgery addresses the femoral and acetabular deformities that lead to impingement. An aspheric femoral head, a shortened and wide femoral neck, coxa vara, and a high-riding greater trochanter are commonly present following the disease course. These residual deformities may lead to joint incongruity, with abnormal loading of the chondrolabral junction and the resultant complex labral and cartilage pathologies.

A 2013 study reported abnormalities of the labrum in 44 of 59 post-LCPD hips (75%).[40] These abnormalities most commonly occurred in the anterolateral aspect of the joint and were highly correlated with cartilaginous abnormalities. Labral abnormalities were found in 97% of patients with an elevated alpha angle, which suggests a loss of sphericity. Treatment should be individualized based on the existing pathology, with the goals of restoring motion and decreasing pain. Surgical dislocation allows for the assessment and treatment of labral pathology and femoral head deformity and for relative femoral neck lengthening via trochanteric advancement to improve the biomechanical efficiency of the abductor muscles.

Femoral head abnormalities can be treated with a variety of techniques. Osteochondroplasty can be used to treat peripheral impingement lesions, although the extent of the resection may be limited by the entrance of the blood supply into the femoral head-neck junction. Central lesions may still be present. It has been suggested that osteochondral autologous transplantation can assist in managing central osteocartilaginous lesions, although this has not been rigorously evaluated, and further studies are needed[41] (**Figure 7**). The central head reduction procedure, which is technically challenging and has evolving indications, may be used to improve sphericity and containment. The central portion of the femoral head is removed and the lateral column is reduced to the medial column with the articular cartilage approximated. Femoral head perfusion is maintained by metaphyseal blood flow to the stable medial portion of the head and flow from the inferior retinacular arteries through the retinacular flap to the lateral column.[42] Short-term studies have reported improvements in sphericity and Harris hip scores, even in hips in advanced Stulberg classes.[19,43]

If instability is present preoperatively or is created by concurrent femoral head-neck osteochondroplasty or central head reduction, a periacetabular osteotomy can be performed to maintain reduction. The authors of a 2015 study reported significant clinical improvement when combined procedures were performed.[44] The median Harris hip score improved from 64 preoperatively to 92 postoperatively ($P < 0.0001$).

In a systematic review that included 138 patients with residual LCPD deformities, the most commonly performed procedures were femoral head-neck osteochondroplasty and relative femoral neck lengthening.[45,46] An intertrochanteric osteotomy was performed in 22.5% of the patients. The complication rate was low (6%), and 75% of patients showed an improvement in symptoms, although 10% of patients still progressed to total hip arthroplasty (THA). Multiplanar deformities resulting from the disease process or hip preservation surgeries create a technical challenge for surgeons who undertake THA in this population. The use of custom implants or modular stems has been discussed.[47,48]

Hip arthroscopy is likely to play an increasing role in the management of LCPD. Osteochondroplasty as well

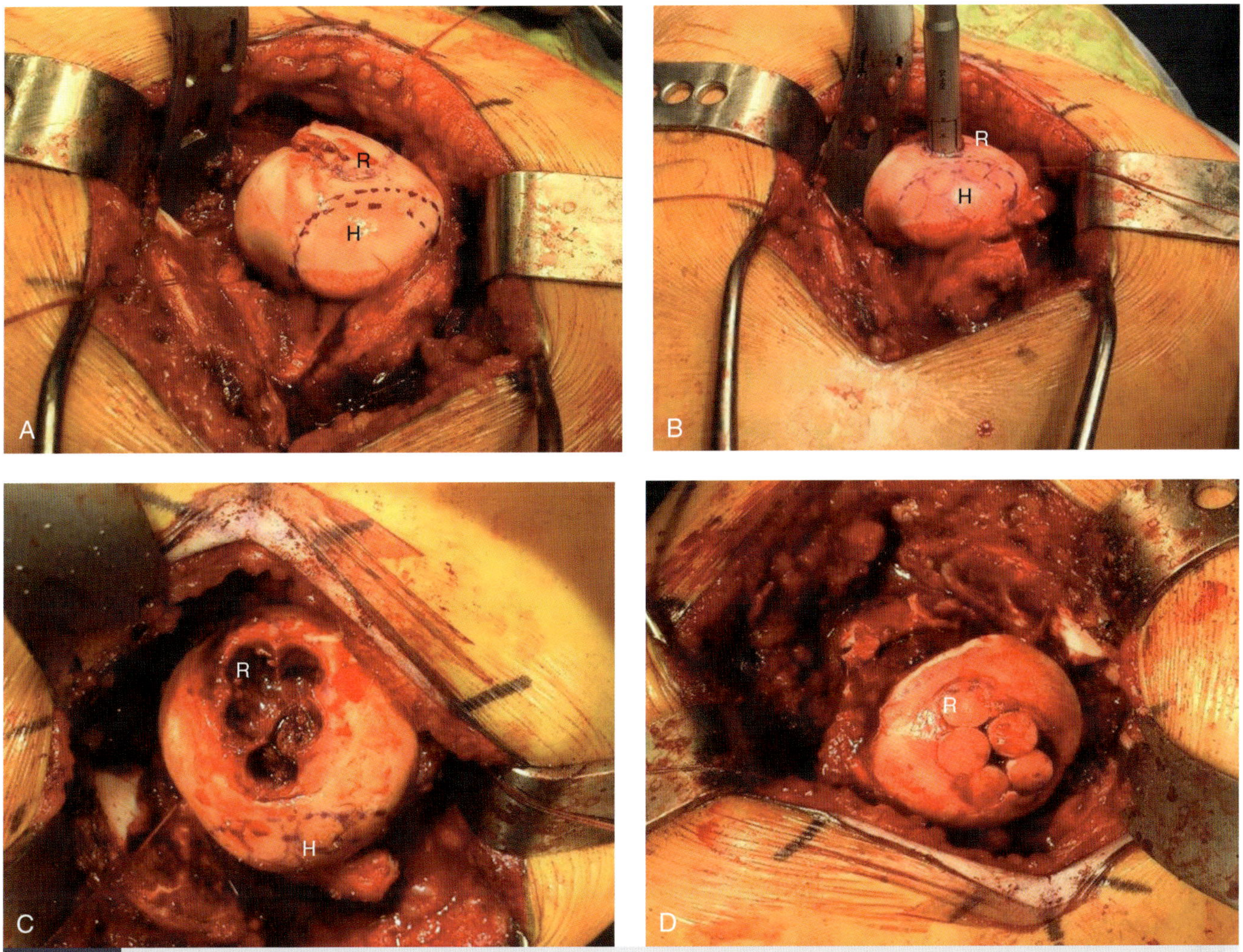

Figure 7 Intraoperative photographs of osteochondral autologous transplantation performed for a large central necrotic defect in a patient with Legg-Calvé-Perthes disease during stage IV. **A,** Healthy osteochondral plugs are transplanted from the anterior impingement region into the central area of necrosis. **B,** The recipient site is prepared by removing necrotic cartilage and bone. **C,** The recipient site after preparation. **D,** The recipient site after transplantation. R = recipient site; H = harvest site.

as labral débridement and loose body removal can be successfully performed. Good short-term improvement in hip scores has been reported.[38]

If osteoarthritis develops, THA remains the mainstay of treatment. Recent large registry series suggest similar survival rates for implants done in patients younger than 40 years with all pathologies and older patients treated with arthroplasty for osteoarthritis.[49,50] In a smaller study specific to LCPD, the cumulative implant survival rate was 96.9% at 15 years.[51] All patients had substantial postoperative improvement in their Harris hip scores. It is important to understand and address the complex deformity innate to the disease and also secondary to previous treatments. Studies within the arthroplasty literature suggest excellent results when modular or custom implants are used to treat a metaphyseal-diaphyseal mismatch.[47,52]

Future Directions

Biologic treatments are currently being investigated in animal models of LCPD, but human clinical evidence is not yet available. The use of diphosphonates to theoretically inhibit initial bone resorption and collapse as well as the use of recombinant human bone morphogenetic protein to augment this process is an appealing treatment approach. However, the biologic mechanisms, safety of the systemic effects, and adverse effects such as local heterotopic ossification must be explored more thoroughly before clinical implementation.

Summary

Because LCPD is ultimately a vascular disease, the ability to shorten the course of the disease and lessen the sequela depends on innovative techniques of promoting efficient revascularization of the epiphysis. Future treatment must be aimed at increasing the speed of revascularization to prevent or decrease damage to the femoral head.

Key Study Points

- The etiology of LCPD is likely caused by the unique characteristics of the blood supply of the femoral head in children and a multifactorial localized ischemia
- The goal of treatment in LCPD is to minimize geometric deformity and maintain congruency of the hip as revascularization occurs and the hip progresses through the stages of this condition.
- The chronic deformity associated with LCPD represents a complex problem that often eventually progresses to osteoarthritis.

Annotated References

1. Loder RT, Skopelja EN: The epidemiology and demographics of Legg-Calvé-Perthes' disease. *ISRN Orthop* 2011.

   This meta-analysis of 144 articles provides updated incidences, demographics, and associations of LCPD with other conditions. The authors found wide-ranging incidences of LCPD from 0.4 to 29.0 per 100,000 individuals. The average age of onset was 6.5 years, with a predilection to boys (81.4%) versus girls (18.6%). Level of evidence: III.

2. Lee ST, Vaidya SV, Song HR, Lee SH, Suh SW, Telang SS: Bone age delay patterns in Legg-Calvé-Perthes disease: An analysis using the Tanner and Whitehouse 3 method. *J Pediatr Orthop* 2007;27(2):198-203.

3. Perry DC, Bruce CE, Pope D, Dangerfield P, Platt MJ, Hall AJ: Perthes' disease of the hip: Socioeconomic inequalities and the urban environment. *Arch Dis Child* 2012;97(12):1053-1057.

   The authors present a retrospective review of 443 children from a national hospital discharge dataset from 2000 to 2010 in Scotland. Variations in the incidence the ICD-10 code for LCPD over time were evaluated as well as between geographic areas and socioeconomic groups using national deprivation indexes. An overall decline in incidence of LCPD over the period studied was reported. The highest incidence of hospital discharges occurred in large urban areas with the lowest deprivation index. Level of evidence: IV.

4. Georgiadis AG, Seeley MA, Yellin JL, Sankar WN: The presentation of Legg-Calvé-Perthes disease in females. *J Child Orthop* 2015;9(4):243-247.

   In a retrospective review of 451 patients with LCPD presenting to a single institution between 1990 and 2014, 18.2% of patients were female (average age of presentation, 6.58 years). Participation in high-impact activities was noted for some female patients, but no statistical significance was found for predilection of one activity over another. Level of evidence: IV.

5. Trueta J: The normal vascular anatomy of the human femoral head during growth. *J Bone Joint Surg Br* 1957;39-B(2):358-394.

6. Holdsworth FW: Epiphyseal growth: Speculations on the nature of Perthes's disease. *Ann R Coll Surg Engl* 1966;39(1):1-16.

7. Hailer YD, Montgomery SM, Ekbom A, Nilsson OS, Bahmanyar S: Legg-Calve-Perthes disease and risks for cardiovascular diseases and blood diseases. *Pediatrics* 2010;125(6):e1308-e1315.

8. Atsumi T, Yamano K, Muraki M, Yoshihara S, Kajihara T: The blood supply of the lateral epiphyseal arteries in Perthes' disease. *J Bone Joint Surg Br* 2000;82(3):392-398.

9. Daniel AB, Shah H, Kamath A, Guddettu V, Joseph B: Environmental tobacco and wood smoke increase the risk of Legg-Calvé-Perthes disease. *Clin Orthop Relat Res* 2012;470(9):2369-2375.

   In this case-control study, 128 age- and sex-matched patients with LCPD were evaluated for exposure to tobacco and wood smoke. The authors found a statistically significant increase in the adjusted odds ratio for those children with indoor use of a wood stove or indoor tobacco smoke exposure. Level of evidence: III.

10. Bahmanyar S, Montgomery SM, Weiss RJ, Ekbom A: Maternal smoking during pregnancy, other prenatal and perinatal factors, and the risk of Legg-Calvé-Perthes disease. *Pediatrics* 2008;122(2):e459-e464.

11. Vosmaer A, Pereira RR, Koenderman JS, Rosendaal FR, Cannegieter SC: Coagulation abnormalities in Legg-Calvé-Perthes disease. *J Bone Joint Surg Am* 2010;92(1):121-128.

12. Sezgin H, Gülman B, Çıraklı A, et al: Effects of circulating endothelial progenitor cells, serum vascular endothelial growth factor and hypogammaglobulinemia in Perthes disease. *Acta Orthop Traumatol Turc* 2014;48(6):628-634.

    This case-control study matched 28 patients with LCPD with 25 healthy age-matched control subjects. High endothelial progenitor cell counts at the fragmentation stage of LCPD and relatively higher counts in bilateral disease suggest that endothelial progenitor cells may be a valuable marker in the diagnosis and follow-up of LCPD. The authors also noted a strong correlation between endothelial progenitor cells and serum vascular endothelial growth factor-A level in the fragmentation stage and in the presence of hypogammaglobulinemia.

13. Talavera-Adame D, Xiong Y, Zhao T, Arias AE, Sierra-Honigmann MR, Farkas DL: Quantitative and morphometric evaluation of the angiogenic effects of leptin. *J Biomed Opt* 2008;13(6):064017.

14. Lee JH, Zhou L, Kwon KS, Lee D, Park BH, Kim JR: Role of leptin in Legg-Calvé-Perthes disease. *J Orthop Res* 2013;31(10):1605-1610.

The authors of this case-control study matched 38 male and 3 female patients with LCPD with 41 healthy age- and sex-matched control patients with fractures. Serum leptin and soluble leptin receptor levels were quantified. The free leptin index (FLI) was defined as the ratio of leptin to soluble leptin receptor levels. Serum leptin levels, soluble leptin receptor levels, and the FLI were compared between groups. Circulating leptin and the FLI were substantially higher in the LCPD group. In addition, leptin, disease severity, and treatment outcomes were associated. This correlation suggests that leptin might play an important role in LCPD pathogenesis.

15. Kamiya N, Yamaguchi R, Adapala NS, et al: Legg-Calvé-Perthes disease produces chronic hip synovitis and elevation of interleukin-6 in the synovial fluid. *J Bone Miner Res* 2015;30(6):1009-1013.

The authors report on 28 patients with stage 1 or 2 LCPD (17 patients managed nonsurgically and 11 treated with proximal femoral varus osteotomy). MRI and synovial fluid analyses were performed. Interleukin-6 was found to be significantly elevated in the affected hip in patients with LCPD compared with the unaffected hip (509.5 pg/mL versus 18.8 pg/mL; $P = 0.0005$).

16. Bowen JR, Schreiber FC, Foster BK, Wein BK: Premature femoral neck physeal closure in Perthes' disease. *Clin Orthop Relat Res* 1982;171:24-29.

17. Jaramillo D, Kasser JR, Villegas-Medina OL, Gaary E, Zurakowski D: Cartilaginous abnormalities and growth disturbances in Legg-Calvé-Perthes disease: Evaluation with MR imaging. *Radiology* 1995;197(3):767-773.

18. Shah H, Siddesh ND, Joseph B: To what extent does remodeling of the proximal femur and the acetabulum occur between disease healing and skeletal maturity in Perthes disease? A radiological study. *J Pediatr Orthop* 2008;28(7):711-716.

19. Tannast M, Hanke M, Ecker TM, Murphy SB, Albers CE, Puls M: LCPD: Reduced range of motion resulting from extra- and intraarticular impingement. *Clin Orthop Relat Res* 2012;470(9):2431-2440.

Motion models for 13 hips with LCPD, 22 hips with femoroacetabular impingement, and 27 normal hips were compared. Range of motion and impingement zones, including internal and external zones were derived from three-dimensional CT modeling of each hip. LCPD was found to have a characteristic pattern of impingement, with intra-articular impingement in flexion and internal rotation between the deformed femoral head and anterosuperior area of the acetabular rim, and extra-articular impingement between the greater trochanter and the supra-acetabular area in abduction. Level of evidence: III.

20. Froberg L, Christensen F, Pedersen NW, Overgaard S: The need for total hip arthroplasty in Perthes disease: A long-term study. *Clin Orthop Relat Res* 2011;469(4):1134-1140.

The authors report on a cohort of 167 patients with LCPD presenting to a single institution between 1941 and 1962. At a mean follow-up of 47 years (range, 37 to 58 years), patients were evaluated for osteoarthritis (defined as joint space width of ≤2.0 mm on plain radiographs) and the presence of THA. In patients with Stulberg class III, IV, or V femoral heads, the odds ratio was increased for THA and radiographic osteoarthritis. Level of evidence: III.

21. Larson AN, Sucato DJ, Herring JA, et al: A prospective multicenter study of Legg-Calvé-Perthes disease: Functional and radiographic outcomes of nonoperative treatment at a mean follow-up of twenty years. *J Bone Joint Surg Am* 2012;94(7):584-592.

A cohort of 56 patients (58 hips) were evaluated at a mean follow-up of 20.4 years (range, 16.3 to 24.5 years) after nonsurgical management of LCPD (involving either range-of-motion exercises or weight-bearing abduction bracing). Four patients had already undergone joint replacement or periacetabular osteotomy, and 41 of 54 hips (76%) not requiring further surgery were at least occasionally painful. Femoroacetabular impingement indicated by physical examination was associated with pain and poorer outcomes on measures including the Iowa Hip Score ($P = 0.0004$), the Medical Outcomes Study 36-Item Short Form ($P = 0.0014$), and the Nonarthritic Hip Score ($P = 0.0007$). Level of evidence: IV.

22. Herring JA, Kim HT, Browne R: Legg-Calve-Perthes disease: Part I. Classification of radiographs with use of the modified lateral pillar and Stulberg classifications. *J Bone Joint Surg Am* 2004;86(10):2103-2120.

23. Rajan R, Chandrasenan J, Price K, Konstantoulakis C, Metcalfe J, Jones S: Legg-Calvé-Perthes: Interobserver and intraobserver reliability of the modified Herring lateral pillar classification. *J Pediatr Orthop* 2013;33(2):120-123.

Thirty-five standard radiographs were reviewed by six senior observers, and the lateral pillar classification was applied. This classification was repeated 6 weeks later. Both the interobserver reliability and intraobserver reliability was found to be fair ($P < 0.01$)

24. Lappin K, Kealey D, Cosgrove A: Herring classification: How useful is the initial radiograph? *J Pediatr Orthop* 2002;22(4):479-482.

25. Park MS, Chung CY, Lee KM, Kim TW, Sung KH: Reliability and stability of three common classifications for Legg-Calvé-Perthes disease. *Clin Orthop Relat Res* 2012;470(9):2376-2382.

The hips of 69 patients with LCPD were classified with the Herring lateral pillar, Catterall, and Salter-Thompson classification systems. The interrater and intrarater reliability of the classification systems was determined by three observers at a minimum of two time points.

26. Stulberg SD, Cooperman DR, Wallensten R: The natural history of Legg-Calvé-Perthes disease. *J Bone Joint Surg Am* 1981;63(7):1095-1108.

27. Wiig O: Perthes' disease in Norway. A prospective study on 425 patients. *Acta Orthop Suppl* 2009;80(333):1-44.

28. Ross JR, Nepple JJ, Baca G, Schoenecker PL, Clohisy JC: Intraarticular abnormalities in residual Perthes and Perthes-like hip deformities. *Clin Orthop Relat Res* 2012;470(11):2968-2977.

Thirty-five patients with residual Perthes and Perthes-like hip deformities were reviewed at a mean age of 8.5 years (range, 10 to 36 years). Patients were reviewed using surgical and radiographic findings. Labral abnormalities were found in 76% of patients, with acetabular chondromalacia in 59% of the hips and femoral head chondromalacia in 81% of the hips. Level of evidence: IV.

29. Shah H, Siddesh ND, Pai H, Tercier S, Joseph B: Quantitative measures for evaluating the radiographic outcome of Legg-Calvé-Perthes disease. *J Bone Joint Surg Am* 2013;95(4):354-361.

In this case-control study, 121 hips treated at a single institution were classified according to the Stulberg system. The mean sphericity deviation scores were found to be significantly lower in Stulberg class 1 hips compared with more involved hips. Class I to II hips had a significantly lower sphericity deviation score ($P < 0.001$). Level of evidence: III.

30. Baunin C, Sanmartin-Viron D, Accadbled F, et al: Prognosis value of early diffusion MRI in Legg Perthes Calvé disease. *Orthop Traumatol Surg Res* 2014;100(3):317-321.

The authors report on 31 patients with unilateral LCPD. Diffusion sequence MRI was performed during the condensation (sclerotic) or the fragmentation phase of the disease. The ADC was calculated as a ratio of the affected side to the unaffected side. The ADC was elevated in all affected epiphyses and metaphyses compared with those of control subjects ($P < 0.001$). Greater metaphyseal ADC was also associated with a higher Herring classification. Level of evidence: III.

31. Yoo WJ, Kim YJ, Menezes NM, Cheon JE, Jaramillo D: Diffusion-weighted MRI reveals epiphyseal and metaphyseal abnormalities in Legg-Calvé-Perthes disease: A pilot study. *Clin Orthop Relat Res* 2011;469(10):2881-2888.

This case-control study evaluated 21 children with unilateral abnormalities of their epiphyses on plain radiographs. Patients also underwent diffusion-weighted MRI, and ADC values were calculated for the affected side. The authors suggest that MRI may be helpful in evaluating ischemic tissue damage.

32. Salter RB: Legg-Perthes disease: The scientific basis for the methods of treatment and their indications. *Clin Orthop Relat Res* 1980;150:8-11.

33. Rich MM, Schoenecker PL: Management of Legg-Calvé-Perthes disease using an A-frame orthosis and hip range of motion: A 25-year experience. *J Pediatr Orthop* 2013;33(2):112-119.

The authors report on 240 patients presenting to a single institution between 1985 and 2001 with LCPD in the necrotic or fragmentation stages. The patients were treated with a protocol aimed at maintaining and achieving good hip abduction and containment through casting, the use of an A-frame orthosis, range-of-motion exercises, and adductor tenotomy if needed. At an average follow-up of 7.8 years (range, 2 to 15.8 years), 89% percent of pillar B and 67% of pillar C hips were spherical and congruent. Level of evidence: IV.

34. Herring JA, Kim HT, Browne R: Legg-Calve-Perthes disease: Part II. Prospective multicenter study of the effect of treatment on outcome. *J Bone Joint Surg Am* 2004;86-A(10):2121-2134.

35. Kim HK, da Cunha AM, Browne R, Kim HT, Herring JA: How much varus is optimal with proximal femoral osteotomy to preserve the femoral head in Legg-Calvé-Perthes disease? *J Bone Joint Surg Am* 2011;93(4):341-347.

Fifty-two patients treated with proximal femoral varus osteotomy for LCPD were evaluated. The change in neck-shaft angle was measured and the association with the Stulberg class at skeletal maturity was determined. Thirty-five percent of the patients had no improvement in the neck-shaft angle after surgery. Findings suggested that a smaller varus change was associated with a greater probability of a lower Stulberg class at final outcome.

36. Kim HT, Gu JK, Bae SH, Jang JH, Lee JS: Does valgus femoral osteotomy improve femoral head roundness in severe Legg-Calvé-Perthes disease? *Clin Orthop Relat Res* 2013;471(3):1021-1027.

This case series evaluated whether VFO improves femoral head roundness, radiographic parameters reflecting hip subluxation, and function. Twenty-five patients were treated with a VFO in the late fragmenting stage, and 7 patients had additional pelvic procedures. VFO was performed at a mean age of 9.8 years. At a minimum follow up of 3.1 years, all femoral head roundness measurements had improved. The mean Iowa hip rating improved from 71 before surgery to 90 at the last follow-up. Overall, in the fragmentation stage, VFO appeared to help the deformed femoral head remodel to fit the acetabulum. Level of evidence: III.

37. Bankes MJ, Catterall A, Hashemi-Nejad A: Valgus extension osteotomy for 'hinge abduction' in Perthes' disease. Results at maturity and factors influencing the radiological outcome. *J Bone Joint Surg Br* 2000;82(4):548-554.

38. Freeman CR, Jones K, Byrd JW: Hip arthroscopy for Legg-Calvè-Perthes disease: Minimum 2-year follow-up. *Arthroscopy* 2013;29(4):666-674.

The authors report on 23 hips treated between 1995 and 2009 for sequelae of LCPD after hip arthroscopy (minimum follow-up, 2 years). Findings during arthroscopy included 18 labral tears, 17 hypertrophic or torn ligamentum teres, 9 femoral and 8 acetabular chondral lesions, 5 loose bodies, 3 osteochondral defects, and 2 cam lesions. The median Harris hip score improved from 56.5 to 85 postoperatively (P <0.01). Level of evidence: IV.

39. Freeman RT, Wainwright AM, Theologis TN, Benson MK: The outcome of patients with hinge abduction in severe Perthes disease treated by shelf acetabuloplasty. *J Pediatr Orthop* 2008;28(6):619-625.

40. Maranho DA, Nogueira-Barbosa MH, Zamarioli A, Volpon JB: MRI abnormalities of the acetabular labrum and articular cartilage are common in healed Legg-Calvé-Perthes disease with residual deformities of the hip. *J Bone Joint Surg Am* 2013;95(3):256-265.

In 54 patients with healed LCPD who underwent noncontrast MRI of the hip at an average follow-up of 8 years after disease onset, abnormalities of the acetabular labrum were found in 75% of the patients and abnormalities of the articular cartilage in 47%. Alpha angles of greater than 55° were found to have the highest association with labral abnormalities. Level of evidence: IV.

41. Khanna V, Tushinski DM, Drexler M, et al: Cartilage restoration of the hip using fresh osteochondral allograft: Resurfacing the potholes. *Bone Joint J* 2014;96-B(11suppl A):11-16.

The authors report on 15 patients who underwent osteochondral allograft treatment for cartilage defects of the femoral head. Two were performed for LCPD. Both patients with LCPD had poor outcomes.

42. Kalhor M, Horowitz K, Gharehdaghi J, Beck M, Ganz R: Anatomic variations in femoral head circulation. *Hip Int* 2012;22(3):307-312.

In a cadaver study of 35 hips, which were injected with colored silicone intravascularly, the medial femoral circumflex artery was found to be the main blood supply to the hip in 29 specimens, and the inferior gluteal artery was found to be the main blood supply in 6 specimens. Retinacular vessels were dominate in the vascularity to the femoral head. Level of evidence: IV.

43. Burian M, Dungl P, Nanka O, et al: Anteromedial wedge reduction osteotomy for the treatment of femoral head deformities. *Hip Int* 2013;23(3):281-286.

The authors report on seven anteromedial wedge reduction osteotomies, six of which were performed for LCPD. At a mean follow-up of 17.4 months, the Harris hip score increased from a mean of 55.4 preoperatively to a mean of 84.8 postoperatively. Level of evidence: IV.

44. Clohisy JC, Nepple JJ, Ross JR, Pashos G, Schoenecker PL: Does surgical hip dislocation and periacetabular osteotomy improve pain in patients with Perthes-like deformities and acetabular dysplasia? *Clin Orthop Relat Res* 2015;473(4):1370-1377.

This case study reports on 16 patients who underwent periacetabular osteotomy and surgical hip dislocation for residual Perthes-like deformity of the proximal femur and associated dysplasia of the acetabulum. All patients with a loss of joint space greater than 50% were excluded. Harris hip scores improved from an average of 62 preoperatively to 87 postoperatively. The lateral center-edge angle and the anterior center-edge angle improved preoperatively to postoperatively (mean of 20° and 19° of correction, respectively). Two clinical failures were reported and involved conversion to THA or a poor Harris hip score. Level of evidence: IV.

45. Novais EN: Application of the surgical dislocation approach to residual hip deformity secondary to Legg-Calvé-Perthes disease. *J Pediatr Orthop* 2013;33(suppl 1):S62-S69.

This review article discusses the indications, technical aspects, and application of surgical hip dislocation to LCPD. Level of evidence: V.

46. Shore BJ, Novais EN, Millis MB, Kim YJ: Low early failure rates using a surgical dislocation approach in healed Legg-Calvé-Perthes disease. *Clin Orthop Relat Res* 2012;470(9):2441-2449.

The authors report on 29 patients with LCPD who underwent surgical hip dislocation during an 8-year period at a single institution for indications such as groin pain with physical activity and pain with hip flexion over long periods. The Western Ontario and McMaster Universities Osteoarthritis Index scores improved postoperatively, with 90% of the patients having improvement in their pain (48% of the patients were pain free). All patients had minimum clinical and radiographic follow-up of 1 year. Level of evidence: IV.

47. Al-Khateeb H, Kwok IH, Hanna SA, Sewell MD, Hashemi-Nejad A: Custom cementless THA in patients with Legg-Calve-Perthes Disease. *J Arthroplasty* 2014;29(4):792-796.

The authors report on 15 primary THAs (14 patients) treated between 1996 and 2003 using custom-made cementless femoral components for advanced osteoarthritis in the setting of LCPD. At a mean follow-up of 10.1 years (range, 5-15 years), the survivorship rate was 100% for femoral components and 79% for acetabular components. Revision arthroplasty of the acetabular component was performed in three hips (21%) at a mean of 8.6 years. In patients with development dysplasia of the hip who had been treated with prior osteotomies, higher rates of stem perforation and difficulty controlling anteversion were reported. Level of evidence: IV.

48. Suzuki K, Kawachi S, Matsubara M, Morita S, Jinno T, Shinomiya K: Cementless total hip replacement after previous intertrochanteric valgus osteotomy for advanced osteoarthritis. *J Bone Joint Surg Br* 2007;89(9):1155-1157.

49. Lehmann TG, Engesaeter IØ, Laborie LB, Lie SA, Rosendahl K, Engesaeter LB: Total hip arthroplasty in

5: Lower Extremity

young adults, with focus on Perthes' disease and slipped capital femoral epiphysis: Follow-up of 540 subjects reported to the Norwegian Arthroplasty Register during 1987-2007. *Acta Orthop* 2012;83(2):159-164.

The authors report on a case series of patients younger than 40 years who underwent THA and were included in the Norwegian Arthroplasty Register between 1987 and 2007. Seventy-two of the included hips had LCPD. The mean self-reported quality-of-life score was significantly lower (74) for those who underwent THA because of LCPD compared with those patients whose primary diagnosis was slipped capital femoral epiphysis (81) (P = 0.008). Level of evidence: IV.

50. Sedrakyan A, Romero L, Graves S, et al: Survivorship of hip and knee implants in pediatric and young adult populations: Analysis of registry and published data. *J Bone Joint Surg Am* 2014;96(suppl 1):73-78.

The authors used data from the Australian Orthopaedic Association National Joint Replacement Registry to analyze the use of THA and total knee arthroplasty in the pediatric population from 1999 to 2012. Compared with older adults, pediatric patients and young adults undergoing THA and total knee arthroplasty had very different diagnoses, including a high prevalence of tumors. Overall, the rate of revision surgery at 5 years was found to be very similar between the groups.

51. Traina F, De Fine M, Sudanese A, Calderoni PP, Tassinari E, Toni A: Long-term results of total hip replacement in patients with Legg-Calvé-Perthes disease. *J Bone Joint Surg Am* 2011;93(7):e25.

Twenty-seven patients (average age, 37.8 years; range, 19 to 65 years) underwent THA for osteoarthritis secondary to LCPD. The mean Harris hip score was 87.5 (range, 73-65) at the last follow-up, which was an improvement from the preoperative mean score of 50.1 (range, 25-75). The cumulative hip survival rate at 15 years was 96.9%, with a complication rate of 12.5%, which included two sciatic nerve palsies in patients who had undergone limb lengthening and one intraoperative fracture. Level of evidence: IV.

52. Seufert CR, McGrory BJ: Treatment of arthritis associated with Legg-Calve-Perthes disease with modular total hip arthroplasty. *J Arthroplasty* 2015;30(10):1743-1746.

Twenty-eight patients with LCPD and Stulberg class III through V hips underwent 35 primary noncemented THAs between 1997 and 2012. The Harris hip score improved on average from 49.8 preoperatively to 93.9 postoperatively at a minimum follow-up of 2 years. One deep infection and one posterior dislocation were reported. Level of evidence: IV.

5: Lower Extremity

Chapter 23

Congenital Dislocations: Knee and Patella

Amy L. McIntosh, MD

Abstract

Congenital dislocation of the knee is a rare condition. It is apparent at birth, and infants usually present with a dramatic hyperextension deformity. Treatment with serial casting should begin as soon as possible in infancy. In knees with more severe quadriceps contractures that prevent effective gradual flexion, a femoral nerve block or botulinum toxin can be a helpful adjunct. A trial of nonsurgical management is appropriate until 12 months of age. Surgical management, including lengthening of the quadriceps mechanism via either V-Y quadricepsplasty or a relative lengthening via an acute femoral shortening (2-3 cm), is indicated in patients who do not respond to casting. Mini-open and percutaneous quadricepsplasty also have been described with good short-term results.

Congenital patellar dislocation is a laterally displaced, hypoplastic patella with severe trochlear dysplasia or an absent trochlea. This condition is often present at birth, but a diagnosis may not be made until years later. If the child has progressive functional decline or developmental milestones are not achieved, surgical treatment should be considered. Extensive lateral release with release of the iliotibial band and occasionally the biceps femoris should be performed. If this release does not allow for centralization of the patella and extensor mechanism, then a V-Y quadricepsplasty or acute femoral shortening should be performed. After centralization, medial imbrication is necessary to maintain reduction.

Keywords: congenital dislocation of the knee; congenital patellar dislocation; pediatrics

Neither Dr. McIntosh nor any immediate family member has received anything of value from or has stock or stock options held in a commercial company or institution related directly or indirectly to the subject of this chapter.

Introduction

This chapter reviews the clinical and radiographic presentations of patients with congenital knee dislocation and congenital patellar dislocation. Treatment strategies, both surgical and nonsurgical, are discussed in detail.

Congenital Dislocation of the Knee

Congenital dislocation of the knee is a rare condition with an incidence of 0.1% or less.[1,2] It is apparent at birth, and infants usually present with a dramatic hyperextension deformity (**Figure 1**). The condition can be diagnosed prenatally with ultrasound.[3] Congenital dislocation of the knee is most commonly associated with female sex, premature birth, and breech delivery. Ipsilateral hip dysplasia and clubfoot are present 70% and 50% of the time, respectively.[4,5] Bilateral congenital dislocation of the knee is almost always syndromic and is associated with laxity conditions such as Larsen, Beals, or Ehlers-Danlos syndromes or neuromuscular conditions such as arthrogryposis or myelodysplasia. If such conditions are suspected, referral to a geneticist and/or a neurologist is necessary.

Clinical Findings

Clinically, the femoral condyles are prominent posteriorly in the popliteal fossa. The foot may be touching the infant's face or shoulder, with marked hyperflexion of the hip. The flexibility of the quadriceps contracture is assessed by applying gentle traction to the tibia while attempting flexion of the knee.

Classification and Radiographic and Anatomic Characteristics

The classification of congenital knee deformity is based on severity. Grade 1 dislocation is defined as hyperextension greater than 15° with full flexion possible and normal radiographic findings. In grade 2 deformity (subluxation), the knee is hyperextended greater than 15°, will not flex beyond neutral extension, and radiographic

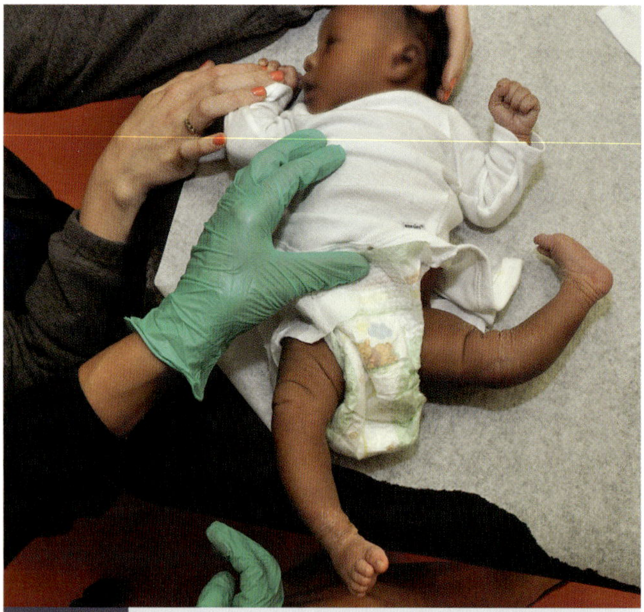

Figure 1 Clinical photograph of an infant with a grade 1 congenital dislocation of the left knee. Note the dramatic hyperextension of the knee. (Copyright Texas Scottish Rite Hospital, Dallas, TX.)

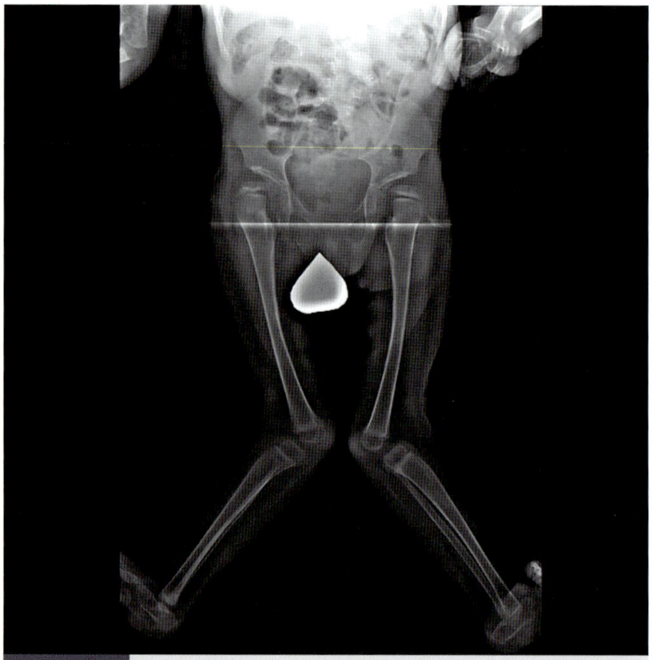

Figure 2 Radiographs of a child with a bilateral grade 2 congenital dislocation of the knee, demonstrating that the tibial and femoral epiphyses are in contact with the anterior translation of the tibia on the femur. (Copyright Texas Scottish Rite Hospital, Dallas, TX.)

findings demonstrate that the tibial and femoral epiphyses are in contact with the anterior translation of the tibia on the femur (**Figure 2**). In grade 3 deformity (dislocation), the knee is hyperextended and passive knee flexion is impossible. Radiographs show that the tibial and femoral epiphyses are not in contact, and the tibia lies anterior to the femur.

Anatomic findings of grade 3 congenital knee dislocation include a shortened and fibrotic quadriceps mechanism, anterior displacement of the hamstring tendons and the iliotibial (IT) band, a contracted anterior capsule, loss of the suprapatellar pouch, redundancy of the posterior capsule, and absence or abnormality of the cruciate ligaments.

Treatment

Treatment should begin as early as possible in infancy. Long leg plaster casting is performed on a serial basis every 7 to 10 days. This process is repeated until the knee can flex more than 90°. At that time, a plastic splint or Pavlik harness can be used until all tendencies for recurrence are overcome. In knees with a more severe quadriceps contracture that prevents effective gradual flexion, a femoral nerve block or botulinum toxin can be a helpful treatment adjunct. The use of botulinum toxin results in long-term quadriceps paralysis that allows gradual stretching to occur.[6] A trial of nonsurgical management is appropriate until the child reaches 12 months of age.

Surgical management is indicated if serial casting is unsuccessful. Surgical treatment includes lengthening of the quadriceps mechanism with either V-Y quadricepsplasty or a relative lengthening via an acute femoral shortening (2-3 cm).[1,7,8] Femoral shortening may be preferred because it minimizes quadriceps dissection and weakening and also decompresses the anterior skin, which lessens skin necrosis. The IT band is often released from its distal insertion, and the anterior capsule and suprapatellar pouch are completely mobilized. Posterolateral and posteromedial capsulorrhaphies should be performed after excision of the redundant capsule. After the capsulorrhaphies, the knee should have a range of motion from 30° to 90° of flexion. No attempt should be made to gain full extension of the knee.

At this point, the knee must be assessed for instability of the anterior cruciate ligament; an anterior drawer test should be performed with the knee flexed to 90°. If the result is unacceptable, the anterior cruciate ligament should be reconstructed with a medial hamstring autograft. The knee should be cast in 45° to 60° of flexion for 8 weeks and then braced to limit full extension for the first 4 months postoperatively.[1]

Minimally invasive treatment of congenital dislocation of the knee (mini-open and percutaneous quadricepsplasty) has been described with good short-term results.[9,10]

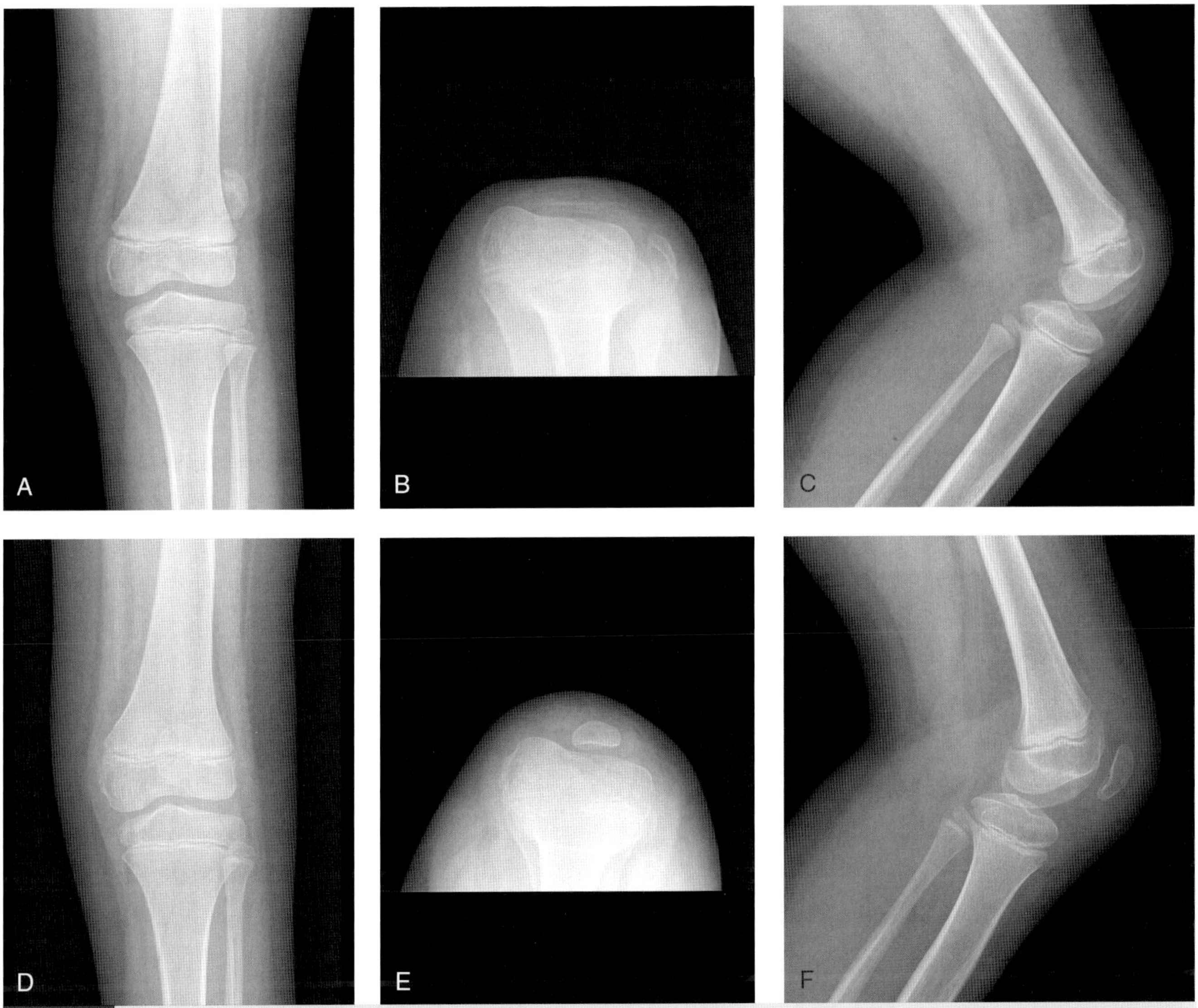

Figure 3 Radiographs show congenital patellar dislocation in a 9-year-old girl before and after surgical reduction and stabilization. AP (**A**), sunrise (**B**), and lateral (**C**) radiographs show the laterally dislocated patella. AP (**D**), sunrise (**E**), and lateral (**F**) radiographs show the patellar position after stabilization. (Reproduced from Polousky JD: Congenital deformities of the knee, in Song KM, ed: *Orthopaedic Knowledge Update: Pediatrics 4*. Rosemont, IL, American Academy of Orthopaedic Surgeons, 2011, pp 195-202.)

Congenital Patellar Dislocation

Congenital patellar dislocation is defined as a laterally displaced, hypoplastic patella with severe trochlear dysplasia or an absent trochlea (**Figure 3**). The condition is often present at birth, but a diagnosis may not be made until years later. It is associated with a knee flexion contracture and valgus external rotation deformity of the tibia.[11,12] Congenital patellar dislocation is also often associated with Down syndrome, Rubinstein-Taybi syndrome, nail-patella syndrome, Larsen syndrome, arthrogryposis, diastrophic dysplasia, and Ellis-van Creveld syndrome. Congenital patellar dislocation should be differentiated from the more common obligatory subluxation, which develops later in childhood and adolescence.[13]

Anatomic and Clinical Characteristics

Anatomic findings include a thickened, tight lateral retinaculum and IT band; a thinned and stretched medial retinaculum and medial patellofemoral ligament; and a lateralized and shortened quadriceps.[14]

Clinically, the child may present with a knee flexion contracture, delayed walking, genu valgum, external tibial torsion, or an associated syndrome or condition. On physical examination, the femoral condyles appear prominent anteriorly. The patella is small and laterally dislocated throughout knee range of motion. Radiographs often demonstrate an empty intercondylar space on Merchant views; however, findings are often unreliable in patients younger than 3 years because of the lack of patellar ossification. MRI or ultrasound may be necessary to confirm the diagnosis.[15]

Treatment

Nonsurgical management cannot correct a congenital patellar dislocation. If the child has progressive functional decline or the inability to achieve developmental milestones, surgical treatment should be considered. Extensive lateral release, with release of the IT band and, occasionally, the biceps femoris should be performed. If this treatment does not allow for centralization of the patella and extensor mechanism, a V-Y quadricepsplasty or an acute femoral shortening should be performed. A medial imbrication is then necessary to maintain reduction. A medial patellofemoral ligament reconstruction can be performed to augment the medial imbrication. There is no need to close or repair the extensive lateral release.[1] Assessment of the distal patellar tendon insertion should then be performed. If distal realignment is deemed necessary, a Roux-Goldthwait transfer or a patellar tendon periosteal sleeve medialization can be performed.[16]

Summary

Congenital knee and patellar dislocations are rare conditions and are often associated with underlying syndromes. Congenital knee dislocation is easily diagnosed during the newborn period because of its dramatic clinical presentation. Treatment with serial casting should begin as soon as possible in infancy. If the result of casting is unsuccessful, surgery is the mainstay of treatment.

Congenital patellar dislocation is more difficult to diagnose than congenital knee dislocation and usually is unrecognized until early childhood when walking milestones are usually achieved. If the child has progressive functional decline or the inability to achieve developmental milestones, surgical treatment should be considered. Acute femoral shortening is an alternative to V-Y quadricepsplasty because it minimizes quadriceps dissection and weakening.

Key Study Points

- Congenital knee and patellar dislocation are rare conditions and are often associated with underlying syndromes.
- Serial casting should begin immediately in the newborn period to treat all grades of congenital knee dislocation.
- Nonsurgical management cannot correct congenital patellar dislocation.
- Surgical treatment of both congenital knee dislocation and congenital patellar dislocation progresses in a stepwise fashion, with the goal of obtaining stability of the tibiofemoral and patellofemoral joints to allow functional gait.

Annotated References

1. Johnston CE II, Oetgen ME: Congenital deformities of the knee, in Scott WN, ed: *Insall & Scott Surgery of the Knee*, ed 5. Philadelphia, PA, Elsevier, 2012, pp 816-841.

   This article includes in-depth descriptions of surgical techniques and intraoperative photographs regarding the treatment of congenital knee dislocation and congenital patellar dislocation.

2. Charif P, Reichelderfer TE: Genu recurvatum congenitum in the newborn: Its incidence, course, treatment, prognosis. *Clin Pediatr (Phila)* 1965;4(10):587-594.

3. Monteagudo A, Kudla MM, Essig M, Santos R, Timor-Tritsch IE: Real-time and 3-dimensional sonographic diagnosis of postural congenital genu recurvatum. *J Ultrasound Med* 2006;25(8):1079-1083.

4. Johnson E, Audell R, Oppenheim WL: Congenital dislocation of the knee. *J Pediatr Orthop* 1987;7(2):194-200.

5. Bensahel H, Dal Monte A, Hjelmstedt A, et al: Congenital dislocation of the knee. *J Pediatr Orthop* 1989;9(2):174-177.

6. Kaissi AA, Ganger R, Klaushofer K, Grill F: The management of knee dislocation in a child with Larsen syndrome. *Clinics (Sao Paulo)* 2011;66(7):1295-1299.

   This article is a case report of a 3-year-old girl who presented with the full clinical and radiographic features of Larsen syndrome. The knee deformity in the child was compatible with a complete (grade 3) anterior dislocation of the tibia on the femur. Treatment included closed reduction by inducing a neuromuscular blockade of the quadriceps using botulinum toxin and percutaneous quadriceps lengthening.

7. Oetgen ME, Walick KS, Tulchin K, Karol LA, Johnston CE: Functional results after surgical treatment for congenital knee dislocation. *J Pediatr Orthop* 2010;30(3):216-223.

8. Johnston CE II: Simultaneous open reduction of ipsilateral congenital dislocation of the hip and knee assisted by femoral diaphyseal shortening. *J Pediatr Orthop* 2011;31(7):732-740.

   This article describes a small case series of five patients who underwent simultaneous reduction for ipsilateral hip dislocation and congenital dislocation of the knee. Treatment also included femoral shortening/plating and capsulorrhaphy of both joints. Level of evidence: III.

9. Abdelaziz TH, Samir S: Congenital dislocation of the knee: A protocol for management based on degree of knee flexion. *J Child Orthop* 2011;5(2):143-149.

   The authors introduce a modified grading system for congenital dislocations of the knee. The treatment protocol was based on the amount of knee flexion that could be obtained. Treatment included casting, percutaneous quadriceps recession, and open V-Y quadricepsplasty.

10. Shah NR, Limpaphayom N, Dobbs MB: A minimally invasive treatment protocol for the congenital dislocation of the knee. *J Pediatr Orthop* 2009;29(7):720-725.

11. Stanisavljevic S, Zemenick G, Miller D: Congenital, irreducible, permanent lateral dislocation of the patella. *Clin Orthop Relat Res* 1976;116:190-199.

12. Gao GX, Lee EH, Bose K: Surgical management of congenital and habitual dislocation of the patella. *J Pediatr Orthop* 1990;10(2):255-260.

13. Weeks KD III, Fabricant PD, Ladenhauf HN, Green DW: Surgical options for patellar stabilization in the skeletally immature patient. *Sports Med Arthrosc* 2012;20(3):194-202.

    The authors present a review article on the treatment of patellar instability in skeletally immature patients.

14. Ghanem I, Wattincourt L, Seringe R: Congenital dislocation of the patella: Part I. Pathologic anatomy. *J Pediatr Orthop* 2000;20(6):812-816.

15. Koplewitz BZ, Babyn PS, Cole WG: Congenital dislocation of the patella. *AJR Am J Roentgenol* 2005;184(5):1640-1646.

16. Langenskiöld A, Ritsilä V: Congenital dislocation of the patella and its operative treatment. *J Pediatr Orthop* 1992;12(3):315-323.

5: Lower Extremity

Chapter 24

Tibial Deformities

Erik C. King, MD John J. Grayhack, MD, MS

Abstract

Orthopaedic surgeons who care for children should be familiar with recent literature published on the developments regarding the etiology, clinical features, and treatment of tibia vara, congenital pseudarthrosis of the tibia, and congenital posteromedial bowing of the tibia.

Keywords: anterolateral tibial bowing; Blount disease; congenital posteromedial bowing of the tibia; congenital pseudarthrosis of the tibia; infantile tibia vara; lower extremity; tibial dysplasia; tibia vara

Introduction

This chapter reviews the recent literature addressing the etiology, clinical features, and treatment of tibia vara, congenital pseudarthrosis of the tibia, and congenital posteromedial bowing of the tibia. In some situations, successful treatment remains challenging. An expanded understanding of tibial deformities may lead to better outcomes for patients.

Tibia Vara

Etiology and Clinical Features

Tibia vara is characterized by varus deformity of the proximal tibia. Tibia vara historically has been classified as infantile, juvenile, or adolescent, based on the patient's age at the time of diagnosis. The infantile form occurs in children younger than 4 years, the juvenile form in children age 4 to 10 years, and the adolescent form in those older than 10 years.[1] Some authors have used the terms early-onset and late-onset, with late-onset tibia vara referring to both the juvenile and adolescent forms. Infantile tibia vara corresponds to the classic description of Blount disease. However, in published studies, the terms tibia vara and Blount disease are used inconsistently, and Blount disease is sometimes applied to patients older than those who should be included in the infantile age range.

Infantile tibia vara is bilateral in 50% of patients. Although both early-onset and late-onset tibia vara are more likely to affect black children, patients with early-onset tibia vara are more likely to have bilateral involvement and are less likely to be black or male compared with patients with late-onset tibia vara.[2] This disease is usually progressive, although spontaneous regression has been noted.[3] The differential diagnosis includes physiologic genu vara, metaphyseal chondrodysplasia, renal osteodystrophy, vitamin D–deficiency rickets, vitamin D–resistant rickets (hypophosphatemic rickets), and focal fibrocartilaginous dysplasia.

The cause of tibia vara is not known. Histologic studies have demonstrated disruption of the normal columnar architecture of the physis, replacement of physeal cartilage by fibrous tissue, and osseous bridging between the epiphysis and metaphysis in patients with advanced disease.[1] Children who have tibia vara are typically overweight or obese. Given the role of vitamin D in bone and growth plate mineralization and regulation, research has been performed to clarify the relationship between tibia vara and vitamin D deficiency. Tibia vara has been found to be more likely in patients with low levels of vitamin D.[4]

Tibia vara is associated with childhood obesity. This finding may be the result of increased compressive forces and growth inhibition at the proximal tibia physis.[5] A recent study investigated whether children with tibia vara had a lower body mass index (BMI) after surgical correction of their lower limb deformity.[6] The relationship of the change in BMI in patients undergoing gradual tibial

Dr. Grayhack or an immediate family member has stock or stock options held in DePuy, Medtronic Sofamor Danek, and Johnson & Johnson and serves as a board member, owner, officer, or committee member of the Pediatric Orthopaedic Society of North America. Neither Dr. King nor any immediate family member has received anything of value from or has stock or stock options held in a commercial company or institution related directly or indirectly to the subject of this chapter.

5: Lower Extremity

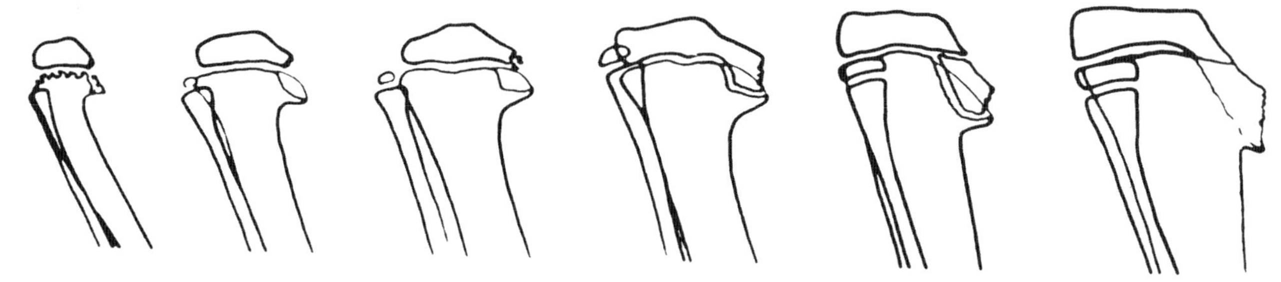

Figure 1 Schematic drawing showing the stages in the Langenskiöld radiographic classification of infantile tibia vara. **A,** Stage I: mild beaking of the tibial metaphysis. **B,** Stage II: beaking with slight depression. **C,** Stage III: depression with early fragmentation. **D,** Stage IV: more severe depression with early bar formation. **E,** Stage V: severely disrupted physis with abnormal growth. **F,** Stage VI: definite bar formation with severe disruption of the articular surface. (Reproduced with permission from Langenskiöld A: Tibia vara: A critical review. *Clin Orthop Relat Res* 1989;9[246]:195-207.)

deformity correction was studied. Of 47 patients undergoing gradual correction with external fixation, 36 (76%) had an increase in their BMI at an average follow-up of 48 months, despite successful correction of varus deformity and limb-length discrepancy along with nutritional counseling. Thus, other strategies are needed to address obesity in these children.

In addition, compared with their peers, children with tibia vara have advanced skeletal maturity.[7] Because advanced skeletal maturity affects the strategy for surgical realignment and the magnitude of planned overcorrection of lower limb deformity, preoperative assessment of bone age should be considered.

Both tibia vara and slipped capital femoral epiphysis (SCFE) are obesity-related bone diseases, but the relationship, if any, between the two entities is unclear. Children with both tibia vara and subsequent SCFE have been reported in the literature.[8] Hypertension also has been shown to be more prevalent in patients with both tibia vara and SCFE. In most patients, hypertension was previously undiagnosed. Because hypertension is a modifiable risk factor, it is plausible that hypertension may represent a modifiable risk factor for both tibia vara and SCFE.[9]

The classic radiographic features of infantile tibia vara are varus angulation at the epiphyseal-metaphyseal junction, a widened and irregular physeal line medially, a medially sloped and irregularly ossified epiphysis, prominent beaking of the medial metaphysis with lucent cartilage islands within the beak, and lateral subluxation of the proximal end of the tibia.[10] The Langenskiöld classification describes the severity of pathologic changes to the proximal tibia epiphysis and metaphysis as seen on radiographs[3] (**Figure 1**). In patients younger than 3 years, it can be difficult to distinguish infantile tibia vara from physiologic genu varum because the classic radiographic features may not yet be present. Historically, a metaphyseal-diaphyseal angle greater than 11° on plain radiographs was used as predictive of an increased risk for the subsequent development of radiographic changes characteristic of infantile tibia vara.[11] There is now a consensus among most authors that metaphyseal-diaphyseal angles less than 9° suggest physiologic genu vara, angles between 9° and 16° are indeterminate and should be monitored, and angles greater than 16° likely indicate infantile tibia vara and should be treated.[12]

Tibia vara also is characterized by procurvatum deformity in the sagittal plane. However, the authors of a recent study reported that clinical evaluation of procurvatum deformity tends to underestimate the true deformity as measured on radiographs.[13] Thus, in planning correction of the three-dimensional deformity, attention should be paid to findings on both coronal and sagittal radiographs.

In addition to bone deformities, abnormalities of the intra-articular structures of the knee occur in tibia vara. As demonstrated in MRI studies, the most severe of these abnormalities occur in the medial compartment of the knee, including increased thickness of the epiphyseal cartilage of the proximal medial aspect of the tibia, increased height and width of the medial meniscus, and abnormal signal in the posterior horn of the medial meniscus[14,15] (**Figure 2**). These morphologic changes may compensate for, or be a consequence of, the diminished height of the ossified portion of the medial proximal aspect of the tibia.

Treatment

Bracing remains the first line of treatment in children when a diagnosis of tibia vara is made before the age of 4 years. Brace treatment is most likely to be effective in children with mild deformity (Langenskiöld stage I and II) and in children younger than 3 years. Bracing is especially effective in patients with unilateral involvement. In children age 4 years or older, surgery should be considered. Traditional surgical techniques include proximal tibial-fibular osteotomy, acute or gradual correction, and hemiepiphysiodesis. In patients with severe or recurrent deformity, epiphysiolysis (physeal bar resection) and medial tibial plateau elevation may be necessary.

Intraoperative neurophysiologic monitoring has been shown to be a useful adjunct in tibial osteotomy surgery, potentially preventing irreversible neurologic damage.[16] A 2013 study confirmed that osteotomy with gradual correction with an external fixator is effective and associated with few complications, even in patients who are obese.[17] Both unilateral external fixators and circular external fixators are safe and effective.[18] If minimal lengthening is needed in addition to angular correction, then osteotomy of the fibula is unnecessary.[19]

Interest in using the growth modulation technique, also known as guided growth, in younger patients has increased. Previously, this technique was reserved for adolescent patients. In growth modulation, a tension band is created across the lateral tibial physis by the extraperiosteal implantation of staples, tension plates, or screws. A 2012 study examined a series of 12 patients with infantile tibia vara (average age, 4.8 years at time of surgery) treated with lateral tension band plating and reported a success rate of 89% with lateral proximal tibial tension band plates.[20]

When used in older children or adolescents, the effectiveness of tension plates is dependent on the magnitude of the varus deformity and the skeletal growth remaining.[21] A 2010 study found that the eight-Plate (Orthofix) effectively treats angular deformities in growing children and is less likely to extrude spontaneously than the Blount staple.[22] Failures and delayed correction were attributed to broken screws and wound infection that required plate removal. Some recurrence of varus deformity occurred in a few patients. After removal of plates, the risk of recurrent varus deformity is attributed to the poor growth potential of the proximal medial tibial physis. Growth modulation does not correct the associated internal tibial rotational deformity in all patients, but this deformity has spontaneously resolved in many patients after coronal plane correction.

Multiple reports have suggested that titanium cannulated screws are prone to breakage in patients with infantile or adolescent tibia vara because of the high BMI of these patients. A 2012 study used biomechanical testing of cyclic loading to failure to compare the strength of two guided-growth devices. With the use of

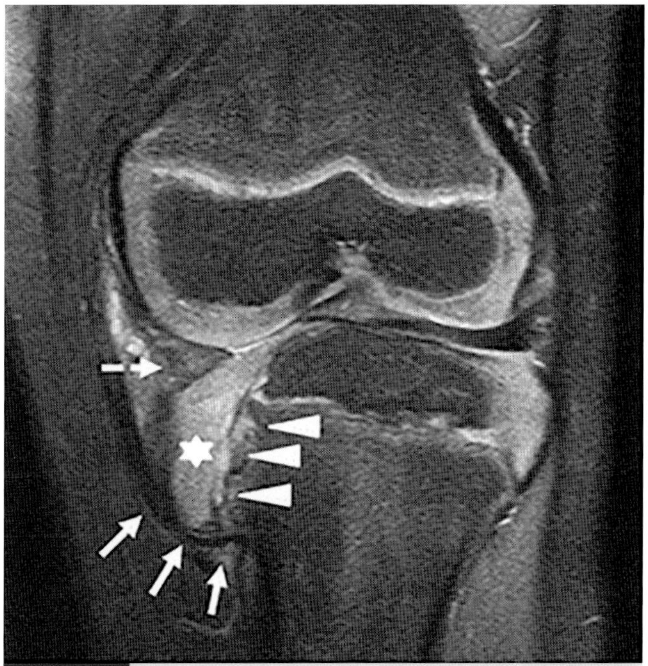

Figure 2 Coronal fat-suppressed spin-echo proton density-weighted MRI from a 3-year-old girl demonstrates downsloping of the medial tibial physis and metaphysis (arrowheads). An enlarged medial meniscus with abnormal signal intensity (interrupted arrow) with an irregular epiphysis (asterisk) that stretches the medial perichondrium (solid arrows) is shown. (Reproduced with permission from Ho-Fung V, Jaimes C, Delgado J, Davidson RS, Jaramillo D: MRI evaluation of the knee in children with infantile Blount disease: Tibial and extra-tibial findings. *Pediatr Radiol* 2013;43[10]:1316-1326.)

titanium cannulated screws, one guided-growth device was found to be significantly stronger than the other ($P = 0.036$).[23] Solid stainless steel screws were shown to be substantially stronger than cannulated screws in both devices. Some authors now recommend stronger implants such as parallel eight-Plates and solid noncannulated stainless steel screws for plate fixation.[24,25]

Medial tibial plateau elevation should be considered in older patients who walk with a large varus thrust and have advanced depression of the medial tibial plateau. Delay in ossification of the medial epiphysis may make the magnitude of medial depression appear greater than it actually is. An intraoperative arthrogram can be useful in determining the true amount of medial plateau depression. Medial tibial plateau elevation can be performed alone or combined with varus correction of the metaphysis (the so-called double osteotomy).[26,27]

Congenital Pseudarthrosis of the Tibia (Tibial Dysplasia)

Etiology and Clinical Features

Congenital pseudarthrosis of the tibia (CPT) is an uncommon disorder that represents a spectrum of disease ranging from anterolateral bowing to fracture pseudarthrosis. Because most patients do not have a true pseudarthrosis at birth, tibial dysplasia is a more accurate term. Approximately 5.7% of children with neurofibromatosis have CPT, and up to 55% of children with CPT have neurofibromatosis type 1.[28,29]

The understanding of CPT etiology is improving. Histologically, the pseudarthrosis site consists of fibrous hamartoma; thick, abnormal periosteum; and fibrovascular tissue. The double inactivation of the *NF1* gene has been suggested as part of the pathologic mechanism, as reported in two recent studies.[30,31] The authors theorize that periosteal cells that have this double inactivation of the *NF1* gene fail terminal osteoblastic differentiation. These abnormal cells proliferate clonally and form the fibrous hamartoma in the tibia that causes pseudarthrosis. It is unknown why this formation is more common in the tibia.

Treatment

Successful management of anterolateral bowing and CPT is difficult and unpredictable. The treatment goal in children who have anterolateral bowing alone is to prevent fracture. To that end, full-time bracing with a custom orthosis during weight-bearing activities should be prescribed until the child reaches skeletal maturity.

After fracture or pseudarthrosis occurs, the treatment goals are to achieve and maintain union while minimizing angular deformity and limb-length discrepancy. Multiple surgeries over many years may be required to achieve these goals. Success is not guaranteed, and amputation remains an ultimate treatment in the most difficult of cases.

Surgical management should address both the biology of CPT and issues of mechanical stability. During the chosen surgical procedure, the abnormal pseudarthrosis bone is resected, the tibial defect is shortened, bone grafting is performed, and the tibia is stabilized. Success rates of each technique reported in the literature have varied.

A variety of surgical techniques have been described, including intramedullary nailing, vascularized fibular grafting, external fixation, and bone transport. Using excision of pseudarthrosis, intramedullary rodding, and cortical bone grafting, a 2011 study found union of the pseudarthrosis was achieved in 9 of 11 children (82%) after the index operation and in the 2 remaining patients after further surgery.[32] At final follow-up, all 11 patients had a soundly united tibia, although persistent fibular pseudarthrosis was present in 10 patients. Ten children underwent 21 secondary operations for various indications. Recently, Fassier-Duval telescopic rods have been used to treat CPT. The effectiveness of these rods has been demonstrated in osteogenesis imperfecta; however, only one study of its efficacy in CPT has been published.[33] The authors concluded that the use of the Fassier-Duval rods is demanding and associated with intraoperative and postoperative complications. Supplemental stabilization in an Ilizarov frame may be beneficial. More studies are needed before the effectiveness of this technique can be determined for patients with CPT.

The effectiveness of circular external fixators in the management of CPT has been reported in several series and substantiated in recent studies.[34,35] A 2011 study suggested a fibular status-based classification and a multitargeted fibular status-based algorithmic approach for osteosynthesis, ankle stabilization, and limb-length equalization.[36] In addition, the Ilizarov technique can be successfully combined with conventional antegrade intramedullary nailing.[37]

Bone transport has shown good short-term results; however, the risk of refracture remains high. A study of long-term outcomes in 12 patients treated with Ilizarov bone transport found that primary consolidation was achieved in 10 patients (83%) at an average follow-up of 24.5 years.[38] Half of these patients had a refracture. At final follow-up, fracture union was achieved in eight patients and fracture nonunion occurred in four patients, including one patient who underwent an amputation. Healed and united bone is often of inferior biological and mechanical quality, so lifetime protection with intramedullary devices, braces, or a combination of both is recommended.

Three approaches to vascularized fibular grafting may be used: transfer of ipsilateral fibula on its intact vascular pedicle, transfer of ipsilateral free vascularized fibula, and transfer of contralateral free vascularized fibula. The latter two approaches require microvascular surgical techniques. The use of ipsilateral free vascularized fibula grafts was reported to achieve union in 73% of patients at an average follow-up of 20.1 months.[39] To enhance union of the free vascularized fibular graft technique, a novel split-tibia coaptation technique was used successfully to achieve bone union in two patients[40] (**Figures 3 and 4**). In this technique, both the proximal and distal stumps of the tibia are split longitudinally and pivoted open to form gutters. The vascularized fibular graft is placed into the tibial gutters and stabilized by external fixation.

In addition to the usual complications of persistent nonunion, refracture, shortening, and angular deformity, the use of the contralateral fibula is associated with donor leg morbidity, most commonly ankle valgus.[41] To minimize ankle valgus, distal tibiofibular joint arthrodesis is recommended, and a distal fibular remnant greater than 5 cm should be retained.[42]

Two recombinant human bone morphogenetic proteins (rhBMPs) are now available for clinical use: rhBMP-2 and rhBMP-7. An important role in early differentiation of mesenchymal progenitor cells to preosteoblast cells is played by rhBMP-2, whereas rhBMP-7 promotes differentiation of preosteoblast cells to osteoblasts. For management of CPT, it seems likely that rhBMP-2 would be effective in the presence of pluripotent cells, such as when autologous bone grafting is performed. In contrast, rhBMP-7 alone would not be as effective until active normal osteoblast cells are present and ready for terminal differentiation. The FDA has not approved labeling rhBMPs for the treatment of CPT.

In a case series of seven patients, the use of rhBMP-2 combined with iliac crest and Williams rodding was shown to lead to earlier union in patients with congenital pseudarthrosis and a higher rate of maintenance of union compared with earlier studies.[43] Similarly, the authors of a 2011 study reported a series of five patients with a mean age of 7.4 years who were treated with rhBMP-2 and intramedullary rodding.[44] Ilizarov external fixation also was used in four of these patients. Radiologic union of the pseudarthrosis was evident in all of the patients at a mean follow-up of 3.5 months postoperatively.

Conversely, rhBMP-7 was evaluated in a 2014 follow-up study in which 20 patients were randomized into two groups.[45] Group 1 received rhBMP-7 along with intramedullary Kirschner wire (K-wire) fixation and autologous bone grafting, and group 2 received only K-wire fixation and grafting. The authors found no substantial difference in healing time between autologous grafting and autologous grafting plus rhBMP-7 at 5 years postoperatively. Similarly, an earlier study reported that the use of rhBMP-7 alone was not sufficient to overcome the poor healing environment associated with congenital pseudarthrosis of the tibia.[46]

Recently, therapy combining rhBMP-2 and a diphosphonate (zoledronic acid) was applied to a mouse model of deficient neurofibromatosis type 1 fracture repair.[47] Surgical repair of fracture that included rhBMP-2 therapy followed by the systemic postoperative administration of zoledronic acid halved the rate of ununited fractures to 37.5%. Only one clinical study using a combination of rhBMP and diphosphonates in humans has been reported. Eight patients with CPT were administered rhBMP-7 at the time of surgery in addition to receiving bone grafting and stabilization, followed by the administration of either pamidronate or zoledronic acid postoperatively.[48] In six of eight patients, primary healing was achieved at an average of 5.5 months after surgery.

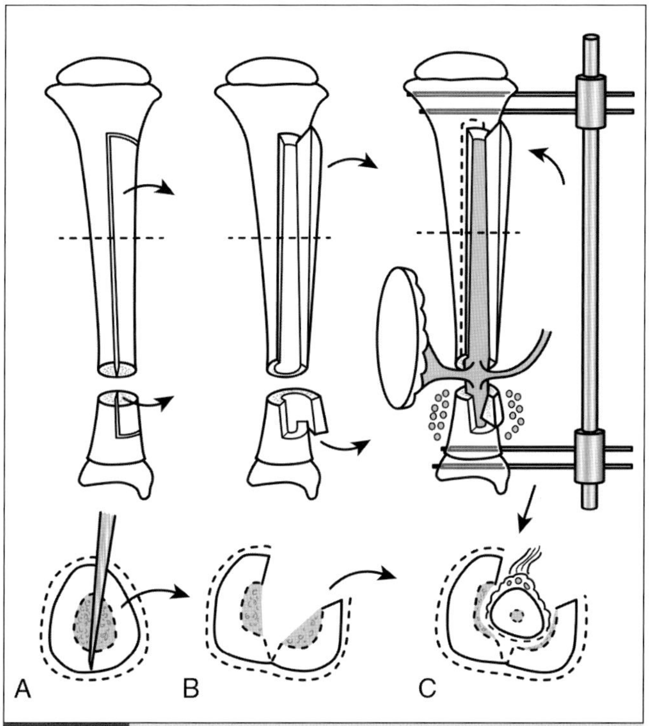

Figure 3 Schematic representation of the split-tibia coaptation technique for free vascularized fibular graft. **A,** Longitudinal and transverse osteotomies are performed at the proximal and the distal tibia. **B,** The medial part of the tibia is opened like a book and gutters are made. **C,** The fibular graft is placed in the gutters and wrapped with the split tibia.

A 2010 study described a two-stage technique in the management of extensive diaphyseal defects by induction of a membrane for bone reconstruction (Masquelet technique, also known as the induced membrane technique).[49] In stage 1, bone débridement is performed, and the defect is filled with bone cement. The cement remains in place for a period of 8 weeks, which allows the formation of induction membrane. In stage 2, the bone cement is gently removed, and the defect is filled with cancellous bone graft. Mixed results have been reported in small case series of patients (including children) with CPT.[50-53] The long-term efficacy of the technique is not yet known.

Given the heterogeneity of CPT and the myriad of treatment options, the European Pediatric Orthopaedic Society performed a multicenter study and proposed a stepwise incremental protocol for the management of CPT. This protocol uses bracing, intramedullary rods, circular frame fixation, and rhBMP-2[54] (**Figure 5**). The goal of this stepwise approach is to optimize pseudarthrosis union while avoiding the use of aggressive limb reconstruction techniques at a young age.

5: Lower Extremity

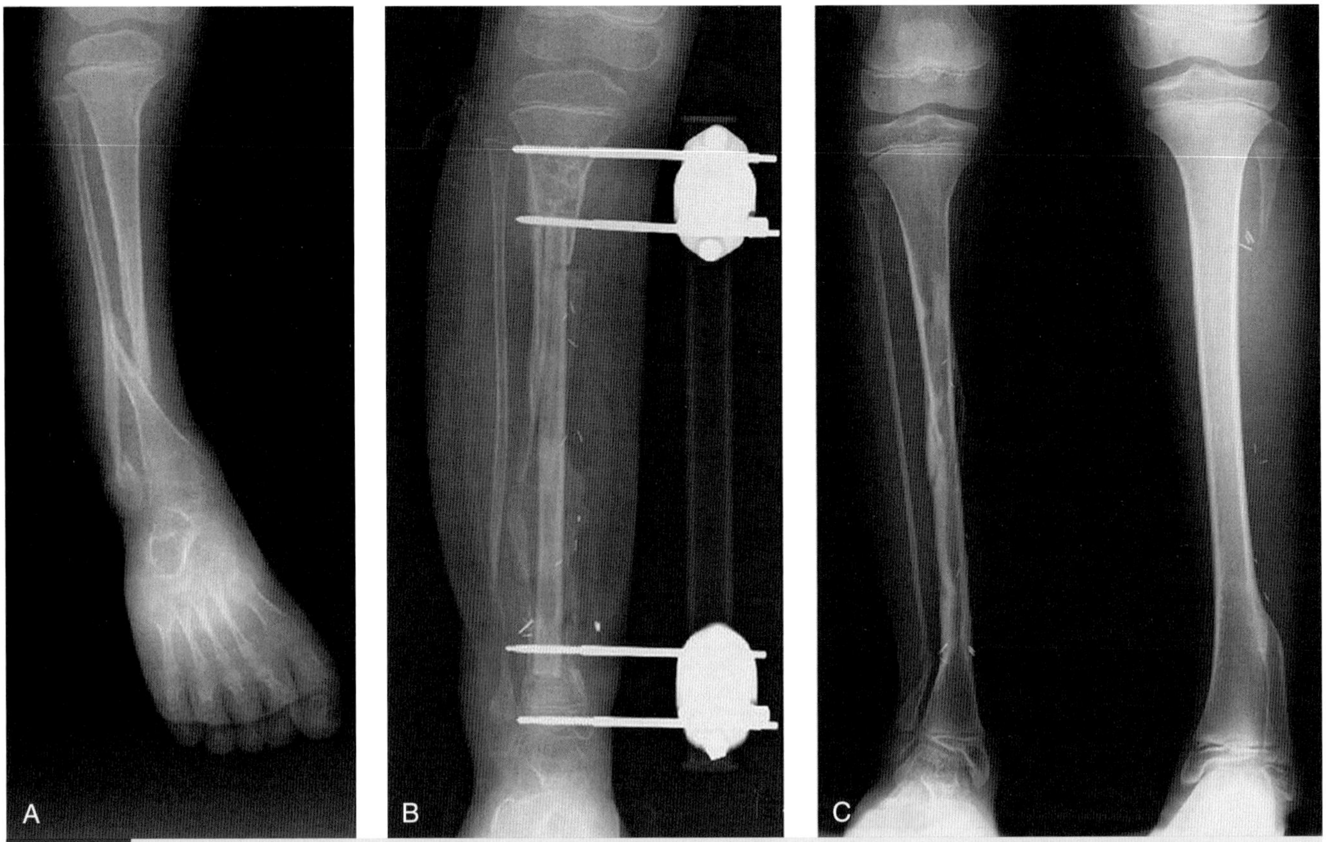

Figure 4 Radiographs from a 5-year-old girl with Boyd type II congenital pseudarthrosis of the tibia. **A,** Preoperative AP radiograph of the affected right tibia. **B,** Postoperative AP radiograph of the affected right tibia. **C,** AP radiograph of both legs at 4 years and 1 month after treatment with a free vascularized fibular graft. The diameter of the graft has enlarged to 83% of the contralateral tibia with no refracture. (Reproduced with permission from Takazawa A, Matsuda S, Fujioka F, Uchiyama S, Kato H: Split tibia vascularized fibular graft for congenital pseudarthrosis of the tibia: A preliminary report of 2 cases. *J Pediatr Orthop* 2011;31[4]:e20-24.)

Congenital Posteromedial Bowing of the Tibia

Etiology and Clinical Features

Congenital posteromedial bowing of the tibia (CPMBT) is a rare condition usually associated with calcaneovalgus foot deformity. Although the deformity in a newborn is distressing to the family, the condition usually resolves spontaneously. CPMBT is most likely caused by intrauterine malpositioning of the leg. In the first year of life, rapid resolution of angulation is noted (**Figure 6**), but the rate of resolution is reduced substantially thereafter. If complete resolution does not occur, the residual deformity consists of tibial shortening and valgus deformity. The degree of residual shortening is directly related to the initial severity of the posteromedial bowing.

Two distinct mechanisms seem to be responsible for resolution of the deformity in CPMBT. One mechanism involves physeal realignment, and the other involves diaphyseal remodeling. A 2009 study reported that physeal realignment occurred at a faster rate than diaphyseal remodeling.[55]

Wedging of the distal tibial epiphysis and fibular hypoplasia with valgus inclination of the distal tibial articular surface occur in some children with CPMBT. Eccentric ossification of the distal tibial epiphysis in early childhood may be a predictor of wedging of the distal tibial epiphysis when the child is older. Periodic follow-up is recommended in children with CPMBT until skeletal maturity is reached to identify those with residual bowing, ankle deformity, muscle weakness, and limb-length inequality. Active surgical intervention may be needed to correct these conditions.

Treatment

Because few studies have been published on CPMBT, there is no strong basis on which to make a recommendation about the age at which surgery should be performed. When treatment is necessary, it usually is aimed

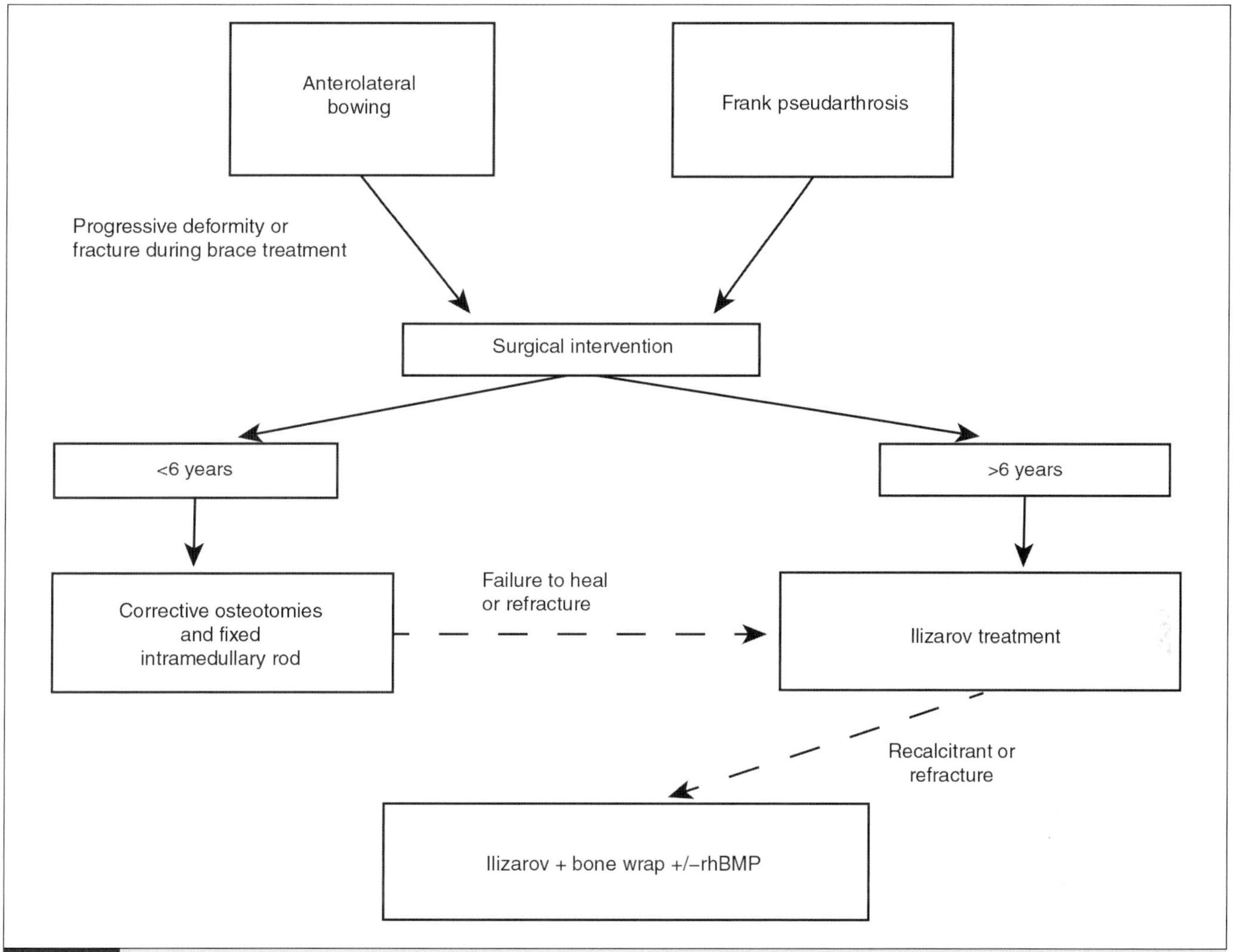

Figure 5 Schematic diagram shows the treatment protocol for the management of congenital pseudarthrosis of the tibia. rhBMP = recombinant bone morphogenetic protein. (Adapted with permission from Nicolaou N, Ghassemi A, Hill RA: Congenital pseudarthrosis of the tibia: The results of an evolving protocol of management. *J Child Orthop* 2013;7[4]:269-276.)

at addressing residual limb-length discrepancy and deformity. If the projected limb-length discrepancy at skeletal maturity is small, then no treatment or contralateral epiphysiodesis should be offered. However, for larger projected limb-length discrepancies, surgical limb lengthening combined with angular correction is indicated.[56]

To correct angulation, single-level tibial and fibular osteotomies may be performed, or multilevel osteotomies may be used if the residual angulation is large or spread over a large segment of bone. A 2014 study reported a series of four patients who were surgically treated for congenital posteromedial bowing of the tibia and fibula exceeding 35° in the coronal plane.[57] In all of the patients, tibial osteotomy was performed at two or three levels accompanied by fibular osteotomy. Intramedullary stabilization was achieved using K-wires or Rush pins. Follow-up ranged from 3 to 7.7 years. Axis correction and bone healing were achieved in all of the patients. A large circumferential periosteal release that accompanied the surgery may have stimulated bone growth, which possibly contributed to limb-length equalization.

Summary

Recent basic science and outcomes research have improved understanding of infantile tibia vara, CPT, and CPMBT. Along with traditional treatment methods, the judicious addition of newer techniques of diagnosis and treatment may result in better outcomes for patients.

5: Lower Extremity

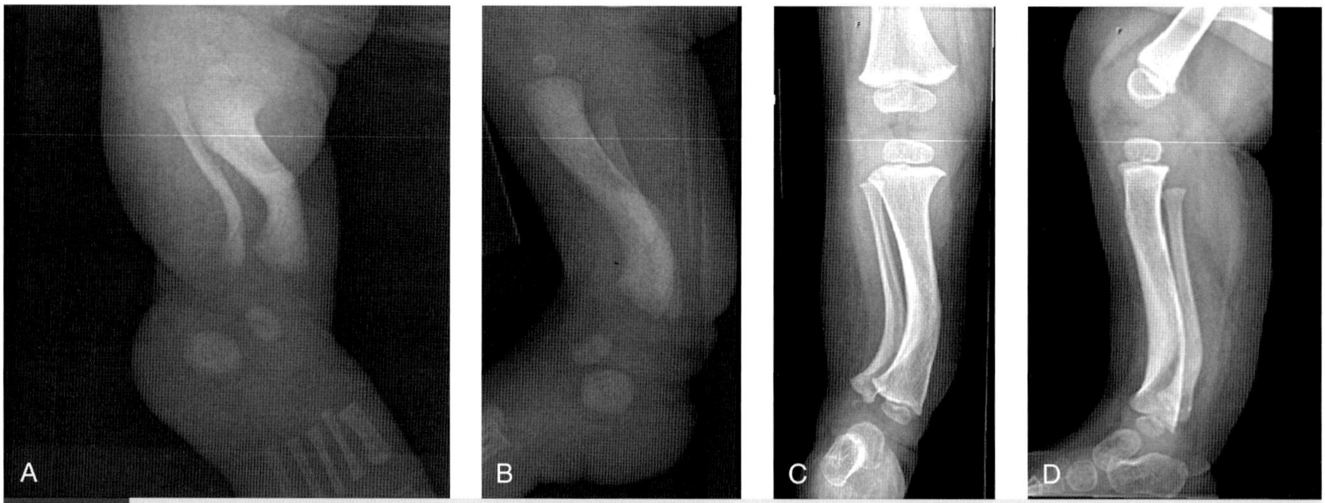

Figure 6 AP (**A**) and lateral (**B**) radiographs of a newborn with congenital posteromedial bowing of tibia. AP (**C**) and lateral (**D**) radiographs taken at 18 months of age show partial resolution of angulation.

Key Study Points

- Tibia vara is characterized by epiphyseal and metaphyseal proximal tibia changes, varus deformity, procurvatum deformity in the sagittal plane, and intra-articular abnormalities in the medial compartment of the knee.
- When bracing is unsuccessful, and for children older than 4 years, tibial osteotomy or growth modulation are effective techniques in managing tibia vara.
- Successful management of CPT remains difficult, although a stepwise incremental protocol may be useful in managing CPT.
- CPMBT usually resolves spontaneously. If CPMBT does not resolve adequately, surgical management of angulation and limb-length discrepancy is recommended.

Annotated References

1. Birch JG: Blount disease. *J Am Acad Orthop Surg* 2013;21(7):408-418.

   The authors present a thorough review of Blount disease.

2. Rivero SM, Zhao C, Sabharwal S: Are patient demographics different for early-onset and late-onset Blount disease? Results based on meta-analysis. *J Pediatr Orthop B* 2015;24(6):515-520.

   The authors present findings from a meta-analysis of 24 published articles on the demographics of early- and late-onset Blount disease. They found that both early- and late-onset Blount disease is more likely to affect black children. The two forms differ substantially in terms of race, sex, and laterality. Patients with early-onset Blount disease are more likely to have bilateral involvement and are less likely to be black or male than patients with late-onset Blount disease.

3. Langenskiöld A: Tibia vara; (osteochondrosis deformans tibiae): A survey of 23 cases. *Acta Chir Scand* 1952;103(1):1-22.

4. Montgomery CO, Young KL, Austen M, Jo CH, Blasier RD, Ilyas M: Increased risk of Blount disease in obese children and adolescents with vitamin D deficiency. *J Pediatr Orthop* 2010;30(8):879-882.

5. Sabharwal S, Zhao C, McClemens E: Correlation of body mass index and radiographic deformities in children with Blount disease. *J Bone Joint Surg Am* 2007;89(6):1275-1283.

6. Sabharwal S, Zhao C, Sakamoto SM, McClemens E: Do children with Blount disease have lower body mass index after lower limb realignment? *J Pediatr Orthop* 2014;34(2):213-218.

   In a study to determine whether children with Blount disease had a lower body mass index after surgical correction of their lower limb deformity, 51 children with Blount disease who underwent lower extremity surgical procedures and nutritional counseling were evaluated. The authors found that despite improvement in limb alignment and limb-length discrepancy after surgery, the BMI mass index of most patients increased. Level of evidence: IV.

7. Sabharwal S, Sakamoto SM, Zhao C: Advanced bone age in children with Blount disease: A case-control study. *J Pediatr Orthop* 2013;33(5):551-557.

   A comparison of the relationship between the bone and chronologic age of 33 children with Blount disease and

33 age-matched and sex-matched control subjects found that children with Blount disease have advanced skeletal maturity. Compared with chronologic age, bone age was advanced 16 months in children with Blount disease and 5 months in the control group. Bone age was advanced 26 months in early-onset Blount disease and 10 months in late-onset Blount disease. Level of evidence: III.

8. Jamil K, Abdul Rashid AH, Ibrahim S: Tibia vara and slipped upper femoral epiphysis: Is there an association? *J Pediatr Orthop B* 2015;24(1):46-49.

   Obesity is a common risk factor in Blount disease and SCFE. The authors present a case report of a child who was treated for bilateral tibia vara at the age of 3 years. SCFE subsequently developed at the age of 13 years.

9. Taussig MD, Powell KP, Cole HA, et al: Prevalence of hypertension in pediatric tibia vara and slipped capital femoral epiphysis. *J Pediatr Orthop* 2015; June9 [Epub ahead of print].

   This study evaluated blood pressure measurements in 44 patients with tibia vara and 127 patients with SCFE. The cohorts were compared with age-matched and sex-matched patients with obesity and without bone disease. The prevalence of prehypertension/hypertension was substantially higher in the tibia vara cohort (64%) and SCFE cohort (64%) compared with the control subjects (43%). The hypothesis that hypertension in conjunction with increased biomechanical forces potentiate the occurrence of SCFE and tibia vara was supported. Level of evidence: III.

10. Johnston CE, Young M: Disorders of the leg, in Herring JA, ed: *Tachdjian's Procedures in Pediatric Orthopaedics: From the Texas Scottish Rite Hospital for Children*, ed 5. Philadelphia, PA, Elsevier, 2014, pp 713-760.

    The authors describe common pediatric leg disorders, including tibia vara, congenital pseudarthrosis of the tibia, and CPMBT.

11. Levine AM, Drennan JC: Physiological bowing and tibia vara: The metaphyseal-diaphyseal angle in the measurement of bowleg deformities. *J Bone Joint Surg Am* 1982;64(8):1158-1163.

12. Feldman MD, Schoenecker PL: Use of the metaphyseal-diaphyseal angle in the evaluation of bowed legs. *J Bone Joint Surg Am* 1993;75(11):1602-1609.

13. Kim SJ, Sabharwal S: Is there a difference in sagittal alignment of Blount's disease between radiographic and clinical evaluation? *Clin Orthop Relat Res* 2014;472(12):3807-3813.

    In a study comparing radiographic measurement of procurvatum deformity in patients with Blount disease with clinical measurements, 43 patients who underwent surgical alignment for Blount disease were evaluated. The authors found that visual inspection of the limb can underestimate the procurvatum deformity of the proximal tibia relative to the measurable deformity on radiographs. Level of evidence: IV.

14. Ho-Fung V, Jaimes C, Delgado J, Davidson RS, Jaramillo D: MRI evaluation of the knee in children with infantile Blount disease: Tibial and extra-tibial findings. *Pediatr Radiol* 2013;43(10):1316-1326.

    A retrospective study compared the knee MRIs of 11 children with infantile Blount disease with an age-matched control group with normal MRI examinations. The most severe abnormalities of infantile Blount disease were noted in the medial compartment of the knee, especially the medial tibial physis and epiphysis.

15. Sabharwal S, Wenokor C, Mehta A, Zhao C: Intra-articular morphology of the knee joint in children with Blount disease: A case-control study using MRI. *J Bone Joint Surg Am* 2012;94(10):883-890.

    A study comparing the preoperative knee MRIs of patients with Blount disease with a control group found that children with Blount disease have increased thickness of the epiphyseal cartilage of the proximal medial tibia, increased height and width of the medial meniscus, and abnormal signals in the posterior horn of the medial meniscus.

16. Jahangiri FR: Multimodality neurophysiological monitoring during tibial/fibular osteotomies for preventing peripheral nerve injuries. *Neurodiagn J* 2013;53(2):153-168.

    In this study, the use of intraoperative neurophysiologic monitoring in 18 pediatric patients undergoing tibial and fibular osteotomies was evaluated. Peroneal nerve signal changes were noted in 4 of 18 patients (22%); causes included peroneal nerve entrapment in 3 patients (17%) and tourniquet pressure in 1 patient (6%).

17. Li Y, Spencer SA, Hedequist D: Proximal tibial osteotomy and Taylor Spatial Frame application for correction of tibia vara in morbidly obese adolescents. *J Pediatr Orthop* 2013;33(3):276-281.

    A retrospective study of patients with Blount disease with a BMI at or above the 99th percentile for age who had undergone gradual tibial deformity correction with a Taylor Spatial Frame (Smith & Nephew) found that the average BMI was 45 kg/m. The authors reported successful treatment in 100% of the patients and a few minor complications. Level of evidence: IV.

18. Oh CW, Kim SJ, Park SK, et al: Hemicallotasis for correction of varus deformity of the proximal tibia using a unilateral external fixator. *J Orthop Sci* 2011;16(1):44-50.

    A study of the efficacy of hemicallotasis using a unilateral external fixator for correction of varus deformity of the proximal tibia included 13 patients. The authors found that surgery corrected the medial proximal tibia angle from a preoperative average of 75.1° to 88.6° at final follow-up. Seven minor complications and one major complication were reported.

19. Sachs O, Katzman A, Abu-Johar E, Eidelman M: Treatment of adolescent Blount disease using Taylor Spatial Frame with and without fibular osteotomy: Is there any difference? *J Pediatr Orthop* 2015;35(5):501-506.

The authors report on two groups of adolescent patients with Blount disease undergoing limb lengthening with Taylor Spatial Frames. Group A was treated with fibular osteotomy and group B was treated without fibular osteotomy. No difference was found between the two groups in terms of quality of correction and complications. Level of evidence: III.

20. Scott AC: Treatment of infantile Blount disease with lateral tension band plating. *J Pediatr Orthop* 2012;32(1):29-34.

    A retrospective chart and radiographic review was performed for 12 children with infantile Blount disease treated with application of lateral proximal tibial tension band plates. The success rate of growth manipulation was 89%. Failures and delayed correction were attributed to wound infection requiring plate removal and broken screws. Some recurrence of varus occurred after plate removal. Level of evidence: IV.

21. Park SS, Gordon JE, Luhmann SJ, Dobbs MB, Schoenecker PL: Outcome of hemiepiphyseal stapling for late-onset tibia vara. *J Bone Joint Surg Am* 2005;87(10):2259-2266.

22. Burghardt RD, Herzenberg JE: Temporary hemiepiphysiodesis with the eight-Plate for angular deformities: Mid-term results. *J Orthop Sci* 2010;15(5):699-704.

23. Stitgen A, Garrels K, Kobayashi H, Vanderby R, McCarthy JJ, Noonan KJ: Biomechanical comparison between 2 guided-growth constructs. *J Pediatr Orthop* 2012;32(2):206-209.

    In this study, the strength to failure between two different tension plates and two different screw types was compared in a solid polyurethane bone model. A substantial increase in strength in one titanium cannulated guided-growth system over another was found. Solid screws were substantially stronger than cannulated screws.

24. Schroerlucke S, Bertrand S, Clapp J, Bundy J, Gregg FO: Failure of Orthofix eight-Plate for the treatment of Blount disease. *J Pediatr Orthop* 2009;29(1):57-60.

25. Burghardt RD, Specht SC, Herzenberg JE: Mechanical failures of eight-plate guided growth system for temporary hemiepiphysiodesis. *J Pediatr Orthop* 2010;30(6):594-597.

26. Gkiokas A, Brilakis E: Management of neglected Blount disease using double corrective tibia osteotomy and medial plateau elevation. *J Child Orthop* 2012;6(5):411-418.

    Eight boys underwent two simultaneous double osteotomies for medial tibial plateau elevation and for correction of tibial deformity. At an average follow-up of 10 years, planned angular correction was achieved and maintained in 100% of the patients. All patients had returned to a higher activity level.

27. Fitoussi F, Ilharreborde B, Lefevre Y, et al: Fixator-assisted medial tibial plateau elevation to treat severe Blount's disease: Outcomes at maturity. *Orthop Traumatol Surg Res* 2011;97(2):172-178.

    In this study, six patients were managed in single-stage surgery consisting of medial tibial plateau elevation osteotomy, lateral epiphysiodesis, and proximal tibia osteotomy to correct varus and rotational deformity. An Ilizarov external fixator was used to achieve fixation. The authors reported good results in six patients, a medium result in one patient, and a poor result in one patient because of incomplete lateral epiphysiodesis. Level of evidence: IV.

28. Crawford AH, Schorry EK: Neurofibromatosis in children: The role of the orthopaedist. *J Am Acad Orthop Surg* 1999;7(4):217-230.

29. Andersen KS: Congenital pseudarthrosis of the leg: Late results. *J Bone Joint Surg Am* 1976;58(5):657-662.

30. Lee DY, Cho TJ, Lee HR, et al: Disturbed osteoblastic differentiation of fibrous hamartoma cell from congenital pseudarthrosis of the tibia associated with neurofibromatosis type I. *Clin Orthop Surg* 2011;3(3):230-237.

    In this study, the mechanism of impaired osteoblastic differentiation of fibrous hamartoma cells was evaluated. Fibroblast-like cells were harvested from the fibrous hamartomas of 11 patients with CPT and neurofibromatosis type 1 and compared with control subjects. The mRNA levels and expression were assayed using quantitative real-time reverse transcription polymerase chain reaction. The authors found that fibrous hamartoma appears to be caused by clonal proliferation of aberrant neurofibromatosis type 1 periosteal cells that are arrested before terminal osteoblastic differentiation.

31. Lee SM, Choi IH, Lee DY, et al: Is double inactivation of the NF1 gene responsible for the development of congenital pseudarthrosis of the tibia associated with NF1? *J Orthop Res* 2012;30(10):1535-1540.

    A study of clonality in fibrous hamartoma tissues by analyzing X-chromosome inactivation patterns included 11 female patients. The authors suggested that double inactivation of the *NF1* gene and subsequent clonal growth could be a pathogenic feature of the fibrous hamartoma tissue in some of the patients with CPT, but may not be essential requirements of its development.

32. Shah H, Doddabasappa SN, Joseph B: Congenital pseudarthrosis of the tibia treated with intramedullary rodding and cortical bone grafting: A follow-up study at skeletal maturity. *J Pediatr Orthop* 2011;31(1):79-88.

    In a study to evaluate the results of the treatment of CPT by excision of the pseudarthrosis, transarticular intramedullary rodding, and autogenous onlay cortical bone grafting, a cohort of children were followed until skeletal maturity. Union of the pseudarthrosis was achieved in 9 of 11 children (82%) after the index procedure and in 2 children (18%) after additional surgery. At final follow-up, 100% of the patients had a soundly united tibia. Persistent fibular pseudarthrosis was present in 10 patients. Ten children underwent 21 secondary surgical procedures for various indications. Level of evidence: IV.

33. Birke O, Davies N, Latimer M, Little DG, Bellemore M: Experience with the Fassier-Duval telescopic rod: First 24 consecutive cases with a minimum of 1-year follow-up. *J Pediatr Orthop* 2011;31(4):458-464.

The authors present a chart and radiographic review of the first 24 consecutive femoral and/or tibial Fassier-Duval telescopic rod insertions in 15 patients (minimum follow-up, 1-year). In two of the patients who had neurofibromatosis type 1 and CPT, several revision procedures were needed because of nonunion, loss of fixation, shortening, migration, and/or joint intrusion.

34. Shabtai L, Ezra E, Wientroub S, Segev E: Congenital tibial pseudarthrosis, changes in treatment protocol. *J Pediatr Orthop B* 2015;24(5):444-449.

Ten children with CPT were treated with resection of pathologic bone, bone grafting, intramedullary rodding, compression with circular frame, simultaneous proximal tibia lengthening, and bone morphogenetic proteins (BMPs). Thirteen surgical procedures were performed to achieve union. Four patients underwent simultaneous lengthening and four patients received rhBMP. Union of the pseudarthrosis was achieved in all of the patients, with lengthening up to 5 cm.

35. Choi IH, Lee SJ, Moon HJ, et al: "4-in-1 osteosynthesis" for atrophic-type congenital pseudarthrosis of the tibia. *J Pediatr Orthop* 2011;31(6):697-704.

The authors report outcomes of the so-called 4-in-1 osteosynthesis, in which all four proximal and distal segments of the tibia and fibula are placed in one healing mass using the Ilizarov technique, for atrophic-type CPT associated with moderate fibular pseudarthrosis. Level of evidence: III.

36. Choi IH, Cho TJ, Moon HJ: Ilizarov treatment of congenital pseudarthrosis of the tibia: A multi-targeted approach using the Ilizarov technique. *Clin Orthop Surg* 2011;3(1):1-8.

A multitargeted approach for the management of CPT using the Ilizarov technique is described. Treatment goals, technical aspects, and complications are discussed.

37. Agashe MV, Song SH, Refai MA, Park KW, Song HR: Congenital pseudarthrosis of the tibia treated with a combination of Ilizarov's technique and intramedullary rodding. *Acta Orthop* 2012;83(5):515-522.

A study of 15 patients with CPT treated with a combination of Ilizarov apparatus and antegrade intramedullary nailing found that 14 patients achieved union. Six patients achieved primary union and eight patients achieved union after secondary procedures. The American Orthopaedic Foot & Ankle Society score improved from a preoperative mean of 40 to 64.

38. Vanderstappen J, Lammens J, Berger P, Laumen A: Ilizarov bone transport as a treatment of congenital pseudarthrosis of the tibia: A long-term follow-up study. *J Child Orthop* 2015;9(4):319-324.

A study of long-term outcomes of 12 consecutive patients treated with Ilizarov bone transport found primary consolidation in 10 patients (83%). Refracture occurred in 50% of these patients. At final follow-up, union occurred in eight patients and nonunion in four patients, including one patient treated with amputation.

39. Tan JS, Roach JW, Wang AA: Transfer of ipsilateral fibula on vascular pedicle for treatment of congenital pseudarthrosis of the tibia. *J Pediatr Orthop* 2011;31(1):72-78.

The long-term results of the use of ipsilateral fibula graft on a vascular pedicle were reviewed. At an average of 20.1 months, union was achieved in 8 of 11 patients (72%). Additional bone grafting procedures were required in four patients with distal nonunions. Three refractures were noted. Four patients eventually underwent amputation, and one patient had a persistent nonunion at final follow-up. Level of evidence: IV.

40. Takazawa A, Matsuda S, Fujioka F, Uchiyama S, Kato H: Split tibia vascularized fibular graft for congenital pseudarthrosis of the tibia: A preliminary report of 2 cases. *J Pediatr Orthop* 2011;31(4):e20-e24.

A split-tibia coaptation technique to improve bone union of free vascularized fibular grafts is described. In two patients, successful bone union was achieved at 12 and 13 weeks postoperatively. Refracture did not occur during the follow-up periods.

41. Iamaguchi RB, Fucs PM, Carlos da Costa A, Chakkour I, Gomes MD: Congenital pseudoarthrosis of the tibia: Results of treatment by free fibular transfer and associated procedures. Preliminary study. *J Pediatr Orthop B* 2011;20(5):323-329.

Sixteen children with CPT treated with contralateral fibular graft were evaluated. Consolidation was achieved after the main surgery in 37% of the patients, and consolidation was achieved in the remaining 63% after multiple procedures. The authors concluded that the proposed procedure leads to a long treatment course with many revisions for correction of possible complications.

42. Iamaguchi RB, Fucs PM, da Costa AC, Chakkour I: Vascularised fibular graft for the treatment of congenital pseudarthrosis of the tibia: Long-term complications in the donor leg. *Int Orthop* 2011;35(7):1065-1070.

In this study, complications in the donor leg after fibula grafting were evaluated. The author found no substantial difference between patients with or without distal tibiofibular joint arthrodesis. Tibiofibular arthrodesis did not prevent ankle valgus. The authors recommended retaining a distal fibular remnant greater than 5 cm to prevent ankle valgus.

43. Richards BS, Oetgen ME, Johnston CE: The use of rhBMP-2 for the treatment of congenital pseudarthrosis of the tibia: A case series. *J Bone Joint Surg Am* 2010;92(1):177-185.

44. Spiro AS, Babin K, Lipovac S, et al: Combined treatment of congenital pseudarthrosis of the tibia, including

recombinant human bone morphogenetic protein-2: A case series. *J Bone Joint Surg Br* 2011;93(5):695-699.

Five patients with CPT treated with rhBMP-2 and intramedullary rodding were evaluated. Ilizarov external fixation was used in four patients. Radiologic union of the pseudarthrosis was evident in 100% of the patients at a mean of 3.5 months postoperatively. The Ilizarov device was removed after a mean of 4.2 months.

45. Das SP, Ganesh S, Pradhan S, Singh D, Mohanty RN: Effectiveness of recombinant human bone morphogenetic protein-7 in the management of congenital pseudoarthrosis of the tibia: A randomised controlled trial. *Int Orthop* 2014;38(9):1987-1992.

    Twenty consecutive patients with CPT and neurofibromatosis type 1 were randomized into two groups. Group 1 received rhBMP-7 along with intramedullary K-wire fixation and autologous bone grafting. Group 2 received only K-wire fixation and grafting. At 5 years postoperatively, no statistical difference in time to primary bone union was noted.

46. Lee FY, Sinicropi SM, Lee FS, Vitale MG, Roye DP Jr, Choi IH: Treatment of congenital pseudarthrosis of the tibia with recombinant human bone morphogenetic protein-7 (rhBMP-7): A report of five cases. *J Bone Joint Surg Am* 2006;88(3):627-633.

47. Schindeler A, Birke O, Yu NY, et al: Distal tibial fracture repair in a neurofibromatosis type 1-deficient mouse treated with recombinant bone morphogenetic protein and a bisphosphonate. *J Bone Joint Surg Br* 2011;93(8):1134-1139.

    The combined use of rhBMP-2 and zoledronic acid in a mouse model of neurofibromatosis type 1–deficient fracture repair is described. When only rhBMP was used to promote repair, 75% of fractures in neurofibromatosis type 1 (±) mice remained ununited at 3 weeks compared with 7% of fractures in control subjects treated with rhBMP-2 and zoledronic acid. Systemic postoperative administration of zoledronic acid halved the rate of ununited fractures to 37.5%.

48. Birke O, Schindeler A, Ramachandran M, et al: Preliminary experience with the combined use of recombinant bone morphogenetic protein and bisphosphonates in the treatment of congenital pseudarthrosis of the tibia. *J Child Orthop* 2010;4(6):507-517.

49. Masquelet AC, Begue T: The concept of induced membrane for reconstruction of long bone defects. *Orthop Clin North Am* 2010;41(1):27-37.

50. Pannier S, Pejin Z, Dana C, Masquelet AC, Glorion C: Induced membrane technique for the treatment of congenital pseudarthrosis of the tibia: Preliminary results of five cases. *J Child Orthop* 2013;7(6):477-485.

    Five patients with CPT were treated with a two-stage surgical technique combining induced membrane, spongy autograft, and intramedullary fixation. Satisfactory bony union of the tibia was achieved in all patients. The authors concluded that this technique avoids external fixation and the technical difficulties of microvascular surgery.

51. Gouron R, Deroussen F, Juvet M, Ursu C, Plancq MC, Collet LM: Early resection of congenital pseudarthrosis of the tibia and successful reconstruction using the Masquelet technique. *J Bone Joint Surg Br* 2011;93(4):552-554.

    The authors report pseudarthrosis excision and the use of the Masquelet technique to reconstruct the bone defect in a child aged 14 months. Consolidation sufficient for complete weight bearing was achieved by 7 weeks. At 2.5 years postoperatively, the child remained asymptomatic.

52. Gouron R, Deroussen F, Plancq MC, Collet LM: Bone defect reconstruction in children using the induced membrane technique: A series of 14 cases. *Orthop Traumatol Surg Res* 2013;99(7):837-843.

    Fourteen children underwent bone reconstruction using the Masquelet (induced membrane) technique in the context of trauma, tumor resection, or congenital pseudarthrosis. The mean age was 10.6 years at the time of reconstruction. Complications included nonunion, wound dehiscence, and graft resorption. Level of evidence: IV.

53. Dohin B, Kohler R: Masquelet's procedure and bone morphogenetic protein in congenital pseudarthrosis of the tibia in children: A case series and meta-analysis. *J Child Orthop* 2012;6(4):297-306.

    The authors report on three cases of CPT in children treated with the Masquelet technique and rhBMP-2. All published cases of CPT that were similarly treated were analyzed. The Masquelet technique did not improve CPT treatment results, but segmental bone reconstruction was possible.

54. Nicolaou N, Ghassemi A, Hill RA: Congenital pseudarthrosis of the tibia: The results of an evolving protocol of management. *J Child Orthop* 2013;7(4):269-276.

    In this retrospective cohort study, the outcomes of a protocol of management based on the recommendations of the European Pediatric Orthopaedic Society multicenter study, using an incremental protocol of bracing, intramedullary rods, and circular frame fixation (with or without BMP-2) was assessed. Ten of 11 patients (91%) successfully healed, and 2 patients (18%) sustained a refracture. All deformity parameters improved. Level of evidence: IV.

55. Shah HH, Doddabasappa SN, Joseph B: Congenital posteromedial bowing of the tibia: A retrospective analysis of growth abnormalities in the leg. *J Pediatr Orthop B* 2009;18(3):120-128.

56. Kaufman SD, Fagg JA, Jones S, Bell MJ, Saleh M, Fernandes JA: Limb lengthening in congenital posteromedial bow of the tibia. *Strategies Trauma Limb Reconstr* 2012;7(3):147-153.

    A study to evaluate 11 patients with congenital posteromedial bowing of the tibia who underwent limb lengthening procedures found a mean preoperative limb-length discrepancy of 3.7 cm. Complications were minor or moderate. The authors concluded that correction and lengthening is an alternative to contralateral epiphysiodesis in select patients.

57. Napiontek M, Shadi M: Congenital posteromedial bowing of the tibia and fibula: Treatment option by multilevel osteotomy. *J Pediatr Orthop B* 2014;23(2):130-134.

The authors review four patients treated surgically for congenital posteromedial bowing of the tibia and fibula. Tibial osteotomy was performed at two or three levels accompanied by fibular osteotomy, and with intramedullary stabilization. Axis correction and bone healing were achieved in all of the patients.

Chapter 25

Congenital Disorders of the Foot

David D. Spence, MD Clayton C. Bettin, MD

Abstract

Congenital deformities of the pediatric foot range in severity from mild, asymptomatic disorders to severe disorders that cause marked functional impairment. The age of affected patients range from newborns to adolescents. Nonsurgical treatment is the initial choice for almost all congenital foot deformities and may include NSAIDs, activity modification, stretching, bracing, and casting. Surgical treatment generally is reserved for patients in whom nonsurgical measures fail to relieve symptoms or improve function.

Keywords: accessory navicular; clubfoot; congenital foot disorders; congenital vertical talus; flatfoot; juvenile hallux valgus; osteochondrosis; pediatric foot; tarsal coalition

Introduction

Deformities of the pediatric foot range from variations in normal anatomy to those causing severe functional impairment. The clinical presentation, diagnosis, and treatment options for the most common pediatric deformities are discussed in this chapter.

Clubfoot

Congenital talipes equinovarus (also known as clubfoot) is an idiopathic foot deformity of unclear etiology more common in males and bilateral in 50% of all patients. It is the most common musculoskeletal birth defect. A genetic etiology has been suggested, with a recent link to the PITX1-TBX4 transcription factor. It is associated with other conditions, including arthrogryposis, myelodysplasia, and tibial hemimelia.

Clubfoot is characterized by numerous bone and soft-tissue abnormalities of variable severity. In general, the major muscle contractures lead to midfoot cavus, forefoot adductus, and relative pronation, in addition to varus and equinus of the hindfoot (**Figure 1**). Specifically, contractures of the Achilles tendon and the posterior tibial tendon lead to hindfoot equinus and varus, with the calcaneus rotated medially around the talus. The posterior tibial contracture also leads to adduction of the forefoot and medial displacement of the navicular with lateral uncovering of the talus. The posteromedial tissues, including the plantar fascia, the spring ligament, the deltoid ligament, the intrinsic muscles of the foot, and the toe flexors, become contracted, leading to midfoot cavus deformity. Deformities of bone also occur, including plantar flexion and medial deviation of the talar neck, wedging of the navicular, and first ray plantar flexion.

The diagnosis usually is made in infancy or, in some patients, before birth on routine prenatal ultrasound. The foot should be inspected to determine (1) the presence and severity of bone and soft-tissue abnormalities and (2) the extent to which these deformities are passively correctable. Skin creases may be noted medially and posteriorly.

The diagnosis of clubfoot is clinical, and radiographs are not routinely obtained. Radiographs may be useful later in the treatment course to confirm that equinus is being corrected at the ankle joint rather than at the midfoot or in cases of recurrence (**Figure 2**).

Treatment options for clubfoot include minimally invasive and extensive surgical methods. There has been a shift away from primary surgical intervention because long-term (>30 years) functional outcomes of extensive soft-tissue releases for idiopathic clubfoot were worse than those reported for patients treated with serial casting. A slightly undercorrected casted foot generally has a better functional outcome than a stiff, surgically corrected foot. A survey of 323 members of the Pediatric Orthopaedic Society of North America (POSNA) showed that 96.7% of the members use the Ponseti treatment method. Patients

Neither of the following authors nor any immediate family member has received anything of value from or has stock or stock options held in a commercial company or institution related directly or indirectly to the subject of this chapter: Dr. Spence and Dr. Bettin.

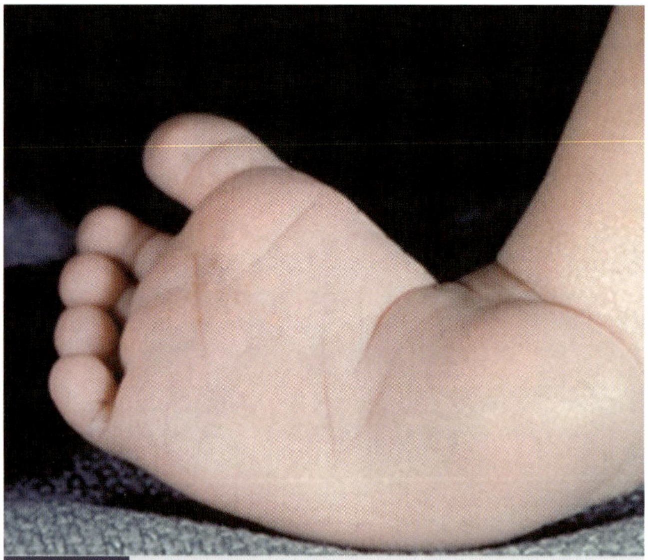

Figure 1 Clinical photograph of congenital clubfoot in a newborn. Multiple deformities are evident: inversion, plantar flexion, internal rotation of the calcaneus, and cavus deformity with a transverse plantar crease. (Reproduced with permission from Kelly DM: Congenital anomalies of the lower extremity, in Canale ST, Beaty JH, eds: *Campbell's Operative Orthopaedics,* ed 12. Philadelphia, PA, Elsevier; 2013, p 995.)

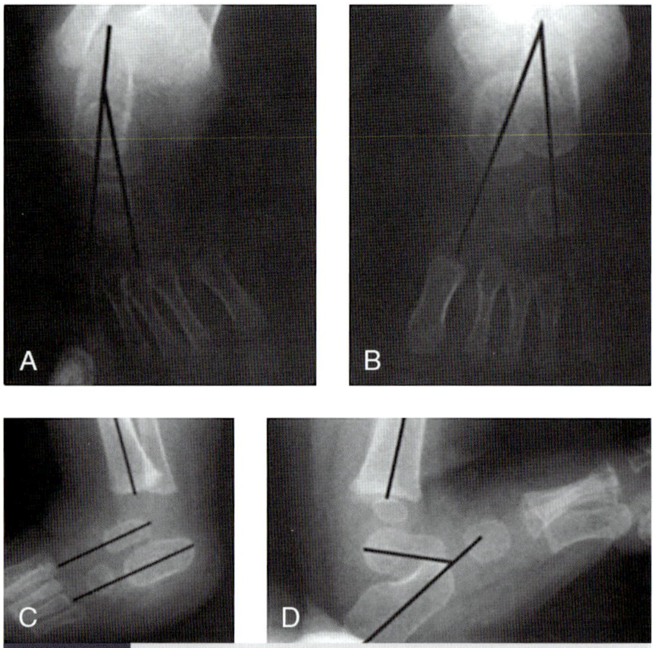

Figure 2 Radiographic images of clubfoot. **A,** AP view of a right clubfoot with a decrease in the talocalcaneal angle and a negative talus-first metatarsal angle. **B,** Talocalcaneal angle on the AP view of a normal left foot. **C,** Talocalcaneal angle of 0° and negative tibiocalcaneal angle on dorsiflexion lateral view of a right clubfoot. **D,** Talocalcaneal and tibiocalcaneal angles on dorsiflexion lateral view of a normal left foot. (Reproduced with permission from Kelly DM: Congenital anomalies of the lower extremity, in Canale ST, Beaty JH, eds: *Campbell's Operative Orthopaedics,* ed 12. Philadelphia, PA, Elsevier, 2013, p 996.)

have an average time to correction of 7.1 weeks, and 81% require an Achilles tenotomy.[1] Those surveyed estimated that they encountered a relapse in 22% of their treated patients, and 7% required comprehensive release. Of interest, 75% of the survey respondents reported that their current treatment approaches differed from those presented in their initial training, and 82% had been trained in the Ponseti method within the past few years. The most common nonsurgical techniques are serial casting (the Ponseti method) and daily stretching and taping by a physical therapist (the French method). The superiority of one method over the other has not been established, and the overall quality of evidence in comparative trials is low.

In the Ponseti method, long-leg plaster casts are applied with manipulation to rotate the foot laterally around a fixed talus. With the first cast, the cavus deformity and relative pronation of the forefoot are corrected by supinating the forefoot to bring it in line with the hindfoot. The knee is casted in 90° of flexion, and casts are changed weekly. Subsequent casts are applied to correct forefoot adduction and hindfoot varus by rotating the calcaneus and the forefoot around the talus, using the talar head as a fulcrum. When the foot can be abducted 70° and the hindfoot is in valgus, the foot must be dorsiflexed at least 15° in the final cast. In more than 90% of patients, this positioning requires a percutaneous Achilles tenotomy.

The final cast remains in place for 3 weeks, which is followed by full-time bracing in a foot abduction orthosis (such as a Denis Browne bar orthosis) that maintains the foot in 70° of external rotation and 15° of dorsiflexion. It is worn 23 hours per day for 3 months after correction, followed by wear during nighttime and naps until the child is 4 years of age.

Poor compliance with brace wear has been correlated with a need for additional surgical procedures.[2] In a 2015 prospective study using a novel pressure sensor to determine actual brace wear, the authors reported decreased actual wear rates for the first, second, and third months of 91.7%, 86.8%, and 77.1%, respectively.[3] At the same time, parents self-reported wear rates of 94.9%, 95.6%, and 94.8%, which calls into question previous assumptions regarding brace compliance. Parents should be instructed on the importance of brace wear in a positive communication style because a physician's communication style affects brace wear and recurrence.[4]

In a prospective randomized study, plaster casts have been demonstrated to have better outcomes than fiberglass casts,[5] and short-leg casts have been shown to be inferior to long-leg casts;[6] equivalent outcomes have been demonstrated when casts are applied by either physical therapists or orthopaedic surgeons.[7] Although initially described for idiopathic clubfoot, the Ponseti method has been applied to patients with arthrogryposis and myelomeningocele. Short-term outcomes suggest that initial correction may be achieved with a longer period of casting than required for idiopathic clubfoot, although the rates of recurrence may be higher.[8,9]

In the French method, a physical therapist performs daily manipulations, and temporary taping instead of casting is applied between therapy sessions. A comparison between the Ponseti and French methods showed them to be equally effective, with 95% initial correction rates in both groups, with correction maintained at 4 years in 84%.[4] Gait analysis showed distinct gait differences between patients treated with these two methods: those with the French method had an equinus gait and foot drop, and the Ponseti group had increased dorsiflexion of the stance phase.[10] This difference was likely attributable to using an Achilles tenotomy in the Ponseti method and the absence of tenotomy in the French method. The French method now has been modified to include tenotomy.[11]

Recurrence in children younger than 2 years usually is correlated with an inability to tolerate bracing and is treated with a trial of repeat casting. For recurrence in children older than 2 years, a repeat trial of casting should be attempted followed by transfer of the anterior tibial tendon to the lateral cuneiform (if ossified) if repeat casting fails. Factors shown to predict increased risk for surgical intervention include brace noncompliance; female sex; and a higher Diméglio score, which correlates with the severity of the clubfoot deformity at the time of the diagnosis and brace application.[2] Surgical intervention generally is reserved for multiple recurrences and residual deformity, typically with dynamic supination and equinus. For dynamic supination, a complete transfer of the anterior tibial tendon to the lateral cuneiform is performed.[12] Anterior tibial tendon transfer has been shown to be effective at preventing additional relapse without affecting long-term foot function.[13]

Lengthening of the Achilles tendon may be required for recurrent equinus. For resistant clubfoot in young children in whom multiple attempts at casting have failed, a posteromedial soft-tissue release with tendon lengthening may be attempted; the extent of soft-tissue release is negatively correlated to long-term foot function. Talonavicular arthrodesis, triple arthrodesis, and talectomy may be required for refractory clubfoot in older patients and as salvage procedures.

Flexible Flatfoot

Pes planus, also known as flatfoot, is a common foot deformity in the pediatric population. Its prevalence has been reported to be as high as 80% in children, but decreases to 10% to 20% in adults. The prevalence has been shown to decrease substantially from 54% of 3-year-old children to 21% of 6-year-old children and is associated with younger age, male sex, ligamentous laxity, and obesity.[14]

In flexible flatfoot, hindfoot valgus and loss of the normal medial longitudinal arch with standing are evident. The talar head may be palpable medially because of its plantarflexed position, and uncovering of the navicular, and associated calluses may be present. The hindfoot shows full passive motion with inversion and eversion; with toe rise, the arch is restored, and the hindfoot rolls into varus to lock the transverse tarsal joints. The range of motion of the tibiotalar joint should be tested, and the Silfverskiöld test should be performed because the condition often is associated with Achilles or gastrocnemius contracture. Many patients are asymptomatic and undergo an orthopaedic evaluation because of parental concerns about the appearance of the foot. Patients who are symptomatic may report medial arch pain, calf pain caused by contracture, and/or lateral sinus tarsi pain caused by calcaneofibular abutment. The entire limb should be inspected for rotational malalignment.

Radiographs should be obtained only if the patient is symptomatic. Weight-bearing AP, lateral, and oblique views are used to evaluate for other potential sources of the planovalgus deformity. On the AP view, the talar head may appear uncovered, and the amount of talonavicular coverage has been shown to be related to the onset of symptoms.[15] On lateral radiographs, the talar declination angle is increased, as is the Meary angle (the angle between the first metatarsal and the axis of the talus). Decreased calcaneal pitch may be observed in patients with contracture of the Achilles tendon.

Nonsurgical measures are the initial treatment choice, beginning with an explanation of the natural history of the condition to both the patient and the family. In 2013, a study of 580 preschool-aged children with flexible flatfoot demonstrated complete resolution in 38% after 1 year.[16] No high-level studies support the treatment of patients who are asymptomatic. In patients with arch pain, a navicular pad, medial arch support, or a University of California Biomechanics Laboratory orthotic may help with symptoms, but it will not correct the deformity or prevent progression in patients who are asymptomatic. Patients with contractures of the Achilles tendon or gastrocnemius muscle should begin a stretching program

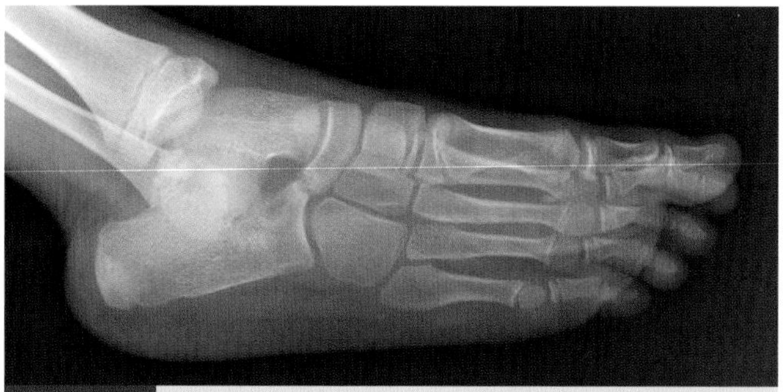

Figure 3 Oblique radiograph of a foot with a calcaneonavicular coalition.

to decrease associated calf pain. In the few patients in whom prolonged nonsurgical measures fail, consideration can be given to lateral column lengthening, either through a calcaneal lengthening osteotomy or a combined calcaneal-cuboid-cuneiform osteotomy.[17] Any surgical intervention needs to be carefully planned to correct all aspects of the deformity. Gastrocnemius recession may be simultaneously considered to treat the associated equinus deformity.[18]

Tarsal Coalition

In patients with a rigid flatfoot, where the arch does not reconstitute with toe rise and the heel does not invert, the most common cause is a tarsal coalition. A tarsal coalition is an abnormal fibrous, cartilaginous, or osseous connection between two bones in the foot that results from abnormal mesenchymal segmentation. This connection blocks normal motion at the subtalar joint and leads to overcompensation by other joints, resulting in a valgus hindfoot, lowering of the arch, and peroneal spasm. The incidence varies between 1% and 5%, and most coalitions are found incidentally, although some are part of genetic syndromes, including Apert syndrome, Muenke syndrome, and fibular deficiency.

Coalitions are most common between the calcaneus and the navicular (age of onset is 8 to 12 years) or the talus and the calcaneus (age of onset is 12 to 15 years). Patients typically have pain that increases with activity around the age that the coalition begins to ossify. Calf pain may result from peroneal muscle spasms, and recurrent ankle sprains may occur because of impaired subtalar mobility. On physical examination, limited subtalar motion is evident and may be associated with contractures of the gastrocnemius-soleus complex. Toe rise should be closely observed to look for reconstitution of the arch and hindfoot inversion, both of which may be impaired in the presence of a coalition.

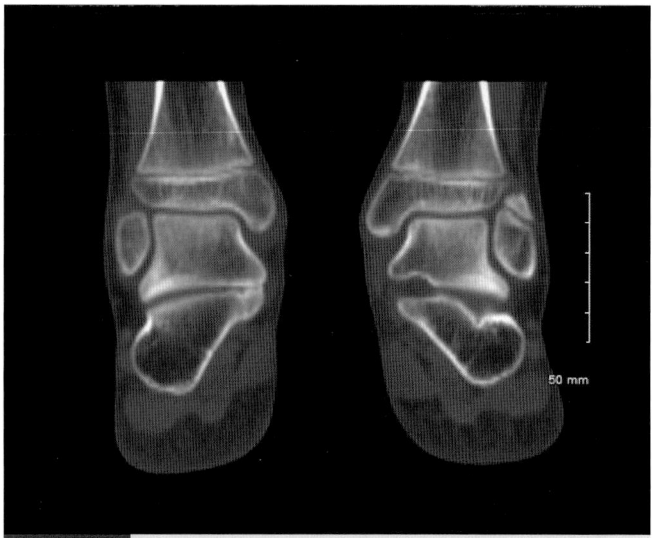

Figure 4 CT scan demonstrates joint space narrowing, articular irregularity, and subchondral cyst formation of the posterior facet of the right foot, which is consistent with a nonosseous talocalcaneal coalition.

Standard radiographic studies should include weight-bearing AP, lateral, 45° oblique, and axial Harris views (**Figure 3**). Cross-sectional imaging with CT or MRI is necessary to evaluate for additional coalitions[19] and guide treatment decisions based on the extent of joint involvement and any signs of surrounding joint degeneration (**Figure 4**). The size of the coalition does not appear to be correlated to the amount of hindfoot valgus or long-term functional outcome.[20]

Nonsurgical measures should be attempted first because many patients with tarsal coalitions are asymptomatic. A period of immobilization, including a cast or walking boot, may provide symptom relief and avoid surgical intervention. Physical therapy also may play a role in relieving pain from secondary issues such as Achilles tendon contractures. If nonsurgical measures fail, surgical interventions range from excision to arthrodesis. Surgical excision of the coalition is done through an oblique sinus tarsi incision just distal to the subtalar joint for a calcaneonavicular coalition; for a talocalcaneal coalition, a medial incision between the flexor digitorum longus and the neurovascular bundle is used. The coalition should be completely excised, and adjacent tissue should be interposed. Commonly used tissues include the extensor digitorum brevis and/or fat graft from anterior to the Achilles tendon. It has been demonstrated that the extensor digitorum brevis was able to fill only 65% of the typical resection gap in calcaneonavicular coalitions, and this deficit, combined with cosmetic issues, led to the adoption of the fat graft for all cases.[21] If substantial

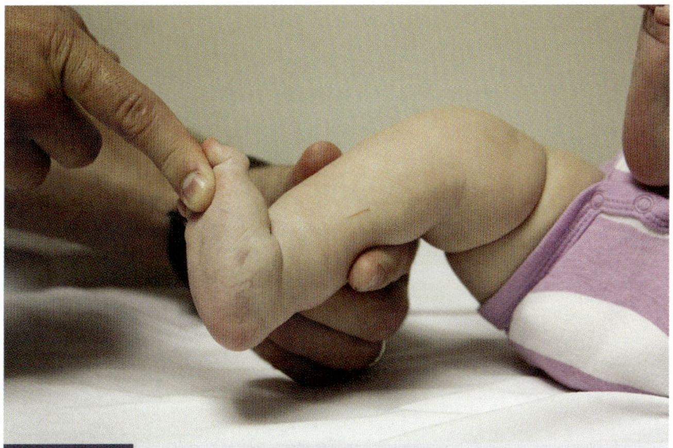

Figure 5 Clinical photograph shows the rocker bottom appearance of the foot of an infant with congenital vertical talus.

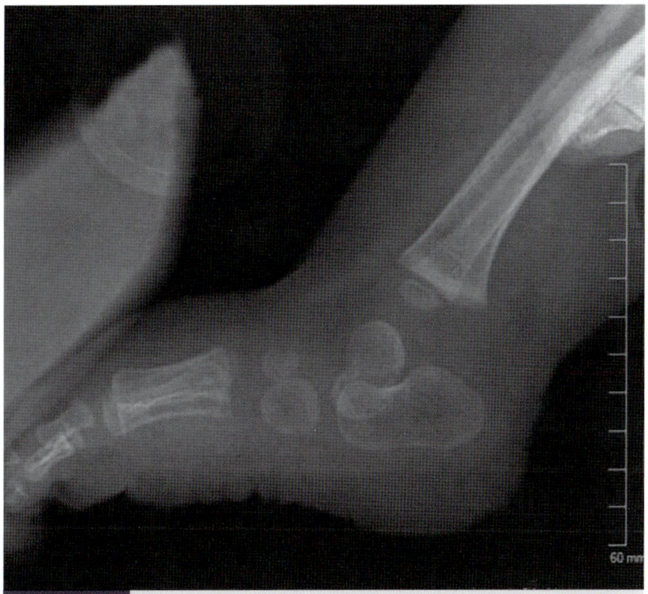

Figure 6 A forced, plantar flexion lateral radiograph of the foot of a patient with congenital vertical talus shows a persistent dorsal dislocation of the talonavicular joint.

hindfoot valgus is present preoperatively, a medial displacement calcaneal osteotomy also may be considered.

The role for arthrodesis is controversial. Traditional guidelines included involvement of more than 30% to 50% of the posterior facet and less than 16° to 21° of hindfoot valgus; however, current literature has suggested that good results can be obtained with joint-preserving procedures, including coalition resection and flatfoot reconstruction even in coalitions involving more than 50% of the posterior talocalcaneal facet.[20,22,23] The goal of surgery is to decrease pain and improve function, but numerous studies have found that normal kinematics are not fully restored after surgery. The exact surgical technique should be based on pain location, the size of the coalition, the health of surrounding joints and the medial facet, the degree of deformity, and any excursion of the heel cord.[24] More than 70% of patients with a surgically treated tarsal coalition did not believe that their activities were limited by foot pain at 4.6 years after surgery, and no substantial difference was found between talocalcaneal and calcaneonavicular coalitions.[25]

Congenital Vertical Talus

Congenital vertical talus is a rare foot deformity consisting of a dorsolateral dislocation of the navicular on the talus that is irreducible and produces a rigid flatfoot deformity. The head of the talus is forced plantarly and medially and is palpable on the medial aspect of the foot. The involved hindfoot shows a fixed equinovalgus posture resulting from contracture of the peroneal and Achilles tendons. Dorsiflexion through the midfoot is caused by the dislocated navicular, and the forefoot is abducted and dorsiflexed by contractures of the anterior tibial, extensor hallucis longus, and extensor digitorum tendons. The talonavicular, posterior ankle, and subtalar joint capsules typically have contractures, and an MRI study showed subtalar joint abnormalities, including lateral translation and eversion of the calcaneus.[26]

One of five patients with congenital vertical talus (**Figure 5**) has a family history of the disorder, and 50% have an associated genetic or neuromuscular disorder. The condition is bilateral in 50% of patients. A mutation has been identified in the homeobox *D10* gene in families with congenital vertical talus, and an autosomal dominant inheritance pattern with incomplete penetrance has been suggested. Associated conditions include chromosomal abnormalities, arthrogryposis, myopathy, and myelodysplasia. Abnormal muscle biopsies are present in 62% of patients, although it is unclear whether this is primary or secondary to the joint deformities.[27]

On a lateral radiograph, the talus is in a vertical position, and the long axis of the talus is plantar to the axis of the first metatarsal-cuneiform axis because of dorsal dislocation of the navicular. Because the navicular typically does not appear on radiographs until age 3 years, the first metatarsal is referenced instead on imaging. A forced plantar flexion lateral radiograph should be obtained and will show a persistent dorsal dislocation of the talonavicular joint (**Figure 6**). In cases of congenital oblique talus, a reduction will be observed on forced plantar flexion lateral radiographs. Cross-sectional imaging of the foot generally is not required; however, additional imaging of the spine may be required if the history and physical examination suggest an associated spinal pathology.

Untreated congenital vertical talus has a poor outcome and is associated with substantial functional deficits because of weak push-off strength, plantar calluses, and difficulty with shoe wear. Initial treatment begins with stretching of the contracted dorsal soft-tissue structures with plantar flexion and inversion of the foot. Traditionally, after a period of stretching, a comprehensive release is done, with open reduction and pinning of the talonavicular joint followed by casting. Regardless of whether a posterior Cincinnati incision or a dorsal approach is used, all contracted tissues must be released, including the peroneal, Achilles, and dorsal extensor tendons. Similar to surgically treated clubfoot, a comprehensive release for congenital vertical talus is associated with stiffness and, in some cases, osteonecrosis of the talus. In an effort to avoid this complication, some centers have started using a rigorous serial casting regimen similar to the Ponseti method for clubfoot to gradually reduce the talonavicular joint.[28,29] Serial casts are applied in the opposite direction used for clubfoot. The casts are followed by pinning the talonavicular joint in a reduced position, with a small arthrotomy if residual reduction is needed, followed by a percutaneous Achilles tenotomy to correct the equinus deformity. A recent retrospective study of 27 patients treated for congenital vertical talus reported better range of motion and lower pain scores in patients treated with a minimally invasion approach compared with an extensive soft-tissue release at an average follow-up of 7 years.[30] However, other researchers reported the use of a minimally invasive technique in a prospective cohort of 21 feet with both idiopathic and teratologic etiologies and noted a 48% recurrence rate.[31] Corrective surgery generally is more successful in younger patients. Salvage procedures may require a naviculectomy to shorten the medial column, a triple arthrodesis, or a talectomy.

Juvenile Hallux Valgus

Hallux valgus that occurs in the preteen or teenage years often is associated with a smaller medial eminence prominence, increased magnitude of the first-second intermetatarsal angle, increased hypermobility of the first tarsometatarsal joint, less pronation, and a higher recurrence rate with surgical intervention than in the adult population.[32] Juveniles are more likely to have bilateral deformities and a family history of hallux valgus as well. Patients may have difficulty with shoe wear, plantar callosities, and transfer metatarsalgia. Nonsurgical management should be considered first in all patients, especially those with ligamentous laxity or neuromuscular disorders, because they have a higher recurrence rate with surgical intervention. Shoes with a wide toe box, toe spacers, and night splints may be used for symptomatic management until physeal closure but are unlikely to correct the deformity. Although patients may dislike the cosmetic deformity, the main indications for surgical intervention are pain and discomfort with shoe wear. Numerous procedures have been described, and determining the appropriate surgical intervention is the subject of much debate. Overarching principles include correction of associated pathology, including first ray hypermobility with arthrodesis of the proximal first ray, increasing the distal metatarsal articular angle with biplanar or double osteotomies, decreasing the intermetatarsal angle with a proximal osteotomy, and avoiding soft-tissue procedures in isolation for incongruent deformities. Arthrodesis of the metatarsophalangeal joint is appropriate in patients with ligamentous laxity (Ehlers-Danlos syndrome), cerebral palsy, Down syndrome, and rheumatoid arthritis.

Metatarsus Adductus

Metatarsus adductus (forefoot adduction with normal hindfoot alignment) may occur in children as part of residual clubfoot or as an isolated deformity. Isolated metatarsus adductus has an unclear etiology and likely results from a combination of intrauterine positioning, hereditary/environmental factors, osseous abnormalities, and muscle imbalance. The Ponseti group reported on 45 feet (32-year follow-up) and found that all the patients with mild to moderate deformity who were treated with observation had good outcomes with deformity resolution.[33] A group of patients with moderate to severe deformity were treated with casting and also had good outcomes, with the exception of three patients with mild residual deformity who experienced mild pain with strenuous activity. This study demonstrates deformity correction in patients with mild to moderate metatarsus adductus with observation only. Patients with flexible deformities that can be passively corrected to midline can be treated at home with serial stretching performed by parents. Rigid deformities can be treated with serial casting or a stretching orthotic to obtain a straight lateral foot border. A recent prospective, randomized trial compared the use of Bebax (Trulife) orthoses with serial casting in 27 infants with resistant metatarsus adductus. The authors found that Bebax orthoses achieved greater improvement in the heel bisector measurement and were substantially less expensive than serial casting; however, the orthosis treatment required more active parental involvement.[34] Patients with persistent metatarsus adductus may be predisposed to the future development of metatarsal stress fractures caused by altered biomechanics and lateral column overload.

Accessory Navicular

An accessory navicular is a normal variant seen in 12% to 14% of patients who are asymptomatic. The navicular ossifies at age 3 years in girls and at age 5 years in boys, with fusion occurring at approximately age 13 years. The navicular tuberosity may have a secondary ossification center (accessory navicular) that begins to ossify at approximately age 8 years and may not fuse, leading to symptom development in some patients. The posterior tibial tendon inserts on the navicular tuberosity medially, and the accessory navicular may appear as a sesamoid bone within the tendon itself (type I). A type II accessory navicular is attached to the tuberosity by a synchondrosis, whereas a type III accessory navicular is a complete bony enlargement of the navicular. Patients report medial arch pain with activity, and a physical examination may show swelling at the plantar-medial aspect of the navicular. Fifty percent of patients have a flexible pes planovalgus deformity as well.

In addition to routine weight-bearing radiographs, an external oblique view will more clearly show the accessory navicular. MRI is useful to evaluate the synchondrosis, rule out concomitant pathology, and assist with surgical planning if initial nonsurgical treatment is unsuccessful.

Initial nonsurgical measures should include NSAIDs, activity modification, and orthotics. A medial-posted orthotic may alleviate some symptoms from forced heel inversion and decrease the pull of the posterior tibial tendon in a patient with a flexible flatfoot; however, the prominence for the support often lies directly under the navicular, so the orthotic may be more irritating than helpful to patients. When used, the orthotic should be constructed with pressure relief in the posteromedial navicular region. Stretching of the Achilles complex also should be done in those with an associated contracture. A short period of cast immobilization also may be beneficial if orthotics fail. Most symptoms will abate after the patient reaches skeletal maturity. In recalcitrant cases, surgical intervention for excision of the accessory navicular may be considered. Frederick Kidner originally described excision of the ossicle with advancement of the posterior tibial tendon to the medial cuneiform, but most authors now advocate ossicle excision with side-to-side repair rather than tendon advancement.[35,36] A generous resection of bone such that the navicular is flush with the medial cuneiform should be performed because the most common cause of persistent pain is inadequate initial excision. In patients approaching skeletal maturity with hindfoot valgus deformity, a lateral column lengthening or a medial displacement osteotomy of the calcaneus are useful adjunctive procedures; however, it is unclear in the literature whether additional procedures result in better clinical outcomes because no comparative studies have been performed.

Osteochondrosis

Osteochondrosis is an aseptic, ischemic necrosis of bone that can occur in any bone of the foot during childhood or adolescence; however, it is more commonly observed in the navicular and the head of the metatarsal.

Köhler Disease

Osteochondrosis of the navicular, also known as Köhler disease, commonly is seen as limping in a child who reports medial-sided foot pain with associated swelling over the navicular, and may be initially misdiagnosed as an infection. First described in 1908, Köhler disease generally occurs in young children and more commonly in boys than girls. Radiographs show flattening of the navicular with sclerotic margins and fragmentation. These findings, along with clinical symptoms, typically resolve in the long term.[37] Treatment includes NSAIDs and activity modification for mild symptoms and immobilization for more severe symptoms. Surgical intervention has no role in this condition.

Freiberg Disease

Osteochondrosis of the second metatarsal head is known as Freiberg disease or infraction. It more commonly occurs in adolescent females and may occur in any metatarsal, although the second metatarsal is most common. Patients typically show pain with weight-bearing activities, swelling of the involved area, and exacerbation of symptoms with distraction and compression of the joint. Depending on the chronicity of the problem, radiographs may show subchondral sclerotic changes in early disease, leading to flattening and joint destruction in late presentations. Initial nonsurgical measures include NSAIDs and a Morton extension orthotic, with immobilization in a cast or a walking boot if orthotics fail.

If prolonged nonsurgical management fails, surgical intervention may be considered, with surgical options including joint débridement, a dorsal closing-wedge osteotomy,[38] osteochondral autograft transplantation,[39] and interpositional devices.[40] In early 2016, a group of researchers reported long-term follow-up of 23 years in 20 patients treated with an intra-articular dorsal wedge osteotomy.[41] The clinical outcomes were excellent in 80% of the patients and good in 20%, with better results observed in patients with less collapse at the time of intervention (Smillie stages II and III). Resection of the metatarsal head should be avoided to prevent the development of transfer metatarsalgia and joint instability.

Apophysitis

Apophysitis refers to inflammation and irritation at an apophysis, which is a secondary ossification center that also is the site of a tendon insertion. Although apophysitis technically can occur at any apophysis, it is most common in the calcaneus and the base of the fifth metatarsal. It typically occurs in young males as part of an overuse injury.

Sever Disease

Calcaneal apophysitis (also known as Sever disease) was first described in 1912 and is most common in children aged 9 to 12 years. It typically presents with a waxing and waning course of pain at the insertion of the Achilles tendon on the calcaneus, along the calcaneal apophysis, or near the insertion of the plantar fascia. Although a direct cause has not been established, pedobarographic analysis has shown an association between symptoms of calcaneal apophysis, high plantar pressures, and hindfoot equinus.[42] Activities such as sports that involve repetitive forceful contraction of the Achilles tendon are bothersome; however, symptoms also may occur with walking.

Sever disease is a clinical diagnosis with a differential diagnosis that includes a stress fracture or a benign bone lesion. Radiographs are not essential to the diagnosis because studies have demonstrated only a 1.4% to 5% rate of abnormal radiographic findings in the workup of this apophysitis;[43] however, a single lateral radiograph is logical in the initial evaluation to assess for occult pathology. Treatment is nonsurgical, with heel cushions, activity modification, stretching of the gastrocnemius-soleus complex, and NSAIDs; symptoms typically resolve with closure of the calcaneal apophysis. The natural history of the disease should be explained to parents, with reassurance frequently provided, because the continuation of symptoms until skeletal maturity can be concerning.

Iselin Disease

Iselin disease also was first described in 1912 as an apophysitis of the fifth metatarsal in an adolescent girl. Apophysitis of the fifth metatarsal appeared radiographically in boys at age 12 years and girls at age 10 years, which are the typical ages of presentation for the disease.[44] Patients may have lateral foot pain from an acute inversion injury or chronic overuse activities and have pain with palpation at the base of the fifth metatarsal. Resistance against eversion of the peroneus brevis reproduces the pain. Because the apophysis may be confused with an avulsion fracture, contralateral radiographs as well as radiographs of the involved foot are useful in the workup. Nonsurgical measures, including rest, ice, immobilization, and NSAIDs, generally are successful in managing symptoms.

Summary

Numerous deformities of the pediatric foot have been identified, and they have varying clinical presentations. Understanding the associated conditions, natural history, and outcomes of nonsurgical and surgical intervention are paramount for managing patient and parent expectations and achieving good clinical outcomes.

Key Study Points

- Nonsurgical treatment is the initial choice for almost all congenital foot deformities and may include stretching, bracing, and casting.
- Clubfoot is the most common musculoskeletal birth defect and may involve numerous bone and soft-tissue abnormalities of varying severity. Generally, treatment with serial casting (the Ponseti method) or daily stretching and taping (the French method) is the preferred treatment, with comprehensive surgical release reserved for recurrent or residual deformities.
- Flexible flatfoot is asymptomatic in most children. If pain or functional limitations persist after prolonged nonsurgical management, lateral column lengthening may be considered.
- Tarsal coalitions are most common between the calcaneus and the navicular or the talus and the calcaneus. A period of cast immobilization may provide pain relief. Surgical options include excision of the coalition, osteotomy, and arthrodesis, depending on pain location, the size of the coalition, the health of surrounding joints, the degree of deformity, and contracture of the heel cord.
- Untreated congenital vertical talus is associated with substantial functional deficits. A rigorous casting regimen has become the initial mode of treatment, followed by minimally invasive surgery; however, more extensive procedures may be required.
- The primary indications for surgical correction of juvenile hallux valgus are pain and discomfort with shoe wear. Surgery should address all underlying pathology.

Annotated References

1. Zionts LE, Sangiorgio SN, Ebramzadeh E, Morcuende JA: The current management of idiopathic clubfoot revisited: Results of a survey of the POSNA membership. *J Pediatr Orthop* 2012;32(5):515-520.

   A survey of 323 POSNA members showed that almost all use the Ponseti method, and a recurrence rate of 22% was estimated. Seven percent of patients ultimately require a comprehensive release. Level of evidence: V.

2. Goldstein RY, Seehausen DA, Chu A, Sala DA, Lehman WB: Predicting the need for surgical intervention in patients with idiopathic clubfoot. *J Pediatr Orthop* 2015;35(4):395-402.

   A review of 134 feet with a minimum 3-year follow-up determined that patients who were noncompliant with bracing were 7.9 times more likely to need surgery. Females were 5.4 times more likely to require surgery, and those with higher Diméglio scores had a higher risk of requiring surgical intervention. Level of evidence: III.

3. Morgenstein A, Davis R, Talwalkar V, Iwinski H Jr, Walker J, Milbrandt TA: A randomized clinical trial comparing reported and measured wear rates in clubfoot bracing using a novel pressure sensor. *J Pediatr Orthop* 2015;35(2):185-191.

   A prospective study with a pressure sensor to determine actual brace wear during a 3-month interval showed wear rates at 1, 2, and 3 months of 91.7%, 86.8%, and 77.1%, respectively. Parents self-reported wear rates at the same intervals of 94.9%, 95.6%, and 94.8%. Level of evidence: II.

4. Richards BS, Faulks S, Rathjen KE, Karol LA, Johnston CE, Jones SA: A comparison of two nonoperative methods of idiopathic clubfoot correction: The Ponseti method and the French functional (physiotherapy) method. *J Bone Joint Surg Am* 2008;90(11):2313-2321.

5. Pittner DE, Klingele KE, Beebe AC: Treatment of clubfoot with the Ponseti method: A comparison of casting materials. *J Pediatr Orthop* 2008;28(2):250-253.

6. Maripuri SN, Gallacher PD, Bridgens J, Kuiper JH, Kiely NT: Ponseti casting for club foot: Above- or below-knee? A prospective randomised clinical trial. *Bone Joint J* 2013;95-B(11):1570-1574.

   A randomized prospective trial in 33 feet showed a 37% recurrence rate with short-leg casts, so the study was stopped early. Level of evidence: II.

7. Janicki JA, Narayanan UG, Harvey BJ, Roy A, Weir S, Wright JG: Comparison of surgeon and physiotherapist-directed Ponseti treatment of idiopathic clubfoot. *J Bone Joint Surg Am* 2009;91(5):1101-1108.

8. Boehm S, Limpaphayom N, Alaee F, Sinclair MF, Dobbs MB: Early results of the Ponseti method for the treatment of clubfoot in distal arthrogryposis. *J Bone Joint Surg Am* 2008;90(7):1501-1507.

9. Gerlach DJ, Gurnett CA, Limpaphayom N, et al: Early results of the Ponseti method for the treatment of clubfoot associated with myelomeningocele. *J Bone Joint Surg Am* 2009;91(6):1350-1359.

10. El-Hawary R, Karol LA, Jeans KA, Richards BS: Gait analysis of children treated for clubfoot with physical therapy or the Ponseti cast technique. *J Bone Joint Surg Am* 2008;90(7):1508-1516.

11. Steinman S, Richards BS, Faulks S, Kaipus K: A comparison of two nonoperative methods of idiopathic clubfoot correction: The Ponseti method and the French functional (physiotherapy) method. Surgical technique. *J Bone Joint Surg Am* 2009;91(suppl 2):299-312.

12. Gray K, Burns J, Little D, Bellemore M, Gibbons P: Is tibialis anterior tendon transfer effective for recurrent clubfoot? *Clin Orthop Relat Res* 2014;472(2):750-758.

    Twenty children with recurrent clubfoot who met the indications for anterior tibial tendon transfer were compared with a control group of patients whose deformity did not recur. At 3 months, no differences in strength, loading, or function were observed, and results were maintained through a 12-month follow-up period. Level of evidence: III.

13. Holt JB, Oji DE, Yack HJ, Morcuende JA: Long-term results of tibialis anterior tendon transfer for relapsed idiopathic clubfoot treated with the Ponseti method: A follow-up of thirty-seven to fifty-five years. *J Bone Joint Surg Am* 2015;97(1):47-55.

    Thirty five patients with idiopathic clubfoot who were treated with the Ponseti method were followed for an average of 47 years. Fourteen of the 35 patients required a tibialis anterior tendon transfer, which was found to be effective at preventing additional relapse of deformity without affecting long-term foot function. Level of evidence: III.

14. Chen KC, Yeh CJ, Tung LC, Yang JF, Yang SF, Wang CH: Relevant factors influencing flatfoot in preschool-aged children. *Eur J Pediatr* 2011;170(7):931-936.

    In 1,598 preschool children, the prevalence of flatfoot decreased from 54% of 3-year-olds to 21% of 6-year-olds. An association was demonstrated between the presence of flatfoot and obesity, younger age, male sex, and joint laxity. Level of evidence: IV.

15. Moraleda L, Mubarak SJ: Flexible flatfoot: Differences in the relative alignment of each segment of the foot between symptomatic and asymptomatic patients. *J Pediatr Orthop* 2011;31(4):421-428.

    In 135 patients with flexible flatfoot, no differences in arch height, forefoot position, lateral column length, or hindfoot alignment were found between symptomatic and asymptomatic patients. The amount of uncoverage of the talus appears to be related to the onset of symptoms. Level of evidence: III.

16. Chen KC, Tung LC, Yeh CJ, Yang JF, Kuo JF, Wang CH: Change in flatfoot of preschool-aged children: A 1-year follow-up study. *Eur J Pediatr* 2013;172(2):255-260.

    Of 580 children with flexible flatfoot who were followed for 1 year, arch height returned to normal in 38%. Level of evidence: III.

17. Moraleda L, Salcedo M, Bastrom TP, Wenger DR, Albiñana J, Mubarak SJ: Comparison of the calcaneo-cuboid-cuneiform osteotomies and the calcaneal lengthening osteotomy in the surgical treatment of symptomatic flexible flatfoot. *J Pediatr Orthop* 2012;32(8):821-829.

    A comparison of two procedures found better improvement of talar head coverage but more complications with calcaneal lengthening osteotomy than combined calcaneo-cuboid-cuneiform osteotomy. Level of evidence: III.

18. Rong K, Ge WT, Li XC, Xu XY: Mid-term results of intramuscular lengthening of gastrocnemius and/or soleus to correct equinus deformity in flatfoot. *Foot Ankle Int* 2015;36(10):1223-1228.

    The Baumann procedure was used as part of the treatment of 35 pediatric patients with equinus deformity and flatfoot with a mean follow-up of 39 months. The average range of motion increased by 13.6° with the knee extended and 9.7° with the knee flexed, with no cases of overcorrection, neurovascular injury, or healing problems. Level of evidence: IV.

19. Masquijo JJ, Jarvis J: Associated talocalcaneal and calcaneonavicular coalitions in the same foot. *J Pediatr Orthop B* 2010;19(6):507-510.

20. Khoshbin A, Law PW, Caspi L, Wright JG: Long-term functional outcomes of resected tarsal coalitions. *Foot Ankle Int* 2013;34(10):1370-1375.

    A retrospective, comparative study of 24 patients (32 feet) with calcaneonavicular and talocalcaneal coalitions treated with excision demonstrated similar long-term results in function and patient satisfaction, even in patients with a talocalcaneal coalition of more than 50% of the posterior facet and hindfoot valgus of more than 16°. Level of evidence: III.

21. Mubarak SJ, Patel PN, Upasani VV, Moor MA, Wenger DR: Calcaneonavicular coalition: Treatment by excision and fat graft. *J Pediatr Orthop* 2009;29(5):418-426.

22. Mosca VS, Bevan WP: Talocalcaneal tarsal coalitions and the calcaneal lengthening osteotomy: The role of deformity correction. *J Bone Joint Surg Am* 2012;94(17):1584-1594.

    Nine feet with unresectable coalitions treated with lateral column lengthening to correct valgus deformity showed short- to intermediate-term pain relief. Level of evidence: IV.

23. Lisella JM, Bellapianta JM, Manoli A II: Tarsal coalition resection with pes planovalgus hindfoot reconstruction. *J Surg Orthop Adv* 2011;20(2):102-105.

    Eight feet treated with coalition resection and flatfoot reconstruction showed increased motion and decreased pain. Level of evidence: IV.

24. Mosca VS: Subtalar coalition in pediatrics. *Foot Ankle Clin* 2015;20(2):265-281.

    This excellent review discusses subtalar tarsal coalition, including inheritance, diagnosis, and nonsurgical and surgical treatment. Level of evidence: V.

25. Mahan ST, Spencer SA, Vezeridis PS, Kasser JR: Patient-reported outcomes of tarsal coalitions treated with surgical excision. *J Pediatr Orthop* 2015;35(6):583-588.

    Sixty-three patients with surgically treated tarsal coalitions were mailed surveys at an average of 4.6 years postoperatively. No substantial differences were found between talocalcaneal and naviculocuneiform coalitions, with 73% of patients reporting that their activities were not limited by foot pain. Level of evidence: IV.

26. Thometz JG, Zhu H, Liu XC, Tassone C, Gabriel SR: MRI pathoanatomy study of congenital vertical talus. *J Pediatr Orthop* 2010;30(5):460-464.

27. Merrill LJ, Gurnett CA, Connolly AM, Pestronk A, Dobbs MB: Skeletal muscle abnormalities and genetic factors related to vertical talus. *Clin Orthop Relat Res* 2011;469(4):1167-1174.

    Muscle biopsies were obtained from 11 of 61 patients affected with vertical talus and associated congenital anomalies and genetic abnormalities and were compared with age-matched control specimens. Abnormalities, including fiber size, type, and predominance, were noted in all 11 of the patients. Level of evidence: III.

28. Dobbs MB, Purcell DB, Nunley R, Morcuende JA: Early results of a new method of treatment for idiopathic congenital vertical talus: Surgical technique. *J Bone Joint Surg Am* 2007;89(suppl 2 pt 1):111-121.

29. Chalayon O, Adams A, Dobbs MB: Minimally invasive approach for the treatment of non-isolated congenital vertical talus. *J Bone Joint Surg Am* 2012;94(11):e73.

    In this case series of 25 feet with nonisolated congenital vertical talus treated with serial casting and limited surgery with follow-up at 2 years, a recurrence rate of 20% was reported. Level of evidence: IV.

30. Yang JS, Dobbs MB: Treatment of congenital vertical talus: Comparison of minimally invasive and extensive soft-tissue release procedures at minimum five-year follow-up. *J Bone Joint Surg Am* 2015;97(16):1354-1365.

    A retrospective review of 27 patients treated for congenital vertical talus was performed. Range of motion, Pediatric Outcomes Data Collection Instrument scores, and radiographs were compared in 16 patients (24 feet) treated with a minimally invasive treatment approach and 11 patients (18 feet) treated with extensive soft-tissue releases. The minimally invasive group achieved better range of motion and lower pain scores at an average follow-up of 7 years. Level of evidence: III.

31. Wright J, Coggings D, Maizen C, Ramachandran M: Reverse Ponseti-type treatment for children with congenital vertical talus: Comparison between idiopathic and teratological patients. *Bone Joint J* 2014;96-B(2):274-278.

    In a prospective cohort study of 21 feet in 13 children undergoing reverse Ponseti casting with percutaneous reduction and fixation, 10 feet had a recurrence. Level of evidence: II.

32. Agrawal Y, Bajaj SK, Flowers MJ: Scarf-Akin osteotomy for hallux valgus in juvenile and adolescent patients. *J Pediatr Orthop B* 2015;24(6):535-540.

    In a case series of 47 juvenile and adolescent feet treated with a Scarf-Akin procedure, the average patient age was 11.7 years. The authors reported a 29.8% radiographic recurrence rate, with 21.3% of patients requiring a revision procedure. Level of evidence: IV.

33. Farsetti P, Weinstein SL, Ponseti IV: The long-term functional and radiographic outcomes of untreated and non-operatively treated metatarsus adductus. *J Bone Joint Surg Am* 1994;76(2):257-265.

34. Herzenberg JE, Burghardt RD: Resistant metatarsus adductus: Prospective randomized trial of casting versus orthosis. *J Orthop Sci* 2014;19(2):250-256.

    A prospective, randomized controlled trial of 43 feet in 27 infants (aged 3 to 9 months) compared serial casting to the Bebax orthosis and found greater improvement in heal bisector measurements and substantially reduced costs with the Bebax orthosis; however, the Bebax treatment requires more active parental cooperation. Level of evidence: II

35. Cha SM, Shin HD, Kim KC, Lee JK: Simple excision vs the Kidner procedure for type 2 accessory navicular associated with flatfoot in pediatric population. *Foot Ankle Int* 2013;34(2):167-172.

    In a prospective study that compared 25 patients treated with excision of the navicular with 25 patients with a Kidner procedure, no important differences were found between the two groups. Level of evidence: II.

36. Pretell-Mazzini J, Murphy RF, Sawyer JR, et al: Surgical treatment of symptomatic accessory navicular in children and adolescents. *Am J Orthop (Belle Mead NJ)* 2014;43(3):110-113.

    In a comparison study of 14 feet treated with excision of the accessory navicular and 18 feet treated with excision and tendon advancement, no substantial differences were found in outcomes, although the authors reported a trend toward more revisions after tendon advancement. Level of evidence: III.

37. Ippolito E, Ricciardi Pollini PT, Falez' F: Köhler's disease of the tarsal navicular: Long-term follow-up of 12 cases. *Pediatr Orthop* 1984;4(4):416-417.

38. Chao KH, Lee CH, Lin LC: Surgery for symptomatic Freiberg's disease: Extraarticular dorsal closing-wedge osteotomy in 13 patients followed for 2-4 years. *Acta Orthop Scand* 1999;70(5):483-486.

39. Tsuda E, Ishibashi Y, Yamamoto Y, Maeda S, Kimura Y, Sato H: Osteochondral autograft transplantation for advanced stage Freiberg disease in adolescent athletes: A report of 3 cases and surgical procedures. *Am J Sports Med* 2011;39(11):2470-2475.

    Osteochondral autograft transplantation for advanced collapse produced good clinical results in three patients. Level of evidence: V.

40. Sansone V, Morandi A, Dupplicato P, Ungaro E: Treatment of late-stage Freiburg's disease using a temporary metal interpositional device. *J Bone Joint Surg Br* 2010;92(6):807-810.

41. Pereira BS, Frada T, Freitas D, et al: Long-term follow-up of dorsal wedge osteotomy for pediatric Freiberg disease. *Foot Ankle Int* 2016;37(1):90-95.

    Patients who were treated with a dorsal wedge osteotomy for pediatric Freiberg disease were very satisfied with pain levels and quality of life at a mean follow-up of 23.4 years. Level of evidence: IV.

42. Becerro de Bengoa Vallejo R, Losa Iglesias ME, Rodríguez Sanz D, Prados Frutos JC, Salvadores Fuentes P, Chicharro JL: Plantar pressures in children with and without Sever's disease. *J Am Podiatr Med Assoc* 2011;101(1):17-24.

    Plantar pressure in 22 boys with apophysitis of the calcaneus was compared with 24 control patients. Results showed a relationship between plantar foot pressures, hindfoot equinus, and pain in the heel. Level of evidence: III.

43. Rachel JN, Williams JB, Sawyer JR, Warner WC, Kelly DM: Is radiographic evaluation necessary in children with a clinical diagnosis of calcaneal apophysitis (Sever disease)? *J Pediatr Orthop* 2011;31(5):548-550.

    Of 96 patients with a chief report of heel pain, 5% were found to have radiographic abnormalities leading to treatment, including immobilization and radiographic follow-up. Level of evidence: IV.

44. Canale ST, Williams KD: Iselin's disease. *J Pediatr Orthop* 1992;12(1):90-93.

Chapter 26

Rotational and Angular Limb Deformity

Ryan D. Muchow, MD

Abstract

Rotational or angular limb deformities are among the most common pediatric orthopaedic concerns. Because such deformities in children generally can be stratified within a physiologic range, it is important for the physician to have a solid understanding of normal growth patterns. Children with rotational problems most commonly have intoeing that has an age-based etiology: metatarsus adductus at birth to age 1 year, internal tibial torsion for toddlers aged 1 to 3 years, and femoral anteversion for children older than 4 years. Children who have angular problems typically have genu varum identified between birth and age 18 to 24 months and genu valgum identified at approximately age 3 to 4 years. In addition to providing the necessary education to parents for the treatment of children with these benign conditions, it is important to provide the context for identifying the pathologic causes of deformity and proper interventions. The history and the physical examination are keys to identifying pathologic deformity and implementing the proper treatment.

Keywords: femoral anteversion; internal tibial torsion; intoeing; outtoeing; physiologic varus; physiologic valgus; rotational profile

Introduction

Rotational or angular limb deformities are common concerns of parents when children are seen in the office of a pediatric orthopaedic surgeon. Although most of these deformities occur in healthy children and will spontaneously resolve, the art of caring for these families lies in understanding expected development and recognizing conditions that may not be within normal boundaries. The history and the physical examination are the mainstays of the physician's tools to determine underlying structural or neurologic abnormalities that may be contributing to the deformity and to educate and provide reassurance to the families of these children.

Neither Dr. Muchow nor any immediate family member has received anything of value from or has stock or stock options held in a commercial company or institution related directly or indirectly to the subject of this chapter.

Rotational Deformity

Normal Development of Femoral Rotation

Femoral rotation, either anteversion or retroversion, is defined by the angle of the femoral neck in the axial plane relative to the femoral shaft. Anteversion is the condition most commonly seen in pediatric patients and results from the normal developmental pathway. Femoral anteversion is greatest in infancy, where the average amount of anteversion is 40°. The degree of anteversion steadily decreases throughout a child's growing years to an average of 16° at maturity.[1,2] Females tend to have greater amounts of anteversion than males, anteversion is typically symmetric, and normal children follow the natural course of decreasing anteversion with age.[3]

In children with femoral anteversion and absence of any other condition, the natural history is benign and improves with age. Various studies have placed an upper limit on the age at which anteversion ceases to improve, which ranges from 8 to 16 years.[1,3-5] When subdivided by children with normal gait, intoeing gait, and outtoeing gait, femoral anteversion decreased at a rate of 1° per year in children with normal gait, decreased 1.6° per year in children with intoeing, and did not change in children with outtoeing.[4] A summary of the literature definitively defines femoral anteversion as a normal developmental finding that improves in most children.[3-9]

Normal Development of Tibial Rotation

Tibial rotation is defined as the inward or outward rotation of the foot relative to the knee. Intrauterine positioning in general forces the hips into an externally rotated position and the foot is internally rotated relative to the knee, thus producing internal tibial torsion. The natural progression of tibial rotation is from internal at birth to slightly external at maturity.[8,10] The transmalleolar axis, the angle formed in the axial plane from a line connecting the malleoli against a line across the femoral condyles, begins at 4° internal in newborns (lateral malleolus anterior to medial malleolus) and progresses to an average of 23° external in adults (lateral malleolus posterior to medial malleolus).[8,10] Similarly, if using the thigh-foot axis, which is the angle between the thigh and the foot in a prone child with the knee flexed to 90°, infants have, on average, 5° of internal tibial torsion, which changes to 10° external by age 10 years.[8,10] It is important to note that a wide range of tibial torsion has been noted throughout development, and the SDs include both internal and external tibial torsion at any given time.[3,8] The natural history of internal tibial torsion, however, is benign and trends external as a child reaches maturity.

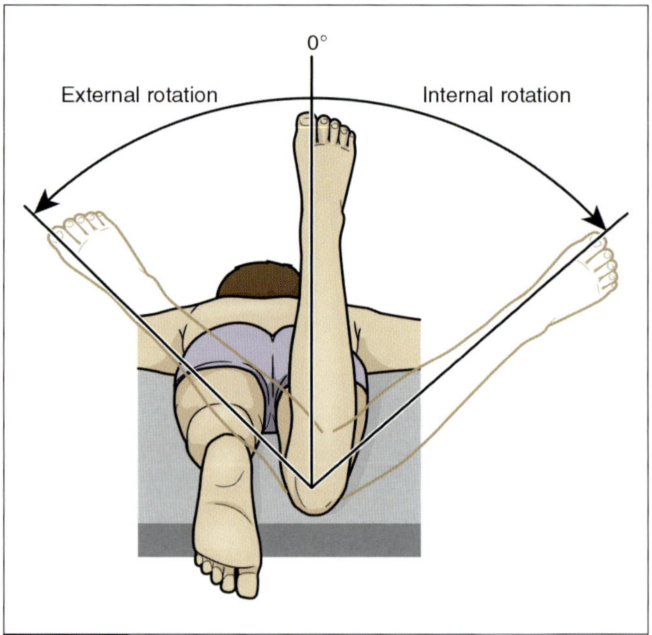

Figure 1 Illustration of the assessment of femoral rotation. The child should lie prone on an examination table with the knees flexed at 90°. The feet are rotated maximally internally and externally.

Evaluation of a Patient With a Rotational Deformity

History

The clinical evaluation begins by assessing the child's development and the history of the deformity. The onset of the deformity, its progression or improvement, and the perceived functional limitations of the child are ascertained from the parents. Coupling this information with birth history, family history, and developmental milestones helps the physician place the child's condition in either a normal category or one where underlying pathology is suspected. All information collected is analyzed against the backdrop of variability in normal development, with the goal being to identify any potential pathologic causes of deformity.

Physical Examination and the Rotational Profile

Observing the child play in the examination room, analyzing his or her gait, and performing a thorough neurologic examination will help confirm or refute suspicions gathered during the history regarding the presence of underlying pathology. From there, a specific assessment of the rotational problem that prompted the chief complaint can be performed. The rotational profile involves examination of gait, the hip, tibia, and feet to identify the location of the torsional abnormality.[8,11]

Gait is observed to note the foot-progression angle, a measure of the degree that the foot turns inward (designated a negative value) or outward (designated a positive value) relative to the axis of the leg. This provides an overview of the rotational deformity and summarizes all the components of the rotational profile. Symmetry and the direction the patellae point also should be noted.

The static evaluation begins with an assessment of hip version. The child is positioned prone on an examination table with the knees bent to 90°. The legs are maximally rotated internally and externally. Internal rotation measuring greater than 70°, with a lesser amount of external rotation, is caused by an increase in femoral anteversion (**Figure 1**). Tibial torsion is assessed with the thigh-foot axis and the transmalleolar axis (**Figure 2**).

The trochanter palpation test is another method of identifying true anteversion.[12] With the child positioned prone and the knee flexed to 90°, the leg is rotated until the prominence of the greater trochanter is palpated most distinctly. Because this represents the most lateral position of the trochanter, the femoral neck is parallel to the floor. Thus, the angle between the vertical and the tibia represents the actual amount of anteversion.

The foot is the final component that contributes to a rotational issue. The heel-bisector line, a line drawn down the axis of the hindfoot through the forefoot, should normally pass through the second web space. Medial or lateral deviations of the line indicate a component

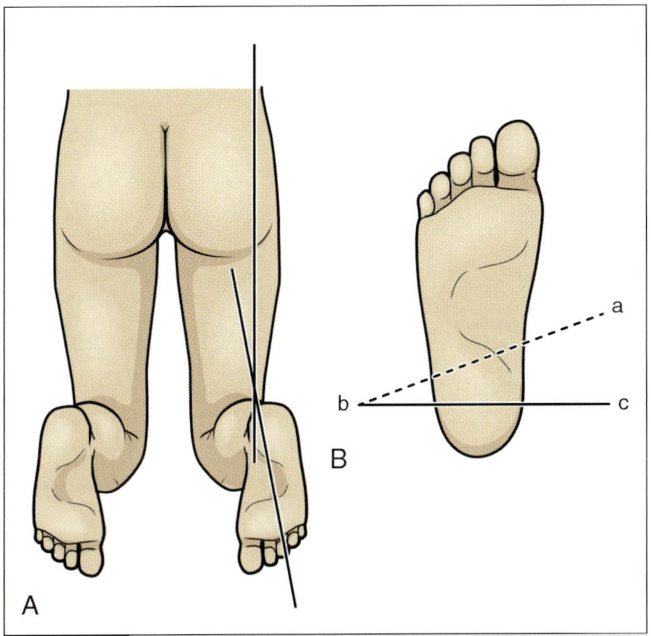

Figure 2 Illustrations for assessing tibial torsion. **A,** For the thigh-foot axis, the child should lie prone on an examination table with the knees flexed at 90°. The angle of the axis of the thigh and the axis of the foot determines internal or external tibial torsion. **B,** The transmalleolar axis is the angle between a line drawn connecting the malleoli (line a-b) and the coronal plane of the tibia (line b-c).

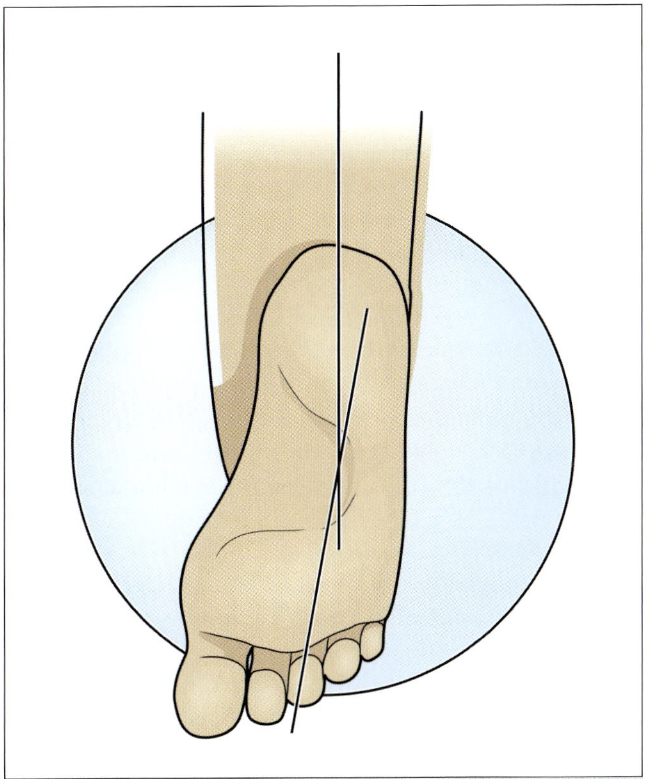

Figure 3 Illustration of the heel-bisector line. The axis of the hindfoot should be parallel to the axis of the forefoot. This illustration shows a mild metatarsus adductus deformity.

of forefoot adduction or abduction, respectively[13] (**Figure 3**).

The results of the rotational profile will allow the physician to identify the location of the rotational deformity. Combining these results with knowledge of normal development, the physician is directed to further evaluate the child radiographically when the deformity exists 2 SDs outside the mean for the child's age.[8] The physical examination will be the key determinant in identifying deformity that requires radiographic evaluation.

Intoeing

The most common age-related causes of intoeing are metatarsus adductus with or without internal tibial torsion from birth to 1 year, internal tibial torsion for toddlers aged 1 to 3 years, and femoral anteversion for children older than 4 years.

Metatarsus Adductus

Most cases of metatarsus adductus are postural in nature and resolve spontaneously with time.[14-16] A natural history of metatarsus adductus was published in 1978 and showed 86% of feet as normal or mildly deformed, 10% as moderately deformed but asymptomatic, and 4% as deformed and stiff at an average of 7 years of age.[16] In terms of prognosis and treatment, it may be helpful to classify the deformity as mild (the foot can be passively corrected beyond neutral), moderate (the foot is passively correctable to neutral), and severe (the foot is unable to be passively corrected).[17] Casting has been advocated to treat moderate and severe cases, with success using either short- or long-leg plaster casts.[18] Surgery is reserved for the most resistant cases of metatarsus adductus. In the literature, viable options with adequate results include lengthening of the abductor hallucis with a medial capsulotomy[19] and an opening wedge osteotomy of the medial cuneiform combined with a closing wedge osteotomy of the cuboid.[20]

Internal Tibial Torsion

Internal tibial torsion is the most common cause of intoeing in children aged 1 to 3 years. Parents may report that the child is clumsy or trips frequently, and the child typically does not have pain. A proper rotational profile confirms the diagnosis, with the thigh-foot axis and the transmalleolar axis demonstrating internal tibial torsion.

Treatment of the condition predominantly involves education, reassurance, and expectant observation. Special shoes, the Denis Browne bar orthosis, twister cables, and shoe inserts have not demonstrated benefit in the treatment of internal tibial torsion.[1,21,22]

Surgical management of internal tibial torsion is rare but may be indicated in a child who has not improved or has intoeing progression, is older than 8 years, has deformity greater than 2 SDs from normal, and has some functional or psychological disability derived from the torsion.[8,9] Gait analysis can be used in this patient population to help identify functional disability.[6] Distal tibia corrective osteotomies are able to improve knee moments and restore many of the kinetic and kinematic values to that of normal controls.[23]

Femoral Anteversion

Femoral anteversion is the most common cause of intoeing in children older than 4 years. Parents may report W-sitting, abnormal running (particularly with compensatory external tibial torsion), and possibly knee pain.

The natural history of an intoeing gait from femoral anteversion is benign. Although parents often note abnormal gait or clumsiness, the physician can reassure them that intoeing tends to resolve in most children. If intoeing persists in some children, it has been demonstrated that the activity level of adolescents with intoeing does not differ from that of their peers.[7]

The development of osteoarthritis is another concern. It has been proposed that femoral anteversion leads to an increase in osteoarthritis of the hip and knee, but this has been refuted in numerous studies.[24-26] Most recently, researchers studied 1,158 cadaver tibiae and femora to determine an association between femoral anteversion and/or tibial torsion and osteoarthritis of the hip or knee. No correlation could be identified.[24] Intoeing secondary to femoral anteversion tends to resolve spontaneously; if it does not, no adverse effect has been found on a child's functional development or long-term health.

Given the benign natural history, parental education and reassurance are the mainstays of treatment, with no role for orthotics, physical therapy, or restriction from W-sitting. Surgical intervention is a rare event; however, indications for corrective osteotomy include a child older than 8 years, persistent deformity with marked functional or cosmetic disability, anteversion greater than 50°, and internal hip rotation greater than 80°.[8,9] Corrective osteotomy may safely be performed proximally in the intertrochanteric region or distally in the supracondylar region. The benefits of a proximal osteotomy include more accurate correction and a decreased requirement for postoperative immobilization[27] versus being able to use a tourniquet, thus limiting blood loss.[28] Another method that has been described is diaphyseal osteotomy with fixation using an intramedullary nail.[29] All three methods report success from a technical and patient-satisfaction perspective and limited complications.

Outtoeing

An external foot-progression angle, also known as outtoeing, occurs less frequently than intoeing, but it may be of no less concern to parents. The benign natural history of this deformity typically allows for treatment that consists of education, reassurance, and expectant observation. However, knowledge of characteristic presentations and a thorough physical examination will allow the physician to differentiate between normal variations and underlying pathology.

Children are typically born with an external rotation contracture of the hip that may exceed the internal rotation and metatarsus adductus present at birth. This is the most common cause of outtoeing in infancy. These children may have an accompanying calcaneovalgus foot, which also will correct itself with time. During the toddler years, children may have external tibial torsion that will trend internal with continued growth. As children get older, they are more likely to have outtoeing secondary to decreased femoral anteversion or planovalgus feet.

Certain conditions occur with outtoeing and should trigger the physician to perform some additional workup. External tibial torsion is associated with cerebral palsy, myelomeningocele, and other neuromuscular disorders. Decreased femoral anteversion is associated with obesity,[30] slipped capital femoral epiphysis, and coxa vara.

Torsional Malalignment Syndrome

Torsional malalignment syndrome (also called miserable malalignment syndrome) may be present in adolescents as the summation of excessive femoral anteversion combined with external tibial torsion. Because of the biomechanical disadvantage this confers on the patellofemoral joint, adolescents often have anterior knee pain. Typically, treatment involves observation of the malrotation and therapy for anterior knee pain. Patients rarely have persistent symptoms that warrant surgical intervention. In the most severe cases, a double osteotomy of the femur and tibia is warranted to correct femoral anteversion and external tibial torsion. Two reports in the literature encompassing 17 patients demonstrated resolution of knee pain and deformity at an average follow-up of 5 and 16 years, respectively.[31,32] Given the complexity of assessing rotation in both segments of the lower extremity, CT assessment of any rotation is recommended before intervention.[32]

Table 1

The Differential Diagnosis for Angular Deformity

Category	Diagnosis
Physiologic	
Idiopathic genu valgum	
Heuter-Volkmann principle	Infantile and adolescent tibia vara
Acquired (insult to the physis)	Trauma, infection, radiation, iatrogenic cause, juvenile inflammatory arthritis, osteochondroma
Congenital (condition affecting the health/growth of the physis)	Skeletal dysplasia, focal fibrocartilaginous dysplasia, osteogenesis imperfecta, multiple hereditary exostosis, Ollier disease, Maffucci syndrome
Metabolic bone disease (the physis is susceptible to the Heuter-Volkmann principle at the age of physiologic angulation: onset younger than age 2 years is varus, and onset older than age 4 to 5 years is valgus)	Rickets, renal osteodystrophy
Adaptive response to a long bone deformity	

Angular Deformity

Normal Development of Lower Extremity Alignment

Understanding the normal physiologic growth patterns in children is fundamental to the evaluation of children with angular deformity. Symmetric varus is the expected angular pattern of growth in children between birth and age 18 to 24 months. This growth transitions to a symmetric valgus alignment that is typically maximal at approximately age 3 to 4 years and ultimately normalizes by age 6 to 8 years. Normal alignment of the lower extremity as a child reaches maturity is 5° to 7° of valgus.[33]

The natural history of angular deformity in the lower extremity depends on its etiology. Physiologic deformity, by definition, will resolve spontaneously. Progressive angular deformity will continue to worsen with time, resulting in gait disturbance, limitations in function, and pain. Regarding the effect of malalignment on osteoarthritis, the literature is decidedly unclear on its association. Various biomechanical and gait studies describe increased force through the medial and lateral compartments, with genu varum and genu valgum, respectively. However, this has not been directly linked to osteoarthritis in any study.[34-37]

Differential Diagnoses

The differential diagnoses for angular deformity are presented in **Table 1**.

Evaluation of a Child With Angular Deformity

The history of presentation is key to working through the differential diagnosis to identify a source for a growth abnormality. Most conditions will be categorized as physiologic, so it is very important to rule out other etiologies and gain a perspective of the onset, duration, and progression of the deformity. Specific events, a history of abnormal growth, or other diseases may help guide the questioning into the large categories of acquired, congenital, or metabolic deformities, respectively. In addition, it is important to gain a sense of the patient's limitations resulting from the deformity and any symptoms that the child may be experiencing.

The physical examination is used to further precisely determine the diagnosis and specifically identify the location of the deformity. An overall assessment of a child should include the child's height, weight, and development. The child's gait should be observed for any abnormalities, including the presence of medial or lateral thrust, joint instability, crouch, or equinus. The musculoskeletal examination is used to identify deformity, assess joints, identify sources of pain, perform a rotational profile, and assess for limb-length discrepancy. The neurologic examination should confirm that the child is developing normally and assess for any underlying neural axis abnormality.

Radiographs are indicated whenever the history and the physical examination create suspicion for true bony deformity. Radiographs are not indicated in cases of physiologic patterns of growth. A standing, full-length AP radiograph that includes both lower limbs is the preferred imaging tool for assessing angular alignment and

Table 2

Normal Values of Alignment

Angle Type	Angle Measurement
Hip	
Neck-shaft angle	130°
Knee	
Lateral distal femoral angle	87°
Medial proximal tibial angle	87°
Posterior distal femoral angle	83°
Posterior proximal tibial angle	81°
Ankle	
Lateral distal tibial angle	89°
Anterior distal tibial angle	80°

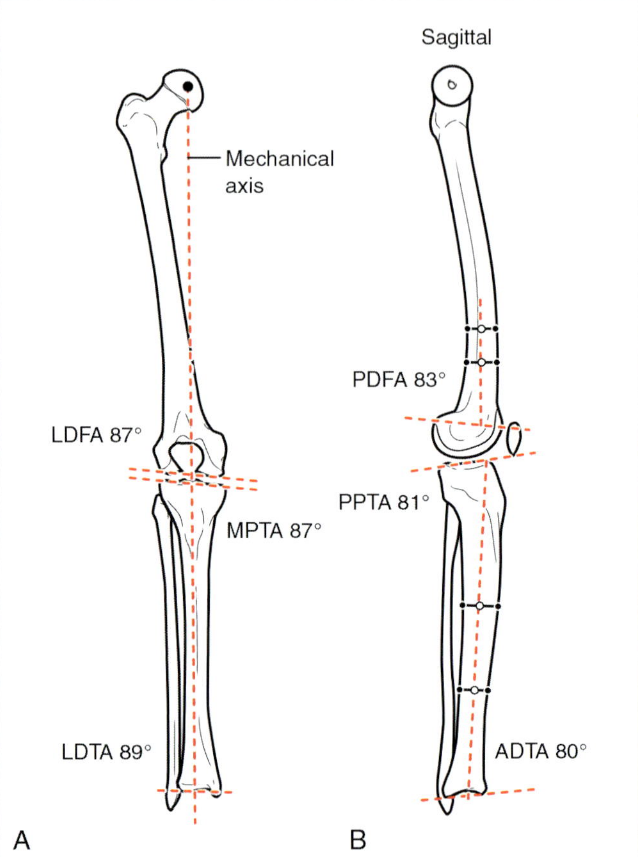

Figure 4 Illustrations of the mechanical axis of the lower limb. A straight line drawn connecting the center of the femoral head to the center of the distal tibia. **A,** The normal angles for the lateral distal femoral angle (LDFA), the medial proximal tibia angle (MPTA), and the lateral distal tibia angle (LDTA) will assist in identifying the location of deformity in the coronal plane. B, The posterior distal femoral angle (PDFA), the posterior proximal tibia angle (PPTA), and the anterior distal tibia angle (ADTA) assist in locating the deformity in the sagittal plane. The ideal degree measurements for each angle type are provided in Table 2.

limb length. Additional biplanar imaging of the involved bones or joints may be necessary for diagnostic purposes, and a bone age test may be helpful for assessing growth remaining. Advanced imaging may be used for evaluating pathology related to the physis or assessing rotational anatomy.

Alignment is assessed by determining the anatomic and mechanical axis of the lower extremity. The anatomic axis is the mid-diaphyseal line of a bone. The mechanical axis represents the weight-bearing alignment of the lower extremity and normally should involve a straight line from the center of the femoral head to the center of the distal tibia passing through the center of the knee. Normal anatomic alignment of the lower extremity produces a femoral-tibial angle of 5° to 7° of valgus at maturity.[38] Normal values of alignment (**Table 2**) are helpful for identifying deformity in a long bone (**Figure 4**).

The center of rotation of angulation is the location of deformity in a long bone. If a single point of deformity exists, the point of intersection between the proximal mechanical axis and the distal mechanical axis is the center of rotation of angulation. Therefore, deformity correction should occur at the center of rotation of angulation to restore the mechanical axis.[38]

The physis should be specifically assessed in a growing child, both as a potential etiology of deformity and as a potential solution for correcting the deformity.

Treatment of Angular Deformity

The indications for treating angular deformity include malalignment that results in pain or functional limitation. Physiologic deformity can be managed with expectant observation. Orthotic management of progressive angular deformity has minimal support in the literature, with perhaps infantile Blount disease having the greatest benefit from bracing.[39-41] Surgical intervention is the mainstay treatment of deformity that causes pain or functional limitation, particularly when the deformity is progressive.

The menu of options for the treatment of angular deformity is extensive and involves three general categories: growth modulation, acute correction, and gradual correction through multiplanar external fixation.[42-44] The technique chosen depends on numerous variables, including physeal growth, the location of the deformity, the age of the patient, any underlying conditions, and the amount of deformity.

Summary

There can be much anxiety associated with a clinic visit for rotational or angular deformities in a child. Given the positive natural history of physiologic growth patterns, parents can take much relief in the knowledge that their child will outgrow the current deformity when it is properly identified. The role of the physician is highly instrumental in determining whether the child's condition is within the normal range or if the underlying etiology will result in progressive and limiting deformity.

Key Study Points

- Femoral anteversion may improve until age 8 years. Long-term functional limitation from persistent femoral anteversion is uncommon.
- Internal tibial torsion is the most common cause of intoeing in toddlers aged 1 to 3 years.
- Physiologic varus is present between birth and age 18 to 24 months, and physiologic valgus is maximal at age 3 to 4 years and should resolve by age 7 years.

Annotated References

1. Fabry G, MacEwen GD, Shands AR Jr: Torsion of the femur: A follow-up study in normal and abnormal conditions. *J Bone Joint Surg Am* 1973;55(8):1726-1738.

2. Shands AR Jr, Steele MK: Torsion of the femur: A follow-up report on the use of the Dunlap method for its determination. *J Bone Joint Surg Am* 1958;40(4):803-816.

3. Jacquemier M, Glard Y, Pomero V, Viehweger E, Jouve JL, Bollini G: Rotational profile of the lower limb in 1319 healthy children. *Gait Posture* 2008;28(2):187-193.

4. Matovinović D, Nemec B, Gulan G, Sestan B, Ravlić-Gulan J: Comparison in regression of femoral neck anteversion in children with normal, intoeing and outtoeing gait: Prospective study. *Coll Antropol* 1998;22(2):525-532.

5. Svenningsen S, Apalset K, Terjesen T, Anda S: Regression of femoral anteversion: A prospective study of intoeing children. *Acta Orthop Scand* 1989;60(2):170-173.

6. Radler C, Kranzl A, Manner HM, Höglinger M, Ganger R, Grill F: Torsional profile versus gait analysis: Consistency between the anatomic torsion and the resulting gait pattern in patients with rotational malalignment of the lower extremity. *Gait Posture* 2010;32(3):405-410.

7. Staheli LT, Lippert F, Denotter P: Femoral anteversion and physical performance in adolescent and adult life. *Clin Orthop Relat Res* 1977;129:213-216.

8. Staheli LT, Corbett M, Wyss C, King H: Lower-extremity rotational problems in children: Normal values to guide management. *J Bone Joint Surg Am* 1985;67(1):39-47.

9. Staheli LT: Torsion: Treatment indications. *Clin Orthop Relat Res* 1989;247:61-66.

10. Staheli LT, Engel GM: Tibial torsion: A method of assessment and a survey of normal children. *Clin Orthop Relat Res* 1972;86:183-186.

11. Staheli LT: Torsional deformity. *Pediatr Clin North Am* 1977;24(4):799-811.

12. Ruwe PA, Gage JR, Ozonoff MB, DeLuca PA: Clinical determination of femoral anteversion. A comparison with established techniques. *J Bone Joint Surg Am* 1992;74(6):820-830.

13. Smith JT, Bleck EE, Gamble JG, Rinsky LA, Pena T: Simple method of documenting metatarsus adductus. *J Pediatr Orthop* 1991;11(5):679-680.

14. Farsetti P, Weinstein SL, Ponseti IV: The long-term functional and radiographic outcomes of untreated and non-operatively treated metatarsus adductus. *J Bone Joint Surg Am* 1994;76(2):257-265.

15. Ponseti IV, Becker JR: Congenital metatarsus adductus: The results of treatment. *J Bone Joint Surg Am* 1966;48(4):702-711.

16. Rushforth GF: The natural history of hooked forefoot. *J Bone Joint Surg Br* 1978;60(4):530-532.

17. Bleck EE: Metatarsus adductus: Classification and relationship to outcomes of treatment. *J Pediatr Orthop* 1983;3(1):2-9.

18. Katz K, David R, Soudry M: Below-knee plaster cast for the treatment of metatarsus adductus. *J Pediatr Orthop* 1999;19(1):49-50.

19. Asirvatham R, Stevens PM: Idiopathic forefoot-adduction deformity: Medial capsulotomy and abductor hallucis lengthening for resistant and severe deformities. *J Pediatr Orthop* 1997;17(4):496-500.

20. McHale KA, Lenhart MK: Treatment of residual clubfoot deformity—the "bean-shaped" foot—by opening wedge medial cuneiform osteotomy and closing wedge cuboid osteotomy: Clinical review and cadaver correlations. *J Pediatr Orthop* 1991;11(3):374-381.

21. Heinrich SD, Sharps CH: Lower extremity torsional deformities in children: A prospective comparison of two treatment modalities. *Orthopedics* 1991;14(6):655-659.

22. Knittel G, Staheli LT: The effectiveness of shoe modifications for intoeing. *Orthop Clin North Am* 1976;7(4):1019-1025.

23. MacWilliams BA, McMulkin ML, Baird GO, Stevens PM: Distal tibial rotation osteotomies normalize frontal plane knee moments. *J Bone Joint Surg Am* 2010;92(17):2835-2842.

24. Weinberg DS, Park PJ, Morris WZ, Liu RW: Femoral version and tibial torsion are not associated with hip or knee arthritis in a large osteological collection. *J Pediatr Orthop* 2015; July 24 [Epub ahead of print]

    In this cadaver study, 1,158 femora and tibiae were assessed for femoral anteversion and tibial torsion and a correlation was made with the development of hip or knee arthritis. The results of multiple regression analysis showed that femoral anteversion and internal tibial torsion were not associated with osteoarthritis. Level of evidence: IV.

25. Hubbard DD, Staheli LT, Chew DE, Mosca VS: Medial femoral torsion and osteoarthritis. *J Pediatr Orthop* 1988;8(5):540-542.

26. Wedge JH, Munkacsi I, Loback D: Anteversion of the femur and idiopathic osteoarthrosis of the hip. *J Bone Joint Surg Am* 1989;71(7):1040-1043.

27. Payne LZ, DeLuca PA: Intertrochanteric versus supracondylar osteotomy for severe femoral anteversion. *J Pediatr Orthop* 1994;14(1):39-44.

28. Hoffer MM, Prietto C, Koffman M: Supracondylar derotational osteotomy of the femur for internal rotation of the thigh in the cerebral palsied child. *J Bone Joint Surg Am* 1981;63(3):389-393.

29. Gordon JE, Pappademos PC, Schoenecker PL, Dobbs MB, Luhmann SJ: Diaphyseal derotational osteotomy with intramedullary fixation for correction of excessive femoral anteversion in children. *J Pediatr Orthop* 2005;25(4):548-553.

30. Galbraith RT, Gelberman RH, Hajek PC, et al: Obesity and decreased femoral anteversion in adolescence. *J Orthop Res* 1987;5(4):523-528.

31. Bruce WD, Stevens PM: Surgical correction of miserable malalignment syndrome. *J Pediatr Orthop* 2004;24(4):392-396.

32. Leonardi F, Rivera F, Zorzan A, Ali SM: Bilateral double osteotomy in severe torsional malalignment syndrome: 16 years follow-up. *J Orthop Traumatol* 2014;15(2):131-136.

    Three patients underwent femoral and tibial osteotomies for torsional malalignment syndrome. CT was recommended for preoperative planning. At an average follow-up of 16 years, successful outcomes were reported with no persistent hip or knee pain. Level of evidence: IV.

33. Salenius P, Vankka E: The development of the tibiofemoral angle in children. *J Bone Joint Surg Am* 1975;57(2):259-261.

34. Bruns J, Volkmer M, Luessenhop S: Pressure distribution at the knee joint: Influence of varus and valgus deviation without and with ligament dissection. *Arch Orthop Trauma Surg* 1993;113(1):12-19.

35. McKellop HA, Llinás A, Sarmiento A: Effects of tibial malalignment on the knee and ankle. *Orthop Clin North Am* 1994;25(3):415-423.

36. Morrison JB: The mechanics of the knee joint in relation to normal walking. *J Biomech* 1970;3(1):51-61.

37. Tetsworth K, Paley D: Malalignment and degenerative arthropathy. *Orthop Clin North Am* 1994;25(3):367-377.

38. Paley D: *Principles of Deformity Correction* .Berlin, Germany, Springer, 2002, pp 1-18.

39. Alsancak S, Guner S, Kinik H: Orthotic variations in the management of infantile tibia vara and the results of treatment. *Prosthet Orthot Int* 2013;37(5):375-383.

    Three different braces were trialed in 22 children with infantile tibia vara to determine effectiveness. The authors concluded that knee-ankle-foot orthoses worn full-time with five points of corrective force along the entire limb were effective at providing deformity correction. Level of evidence: III.

40. Raney EM, Topoleski TA, Yaghoubian R, Guidera KJ, Marshall JG: Orthotic treatment of infantile tibia vara. *J Pediatr Orthop* 1998;18(5):670-674.

41. Zionts LE, Shean CJ: Brace treatment of early infantile tibia vara. *J Pediatr Orthop* 1998;18(1):102-109.

42. Stevens PM, Maguire M, Dales MD, Robins AJ: Physeal stapling for idiopathic genu valgum. *J Pediatr Orthop* 1999;19(5):645-649.

43. Stevens PM: Guided growth for angular correction: A preliminary series using a tension band plate. *J Pediatr Orthop* 2007;27(3):253-259.

44. Métaizeau JP, Wong-Chung J, Bertrand H, Pasquier P: Percutaneous epiphysiodesis using transphyseal screws (PETS). *J Pediatr Orthop* 1998;18(3):363-369.

Chapter 27

Limb-Length Discrepancy, Limb Deficiency, and Amputation

Janet L. Walker, MD

Abstract

Children with lower limb-length discrepancy can be managed with epiphysiodesis, limb shortening, and limb lengthening. It is helpful to be familiar with the most common types of lower limb deficiencies and their orthopaedic management along with surgical and prosthetic techniques when lower limb amputation is necessary.

Keywords: amputations in children; epiphysiodesis; femoral deficiency; fibular deficiency; limb lengthening; limb-length inequality; tibial deficiency; transverse deficiency

Introduction

This chapter reviews the general management of limb-length discrepancy, including epiphysiodesis, shortening, and lengthening. It discusses the classifications and treatment of the most common lower limb deficiencies—fibular, femoral, and tibial—and presents general surgical and prosthetic considerations for children with amputations.

Limb-Length Discrepancy

Length discrepancy in the lower limbs is very common, with some studies demonstrating small degrees of limb-length inequality in more than half of the US population. A limb-length discrepancy of 2 cm or more was found in 7% of typical 8- to 12-year-old children.[1] Gait patterns may be altered when discrepancies are 2 cm or greater. Finite element models show increased sacroiliac joint loading, with peak stresses that progressively increase with discrepancies from 1 to 3 cm.[2] These models propose a mechanism by which limb-length discrepancies may lead to low back pain. Long-term studies about the relationship between limb-length discrepancies and osteoarthritis do not exist, but adults with knee osteoarthritis report pain more commonly in the apparent short leg.[3] For children with a limb-length discrepancy, their parents reported no difference in Pediatric Outcomes Data Collection Instrument (PODCI) scores related to the amount of their child's discrepancy.[4] For those with a limb-length discrepancy greater than 2 cm, parents were less satisfied with their child's appearance and more concerned about possible surgery in the future. They thought that the happiness of their child was adversely affected by the limb-length discrepancy, and for larger degrees of discrepancy, parents were more willing to seek surgical treatment.

Neither Dr. Walker nor any immediate family member has received anything of value from or has stock or stock options held in a commercial company or institution related directly or indirectly to the subject of this chapter.

Assessment

Direct clinical measurement of limb-length inequality with a tape measure, which is designed to measure differences in the distances between bony landmarks, can be performed in both the supine and standing positions. Indirect clinical measurement of limb-length discrepancy can be determined with the patient standing with blocks under the short leg until the iliac crests are level. Radiographic techniques include orthoradiography, scanography, and CT. Scanography measures only limb lengths. Orthoradiography and CT assess both length and limb alignment. CT has a lower radiation dosage than orthoradiography, but it is less accessible at most medical centers.[5-7] Although supine tape measurements of limb lengths have excellent interrater and intrarater reliability compared with CT,[5] most centers rely on some objective form of documentation. Many centers are switching to digital radiography systems because they have been shown to produce reliable measurements that are comparable with hard-copy long-leg radiographs.[6,8] Low-dose, upright biplanar radiographic imaging using highly sensitive gaseous photon detectors has been shown to produce reliably accurate limb-length measurements compared with teleoroentgenograms and CT scans and has less radiation exposure.[6] Biplanar imaging also allows for measurements of limb alignment and torsion but requires a standing position (**Figure 1**). In all cases, length calculations must take into account joint contractures, foot deficiency or deformity, pelvic anomalies, and/or hip dysplasia that might affect overall limb length.

Clinical Decision Making

In general, treatment decisions about limb equalization are based on the projected limb-length discrepancy at maturity. Observation or shoe modification is recommended for discrepancies of 2 cm or less. Discrepancies ranging from 2 to 5 cm are amenable to shortening procedures by either epiphysiodesis before maturity or femoral shortening at maturity. Greater degrees of shortening can result in a disproportionate body appearance. Limb lengthening is used for discrepancies of 5 cm or more. Combining shortening or epiphysiodesis with lengthening can reduce the amount of lengthening needed. For patients with discrepancies greater than 20 cm or those with a limb that cannot tolerate lengthening, amputation and prosthetic fitting should be considered.

Many other factors also need to be considered. A child who is already below normal in height may not want to accept a treatment that results in further loss of stature. Greater degrees of shortening or epiphysiodesis may be appropriate if the abnormal leg is too long (for example, hemihypertrophy). Associated deformities that require corrective surgery can be combined with lengthening to correct milder degrees of limb-length discrepancy. Limbs with unstable joints, contracted soft tissues, or neurovascular problems may be poor candidates for lengthening; alternatives such as amputation or contralateral shortening may be more acceptable, even if a disproportionate appearance results.

Four widely used methods estimate lower limb growth and predict limb-length inequality. The arithmetic method combines the rate of growth of the distal femur (0.375 inch or 9.5 mm per year) and the proximal tibia (0.25 inch or 6.4 mm per year) with chronologic age and the assumption of maturity at 16 years for boys and 14 years for girls.[9] The growth remaining method uses growth remaining graphs and skeletal age.[10] The straight-line graph method[11] simplifies the estimation process of the growth remaining method.[10] The multiplier method uses chronologic age and data from several limb-length

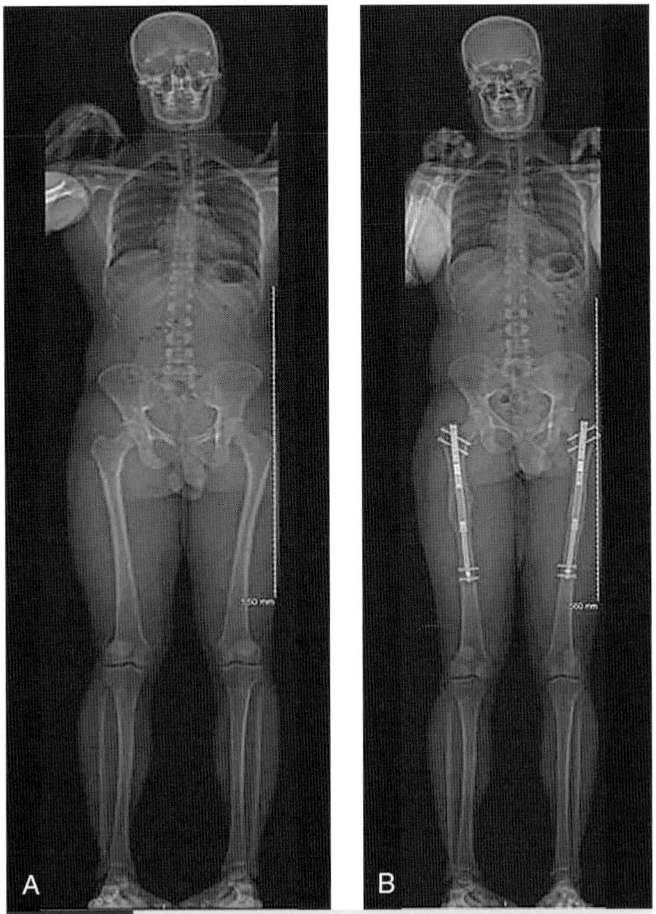

Figure 1 EOS radiographic images accurately measure limb length and alignment. **A,** Image before limb lengthening performed because of the short stature of the patient. **B,** Image after limb lengthening was performed using the PRECICE intramedullary lengthener. (Reproduced with permission from Paley D, Harris M, Debiparshad K, Prince D: Limb lengthening by implantable limb lengthening devices. *Tech Orthop* 2014;29[2]:72-85.)

databases.[12] In 2012, researchers found that for children of all ages, the multiplier method, using chronologic age, had standard errors of less than 5 cm. However, for older children in the adolescent growth spurt who were Sanders digital age stage II or greater, skeletal age maturity determinations were superior to the multiplier method using chronologic age and had standard errors of less than 2 cm.[13]

Epiphysiodesis or Shortening

Epiphysiodesis is a commonly used procedure to achieve limb-length equalization by maturity and has a low morbidity rate. It is generally recommended for predicted limb-length discrepancies of 2 to 6 cm at maturity. The original technique for epiphysiodesis required an open bone block (Phemister technique) and had good and predictable results. Currently, percutaneous techniques have been popularized because of reduced morbidity and scarring.[14] Radiostereometric analysis has demonstrated that growth arrest can be expected within 12 weeks when using percutaneous drilling and curettage.[15] Implants to tether, rather than arrest, growth have been described using transphyseal screws and physeal plates. They are an attractive option when the timing of growth arrest is unpredictable. Implant removal can reverse the tether when length equality is achieved. Recent studies, however, have shown that medial and lateral physeal plates are less effective than epiphysiodesis using drilling and curettage.[16] In addition, transphyseal screws achieved only 66% of the expected growth retardation from the preoperative prediction.[17]

Limb shortening after maturity is most commonly performed in the femoral segment because of fewer neurovascular concerns. Open and closed intramedullary techniques produce shortening of accurately defined amounts of up to 5 cm or 10% of bone length. Greater degrees of shortening produce a disproportionate appearance and excessive weakness, especially of the quadriceps, and are not recommended.

Limb Lengthening

Distraction osteogenesis is the most accepted method of limb lengthening, especially for deficits greater than 2.5 cm.[18] The process consists of a low-energy corticotomy or osteotomy of the bone and a latency period of 5 to 7 days to allow for early fracture healing. This process is then followed by a gradual stretching of the distraction gap of 1 mm per day, which is divided into 0.25 mm or smaller increments. External fixators or intramedullary lengthening nails facilitate the distraction process. When sufficient distraction has occurred, the regenerate bone is allowed to heal. Lengthening of 3 to 6 cm or 20% of bone length is usually accomplished with few major complications. Greater amounts of lengthening are associated with an exponential increase in complications.

Overall, studies report that limb lengthening is associated with substantial rates of complications that range from 50% to 100%.[18,19] Complications are so frequent that authors have tried to classify them by severity, the need for further surgery, prolongation of treatment, or lasting sequelae. To help assess the complexity of limb lengthening for an individual patient, the Limb Lengthening and Reconstruction Society developed the LLRS AIM Index (a mnemonic indicating seven pretreatment domains: location and number of deformities, leg-length inequality at maturity, risk factors, soft-tissue coverage, angular deformity, infection/bone quality, and motion/stability of the joints above and below),[20] which serves to quantify the severity of lower limb deformities (**Table 1**). The index provides a method for communicating the complexity of a deformity by a scale that is reliable and has good interrater and intraobserver validity. However, based on expert opinion, the LLRS AIM Index does not separate congenital versus acquired etiologies and has not yet been tested to prove that it correlates with the difficulty of lengthening. In children, unlike in patients of other ages, concomitant deformity does not always influence the complication rate. In a 2014 study, only the proportion of limb-length discrepancy-predicted complications were reported.[19] The techniques of lengthening continue to evolve to address potential complications.

External fixation systems are frequently used to provide distraction in limb lengthening. Lengthening fixators consisting of monolateral frames and lengthening rails are easy to apply and are less cumbersome for patients. However, they have limited ability to progressively correct deformities. Circular external fixator systems, originally popularized for lengthening by Ilizarov, allow the progressive correction of deformities in multiple planes and can be adjusted during the lengthening process. They also can be extended across joints to protect them from subluxation. Originally described with transfixing fine wires, modifications that use half pins have decreased soft-tissue complications and improved frame stability. Distraction and deformity correction occur by adjusting the uprights and hinges attached to the frames in a particular order. Newer computer-assisted distraction and deformity correction systems use struts attached to the circular external fixator that can be adjusted, based on computer calculations, to simultaneously correct length, angulation, translation, and rotation, thereby reducing the time required for the correction while increasing the correction accuracy.[21]

Pins and wires may cause neurovascular injury when they are placed percutaneously. However, detailed knowledge of the cross-sectional anatomy and the use of nerve stimulators will reduce neurovascular risks. The complications are associated with pin infections and usually can be managed with antibiotics. In the long term, pins and wires may loosen or break if stress levels are exceeded, but sturdy constructs will minimize this risk. In most designs, the fixation system is strong enough to allow for weight bearing, thereby facilitating bone formation.

To address complications of external fixation, the length of time in the external device can be reduced by also using internal fixation, intramedullary nails, or plates. Because of the concern about deep infection with such

Table 1

Limb Lengthening and Reconstruction Society AIM Index for Limb Deformity[a]

Index Category	Points
Location (number of deformities per limb ≥ 10° angulation in separate planes and rotation all count as separate deformities)	
No deformity	0
One deformity	1
Two deformities	2
Three deformities	3
More than three deformities	4
Leg-length inequality (estimate at skeletal maturity)	
0-2 cm	0
>2-5 cm	1
>5-10 cm	2
>10-15 cm	3
>15 cm	4
Risk factors (assess clinically)	
None	0
Age younger than 5 or older than 40 years	Add 1 point
Smoking history	Add 1 point
Obesity	Add 1 point
Other disease (for example, diabetes)	Add 1 point
Soft-tissue coverage	
Normal	0
Bruising/contusion	1
Scarring/open grade I	2
Poor coverage/open grade II	3
Inadequate coverage/open grade III	4

Continued on next column

Index Category	Points
Angular deformity (measure and assign greatest primary deformity)	
0°-10°	0
>10°-20°	1
>20°-40°	2
>40°-60°	3
>60°	4
Infection/bone quality (select most severe)	
Normal	0
Osteoporotic	1
Dysplastic	2
Infection	3
Combination	4
Motion/stability of the joints above and below	
Normal	0
Decreased motion (<60% of normal)	1
Subluxation of joint	2
Dislocation of joint	3
More than 1 joint affected	4
Scoring (AIM Index scores range from a minimum of 0 to a maximum of 28)	**Score**
Normal	0
Minimal complexity	1-5
Moderate complexity	6-10
Substantial complexity	11-15
High complexity	16-28

[a]LLRS AIM is a mnemonic of the seven criteria that are required to determine the index (see text).

Adapted with permission from McCarthy JJ, Iobst CA, Rozbruch SR, Sabharwal S, Eismann EA: Limb Lengthening and Reconstruction Society AIM index reliably assesses lower limb deformity. *Clin Orthop Relat Res* 2013;471(2):621-627.

hybrid systems, a completely implanted intramedullary lengthener has been developed. The two FDA-approved devices for intramedullary lengthening are the Intramedullary Skeletal Kinetic Distractor (ISKD; Orthofix) and the PRECICE nail (Ellipse Technology).[22] The ISKD has a clutch mechanism that is triggered by limb rotation of 3° to 7° to achieve elongation. Control of distraction has been reported as being inconsistent (either going too fast or too slowly) and cannot be reversed. The PRECICE nail has a magnetic actuator drive that uses an external electromagnetic activator to control the rate and direction of the nail telescoping. Both nail systems lengthen along the anatomic axis and have potential mechanical complications. In the femur, where the mechanical axis is substantially different from the anatomic axis, lengthening can result in valgus deformity that may require other corrective procedures. One centimeter of femoral lengthening results in a 1° increase of genu valgum.[23] Results show that the ISKD may be inferior to lengthening with an external fixator over an intramedullary nail.[24] Compared with reported complications when lengthening with external fixation, the PRECICE nail had excellent control of distraction, a better healing index, and improved range of motion[25] (**Figure 1**). Joint subluxation, however, was still a problem.

Loss of joint motion frequently occurs during limb lengthening. Physical therapy, splinting, and botulinum toxin injections are used to avoid contractures and loss of motion while the soft tissues are being stretched. Loss of motion may signal joint subluxation. Preventing joint subluxation may require preoperative reconstructive surgery to increase the stability of the joints, and external frames may need to be extended, with hinges across the joints. This modification is especially crucial with lengthening as the result of a congenital deficiency. The lengthening process may need to be slowed if loss of motion or joint subluxation occurs. Secondary soft-tissue releases for the hip adductors, the quadriceps, the hamstrings, and the gastrocnemius may be needed. Joint motion may improve up to 2 years after lengthening, but aggressive physical therapy and splinting during the process is required.

In 2013, researchers found electrophysiologic evidence of nerve dysfunction during lengthening in 7 of 36 patients, which also was more common when lengthening was being performed for congenital etiologies.[26] Nerve changes may not be correlated with the amount of lengthening but rather the rate of distraction or double-level lengthening. Neurologic signs were found in three patients with electromyographic changes. The peroneal nerve was more susceptible than the tibial nerve, especially in tibial lengthening. Twenty-five percent of the patients undergoing lengthening after a traumatic event had preoperative electromyographic changes not detected clinically, and the electromyographic changes were found to deteriorate with lengthening. If the distraction is slowed or stopped, nerve symptoms usually are resolved. Nerve decompression before lengthening may prevent complications.

Bone healing complications occur with premature or delayed consolidation, angular displacement, fractures, and bending of the regenerated bone. Fractures occur most often after lengthening for a congenital deficiency in children younger than 9 years with lengthening greater than 15% and a latency period of less than 7 days.[27] Bone consolidation must be followed closely, and the rate of distraction should be adjusted accordingly. Proven techniques do not exist for predicting the strength of the regenerated bone or determining the time for fixator removal. Intramedullary nails and submuscular plates can provide supplemental stability. Bone formation enhancement techniques have included low-intensity pulsed ultrasound, pulsed electromagnetic fields, and the use of diphosphonates and bone morphogenetic proteins,[28] all of which are off-label uses for pediatric applications. Cultured, expanded bone marrow and platelet-rich plasma injections seem to produce encouraging results, but they require additional surgical procedures and specialized capabilities for processing the cells.

Limb Deficiencies

Prenatal ultrasound can detect most upper and lower limb deficiencies, but they will be undiagnosed in 20% to 25% of prenatal patients.[29] In 2014, researchers found detection rates of 52% for femoral deficiency, 23% for fibular deficiency, and 30% for combined femoral and fibular deficiencies.[30] These researchers stressed the importance of checking both femoral and tibial lengths to increase the chances of detection. They also found that 65% of mothers preferred to have prenatal detection to allow for prenatal counseling.

The genetic mechanisms involved in limb deficiencies are areas of active research. From animal studies, the gene *FGF10* is known to be necessary for limb development. *FGF10* induces formation of the apical ectodermal ridge. In a 2012 population-based study of limb deficiencies without known cause, researchers found that, in non-Hispanic Caucasian infants, variants of *FGF10* increased the risk for a wide range of nonsyndromic limb deficiencies.[31] Recent epidemiologic studies have linked slightly increased risks for limb deficiency to maternal active smoking and passive exposure to cigarette smoke, increased nitrates in drinking water, and increased maternal dietary consumption of caffeine.

Fibular Deficiency

Fibular deficiency is the most common lower limb deficiency and has a prevalence of 7 to 20 per 1 million births.[32] Fibular deficiency is part of a spectrum of anomalies believed to be related to a defect in the so-called femoral-fibular-ulnar developmental field[33] (**Figure 2**). It is associated with femoral hypoplasia, including proximal femoral focal deficiency (PFFD), genu valgum, lateral femoral condylar hypoplasia, cruciate ligament deficiency, tibial bowing and shortening, ankle instability, tarsal coalition, deficient lateral foot rays, and ulnar deficiency in the upper limb. The most common classification is based on radiologic findings of deficiency.[33] However, this system has poor correlation with treatment. Other researchers have proposed a classification system based on the clinical deformity, which helps direct treatment[34] (**Figure 3**). Salvage of the foot is considered in patients who have three or more foot rays that are stable enough for weight bearing. Because upper limb anomalies are common, upper limb function also must be considered before foot amputation.

Milder degrees of limb shortening can be managed with epiphysiodesis, although linear growth inhibition patterns are seen in 82% of patients, making such predictions less precise.[32,35] Limb lengthening may be used to correct greater degrees of shortening, but the process is fraught with a high rate of complications, including tibial bowing and ankle displacement. Resection of the fibular anlage has been demonstrated to reduce the recurrence of genu valgum, valgus tibial deformity, and lateral ankle displacement with lengthening procedures.[36] Reconstruction of the lateral malleolus has been described using the cartilaginous fibular remnant or the contralateral proximal fibula.[37,38] Reorientation of the valgus deformity in the distal tibial epiphysis and/or the subtalar joint can be managed with osteotomies and facilitates a stable weight-bearing ankle.

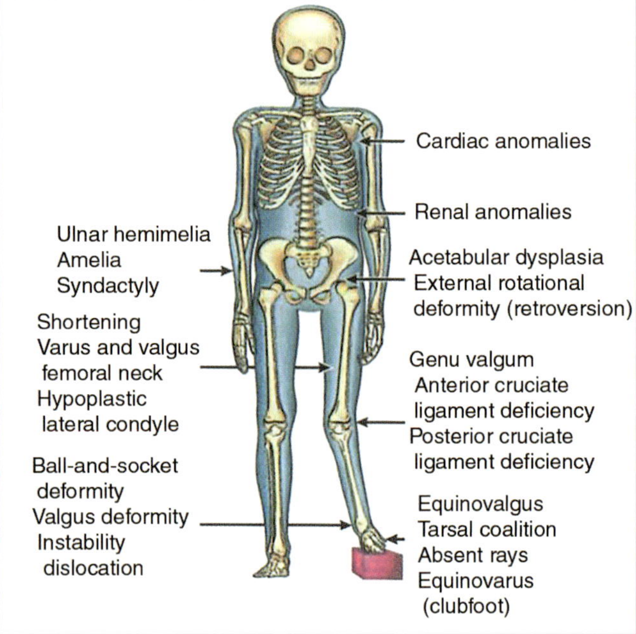

Figure 2 Illustration shows fibular deficiencies and associated anomalies.

Regardless of how the limb-length inequality is treated, fibular deficiency is frequently associated with progressive genu valgum that may require additional treatment. If identified and sufficient growth remains, hemiepiphysiodesis can correct the deformity.[39] Recurrence after osteotomy or hemiepiphysiodesis frequently occurs if growth is remaining, and overcorrection may be appropriate to compensate for the expected recurrence.

Although cruciate ligament deficiency accompanies knee concerns for many patients, a long-term follow-up study showed that only 20% of the patients had occasional instability during sporting activities, and none required bracing or surgery.[40] Previous studies have suggested hypertrophy of the ligament of Humphrey provides extra stability in the absence of the cruciate ligaments.

Femoral Deficiency

As discussed previously, femoral deficiency may be part of a spectrum of disorders with fibular deficiency because they frequently occur together. The classification of PFFD alone has been expanded to include the spectrum of femoral deficiency and is primarily radiographic in design. A recent classification system has incorporated this wide spectrum of femoral deficiency with an approach to treatment[41] (**Figure 4**). Considerations for the treatment of limb-length discrepancy depend on the stability and mobility of the hip (either primarily or with reconstruction), the integrity of the foot and ankle, knee function, and the projected discrepancy. With a good hip, minor deformity, and mild limb-length discrepancy, epiphysiodesis may be the only treatment needed. Contralateral

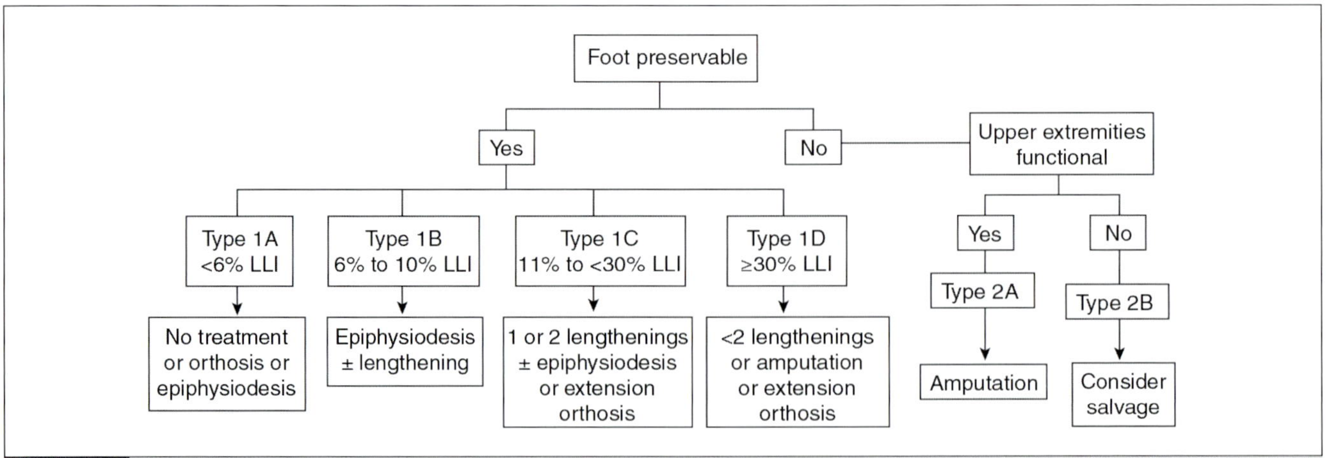

Figure 3 Flowchart shows the Birch classification and algorithm for the treatment of fibular deficiency. LLI = limb-length inequality.

femoral shortening may be considered at maturity for discrepancies of 2 to 5 cm. Femoral deformity resulting from coxa vara, femoral shaft varus, or distal femoral valgus may require an osteotomy. Knee function and stability are important factors because 95% of patients with PFFD have abnormal cruciate ligaments. The combined absence of the anterior cruciate ligament and the posterior cruciate ligament is the most common pattern. However, the severity of the cruciate ligament dysplasia did not correlate with the severity of PFFD. Additional reconstruction and protection of knee stability are needed if femoral lengthening is to be performed.

A Van Nes rotationplasty is a viable alternative for initial treatment of PFFD or can be used after failed limb reconstruction for PFFD.[42,43] This procedure fuses the short femur to the tibia, thus creating a combined thigh bone, and rotates the ankle 90° into the plane to function as a knee. Despite the unusual appearance of the limb with the foot rotated, no differences were found in the long-term Medical Outcomes Study 36-Item Short Form (SF-36) or other health-related quality-of-life measures.[42] A literature review demonstrated good to excellent results in 56 of 59 patients.[43] Those with poor results had associated fibular deficiency and three foot rays or fewer, thus indicating that good foot and ankle function is necessary for a good outcome.

If the hip in femoral deficiency cannot be stabilized, lengthening and rotationplasty options are rarely considered. Many patients may consider an extension prosthesis that fits over the foot without surgery. Alternatively, surgery with fusion of the residual femur to the tibial segment produces a combined bone that serves as a thigh segment. Amputation of the foot then facilitates prosthetic fitting with a transfemoral prosthesis.

Tibial Deficiency

Tibial deficiency is the least common lower limb deficiency and has a prevalence of one per 1 million births.[44] In some families, tibial deficiencies may be inherited, often as an autosomal dominant trait. Associated anomalies, such as great toe polydactyly, toe syndactyly, absent foot rays, tarsal coalition, hip dysplasia, femoral duplication, cleft hand or foot, radial deficiency, thumb hypoplasia, congenital scoliosis, tethered cord, and spinal dysraphism, occur in 78% of patients with tibial deficiency. Unlike fibular deficiency, other organ systems are frequently involved. Patients may have cardiopulmonary, gastrointestinal, and genitourinary anomalies; hydrocephalus; blindness; and ear malformations.

The four-part Jones classification is the most accepted classification system and is based on the presence or absence of the proximal or distal tibia (**Figure 5, A**). Based

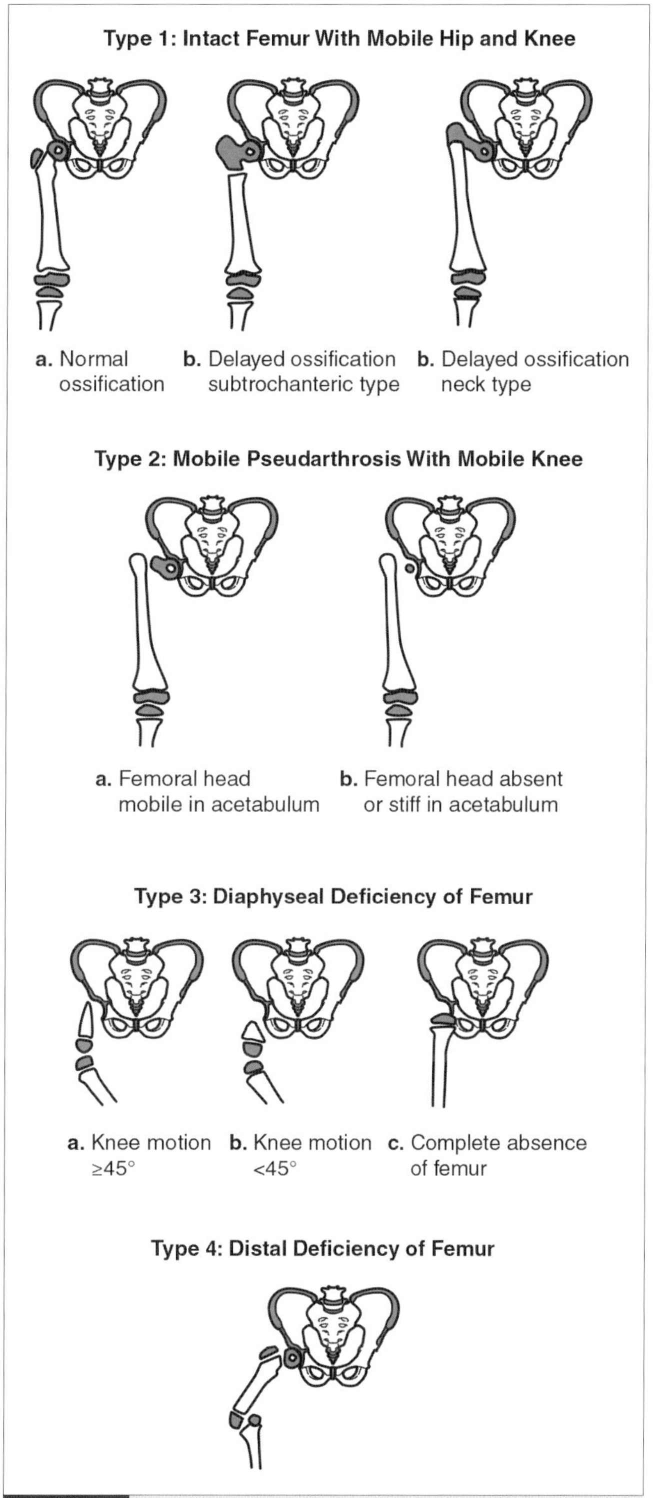

Figure 4 Illustration of the Paley classification system of congenital femoral deficiency. **A,** Type 1: intact femur with a mobile hip and knee. **B,** Type 2: proximal femoral pseudarthrosis with a mobile hip and knee. **C,** Type 3: diaphyseal deficiency of the femur with an absent hip joint and a mobile knee. **D,** Type 4: distal femoral deficiency.

5: Lower Extremity

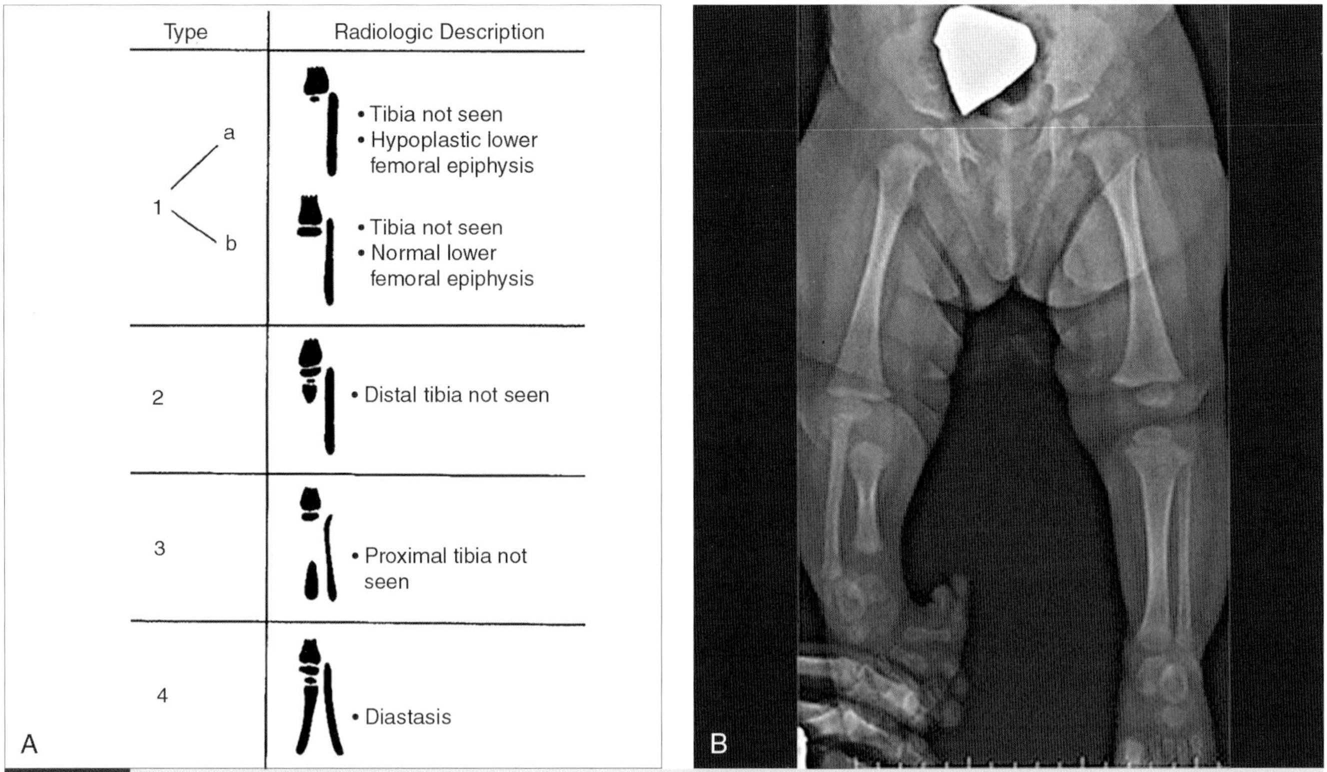

Figure 5 **A,** Illustration of the four-part Jones classification of tibial deficiency. **B,** AP radiograph of the tibiae of a patient with the proposed type 5 classification characterized by hypoplasia of the tibia; however, both the proximal and distal tibial physes are present. (Panel A reproduced with permission from Jones D, Barnes J, Lloyd-Roberts GC: Congenital aplasia and dysplasia of the tibia with intact fibula: Classification and management. *J Bone Joint Surg Br* 1978;60:31-39, and panel B reproduced with permission from Clinton R, Birch JG: Congenital tibial deficiency: A 37 year experience at one institution. *J Pediatr Orthop* 2015;35[4]:385-390.)

on a 2015 review of 95 patients with tibial deficiency, an additional classification (type 5) was proposed, wherein there is hypoplasia of the tibia, but both the proximal and distal tibial physes are present[44] (**Figure 5, B**).

Treatment depends on the presence or absence of active knee extension and knee stability. Reconstruction without active knee extension, by centralizing the fibula (Brown procedure) is unsuccessful, and knee disarticulation is recommended. With active knee extension, a vestigial proximal tibial segment can be elongated by synostosis to the fibula. A modified Syme ankle disarticulation or a Boyd amputation at the end of the fibula can facilitate prosthetic fitting with below-knee prostheses. Patients with some preservation of the distal tibia may be candidates for lengthening and reconstruction of the ankle with preservation of the foot.

Transverse Deficiency

Congenital transverse deficiency is much less common in the lower limbs compared with the upper limbs. It is important to distinguish congenital transverse deficiencies from congenital amputations resulting from amniotic bands. Congenital deficiencies are suspected if nubbins caused by failure formation are present. Nubbins may have an indentation but no band where they attach to the limb and may have small nail remnants (**Figure 6**). Amputations caused by amniotic band syndrome frequently have manifestations of bands elsewhere in the limb or the body. Congenital deficiencies are associated with increased risks for other anomalies, and screening renal ultrasounds should be obtained to look for silent urogenital anomalies. In addition, terminal overgrowth problems seen with transosseous amputations caused by amniotic bands do not occur in congenital transverse deficiencies. As such, congenital transverse deficiencies can be managed with a prosthetic fitting based on the level of the deficiency.

Amputations and Prosthetics

Surgical Techniques

In children, amputations through joints are preferred to avoid the complication of terminal overgrowth. The biologically active skeleton of children produces bone spikes and extensions after transosseous amputations, producing pain and bony protrusions through the skin. Multiple surgeries may be needed to treat these protrusions throughout the growing years. Why this problem is avoided with disarticulations in children is not completely clear. The concept of a protective cartilage cap is used to manage overgrowth, which may explain why terminal overgrowth does not occur in disarticulations. If a transosseous amputation is needed, using a cartilaginous remnant, such as a metatarsal or a proximal/distal fibula as a plug in the distal canal, may reduce overgrowth. The proximal fibula can be used in transtibial amputations as a secondary procedure to reduce the frequency of revisions needed for bony overgrowth.[45]

Although maintaining bone length is important for function, insufficient soft-tissue coverage with skin grafts may result in a limb that cannot tolerate prosthetic wear. The most durable grafts are composed of full-thickness skin and subcutaneous fat, which is mobile. At the ankle, maintaining the heel pad is particularly helpful and allows for end bearing. Maintaining muscle coverage and attachment also may preserve function, particularly in transfemoral amputations. In partial foot amputations, there may be an imbalance of muscle pull. Reattachment of the remnants of muscles or tendons to more proximal locations may help maintain balance. For example, reattaching the anterior tibialis tendon to the talus in a midfoot-level amputation prevents the gastrocnemius from being unopposed, resulting in equinus.

Even though disarticulations are preferred in children, they are poorly tolerated in adults because ample space is not available for prosthetic componentry if the limbs are the same length. Congenital deficiencies usually have enough limb hypoplasia, so space for prosthetic componentry is not a problem. However, children whose bones are expected to grow fully, for example, those sustaining a posttraumatic amputation, may have to undergo additional growth-retarding procedures to enhance prosthetic componentry options at maturity. A 10-cm limb-length discrepancy is needed for standard knee and foot components, and newer component designs may require more space.

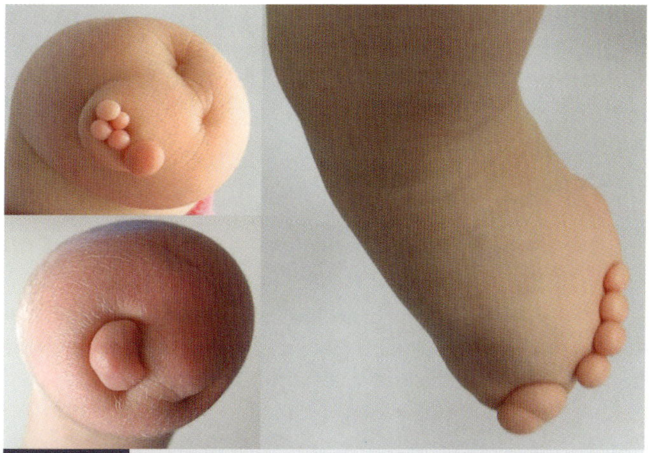

Figure 6 **A** through **C,** Clinical photographs of nubbins caused by failure of formation resulting from limb deficiency, not by amputation caused by amniotic bands.

Prosthetic Management

Children should be fitted with lower limb prostheses when they begin to pull to stand. Historically, the initial prosthetic knee did not have a joint or the joint was permanently locked to provide stability while the child was learning to ambulate. Early fitting with an articulating knee, however, has been shown to reduce the adoption of clearance adaptations, especially circumduction, as ambulation develops.[46] Most children with lower limb amputations respond to physical therapy and adapt quickly. Those with unilateral lower limb amputation will have diminished walking speed, distance, and functional balance compared with control subjects. Improved postural control and balance are associated with faster walking speeds. Because many children with limb deficiencies have associated deformities, the prosthesis may need to be adjusted to compensate for and maintain appropriate mechanical alignment. Children undergoing guided growth treatment may need prosthetic components that allow for adjustment as bony alignment changes. Radiographs can be helpful in correctly aligning the prosthesis.[47]

Prosthetic designs for adults are rapidly improving, and some of these features are beneficial for the pediatric population. A wide variety of suspension silicone/gel liners, especially those that do not require additional length for prosthetic attachment, have greatly improved prosthetic suspension in this very active population. Increased durability of the components, complex foot systems with vertical loading, energy storage and return, and multiaxial rotation and deflection also are important prosthetic improvements that are applicable for both adult and pediatric patients. Dynamic response and energy return are important for children. Many children participate in high-level physical activities, and prosthetic feet specifically designed for high-level sporting activities are becoming available in pediatric sizes. A 2014 study showed that, although high-performance prosthetic feet may improve gait mechanics, they do not affect patient measurements on sports/physical functioning or happiness scales of the PODCI. Both scales were noted to decline when comparing children 4 to 9 years of age with adolescents 10 to 19 years of age.[48] Microprocessor-controlled components for prosthetic knee and ankle joints are available for the adolescent population and allow greater gait adaptation for a variety of real-world situations.

Outcomes

Amputation often is considered a failure of medical science. In treatment discussions, patients and physicians must carefully weigh all the risks and benefits of amputation versus reconstruction. Children with limb loss have participation and health-related quality-of-life goals equal to children without limb loss.[49] However, adolescents with lower limb loss often have less diverse participation and less interaction in social and skill-based activities. If amputation is required, the family should be advised that children who undergo multiple surgical attempts at reconstruction before amputation have lower global function, more pain, and poorer adjustment to their limitations compared with those having amputation as an initial procedure.[50] Adults who had amputations for fibular deficiency as children have an average to above average quality of life when compared with the able-bodied adult population.[51] Most individuals with a congenital limb deficiency live ordinary lives. However, adults do report increased prevalence of chronic pain and early retirement.

Summary

Lower limb-length discrepancy can be associated with altered gait, increased knee pain, and less parental satisfaction concerning the child's condition. Radiographic assessment methods have improved and now offer reduced radiation exposure. These assessments can aid in measuring and predicting lower limb-length discrepancy. Percutaneous drilling is preferred over implant-only techniques for epiphysiodesis. Techniques for limb lengthening are evolving with the use of intramedullary devices to reduce the high complication rates of limb lengthening. Limb-length equalization techniques are often used in the treatment of lower limb deficiencies. Improvements in ultrasound have increased the prenatal detection rate of limb deficiencies. Refinements in the classification systems for fibular, femoral, and tibial deficiency are helpful in clinical decision making. In children with congenital limb loss, the presence of nubbins predicts congenital deficiency instead of amputation by amniotic bands. In children who have amputations to manage limb anomalies, tumors, or trauma, disarticulation or cartilage capping procedures should be considered to reduce terminal overgrowth. Children with lower limb amputation can expect a high quality of life because of improving prosthetic designs.

Key Study Points

- Skeletal age is important in the accurate estimation of lower limb length discrepancy and timing of epiphysiodesis, especially during the adolescent growth spurt.
- Percutaneous drilling techniques are preferred over those with implants only for epiphysiodesis.
- Lower limb lengthening using implantable lengthening nails is still associated with high but improved complication rates compared with external fixation.
- Improving classification systems in fibular, femoral, and tibial deficiencies can help guide clinical decision making.
- The presence of nubbins indicates a congenital deficiency, not amputation caused by amniotic bands.

Annotated References

1. Drnach M, Kreger A, Corliss C, Kocher D: Limb length discrepancies among 8- to 12-year-old children who are developing typically. *Pediatr Phys Ther* 2012;24(4):334-337.

   Limb lengths were measured with a tape measure in 43 girls and 62 boys. Discrepancies of greater than 2 cm were found in seven children.

2. Kiapour A, Abdelgawad AA, Goel VK, Souccar A, Terai T, Ebraheim NA: Relationship between limb length discrepancy and load distribution across the sacroiliac joint: A finite element study. *J Orthop Res* 2012;30(10):1577-1580.

   A finite element analysis showed that the load and peak stresses across the sacroiliac joint progressively increased as the limb-length discrepancy increased from 1 to 3 cm.

3. Noll DR: Leg length discrepancy and osteoarthritic knee pain in the elderly: An observational study. *J Am Osteopath Assoc* 2013;113(9):670-678.

   In 32 patients with knee pain, 28 women and 4 men reported that pain was more frequent in the apparent short leg.

4. Lee KM, Chung CY, Gwon DK, et al: Parental perspectives on leg length discrepancy. *J Pediatr Orthop B* 2012;21(2):146-149.

   Fifty-eight parents of children with limb-length discrepancy were surveyed, and the results showed that a discrepancy greater than 2 cm was associated with less satisfaction with appearance and happiness but no difference in pain or function.

5. Neelly K, Wallmann HW, Backus CJ: Validity of measuring leg length with a tape measure compared to a

computed tomography scan. *Physiother Theory Pract* 2013;29(6):487-492.

Thirty patients who had tape measure and CT assessments of limb-length discrepancy showed excellent validity of the tape measurement compared with CT.

6. Khakharia S, Bigman D, Fragomen AT, Pavlov H, Rozbruch SR: Comparison of PACS and hard-copy 51-inch radiographs for measuring leg length and deformity. *Clin Orthop Relat Res* 2011;469(1):244-250.

   Forty patients who had both hard-copy 51-inch radiographs and digital radiographs showed comparable reliability of limb-length measurements. Level of evidence: III.

7. Aaron A, Weinstein D, Thickman D, Eilert R: Comparison of orthoroentgenography and computed tomography in the measurement of limb-length discrepancy. *J Bone Joint Surg Am* 1992;74(6):897-902.

8. Escott BG, Ravi B, Weathermon AC, et al: EOS low-dose radiography: A reliable and accurate upright assessment of lower-limb lengths. *J Bone Joint Surg Am* 2013;95(23):e1831-e1837.

   EOS (EOS Imaging) measurements of a phantom limb showed that this type of radiography is more accurate than CT scanography and has less radiation exposure.

9. Westh RN, Menelaus MB: A simple calculation for the timing of epiphysial arrest: A further report. *J Bone Joint Surg Br* 1981;63(1):117-119.

10. Anderson M, Green WT, Messner MB: Growth and predictions of growth in the lower extremities. *J Bone Joint Surg Am* 1963;45:1-14.

11. Moseley CF: A straight-line graph for leg-length discrepancies. *J Bone Joint Surg Am* 1977;59(2):174-179.

12. Paley D, Bhave A, Herzenberg JE, Bowen JR: Multiplier method for predicting limb-length discrepancy. *J Bone Joint Surg Am* 2000;82(10):1432-1446.

13. Sanders JO, Howell J, Qiu X: Comparison of the Paley method using chronological age with use of skeletal maturity for predicting mature limb length in children. *J Bone Joint Surg Am* 2011;93(11):1051-1056.

    Among 24 patients, the Paley method with chronologic age predicts less than or equal to 5 cm of limb discrepancy with all ages, but skeletal age may be better for predictions during the adolescent growth spurt.

14. Canale ST, Christian CA: Techniques for epiphysiodesis about the knee. *Clin Orthop Relat Res* 1990;255:81-85.

15. Horn J, Gunderson RB, Wensaas A, Steen H: Percutaneous epiphysiodesis in the proximal tibia by a single-portal approach: Evaluation by radiostereometric analysis. *J Child Orthop* 2013;7(4):295-300.

    Radiostereometric analysis showed physeal closure within 12 weeks with a single portal drill and curettage epiphysiodesis in the proximal tibia.

16. Stewart D, Cheema A, Szalay EA: Dual 8-plate technique is not as effective as ablation for epiphysiodesis about the knee. *J Pediatr Orthop* 2013;33(8):843-846.

    In 16 physeal ablations versus 11 dual eight-plate epiphysiodeses of the knee, significantly superior results (P <0.001) were reported with ablation. Level of evidence: III.

17. Ilharreborde B, Gaumetou E, Souchet P, et al: Efficacy and late complications of percutaneous epiphysiodesis with transphyseal screws. *J Bone Joint Surg Br* 2012;94(2):270-275.

    Forty-five patients with percutaneous epiphysiodesis using transphyseal screws achieved only 66% of the predicted growth retardation.

18. Hasler CC, Krieg AH: Current concepts of leg lengthening. *J Child Orthop* 2012;6(2):89-104.

    The authors review the historical and current methods of limb lengthening.

19. Oostenbroek HJ, Brand R, van Roermund PM, Castelein RM: Paediatric lower limb deformity correction using the Ilizarov technique: A statistical analysis of factors affecting the complication rate. *J Pediatr Orthop B* 2014;23(1):26-31.

    Thirty-seven children with limb lengthening showed that the percentage of limb-length discrepancy was the only predictor of the complication rate.

20. McCarthy JJ, Iobst CA, Rozbruch SR, Sabharwal S, Eismann EA: Limb Lengthening and Reconstruction Society AIM Index reliably assesses lower limb deformity. *Clin Orthop Relat Res* 2013;471(2):621-627.

    This article describes an index derived by consensus of the Limb Lengthening and Reconstruction Society for assessing lower limb deformity and the difficulty of reconstruction.

21. Solomin LN, Paley D, Shchepkina EA, Vilensky VA, Skomoroshko PV: A comparative study of the correction of femoral deformity between the Ilizarov apparatus and Ortho-SUV Frame. *Int Orthop* 2014;38(4):865-872.

    This study compared 123 patients with femoral deformities. Seventy-eight patients were treated with Ilizarov fixation and 45 with six-axis frames. Results showed that the six-axis frames were faster and more accurate for correcting femoral deformity.

22. Rozbruch SR, Birch JG, Dahl MT, Herzenberg JE: Motorized intramedullary nail for management of limb-length discrepancy and deformity. *J Am Acad Orthop Surg* 2014;22(7):403-409.

    The authors review motorized intramedullary nails for lengthening and surgical techniques.

23. Burghardt RD, Paley D, Specht SC, Herzenberg JE: The effect on mechanical axis deviation of femoral lengthening with an intramedullary telescopic nail. *J Bone Joint Surg Br* 2012;94(9):1241-1245.

Lengthening of the femur along the anatomic axis resulted in a shift of the mechanical axis by 1° for each centimeter of lengthening.

24. Mahboubian S, Seah M, Fragomen AT, Rozbruch SR: Femoral lengthening with lengthening over a nail has fewer complications than intramedullary skeletal kinetic distraction. *Clin Orthop Relat Res* 2012;470(4):1221-1231.

The hybrid technique of limb lengthening of the femur with an external fixator over an intramedullary nail had fewer complications than the internal ISKD. Level of evidence: III.

25. Shabtai L, Specht SC, Standard SC, Herzenberg JE: Internal lengthening device for congenital femoral deficiency and fibular hemimelia. *Clin Orthop Relat Res* 2014;472(12):3860-3868.

In 18 patients who underwent limb lengthening with the PRECICE nail, the authors reported better control of lengthening and better range of motion than with external fixation. Joint subluxation developed in 1 of the 18 patients. Level of evidence: IV.

26. Simpson AH, Halliday J, Hamilton DF, Smith M, Mills K: Limb lengthening and peripheral nerve function-factors associated with deterioration of conduction. *Acta Orthop* 2013;84(6):579-584.

Electrophysiologic testing in 36 patients undergoing limb lengthening showed that preoperative asymptomatic findings deteriorated during lengthening, and changes that occurred during lengthening were more common in those with a discrepancy with a congenital etiology.

27. Launay F, Younsi R, Pithioux M, Chabrand P, Bollini G, Jouve JL: Fracture following lower limb lengthening in children: A series of 58 patients. *Orthop Traumatol Surg Res* 2013;99(1):72-79.

Fractures occurred in 20 of 58 patients undergoing limb lengthening. They occurred more frequently in those who had congenital etiologies, were younger than 9 years, had greater than 15% lengthening, and had latency periods of less than 7 days. Level of evidence: IV.

28. Sabharwal S: Enhancement of bone formation during distraction osteogenesis: Pediatric applications. *J Am Acad Orthop Surg* 2011;19(2):101-111.

This article reviews bone formation enhancement techniques during limb lengthening.

29. Dicke JM, Piper SL, Goldfarb CA: The utility of ultrasound for the detection of fetal limb abnormalities: A 20-year single-center experience. *Prenat Diagn* 2015;35(4):348-353.

A 20-year review of prenatal ultrasounds for limb anomalies demonstrates that 20% to 25% of cases will escape prenatal diagnosis.

30. Radler C, Myers AK, Hunter RJ, Arrabal PP, Herzenberg JE: Prenatal diagnosis of congenital femoral deficiency and fibular hemimelia. *Prenat Diagn* 2014;34(10):940-945.

A survey of mothers of children with femoral and fibular deficiencies found that 63% preferred prenatal diagnosis even though the ultrasounds did not always detect their child's anomaly.

31. Browne ML, Carter TC, Kay DM, et al: Evaluation of genes involved in limb development, angiogenesis, and coagulation as risk factors for congenital limb deficiencies. *Am J Med Genet A* 2012;158A(10):2463-2472.

In a population-based case control study of single nucleotide polymorphous symptoms in 389 infants with limb deficiencies compared with 980 control subjects, anomalies in *FGF10* were found to be statistically significant in those with limb deficiencies.

32. Lewin SO, Opitz JM: Fibular a/hypoplasia: Review and documentation of the fibular developmental field. *Am J Med Genet Suppl* 1986;2(suppl):215-238.

33. Achterman C, Kalamchi A: Congenital deficiency of the fibula. *J Bone Joint Surg Br* 1979;61(2):133-137.

34. Birch JG, Lincoln TL, Mack PW, Birch CM: Congenital fibular deficiency: A review of thirty years' experience at one institution and a proposed classification system based on clinical deformity. *J Bone Joint Surg Am* 2011;93(12):1144-1151.

This review of 104 patients with fibular deficiency proposes a new classification system that directs treatment.

35. Hamdy RC, Makhdom AM, Saran N, Birch J: Congenital fibular deficiency. *J Am Acad Orthop Surg* 2014;22(4):246-255.

This general review article on congenital fibular deficiency discusses classification systems, assessment, and management.

36. Radler C, Antonietti G, Ganger R, Grill F: Recurrence of axial malalignment after surgical correction in congenital femoral deficiency and fibular hemimelia. *Int Orthop* 2011;35(11):1683-1688.

Recurrent valgus deformity was found in 23 of 43 limbs undergoing lengthening or deformity correction. The deformity was worse in those with more severe femoral deficiencies and those fibular deficiencies that did not have fibular anlage resection.

37. El-Tayeby HM, Ahmed AA: Ankle reconstruction in type II fibular hemimelia. *Strategies Trauma Limb Reconstr* 2012;7(1):23-26.

This article describes ankle reconstruction using advancement of the cartilaginous fibular remnant and fixation to the tibia.

38. Cavadas PC, Thione A: Reconstruction of the lateral malleolus in a type-Ib fibular hemimelia with a microvascular

proximal fibular flap: A case report. *J Pediatr Orthop B* 2015;24(4):370-372.

This case report demonstrates the use of microvascular transfer of the contralateral proximal fibula to reconstruct the ankle and fibular deficiencies.

39. Gyr BM, Colmer HG IV, Morel MM, Ferski GJ: Hemiepiphysiodesis for correction of angular deformity in pediatric amputees. *J Pediatr Orthop* 2013;33(7):737-742.

Hemiepiphysiodesis in 23 patients with either a Syme ankle disarticulation or transtibial amputation provided reliable correction of their angular deformity. Level of evidence: IV.

40. Crawford DA, Tompkins BJ, Baird GO, Caskey PM: The long-term function of the knee in patients with fibular hemimelia and anterior cruciate ligament deficiency. *J Bone Joint Surg Br* 2012;94(3):328-333.

A survey of 11 patients with fibular deficiency and associated anterior cruciate ligament deficiency found that these patients live active lives without any substantial differences in SF-36 scores.

41. Paley D, Standard SC: Lengthening reconstruction surgery: For congenital femoral deficiency, in Rozbruch SR, Ilizarov S, eds: *Limb Lengthening and Reconstruction Surgery*. New York, NY, Informa Healthcare USA, 2007, pp 393-428.

42. Ackman J, Altiok H, Flanagan A, et al: Long-term follow-up of Van Nes rotationplasty in patients with congenital proximal focal femoral deficiency. *Bone Joint J* 2013;95-B(2):192-198.

A follow-up of 12 patients treated with Van Nes rotationplasty found no differences in their SF-36 and health-related quality-of-life scores compared with control subjects.

43. Canavese F, Samba A, Khan A, Dechelotte P, Krajbich JI: Rotationplasty as a salvage of failed primary limb reconstruction: Up to date review and case report. *J Pediatr Orthop B* 2014;23(3):247-253.

This case report (1 patient) and review of the literature (58 patients) suggest that patients have good or excellent results with rotationplasty as a salvage for limb reconstruction; however, fibular deficiency occurred in 3 patients who had three or fewer foot rays.

44. Clinton R, Birch JG: Congenital tibial deficiency: A 37-year experience at 1 institution. *J Pediatr Orthop* 2015;35(4):385-390.

This review examines 125 limbs in 95 patients with tibial deficiency and the proposed modification to the Jones classification to include type 5 in which global tibial deficiency is present but with both proximal and distal physes. Level of evidence: IV.

45. Fedorak GT, Watts HG, Cuomo AV, et al: Osteocartilaginous transfer of the proximal part of the fibula for osseous overgrowth in children with congenital or acquired tibial amputation: Surgical technique and results. *J Bone Joint Surg Am* 2015;97(7):574-581.

A study of autologous osteocartilaginous capping with the proximal part of the fibula to the distal tibia in children with transtibial amputations demonstrated that 90% did not have recurrent overgrowth after a mean follow-up of 7.2 years. Level of evidence: IV.

46. Geil M, Coulter C: Analysis of locomotor adaptations in young children with limb loss in an early prosthetic knee prescription protocol. *Prosthet Orthot Int* 2014;38(1):54-61.

Fitting toddlers with an early prosthetic knee reduced the adoption of clearance adaptations while walking ability was developing.

47. Mooney R, Carry P, Wylie E, et al: Radiographic parameters improve lower extremity prosthetic alignment. *J Child Orthop* 2013;7(6):543-550.

Long-leg radiographs were shown to substantially improve prosthetic fitting alignment from 20% to 77% in the construction of 45 prostheses for patients with congenital or acquired limb deficiencies.

48. Jeans KA, Karol LA, Cummings D, Singhal K: Comparison of gait after Syme and transtibial amputation in children: Factors that may play a role in function. *J Bone Joint Surg Am* 2014;96(19):1641-1647.

Sixty-four patients with unilateral below-knee prostheses showed that increased ankle motion associated with high-performance dynamic prosthetic feet did not improve the PODCI sports/physical functioning subscale. Level of evidence: III.

49. Michielsen A, van Wijk I, Ketelaar M: Participation and health-related quality of life of Dutch children and adolescents with congenital lower limb deficiencies. *J Rehabil Med* 2011;43(7):584-589.

Fifty-six children with congenital lower limb deficiencies showed that their participation and overall health-related quality of life did not differ from typical children, but adolescent activities showed less diversity and less interaction with social and skill-based activities.

50. Dabaghi A, Haces F, Cadevila R: Is there a difference in function, outcome, satisfaction and adjustment to having a prosthesis in primary transtibial amputations versus multiple previous reconstructive procedures prior to amputation? *J Prosthet Orthot* 2015;27(2):40-43.

Twenty-five patients treated initially with amputation were compared with 34 patients who underwent multiple reconstructive surgeries before amputation. Improved transfers, pain, global function, and adjustment to limitation were found in those with primary amputation.

51. Walker JL, Knapp D, Minter C, et al: Adult outcomes following amputation or lengthening for fibular deficiency. *J Bone Joint Surg Am* 2009;91(4):797-804.

5: Lower Extremity

Section 6

Spine

SECTION EDITOR:
James O. Sanders, MD

Chapter 28

Early-Onset Scoliosis and Congenital Spine Disorders

Michael Glotzbecker, MD Daniel J. Hedequist, MD John B. Emans, MD

Abstract

Early-onset idiopathic scoliosis and congenital spine anomalies present unique treatment challenges because of the need to balance control of spinal and chest deformities while allowing growth of the spine and chest. To provide optimal care to patients, it is helpful to review treatment principles common to these conditions and understand the natural history, clinical and radiographic evaluations, nonsurgical and surgical treatment options, clinical outcomes, and complications related to these diagnoses.

Keywords: congenital scoliosis; early-onset idiopathic scoliosis; early-onset scoliosis; thoracic insufficiency syndrome

Introduction

Early-onset scoliosis (EOS) is an all-encompassing term, and it is inclusive of all etiologies of scoliosis in patients younger than 10 years.[1] The use of this age-based separation reflects the potential physiologic consequences of spinal deformity at a young age and the shared goals of treatment. A consideration uniquely important in this age group is the development of the lungs in the setting of a growing and changing thoracic cavity. This chapter discusses the most commonly encountered forms of EOS: early-onset idiopathic scoliosis (EOIS) and congenital scoliosis.

Spine Growth and Lung Development

The bony anatomy of the spinal column forms in utero at 3 to 5 weeks of gestation, and segmentation occurs between weeks 6 and 8.[2] Other organ systems are formed concurrently, which explains why abnormalities in these organ systems are commonly encountered in patients with congenital scoliosis.

Two-thirds of adult sitting height is achieved by age 5 years, 50% of the adult thoracic volume is achieved by age 10 years, and the most rapid increase in the number and volume of alveoli occur from birth to age 3 years.[3] For this reason, spinal deformity at a young age has been associated with pulmonary dysfunction, which in its most severe form presents as thoracic insufficiency syndrome.[4] Pulmonary function is dependent on adequate thoracic volume (height, width, and depth) and thoracic function (chest expansion and diaphragm contraction). For these reasons, treatment goals and strategies in EOS are directed at preserving growth of the spine and thoracic cavity to maximize lung function.

Definitions

The use of the term early onset is meant to distinguish patients who have substantial remaining growth of the spine and thorax such that this growth must be accounted for when making treatment decisions. EOS includes all etiologies (congenital, neuromuscular, syndromic, and idiopathic). The traditional classification of idiopathic scoliosis divided patients into groups based on age: infantile, younger than 3 years; juvenile, age 3 years to

Dr. Glotzbecker or an immediate family member serves as a paid consultant to or is an employee of DePuy and Medtronic and has received research or institutional support from Synthes. Dr. Hedequist or an immediate family member serves as a board member, owner, officer, or committee member of the American Academy of Orthopaedic Surgeons and the Pediatric Orthopaedic Society of North America. Dr. Emans or an immediate family member has received royalties from Synthes; serves as a paid consultant to or is an employee of Medtronic Sofamor Danek and Synthes; and serves as an unpaid consultant to Medtronic Sofamor Danek and Synthes.

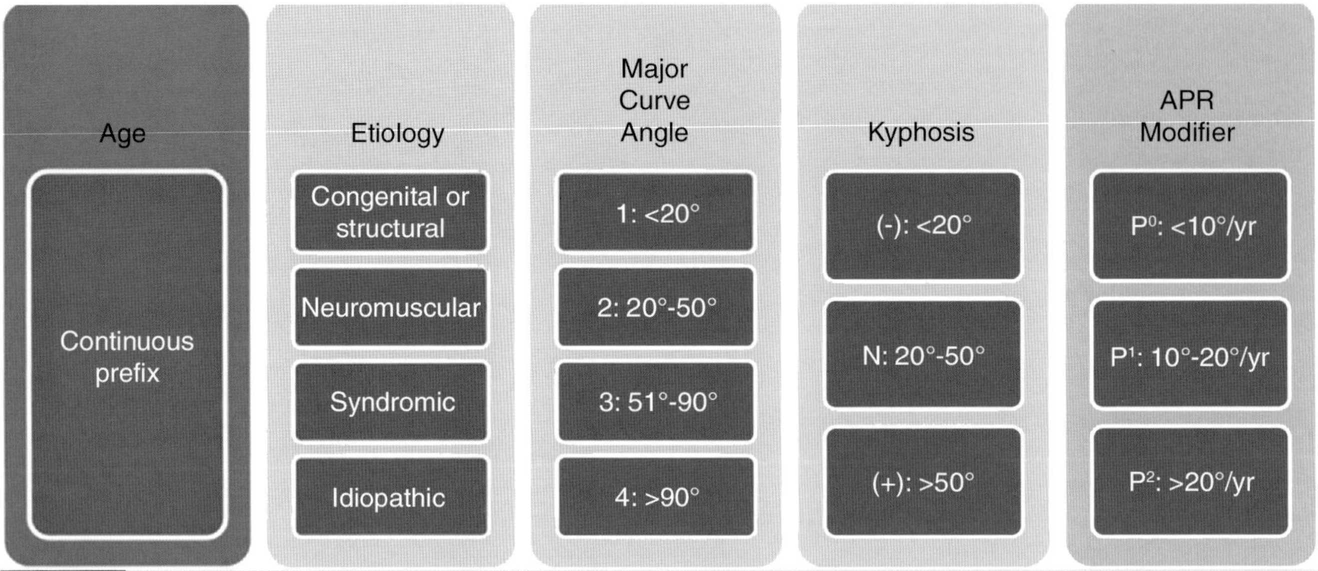

Figure 1 Illustration of the Classification of Early-Onset Scoliosis (C-EOS). This classification system consists of a continuous prefix (age), three core variables (etiology, major curve angle, and kyphosis), and an optional modifier (curve progression). APR = annual progression ratio; (–), N, and (+) are kyphosis variables; P = progression modifier. (Adapted with permission from Williams BA, Matsumoto H, McCalla DJ, et al: Development and initial validation of the Classification of Early-Onset Scoliosis (C-EOS). *J Bone Joint Surg Am* 2014;96[16]:1359-1367.)

younger than 10 years; and adolescent, 10 years and older. Although this terminology is still used, the treatment considerations are similar in the first two groups; therefore, it is probably more useful to consider both of those groups as having EOIS. A recent position statement grouped all patients younger than 10 years as having EOS.[1] However, because many studies have used the more historical terminology, that terminology will be used in this chapter.

Thoracic insufficiency syndrome is defined as the inability of the thorax to support normal respiration and growth.[4] The most common scenario for this diagnosis is encountered in patients with congenital scoliosis with a shortened spine, fused ribs, and a constricted hemithorax. The shortened spine and fused ribs lead to a reduction in thoracic volume and abnormal thoracic cage motion. However, the term thoracic insufficiency syndrome can be used for any patient with substantial spinal or thoracic deformity leading to inadequate pulmonary function. The thoracic lordosis associated with many types of spinal deformity can lead to a reduction in anteroposterior chest depth as the spine moves toward the sternum. The clinical signs associated with thoracic insufficiency syndrome include loss of chest wall expansion, failure to thrive (delayed growth and poor weight gain), worsening thoracic deformity based on three-dimensional imaging studies, and a decline in pulmonary function. The patient may have restrictive lung disease, with a reduction in vital capacity and total lung capacity, leading to alveolar hypoventilation, hypoxic vasoconstriction, and eventually pulmonary artery hypertension or cor pulmonale.[5]

Given the heterogeneity of individuals with EOS, there have been recent attempts to create a classification system.[6] The Classification of Early-Onset Scoliosis (C-EOS) system categorizes patients based on age, etiology, major Cobb angle, kyphosis, and progression (**Figure 1**). The C-EOS has excellent interobserver reliability and is being used in current research efforts to standardize communication as well as for correlation of patient characteristics with outcome data.

General Principles

Outcome Measures

Choosing the appropriate outcome measures in this patient population is challenging. Most research has focused on reporting changes in spinal and thoracic growth, such as the Cobb angle and the thoracic height before and after treatment.[7] However, it is unclear whether maintaining or improving spinal growth actually leads to better clinical outcomes. The Early-Onset Scoliosis Questionnaire (EOSQ) has been developed and can be used as a disease-specific outcome measure.[8,9] Combining patient-reported outcomes with radiographic and pulmonary functional data will likely aid in understanding the effects of treatment and observation on disease.

Treatment

The current treatment goals in EOS are to maximize thoracic volume and function, increase spine length, and maintain spine mobility throughout the child's growth while minimizing complications. Treatment decisions include both the type of treatment and the timing of intervention. Because the spinal deformity often includes a large portion of the spine, early definitive fusion is associated with poor outcomes.[10] Even in the absence of comorbid cardiac or pulmonary disease, patients with severe scoliosis who are younger than 5 years are at risk for long-term cardiopulmonary complications.[11,12]

Faced with a progressive deformity, a choice is often made between the effect of untreated progressive deformity versus the pulmonary growth restriction and loss of spinal height associated with spinal fusion. Less invasive options, such as bracing or casting, may slow deformity progression and delay the need for surgery. Surgical intervention using growth-friendly instrumentation such as the Vertical Expandable Prosthetic Titanium Rib (VEPTR; DePuy Synthes), growing rods such as MAGEC rods (Ellipse Technologies), tethers, or the SHILLA (Medtronic) growth guidance system can control a curve while preserving growth of the spine and thoracic cavity. Earlier intervention may result in more complications but may be required if the deformity is causing irreversible pulmonary damage.[13,14] The development of the thorax should be the most heavily weighed factor in decision making. Although spinal imbalance and deformity can be improved at the end of growth, no such strategy exists to correct thoracic shape and dysfunction resulting from EOS.

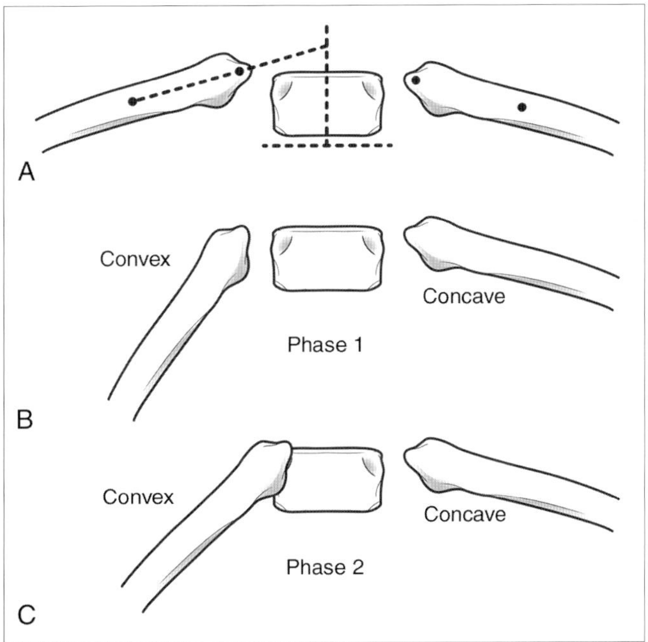

Figure 2 **A,** Illustration demonstrates the elements in the calculation of the rib-vertebral angle difference (RVAD). A line is drawn perpendicular to the end plate of the apical vertebra. A line is then drawn from the midpoint of the head of the rib to the midpoint of the neck of the rib on the convex side, and the created angle is calculated. The angle is calculated with the same method on the concave side. The difference between the two measurements is the RVAD. **B,** Illustration of the phase 1 relationship between the rib head and vertebra body demonstrating no overlap; an RVAD can be calculated. **C,** Illustration of the phase 2 relationship between the rib head and vertebra body with overlap of the rib on the vertebra, which is indicative of curve progression.

Early-Onset Idiopathic Scoliosis

Etiology

Because EOIS is less common than adolescent idiopathic scoliosis (AIS), it is important to rule out other causes of scoliosis such as neuromuscular or genetic conditions or an underlying spinal cord anomaly. By definition, EOIS has no clear underlying etiology. Intrauterine molding, a supine sleep position, and an undefined genetic contribution have all been postulated as causative factors. Previous terminology has divided the patient population into infantile (younger than 3 years) and juvenile (3 years to younger than 10 years) idiopathic scoliosis, but more current terminology combines these groups under the umbrella classification of EOIS, which includes all patients younger than 10 years.[1]

Natural History

Curves may resolve in many patients, but may progress in some patients. A systematic review of the literature found that infantile scoliosis curves resolved in 573 patients, whereas the curves progressed in 333 patients.[15] Younger age and single curves have been postulated as predictive factors for progression, but the rib-vertebral angle difference (RVAD) is the most reliable indicator of curve progression[15,16] (**Figure 2**). When the RVAD is less than 20°, 83% of patients had resolution of the scoliosis. When the RVAD was greater than 20°, 84% of the patients had progressive curves. Subsequent studies have confirmed the usefulness of the RVAD in predicting curve progression in patients in this age group. The RVAD has traditionally been used for patients with infantile scoliosis and has not been applied to older patients with EOS (3 years to younger than 10 years).

Clinical Evaluation

Patients with EOIS are more commonly males than females, especially patients younger than 3 years. Although

6: Spine

left-sided curves are considered atypical in AIS, left-sided thoracic curves occur more frequently. Each patient with a possible spinal deformity should have a complete neurologic examination, including gait, patellar and Achilles reflexes, sensation, and abdominal reflexes. A skin examination should evaluate for cutaneous manifestations of a systemic condition or spinal dysraphism. Associated conditions include developmental dysplasia of the hip, inguinal hernia, and congenital heart disease.

Imaging

Standard radiographic examination includes full-length PA and lateral radiographs. Measurement of the Cobb angle and RVAD will help direct treatment decisions. The radiographic position should be considered when assessing curve progression. For example, a radiograph taken upright after the infant begins walking may cause a curve to appear larger than a previously obtained supine radiograph. Bending or traction radiographs are generally reserved for assessing flexibility and surgical planning. In patients with EOIS, MRI can be used to rule out associated neural axis abnormalities such as Chiari I malformation, syrinx, or tethered cord. In patients with EOIS who are younger than 3 years and have a curve greater than 20°, the rates of neural axis abnormality range from 13% to 22% despite normal neurologic examination findings and the absence of associated syndromes.[17,18] However, when identified, these anomalies frequently require neurosurgical intervention. Early recognition of these anomalies is clinically important because they may cause irrevocable spine deformity progression. Recognition of tethering lesions is most accurately achieved by MRI, but spinal ultrasound performed before 6 to 8 weeks of age will identify low conus, lipoma, and major anomalies of the filum while avoiding the need for anesthesia in very young patients. If there are neurologic abnormalities, deformed feet, urinary incontinence, or major spinal anomalies (such as diastematomyelia or congenital spinal dislocation), MRI is always indicated. In the setting of normal ultrasound findings, an MRI should be pursued at a later date in a patient with a progressing curve.

Nonsurgical Treatment

In patients with a low RVAD, careful follow-up to assess for curve resolution is appropriate. In patients with an RVAD greater than 20°, there is a high likelihood of progression, and treatment should be considered. Options for nonsurgical management include casting, bracing, or both.

In patients with a curve that is predicted to be progressive, bracing or casting should be considered. Although bracing has proved effective in a prospective randomized controlled trial of patients with AIS,[19] the efficacy of bracing in younger patients is not supported by level I or level II evidence. However, other noninvasive treatments have recently gained popularity. Casting for EOS can be curative, or at a minimum delay the need for surgical intervention.[20] The rationale for cast treatment includes its ability to harness the rapid growth velocity that is common in young patients. It seems that patients with smaller Cobb angles who are treated at a younger age have a greater chance of a successful outcome.[20,21] The flexibility of the curve or the quality of the cast may affect success rates. The goal of casting should be understood when initiating treatment. Although some patients (those with a smaller curve or younger age) treated with casting may be cured, there are many instances when a cure is not expected. However, casting can be used as a means to delay surgery in patients with larger curves so that surgical treatment can be initiated at an older age.[22]

Surgical Treatment

Growth-Friendly Instrumentation

There are multiple technologies used to treat patients with EOIS when nonsurgical treatment has been unsuccessful. All of these technologies attempt to maximize spinal and thoracic growth while controlling spinal deformity and minimizing complications. Because early spinal fusion has been associated with poor outcomes, growth-friendly strategies are currently accepted.

The traditional dual growing rod technique uses localized fusion with spine anchors at the top and the bottom of the curve and leaves the middle of the spine untouched to allow for serial distractions. Variations on this method include the use of rib anchors rather than spine anchors. The SHILLA system uses a strategy in which there is an apical fusion and correction at the area of deformity, with nonfusion/gliding implants proximally and distally that allow for guided growth through the "normal" spine segments.[23] The relative merit of this system is the avoidance of repetitive surgeries for routine surgical lengthening. New technologies that use a variety of convex tethers may provide another option for guided correction and growth.[24] Another new technology is the MAGEC rod, which allows for magnetic lengthening through a device exterior to the skin.[25] Comparative studies and long-term outcomes are lacking for these treatments to determine which strategy is best.

Outcomes and Complications

Except for young patients with EOIS who are "cured" with casting, a normal spine at the end of growth is achieved in only a few patients. After treatment with growth-friendly instrumentation, most patients require definitive fusion when they reach an appropriate age. In addition, junctional kyphosis is a frequently encountered complication. Junctional kyphosis is common in growth-friendly implants and is likely related to both the high underlying incidence of preoperative kyphosis and the mechanism by which the rods are lengthened, with posterior distraction promoting kyphosis.[26] Rod breakage or implant dislodgement is common and expected at some point during treatment.[27] Although growth-friendly surgical treatment may lessen the deformity at final fusion, spontaneous fusion during the lengthening treatment and curve stiffness present challenging obstacles at the time of final fusion or may bring a premature end to growth-friendly treatment.[28]

The repetitive use of anesthetics often required along with the iatrogenic radiation exposure associated with treatment started at a young age may have detrimental effects on patient outcomes, such as psychological disturbances and the role of radiation exposure in the development of secondary malignancies.[29,30] Also, early treatment may lead to a decrease in the effectiveness of repeated surgical lengthenings over time (the law of diminishing returns).[31] In the event of severe complications such as infection or spontaneous fusion, treatment may be ended before adequate space for lung development has been achieved.[32] The delicate balance between early intervention and curve control versus the complications associated with growth-friendly treatments is not yet established; however, it is hoped that data gathered from patient-reported outcome measures will help distinguish between treatment options.

Congenital Scoliosis

Etiology

Similar to EOIS, congenital scoliosis has no clear etiology. Multiple environmental and genetic causes have been proposed but are unproved. Most cases are sporadic and have a low familial recurrence rate. Discovery of mutations in the genes of the notch family and their association with Alagille syndrome and spondylocostal dyostosis adds support to theories that genetic factors have a role in the etiology. The importance of *HOX* genes in the creation of the axial and appendicular skeleton offer further reasons to suspect a genetic etiology.[2]

Classification

Congenital spinal anomalies are classified as a failure of formation (**Figure 3**), a failure of segmentation (**Figure 4**), or a combination of both types.[33] In a failure of formation, the extent to which the vertebral body is not formed defines the deformity. A wedge vertebra has pedicles on both sides but asymmetric formation and growth of the vertebral body on one side, whereas a hemivertebra represents a complete unilateral failure of formation. Depending on the relationship to adjacent vertebrae and the number of disks present, the hemivertebrae can be defined as nonsegmented, partially segmented, or fully segmented. A hemimetameric shift describes a spine with balanced deformities and growth potential on both sides of the spine, with similar hemivertebrae situated on opposite sides. With a failure of segmentation, adjacent vertebrae are inappropriately connected. In its most benign form, a block vertebra is symmetrically fused to an adjacent vertebra. On the severe end of the spectrum is a unilateral bar, in which one side of the vertebral bodies are fused, which allows for unchecked growth on the contralateral side. Fused ribs are commonly associated with congenital scoliosis. Many congenital spine deformities are more complex than can be described by this classification, with nonconcordance between anterior and posterior elements in the congenital spinal anomaly.

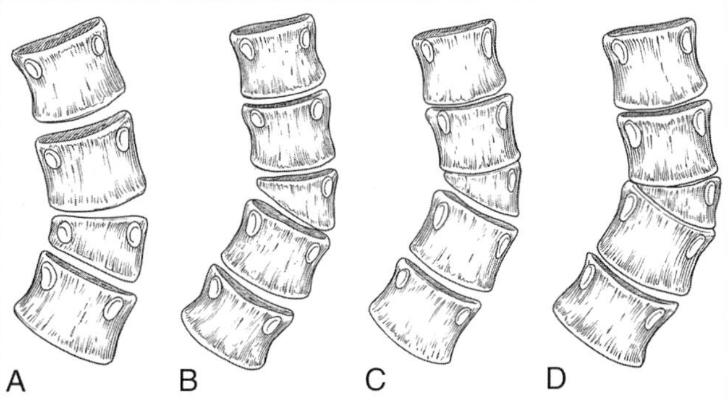

Figure 3 Illustrations of formation defects. **A,** Wedge vertebra. **B,** Fully segmented hemivertebra. **C,** Partially segmented hemivertebra. **D,** Unsegmented hemivertebra. (Reproduced from Hedequist D, Emans J: Congenital scoliosis. *J Am Acad Orthop Surg* 2004;12[4]:266-275.)

Natural History

The presence of deformity and the likelihood of progression are dependent on the location and type of congenital abnormality. The anatomic deformity can result in immediate asymmetry in the spine, but the relative risk of progression is related to the comparative growth potential of the two sides of the spine and the presence of tethering structures. The progression of various congenital abnormalities was characterized by McMaster and Ohtsuka[34] (**Figure 5**). The risk of progression is highest for a unilateral bar with contralateral hemivertebrae, followed by a unilateral bar, a hemivertebra, a wedged vertebra, and a block vertebra. Unbalanced congenital

6: Spine

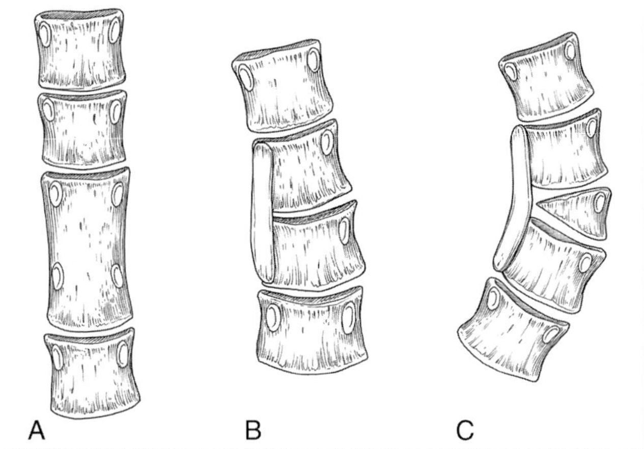

Figure 4 Illustrations of segmentation defects. **A,** Block vertebra. **B,** Unilateral segmentation (bar) defect. **C,** Unilateral bar with a contralateral hemivertebra. (Reproduced from Hedequist D, Emans J: Congenital scoliosis. *J Am Acad Orthop Surg* 2004;12[4]:266-275.)

abnormalities that are present at junctional areas of the spine (such as cervicothoracic, thoracolumbar, and lumbosacral areas) are more likely to be clinically apparent. Progression typically occurs during rapid growth, either during the first 3 years of life or during the growth spurt in early adolescence.

Clinical Features

Patients with congenital scoliosis should be assessed with a full neurologic examination, including an evaluation of reflexes. Sagittal and coronal balance and rib cage deformity should be assessed. A thorough skin examination for evidence of spinal dysraphism as well as inspection for foot deformity or other neurologic dysfunction should be performed given the associated neural axis abnormalities. Exercise tolerance as well as inspiratory and expiratory capacity should be assessed because of the possible negative effect of chest wall and spinal deformity on pulmonary function. The presence of substantial rib fusions in the setting of congenital scoliosis may present as thoracic insufficiency syndrome.

As previously discussed, the formation of the spine occurs concurrently with other organ systems. Associated conditions include vertebral-anal-cardiac-tracheal-esophageal-renal-limb (VACTERL) association, which is representative of the other organ systems commonly affected in patients with congenital scoliosis. Other musculoskeletal abnormalities include radial hypoplasia, hip dysplasia, and clubfoot and those seen in Klippel-Feil syndrome and Sprengel deformity. Congenital heart disease (such as a ventricular septal defect, an atrial septal defect, tetralogy of Fallot, or transposition of great vessels) is present in as many as 25% of patients with congenital scoliosis. A urologic or müllerian duct abnormality (such as horseshoe kidney, renal aplasia, duplicate ureters, or hypospadias) is seen in up to 33% of patients.[2] Many of these associated conditions are readily apparent, but renal obstruction and unilateral hearing loss are easily missed unless screening is performed.

Imaging

Imaging begins with standard PA and lateral radiographs. In a nonambulatory patient, supine or sitting radiographs can be used. When a patient transitions to ambulatory status, any change in the deformity noted on radiographs must be interpreted in the context of the change in the radiographic position (for example, supine versus upright). Measuring a Cobb angle may be more difficult in these patients, and quantifying the amount of chest deformity is challenging. Similar landmarks should be used when comparing sequential radiographs. Even in the absence of neurologic abnormalities on examination, a screening MRI is generally recommended to rule out associated neural axial abnormalities, which are found in up to 35% of patients with congenital scoliosis.[2] However, anesthetic risks (including the unclear effects on the developing brain) associated with the patient's age should be weighed when determining the timing of radiologic studies. As previously mentioned, a spine ultrasound can identify certain conditions and avoids the use of anesthesia in very young patients. However, immediate MRI is indicated depending on the presence of certain symptoms and/or the severity of the spinal anomaly. Substantial progression of curvature in a normally segmented spine requires MRI. CT should be used preoperatively to define the anatomy because posterior abnormalities may not correlate with findings on plain radiographs and there is frequent discordance of anterior and posterior anomalies.[35]

Nonsurgical Treatment

Observation is warranted for many congenital curves that have limited deformity or progression over time. Many congenital abnormalities may have relatively balanced growth and will not require treatment. Bracing is generally viewed as ineffective treatment for congenital curves; however, it may be used for compensatory curves of a normally segmented spine. Casting or bracing congenital curves as a tactic to delay the need for surgery has been advocated; however, it is expected that this strategy is less successful in managing patients with congenital curves than those with normally segmented spines. In patients with associated chest wall and rib anomalies, casting and bracing may have negative consequences, which are not well understood.

Site of Curvature	Type of Congenital Anomaly					
	Block Vertebra	Wedged Vertebra	Hemivertebra: Single	Hemivertebra: Double	Unilateral Unsegmented Bar	Unilateral Unsegmented Bar and Contralateral Hemivertebrae
Upper thoracic	<1°–1°	★ –2°	1°–2°	2°–2.5°	2°–4°	5°–6°
Lower thoracic	<1°–1°	2°–2°	2°–2.5°	2°–2.5°	5°–6.5°	6°–7°
Thoracolumbar	<1°–1°	1.5°–2°	2°–3.5°	5°– ★	6°–9°	>10°– ★
Lumbar	★	<1°– ★	<1°–1°	★	>5°– ★	★
Lumbosacral	★	★	<1°–1.5°	★	★	★

No treatment required   May require spinal fusion   Require spinal fusion

★ Too few or no curves

Figure 5 Illustration summarizing the natural history of congenital curves by the type of vertebral anomaly and curve location for a series of 251 patients. Median yearly deterioration is given for children younger than 10 years on the left and for children 10 years and older on the right of each cell. (Reproduced with permission from McMaster MJ, Ohtsuka K: The natural history of congenital scoliosis: A study of two hundred and fifty-one patients. *J Bone Joint Surg Am* 1982;64[8]:1128-1147.)

Surgical Treatment

As in patients with EOIS, the surgical treatment goals in patients with congenital deformity are to maximize spine and chest growth, control chest wall and spinal deformity, and minimize patient complications and distress. It is safe to use spinal instrumentation in these patients.[36] The use of preoperative traction can help with gradual, partial correction of severe deformity (with or without an anterior release).[37] Balancing early versus late intervention is challenging. It is known that early fusion leads to poor outcomes with regard to pulmonary function; therefore, other treatment strategies should be considered.[10] Because the types of deformity are broad, so are the possible treatment options.

If a small section of the spine is affected by a minimal deformity, an in situ fusion may prevent curve progression without detriment to the growing lungs. This is not a treatment option if the deformity is substantial enough that it requires more acute correction or if the deformity spans a large segment of spine because in situ fusion would prevent adequate spinal growth. Hemiepiphyseodesis offers the potential for gradual deformity correction by slowing growth on the convex side and allowing the concave side to grow. Although historical results have been mixed, the more recent literature has documented promising outcomes.[38]

If an isolated hemivertebra is causing coronal or sagittal imbalance, a hemivertebra excision offers an attractive surgical option. The most common hemivertebrae requiring this approach are fully segmented deformities at transition zones of the spine. When successful, spinal balance can be restored and the progression of adjacent compensatory curves can be prevented. Although historical reports include anterior and posterior resections, posterior-only approaches are currently advocated.[39]

In patients with adequate thoracic volume but an unacceptable coronal or sagittal deformity, an acute fusion with deformity correction is a reasonable option. If bending radiographs fail to demonstrate adequate flexibility for acceptable correction, treatment options include anterior and posterior approaches as well as posterior-based approaches such as pedicle subtraction osteotomies or vertebral column resection. The selected approach depends on the magnitude and location of the deformity.

Growth-friendly strategies are commonly used in the treatment of congenital scoliosis. Traditional growing rods are probably the most indicated instrumentation for patients with spinal deformity without substantial rib fusions or chest wall abnormality. Growing rods have been shown to increase spinal growth, control spinal curvature, and improve space available for lungs in patients

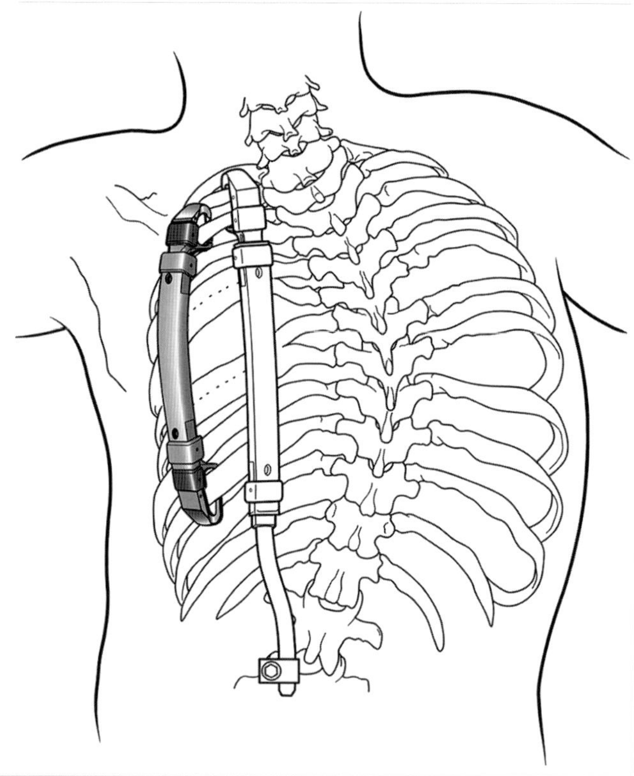

Figure 6 Schematic representation of Vertical Expandable Prosthetic Titanium Rib devices used after an opening wedge thoracostomy in patients with congenital vertebral anomalies and fused ribs. A rib-rib device (shaded) or a hybrid rib prosthesis (unshaded) may be used to promote thoracic growth by lengthening the concave hemithorax. (Adapted with permission from Campbell RM Jr, Smith MD, Hell-Vocke AK: Expansion thoracoplasty: The surgical technique of opening-wedge thoracostomy. Surgical technique. *J Bone Joint Surg Am* 2004;86[suppl 1]:51-64.)

with congenital scoliosis.[40] The use of VEPTR has been one of the most commonly adopted implant strategies for the treatment of congenital scoliosis (**Figure 6**). The ideal candidate for a VEPTR implant has progressive congenital spinal deformity, an associated hemithoracic constriction, and multiple fused ribs. In these patients, expansion thoracostomy and placement of a VEPTR expands the chest and controls deformity.[14,41] The VEPTR can be connected to the pelvis, spine, or ribs.

Less commonly, the SHILLA system has been used to correct the apical abnormality and allow guided growth cephalad and caudal to the deformity.[23]

Outcomes and Complications

Although chest wall expansion has been shown to increase the space available for lungs, a systematic review failed to demonstrate an improvement in pulmonary function.[42] Understanding the appropriate outcomes is challenging. Ultimately, improvement and maintenance of pulmonary function is the most important outcome. Because of substantial obstacles to obtaining meaningful pulmonary function tests in very young children, surrogate means such as radiographic measurements of spinal length and chest width are used to evaluate pulmonary function; however, it is unclear how well these measurements correlate with actual pulmonary function.[7] Better outcome measures are needed, specifically to understand the effects of treatment on pulmonary function. Patient-reported outcomes and cost-effectiveness studies will become increasingly important in evaluating treatment strategies.

Complications with the use of growth-friendly strategies for patients with scoliosis are common. Device migration, infection, and brachial plexus palsy have been reported with use of the VEPTR.[43,44] The C-EOS may be helpful in predicting complications such as anchor failure.[45] Complications may be more common in patients treated at a younger age, which is likely related to the severity of disease and the number of surgical treatments.[13] Junctional kyphosis is also an unsolved but common complication.[46]

Summary

Both EOIS and congenital scoliosis present challenging clinical situations. Treatment goals common to patients with either diagnosis include maximizing spinal growth and pulmonary function while avoiding complications. Repetitive use of anesthetics and iatrogenic radiation exposure are problematic. Many treatments options are available, including a variety of growth-friendly implants.

Major challenges exist in understanding the disease and the effects of treatment on the disease. Junctional kyphosis, surgical site infection, and implant failure are common complications and areas of current research interest. Traditionally reported radiographic outcomes may not be good surrogates for actual patient outcomes or improvement in pulmonary function. Patient-reported outcomes require further study and correlation with traditionally collected radiographic outcomes.

Key Study Points

- EOS is an all-encompassing term, and it is inclusive of all etiologies of scoliosis in patients younger than 10 years.
- Lung development in patients with a growing and changing thoracic cavity is uniquely important in this population.
- Treatment goals and strategies in patients with EOS are directed at preserving the growth of the spine and thoracic cavity to maximize lung function.
- Less invasive treatment options, such as bracing and casting, may slow deformity progression and delay the need for surgery.
- Surgical interventions using growth-friendly instrumentation, tethers, or a growth guidance system can control a curve while preserving growth of the spine and thoracic cavity.

Annotated References

1. Skaggs DL, Guillaume T, El Hawary L, et al: Early Onset Scoliosis Consensus Statement, SRS Growing Spine Committee, 2015. *Spine Deform* 2015;3(2):107.

   EOS refers to spinal deformity that is present in patients before 8 to 10 years of age. EOS is further organized to reflect etiology as applicable.

2. Hensinger RN: Congenital scoliosis: Etiology and associations. *Spine (Phila Pa 1976)* 2009;34(17):1745-1750.

3. Dimeglio A: Growth in pediatric orthopaedics. *J Pediatr Orthop* 2001;21(4):549-555.

4. Campbell RM Jr, Smith MD, Mayes TC, et al: The characteristics of thoracic insufficiency syndrome associated with fused ribs and congenital scoliosis. *J Bone Joint Surg Am* 2003;85(3):399-408.

5. Gillingham BL, Fan RA, Akbarnia BA: Early onset idiopathic scoliosis. *J Am Acad Orthop Surg* 2006;14(2):101-112.

6. Williams BA, Matsumoto H, McCalla DJ, et al: Development and initial validation of the Classification of Early-Onset Scoliosis (C-EOS). *J Bone Joint Surg Am* 2014;96(16):1359-1367.

   Using formal consensus-building methods in a large group of surgeons experienced in treating EOS, a novel classification system for EOS was developed.

7. Glotzbecker M, Johnston C, Miller P, et al: Is there a relationship between thoracic dimensions and pulmonary function in early-onset scoliosis? *Spine (Phila Pa 1976)* 2014;39(19):1590-1595.

   Traditional two-dimensional measurements of thoracic dimension (T1-T12 height) were used to determine outcomes in patients with EOS. These measurements were found to be weak predictors of pulmonary function outcomes. However, better outcome measures need to be developed. Level of evidence: III.

8. Vitale MG, Corona J, Matsumoto H, et al: Development and initial validation of a disease specific outcome measure for early onset scoliosis. *Stud Health Technol Inform* 2010;158:172-176.

9. Corona J, Matsumoto H, Roye DP, Vitale MG: Measuring quality of life in children with early onset scoliosis: Development and initial validation of the early onset scoliosis questionnaire. *J Pediatr Orthop* 2011;31(2):180-185.

   The EOSQ reflects quality of life and caregiver burden in the EOS population. The EOSQ will expand options for outcome assessment in these children.

10. Karol LA, Johnston C, Mladenov K, Schochet P, Walters P, Browne RH: Pulmonary function following early thoracic fusion in non-neuromuscular scoliosis. *J Bone Joint Surg Am* 2008;90(6):1272-1281.

11. Pehrsson K, Larsson S, Oden A, Nachemson A: Long-term follow-up of patients with untreated scoliosis: A study of mortality, causes of death, and symptoms. *Spine (Phila Pa 1976)* 1992;17(9):1091-1096.

12. Branthwaite MA: Cardiorespiratory consequences of unfused idiopathic scoliosis. *Br J Dis Chest* 1986;80(4):360-369.

13. Upasani VV, Miller PE, Emans JB, et al; Children's Spine Study Group: VEPTR implantation after age 3 is associated with similar radiographic outcomes with fewer complications. *J Pediatr Orthop* 2015; Feb 26 [Epub ahead of print].

    VEPTR treatment resulted in similar deformity control and thoracic growth in patients younger than 3 years and in those 3 to 6 years of age. Lower complication rates were reported in the older age group. Level of evidence: III.

14. Campbell RM Jr, Smith MD, Mayes TC, et al: The effect of opening wedge thoracostomy on thoracic insufficiency syndrome associated with fused ribs and congenital scoliosis. *J Bone Joint Surg Am* 2004;86(8):1659-1674.

15. Fernandes P, Weinstein SL: Natural history of early onset scoliosis. *J Bone Joint Surg Am* 2007;89(suppl 1):21-33.

16. Mehta MH: The rib-vertebra angle in the early diagnosis between resolving and progressive infantile scoliosis. *J Bone Joint Surg Br* 1972;54(2):230-243.

17. Pahys JM, Samdani AF, Betz RR: Intraspinal anomalies in infantile idiopathic scoliosis: Prevalence and role

of magnetic resonance imaging. *Spine (Phila Pa 1976)* 2009;34(12):E434-E438.

18. Gupta P, Lenke LG, Bridwell KH: Incidence of neural axis abnormalities in infantile and juvenile patients with spinal deformity: Is a magnetic resonance image screening necessary? *Spine (Phila Pa 1976)* 1998;23(2):206-210.

19. Dolan LA, Wright JG, Weinstein SL: Effects of bracing in adolescents with idiopathic scoliosis. *N Engl J Med* 2014;370(7):681.

    Bracing substantially decreased the progression of high-risk curves to the threshold for surgery in patients with AIS. The benefit increased with longer hours of brace wear.

20. Mehta MH: Growth as a corrective force in the early treatment of progressive infantile scoliosis. *J Bone Joint Surg Br* 2005;87(9):1237-1247.

21. Iorio J, Orlando G, Diefenbach C, et al: Serial casting for infantile idiopathic scoliosis: Radiographic outcomes and factors associated with response to treatment. *J Pediatr Orthop* 2015; Sep 22 [Epub ahead of print].

    The authors report on 21 patients with an average age of 2.1 years who underwent serial casting for EOS. The patient's body mass index and age younger than 1.8 years at the initiation of casting were important predictors of success. Level of evidence: IV.

22. Waldron SR, Poe-Kochert C, Son-Hing JP, Thompson GH: Early onset scoliosis: The value of serial Risser casts. *J Pediatr Orthop* 2013;33(8):775-780.

    Serial Risser casting is a safe and effective intermediate treatment of EOS. It can stabilize relatively large curves in young children and allows the child to reach a more suitable age for other forms of treatment. Level of evidence: IV.

23. McCarthy RE, McCullough FL: Shilla growth guidance for early-onset scoliosis: Results after a minimum of five years of follow-up. *J Bone Joint Surg Am* 2015;97(19):1578-1584.

    This study presents a 5-year follow-up evaluation of 40 patients with EOS treated with SHILLA growth guidance. The complication rate was high (73%), but acceptable. The authors concluded that children with a wide variety of diagnoses can be safely treated with the SHILLA procedure.

24. Jain V, Lykissas M, Trobisch P, et al: Surgical aspects of spinal growth modulation in scoliosis correction. *Instr Course Lect* 2014;63:335-344.

    Spinal growth modulation for scoliosis correction is a technique for slowing growth on the convex side of the curve and enhancing growth on the concave side by using the Heuter-Volkmann principle. The authors review current available techniques.

25. Hickey BA, Towriss C, Baxter G, et al: Early experience of MAGEC magnetic growing rods in the treatment of early onset scoliosis. *Eur Spine J* 2014;23(suppl 1):S61-S65.

    The MAGEC growing rod system effectively controls EOS when used as either a primary or revision procedure. Although implant-related complications are common, the avoidance of multiple surgeries after implantation is beneficial.

26. Shah SA, Karatas AF, Dhawale AA, et al; Growing Spine Study Group: The effect of serial growing rod lengthening on the sagittal profile and pelvic parameters in early-onset scoliosis. *Spine (Phila Pa 1976)* 2014;39(22):E1311-E1317.

    This study examined the effect of repeated lengthenings with growing rods on the sagittal and pelvic profile in patients with EOS. Thoracic kyphosis decreased after the index surgery and increased between the index surgery and the latest follow-up, and it was accompanied by an increase in lumbar lordosis. Level of evidence: IV.

27. Yang JS, Sponseller PD, Thompson GH, et al; Growing Spine Study Group: Growing rod fractures: Risk factors and opportunities for prevention. *Spine (Phila Pa 1976)* 2011;36(20):1639-1644.

    Risk factors for rod fractures include prior fracture, single rods, stainless steel rods, small diameter rods, proximity to tandem connectors, short tandem connectors, and preoperative ambulation. Repeat fractures are common, especially with single rods.

28. Flynn JM, Tomlinson LA, Pawelek J, Thompson GH, McCarthy R, Akbarnia BA; Growing Spine Study Group: Growing-rod graduates: Lessons learned from ninety-nine patients who completed lengthening. *J Bone Joint Surg Am* 2013;95(19):1745-1750.

    Most patients in this study who completed treatment with a growing rod underwent rod removal and final instrumented fusion. The final fusion often included the same levels spanned by the growing rods and usually achieved less than 50% in additional correction of the deformity remaining at the end of growing rod management. Level of evidence: IV.

29. Flynn JM, Matsumoto H, Torres F, Ramirez N, Vitale MG: Psychological dysfunction in children who require repetitive surgery for early onset scoliosis. *J Pediatr Orthop* 2012;32(6):594-599.

    Clinicians caring for children with EOS should have a heightened awareness for possible adverse psychological outcomes and should consider early referral for appropriate psychological assessment and care. Additional studies are necessary to further qualify and quantify the psychological effects of multiple anesthesia surgeries. Level of evidence: III.

30. Khorsand D, Song KM, Swanson J, Alessio A, Redding G, Waldhausen J: Iatrogenic radiation exposure to patients with early onset spine and chest wall deformities. *Spine (Phila Pa 1976)* 2013;38(17):E1108-E1114.

    Children managed for thoracic insufficiency syndrome using a consistent protocol received iatrogenic radiation doses that were on average four times the estimated average US background radiation exposure of 3 mSv/yr.

Radiation from CT accounted for 74% of the total dose. Level of evidence: III.

31. Sankar WN, Skaggs DL, Yazici M, et al: Lengthening of dual growing rods and the law of diminishing returns. *Spine (Phila Pa 1976)* 2011;36(10):806-809.

There appears to be a law of diminishing returns with repeated lengthenings with dual growing rods. Repeated lengthenings still result in a net T1-S1 increase; however, this gain tends to decrease with each subsequent lengthening and over time.

32. Kabirian N, Akbarnia BA, Pawelek JB, et al; the Growing Spine Study Group: Deep surgical site infection following 2344 growing-rod procedures for early-onset scoliosis: Risk factors and clinical consequences. *J Bone Joint Surg Am* 2014;96(15):e128. [Epub ahead of print].

The prevalence of deep surgical site infection (7.7%) associated with growing rod surgery is higher than that associated with standard pediatric spinal fusion (historical data). Nonambulatory status, more revisions, and stainless steel implants increased the risk of deep surgical site infection. Level of evidence: IV.

33. Hedequist D, Emans J: Congenital scoliosis: A review and update. *J Pediatr Orthop* 2007;27(1):106-116.

34. McMaster MJ, Ohtsuka K: The natural history of congenital scoliosis: A study of two hundred and fifty-one patients. *J Bone Joint Surg Am* 1982;64(8):1128-1147.

35. Hedequist DJ, Emans JB: The correlation of preoperative three-dimensional computed tomography reconstructions with operative findings in congenital scoliosis. *Spine (Phila Pa 1976)* 2003;28(22):2531-2534, discussion 1.

36. Hedequist DJ, Hall JE, Emans JB: The safety and efficacy of spinal instrumentation in children with congenital spine deformities. *Spine (Phila Pa 1976)* 2004;29(18):2081-2086, discussion 2087.

37. Rinella A, Lenke L, Whitaker C, et al: Perioperative halo-gravity traction in the treatment of severe scoliosis and kyphosis. *Spine (Phila Pa 1976)* 2005;30(4):475-482.

38. Demirkiran G, Dede O, Ayvaz M, Bas CE, Alanay A, Yazici M: Convex instrumented hemiepiphysiodesis with concave distraction: A treatment option for long sweeping congenital curves. *J Pediatr Orthop* 2015; Mar 24 [Epub ahead of print].

Convex instrumented hemiepiphysiodesis with concave distraction resulted in good curve correction while maintaining the growth of the thorax. The correction of the anomalous segment improved over time, proving the effectiveness of the hemiepiphysiodesis.

39. Hedequist D, Emans J, Proctor M: Three rod technique facilitates hemivertebra wedge excision in young children through a posterior only approach. *Spine (Phila Pa 1976)* 2009;34(6):E225-E229.

40. Elsebai HB, Yazici M, Thompson GH, et al: Safety and efficacy of growing rod technique for pediatric congenital spinal deformities. *J Pediatr Orthop* 2011;31(1):1-5.

Growing rods are a safe and effective treatment technique in selected patients with congenital spinal deformities. The deformity, spinal growth, and space available for lungs improved. Level of evidence: IV.

41. Flynn JM, Emans JB, Smith JT, et al: VEPTR to treat nonsyndromic congenital scoliosis: A multicenter, mid-term follow-up study. *J Pediatr Orthop* 2013;33(7):679-684.

A multicenter study of 24 patients demonstrated that VEPTR insertion with expansion thoracoplasty represents a successful treatment paradigm for nonsyndromic congenital spinal deformities. Level of evidence: IV.

42. Sponseller PD, Yazici M, Demetracopoulos C, Emans JB: Evidence basis for management of spine and chest wall deformities in children. *Spine (Phila Pa 1976)* 2007;32(19suppl):S81-S90.

43. Emans JB, Caubet JF, Ordonez CL, Lee EY, Ciarlo M: The treatment of spine and chest wall deformities with fused ribs by expansion thoracostomy and insertion of vertical expandable prosthetic titanium rib: Growth of thoracic spine and improvement of lung volumes. *Spine (Phila Pa 1976)* 2005;30(17suppl):S58-S68.

44. Garg S, LaGreca J, St Hilaire T, et al: Wound complications of vertical expandable prosthetic titanium rib incisions. *Spine (Phila Pa 1976)* 2014;39(13):E777-E781.

The incidence of infection in patients with four or more VEPTR lengthenings was 24% and did not differ across various incision locations. Level of evidence: III.

45. Park HY, Matsumoto H, Feinberg N, et al: The classification for early-onset scoliosis (C-EOS) correlates with the speed of vertical expandable prosthetic titanium rib (VEPTR) proximal anchor failure. *J Pediatr Orthop* 2015; Nov 13 [Epub ahead of print].

Analyzing C-EOS classes with more than three individuals, survival analysis demonstrated that the C-EOS discriminates low-, medium-, and high-speed VEPTR anchor failure. This supports the validity of the C-EOS and its potential use in guiding decision making. Level of evidence: III.

46. El-Hawary R, Sturm P, Cahill P, et al: What is the risk of developing proximal junctional kyphosis during growth friendly treatments for early-onset scoliosis? *J Pediatr Orthop* 2015; Jul 17 [Epub ahead of print].

The risk of developing proximal junctional kyphosis during distraction-based, growth-friendly treatment of EOS was 20% immediately after implantation and 28% at a minimum 2-year follow-up, with no difference observed between rib-based and spine-based treatment groups. Level of evidence: III.

Chapter 29

Adolescent Idiopathic Scoliosis

Matthew E. Oetgen, MD, MBA   Benjamin D. Martin, MD

Abstract

Adolescent idiopathic scoliosis is a three-dimensional deformity of the spine affecting approximately 2% to 3% of children. Treatment goals are aimed at minimizing patient deformity and maximizing functional outcome throughout life. The risk of progression of scoliosis is affected by the magnitude of the deformity and growth potential, with younger children and larger deformities at higher risk of progression. Traditional treatment options include observation, brace treatment, and surgical intervention consisting of spinal fusion. More recent alternative treatments, such as scoliosis-specific physical therapy protocols and motion-preserving growth modulation surgery, are generating increasing interest from the public and the medical community. Although surgical techniques have evolved over time with more powerful correction ability, limited data exist regarding the changes in functional and patient-reported health-related outcomes associated with these changes in surgical technique. Future investigation into the outcomes of patients with adolescent idiopathic scoliosis will be important to determine the optimal cost-benefit decisions for nonsurgical and surgical treatment of this disease.

Keywords: adolescent idiopathic scoliosis; nonsurgical treatment; spinal fusion

Dr. Oetgen or an immediate family member serves as a board member, owner, officer, or committee member of the American Academy of Orthopaedic Surgeons, the Pediatric Orthopaedic Society of North America, and the Scoliosis Research Society. Dr. Martin or an immediate family member serves as a board member, owner, officer, or committee member of the Pediatric Orthopaedic Society of North America and the United States Bone and Joint Initiative.

Introduction

Adolescent idiopathic scoliosis (AIS) is a three-dimensional deformity of the spine with a coronal curve magnitude of greater than 10°. Although the deviation in the coronal plane was traditionally the focus of this disease, more recently, the importance of the three dimensional aspect of scoliosis has been realized, and the deformities in the sagittal and axial planes also have been recognized.[1,2] In the sagittal plane, there is often a loss of kyphosis that produces a relative "hypokyphotic" sagittal alignment. In the axial plane, there is substantial deformity with maximal rotation of the apical vertebral body toward the coronal deformity. Taken together, these spinal malalignments produce the typical appearance of AIS.

Classification

The most basic classification system for AIS is a simple descriptive system indicating the location of the deformity (cervicothoracic, thoracic, thoracolumbar, or lumbar) and the magnitude of the deformity. A more structured classification system based on the radiographic description of the curve location introduced in 1983 by King and Moe sought to determine when selective thoracic instrumentation was warranted by dividing thoracic curves into five types. However, because of some shortcomings in the King-Moe system, a more robust (and more complex) classification system was developed by Lenke and colleagues in 1997. In an attempt to improve surgical planning, the Lenke system focuses mainly on surgically treatable scoliosis deformities.

The Lenke classification of AIS consists of six main categories defined by the location of the major spinal deformity (defined as the largest magnitude curve) and the location of any compensatory spinal deformities (defined as a curve with less than 25° of residual magnitude on bending radiographs).[3] In addition, the classification contains two modifiers: one for the lumbar curvature and one for the sagittal plane deformity (**Figure 1**). This system allows for reproducible categorization of AIS and helps in surgical decision making.[4] Using the Lenke classification, the most common location of spinal deformity in patients

Curve Type	Proximal Thoracic	Main Thoracic	Thoracolumbar/Lumbar	Description
1	Nonstructural	Structural[a]	Nonstructural	Main thoracic (MT)
2	Structural[†]	Structural[a]	Nonstructural	Double thoracic (DT)
3	Nonstructural	Structural[a]	Structural[b]	Double major (DM)
4	Structural[†]	Structural[c]	Structural[c]	Triple major (TM)
5	Nonstructural	Nonstructural	Structural[a]	Thoracolumbar/lumbar (TL/L)
6	Nonstructural	Structural[b]	Structural[a]	Thoracolumbar/lumbar–main thoracic (TL/L-MT)

[a]Major curve: largest Cobb measurement, always structural [b]Minor curve: remaining structural curves [c]Type 4: MT or TL/L can be the major curve.

Structural Criteria
(Minor curves)

Proximal thoracic - Side-bending Cobb angle ≥25°
- T2-T5 kyphosis ≥+20°

Main thoracic - Side-bending Cobb angle ≥25°
- T10-L2 kyphosis ≥+20°

Thoracolumbar/lumbar - Side-bending Cobb angle ≥25°
- T10-L2 kyphosis ≥+20°

Location of Apex
(Scoliosis Research Society definition)

Curve	Apex
Thoracic	T2 to T11-12 disk
Thoracolumbar	T12-L1
Lumbar	L1-2 disk to L4

Modifiers

Lumbar Coronal Modifier	Center Sacral Vertical Line to Lumbar Apex
A	Between pedicles
B	Touches apical body(ies)
C	Completely medial

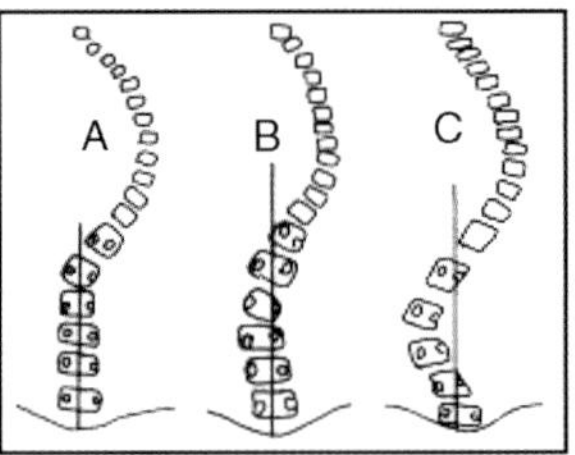

Thoracic Sagittal Profile (T5-T12)	
Modifier	Cobb Angle
– (hypo)	<10°
N (normal)	10° - 40°
+ (hyper)	>40°

Curve type (1-6) + Lumbar coronal modifier (A, B, C) + Thoracic sagittal modifier (–, N, +) = curve classification (eg, 1B+): _______

Figure 1 Charts show the Lenke classification system for adolescent idiopathic scoliosis. (Adapted with permission from Lenke LG, Betz RR, Harms J, et al: Adolescent idiopathic scoliosis: A new classification to determine the extent of spinal arthrodesis. *J Bone Joint SurgAm* 2001;83(8):1169-1181.)

with AIS is in the thoracic spine, with approximately 60% of deformities located in this region.[5]

Treatment Concepts

The treatment goals of AIS are the prevention of spinal deformity progression and the avoidance of physical impairment, pain, and disfigurement. The flexibility and movement of the spine should be maximized over time, and malalignment should be avoided because it can lead to future spondylotic degeneration. Traditionally, there are three mainstays of treatment of scoliosis depending on the age and skeletal maturity or growth potential of a patient. In patients with substantial remaining growth, observation of the spinal deformity is indicated when the deformity is less than 20°, a spinal orthotic is used to decrease progression when the deformity is between 20° and 45°, and surgery is indicated for progressive deformities with magnitudes greater than 50°. Patients with little growth remaining or those who have reached skeletal maturity are typically not candidates for brace treatment, so observation and reassurance are indicated unless the deformity is greater than 50°, at which point surgical intervention should be considered. Although these are the traditional methods of treatment, this general algorithm has developed with little understanding of the long-term repercussions and natural history of untreated scoliosis. As more focus is placed on objective measures of patient health as they relate to scoliosis (such as pulmonary function) and data regarding patient-reported outcomes become available, there will likely be important changes in these traditional treatment plans.

Alternative nonsurgical treatment modalities have been suggested to prevent scoliosis progression and, in some instances, to decrease the deformity; however, there is little evidence to support these treatments. Numerous physical therapy methods and protocols have been designed to prevent and reverse spinal deformity; however, few scientific data exist to support these treatment modalities compared with nature history.[6] Caution is indicated, however, when assessing the role of physical therapy in the treatment of scoliosis, because a lack of evidence should not necessarily be taken to indicate a lack of effectiveness. Further investigations into the role of scoliosis-specific exercises are warranted and should include well-controlled, scientifically rigorous studies. Only when additional data are obtained can a clearer picture of the effectiveness and potential indications for this treatment be determined. The treatment of spinal deformity with chiropractic manipulation, electrical stimulation, and traction have all been investigated, but there is no evidence to support their efficacy.[7]

Etiology

A variety of possible pathogenetic factors have been suggested to explain AIS, including factors related to genetic susceptibility, biomechanics, and neurologic control of the body.[8] The underlying causes of AIS are being elucidated through experimental research. Population-based genetic studies comparing patients with idiopathic scoliosis to control subjects have identified DNA sequence variations that are associated with disease susceptibility. Such genome-wide association studies have effectively implicated several candidate genes and the biochemical functions of their encoded proteins in AIS. These genes include *CHL1*, *DSCAM*, and *CNTNAP2*, which participate in axon guidance;[9] *LBX1* and *PAX1*, which are important in muscle and spine pattern formation;[10-12] and *GPR126*, which is important in various processes such as myelination and disk chondrogenesis.[13] Importantly, *LBX1*, *PAX1*, and *GPR126* have been associated with AIS in both Asian and non-Hispanic white populations, and *PAX1* is specifically associated in females but not males, providing a first clue to the female prevalence of this disease. A recent gene-targeting study in which *GPR126* was specifically removed from chondrocytes produced an idiopathic scoliosis in a mouse.[14] This is the first report of a genetically defined mouse model for AIS and opens the way for mechanistic studies to define its etiology. Although AIS is likely a multifactorial condition as opposed to being caused by a single gene,[15] continued genomic investigations of AIS using new and advanced techniques show promise for further understanding of this condition.

There appears to be evidence for inheritance of this disorder, with an increased prevalence in future generations, but the penetrance of scoliosis is variable. There is a relationship between AIS and sex, with an equal prevalence between males and females for small curves and an increasing prevalence of deformity in females as curve magnitude increases.

The prevalence of AIS has remained relatively constant over time, and it is present in approximately 2% of children aged 10 to 14 years. In this affected population, approximately 10% have progressive deformities of more than 20°, and 0.1% have deformities that progress to more than 50°.[16]

Progression of this disease is known to be affected by patient growth. In general, as the patient grows, there is a risk of spinal deformity progression, with the highest risk during the time of most rapid growth. Various clinical markers are used to assess growth and the risk of deformity progression. The Risser sign is a classic marker for skeletal maturity and is defined as the radiographic ossification of the iliac apophysis. This apophysis progressively ossifies from anterior to posterior and is graded from 0 (no ossification) to 5 (a fully fused apophysis), with interval measurements based on the progression of the appearance of the apophysis from anterior to posterior. The menarchal status in females is another marker used to indicate growth potential, although this has variable predictive ability in regards to growth remaining. Menarche typically occurs following the peak height velocity, but the growth potential following the start of menarche is quite variable and ranges from 2.5 years to no growth remaining.

The peak height velocity, which is defined as the maximum change in skeletal growth of a child over time, also can be used to assess skeletal growth. The peak height velocity is reported to be approximately 8 cm per year for girls and 9.5 cm per year for boys. Although these markers are useful, many are not apparent until after the peak height velocity has occurred, which limits their usefulness during the time of maximal risk of deformity progression.[17] Evaluation of the skeletal maturation of the hand has been investigated and is suggested to be a better marker for growth velocity and the risk of scoliosis progression.[18]

Natural History

After an adolescent reaches skeletal maturity, the natural history of scoliosis appears to be dependent on the magnitude of the deformity. A study at the University of Iowa reported little deformity progression over time if the curvature was less than 30° at skeletal maturity and a maximal risk of progression of deformity with curvatures greater than 50° at the time of skeletal maturity.[19] In a study consisting of 102 patients with an average follow-up o 40 years, the authors reported that the average progression of deformity over the follow-up period was 2.6° for thoracic curves of less than 30° at skeletal maturity, 10.2° for thoracic curves 30° to 50° at skeletal maturity, and 29.4° for curves 50° to 75° at skeletal maturity.[20] This pattern was also found in lumbar curves, with an average progression of 0°, 15.4°, and 18.5° for those curves measuring less than 30°, 30° to 50°, and 50° to 75° at skeletal maturity, respectively.

Based on the University of Iowa data, recommendations for surgery have evolved, with a general indication for surgery being a deformity greater than 50° because of the risk of progressive deformity into adulthood. Outcomes for patients with curves between 30° and 50° at skeletal maturity appear to be dependent on the location of the deformity, with lumbar curves being at increased risk for progression compared with thoracic curves.

More recent long-term data has focused on the clinical and radiographic outcomes of AIS. These data suggest the clinical effect of slowly progressing thoracic scoliosis continuing into adulthood may not be as important as originally suspected.[21] In addition, even moderate progression of smaller magnitude lumbar scoliosis into adulthood may be associated with more negative functional outcomes, such as increasing back pain, than previously believed. Despite this lack of data, there may be as yet unappreciated physiologic consequences of untreated thoracic scoliosis. A 2011 study reported that up to 19% of patients with AIS have moderately impaired pulmonary function (<65% predicted forced expiratory volume in 1 second) preoperatively, with those patients with this moderate pulmonary dysfunction having a mean thoracic curve magnitude of 70°.[22] The authors concluded that, given the normally accepted age-related decline in pulmonary function, these patients are at substantial risk for serious pulmonary morbidity. Specific investigation of the changes in pulmonary function in this patient population after surgical intervention are needed.

Investigation of long-term functional outcomes (as defined by physiologic, psychological, and appearance-related patient-reported outcome measures) of various-sized AIS deformities at the time of skeletal maturity is needed to help redefine treatment algorithms during the adolescent period. In the absence of these data, current treatment algorithms are based on the skeletal maturity of the patient and the magnitude of the deformity, as was previously discussed.

Given the lack of clear data regarding the long-term health risks of slowly progressive scoliosis through adulthood, it is worth reassessing the decision-making process in regards to surgical correction of this deformity. Although there is evidence that larger deformities will progress, an absolute correlation with decreased health is lacking. Other factors such as the risk of back pain, functional disability, and the disfiguring effects of spinal deformity must also factor into the decision for surgical correction; however, these factors may have different weights in different individuals. As such, the decision to proceed with surgical correction of scoliosis should ultimately be made in a shared-decision process with the physician providing the current knowledge of the long-term outcomes of both surgical intervention and observation and the patient and patient's family providing their preference for treatment.

Diagnosis and Presentation

AIS is often discovered by primary care physicians during a yearly well-child evaluation. The Adams forward bend test is the most common assessment test in this setting. The test is performed by having the patient bend forward at the waist until the back is horizontal to the ground. Spinal deformity is assessed by looking for asymmetry of the back, with an elevation of one side suggestive of the axial plane trunk deformity commonly seen in AIS (**Figure 2**). Use of a scoliometer adds a quantitative element to this examination, with varying suggestions regarding the threshold of rotational deformity that should trigger an orthopaedic referral. A threshold scoliometer value of 7° appears to be a suitable measurement to avoid missing deformities that could be braced and to limit unnecessary referrals.[23] Digital measurement of trunk rotation with a smart phone is possible using a scoliometer application and has been shown to be as accurate as classic scoliometer measurements in a recent comparison.[24]

The cost versus benefit effectiveness of routine school-based scoliosis screening programs is controversial. Originally started as a program to detect spinal deformity associated with tuberculosis and polio, screening programs became increasingly recommended in the United States, with 21 states mandating screening and an additional 12 recommending screening as of 2003. However, the US Preventive Services Task Force published a recommendation in 2004 against routine school-based scoliosis screening because of the ineffectiveness of these programs. Since that recommendation was made, several states have reversed their recommendation for routine school-based screenings. Given the recent findings on the effectiveness of bracing for scoliosis to prevent progressive spinal deformity, renewed interest in school screening programs for scoliosis has been demonstrated, and the Pediatric Orthopaedic Society of North America, the Scoliosis Research Society (SRS), and the American

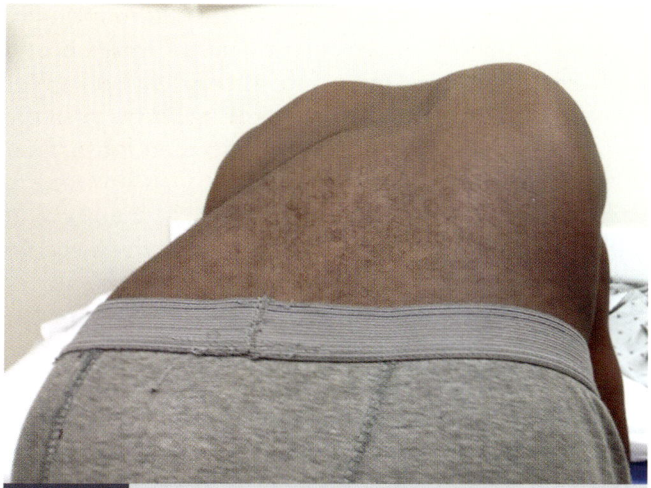

Figure 2 Clinical photograph of a patient with adolescent idiopathic scoliosis performing the Adam forward bend test. Note the rotational trunk deformity indicated by the asymmetry of the ribs, with the right rib cage being more prominent than the left.

Academy of Pediatrics have declared joint support for these programs.[25]

Physical Examination

Examination of a child with suspected idiopathic scoliosis is performed to define the appearance of the deformity and assess for signs of nonidiopathic scoliosis. Because AIS is a diagnosis of exclusion, other causes of spinal deformity must be ruled out through examination and imaging findings. The patient should be clothed in an examination gown to allow full assessment. Inspection of the skin is important to identify cutaneous stigmata of other diseases, specifically café-au-lait spots, sacral dimples, or hairy patches overlying the spine. Careful inspection of the entire patient, including the limbs, should be performed to look for subtle examination findings that may be associated with scoliosis-associated syndromes such as arachnodactyly and Marfan syndrome. With the patient standing, the shoulders, the pelvis, and trunk symmetry should be assessed and overall alignment documented. The Adams forward bend test is used to document axial plane trunk rotation, and gait assessment is important to document subtle neurologic deficits or muscle weakness. A full neurologic assessment of the upper and lower extremities is required, with documentation of the strength and sensation of all nerve root distributions as well as a complete reflex examination, including the presence of symmetric abdominal reflexes, which, if abnormal, can indicate associated intraspinal abnormalities.

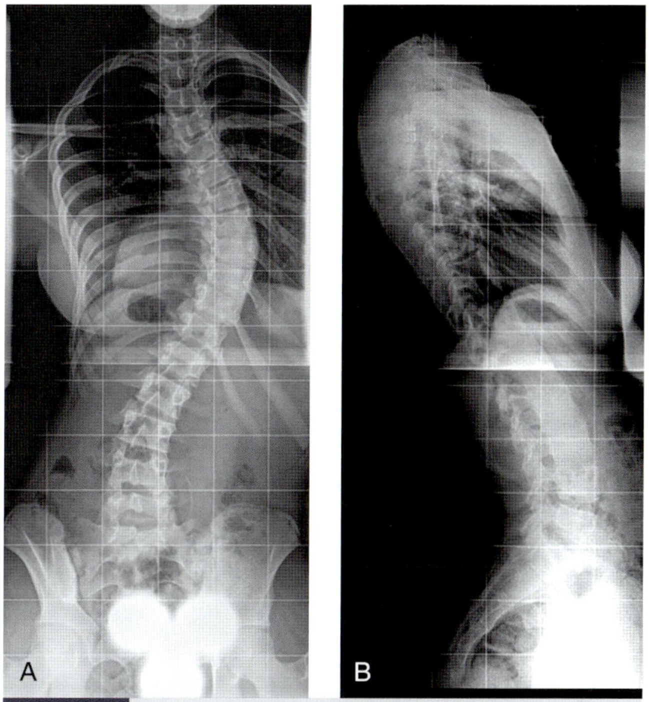

Figure 3 Appropriate full-length PA (**A**) and lateral (**B**) radiographs are used in the assessment of idiopathic scoliosis. A 55° right thoracic curve is shown.

Imaging

Radiographic assessment of patients with suspected spinal deformity should start with PA and lateral radiographs performed on a full-length (36 × 14 inch) cassette in the standing position (**Figure 3**). Appropriate breast and gonadal shielding should be used to limit radiation exposure to these radiosensitive areas. Recent concerns regarding the cumulative effects of radiation exposure in immature patients and the future risk of malignancy has led to advances in lower dose imaging modalities. Digital radiography is the current standard in radiographic imaging because it leads to a substantial decrease in radiation exposure.[26] A recently introduced, novel imaging system using biplanar digital slot scanning substantially further decreases radiation exposure compared with traditional digital radiography, with no difference in image quality.[27] Nonradiation-based imaging systems such as surface imaging and ultrasound have been assessed, but their use is limited.

MRI is used to assess the spinal cord for evidence of intraspinal abnormalities in patients with abnormal physical examination findings or, occasionally, for patients with substantial scoliosis-related pain. Routine evaluation of the spinal cord using MRI before surgical intervention in patients with normal physical examination or radiographic findings is a debated issue. Proponents of routine MRI point to the fact that the incidence of intraspinal abnormality in patients with suspected AIS can be up to 10%; however, others physicians argue that very few cases of intraspinal abnormality require neurosurgical intervention before spinal deformity correction, thus demonstrating the limited clinical effect of routine MRI evaluation.[28,29] Some findings, including limited axial plane rotation, abnormal reflexes on examination, lack of thoracic hypokyphosis, atypical curve direction (left thoracic or right thoracolumbar/lumbar), rapid deformity progression, and substantial back or radicular pain, warrant further investigation of the spine with MRI to assess for associated causative intraspinal abnormalities.

Treatment

Prediction

Treatment decisions for those with AIS are based mainly on the maturity of the patient and the size of the curve. Immature patients with substantial remaining growth have a higher risk of curve progression than more mature patients with the same size curve. Curve magnitude, in the context of maturity, is important in the decision-making process. Curve magnitudes greater than 20° have approximately a threefold increased risk of progression compared with curves less than 20° in patients with Risser grade 0, 1, or 2 skeletal maturity.[30]

Several genetic markers of AIS have been identified. Currently, there is only one commercial test available that attempts to stratify patients for progression risk.[31,32] Although promising in theory, clinical investigation of this test has been disappointing, with little evidence to confirm that it can predict progressive curves in the at-risk cohort of children.

Observation

Observation is indicated for curves of less than 20° because of the relatively low risk of progression. Examination of skeletally immature children at 4- to 6-month intervals allows active treatment to be initiated when progression becomes clear. The exact definition of progression varies slightly among authors, but it is generally accepted that an increase greater than 5° is outside the range of interobserver and intraobserver measurement error. Despite this generally accepted value of progression, clinicians should be mindful of the long-term changes in scoliosis magnitude because single measurements have been shown to be variable. Diurnal variations in the Cobb angle have been shown to be up to 5°, so decisions regarding treatment based on curve progression should be made based on a broader deformity evaluation.[33]

Bracing

Bracing is the mainstay of nonsurgical treatment of scoliosis. The SRS criteria for bracing are curves 25° to 45° in patients who are Risser grade 0, 1, or 2 and less than 1 year postmenarchal if female. Recently, a randomized controlled study reported that bracing was successful at avoiding progression past 50° in 72% of patients, compared with 48% of patients who were observed only.[34] The study was stopped early because of the clearly superior efficacy of bracing compared with observation. The number of hours of brace wear is important to success, with those wearing the brace more than 12 hours per day having a greater than 80% chance of avoiding curve progression.[34,35] Treating approximately three patients with bracing will avoid one surgical procedure,[34,36] assuming that the patients are compliant with bracing protocols. Compliance is the main impediment to successful treatment. Most current studies use compliance monitors inside the brace to accurately measure time in the brace. These monitors are mainly used for research but are relatively inexpensive and are being adopted in clinical practices to monitor patient compliance.

A thoracolumbosacral orthosis is generally prescribed for treatment and is intended to be a full-time brace. As previously noted, the total number of hours of brace wear influences success. Bracing is not effective for curves with an apex above T7.

The Charleston or Providence nighttime braces are bending braces that are used as an alternative to a full-time thoracolumbosacral orthosis. The goal of this type of nighttime brace is to create opposing forces about the apex of the curve and push it toward the midline or past it. Although data exist demonstrating their effectiveness, current high-level studies comparing these two bracing techniques are lacking.

A dynamic, flexible brace was developed as an alternative to rigid braces. The goal of the SpineCor brace (The Spine Corporation) is to use neurologic feedback to rebalance abnormal muscles to prevent progression. A prospective, randomized controlled study indicated a higher rate of progression in patients treated in the SpineCor brace compared with rigid bracing.[37]

After patients have adapted to their brace, a radiograph is taken with the patient in the brace to evaluate brace quality. Ideally, a thoracolumbosacral orthosis will reduce the curve approximately 50%, whereas a nighttime brace will achieve closer to 80% to 90% curve correction. Children are monitored every 6 months, usually with a radiograph taken when out of the brace, to evaluate for progression. Bracing in females is discontinued approximately 18 to 24 months after menarche when the patient is at Risser grade 4 or when growth has plateaued. Because males often continue to grow after Risser grade 4, height gain should be followed to determine when bracing should be discontinued.[38] Most physicians agree that bracing has substantial effects on both the patient and his or her family; however, there are limited data evaluating the extent of the psychological effect.[39]

Surgery

For adolescents presenting with curves greater than 50° or curves progressing past 45° in immature patients, posterior spinal fusion is recommended. Curves of this magnitude tend to progress 1° per year even after skeletal maturity.[20] The primary goal of surgery is to prevent further progression by obtaining fusion while maintaining spinal balance in the coronal and sagittal planes. Secondary goals include decreasing the size of the curve and reducing the associated deformities such as trunk shift, waist asymmetry, shoulder height differences, and rotational prominences on the back. As few motion segments as necessary should be fused to achieve these goals.

The Lenke classification provides guidance on the selection of fusion levels in the surgical treatment of AIS.[3] As opposed to the classic King-Moe classification, the Lenke classification includes curves with the major component in the thoracolumbar and lumbar spine and highlights the importance of the sagittal plane. The classification includes 6 curve types, 3 lumbar modifiers, and 3 sagittal modifiers, resulting in 42 different possible patterns. Supine bending films are required to use the classification system to distinguish structural (curves that do not bend out to <25°) from nonstructural curves (curve that bend out to <25°). Despite the purpose of the Lenke classification in regards to standardizing surgical planning, controversy still exists in regards to which curves require fusion, the exact choice of fusion levels, and the appropriateness of fusing into the lower lumbar spine.

The most common curve patterns are Lenke types 1A and 1B. For these curves, the upper instrumented vertebra is typically the proximal end vertebra (often T4) (**Figure 4**). The choice of the lowest instrumented vertebra is not as clear, but the lowest vertebra that is substantially touched by the center sacral vertical line is commonly the lowest instrumented vertebra. If the proximal thoracic curve is structural (Lenke type 2), the left shoulder is elevated, or there is kyphosis greater than 20° from T2 through T5, then T2 or T3 should be considered for the upper instrumented vertebra because this allows correction of the structural upper thoracic curve, which theoretically improves the ability to level the upper thoracic vertebrae with the goal of improving shoulder balance. Thoracolumbar and lumbar curves (Lenke type 5) are typically fused from the proximal end vertebra to the distal end vertebra.

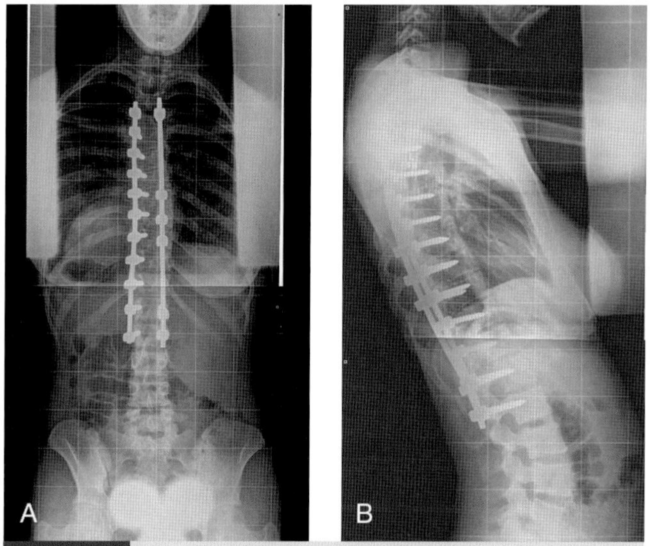

Figure 4 PA (**A**) and lateral (**B**) radiographs of the patient shown in Figure 3 taken 2 years after a T4-L2 posterior spinal fusion for adolescent idiopathic scoliosis shows correction of the deformity from 55° preoperatively to 14° postoperatively.

Selective thoracic fusions are appealing for the preservation of lumbar motion. Having more available motion segments in the lumbar spine after fusion will allow for greater distribution of functional motion.[40] In addition, it seems intuitive that a curved, flexible spine offers a better long-term outcome than a straight, fused spine. However, there is no definitive connection between long fusions and symptomatic distal facet or disk degeneration. Historically, selective thoracic fusions were used for King-Moe type II curves in which the lumbar curve was considered compensatory. Lenke type 1B and 1C patterns include these curve types. Spontaneous lumbar correction occurs with correction of the thoracic curve.[41] However, over time, the use of selective thoracic fusion has evolved to include Lenke type 3C curves.[42,43]

Commonly used criteria for selective fusion include a thoracic-to-lumbar curve magnitude ratio greater than 1.2, an apical vertebral translation ratio greater than 1.2, and a preoperative lumbar curve less than 45°[42] (**Figure 5**). In a 20-year follow-up study that included Lenke type 1B, 1C, and 3C curves, lumbar curve correction and overall balance was maintained over time; however, the patients had lower scores in self-image on the SRS-24 questionnaire compared with patients treated with fusions that included the lumbar spine.[44] Specifically, for Lenke type 3C patterns, patients with long fusions tend to have better balance and radiographic parameters than patients treated with selective fusions at 2-year follow-ups;[43] however, concerns remain about long-term function as patients age.

Most spinal fusions are now performed using a posterior approach. Historically, lumbar and thoracolumbar curves were approached anteriorly to decrease the number of levels needed to obtain correction. The use of pedicle screws that provide three-column fixation combined with wide posterior releases allow the posterior approach to provide similar radiographic outcomes as achieved with the anterior approach.[45,46]

Pedicle screws have become the standard implant for AIS correction because they provide more control of the vertebral body, allow for better three-dimensional correction, increase the strength of the construct, and are helpful in avoiding entry into the spinal canal. However, the cost of pedicle screws is substantially higher than other implants. Although radiographic correction may be better than with hybrid constructs, no study has shown a difference in patient outcomes. Given that the costs of modern implants approaches 30% of the total cost for primary AIS surgical care,[47] there is interest in determining the clinical difference between implants with high- and low-density constructs.[48,49] More research is needed to better understand the appropriate balance between cost, implant density, curve correction, and clinical outcomes.

An ideal treatment of AIS would allow for curve correction without sacrificing motion. Anterior vertebral body tethering is a new technique that strives to achieve this goal.[50] The two-year results of 11 patients with Lenke type 1 curves treated with anterior vertebral body tethering were recently published.[51] In the first five patients the tethers were placed through an open approach, and in the remaining six patients the tethers were inserted thoracoscopically. The average Cobb angle improved from 44° to 13° at 2 years. These patients had no substantial change in thoracic kyphosis, but the scoliometer rotation measure improved over time. Currently, there is no consensus on the appropriate indication or physiologic timing for this intervention. More research is needed to better understand the long-term outcomes and potential complications of vertebral body tethering.

The overall complication rate for the surgical treatment of AIS is relatively low.[52] An infection within the first 3 months occurs in approximately 1% of patients and most commonly results from *Staphylococcus aureus*. Late infections may require hardware removal. The risk of spinal cord injury is less than 1%, but the risk is higher in revision settings and if osteotomies are performed.[52] Most spinal cord injuries are thought to be vascular in nature and result from the correction. Pseudarthrosis is uncommon in young, healthy patients undergoing spinal fusion.

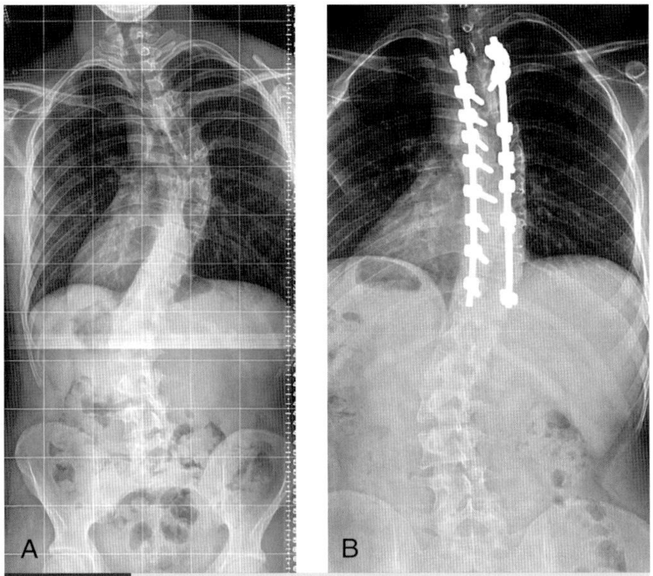

Figure 5 **A,** Preoperative radiograph of a patient with adolescent idiopathic scoliosis with a 55° right thoracic curve and a 45° left lumbar deformity. **B,** PA radiograph taken 3 years after a selective thoracic fusion. The postoperative radiograph show correction of the right thoracic curve to 30° with spontaneous correction of the lumbar deformity to 26°.

Outcomes

Long-term studies investigating the natural history of AIS have demonstrated relatively few functional limitations in patients who were treated only with observation or bracing.[53] In general, these studies have shown that spinal deformities tend to progress but the risk of severe pulmonary or cardiac disease is limited; patients seem to lead functional lives without excessive pain; and social function is normal, with only self-image being consistently lower in patients with scoliosis compared with normal control subjects.[53-56] Although short-term studies have demonstrated improvements in patient-reported outcomes after surgery for AIS, midterm outcome investigations have shown that these results change over time.[57]

Questions remain regarding the incremental improvements in health-related quality of life with modern advancements in surgical techniques. Given the substantial increase in the cost associated with modern surgical interventions,[58] which are mainly associated with modern pedicle screw instrumentation, future studies are critically needed to determine the cost-benefit ratios of nonsurgical and surgical treatment options for AIS using patient-specific health-related outcome measures. The currently used scoliosis-specific patient-reported outcomes measure, the SRS-22, has been assessed and shows variable ability to discriminate between curve magnitudes. Although this tool has shown good discriminative validity between small nonoperative curves and large preoperative curves, this was shown only in a few domains of the tool. In addition, few differences were noted within moderate size curves.[59] This variable discriminative validity of the current scoliosis-specific patient-reported outcomes measure highlights the need for future improvements in the design of these outcomes measures.

Summary

AIS affects approximately 2% to 3% of patients between the ages of 10 and 14 years. Accurate diagnosis and prediction of the likelihood of deformity progression is important to determine optimal treatment strategies. Observation, scoliosis-specific exercises, brace treatment, and surgical intervention may be indicated based on the maturity of the patient and the magnitude of the deformity. Future investigations of patient outcomes after different treatments will be important in optimizing cost-effective treatments.

Key Study Points

- AIS is a three-dimensional spinal deformity producing deviations in the coronal, sagittal, and axial planes, and it affects 2% to 3% of children.
- Treatment of AIS is based on the magnitude of the deformity and the skeletal maturity of the patient. In patients with substantial remaining growth, the basic treatment guidelines are observation for curves less than 20°, brace treatment for curves 20° to 45°, and spinal fusion for curves greater than 50°.
- Long-term studies for patients with untreated AIS have demonstrated relatively few functional differences compared with normal control subjects. Future investigations into the functional benefits of surgery for idiopathic scoliosis using detailed patient-reported health-related outcome tools will be important in optimizing treatment algorithms.

Annotated References

1. Labelle H, Aubin CE, Jackson R, Lenke L, Newton P, Parent S: Seeing the spine in 3D: How will it change what we do? *J Pediatr Orthop* 2011;31(1suppl):S37-S45.

   The authors present a systematic review that assesses the current ability to classify idiopathic scoliosis with a three-dimensional radiographic system. Level of evidence: III.

2. Newton PO, Fujimori T, Doan J, Reighard FG, Bastrom TP, Misaghi A: Defining the "three-dimensional sagittal plane" in thoracic adolescent idiopathic scoliosis. *J Bone Joint Surg Am* 2015;97(20):1694-1701.

   This prospective study of patients with AIS used three-dimensional imaging to assess true segmental axial plane and sagittal plane deformity and correction before and after posterior spinal fusion. Level of evidence: IV.

3. Lenke LG, Betz RR, Harms J, et al: Adolescent idiopathic scoliosis: A new classification to determine extent of spinal arthrodesis. *J Bone Joint Surg Am* 2001;83(8):1169-1181.

4. Richards BS, Sucato DJ, Konigsberg DE, Ouellet JA: Comparison of reliability between the Lenke and King classification systems for adolescent idiopathic scoliosis using radiographs that were not premeasured. *Spine (Phila Pa 1976)* 2003;28(11):1148-1156, discussion 1156-1157.

5. Lenke LG, Betz RR, Clements D, et al: Curve prevalence of a new classification of operative adolescent idiopathic scoliosis: Does classification correlate with treatment? *Spine (Phila Pa 1976)* 2002;27(6):604-611.

6. Romano M, Minozzi S, Bettany-Saltikov J, et al: Exercises for adolescent idiopathic scoliosis. *Cochrane Database Syst Rev* 2012;8:CD007837.

   A systematic review of the effects of physical therapy treatment of AIS found very low-quality studies with little support for treatment of scoliosis with physical therapy. Level of evidence: III.

7. Płaszewski M, Bettany-Saltikov J: Non-surgical interventions for adolescents with idiopathic scoliosis: An overview of systematic reviews. *PLoS One* 2014;9(10):e110254.

   A systematic review of nonsurgical treatment of AIS found little high-quality evidence to support these modalities in the treatment of idiopathic scoliosis. Level of evidence: III.

8. Dayer R, Haumont T, Belaieff W, Lascombes P: Idiopathic scoliosis: Etiological concepts and hypotheses. *J Child Orthop* 2013;7(1):11-16.

   A review of current understanding of etiologic possibilities for idiopathic scoliosis is presented. Level of evidence: V.

9. Sharma S, Gao X, Londono D, et al: Genome-wide association studies of adolescent idiopathic scoliosis suggest candidate susceptibility genes. *Hum Mol Genet* 2011;20(7):1456-1466.

   The authors present a genome-wide association study of approximately 327,000 single nucleotide polymorphisms in 19 families with AIS. They found a possible correlation between axon guidance pathways and AIS susceptibility. Level of evidence: III.

10. Takahashi Y, Kou I, Takahashi A, et al: A genome-wide association study identifies common variants near LBX1 associated with adolescent idiopathic scoliosis. *Nat Genet* 2011;43(12):1237-1240.

A genome-wide association study of 1,376 Japanese female subjects with AIS and 11,297 female control subjects identified a single nucleotide polymorphism on chromosome 10 near *LBX1* associated with AIS susceptibility. Level of evidence: III.

11. Londono D, Kou I, Johnson TA, et al; TSRHC IS Clinical Group; International Consortium for Scoliosis Genetics; Japanese Scoliosis Clinical Research Group: A meta-analysis identifies adolescent idiopathic scoliosis association with LBX1 locus in multiple ethnic groups. *J Med Genet* 2014;51(6):401-406.

    The authors present the results of a meta-analysis of the *LBX1* locus in a number of ethnic groups that was performed to assess the importance of the association of this locus with AIS susceptibility. The authors confirmed the importance of this locus as a major susceptibility locus for AIS in both Asian and non-Hispanic white ethnic groups. Level of evidence: III.

12. Sharma S, Londono D, Eckalbar WL, et al; TSRHC Scoliosis Clinical Group; Japan Scoliosis Clinical Research Group: A PAX1 enhancer locus is associated with susceptibility to idiopathic scoliosis in females. *Nat Commun* 2015;6:6452.

    The authors report on a genome-wide association study in which they found a locus distal to *PAX1* to be associated with scoliosis susceptibility in females but not males from the United States and Japan. Level of evidence: III.

13. Kou I, Takahashi Y, Johnson TA, et al: Genetic variants in GPR126 are associated with adolescent idiopathic scoliosis. *Nat Genet* 2013;45(6):676-679.

    A genome-wide association study of 1,819 Japanese subjects with AIS and 25,939 control subjects identified a new single nucleotide polymorphism on chromosome 6 near *GPR126* associated with AIS susceptibility. Level of evidence: III.

14. Karner CM, Long F, Solnica-Krezel L, Monk KR, Gray RS: Gpr126/Adgrg6 deletion in cartilage models idiopathic scoliosis and pectus excavatum in mice. *Hum Mol Genet* 2015;24(15):4365-4373.

    The authors demonstrate knock-out of *GPR126* in a mouse model resulted in post-natal development of scoliosis and malformation of vertebral bodies. This animal knock-out model suggested loss of function of *GPR126* could be a genetic cause of scoliosis. Level of evidence: III.

15. Gorman KF, Julien C, Moreau A: The genetic epidemiology of idiopathic scoliosis. *Eur Spine J* 2012;21(10):1905-1919.

    The authors present a current review of the genetic associations with idiopathic scoliosis.

16. Negrini S, Aulisa AG, Aulisa L, et al: 2011 SOSORT guidelines: Orthopaedic and rehabilitation treatment of idiopathic scoliosis during growth. *Scoliosis* 2012;7(1):3.

    Current conservative treatments of idiopathic scoliosis are reviewed. Level of evidence: V.

17. Busscher I, Kingma I, de Bruin R, Wapstra FH, Verkerke GJ, Veldhuizen AG: Predicting the peak growth velocity in the individual child: Validation of a new growth model. *Eur Spine J* 2012;21(1):71-76.

    The authors describe a novel mathematical model for demonstrating an accurate method to predict the age and magnitude of the peak height velocity in adolescents. Level of evidence: IV.

18. Sanders JO, Khoury JG, Kishan S, et al: Predicting scoliosis progression from skeletal maturity: A simplified classification during adolescence. *J Bone Joint Surg Am* 2008;90(3):540-553.

19. Weinstein SL, Zavala DC, Ponseti IV: Idiopathic scoliosis: Long-term follow-up and prognosis in untreated patients. *J Bone Joint Surg Am* 1981;63(5):702-712.

20. Weinstein SL, Ponseti IV: Curve progression in idiopathic scoliosis. *J Bone Joint Surg Am* 1983;65(4):447-455.

21. Weinstein SL, Dolan LA, Spratt KF, Peterson KK, Spoonamore MJ, Ponseti IV: Health and function of patients with untreated idiopathic scoliosis: A 50-year natural history study. *JAMA* 2003;289(5):559-567.

22. Johnston CE, Richards BS, Sucato DJ, Bridwell KH, Lenke LG, Erickson M; Spinal Deformity Study Group: Correlation of preoperative deformity magnitude and pulmonary function tests in adolescent idiopathic scoliosis. *Spine (Phila Pa 1976)* 2011;36(14):1096-1102.

    The authors present the results of a study of a large multicenter prospective scoliosis database correlating preoperative pulmonary function to curve magnitude in patients with AIS. The authors found impaired pulmonary function of less than 65% predicted forced expiratory volume in 1 second in those patients with a larger curve magnitude (mean, 70°), worse apical rotation, and hypokyphosis.

23. Korovessis PG, Stamatakis MV: Prediction of scoliotic Cobb angle with the use of the scoliometer. *Spine (Phila Pa 1976)* 1996;21(14):1661-1666.

24. Balg F, Juteau M, Theoret C, Svotelis A, Grenier G: Validity and reliability of the iPhone to measure rib hump in scoliosis. *J Pediatr Orthop* 2014;34(8):774-779.

    This prospective study demonstrated the excellent intraobserver and interobserver reliability and accuracy of the Scoligauge (Ockendon) iPhone (Apple) application for measuring the rib hump in scoliosis. Level of evidence: I.

25. Richards BS, Vitale MG: Screening for idiopathic scoliosis in adolescents: An information statement. *J Bone Joint Surg Am* 2008;90(1):195-198.

26. Grieser T, Baldauf AQ, Ludwig K: Radiation dose reduction in scoliosis patients: Low-dose full-spine radiography with digital flat panel detector and image stitching system. *Rofo* 2011;183(7):645-649.

This cohort study measured the patient radiation dose during spine radiography using digital imaging equipment. The authors reported a substantial reduction in exposure compared with traditional imaging methods. Level of evidence: III.

27. Ilharreborde B, Ferrero E, Alison M, Mazda K: EOS microdose protocol for the radiological follow-up of adolescent idiopathic scoliosis. *Eur Spine J* 2015.

    The authors present a prospective study of the EOS (EOS Imaging) microdose protocol assessing dose exposure and image quality. A substantial decrease in patient radiation dose without image quality degradation was reported. Level of evidence: III.

28. Nakahara D, Yonezawa I, Kobanawa K, et al: Magnetic resonance imaging evaluation of patients with idiopathic scoliosis: A prospective study of four hundred seventy-two outpatients. *Spine (Phila Pa 1976)* 2011;36(7):E482-E485.

    A prospective assessment of 472 consecutive patients with idiopathic scoliosis using MRI is presented. The authors found a rate of 3.8% for neural axis abnormalities. Level of evidence: IV.

29. Richards BS, Sucato DJ, Johnston CE, et al; Spinal Deformity Study Group: Right thoracic curves in presumed adolescent idiopathic scoliosis: Which clinical and radiographic findings correlate with a preoperative abnormal magnetic resonance image? *Spine (Phila Pa 1976)* 2010;35(20):1855-1860.

30. Lonstein JE, Carlson JM: The prediction of curve progression in untreated idiopathic scoliosis during growth. *J Bone Joint Surg Am* 1984;66(7):1061-1071.

31. Ogura Y, Takahashi Y, Kou I, et al: A replication study for association of 5 single nucleotide polymorphisms with curve progression of adolescent idiopathic scoliosis in Japanese patients. *Spine (Phila Pa 1976)* 2013;38(7):571-575.

    The authors report on a genetic determinant of AIS in the Japanese population. Level of evidence: III.

32. Tang QL, Julien C, Eveleigh R, et al: A replication study for association of 53 single nucleotide polymorphisms in ScoliScore test with adolescent idiopathic scoliosis in French-Canadian population. *Spine (Phila Pa 1976)* 2015;40(8):537-543.

    Fifty-two previously identified single nucleotide polymorphisms associated with scoliosis and used in the ScoliScore test were evaluated in a French-Canadian cohort. The authors found none of these single nucleotide polymorphisms were associated with idiopathic scoliosis curve progression or occurrence in this population. Level of evidence: IV.

33. Beauchamp M, Labelle H, Grimard G, Stanciu C, Poitras B, Dansereau J: Diurnal variation of Cobb angle measurement in adolescent idiopathic scoliosis. *Spine (Phila Pa 1976)* 1993;18(12):1581-1583.

34. Weinstein SL, Dolan LA, Wright JG, Dobbs MB: Effects of bracing in adolescents with idiopathic scoliosis. *N Engl J Med* 2013;369(16):1512-1521.

    This randomized, controlled trial investigated the effectiveness of brace treatment for patients with idiopathic scoliosis at risk for progression. The authors found that brace therapy substantially decreased deformity progression. Level of evidence: I.

35. Katz DE, Herring JA, Browne RH, Kelly DM, Birch JG: Brace wear control of curve progression in adolescent idiopathic scoliosis. *J Bone Joint Surg Am* 2010;92(6):1343-1352.

36. Sanders JO, Newton PO, Browne RH, Katz DE, Birch JG, Herring JA: Bracing for idiopathic scoliosis: How many patients require treatment to prevent one surgery? *J Bone Joint Surg Am* 2014;96(8):649-653.

    The authors of this prospective cohort study on the effectiveness of brace treatment of idiopathic scoliosis found that brace treatment was effective at preventing radiographic progression of scoliosis. Brace treatment of three patients led to the avoidance of one surgery. Level of evidence: II.

37. Guo J, Lam TP, Wong MS, et al: A prospective randomized controlled study on the treatment outcome of SpineCor brace versus rigid brace for adolescent idiopathic scoliosis with follow-up according to the SRS standardized criteria. *Eur Spine J* 2014;23(12):2650-2657.

    This randomized controlled trial compared the effectiveness of the SpineCor brace versus a rigid brace for prevention of scoliosis progression. The curve progression rate was found to be substantially higher in the SpineCor group. Level of evidence: I.

38. Karol LA, Johnston CE II, Browne RH, Madison M: Progression of the curve in boys who have idiopathic scoliosis. *J Bone Joint Surg Am* 1993;75(12):1804-1810.

39. Negrini S, Minozzi S, Bettany-Saltikov J, et al: Braces for idiopathic scoliosis in adolescents. *Cochrane Database Syst Rev* 2015;6:CD006850.

    The authors present a systematic review of the effectiveness of brace treatment of AIS. Level of evidence: III.

40. Marks M, Newton PO, Petcharaporn M, et al: Postoperative segmental motion of the unfused spine distal to the fusion in 100 patients with adolescent idiopathic scoliosis. *Spine (Phila Pa 1976)* 2012;37(10):826-832.

    The authors found that preservation of distal unfused levels allowed greater distribution of motion across unfused levels in this prospective study of patients treated with posterior spinal fusion for AIS. Level of evidence: IV.

41. Lenke LG, Betz RR, Bridwell KH, Harms J, Clements DH, Lowe TG: Spontaneous lumbar curve coronal correction after selective anterior or posterior thoracic fusion in adolescent idiopathic scoliosis. *Spine (Phila Pa 1976)* 1999;24(16):1663-1671, discussion 1672.

42. Schulz J, Asghar J, Bastrom T, et al; Harms Study Group: Optimal radiographical criteria after selective thoracic fusion for patients with adolescent idiopathic scoliosis with a C lumbar modifier: Does adherence to current guidelines predict success? *Spine (Phila Pa 1976)* 2014;39(23):E1368-E1373.

The assessment of patients with lumbar modifier C scoliosis who underwent selective thoracic fusion to determine optimal outcomes for this treatment is presented. Optimal treatment goals were determined to be a lumbar Cobb angle less than 26°, coronal balance of 2 cm or less, a deformity-flexibility quotient less than 4, lumbar correction more than 37%, and trunk shift less than 1.5 cm. Level of evidence: IV.

43. Singla A, Bennett JT, Sponseller PD, et al: Results of selective thoracic versus nonselective fusion in Lenke type 3 curves. *Spine (Phila Pa 1976)* 2014;39(24):2034-2041.

The authors present a retrospective comparison of Lenke type 3 deformities treated with selective versus nonselective spinal fusion. Better radiographic results in the nonselective fusion group were reported at the 2-year follow-up. Level of evidence: III.

44. Larson AN, Fletcher ND, Daniel C, Richards BS: Lumbar curve is stable after selective thoracic fusion for adolescent idiopathic scoliosis: A 20-year follow-up. *Spine (Phila Pa 1976)* 2012;37(10):833-839.

The authors present a long-term follow-up study of a cohort of patients who underwent selective thoracic fusion. Results showed stable lumbar curve correction after 20 years. Level of evidence: IV.

45. Geck MJ, Rinella A, Hawthorne D, et al: Comparison of surgical treatment in Lenke 5C adolescent idiopathic scoliosis: Anterior dual rod versus posterior pedicle fixation surgery. A comparison of two practices. *Spine (Phila Pa 1976)* 2009;34(18):1942-1951.

46. Shufflebarger HL, Geck MJ, Clark CE: The posterior approach for lumbar and thoracolumbar adolescent idiopathic scoliosis: Posterior shortening and pedicle screws. *Spine (Phila Pa 1976)* 2004;29(3):269-276, discussion 276.

47. Kamerlink JR, Quirno M, Auerbach JD, et al: Hospital cost analysis of adolescent idiopathic scoliosis correction surgery in 125 consecutive cases. *J Bone Joint Surg Am* 2010;92(5):1097-1104.

48. Bharucha NJ, Lonner BS, Auerbach JD, Kean KE, Trobisch PD: Low-density versus high-density thoracic pedicle screw constructs in adolescent idiopathic scoliosis: Do more screws lead to a better outcome? *Spine J* 2013;13(4):375-381.

A retrospective study of 91 Lenke type 1 curves treated with low-density versus high-density screw constructs found that radiographic results at an average of 2 years after surgery showed no difference between the groups. Level of evidence: III.

49. Larson AN, Polly DW Jr, Diamond B, et al; Minimize Implants Maximize Outcomes Study Group: Does higher anchor density result in increased curve correction and improved clinical outcomes in adolescent idiopathic scoliosis? *Spine (Phila Pa 1976)* 2014;39(7):571-578.

A retrospective study of 521 Lenke type 1, 2, and 5 curves treated with low-density versus high-density screw constructs found that patients with the high-density constructs showed improved deformity correction and had small but better patient-reported outcomes compared with those treated with the low-density constructs. Level of evidence: III.

50. Samdani AF, Ames RJ, Kimball JS, et al: Anterior vertebral body tethering for immature adolescent idiopathic scoliosis: One-year results on the first 32 patients. *Eur Spine J* 2015;24(7):1533-1539.

The authors present the 1-year results of a cohort of patients treated with anterior thoracic tethering. This study demonstrated improvements in the deformities with few complications. Level of evidence: IV.

51. Samdani AF, Ames RJ, Kimball JS, et al: Anterior vertebral body tethering for idiopathic scoliosis: Two-year results. *Spine (Phila Pa 1976)* 2014;39(20):1688-1693.

The authors report the 2-year follow-up data on 11 patients treated with anterior vertebral body tethering. At 2 years, the average thoracic curve correction was 70%. Two patients needed revision surgery to loosen the tether to prevent overcorrection. Level of evidence: IV.

52. Reames DL, Smith JS, Fu KM, et al; Scoliosis Research Society Morbidity and Mortality Committee: Complications in the surgical treatment of 19,360 cases of pediatric scoliosis: A review of the Scoliosis Research Society Morbidity and Mortality database. *Spine (Phila Pa 1976)* 2011;36(18):1484-1491.

The authors report on the SRS morbidity and mortality data for pediatric scoliosis. Level of evidence: IV.

53. Danielsson AJ, Hasserius R, Ohlin A, Nachemson AL: Health-related quality of life in untreated versus brace-treated patients with adolescent idiopathic scoliosis: A long-term follow-up. *Spine (Phila Pa 1976)* 2010;35(2):199-205.

54. Simony A, Hansen EJ, Carreon LY, Christensen SB, Andersen MO: Health-related quality-of-life in adolescent idiopathic scoliosis patients 25 years after treatment. *Scoliosis* 2015;10:22.

At the 25-year follow-up of a group of patients treated with a brace or Harrington instrumentation for scoliosis, no differences were noted in health-related quality of life between either of the treatment groups and age-matched, normal control subjects. Level of evidence: II.

55. Rushton PR, Grevitt MP: Comparison of untreated adolescent idiopathic scoliosis with normal controls: A review and statistical analysis of the literature. *Spine (Phila Pa 1976)* 2013;38(9):778-785.

A meta-analysis of studies reporting health-related quality of life for patients treated for scoliosis found pain and self-image scores were lower in scoliosis patients compared with normal control subjects. Level of evidence: III.

56. Danielsson AJ: Natural history of adolescent idiopathic scoliosis: A tool for guidance in decision of surgery of curves above 50°. *J Child Orthop* 2013;7(1):37-41.

A review of the natural history of patients with scoliosis greater the 50° is presented. Level of evidence: Level of evidence: V.

57. Ghandehari H, Mahabadi MA, Mahdavi SM, Shahsavaripour A, Seyed Tari HV, Safdari F: Evaluation of patient outcome and satisfaction after surgical treatment of adolescent idiopathic scoliosis using Scoliosis Research Society-30. *Arch Bone Jt Surg* 2015;3(2):109-113.

The authors present a prospective cohort study of 135 patients treated with posterior spinal fusion for AIS. Preoperative and postoperative SRS-30 questionnaires were recorded and the authors found postoperative improvements in the self-reported scores. A positive correlation between reported outcome and radiographic correction was noted. Level of evidence: III.

58. Martin CT, Pugely AJ, Gao Y, et al: Increasing hospital charges for adolescent idiopathic scoliosis in the United States. *Spine (Phila Pa 1976)* 2014;39(20):1676-1682.

The results of an investigation into the hospital charges associated with posterior spinal fusion for AIS are reported. The authors found a rising cost for posterior spinal fusion despite a stable volume of procedures. The biggest contributor to increasing costs was the cost of the implants. Level of evidence: IV.

59. Berliner JL, Verma K, Lonner BS, Penn PU, Bharucha NJ: Discriminative validity of the Scoliosis Research Society 22 questionnaire among five curve-severity subgroups of adolescents with idiopathic scoliosis. *Spine J* 2013;13(2):127-133.

The authors present a retrospective review of the ability of the SRS-22 questionnaire to differentiate between patients with different curve magnitudes. The authors found the SRS-22 to be able to discriminate between small magnitude curves and large magnitude curves, but there was little discriminative validity between groups with small curve magnitude differences.

Chapter 30

Neuromuscular Spine Deformity

Amanda T. Whitaker, MD Brian Snyder, MD, PhD

Abstract

Spinal deformity (scoliosis and/or kyphosis) commonly affects children with neuromuscular maladies such as cerebral palsy, muscular dystrophy, spinal muscular atrophy, hereditary motor neuropathy (Charcot-Marie-Tooth disease), Rett syndrome, myelodysplasia, Friedreich ataxia, arthrogryposis, and spinal cord injury. The severity of the spinal deformity is often related to the extent of the neurologic impairment and the age of the child at presentation. Many comorbidities are associated with neuromuscular scoliosis, including hip instability, thoracic insufficiency, and cardiopulmonary compromise. Large curves in patients with the most involved and medically complicated disease are treated surgically, although risks are high and the perceived benefits may be limited. However, improvements in measuring outcomes and quality of life in patients with neuromuscular deformities may better demonstrate the benefits of surgical treatment.

Keywords: kyphosis; neuromuscular; scoliosis; spine; spinal deformity

Introduction

Spinal deformity (scoliosis and/or kyphosis) commonly affects children with neuromuscular diseases such as cerebral palsy, muscular dystrophy, spinal muscular atrophy (SMA), hereditary motor neuropathy (Charcot-Marie-Tooth disease), Rett syndrome, myelodysplasia, Friedreich ataxia, arthrogryposis, and spinal cord injury[1,2] (**Table 1**). The severity of a spinal deformity is often related to the extent of the neurologic impairment and the age of the child at the initial medical consultation regarding disfigurement. In children with more severe disease, a larger curve is often seen at a younger age. The likelihood of curve progression increases as a function of a child's statural growth remaining.[3]

Risk factors for the development of neuromuscular spine deformity include truncal hypotonia, spasticity/dystonia, impaired sitting balance, and nonambulatory status.[4-6] Large lumbar curves are associated with pelvic obliquity and hip instability, whereas large thoracic curves are associated with thoracic insufficiency and cardiopulmonary compromise.[5-7] Unlike in patients with adolescent idiopathic scoliosis, nonsurgical interventions (bracing, physical therapy, and/or wheelchair modifications) have not been demonstrated to ameliorate long-term curve progression in children with neuromuscular spinal deformity.[8,9] Surgical interventions that stabilize or correct spinal deformity can reduce curve magnitude and associated pelvic obliquity and increase thoracic volume. These corrections contribute to improved sitting posture, reduced dependence on external supports, and improved pulmonary function.[10] However, the rate of complications associated with the surgical treatment of neuromuscular spinal deformity is high because of the frail health of these children, who frequently have complex medical comorbidities.[11]

In this era of needing to establish the quality and value of treatment interventions, the appropriate metrics to prove the success of treating neuromuscular scoliosis have not yet been defined. Patient-related outcome measures such as quality of life (QOL) assessments are difficult to directly ascertain in these patients, who are often limited by cognitive and physical impairments. The few prospective and retrospective studies that have evaluated QOL based on feedback from patients and caregivers have provided mixed results.[12,13] Assessment of the real cost of these treatments remains elusive.

Dr. Whitaker or an immediate family member is an employee of Lumenis and has received research or institutional support from the Orthopaedic Research and Education Foundation. Dr. Snyder or an immediate family member serves as an unpaid consultant to Orthopediatrics and serves as a board member, owner, officer, or committee member of the American Academy of Orthopaedic Surgeons, the Orthopaedic Research Society, the Pediatric Orthopaedic Society of North America, and the Scoliosis Research Society.

Table 1

Incidence of Scoliosis in Neuromuscular Conditions

Diagnosis	Incidence (%)	Etiology	Presentation
Cerebral palsy	25-100	Brain injury	Spastic, dyskinetic, ataxic, and mixed variants that can affect all or part of the body, with varying severity of involvement
Charcot-Marie-Tooth disease Hereditary motor and sensory neuropathy	30	Genetic defect in axon or myelin composition (90% in *PMP22, MPZ, GJB1* or *MFN2* gene)	Peripheral neuropathy with variable penetrance manifested by cavovarus feet, loss of intrinsics, and loss of proprioception
Spina bifida	60-100	Folate deficiency	Neural tube defects ranging in level and severity of involvement
Rett syndrome	64	*MeCP2* gene mutation	Regression of milestones between 6 and 18 months of age
Spinal muscular atrophy	70	*SMN1 gene mutation* *SMN2 gene number modifies severity*	Death of anterior horn cells of the spinal cord
Friedreich ataxia	80	*FXN* gene (fraxin) trinucleotide repeats	Onset of ataxia, weakness, stiffness, cardiomyopathy, diabetes, hearing loss, and impaired vision at puberty
Duchenne muscular dystrophy	90	Mutation in gene for dystrophin	X-linked disorder appearing in early childhood, with muscle weakness, pseudohypertrophy, and delayed achievement of developmental milestones
Spinal cord injury	100	Trauma	Trauma to the spinal cord with neurologic injury

Patient Assessment

The evaluation of a patient with neuromuscular scoliosis should consider the child's physiologic age, the magnitude and location of the spinal deformity, the underlying neuromuscular disease, associated medical comorbidities, and functional status. These findings will aid in the development of a rational treatment strategy based on the patient's prognosis, expected rate of curve progression, and exacerbation of musculoskeletal and medical ailments related to the scoliosis. Curve magnitudes of less than 45° do not impair functional mobility, aggravate ischial decubiti, decrease oxygen saturation, or alter heart rate. Curve magnitudes greater than 45° compromise sitting posture, which interferes with trunk balance and positioning.[7] Large (>70°) thoracic curves are often associated with rib cage distortion that contributes to thoracic insufficiency syndrome and restricted pulmonary function. Large thoracolumbar and lumbar curves are often associated with pelvic obliquity, which contributes to hip instability and infrapelvic deformity from soft-tissue contractures.[14,15] However, the causal relationship between hip and spine deformity has not been established.[16] In nonambulatory children with unilateral hip instability, a compensatory lumbar curve may develop. As the lumbar curve and pelvic obliquity increase, the hip on the concave side becomes adducted and the hip on the convex side becomes abducted, creating a "windswept" posture. Increasing pelvic obliquity exacerbates the risk of hip subluxation and dislocation; however, posterolateral hip displacement also may be induced by flexion and adduction contractures about the hip rather than by the scoliosis itself.[17,18]

Spinal deformity will progress in 85% of children with cerebral palsy and scoliosis who present with a curve greater than 40° and who are younger than 15 years.[3] In this patient cohort, the severity of the spinal deformity and the likelihood of progression is predicted by the child's age (growth remaining) and functional status as measured by the Gross Motor Function Classification System (GMFCS) (**Figure 1**). The risk of development of a substantial spinal deformity (Cobb angle >50°) in children at GMFCS levels I and II is similar to that of children without cerebral palsy, whereas children at GMFCS level V are at highest risk (relative risk = 34.99).[16] Unlike adolescent idiopathic scoliosis, spinal deformity in nonambulatory

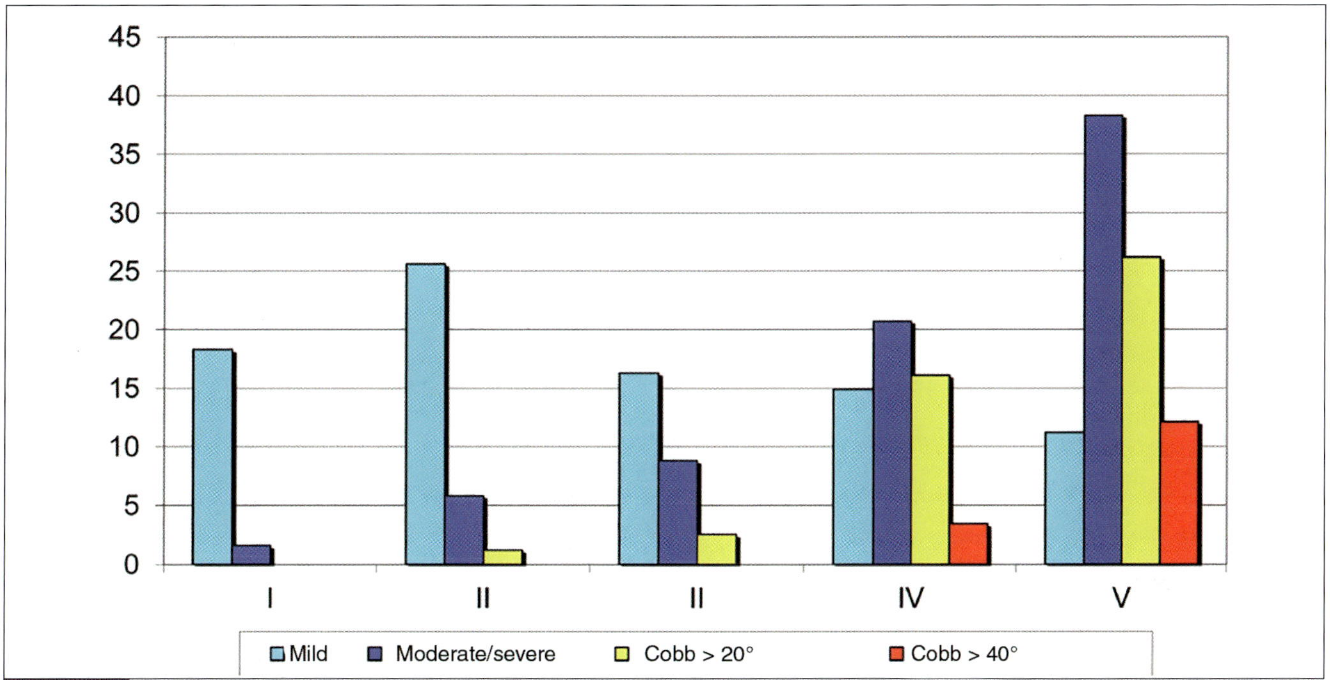

Figure 1 Bar graph showing the incidence and severity of scoliosis based on the Gross Motor Function Classification System. Distribution of scoliosis is based on the clinical and initial radiographic examinations. Patients with a Cobb angle of greater than 40° are also included in the group with a Cobb angle of greater than 20°. (Reproduced with permission from Persson-Bunke M, Hägglund G, Lauge-Pedersen H, Wagner P, Westbom L: Scoliosis in a total population of children with cerebral palsy. *Spine* 2012;37[12]:e708-e713.)

children with neuromuscular scoliosis may continue to progress after skeletal maturity. Curve progression has been reported to be 0.8° per year in curves less than 50° at skeletal maturity and 1.4° per year in curves greater than 50° at skeletal maturity.[19] The per annum risk of curve progression also is predicted by the GMFCS. Scoliosis in ambulatory children with cerebral palsy (GMFCS levels I through III) does not substantially increase, whereas nonambulatory children with cerebral palsy (GMFCS levels IV and V) may have a 3.5° per year increase in curve magnitude (thoracic kyphosis increases 2.2° per year and the apical vertebra translates laterally 5.4 mm per year).[4]

The likelihood of the development of scoliosis is not related to the subtype of cerebral palsy (spastic, ataxic, or dyskinetic).[16] However, ataxia before age 10 years and scoliosis before age 15 years are associated with curve progression in patients with Friedreich ataxia.[20,21] Substantial and progressive scoliosis will develop in nearly all children with acquired quadriplegia or paraplegia as a consequence of spinal cord injury sustained before age 12 years.[22] By 4 to 6 years of age, early-onset scoliosis, pelvic obliquity, and hip instability will develop in children with severe muscle weakness and truncal hypotonia resulting from muscle dystrophy, myopathy, or neuropathy. The scoliosis is rapidly progressive (8°/yr) and severely compromises pulmonary function (relative vital capacity of 54% predicted at age 4 to 6 years).[5,6] Glucocorticoid treatment has decreased the rate of progressive scoliosis and the need for spinal fusion in children with Duchenne muscular dystrophy (DMD).[23] In patients with spina bifida, the level of the posterior spinal element defect correlates with the incidence of scoliosis and the orthopaedic manifestation[24] (**Table 2**).

Nonsurgical Interventions

Braces, serial Risser or Mehta casts, and wheelchair modifications have been used to improve sitting posture and trunk balance in patients with neuromuscular spinal deformity. However, although these interventions may slow the advancement of spinal deformity, they will not prevent progression.[9,20] A 70% to 80% failure rate has been reported with the use of a rigid thoracolumbosacral orthosis to correct neuromuscular scoliosis; this high failure rate may be attributable to incorrect implementation of the appliance and poor patient compliance.[8,9] A semirigid thoracolumbosacral orthosis with an anterior opening improves wear tolerance (10 to 12 hr/d) and sitting posture and makes breathing easier.[16,25] It is especially important that the brace include a large anterior window sufficient to accommodate the presence of a gastrostomy tube to allow for abdominal distension during feeding and

Table 2

Level of Function and Clinical Manifestations of Spina Bifida Based on the Spinal Level of Involvement

Level	Function	Clinical Manifestations
Thoracic	Sitter	Spinal deformities Seating devices Mobility devices
Upper lumbar	Independent sitter, hands-free, possible household ambulator with hip-knee-ankle-foot orthosis	Spinal deformity Seating devices Mobility devices Hip flexion deformity
Midlumbar	Household ambulator, possibly community ambulator with knee-ankle-foot orthosis or ankle-foot orthosis (requires strong quadriceps)	Hip flexion and adduction deformity Hip subluxation/dislocation
Lower lumbar	Community ambulator with ankle-foot orthosis	Foot deformities Foot ulcerations
Sacral	Community ambulator	Cavovarus feet Claw toes Foot ulcers Urologic problems

to facilitate diaphragmatic breathing. Younger patients with smaller Cobb angles and long sweeping curves respond best to bracing, which indicates that patient age, the extent of deformity, the number of vertebrae forming the scoliosis, and the flexibility of the curve correlate with the extent of in-brace curve correction.[26] Children with scoliosis as a consequence of spinal cord injury with curve magnitudes less than 40° may respond to bracing; however, a consistent response to bracing has not been demonstrated in patients with curves greater than 40°.[27] Although brace wear (>13 hr/d) and the extent of in-brace correction (50%) have been used as predictors of successful bracing in patients with adolescent idiopathic scoliosis, no such parameters have been shown to be predictive of effective brace treatment in those with neuromuscular scoliosis.[8] Serial Mehta or Risser casts have been used to control scoliosis progression in patients with early-onset scoliosis who have an underlying neuromuscular disease, but this approach should be used with caution, especially in patients with spasticity or dystonia. Wheelchair modifications using pummels, wedges, lateral trunk supports, hip blocks, or customized molded seat backs to accommodate hyperlordosis can improve sitting posture and increase patient comfort and function; however, these modifications do not treat the underlying spinal deformity.

Surgical Intervention

Decision Making

If nonsurgical management is unsuccessful, surgical treatment is indicated for a severe (>50°), progressive, neuromuscular spinal deformity that is causing pain, interfering with sitting balance, contributing to ischial decubiti, inducing hip instability, or compromising cardiopulmonary function (thoracic insufficiency syndrome). The decision to surgically treat a patient with neuromuscular scoliosis requires consideration of many patient-related factors that influence the risks of surgery, the expected benefits from the intervention, the likelihood of success, and the potential for complications. The goals of surgery are to achieve solid arthrodesis to decrease progression of spinal deformity; relieve pain from costoiliac impingement syndrome; prevent decubiti by eliminating pelvic obliquity; improve sitting balance and wheelchair tolerance; enhance the ability for social interaction by aligning the head midline over level shoulders and pelvis; create a stable, balanced, upright torso to minimize use of the upper limbs for auxiliary trunk support; facilitate daily care; decrease the need for assistance during activities of daily living; diminish thoracic distortion; and increase thoracic height to facilitate diaphragmatic excursion and pulmonary function. The benefits of surgery must outweigh the risks and improve on the natural history of the disease if the scoliosis remains untreated. To aid parents in deciding whether surgical treatment or palliative care is the appropriate choice for their child, a shared decision-making aid is available.[28] Caregivers should be provided with information about the risks and benefits of surgery and the expected issues that will likely be encountered during the perioperative and postoperative periods.

Minimizing Preoperative Risks

Compared with patients with adolescent idiopathic scoliosis, children with neuromuscular scoliosis who undergo surgical treatment have complex medical issues that may extend their hospitalization (6.1 versus 9.2 days, respectively), increase the need for prolonged admission to the intensive care unit (ICU), and increase the probability of postoperative complications.[29] Common comorbidities include recurrent aspiration pneumonias from gastroesophageal reflux, the inability to manage oral secretions, respiratory failure from thoracic insufficiency syndrome, restrictive lung disease, cardiomyopathy (for example, mitochondrial and syndromic diseases in patients with DMD), poor gastrointestinal function (reflux, constipation, malabsorption), malnutrition, seizures (in patients with cerebral palsy and Rett syndrome), coagulopathies (in patients with DMD and those taking antiseizure drugs), compromised immune function, and osteopenia (disuse, vitamin D deficiency).[29] A careful evaluation by a multidisciplinary team of specialists and the institution of systematic protocols for anticipating and managing these comorbidities perioperatively may avoid many postoperative complications.

Comprehensive pulmonary function tests are often difficult to perform in children with neuromuscular scoliosis because of their inability to cooperate. A 2011 study of 74 patients with neuromuscular scoliosis reported that postoperative pulmonary complications were probable in adolescents older than 16.5 years who have severe scoliosis (Cobb angle >69°) and a preoperative forced vital capacity (FVC) of less than 39.5% of predicted value and a forced expiratory volume at 1 second (FEV_1) of less than 40% of predicted value.[30] An FEV_1 less than 40% of predicted value was prognostic for prolonged mechanical ventilation after surgery.[31] For patients with neurogenic scoliosis and compromised pulmonary function (FVC <30% to 40% of predicted value), pulmonary complications can be avoided by implementing pulmonary training before and after surgery.[32] This training can include noninvasive positive pressure ventilation to compensate for intrinsic respiratory muscle weakness and mechanical insufflation-exsufflation to augment mucous clearance.

Patients with Rett syndrome and scoliosis were found to have higher rates of postoperative complications compared with patients with cerebral palsy, with respiratory problems being the most severe complication.[33] Tracheostomy before spinal surgery should be considered in patients with severe pulmonary insufficiency, poor pulmonary toilet, dependence on continuous positive airway pressure and bilevel positive airway pressure assistance, and a history of frequent intubation and/or prolonged time to extubation. Prophylactic tracheostomy expedites recovery of respiratory function, facilitates pulmonary toilet, and eliminates the need for urgent tracheostomy weeks after spinal surgery in a debilitated patient who has undergone multiple failed attempts at extubation.

Muscular dystrophies are often associated with cardiomyopathy and/or conduction abnormalities. An electrocardiogram and echocardiogram should be obtained preoperatively for these patients. A left ventricular ejection fraction less than 50% may be a relative contraindication to surgery. Consultation with a cardiologist to guide perioperative management is recommended. Transesophageal echocardiography and/or use of a Swan-Ganz catheter to monitor atrial filling pressures enables the intraoperative evaluation of cardiac function. Hypotensive anesthesia should be avoided. Fluid replacement with blood products and colloid (rather than crystalloid) helps to maximize the Starling curve.

Many children with neuromuscular scoliosis also have epilepsy. Some anticonvulsant medications adversely affect clotting (for example, valproic acid has a qualitative effect on platelet function that resolves over 4 to 6 weeks).[34] Postoperative ileus and delayed gastric motility can affect the serum concentration of anticonvulsant drugs administered enterically, but several of these medications are unavailable for parental administration. Therefore, a neurologist should be consulted weeks before the surgery to adjust antiepileptic medications to avoid excess bleeding and decrease the risk of postoperative seizures. In addition, it is recommended that bleeding time be determined. Aspirin and NSAIDs should be avoided. If platelet function is abnormal, a hematology consultation is recommended in addition to having platelets and blood available for the procedure.[35] For children with ventricular-peritoneal shunts, the functionality of the shunt should be assessed using appropriate imaging studies; preoperative clearance by a neurosurgeon should be obtained.

Osteopenia is common across the spectrum of neuromuscular diseases because of poor nutrition, the long-term administration of anticonvulsant drugs, and the limited weight-bearing status of patients. Low bone mineral density decreases bone stiffness and strength and increases the risk of fragility fractures and the failure of bone anchor fixation. Proper diagnostic studies to determine the cause of osteopenia are required because osteoporosis (normal bone tissue mineralization but low bone mass) is treated differently than osteomalacia (low bone tissue mineralization as a consequence of vitamin D deficiency, poor nutrition, malabsorption, anticonvulsant drug induction of p450 microenzymes, renal or hepatic failure, steroid administration, or endocrinopathy). Dietary modifications to increase calcium and vitamin D intake in patients at risk for osteomalacia may be supplemented with bisphosphonates (also known as diphosphonates) to improve bone quality in patients with osteoporosis by decreasing osteoclastic bone resorption. The intravenous administration of zoledronate over a 2-year period was found to increase bone mineral density and improve vertebral morphology.[36] In anticipation of spinal fusion, a consultation with an endocrinologist can be considered so that a bisphosphonate can be administered 9 to 12 months prior to surgery to allow for the maximization of bone anchor stability. Zoledronate administration in adults with osteoporosis undergoing lumbar spinal fusion decreased the time to fusion, increased the fusion rate, decreased the number of adjacent compression fractures, and improved clinical outcomes; no deleterious effects such as decreased fusion mass were reported.[37,38] Bisphosphonate administration improves screw fixation in the spine and in osteoporotic bone.[39,40]

Higher infection rates have been reported in patients who have cerebral palsy and poor nutritional status (albumin <3.5 mg/dL and total lymphocyte count <1,500 cells/mm^3) who underwent surgery for scoliosis.[41] Discussion with a nutritionist and insertion of a nasogastric tube or gastrostomy tube to augment enteral feeding weeks before surgery should be considered. Gastrointestinal problems such as postoperative ileus, pancreatitis, gastroesophageal reflux, and constipation can complicate the postoperative course and lengthen the hospital stay. A bowel preparation (laxatives, enema) administered before surgery may improve gastrointestinal mobility, decrease constipation, and accelerate enteral feeding after surgery.

Urinary and bowel incontinence increase the risk of surgical site infections.[42] The likelihood of a postoperative wound infection was increased in patients with myelomeningocele and a positive preoperative urine culture, thereby supporting the importance of prophylactic antibiotic treatment before surgery.[43] Quality and safety guidelines to mitigate the risk of surgical site infection in patients with neuromuscular spinal deformity undergoing spinal fusion endorse routine methicillin-resistant *Staphylococcus aureus* screening (nares, axilla, and groin), surgical site hair removal with clippers, the administration of gram-positive and gram-negative antibiotics within 1 hour of skin incision, and chlorhexidine skin preparation.[44]

Planning

The goal of spine surgery in patients with neuromuscular spinal deformity is to create a balanced spine, with the head centered over level shoulders and pelvis to improve sitting balance. In addition to frontal plane alignment, the sagittal spine contour should allow for sufficient thoracic kyphosis to lessen the likelihood of proximal junction kyphosis at the cervical thoracic junction and provide for sufficient lumbar lordosis to compensate for weak hip girdle muscles by aligning the trunk center of gravity at or slightly behind the hip joints. Because adequate hip range of motion is a prerequisite to facilitate sitting, transfers, toileting, and hygiene, intrapelvic and infrapelvic pathology (for example, windswept deformity) related to hip instability and/or contractures (psoas, adductors, tensor fascia lata, hamstrings) should be addressed before or coincident with spinal instrumentation. A fixed hip flexion contracture can increase lumbar lordosis, whereas a fixed proximal hamstring contracture can decrease lumbar lordosis, which will affect the sagittal alignment of a fused spine. A salvage hip procedure such as a Chiari iliac osteotomy may be difficult to perform after spinal instrumentation is fixed to the pelvis with iliac screws. Careful preoperative planning that considers the age of the patient (spine and thoracic growth remaining), the flexibility of the spinal deformity, the causal pathophysiology, and associated intraspinal pathology (Chiari malformation, syrinx, or tethered cauda equina) will aid in the selection of growth-friendly spine implants versus definitive spinal fusion, the use of preoperative and/or intraoperative halo traction with or without femoral traction, and the choice of appropriate methods for intraoperative neuromonitoring, blood management, and spinal fixation.

Sitting (or standing) AP and lateral spine radiographs obtained on a single cassette that includes the head, neck, and pelvis will show the full scope of the spinal and trunk deformities requiring correction and will help identify the extent that associated hip pathology and/or pelvic obliquity and cervical spinal deformity (torticollis, laterocollis) are related to the overall deformity of the axial skeleton. Supine, push-pull longitudinal traction; right and left bending; and sagittal prone-supine bending (over a fulcrum) radiographs will demonstrate the flexibility of the spinal deformity (**Figures 2** and **3**). Syndromic patients (those with storage diseases, Larsen syndrome, Down syndrome, Klippel-Feil syndrome, or arthrogryposis) should have static (AP, lateral, and open-mouth) and dynamic (lateral flexion-extension) views of the cervical spine to evaluate for associated axial and subaxial cervical spinal

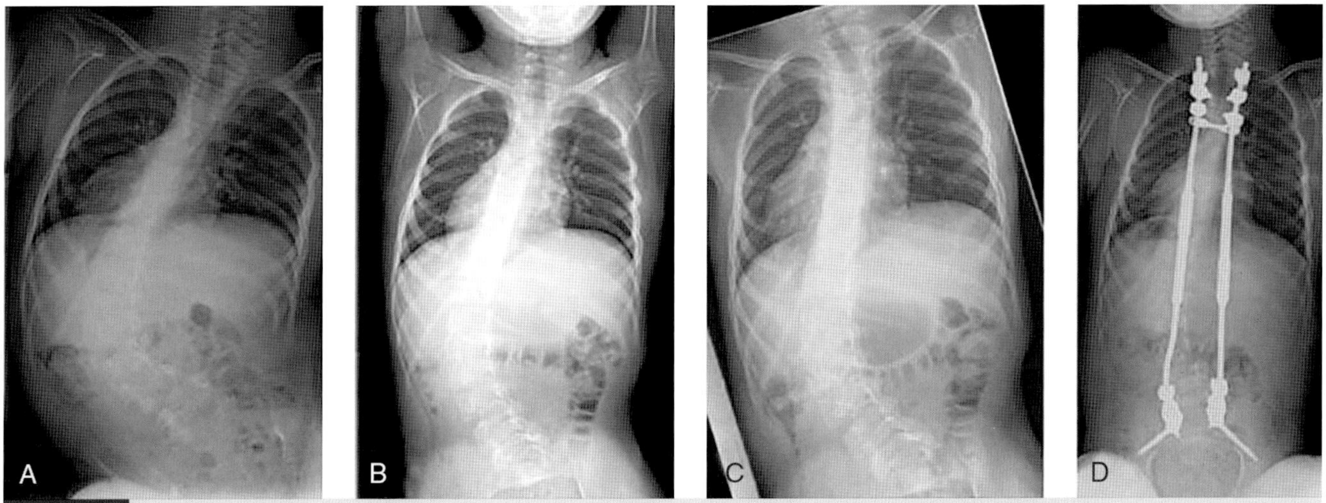

Figure 2 Radiographs from an 8-year-old boy with type II spinal muscular atrophy. **A,** Standard upright PA scoliosis radiograph shows a major curve measuring 82°. **B,** Supine traction PA scoliosis radiograph shows reduction in the major curve to 42°. **C,** Supine left bending (lumbar curve) PA scoliosis radiograph demonstrates approximately the same amount of correction (to 45°). **D,** PA upright radiograph after magnetic growing rod insertion shows that the major curve measures 41°, similar to the curve measurement in the traction radiograph.

deformity that may contribute to occult mechanical instability and the risk of cervical spinal cord injury.

Serial transaxial CT of the entire spine and rib cage with two- and three-dimensional tomographic reconstructions is indicated to evaluate abnormal osseous anatomy related to congenital vertebral anomalies, neurofibromatosis, pathologic fractures, tumors, complex or unusual spinal deformity, and the morphology of the pedicles to accommodate pedicle screw anchors. MRI of the entire spine from the foramen magnum to the sacrum is required in rapidly progressing spinal deformities (>15° in a 1-year period), in myelomeningocele, in left thoracic curves or unusual patterns of spinal deformity, and in abnormally progressing foot deformity (equinovarus-cavovarus) to evaluate for Chiari malformation or intraspinal pathology.[45]

Preoperative halo-gravity traction applied full time for several weeks before spine instrumentation can be considered for the treatment of large, stiff curves (Cobb angle >60° on bending or traction radiographs).[46] The child must have no cervical spine instability, and spasticity and/or seizures must be well controlled. The traction weight is increased incrementally to up to 50% of the child's body weight, with careful neurologic evaluation every 4 to 8 hours of the cranial nerves (especially the abducens nerve), cervical sympathetic chain (pupillary dilation), deviations in motor or sensory functions for dermatomes or myotomes C5-T1 and L1-S1, and changes in bowel and bladder function from baseline levels.[46] Anterior release (open or thoracoscopic) of the anterior longitudinal ligament and intervertebral disk may be considered for excessive thoracic kyphosis (>65°) and/or a rigid scoliosis that failed to substantially improve with halo traction. Intraoperative halo-pelvic or halo-femoral traction in which the distal traction is applied to the concave side or the elevated hemipelvis facilitates deformity correction by viscoelastic creep that gradually stretches the soft-tissue connections. The total traction force (approximately 50% of body weight) is equally distributed between the halo and the lower extremity.

Neuromonitoring is recommended when correcting a neuromuscular scoliosis because loss of residual bowel, bladder, motor, or sensory functions can substantially affect the patient's QOL. Most of these patients will be unable to cooperate with a wake-up test. In a patient who is incontinent and has spastic quadriplegia, a spinal cord injury may result in urinary and bowel retention that negatively alters daily care activities, with the need for catheterization and a bowel regimen requiring digital stimulation. Spinal somatosensory-evoked potentials (SSEPs) may be unreliable in neuromuscular scoliosis.[47] Transcranial motor-evoked potentials improve reliability when combined with SSEPs. In a study that included 39 patients with cerebral palsy, the responses to at least one modality could be monitored in 86% of the patients.[48] Stimulation to measure transcranial motor-evoked potentials does not elicit seizure activity or increase postoperative seizure activity.[49] In patients with DMD or SMA, motor-evoked potentials may be absent but SSEPs are often present. Electromyographic stimulation of each pedicle screw can be helpful in determining pedicle wall perforation and contact with the spinal cord or a nerve root.

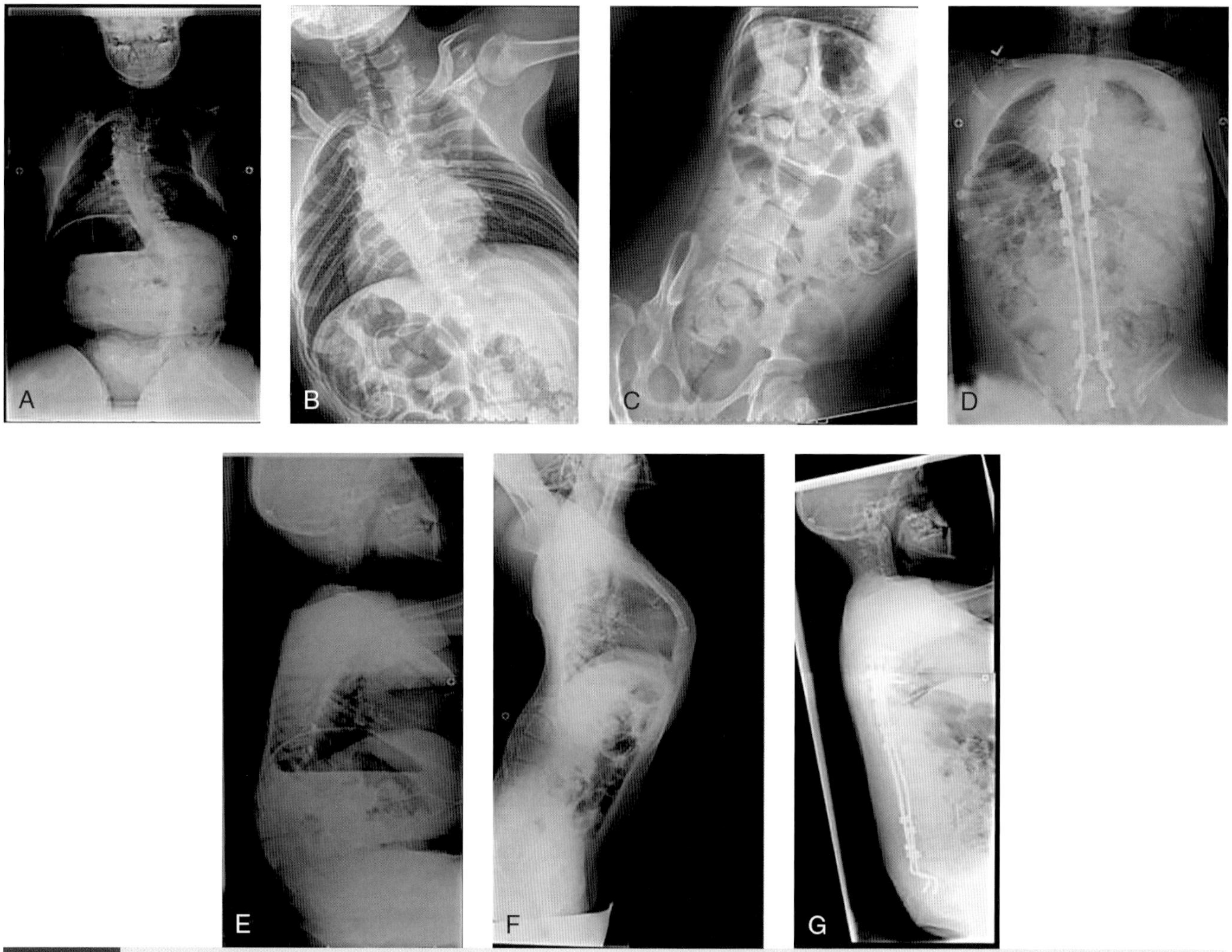

Figure 3 Radiographs from a 14-year-old boy with myelomeningocele. **A,** Sitting upright PA scoliosis radiograph shows a 57° main thoracic curve and a 44° lumbar curve. **B,** Supine left bending (thoracic curve) PA scoliosis radiograph shows main thoracic curve reduction to 11°, not including the congenital upper thoracic anomalies. **C,** Supine right bending (lumbar curve) PA scoliosis radiograph shows lumbar curve reduction to 3°. Sitting PA radiograph (**D**) and sitting lateral scoliosis radiograph (**E**) show 88° of lumbar kyphosis. **F,** Supine lateral radiograph taken with a bolster over the kyphosis shows residual kyphosis of 46°. **G,** Lateral radiograph after fusion and L1 vertebrectomy shows 18° of lumbar kyphosis.

Controlling for the number of levels fused and patient weight, those with neuromuscular disease have a substantially higher amount of intraoperative blood loss during spinal fusion than patients with idiopathic scoliosis. Modifiable coagulopathies must be considered. Continual exudate of blood from osteoporotic bone is commonplace in children with neurogenic spinal deformity. An intraoperative coagulopathy often develops in children with DMD who have normal prothrombin time or partial thromboplastin time. Children taking valproic acid have qualitative platelet dysfunction. The overly aggressive administration of crystalloid solution to treat intraoperative blood loss further dilutes coagulation factors. Early judicious replacement with fresh frozen plasma and/or cryoprecipitate is required to prevent excessive exsanguination. Point-of-care devices and platelet mapping are used to determine coagulopathy and guide treatment, such as the use of fresh frozen plasma to treat hypofibrinogenemia (fibrinogen <1.5 g/L) and low factor XIII.[50] An arterial line facilitates continual monitoring of blood pressure with the goal of maintaining an intraoperative mean arterial pressure of 65 mm Hg. Insertion of a large-bore (≥18-gauge) central line or a peripherally inserted central catheter line with the tip at the superior vena cava allows for improved venous access for the administration of blood products and the intraoperative assessment of central venous pressure to evaluate hypovolemia.

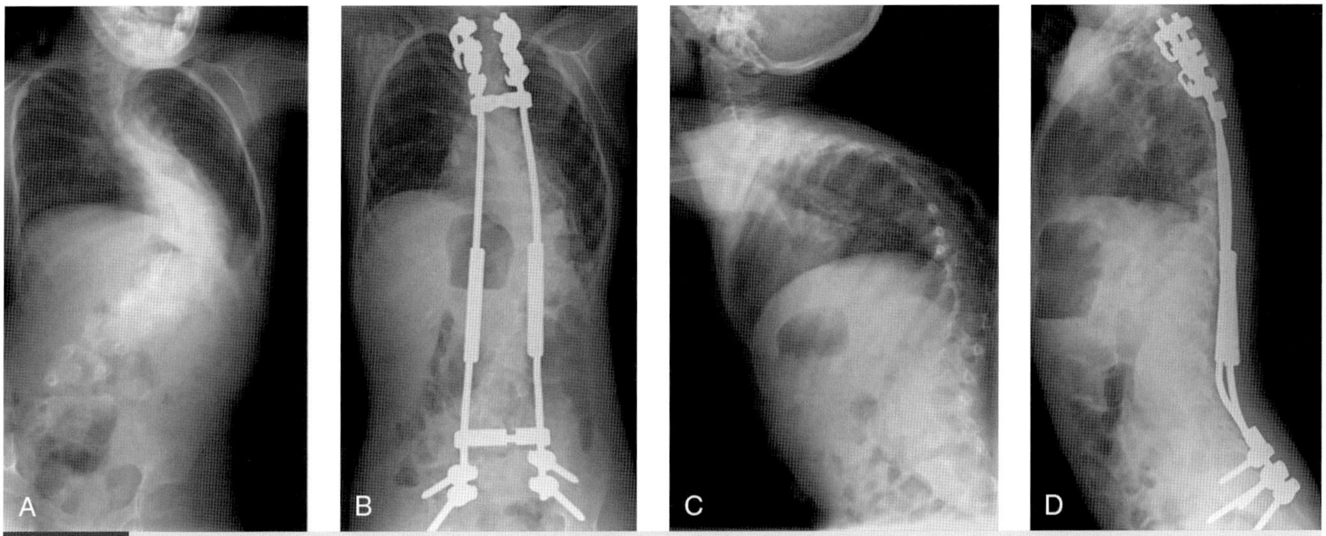

Figure 4 Radiographic images from a patient with neuromuscular scoliosis who was treated with growing rods, a hook-screw hybrid construct, and iliac screws. **A,** Preoperative PA scoliosis radiograph. **B,** Postoperative PA scoliosis radiograph shows the growing rod construct with hooks, cross-links, and iliac screws. **C,** Lateral preoperative scoliosis radiograph. **D,** Lateral postoperative scoliosis radiograph shows improvement in thoracic kyphosis and lumbar lordosis after treatment.

The intraoperative administration of antifibrinolytic agents such as tranexamic acid and aminocaproic acid has been shown to substantially decrease intraoperative blood loss. Tranexamic acid is given as a bolus (100 mg/kg before incision) and followed by an infusion (10 mg/kg/hr) until wound closure.[51] Additional measures to decrease blood loss include dermal injection of 1:500,000 dilution of epinephrine along and deep to the skin incision, soft-tissue dissection with electrocautery, placing a tamponade by packing sponges along the lateral gutter deep to the paraspinal muscles (Hibb technique), packing decorticated bone and exposed dura with collagen sponges, injecting hemostatic matrix into pedicle tracks, using bipolar radiofrequency hemostatic sealer to coagulate bleeding muscle and bone, and suctioning blood and recycling it with a cell saver.

Technique

Nonfusion Constructs

The previous paradigm of making a "crooked" spine "straight" by instrumenting multiple levels and fusing the spine early has been shown to inhibit lung growth and development and decrease pulmonary function. Devices for preserving and potentially modulating spinal and thoracic growth are now approved for use in growing children. Severe, progressive spine deformity in children younger than 10 years who are unresponsive to bracing is an indication for the use of a posteriorly placed, expandable rod system that spans the entire scoliosis and functions as an internal corrective splint (**Figure 4**). Compared with single-rod constructs, dual-rod systems offer better structural stability and curve correction.[52] The rods, placed above the paravertebral muscles, are fixed proximally to the spine or ribs and distally to the spine and/or pelvis using a variety of anchors, including sublaminar hooks, pedicle screws, rib cradles, and iliac crest S-hooks (**Figure 5**). In particular, the Vertical Expandable Prosthetic Titanium Rib (VEPTR; DePuy Synthes) fastened proximally with rib cradles and distally with Dunn-McCarthy S-hooks over the ilium has been effective in treating myelodysplasia in young patients with spina bifida and in obviating the need for early kyphectomy and fusion.[53] Sequential distraction of the implant through a limited surgical exposure is performed every 6 to 9 months to progressively correct the scoliosis and maintain growth of the spine. This results in slightly less than expected axial spine growth of approximately 1.8 cm per year.[54] The frequency of sequential lengthening of the implants is controversial because more frequent lengthening increases infection risk but decreases stress on the implants.[52] Dynamic implant systems such as the Magnetic Expansion Control (MAGEC; Ellipse Technologies) device can be lengthened (or shortened) noninvasively by virtue of a magnetic, screw-driven actuator in series with the rod. This device eliminates the need for open procedures to manually distract the rod. Sequential rod expansion is well tolerated by patients and can be performed without anesthesia in an office setting.[55]

The SHILLA growth guidance system (Medtronic) is predicated on the so-called Luque trolley concept of using multiple sublaminar wires as segmental anchors to align

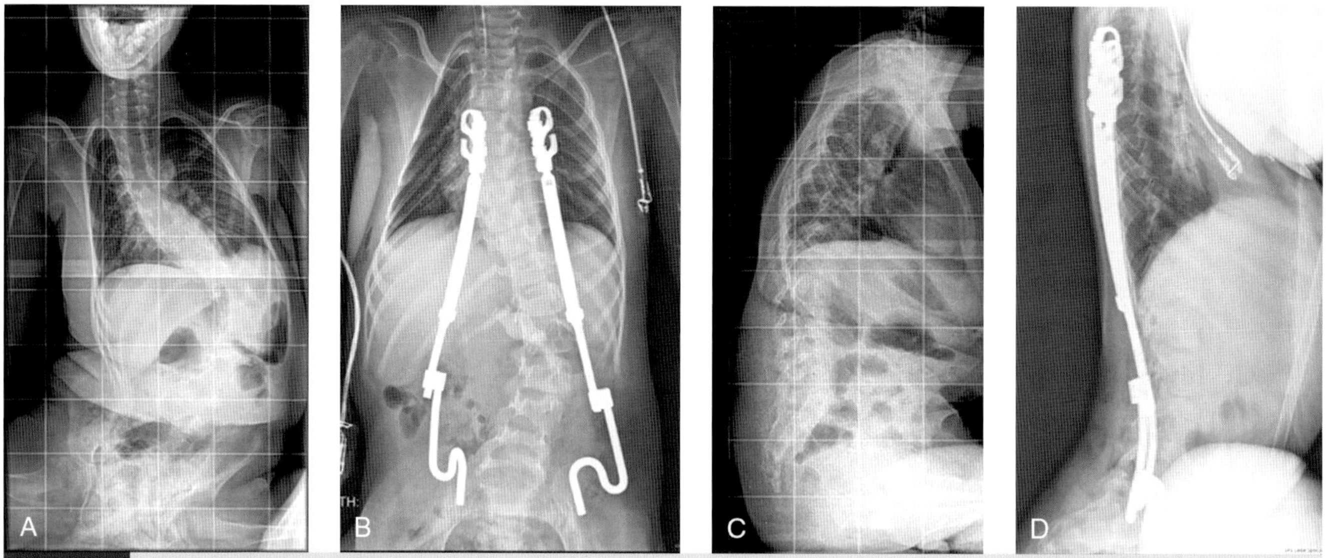

Figure 5 Radiographic images from a patient with neuromuscular scoliosis treated with the Vertical Expandable Prosthetic Titanium Rib (VEPTR), growing rods, and S-rod pelvic fixation. **A,** Preoperative PA scoliosis radiograph. **B,** Postoperative PA scoliosis radiograph shows the VEPTR proximally, S-rod pelvic fixation distally, and growing rods. **C,** Preoperative lateral scoliosis radiograph. **D,** Postoperative lateral scoliosis radiograph demonstrates improvement in lumbar lordosis.

the contorted vertebrae along dual posteriorly placed rods spanning the scoliosis. The rods act as rails for the wires to slide along. This current iteration uses pedicle screws with locking set screws to fix the vertebrae at the apex of the deformity to dual rods that span the scoliosis. This technique achieves immediate deformity correction and local arthrodesis. Vertebrae proximal and distal to the apex of the deformity are captured using multiaxial pedicle screws with nonlocking, flanged set screws that slide along the rods. This approach allows guided longitudinal growth while maintaining alignment of the nonfused vertebrae.[56] The law of diminishing growth associated with distraction-based systems is avoided because sequential rod lengthening to correct the scoliosis and maintain spinal growth is not required.[57] A 5-year, single-surgeon cohort demonstrated increased spinal growth by 15.8 cm/yr, increased space available for the lung by 29.1%, and a 73% complication rate.[58]

Early results with magnetic rods demonstrated improved scoliosis correction and higher FVC and FEV_1 values.[59] However, the use of rib-based (VEPTR) versus spine-based anchors for fixation to the thorax did not improve the “parasol rib deformity” in patients with hypotonic neuromuscular scoliosis.[60] Posteriorly placed, nonfusion systems have a 46% complication rate related to infection and wound dehiscence, which is exacerbated by multiple, open, manual lengthening procedures in addition to device failures.[52] These implants must serve multiple functions, including maintaining correction of the spinal deformity and modulating axial growth, without failing mechanically for an indeterminate number of years in a semimobile patient. Device fatigue fracture can be prevented by using the largest rod diameter possible. Minimizing the number of rod connectors helps prevent stress risers and crevice corrosion. The applied stress to each bone anchor is reduced by distributing the load among six bone anchors (three pedicle screws, sublaminar hooks, and/or rib cradles per rod) at the upper and lower end of each dual-rod construct.[61] To achieve the same gain in spine height over 2 years, lengthening a dual-rod system every 2 months decreases the resulting rod stress by 50% to 75% compared with lengthening every 6 months. This approach is now easily achievable using magnetic rod systems.[54]

Fusion Constructs

A dual-rod construct fixed with multiple vertebral bone anchors spanning the entire spinal deformity is essential to distribute corrective forces and moments in osteoporotic bone. Sagittal balance is as important as coronal plane correction to enable head control and sitting balance. Instrumentation should extend proximal to T4 to avoid upper thoracic junctional kyphosis. Sufficient lumbar lordosis (approximately 45°) is recommended to avoid pressure on the coccyx and ischium and transfer weight to the thighs while sitting. If the child is ambulatory, lumbosacral mobility should be preserved for walking and sitting; therefore, distal fixation proximal to L5 is

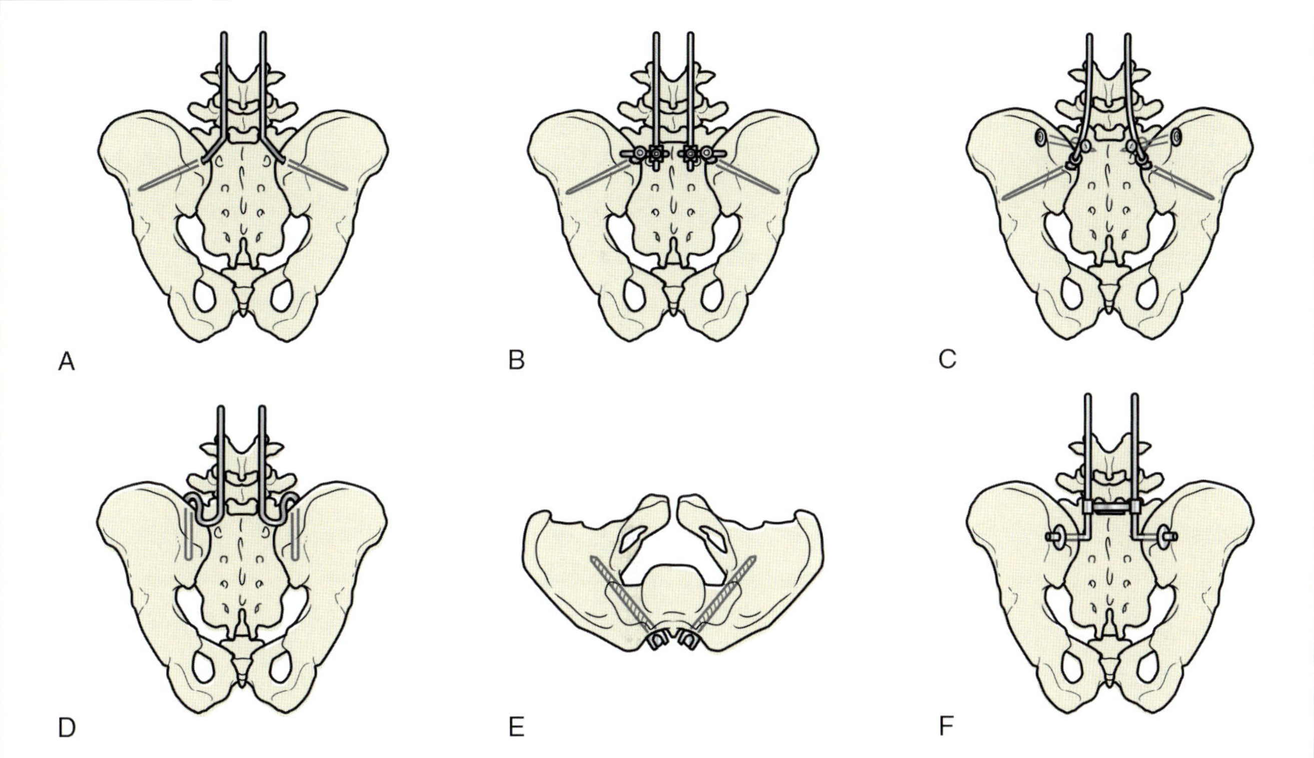

Figure 6 Illustrations of techniques to achieve sacropelvic fixation in patients with neuromuscular scoliosis. **A,** Galveston technique. **B,** Iliac screw technique. **C,** Technique using a maximum-width construct. **D,** S-rod (Dunn-McCarthy) technique. **E,** Technique using sacral alar iliac screws. **F,** Spinopelvic transiliac fixation technique.

indicated in an ambulatory patient whose spinal deformity is proximal to L5 and who has a level pelvis and stable hips.[62] Fixation to L5 is indicated in a nonambulatory patient with a spinal deformity that extends to L5, a level pelvis (obliquity <15°), and stable hips. Fixation to the pelvis is indicated in a nonambulatory patient lacking independent trunk support whose spinal deformity includes the pelvis or who has a collapsing curve so that the C7 plumb line projects lateral to the sacroiliac joint or who has hypolordosis (<15°), excessive pelvic obliquity (>15°), or a structural defect (deficient pars, absent L5 neural arch). Vertebral bone anchors include fixed- or variable-angle pedicle screws, sublaminar hooks, sublaminar Luque wires, cables, and bands. Pedicle screws provide rigid three-column fixation that enables improved deformity correction, potentially obviating the need for anterior procedures, which reduces blood loss and surgical time. Hybrid systems that combine pedicle screws, hooks, and/or sublaminar wires allow adequate curve correction, are less expensive than all-pedicle screw constructs, but do not reduce surgical time or blood loss.[63]

Many techniques exist to achieve sacropelvic fixation[64] (**Figure 6**). A Galveston construct using dual-rod constructs or iliac screws extends distal lever-arm fixation to better counteract the flexion moment created by the long spinal construct above. The authors of a 2015 study reported that at least six points of lumbar-sacral-pelvic fixation are required to achieve satisfactory stability.[65] Thirty-five percent of constructs with less than six bone anchors failed at 18 months, whereas constructs with at least six bone anchors remained intact at 28 months.

After release of the posterior interspinous ligaments (with or without the ligamentum flavum) and bilateral facetectomies, large rigid curves associated with excessive pelvic obliquity, thoracic kyphosis, or lumbar hyperlordosis may require Ponte or Smith-Petersen osteotomies at multiple segments or pedicle subtraction or vertebral column resection at a specific level to sufficiently destabilize the spine to permit adequate realignment[66] (**Table 3**). In patients with myelodysplasia, pedicle subtraction vertebrectomy for collapsing C-shaped kyphosis or kyphectomy for rigid myelokyphosis (lumbar kyphosis and thoracic lordosis) may be necessary. Anterior ligamentous release with intervertebral disk resection and possible partial corpectomy may be indicated to improve the mobility of an inflexible hyperkyphotic spinal deformity or to facilitate arthrodesis in patients with

Table 3

Spine Osteotomies

Osteotomy	Deformity	Columns Resected	Hinge	Illustration
Smith-Petersen	Mild	Lamina	Disk	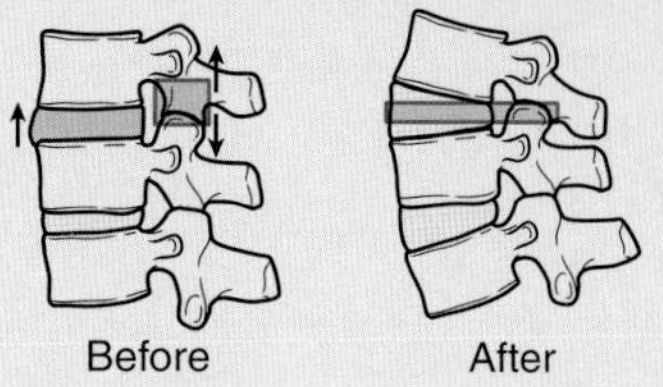
Pedicle subtraction	Kyphosis	Posterior middle Anterior (partial)	Anterior vertebral cortex	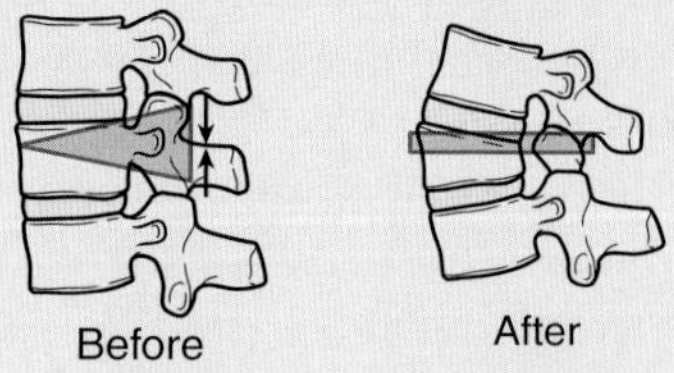
Vertebral column resection	Severe	Posterior middle Anterior multiple segments	Pivot where needed	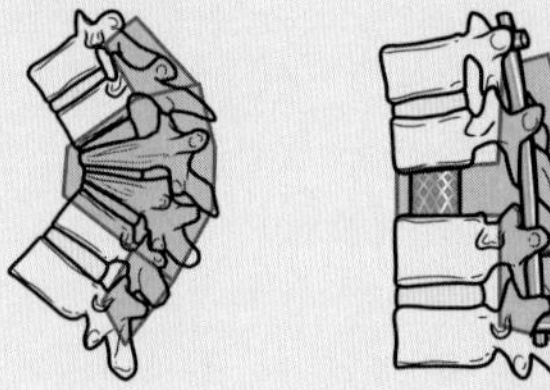

neurofibromatosis, connective tissue disorders, or those at risk for compromised bone healing. In skeletally immature patients, fusing the anterior spine prevents the crankshaft phenomenon. If both anterior and posterior procedures are required, controversy exists regarding the staging of the procedures. Some authors report more complications with single-stage anterior-posterior surgery but less morbidity, better correction, and reduced cost. Some authors claim comparable results and complication rates for single- and multiple-staged procedures. Other authors claim that staging the procedures is associated with less blood loss, shorter surgical times, decreased complication rates, and no increase in the length of stay in the ICU or the hospital.[67-71]

The primary purpose of the procedure is to attain a stable, fused spine. After instrumentation, the lamina, facets, and transverse processes should be decorticated. Arthrodesis is induced by using local autologous bone graft obtained from resection of the facets, spinous processes, and lamina, and is supplemented by autologous iliac crest or allogenic cancellous bone graft. Excellent fusion rates are obtained using allogenic bone graft.[72] The use of bone morphogenetic protein-2 is rarely indicated in primary spinal procedures.

Complications

Historically, complication rates vary from 44% to 80%, with pulmonary issues predominating (pneumonia, atelectasis, aspiration, pneumothorax).[11] Death has been reported in up to 7% of patients. In a meta-analysis of 15,218 patients with neuromuscular scoliosis, the prevalence of complications was as follows: 22.7% pulmonary, 12.5% implant-related, 10.9% infection, 3.0% neurologic, and 1.9% pseudarthrosis.[73]

In most neuromuscular diseases, spinal deformity is concomitant with intrinsic intercostal muscle weakness and restricted growth of the thoracic cavity, which compromise respiratory function by limiting excursion of the diaphragm and restricting inspiratory expansion of the rib cage.[74] Aggressive postoperative pulmonary toilet, including postural drainage, use of a vibrating vest and cough-assisting device to mobilize mucous plugs, and use of continuous positive airway pressure and bilevel positive airway pressure assistance to prevent atelectasis can ameliorate these problems.

Increased infection risk has been related to inadequate prophylactic antibiotic dosing, the length of the construct, the type of pelvic fixation, the duration of hospitalization, and patient comorbidities.[75] A multifaceted approach may help reduce the incidence of surgical site infections. Such an approach can include preoperative assessment of patient nutrition with appropriate intervention, diligent use of preoperative skin cleansing, prophylactic use of perioperative antibiotics to cover methicillin-resistant *S aureus* and gram-negative bacteria, use of titanium instrumentation, meticulous handling of soft tissues, débridement of devitalized tissues, wound lavage with dilute povidone iodine, instillation of vancomycin powder into the wound at closure, and careful postoperative wound care.

Malnutrition, constipation, and ileus can be effectively treated by parental hyperalimentation until bowel motility returns and by enteral feedings with a nasogastric, gastric, or jejunum tube. Neuromonitoring can help anticipate neurologic injuries. Intraoperative CT transaxial imaging allows confirmation of proper placement of pedicle screws and decreases the likelihood of encroachment on neurologic or vascular structures. Device fatigue failure can be prevented by using the largest possible rod diameter. Implant failure is particularly associated with thoracic hyperkyphosis, which can be mitigated by anterior release; the use of rigid, multilevel segmental fixation using pedicle screws and/or sublaminar hook-claw constructs; and the use of an in situ rod bent to accommodate the kyphosis.

In patients with Friedreich ataxia, proximal junctional kyphosis has been reported to occur with fusion to T4, but was prevented when fusion was done above T4.[20] In general, instrumentation to T2 or T3 and care to preserve the tension band created by the interspinous ligaments and facet joint capsule proximally helps to mitigate the risk of proximal junctional kyphosis.

The Value of Treating Neuromuscular Scoliosis

Outcomes

Treatment of neuromuscular scoliosis by spinal instrumentation and fusion is sufficiently successful in correcting spinal deformity and pelvic obliquity to create a balanced spine over a level pelvis.[10] However, spinal deformity progresses in 10% to 30% of patients after fusion.[76] Tools to assess the QOL of patients with neuromuscular scoliosis have been developed. The Caregiver Priorities and Child Health Index of Life With Disabilities (CPCHILD; Narayanan, Weil, and Fehlings) questionnaire was specifically designed and validated to evaluate patients with cerebral palsy.[77] Measuring QOL after scoliosis surgery is difficult because many patients are incapable of independently responding to QOL questionnaires. The responses of caregivers to these surveys may reflect positive or negative bias. Caregivers report high satisfaction after spinal fusion for neuromuscular scoliosis, despite no change in pain, incidence of decubiti, function, or time required for daily care.[13,78,79] A prospective study of severely affected, nonambulatory children with cerebral palsy (GMFCS levels IV and V) and scoliosis demonstrated clinically significant improvements in five of six domains on the CPCHILD questionnaire 1 year after spinal surgery; however, there was little change in caregiver burden.[13] Although spinal fusion improved coronal alignment in patients with myelodysplasia, the rate of postoperative spine infections was high (32.4%), and the overall QOL in adulthood was unchanged compared with patients treated nonsurgically.[80]

Cost

Compared with the treatment of adolescent idiopathic scoliosis, the expenditure for healthcare and resource utilization is substantially higher for patients with neuromuscular spinal deformity.[29] The increased number of bone anchors accounts for most of the expense of neuromuscular spinal fusion, followed by the costs associated with ICU admission and inpatient care. The length of hospitalization accounts for a large variability in costs.[81] The implants range in cost from approximately $30 for Luque wire to $275 for cable, $493 for a hook, and $673 for a pedicle screw, with pedicle screws offering improved curve correction.[82,83] Often unaccounted for in real cost analyses is the time caregivers take off from work to care for their children in the hospital and after discharge. These analyses also fail to account for potential cost savings related to decreased emergency care visits and hospitalizations for pulmonary complications related to a severe spinal deformity.

Ethics

Treating patients with neuromuscular scoliosis entails complex clinical decisions that account for medical indications, patient preferences, QOL, and contextual features.[84] As previously mentioned, a shared decision-making aid has been developed to properly educate caregivers and engage them in the decision-making process when choosing how to manage a patient with a neuromuscular spinal deformity.[28] However, the inability to directly measure a patient's QOL obscures the true benefit of restoring an upright posture to a patient with a distorted spine.

Summary

Neuromuscular scoliosis associated with cerebral palsy, muscular dystrophies, and myelodysplasia is typically characterized by long, collapsing C-shaped curves associated with pelvic obliquity and kyphosis. The scope and magnitude of the deformity are inversely related to the patient's gross motor function and directly related to the severity of the disease or the neurologic level. However, each disease entity is associated with different levels of patient functionality, different natural histories for curve progression, different surgical risk profiles, and has inconsistent evidence for or against surgical treatment. In general, high rates of curve progression are associated with younger patients with more severe spinal deformities. Bracing and other nonsurgical measures are ineffective in ameliorating curve progression in the long term, but can be used as a temporizing strategy until the child is sufficiently healthy and/or attains skeletal maturity and can undergo definitive spinal fusion.

Nonfusion, growth-friendly instrumentation systems have been shown to effectively correct spinal deformity and improve thoracic volume in young children with a rapidly progressing spinal deformity that is unresponsive to bracing. The assistance of a multidisciplinary team preoperatively can decrease modifiable risks related to cardiopulmonary, gastrointestinal, and neurologic comorbidities. Careful preoperative planning can decrease intraoperative complications and improve postoperative deformity correction. The goals of surgery are to establish a stable, balanced, painless spinal fusion. The surgical approach and instrumentation must be individualized based on the severity and stiffness of the curve, the extent of neurologic impairment, and the patient's skeletal maturity and baseline functional status.

New outcome tools are being developed to assess patient and caregiver QOL and satisfaction. Increased quality, decreased cost, and shared decision making will increase the value of spinal fusion in patients with neuromuscular scoliosis.

Key Study Points

- Spinal deformity is proportional to the extent of neurologic disability.
- Nonsurgical care of spinal deformity is palliative.
- The goal of surgery is to establish a stable, balanced, painless spinal fusion. The surgical approach and instrumentation must be individualized based on the patient's curve severity and stiffness, extent of neurologic impairment, skeletal maturity, and baseline functional status.
- Preoperative medical comorbidities increase the risk of postoperative complications. A multidisciplinary team is required to anticipate and minimize complications.
- With appropriate anticipatory medical management and fourth-generation spinal instrumentation, prospective and retrospective outcome studies suggest that improved long-term benefits in life expectancy, lung function, sitting balance, and QOL are associated with spinal fusion.

Acknowledgment

The authors thank Alexandra Grzywna for her contributions to the literature search and assembly of this chapter.

Annotated References

1. Canavese F, Rousset M, Le Gledic B, Samba A, Dimeglio A: Surgical advances in the treatment of neuromuscular scoliosis. *World J Orthop* 2014;5(2):124-133.

   The authors present a review of neuromuscular scoliosis. Level of evidence: V.

2. Harrison DJ, Webb PJ: Scoliosis in the Rett syndrome: Natural history and treatment. *Brain Dev* 1990;12(1):154-156.

3. Saito N, Ebara S, Ohotsuka K, Kumeta H, Takaoka K: Natural history of scoliosis in spastic cerebral palsy. *Lancet* 1998;351(9117):1687-1692.

4. Lee SY, Chung CY, Lee KM, Kwon SS, Cho KJ, Park MS: Annual changes in radiographic indices of the spine in cerebral palsy patients. *Eur Spine J* 2016;25(3):679-686.

   This retrospective review of 184 patients with cerebral palsy and scoliosis who were followed for 1 year found no curve progression in patients at GMFCS levels I through III. In patients at GMFCS levels IV and V, there was a

3.5° change per year, thoracic kyphosis increased by 2.2°, and the apical vertebrae shifted 5.4 mm per year. Level of evidence: IV.

5. Fujak A, Raab W, Schuh A, Richter S, Forst R, Forst J: Natural course of scoliosis in proximal spinal muscular atrophy type II and IIIa: Descriptive clinical study with retrospective data collection of 126 patients. *BMC Musculoskelet Disord* 2013;14:283.

   This retrospective study included 126 patients with SMA type II (n = 99) and SMA type IIIA (n = 27). The patients with SMA type II had scoliosis and pelvic obliquity at a young age and reduction of relative vital inspiratory capacity to 54% by 4 to 6 years of age, which progressively decreased with age. Level of evidence: III.

6. Granata C, Merlini L, Magni E, Marini ML, Stagni SB: Spinal muscular atrophy: Natural history and orthopaedic treatment of scoliosis. *Spine (Phila Pa 1976)* 1989;14(7):760-762.

7. Kalen V, Conklin MM, Sherman FC: Untreated scoliosis in severe cerebral palsy. *J Pediatr Orthop* 1992;12(3):337-340.

8. Weinstein SL, Dolan LA, Wright JG, Dobbs MB: Effects of bracing in adolescents with idiopathic scoliosis. *N Engl J Med* 2013;369(16):1512-1521.

   This randomized controlled trial evaluated the effects of bracing in 116 patients with adolescent idiopathic scoliosis who were randomly assigned to bracing or no bracing and an additional 126 patients who were given the choice of bracing or observation. The authors found 72% of the patients treated with bracing had curve progression to less than 50° compared with 48% without bracing. The success of bracing correlated with the amount of time in the brace. Level of evidence: I.

9. Olafsson Y, Saraste H, Al-Dabbagh Z: Brace treatment in neuromuscular spine deformity. *J Pediatr Orthop* 1999;19(3):376-379.

10. Larsson EL, Aaro SI, Normelli HC, Oberg BE: Long-term follow-up of functioning after spinal surgery in patients with neuromuscular scoliosis. *Spine (Phila Pa 1976)* 2005;30(19):2145-2152.

11. Benson ER, Thomson JD, Smith BG, Banta JV: Results and morbidity in a consecutive series of patients undergoing spinal fusion for neuromuscular scoliosis. *Spine (Phila Pa 1976)* 1998;23(21):2308-2317, discussion 2318.

12. Suk KS, Baek JH, Park JO, et al: Postoperative quality of life in patients with progressive neuromuscular scoliosis and their parents. *Spine J* 2015;15(3):446-453.

    This retrospective review of 58 patients with neuromuscular scoliosis evaluated QOL data for patients who underwent spinal fusion and their caregivers. There was improvement in patient balance, pain, and social functioning, but no improvement in caregiver QOL. Level of evidence: III.

13. Difazio RL, Vessey JA, Zurakowski D, Snyder BD: Differences in health-related quality of life and caregiver burden after hip and spine surgery in non-ambulatory children with severe cerebral palsy. *Dev Med Child Neurol* 2016;58(3):298-305.

    The caregiver's perceptions of their child's health-related QOL demonstrated an improvement from baseline to 12 months (*P* <0.001). Patients who had spine surgery demonstrated a steady improvement over time, whereas patients who had hip surgery had decreased improvement at 6 weeks, followed by steady improvement. Improvements were noted in five of six of the CPCHILD domains, with no changes in the QOL domain. No changes were noted in any of the Assessment of Caregiver Experience With Neuromuscular Disease domains. Level of evidence: II.

14. Madigan RR, Wallace SL: Scoliosis in the institutionalized cerebral palsy population. *Spine (Phila Pa 1976)* 1981;6(6):583-590.

15. Campbell RM Jr, Smith MD, Mayes TC, et al: The characteristics of thoracic insufficiency syndrome associated with fused ribs and congenital scoliosis. *J Bone Joint Surg Am* 2003;85(3):399-408.

16. Persson-Bunke M, Hägglund G, Lauge-Pedersen H, Wagner P, Westbom L: Scoliosis in a total population of children with cerebral palsy. *Spine (Phila Pa 1976)* 2012;37(12):E708-E713.

    This prospective cohort of children in Sweden with cerebral palsy reported that the prevalence and severity of scoliosis increased with the GMFCS level. Level of evidence: II.

17. Cooke PH, Cole WG, Carey RP: Dislocation of the hip in cerebral palsy: Natural history and predictability. *J Bone Joint Surg Br* 1989;71(3):441-446.

18. Lonstein JE, Beck K: Hip dislocation and subluxation in cerebral palsy. *J Pediatr Orthop* 1986;6(5):521-526.

19. Thometz JG, Simon SR: Progression of scoliosis after skeletal maturity in institutionalized adults who have cerebral palsy. *J Bone Joint Surg Am* 1988;70(9):1290-1296.

20. Tsirikos AI, Smith G: Scoliosis in patients with Friedreich's ataxia. *J Bone Joint Surg Br* 2012;94(5):684-689.

    This retrospective review of 31 patients with Friedreich ataxia and scoliosis from 1978-2008 reported that in the 17 patients who underwent surgery, there was 1 death, 1 revision, 4 cases of proximal junctional kyphosis, no neurologic complications, and no wound issues. Level of evidence: IV.

21. Labelle H, Tohmé S, Duhaime M, Allard P: Natural history of scoliosis in Friedreich's ataxia. *J Bone Joint Surg Am* 1986;68(4):564-572.

22. Mulcahey MJ, Gaughan JP, Betz RR, Samdani AF, Barakat N, Hunter LN: Neuromuscular scoliosis in

children with spinal cord injury. *Top Spinal Cord Inj Rehabil* 2013;19(2):96-103.

In this retrospective review of 217 children with spinal cord injury, 100% had scoliosis. The children younger than 12 years were 3.7 times more likely to undergo spinal fusion than the older children. Neurologic level, motor level, and injury severity were not predictors of the need for spinal fusion. Level of evidence: IV.

23. Lebel DE, Corston JA, McAdam LC, Biggar WD, Alman BA: Glucocorticoid treatment for the prevention of scoliosis in children with Duchenne muscular dystrophy: Long-term follow-up. *J Bone Joint Surg Am* 2013;95(12):1057-1061.

In this prospective observational study of 54 boys with DMD, 30 received glucocorticoids. Of those receiving glucocorticoids, 20% required spinal fusion compared with 92% in the nonglucocorticoid group. Level of evidence: II

24. Sharrard WJ: The segmental innervation of the lower limb muscles in man. *Ann R Coll Surg Engl* 1964;35:106-122.

25. Letts M, Rathbone D, Yamashita T, Nichol B, Keeler A: Soft Boston orthosis in management of neuromuscular scoliosis: A preliminary report. *J Pediatr Orthop* 1992;12(4):470-474.

26. Nakamura N, Uesugi M, Inaba Y, Machida J, Okuzumi S, Saito T: Use of dynamic spinal brace in the management of neuromuscular scoliosis: A preliminary report. *J Pediatr Orthop B* 2014;23(3):291-298.

The authors of this retrospective study of the use of a dynamic spinal brace in 52 patients with neuromuscular scoliosis found that the brace was more effective in younger patients with longer curves. Overall improvement was reported in sitting ability and caregiver satisfaction. Level of evidence: IV.

27. Mehta S, Betz RR, Mulcahey MJ, McDonald C, Vogel LC, Anderson C: Effect of bracing on paralytic scoliosis secondary to spinal cord injury. *J Spinal Cord Med* 2004;27(suppl 1):S88-S92.

28. Shirley E, Bejarano C, Clay C, Fuzzell L, Leonard S, Wysocki T: Helping families make difficult choices: Creation and implementation of a decision aid for neuromuscular scoliosis surgery. *J Pediatr Orthop* 2015;35(8):831-837.

This prospective evaluation of a shared decision-making aid for neuromuscular scoliosis showed improvement in knowledge, satisfaction, and decision conflict among caregivers. Level of evidence: II.

29. Murphy NA, Firth S, Jorgensen T, Young PC: Spinal surgery in children with idiopathic and neuromuscular scoliosis: What's the difference? *J Pediatr Orthop* 2006;26(2):216-220.

30. Kang GR, Suh SW, Lee IO: Preoperative predictors of postoperative pulmonary complications in neuromuscular scoliosis. *J Orthop Sci* 2011;16(2):139-147.

This retrospective review of 74 patients found that a postoperative pulmonary complication was more likely to develop in patients with a preoperative FVC less than 39.5% of predicted value, an FEV_1 less than 40% of predicted value, a Cobb angle greater than 69°, or in those older than 16.5 years. Level of evidence: IV.

31. Yuan N, Skaggs DL, Dorey F, Keens TG: Preoperative predictors of prolonged postoperative mechanical ventilation in children following scoliosis repair. *Pediatr Pulmonol* 2005;40(5):414-419.

32. Khirani S, Bersanini C, Aubertin G, Bachy M, Vialle R, Fauroux B: Non-invasive positive pressure ventilation to facilitate the post-operative respiratory outcome of spine surgery in neuromuscular children. *Eur Spine J* 2014;23(suppl 4):S406-S411.

This prospective study reported on 13 patients who participated in a preoperative respiratory training program before spinal surgery. The program included noninvasive positive pressure ventilation and mechanical insufflation-exsufflation. The patients had no postoperative respiratory complications. Level of evidence: IV.

33. Gabos PG, Inan M, Thacker M, Borkhu B: Spinal fusion for scoliosis in Rett syndrome with an emphasis on early postoperative complications. *Spine (Phila Pa 1976)* 2012;37(2):E90-E94.

This retrospective case-control study reported on early postoperative complications in 16 patients with Rett syndrome who underwent spinal fusion. A high rate of early complications (28 major and 37 minor) was reported. Major respiratory complications occurred in 63% of the patients and gastrointestinal complications in 61%. Level of evidence: III.

34. Chambers HG, Weinstein CH, Mubarak SJ, Wenger DR, Silva PD: The effect of valproic acid on blood loss in patients with cerebral palsy. *J Pediatr Orthop* 1999;19(6):792-795.

35. Carney BT, Minter CL: Is operative blood loss associated with valproic acid? Analysis of bilateral femoral osteotomy in children with total involvement cerebral palsy. *J Pediatr Orthop* 2005;25(3):283-285.

36. Simm PJ, Johannesen J, Briody J, et al: Zoledronic acid improves bone mineral density, reduces bone turnover and improves skeletal architecture over 2 years of treatment in children with secondary osteoporosis. *Bone* 2011;49(5):939-943.

A prospective study of 20 patients with secondary osteoporosis found intravenous zoledronic acid used over 2 years improved bone mineral density and content without any serious adverse effects. Level of evidence: IV.

37. Chen F, Dai Z, Kang Y, Lv G, Keller ET, Jiang Y: Effects of zoledronic acid on bone fusion in osteoporotic patients after lumbar fusion. *Osteoporos Int* 2016;27(4):1469-1476.

This randomized controlled trial reported on patients with osteoporosis who underwent single-level fusions for degenerative spondylolisthesis. Patients were assigned to zoledronic acid or saline infusions after spinal surgery. Those who received the zoledronic acid demonstrated more bridging bone ($P < 0.05$), no vertebral compression fractures ($P < 0.05$), and prevention of decline in bone mineral density compared with the control group. Level of evidence: I.

38. Park YS, Kim HS, Baek SW, Kong DY, Ryu JA: The effect of zoledronic acid on the volume of the fusion-mass in lumbar spinal fusion. *Clin Orthop Surg* 2013;5(4):292-297.

    This retrospective case-controlled study of 44 patients treated with one- and two-level spinal fusions compared outcomes in those treated with and without zoledronic acid and with and without autograft. No difference in spinal fusion mass or outcomes was found among the groups. Level of evidence: III.

39. Moroni A, Faldini C, Hoang-Kim A, Pegreffi F, Giannini S: Alendronate improves screw fixation in osteoporotic bone. *J Bone Joint Surg Am* 2007;89(1):96-101.

40. Xue Q, Li H, Zou X, et al: Alendronate treatment improves bone-pedicle screw interface fixation in posterior lateral spine fusion: An experimental study in a porcine model. *Int Orthop* 2010;34(3):447-451.

41. Jevsevar DS, Karlin LI: The relationship between preoperative nutritional status and complications after an operation for scoliosis in patients who have cerebral palsy. *J Bone Joint Surg Am* 1993;75(6):880-884.

42. Perry JW, Montgomerie JZ, Swank S, Gilmore DS, Maeder K: Wound infections following spinal fusion with posterior segmental spinal instrumentation. *Clin Infect Dis* 1997;24(4):558-561.

43. Hatlen T, Song K, Shurtleff D, Duguay S: Contributory factors to postoperative spinal fusion complications for children with myelomeningocele. *Spine (Phila Pa 1976)* 2010;35(13):1294-1299.

44. Glotzbecker MP, Riedel MD, Vitale MG, et al: What's the evidence? Systematic literature review of risk factors and preventive strategies for surgical site infection following pediatric spine surgery. *J Pediatr Orthop* 2013;33(5):479-487.

    The authors report on a systematic review of the literature on surgical site infection risk factors and evidence-based practices to reduce surgical site infections in pediatric spinal surgery. Level of evidence: V.

45. Schwend RM, Hennrikus W, Hall JE, Emans JB: Childhood scoliosis: Clinical indications for magnetic resonance imaging. *J Bone Joint Surg Am* 1995;77(1):46-53.

46. Sink EL, Karol LA, Sanders J, Birch JG, Johnston CE, Herring JA: Efficacy of perioperative halo-gravity traction in the treatment of severe scoliosis in children. *J Pediatr Orthop* 2001;21(4):519-524.

47. Ashkenaze D, Mudiyam R, Boachie-Adjei O, Gilbert C: Efficacy of spinal cord monitoring in neuromuscular scoliosis. *Spine (Phila Pa 1976)* 1993;18(12):1627-1633.

48. DiCindio S, Theroux M, Shah S, et al: Multimodality monitoring of transcranial electric motor and somatosensory-evoked potentials during surgical correction of spinal deformity in patients with cerebral palsy and other neuromuscular disorders. *Spine (Phila Pa 1976)* 2003;28(16):1851-1855, discussion 1855-1856.

49. Salem KM, Goodger L, Bowyer K, Shafafy M, Grevitt MP: Does transcranial stimulation for motor evoked potentials (TcMEP) worsen seizures in epileptic patients following spinal deformity surgery? *Eur Spine J* 2015; May 15 [Epub ahead of print].

    Twelve patients with seizure disorder who underwent spinal fusion and had transcranial stimulation for motor-evoked potentials had no seizure activity while in the hospital and no increased seizure activity for an average of 23 months postoperatively. Level of evidence: IV.

50. Theusinger OM, Spahn DR: Perioperative blood conservation strategies for major spine surgery. *Best Pract Res Clin Anaesthesiol* 2016;30(1):41-52.

    Blood conservation strategies in spine surgery are reviewed. Level of evidence: III.

51. Thompson GH, Florentino-Pineda I, Poe-Kochert C, Armstrong DG, Son-Hing J: Role of Amicar in surgery for neuromuscular scoliosis. *Spine (Phila Pa 1976)* 2008;33(24):2623-2629.

52. Akbarnia BA, Breakwell LM, Marks DS, et al; Growing Spine Study Group: Dual growing rod technique followed for three to eleven years until final fusion: The effect of frequency of lengthening. *Spine (Phila Pa 1976)* 2008;33(9):984-990.

53. Flynn JM, Ramirez N, Emans JB, Smith JT, Mulcahey MJ, Betz RR: Is the Vertebral Expandable Prosthetic Titanium Rib a surgical alternative in patients with spina bifida? *Clin Orthop Relat Res* 2011;469(5):1291-1296.

    The authors of a prospective evaluation of 16 nonambulatory children with myelodysplasia treated with VEPTR reported improved spinal growth, improved pulmonary function in 11 patients, and 14 complications. Level of evidence: IV.

54. Agarwal A, Zakeri A, Agarwal AK, Jayaswal A, Goel VK: Distraction magnitude and frequency affects the outcome in juvenile idiopathic patients with growth rods: Finite element study using a representative scoliotic spine model. *Spine J* 2015;15(8):1848-1855.

    A scoliosis model was used to measure the distraction forces in growing rod constructs at different lengthening intervals. Less stress was found with distractions performed every 2 months than with distractions performed once yearly. Level of evidence: V.

55. Akbarnia BA, Cheung K, Noordeen H, et al: Next generation of growth-sparing techniques: Preliminary clinical results of a magnetically controlled growing rod in 14 patients with early-onset scoliosis. *Spine (Phila Pa 1976)* 2013;38(8):665-670.

This prospective multicenter case study evaluated the use of magnetic growing rods in 14 patients, 4 of whom had neuromuscular scoliosis. No neurologic complications and an average of 3.09 mm of growth per month were reported for those treated with dual-rod constructs. Level of evidence: IV.

56. McCarthy RE, Luhmann S, Lenke L, McCullough FL: The Shilla growth guidance technique for early-onset spinal deformities at 2-year follow-up: A preliminary report. *J Pediatr Orthop* 2014;34(1):1-7.

At the 2-year follow-up, 10 patients treated with the Shilla technique had curve improvement, an increase in space available for the lungs, and an increase in truncal height. Five complications required surgery. Level of evidence: IV.

57. Noordeen HM, Shah SA, Elsebaie HB, Garrido E, Farooq N, Al-Mukhtar M: In vivo distraction force and length measurements of growing rods: Which factors influence the ability to lengthen? *Spine (Phila Pa 1976)* 2011;36(26):2299-2303.

Prospective measurements of growing rod distraction forces in 26 patients showed increased force was required with increased lengthening, and diminished returns occurred with each lengthening procedure. Level of evidence: III.

58. McCarthy RE, McCullough FL: Shilla growth guidance for early-onset scoliosis: Results after a minimum of five years of follow-up. *J Bone Joint Surg Am* 2015;97(19):1578-1584.

In a retrospective 5-year follow-up of 40 patients who were treated with Shilla growth guidance for spinal deformity, the 16 patients with neuromuscular scoliosis had improved curves, more lung space, and increased spinal column growth. Level of evidence: IV.

59. Yoon WW, Sedra F, Shah S, Wallis C, Muntoni F, Noordeen H: Improvement of pulmonary function in children with early-onset scoliosis using magnetic growth rods. *Spine (Phila Pa 1976)* 2014;39(15):1196-1202.

The authors of a retrospective review of six patients with neuromuscular scoliosis treated with magnetic growing rods found improvement in coronal deformity and the percentages of FVC and FEV_1 predicted values over a 2-year period. Level of evidence: IV.

60. Livingston K, Zurakowski D, Snyder B; Growing Spine Study Group; Children's Spine Study Group: Parasol rib deformity in hypotonic neuromuscular scoliosis: A new radiographical definition and a comparison of short-term treatment outcomes with VEPTR and growing rods. *Spine (Phila Pa 1976)* 2015;40(13):E780-E786.

Forty-four patients with hypotonic neuromuscular scoliosis were treated with growing rods and VEPTR. The authors reported that the parasol score correlated with the assisted ventilation rating. Parasol scores worsened with VEPTR and stayed same in those treated with growing rods. The assisted ventilation rating stayed the same. Level of evidence: IV.

61. Vitale MG, Matsumoto H, Feinberg N, et al; Children's Spine Study Group; Growing Spine Study Group: Proximal rib vs proximal spine anchors in growing rods: A multicenter prospective cohort study. *Spine Deform* 2015;3(6):626-627.

This prospective observational study of 106 patients (aged 3 to 9 years) with scoliosis greater than 40° showed that five or more proximal anchors was protective against proximal rod migration. Level of evidence: II.

62. Dubousset J: Pelvic obliquity: A review. *Orthopedics* 1991;14(4):479-481.

63. Mattila M, Jalanko T, Puisto V, Pajulo O, Helenius IJ: Hybrid versus total pedicle screw instrumentation in patients undergoing surgery for neuromuscular scoliosis: A comparative study with matched cohorts. *J Bone Joint Surg Br* 2012;94(10):1393-1398.

Sixty-six patients with neuromuscular scoliosis were treated with spinal surgery: 33 with hybrid instrumentation and 33 with all-pedicle screw instrumentation. Those treated with all-pedicle screw instrumentation had shorter surgical times, better correction, and less blood loss than those in the hybrid group. No difference in outcomes occurred based on the Scoliosis Research Society-24 questionnaire. Level of evidence: III.

64. Dayer R, Ouellet JA, Saran N: Pelvic fixation for neuromuscular scoliosis deformity correction. *Curr Rev Musculoskelet Med* 2012;5(2):91-101.

A review of pelvic fixation techniques in neuromuscular scoliosis is presented. Level of evidence: V.

65. Myung KS, Lee C, Skaggs DL: Early pelvic fixation failure in neuromuscular scoliosis. *J Pediatr Orthop* 2015;35(3):258-265.

Forty-one patients with neuromuscular scoliosis underwent posterior-only spinal fusion and pelvic fixation. The authors reported a 29% failure rate for pelvic fixation at a mean follow-up of 18 months. No failures of fixation occurred with constructs that had at least six screws in L5, S1, and the pelvis. Level of evidence: III.

66. Diab MG, Franzone JM, Vitale MG: The role of posterior spinal osteotomies in pediatric spinal deformity surgery: Indications and operative technique. *J Pediatr Orthop* 2011;31(1suppl):S88-S98.

A review of posterior osteotomies for the correction of pediatric spinal deformity is presented. Level of evidence: V.

67. McDonnell MF, Glassman SD, Dimar JR II, Puno RM, Johnson JR: Perioperative complications of anterior procedures on the spine. *J Bone Joint Surg Am* 1996;78(6):839-847.

68. Shufflebarger HL, Grimm JO, Bui V, Thomson JD: Anterior and posterior spinal fusion: Staged versus same-day surgery. *Spine (Phila Pa 1976)* 1991;16(8):930-933.

69. Powell ET IV, Krengel WF III, King HA, Lagrone MO: Comparison of same-day sequential anterior and posterior spinal fusion with delayed two-stage anterior and posterior spinal fusion. *Spine (Phila Pa 1976)* 1994;19(11):1256-1259.

70. O'Brien T, Akmakjian J, Ogin G, Eilert R: Comparison of one-stage versus two-stage anterior/posterior spinal fusion for neuromuscular scoliosis. *J Pediatr Orthop* 1992;12(5):610-615.

71. Tsirikos AI, Chang WN, Dabney KW, Miller F: Comparison of one-stage versus two-stage anteroposterior spinal fusion in pediatric patients with cerebral palsy and neuromuscular scoliosis. *Spine (Phila Pa 1976)* 2003;28(12):1300-1305.

72. Price CT, Connolly JF, Carantzas AC, Ilyas I: Comparison of bone grafts for posterior spinal fusion in adolescent idiopathic scoliosis. *Spine (Phila Pa 1976)* 2003;28(8):793-798.

73. Sharma S, Wu C, Andersen T, Wang Y, Hansen ES, Bünger CE: Prevalence of complications in neuromuscular scoliosis surgery: A literature meta-analysis from the past 15 years. *Eur Spine J* 2013;22(6):1230-1249.

The prevalence rates of complications in 15,218 patients with neuromuscular scoliosis treated with spinal fusion were as follows: 22.7% pulmonary, 12.5% implant related, 10.9% infection, 3.0% neurologic, and 1.9% pseudarthrosis. Level of evidence: IV.

74. Horacek O, Chlumsky J, Mazanec R, Kolar P, Andel R, Kobesova A: Pulmonary function in patients with hereditary motor and sensory neuropathy: A comparison of patients with and without spinal deformity. *Neuromuscul Disord* 2012;22(12):1083-1089.

Pulmonary function test results were compared in cohorts of patients with and without spinal deformity and with and without neuropathy. The authors concluded that respiratory muscle weakness is the main pathology for pulmonary dysfunction in patients with hereditary motor sensory neuropathy. Level of evidence: II.

75. Ramo BA, Roberts DW, Tuason D, et al: Surgical site infections after posterior spinal fusion for neuromuscular scoliosis: A thirty-year experience at a single institution. *J Bone Joint Surg Am* 2014;96(24):2038-2048.

Surgical site infection was more common in patients with spina bifida than in those with other diagnoses. Other factors associated with surgical site infection were a body mass index greater than 25 kg/m^2, incontinence, inadequate prophylactic antibiotic dosing, length of fusion, pelvic fixation, length of hospital stay, and the presence of other complications. Level of evidence: III.

76. Comstock CP, Leach J, Wenger DR: Scoliosis in total-body-involvement cerebral palsy: Analysis of surgical treatment and patient and caregiver satisfaction. *Spine (Phila Pa 1976)* 1998;23(12):1412-1424, discussion 1424-1425.

77. Narayanan UG, Fehlings D, Weir S, Knights S, Kiran S, Campbell K: Initial development and validation of the Caregiver Priorities and Child Health Index of Life with Disabilities (CPCHILD). *Dev Med Child Neurol* 2006;48(10):804-812.

78. Askin GN, Hallett R, Hare N, Webb JK: The outcome of scoliosis surgery in the severely physically handicapped child: An objective and subjective assessment. *Spine (Phila Pa 1976)* 1997;22(1):44-50.

79. Cassidy C, Craig CL, Perry A, Karlin LI, Goldberg MJ: A reassessment of spinal stabilization in severe cerebral palsy. *J Pediatr Orthop* 1994;14(6):731-739.

80. Khoshbin A, Vivas L, Law PW, et al: The long-term outcome of patients treated operatively and non-operatively for scoliosis deformity secondary to spina bifida. *Bone Joint J* 2014;96-B(9):1244-1251.

The authors compared 34 adults treated surgically and 11 treated nonsurgically in childhood for scoliosis secondary to spina bifida. At an average follow-up of 14.1 years, the surgically treated patients had improvement in coronal deformity; however, no difference in health-related QOL or sitting balance was found between the groups. The surgical group had a 32.4% rate of postoperative infections. Level of evidence: III.

81. Diefenbach C, Ialenti MN, Lonner BS, Kamerlink JR, Verma K, Errico TJ: Hospital cost analysis of neuromuscular scoliosis surgery. *Bull Hosp Jt Dis (2013)* 2013;71(4):272-277.

A hospital cost analysis was done for 74 patients with neuromuscular scoliosis who received surgical treatment. The cost calculation was based on the surgical correction, the hospital stay, and postoperative care. Total costs were \$50,096 ± \$23,998. Twenty-four percent of the costs were attributable to implants, 22% to inpatient and ICU care, and 11% to bone grafts. Level of evidence: III.

82. Ritter MA, Lutgring JD, Davis KE, Berend ME, Meding JB: A clinical, radiographic, and cost comparison of cerclage techniques: Wires vs cables. *J Arthroplasty* 2006;21(7):1064-1067.

83. Kim YJ, Lenke LG, Cho SK, Bridwell KH, Sides B, Blanke K: Comparative analysis of pedicle screw versus hook instrumentation in posterior spinal fusion of adolescent idiopathic scoliosis. *Spine (Phila Pa 1976)* 2004;29(18):2040-2048.

84. Whitaker AT, Sharkey M, Diab M: Spinal fusion for scoliosis in patients with globally involved cerebral palsy: An ethical assessment. *J Bone Joint Surg Am* 2015;97(9):782-787.

An ethical assessment and review of the literature was performed regarding spinal fusion in patients with GMFCS level V cerebral palsy. A four-topic model was used. Level of evidence: V.

Chapter 31

Kyphosis

Matthew E. Oetgen, MD, MBA

Abstract

Kyphosis is a common deformity in children. Normally, sagittal alignment changes with age, with thoracic kyphosis decreasing and lumbar lordosis increasing, until normal adult spinal and sagittal pelvic alignment is achieved. Abnormal sagittal spinal alignment in pediatric patients can occur as the result of a variety of conditions, which are often associated with developmental structural abnormalities of the vertebral bodies. Regardless of the etiology, is important to assess the neurologic status of patients with kyphosis because this spinal deformity is associated with the possibility of neurologic injury. Treatment depends on the age of the patient, the magnitude of the deformity, and the underlying etiology. Treatment options consist of observation, brace treatment, and spinal fusion. Long-term patient satisfaction and functional outcome may be improved with normal sagittal spinal alignment, which demonstrates the importance of treatment of pathologic kyphosis in this patient population.

Keywords: congenital kyphosis; kyphosis; sagittal spinal alignment; Scheuermann kyphosis

Introduction

The sagittal alignment of the skeletally mature spine is relatively well understood, with the normal values of cervical lordosis, thoracic kyphosis, lumbar lordosis, and pelvic parameters previously reported.[1] Despite this understanding of the adult spine, the normal development of spinal sagittal alignment throughout childhood and adolescence remains less clearly defined. It is particularly important to better define the effects of the many pediatric conditions that can result in pathologic sagittal spinal alignment and better monitor the growth of children with these conditions to assist in determining when intervention is needed.[2] A thorough understanding of the development of the sagittal plane may be important in optimizing long-term outcomes because it will aid surgeons in determining when surgical interventions, such as contouring sagittal spinal alignment using modern segmental spinal instrumentation, are appropriate.

Despite its apparent importance, there is a relative paucity of information about the development of sagittal spinal alignment in children. An analysis of the normative sagittal spinal alignment of 121 children aged 3 to 15 years who were stratified into four age groups showed that the total global kyphosis measured from T1-T12 averaged 44.9° to 53.3° and was larger than adult normative values.[3] The total lumbar lordosis averaged −44.7° to −57.3° and was smaller than adult normative values. The average thoracic apex was the T7-T8 disk, and the lumbar apex was the L4 vertebra, which were both similar compared with these parameters in adults; however, there was an average of 3.6° of kyphosis across the thoracolumbar junction (T10-L2) in children. These findings suggest a more gradual transition from thoracic kyphosis to lumbar lordosis at the thoracolumbar junction, with greater kyphosis in this region in children compared with adults. This finding challenges the widely held belief that this area is essentially neutral in alignment. A change in alignment during growth also was found, with a notable decrease in global kyphosis and an increase in lumbar lordosis in children in the 10- to 12-year age group, with a later increase in kyphosis and decrease in lordosis in children in the 13- to 15-year age group. It was postulated that this change resulted from the adolescent growth spurt with disproportionate anterior vertebral growth[3] (**Figure 1**). A 2015 study reported that the normative sagittal spinal alignment of children in a sitting position showed less thoracic kyphosis and lumbar lordosis compared with normative standing sagittal alignment values.[4]

Recently, a better understanding of the relationship between the sagittal spinal alignment and sagittal pelvic

Dr. Oetgen or an immediate family member serves as a board member, owner, officer, or committee member of the American Academy of Orthopaedic Surgeons, the Pediatric Orthopaedic Society of North America, and the Scoliosis Research Society.

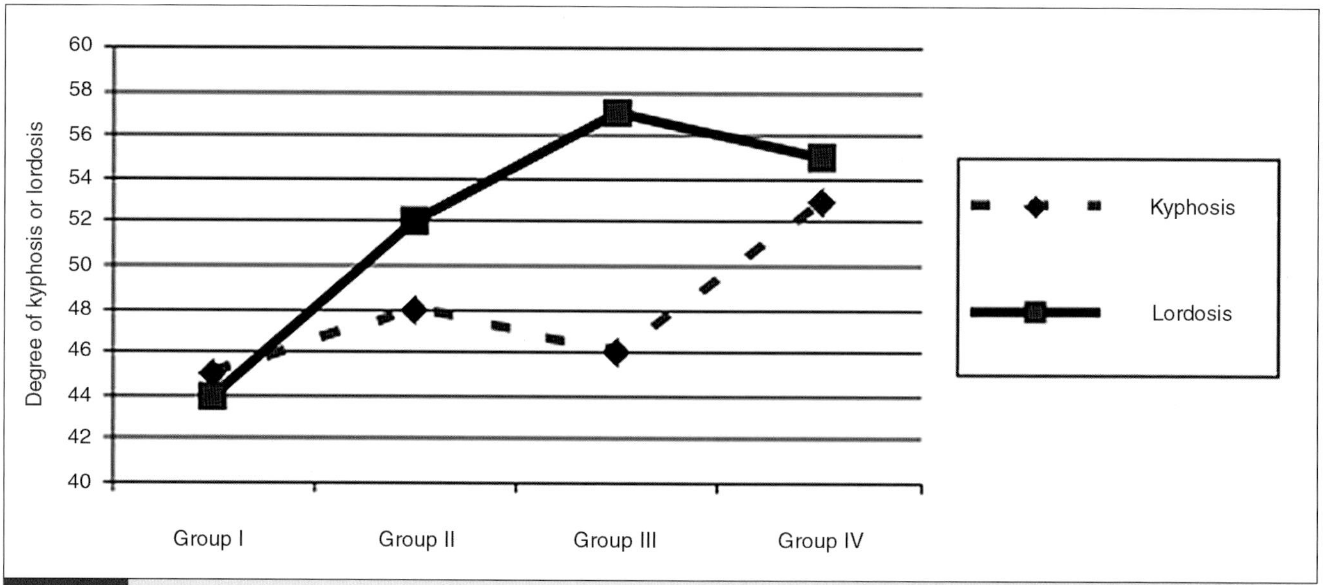

Figure 1 The line graph depicts the age-related changes in thoracic kyphosis and lumbar lordosis found in a study of radiographic sagittal spinal alignment in 151 normal children without musculoskeletal abnormalities. The children were divided into four groups based on age: group I: age 3 to 6 years; group II: age 7 to 9 years; group III: age 10 to 12 years; group IV: age 13 to 15 years.

alignment has emerged, with multiple investigations demonstrating that the interaction of these two areas leads to global sagittal balance (**Figure 2**). Although few data exist demonstrating normative sagittal pelvic values in children and the progressive changes that take place during development, these parameters in children were investigated in a 2004 study.[5] The authors found that the complex interaction between the sagittal spinal and pelvic parameters exists in children as it does in adults. In children, the pelvic incidence increases linearly from age 4 to 18 years; this was hypothesized to correlate with changing sagittal spinal alignment to maintain a constant sagittal balance.[5]

In general, it appears likely that global and segmental sagittal spinal alignment and sagittal pelvic alignment in a growing child is quite dynamic and should be carefully considered when planning a surgical intervention.

Physiologic Consequences of Kyphosis

Excessive thoracic kyphosis and abnormal global sagittal plane alignment has been shown to lead to a variety of physiologic effects, including the potential association with adolescent back pain, the risk of neurologic injury, and a decrease in self-reported patient satisfaction. In a cross-sectional study of Flemish adolescents, a correlation was found between poor sagittal standing posture and back and neck pain; however, this study used observational sagittal alignment of patients rather than radiographic parameters of spinal alignment.[6] A systemic review of patients with thoracic spine pain reported poor posture as a potential factor associated with pain, although the study authors found that there were many variables associated with spine pain in the pediatric population.[7]

Neurologic injury associated with excessive kyphosis in pediatric patients has been widely reported in the literature. In general, neurologic injury is suspected to occur as a result of excessive compression of the spinal cord when it is draped over a curve with a substantial kyphotic thoracic angle. Neurologic involvement has been most often reported in patients with congenital kyphotic deformities or those with rapidly progressing sharp kyphotic deformities such as those that occur in patients with neurofibromatosis type-1.[8] Patients with a substantial kyphotic deformity may be at greater risk for neurologic injury when undergoing lower limb surgery. A 2015 case report described the development of paraplegia in two children with skeletal dysplasia and associated thoracic kyphosis who were surgically treated for a lower limb deformity.[9] These outcomes highlight the need to take precautions to avoid iatrogenic spinal cord injury in patients with hyperkyphosis.

Patient-reported outcomes appear to be negatively associated with increased thoracic kyphosis. Evaluation of a prospectively collected spinal deformity database demonstrated worse self-reported values in all domains of the Scoliosis Research Society-22 questionnaire in patients with Scheuermann kyphosis compared with patients

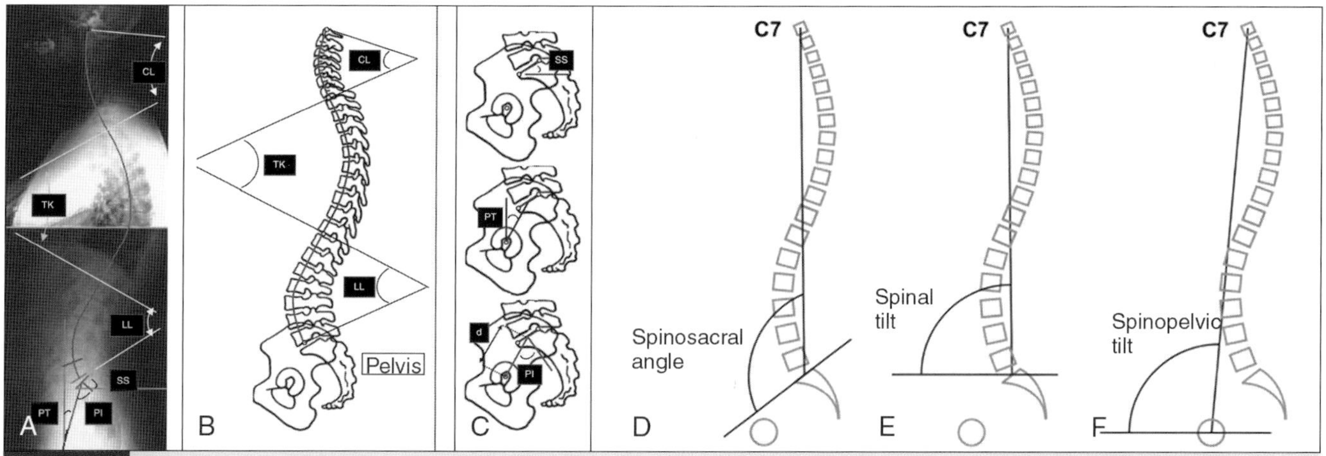

Figure 2 **A** through **C,** Techniques for measuring spinal sagittal plane alignment and pelvic parameters. **A,** Sagittal radiograph of the spine and pelvis show the simplified curve model of the spine and the shape and orientation parameters of the pelvis. **B,** Illustration of the spine with the shape parameters delineated. **C,** Illustration of the pelvis with its shape and orientation parameters delineated. CL = cervical lordosis, TK = thoracic kyphosis, LL = lumbar lordosis, SS = sacral slope, PT = pelvic tilt, PI = pelvic incidence, d = distance from center of sacral plate to femoral head axis of rotation. The relationship of the pelvic parameters is PI = PT + SS. Illustration of techniques for measuring the global spinal sagittal alignment include measurement of the spinosacral angle (**D**), spinal tilt (**E**), and spinopelvic tilt (**F**). (Panels A, B, C reproduced with permission from Berthonnaud E, Dimnet J, Roussouly P, Labelle H: Analysis of the sagittal balance of the spine and pelvis using shape and orientation parameters. *J Spinal Disord Tech* 2005;18:40-47 and panels D, E, F reproduced with permission from Mac-Thiong JM, Labelle H, Roussouly P: Pediatric sagittal alignment. *Eur Spine J* 2011;20[suppl 5]:586-590.)

with scoliosis and normal control subjects. The self-image domain had the highest negative correlation with increasing kyphosis.[10] This negative correlation also was demonstrated in patients with thoracic hyperkyphosis (>45°) that was not associated with Scheuermann kyphosis.[11]

Patient Presentation and Assessment

The typical presentation of kyphosis varies based on the age of the patient and the location of the deformity. In infants and children who are not yet of walking age, excessive thoracic or thoracolumbar kyphosis is often appreciated as an obvious gibbus with inspection of the back. Commonly, this is a flexible deformity that is easily straightened with gentle three-point bending of the spine and is likely associated with relatively weak core strength in patients in this young age group. In older children of walking age, the presentation of kyphosis is dependent on the location of the deformity and the underlying etiology. Congenital kyphosis or kyphosis associated with underlying conditions that lead to structural abnormalities of the vertebral bodies often present as relatively short, sharp deformities of the spine. Overall sagittal spinal alignment is affected by the location of the kyphosis. Excessive thoracic kyphosis is often associated with increased lumbar lordosis, which is used as a compensatory mechanism to improve global alignment, whereas thoracolumbar kyphosis is associated with a compensatory thoracic lordosis or a mild crouching gait to compensate for global alignment.

Given the rare but reported occurrence of progressive myelopathy in pediatric patients with excessive kyphosis, a thorough neurologic assessment, including strength, sensation, and reflex testing, should be included in the evaluation of all patients presenting with kyphosis. Any evidence of abnormalities on examination should be further evaluated with MRI to assess for evidence of spinal cord compression or other neural axis anomalies.

Radiologic assessment of patients with kyphosis typically starts with upright, full-length radiographs of the spine. Positioning of the arms to move them out of the way of the spine when obtaining lateral radiographs has been shown to affect overall spinal alignment. Although a variety of techniques exist to limit this effect, it appears that passively supporting the arms in approximately 30° of forward flexion limits the amount of shifting of the sagittal vertical axis when compared with the arms-at-the-sides position.[12] Including the area from the pelvis to the femoral heads on lateral radiographs allows for the simultaneous measurement of sagittal pelvic parameters.

Cross-sectional imaging is useful in certain circumstances to further assess the spine. CT is helpful in defining bony anatomy, particularly for preoperative planning. MRI is useful in assessing intraspinal anomalies and the health of the spinal cord in patients with substantial angular kyphosis.

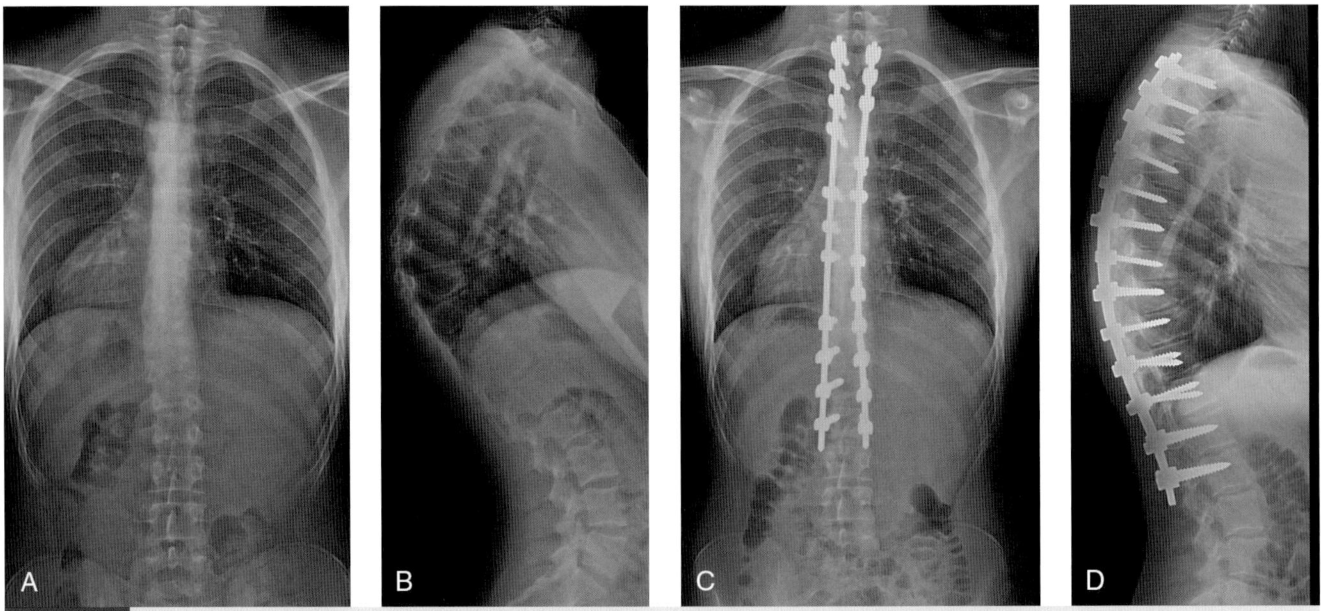

Figure 3 Preoperative PA (**A**) and lateral (**B**) radiographs of the spine of a 16-year-old boy with Scheuermann kyphosis measuring 93°. Postoperative AP (**C**) and lateral (**D**) radiographs after kyphosis correction using a segmental pedicle screw construct and multiple Ponte osteotomies.

Conditions of Pediatric Kyphosis

Physiologic Round-Back Deformity or Postural Kyphosis

Postural kyphosis is a nonpathologic condition of excessive kyphotic alignment. It is often a relatively flexible deformity that can be passively corrected by active spinal extension by the patient. When viewed from the side, the patient often demonstrates a relatively gentle kyphotic alignment on forward bending as opposed to a sharp, angular kyphosis seen in other conditions. Other than the excessive kyphosis, radiographic findings are normal, with no evidence of abnormal development of the vertebral bodies. Treatment is directed at educating the patient and family about the condition and providing reassurance. Postural exercises consisting of paraspinal and core muscle strengthening to improve postural alignment are prescribed. Brace treatment or surgical intervention is rarely, if ever, indicated for postural kyphosis.

Scheuermann Kyphosis

Scheuermann kyphosis is a pathologic condition of excessive kyphosis most often seen in adolescents. This condition is diagnosed when excessive clinical kyphosis is associated with the radiographic finding of excessive anterior wedging of 5° or more of at least three adjacent vertebral bodies. Additional radiologic characteristics may include Schmorl nodules, narrowing of intervertebral disk spaces, and vertebral end plate irregularities[13] (**Figure 3**). Scheuermann kyphosis is commonly associated with dull back pain over the apex of the deformity and tight hamstrings on physical examination; in approximately one-third of patients, a mild degree of scoliosis is present.[14]

Outcomes

The natural history of both treated and untreated Scheuermann kyphosis is poorly documented in the medical literature. In a 1993 report on the long-term follow-up of 67 patients with Scheuermann kyphosis and an age- and sex-matched control group, it was found that patients in the Scheuermann group tended to have more back pain, jobs requiring lower-activity levels, and less range of motion and strength of the trunk compared with the control group.[15] No differences in the groups were found regarding educational levels, the extent of pain interference with activities of daily living, self-consciousness, self-esteem, or social limitations. Some degree of restrictive pulmonary disease was seen in those individuals with greater than 100° of kyphosis. These long-term results are interesting in light of the lower levels of self-reported outcomes in patients with Scheuermann kyphosis compared with normal control subjects noted in a recent 2013 study.[10] The reasons for this discrepancy may be that outcomes of the cohort in the 1993 study were not generalizable; the natural history of patients in that study were not typical of patients with Scheuermann kyphosis; or differences exist between younger patients with Scheuermann kyphosis and older patients, with the inferior outcomes reported by younger patients improving over time. A 2012 report of long-term outcomes demonstrated increased odds for back pain and functional disability in patients with Scheuermann kyphosis; however, the amount of pain and disability was not related to the degree of kyphosis.[16] Given these discrepancies in reported outcomes, additional and longer-term follow-up studies are needed.

Treatment

Treatment options consist of observation, physical therapy, bracing, and surgical intervention. Physical therapy, consisting of hamstring stretching and core and paraspinal muscle strengthening, has been shown to improve symptomatic pain but does not affect the degree of kyphosis.[17] Brace treatment of Scheuermann kyphosis has been demonstrated to be effective at improving the spinal deformity in patients with less rigid curves. Bracing is considered for those with less severe deformity (<65°) who have at least 1 year of growth remaining. Despite the radiographic improvement seen with brace wear in this population, there is a high degree of deformity recurrence (up to 30% of patients) after bracing is discontinued.[14]

Because of the relatively benign long-term results reported for patients with Scheuermann kyphosis, surgical intervention is controversial and there is little evidence-based material defining surgical indications. Relative surgical indications include progressive deformity greater than 70°, disabling back pain that is recalcitrant to nonsurgical treatment, and serious cosmetic concerns expressed by the patient.[14] Given the relatively low percentage of patients with uncontrolled deformity progression and severe back pain, cosmetic concerns of the patient are often the most influential consideration in surgical decision making.

The surgical treatment of Scheuermann kyphosis has changed over time. Currently, the most popular approach is a posterior spinal fusion with posterior column shortening osteotomies. Although a combined anterior-posterior approach is effective, recent studies have demonstrated equivalent correction and decreased complications with the posterior-only approach.[18,19] Although the current method of surgical treatment of this condition is generally considered safe, it has been shown to have a higher complication rate than treatment for adolescent idiopathic scoliosis. A recent comparison of patients treated for Scheuermann kyphosis and those treated for adolescent idiopathic scoliosis showed a higher rate of postoperative neurologic injury (2.1% versus 0.13%), instrumentation complications (3.1% versus 0.63%), and surgical site infection (10.3% versus 0.75%) in the patients with Scheuermann kyphosis than in those with idiopathic scoliosis, respectively.[10] In addition, subtle preoperative neurologic abnormalities are present in up to 9% of patients with Scheuermann kyphosis, so careful preoperative assessment and judicious use of neurologic imaging is needed.[20]

Congenital Kyphosis

Congenital kyphosis is a varied group of spinal deformities, with abnormal embryologic formation of the vertebral bodies being the common etiology. This group of deformities is broadly categorized into those with a failure of vertebral formation, a failure of vertebral segmentation, or a mix of these two conditions.[21] Congenital kyphosis should be distinguished from postural, early upper lumbar kyphosis seen in some children before walking age, which is likely associated with poor muscle tone of the trunk. Postural kyphosis is commonly seen without evidence of vertebral body abnormality (as opposed to congenital kyphosis or the vertebral body anterior-inferior beaking seen in patients with mucopolysaccharidoses) and will typically resolve with time and normal motor development. In addition, early infantile kyphosis resulting from mild anterior-superior upper lumbar body hypoplasia has been described and has been shown to resolve spontaneously with growth.[22]

The natural history of congenital kyphosis is variable and mainly influenced by the location and type of deformity and the number of vertebral levels involved. In general, progressive kyphotic deformity is typical, with progression seen most commonly during periods of rapid spinal growth.

A three-part classification system is used to describe congenital kyphosis based on the type of vertebral anomaly associated with the deformity[21,23] (**Figure 4**). Patients with kyphosis involving failures of vertebral body formation (type 1) typically have rapid progression during periods of growth and are at higher risk for neurologic deterioration because of the typically short, sharp deformity pattern (**Figure 5**). Type 2 deformities are associated with failures of vertebral body segmentation and often progress less rapidly and are rarely associated with progressive neurologic deterioration because the deformity is less sharply angulated. Mixed pattern deformities (type 3) and those associated with congenital vertebral dislocation have the most aggressive natural history, with deformity progression and neurologic deterioration almost assured without intervention.

Treatment of congenital kyphosis is dependent on patient age, neurologic status, and progression of the deformity. Management typically involves observation, with radiographic and neurologic examinations performed at regular intervals. Brace treatment has not been shown to be efficacious in this condition. Surgical intervention is

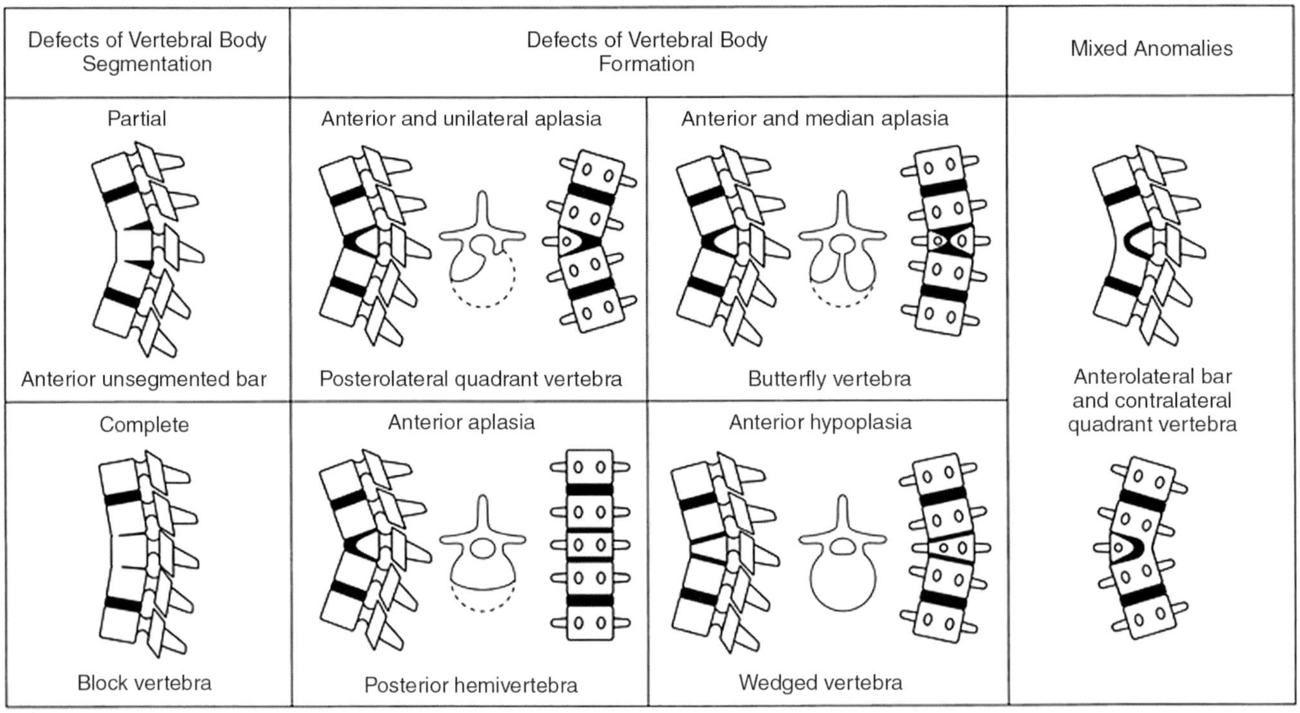

Figure 4 Illustration of a three-part classification system used to describe congenital kyphosis based on the type of vertebral body anomaly associated with the deformity.

required if deformity progression is noted or neurologic deterioration is found.

In patients with congenital kyphosis associated with failures of formation, posterior arthrodesis can lead to progressive correction of the deformity over time via anterior spinal column growth. This treatment is more successful in patients younger than 5 years and those with a deformity of less than 50°. Anterior and posterior arthrodesis is indicated in patients with progressive congenital kyphosis who are older than 5 years or have a curve magnitude greater than 50°. The anterior surgery can be performed through a separate anterior approach, via a costotransversectomy, or through an all-posterior approach, depending on the need for anterior decompression and the skill and comfort level of the treating surgeon.[24,25]

Other Conditions Associated With Kyphosis

Mucopolysaccharidosis

Mucopolysaccharidosis is a family of six genetic disorders defined by abnormal lysosomal storage caused by deficiency of enzymes required for degradation of intracellular gylcosaminoglycans.[26] Although these conditions have a multitude of musculoskeletal manifestations, acute thoracolumbar kyphosis associated with abnormalities of vertebral development (inferior L1-L2 vertebral body beaking) is considered pathognomonic for this condition[26] (**Figure 6**). Although nonsurgical management can be considered as a method to delay definitive treatment in patients with deformity progression, long-term outcomes of brace or cast treatment of kyphosis associated with mucopolysaccharidosis are unproven. Progressive deformity is definitively treated with circumferential spinal fusion to achieve maximal correction with the lowest risk of recurrent deformity.[27,28]

Achondroplasia

Achondroplasia is the most common skeletal dysplasia, with an incidence of approximately 1 in 30,000 live births each year.[29] The disorder is characterized by abnormal enchondral ossification of long bones caused by a mutation in the fibroblast growth factor receptor-3 gene (*FGFR3*). One of the most common skeletal manifestations of achondroplasia is the development of thoracolumbar kyphosis, with a reported prevalence of 87% in patients younger than 2 years, 39% in patients aged 2 to 5 years, and 11% in patients older than 5 years.[29] The most common clinical course is one of gradual improvement as the child matures and trunk and core strength increase with growth and progressing functional development (from sitting to standing to walking). Risk factors for progressive kyphosis have

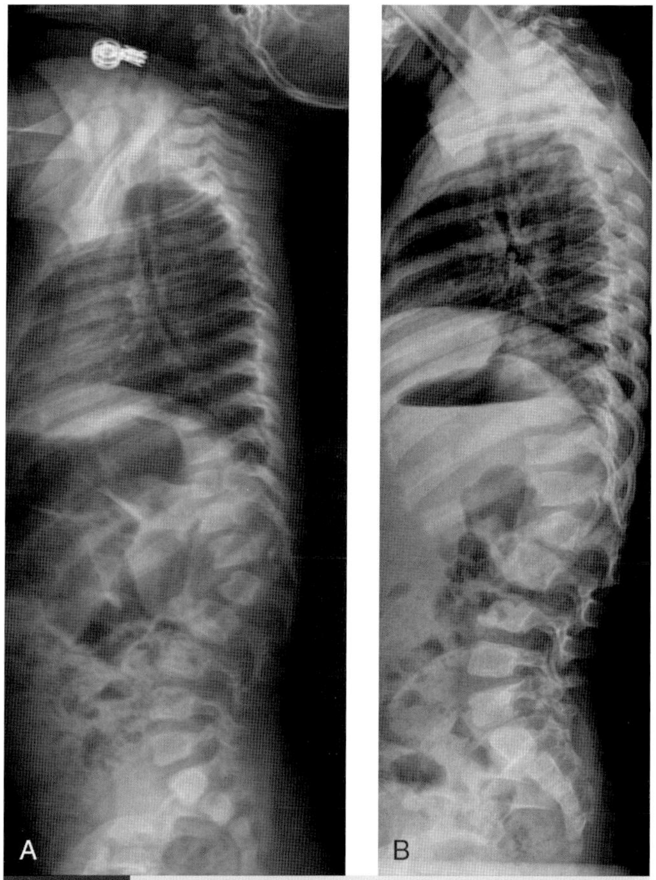

Figure 5 **A,** Sitting lateral radiograph of the spine of a 2-year-old boy with 32° of congenital thoracolumbar kyphosis resulting from a type 1 defect in the L1 vertebral body. **B,** Sitting lateral radiograph obtained at age 3 years shows continued thoracolumbar kyphosis of 32° resulting from the failure of anterior vertebral body formation at L1.

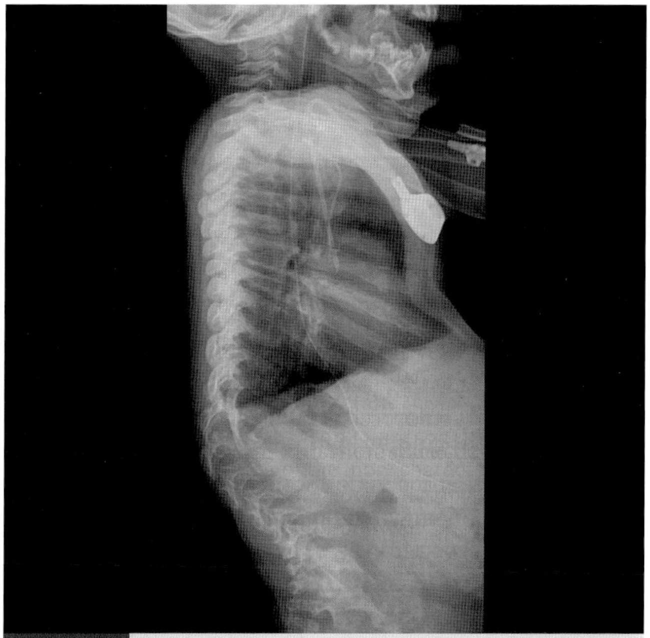

Figure 6 Lateral standing radiograph of a 2-year-old patient with type 1 mucopolysaccharidosis. The patient has 48° of kyphosis with an apex at L1. Note the anterior vertebral body beaking that is pathognomonic for this condition.

been reported with delayed motor development, initial kyphosis greater than 25°, and a greater percentage of apical vertebral wedging and translation.[30] In patients with persistent or progressive thoracolumbar kyphosis after walking age, a brace has been suggested to improve alignment and possibly help correct the deformity by allowing improved anterior vertebral body growth and development[31] (**Figure 7**). Although the natural history of thoracolumbar kyphosis in patients with achondroplasia has not been thoroughly documented, surgery has been proposed for patients with persistent or progressive deformity because of concerns about poor long-term function. In general, persistent thoracolumbar kyphosis greater than 50° after age 5 years is considered an indication for corrective spinal fusion. A combined anterior-posterior approach or posterior-only fusion have both been shown to be effective methods of treatment.[29]

Iatrogenic Kyphosis

Proximal junctional kyphosis and distal junctional kyphosis are complications seen after spinal instrumentation in pediatric patients. Although no clear definition exists, this type of kyphosis is typically characterized by a progression of deformity of greater than 5° to 10° at the proximal or distal end of a fusion.[32] The difficulty in determining the existence of this complication is further accentuated by the difficulty in obtaining accurate radiographic measurements. Multiple studies have demonstrated a high degree of variability in measurements and poor interclass correlation between practitioners measuring proximal junction kyphosis in patients with adolescent idiopathic scoliosis or early-onset scoliosis.[33,34]

The prevalence of junctional kyphosis is varied and depends on the underlying spinal pathology, the underlying condition of the patient, the age of the patient, and the amount of postoperative deformity correction.[35] Techniques to prevent junctional kyphosis include planning deformity correction to achieve appropriate global sagittal balance, which may be predicted by baseline sagittal pelvic parameters; choosing appropriate proximal and distal end vertebrae in surgical planning; and using proper surgical techniques to minimize disruption of adjacent nonfused facet joint capsules and interspinous ligaments, which provide inherent junctional stability.[35-37]

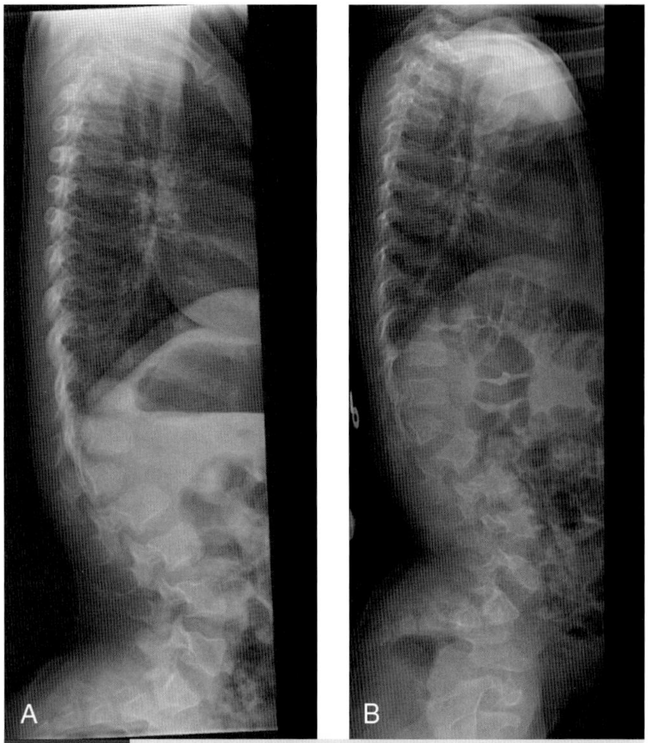

Figure 7 **A,** Standing lateral radiograph of a 2.5-year-old girl with achondroplasia shows a 44° thoracolumbar kyphosis with an apex at L1. **B,** Standing lateral radiograph shows some improvement of the kyphosis to 38° in a thoracolumbar orthosis.

Summary

Patients with normal sagittal spinal alignment have been shown to have better long-term outcomes compared with patients with excessive spinal kyphosis. Increased back pain, poorer self-image, and possible neurologic deterioration over time can be seen with excessive kyphosis, which demonstrates the importance of diagnosis and proper treatment of this condition. A variety of underlying conditions are associated with kyphosis in the pediatric population, so a thorough evaluation and appropriate imaging are needed when this spinal deformity is encountered. Treatment aimed at correcting and maintaining sagittal alignment is important and should be undertaken within the context of the underlying condition of the individual patient.

Key Study Points

- Normal pediatric sagittal spine alignment is dynamic and changes as children develop. Thoracic kyphosis decreases and lumbar lordosis increases until normal adult sagittal plane alignment is achieved. The pelvic incidence appears to increase during development to maintain overall global alignment based on changes in the spinal alignment.
- Abnormal sagittal plane alignment resulting from excessive thoracic kyphosis has been associated with increased back pain and possible delayed neurologic injury. Long-term patient-reported satisfaction and functional outcomes are better in those with normal sagittal spinal alignment compared with patients with abnormal sagittal alignment.
- Pathologic kyphosis is associated with a variety of pediatric conditions. The most common cause is Scheuermann kyphosis, which can be treated with observation, brace treatment, or surgery, depending on the magnitude of the deformity and skeletal maturity of the patient.
- Other conditions associated with abnormal kyphosis include congenital kyphosis, skeletal dysplasia, mucopolysaccharidosis, and iatrogenic junctional kyphosis after surgical intervention. A thorough patient and radiographic evaluation is needed when a diagnosis of kyphosis is made.

Annotated References

1. Vialle R, Levassor N, Rillardon L, Templier A, Skalli W, Guigui P: Radiographic analysis of the sagittal alignment and balance of the spine in asymptomatic subjects. *J Bone Joint Surg Am* 2005;87(2):260-267.

2. Mac-Thiong JM, Labelle H, Roussouly P: Pediatric sagittal alignment. *Eur Spine J* 2011;20(suppl 5):586-590.

   The authors review pediatric spinal alignment and the developmental relationship of sagittal segmental spinal and spinopelvic parameters. Level of evidence: V.

3. Cil A, Yazici M, Uzumcugil A, et al: The evolution of sagittal segmental alignment of the spine during childhood. *Spine (Phila Pa 1976)* 2005;30(1):93-100.

4. Kamaci S, Yucekul A, Demirkiran G, Berktas M, Yazici M: The evolution of sagittal spinal alignment in sitting position during childhood. *Spine (Phila Pa 1976)* 2015;40(13):E787-E793.

   This cross-sectional study of spinal alignment in children in a sitting position showed the development of segmental sagittal spinal alignment. Overall, the authors found less thoracic kyphosis and lumbar lordosis in children in a sitting position compared with children in a standing position. Level of evidence: IV.

5. Mac-Thiong JM, Berthonnaud E, Dimar JR II, Betz RR, Labelle H: Sagittal alignment of the spine and pelvis during growth. *Spine (Phila Pa 1976)* 2004;29(15):1642-1647.

6. Dolphens M, Cagnie B, Coorevits P, et al: Sagittal standing posture and its association with spinal pain: A school-based epidemiological study of 1196 Flemish adolescents before age at peak height velocity. *Spine* 2012;37(19):1657-1666.

   In an investigation of the association between observational trunk alignment, low back pain, and neck pain, the authors describe the results of their assessment of a cross-sectional baseline data set on standing sagittal postures in Flemish adolescents Level of evidence: IV.

7. Briggs AM, Smith AJ, Straker LM, Bragge P: Thoracic spine pain in the general population: Prevalence, incidence and associated factors in children, adolescents and adults. A systematic review. *BMC Musculoskelet Disord* 2009;10:77.

8. Zhang Z, Wang H, Liu C: Compressive myelopathy in severe angular kyphosis: A series of ten patients. *Eur Spine J* 2015.

   The authors describe the results of a case series of patients with severe kyphosis in whom compressive myelopathy developed. Nine of the 10 patients had improved neurologic function after surgical kyphosis correction. Level of evidence: IV.

9. Pruszczynski B, Mackenzie WG, Rogers K, White KK: Spinal cord injury after extremity surgery in children with thoracic kyphosis. *Clin Orthop Relat Res* 2015;473(10):3315-3320.

   A case report is presented of two patients with skeletal dysplasia in whom paraplegia developed after they underwent lower limb surgery. The underlying severe thoracic kyphosis was associated with the development of paraplegia. Level of evidence: IV.

10. Lonner B, Yoo A, Terran JS, et al: Effect of spinal deformity on adolescent quality of life: Comparison of operative Scheuermann kyphosis, adolescent idiopathic scoliosis, and normal controls. *Spine (Phila Pa 1976)* 2013;38(12):1049-1055.

    The authors present the results of a retrospective review of a prospectively collected database assessing patient-reported outcomes using the Scoliosis Research Society-22 questionnaire in patients with Scheuermann kyphosis. Patients with kyphosis had worse outcomes compared with normal control subjects or those with scoliosis. Level of evidence: III.

11. Petcharaporn M, Pawelek J, Bastrom T, Lonner B, Newton PO: The relationship between thoracic hyperkyphosis and the Scoliosis Research Society outcomes instrument. *Spine (Phila Pa 1976)* 2007;32(20):2226-2231.

12. Marks M, Stanford C, Newton P: Which lateral radiographic positioning technique provides the most reliable and functional representation of a patient's sagittal balance? *Spine (Phila Pa 1976)* 2009;34(9):949-954.

13. Tribus CB: Scheuermann's kyphosis in adolescents and adults: Diagnosis and management. *J Am Acad Orthop Surg* 1998;6(1):36-43.

14. Tsirikos AI, Jain AK: Scheuermann's kyphosis: Current controversies. *J Bone Joint Surg Br* 2011;93(7):857-864.

    This review article details the latest evidence-based medicine regarding Scheuermann kyphosis. Level of evidence: V.

15. Murray PM, Weinstein SL, Spratt KF: The natural history and long-term follow-up of Scheuermann kyphosis. *J Bone Joint Surg Am* 1993;75(2):236-248.

16. Ristolainen L, Kettunen JA, Heliövaara M, Kujala UM, Heinonen A, Schlenzka D: Untreated Scheuermann's disease: A 37-year follow-up study. *Eur Spine J* 2012;21(5):819-824.

    The results of a long-term follow-up study on 80 patients with Scheuermann kyphosis are presented. Overall, the authors found that patients with Scheuermann kyphosis had a higher risk for back pain and functional disability compared with control subjects. Level of evidence: IV.

17. Weiss HR, Dieckmann J, Gerner HJ: Effect of intensive rehabilitation on pain in patients with Scheuermann's disease. *Stud Health Technol Inform* 2002;88:254-257.

18. Etemadifar M, Ebrahimzadeh A, Hadi A, Feizi M: Comparison of Scheuermann's kyphosis correction by combined anterior-posterior fusion versus posterior-only procedure. *Eur Spine J* 2015.

    The authors report on a randomized controlled trial of patients with Scheuermann kyphosis who underwent an anterior-posterior or a posterior-only approach to surgery. Clinical and radiologic parameters were similar between groups. A higher rate of complications was found in the group treated with the anterior-posterior approach. Level of evidence: II.

19. Tsutsui S, Pawelek JB, Bastrom TP, Shah SA, Newton PO: Do discs "open" anteriorly with posterior-only correction of Scheuermann's kyphosis? *Spine (Phila Pa 1976)* 2011;36(16):E1086-E1092.

    The authors present the results of a comparison of the degree of correction in patients with Scheuermann kyphosis treated with posterior fusion with and without anterior release. The amount of correction was similar in both groups. Level of evidence: III.

20. Cho W, Lenke LG, Bridwell KH, et al: The prevalence of abnormal preoperative neurological examination in Scheuermann kyphosis: Correlation with X-ray, magnetic resonance imaging, and surgical outcome. *Spine (Phila Pa 1976)* 2014;39(21):1771-1776.

The authors report that 9% of patients with Scheuermann kyphosis have abnormal findings on preoperative neurologic examinations. Level of evidence: IV.

21. McMaster MJ, Singh H: Natural history of congenital kyphosis and kyphoscoliosis: A study of one hundred and twelve patients. *J Bone Joint Surg Am* 1999;81(10):1367-1383.

22. Campos MA, Fernandes P, Dolan LA, Weinstein SL: Infantile thoracolumbar kyphosis secondary to lumbar hypoplasia. *J Bone Joint Surg Am* 2008;90(8):1726-1729.

23. Winter RB, Moe JH, Wang JF: Congenital kyphosis: Its natural history and treatment as observed in a study of one hundred and thirty patients. *J Bone Joint Surg Am* 1973;55(2):223-256.

24. Spiro AS, Rupprecht M, Stenger P, et al: Surgical treatment of severe congenital thoracolumbar kyphosis through a single posterior approach. *Bone Joint J* 2013;95-B(11):1527-1532.

 The authors present the results of a case series of 10 patients who underwent posterior-only surgery for correction of severe kyphosis. Overall excellent correction was achieved without complications. Level of evidence: IV.

25. Zeng Y, Chen Z, Qi Q, et al: The posterior surgical correction of congenital kyphosis and kyphoscoliosis: 23 cases with minimum 2 years follow-up. *Eur Spine J* 2013;22(2):372-378.

 The authors present the results of a case series of 23 patients who underwent posterior-only surgery for correction of severe kyphosis. Overall excellent correction was achieved without complications. Level of evidence: IV.

26. White KK, Sousa T: Mucopolysaccharide disorders in orthopaedic surgery. *J Am Acad Orthop Surg* 2013;21(1):12-22.

 This article describes the orthopaedic manifestations of mucopolysaccharidosis and treatment. Level of evidence: V.

27. Abelin Genevois K, Garin C, Solla F, Guffon N, Kohler R: Surgical management of thoracolumbar kyphosis in mucopolysaccharidosis type 1 in a reference center. *J Inherit Metab Dis* 2014;37(1):69-78.

 Good clinical and radiographic outcomes were reported in this case series of 14 patients with mucopolysaccharidosis and thoracolumbar kyphosis who were treated with circumferential fusion. Level of evidence: IV.

28. Garrido E, Tomé-Bermejo F, Adams CI: Combined spinal arthrodesis with instrumentation for the management of progressive thoracolumbar kyphosis in children with mucopolysaccharidosis. *Eur Spine J* 2014;23(12):2751-2757.

 Good clinical and radiographic outcomes were reported in this case series of four patients with mucopolysaccharidosis and thoracolumbar kyphosis who were treated with circumferential fusion with pedicle screw constructs. Level of evidence: IV.

29. Shirley ED, Ain MC: Achondroplasia: Manifestations and treatment. *J Am Acad Orthop Surg* 2009;17(4):231-241.

30. Borkhuu B, Nagaraju DK, Chan G, Holmes L Jr, Mackenzie WG: Factors related to progression of thoracolumbar kyphosis in children with achondroplasia: A retrospective cohort study of forty-eight children treated in a comprehensive orthopaedic center. *Spine (Phila Pa 1976)* 2009;34(16):1699-1705.

31. Pauli RM, Breed A, Horton VK, Glinski LP, Reiser CA: Prevention of fixed, angular kyphosis in achondroplasia. *J Pediatr Orthop* 1997;17(6):726-733.

32. Cho SK, Kim YJ, Lenke LG: Proximal junctional kyphosis following spinal deformity surgery in the pediatric patient. *J Am Acad Orthop Surg* 2015;23(7):408-414.

 This review article describes the current understanding and treatment of proximal junctional kyphosis after spinal deformity surgery in pediatric patients. Level of evidence: V.

33. Barrett KK, Andras LM, Tolo VT, Choi PD, Skaggs DL: Measurement variability in the evaluation of the proximal junction in distraction-based growing rods patients. *J Pediatr Orthop* 2015;35(6):624-627.

 A high degree of interobserver and intraobserver variability was reported in radiographic measurement of proximal junctional kyphosis and early-onset scoliosis in patients treated with growing rods. Level of evidence: III.

34. Basques BA, Long WD III, Golinvaux NS, et al: Poor visualization limits diagnosis of proximal junctional kyphosis in adolescent idiopathic scoliosis. *Spine J* 2015.

 The authors reported a high degree of interobserver and intraobserver variability in radiographic measurements of proximal junctional kyphosis in patients with adolescent idiopathic scoliosis. Level of evidence: III.

35. Kim YJ, Lenke LG, Bridwell KH, et al: Proximal junctional kyphosis in adolescent idiopathic scoliosis after 3 different types of posterior segmental spinal instrumentation and fusions: Incidence and risk factor analysis of 410 cases. *Spine (Phila Pa 1976)* 2007;32(24):2731-2738.

36. Cho KJ, Lenke LG, Bridwell KH, Kamiya M, Sides B: Selection of the optimal distal fusion level in posterior instrumentation and fusion for thoracic hyperkyphosis: The sagittal stable vertebra concept. *Spine (Phila Pa 1976)* 2009;34(8):765-770.

37. Denis F, Sun EC, Winter RB: Incidence and risk factors for proximal and distal junctional kyphosis following surgical treatment for Scheuermann kyphosis: Minimum five-year follow-up. *Spine (Phila Pa 1976)* 2009;34(20):E729-E734.

Chapter 32

Pediatric Cervical Spine Disorders

Firoz Miyanji, MD, FRCSC

Abstract

The diagnosis and management of pediatric cervical spine disorders pose many unique challenges for the treating physician. To optimize care for these children, it is critical to have a clear understanding of the variations in normal growth and development and the disparate presentations of the many disorders of the pediatric cervical spine from infancy through adolescence.

Keywords: cervical spine; dysplasia; subluxation; synchondrosis

Introduction

The unique growth and development of the pediatric cervical spine lends itself to a spectrum of disorders not commonly seen in the adult population. The spectrum of disease, patterns of injury, and any nontraumatic instability also may be different from infancy through childhood and into adolescence. Many congenital syndromes and skeletal dysplasias have pathognomonic involvement of the cervical spine, which is important for the pediatric orthopaedic surgeon to recognize. Understanding variations of normal in the developing cervical spine may aid in understanding the natural history of disease. This chapter highlights important principles of the growing pediatric cervical spine, common osseoligamentous afflictions, challenges in diagnoses, and treatment options.

Embryology and Developmental Anatomy

Embryologic formation of the spine (and the spinal cord) progresses in an organized manner beginning with the formation of the primitive streak, the notochord, somites, and sclerotomes. Initial spine development begins during the third week of gestation, with the axial skeleton arising from somites. Paired somites appear approximately on gestational day 20. They arise from the paraxial mesoderm in a cranial-to-caudal fashion at a rate of approximately three to four somites per day. Initially, 42 to 44 somite pairs flank the notochord, forming the base of the skull, and extend caudally. The basiocciput develops from somites 1 to 4, the atlantoaxial column from somites 5 to 7, and the subaxial spine from somites 7 to 12.

The somites then separate into sclerotomes, which ultimately form the bony spinal column. After sclerotome division is complete, the caudal half of the supra-adjacent sclerotome merges with the cranial half of the subadjacent sclerotome, forming the vertebra precursor. The division and subsequent refusion explains why eight cervical nerves but only seven cervical vertebrae are present. The cranial division of the first cervical sclerotome (the proatlas) contributes to form the base of the occiput and the tip of the odontoid process, whereas the caudal division of the first cervical sclerotome and the cranial division of the second cervical sclerotome forms the first cervical vertebra. The ventral sclerotome forms the vertebral body, and the dorsal sclerotome becomes the ventral arch (**Figure 1**).

Atlas

The first cervical vertebra has several morphologic characteristics that distinguish it from the other cervical vertebrae. It is incompletely ossified at birth and develops from three ossification centers. The two posterolateral ossification centers (which give rise to the lateral masses and the posterior arch) are present at birth, and the anterior ossification center (the anterior arch) appears between 6 months and 2 years of age. The age at which closure of the synchondroses occurs remains controversial. It was initially reported in 1937 that the posterior midline synchondrosis fuses by 3 to 5 years of age, whereas the two anterior synchondroses fuse by 7 to 9 years of age.[1] Later, it was reported the posterior synchondrosis closed by age 5 years, and the anterior synchondroses closed by age 6 years.[2] A recent study found that the median age of complete ossification of the anterior synchondroses was 8.5 years, with an interquartile range (IQR)

Dr. Miyanji or an immediate family member has received research or institutional support from DePuy.

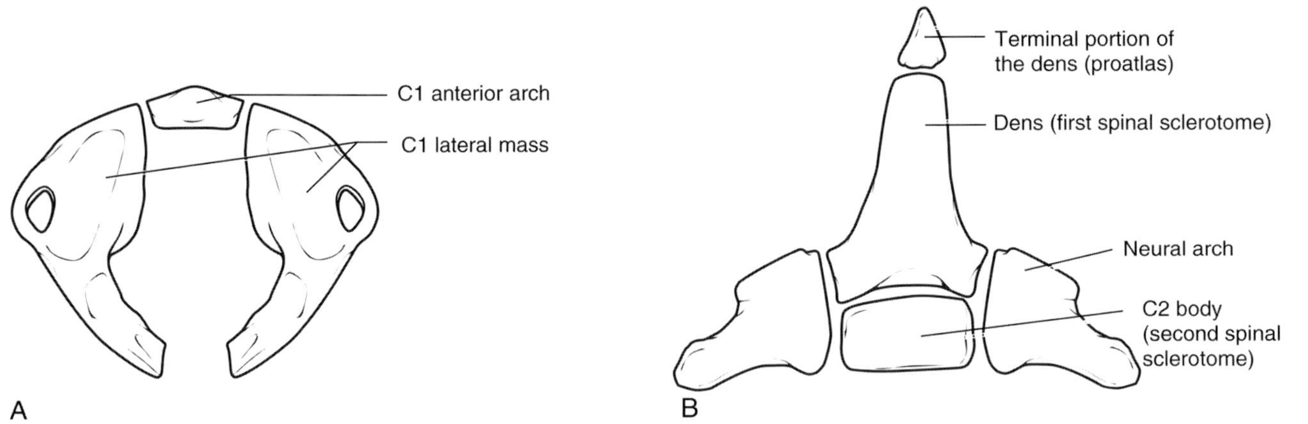

Figure 1 Schematic drawings of the developmental anatomy of C1 and C2. **A,** Cross-sectional view of C1. **B,** Anterior view of C2. (Adapted from Miyanji F: Cervical abnormalities, back pain, and the surgical treatment of spondylolysis and spondylolisthesis, in Song KM, ed: *Orthopaedic Knowledge Update: Pediatrics 4*, Rosemont, IL, American Academy of Orthopaedic Surgeons, 201l, pp 293-313.)

of 5.5 to 13 years; however, approximately 45% of the patients showed incomplete ossification at age 10 years.[3] A 2013 quantitative, age-dependent, cross-sectional analysis of the closure of the C1 synchondroses noted complete closure of the posterior synchondrosis by age 3 years in all but 1 of 54 patients (1.9%). Also in the series, closure of the anterior synchondroses was generally found after age 3 years, and it was observed that the widths of the synchondroses decreased linearly with age as ossification progressed.[4] An analysis of 841 CT studies of the atlas also confirmed the universal features of the development of C1, notably the three ossification centers with two anterolateral synchondroses and one posterior midline synchondrosis.[2] The authors, however, noted an anterior midline synchondrosis in up to 20% of cases, highlighting the fact that the anterior arch may develop from a pair of symmetric ossification centers, not from a single anterior ossification center in some instances.[3]

In a retrospective review of CT scans of patients younger than 8 years, a group of authors found up to 21% with multiple anterior ossification centers, with incomplete ossification of the anterior arch in 46% of those aged 7 to 8 years.[5] The authors also noted incomplete ossification of the posterior synchondrosis in 16% of those older than 5 years, highlighting the variability present in C1 ossification patterns and the timing of synchondrosis fusion.

Axis

The axis is formed from five ossification centers: paired neural arch ossification centers (lateral masses), a basal central ossification center (body), a dentate center (dens), and an apical center (the odontoid tip). In fetal life, the dens arises from paired ossification centers that are symmetric about the sagittal midline plane. Although by birth these centers have usually fused and all that remains is a sagittally oriented cleft at the tip of the ossifying odontoid, some authors believe that the fusion may occur within the first 3 months of life.[6] The C2 body appears by the fifth fetal month and is separated from the dens by the dentocentral synchondrosis, which fuses at 3 to 6 years of age. A more recent CT study of 835 patients noted that the dentocentral synchondrosis closure occurred earlier than previously reported.[3] Most of the patients in the study with complete radiolucency of the dentocentral synchondrosis were younger than 3.3 years. The authors noted that beyond this age, sclerotic traces of the synchondrosis remained visible.

Historically, the ossiculum terminale at the tip of the dens has been reported to appear in children aged 5 to 8 years, with fusion to the dens between the ages of 10 and 13 years.[7] More recently, however, researchers have found that the ages of initial ossification and fusion are younger than what had been previously suggested,[3] with a median age at initial ossification of the apical center of 2.7 years (IQR, 1.9 to 3.6 years). The oldest child in this study with no ossification in the apical center was 12.8 years. The authors found that the median age of incorporation of the apical center was 8.2 years (IQR, 7.1 to 9.9 years). The neural arch ossification centers appear bilaterally at fetal age 7 months and fuse posteriorly by age 3 years. The estimated median age of initial ossification of the neurocentral synchondroses was reported to be 3.8 years (IQR, 2.9 to 4.6 years).[3] It also is well recognized that the superior portion of the neurocentral synchondrosis (between the neural arches and the odontoid) closes later than the inferior portion (between the arches and the C2 body).

Lower Cervical Vertebrae

The lower cervical vertebrae are formed from two lateral ossification centers and a third one for the body. The neural arches appear by fetal age 7 to 9 weeks, and the body appears by fetal age 5 months. The neurocentral synchondroses separating the lateral masses from the body close between 3 and 6 years of age. The posterior synchondrosis usually unites by 2 to 4 years of age. The superior and inferior epiphyseal rings appear at puberty and unite with the body at about age 25 years and are responsible for the vertical growth of the body.

Imaging Parameters and Evaluation

Craniometry

Numerous lines, angles, and measurements have been applied to diagnostic images to assess the craniocervical junction. As shown in **Figure 2**, the most widely used craniometric measurements include the McRae line, Chamberlain line, the Wackenheim clivus baseline, the Welcher basal angle, the Powers ratio, the anterior atlantodens interval (AADI), and the posterior atlantodens interval (PADI).

Although AP, lateral, and open-mouth odontoid plain radiographs are traditionally obtained to evaluate the cervical spine, the routine use of open-mouth odontoid radiographs in children remains questionable. In 2000, researchers reported on 51 children with cervical spine injuries and found that the open-mouth odontoid radiographs were not useful, especially for children younger than 9 years.[7]

The Chamberlain line is useful for identifying basilar invagination; however, as a normal variant, the dens may project a few millimeters (1 mm ± 3.6 to 6.6 mm) above the line.[8] If the opisthion is not clearly visualized in very young children, the McGregor line may be useful by connecting the posterior pole of the palate to the lowest point of the occipital squamosal surface. The Wackenheim clivus baseline can be used to identify basilar invagination, atlantoaxial dislocation, and atlanto-occipital dislocation. The angle formed by the Wackenheim clivus line with a line drawn along the posterior surface of the odontoid is called the craniovertebral angle and varies from 150° to 180° with flexion and extension, respectively.[8] The Welcher basal angle should always be less than 140°. Platybasia is associated with an increase in this angle.

Other useful parameters to assess atlanto-occipital instability include the Powers ratio, the basion-axial interval (BAI), the basion-dens interval (BDI), and the atlanto-occipital joint space (**Figure 2**). Although studies have reported the Powers ratio to be 33% to 60% sensitive, the BDI to be 50% sensitive, and the BAI to be close to 100% sensitive in children, these radiographic parameters have been difficult to assess because of the inherent challenges of visualizing the anatomic structures on plain radiographs in very young patients or those with anatomic abnormalities.[9] More recent studies have encouraged the use of CT scans in this setting and report improvements in sensitivity, specificity, and positive and negative predictive values in diagnosing atlanto-occipital instability compared with plain radiographs. In 2005, a BDI of greater than 10 mm on a CT scan was considered to be diagnostic of atlanto-occipital dissociation.[10]

The AADI has commonly been used to assess motion at C1-C2 and is emphasized as a marker for predicting potential cord compression at the atlantoaxial junction. In children younger than 8 years, it is agreed that an AADI of up to 5 mm is acceptable because of the increased cartilage content of the odontoid and the ring of the atlas in very young children. In addition, overriding of the anterior arch of the atlas on top of the odontoid can be seen in up to 20% of children.[11] In patients older than 8 years, an AADI of less than 3 mm between flexion and extension excursion is considered normal. A longitudinal study reported that the AADI in patients with normal anatomy averaged 1.9 mm in very young children and reached 2.45 mm in adolescents.[12] It remains unclear whether AADI values beyond these are predictive of cord compression. Some researchers believe that a minimal sagittal diameter is important in the development of myelopathy, whereas others argue that the degree of instability is more important.

The concept of the space available for the cord is considered most indicative for identifying patients at increased risk for the development of important neurologic symptoms, particularly in chronic conditions. It represents the diameter of the spinal cord, surrounding cerebrospinal fluid, and the dura mater at the level of C1 and was established with MRI. Conceptually, the space available for the cord is represented by the PADI, which can be measured on plain lateral radiographs. In adults, absolute stenosis is defined as a flexion PADI of less than 10 mm, whereas relative stenosis is considered to be between 10 and 13 mm. In children, however, the amount of narrowing of the canal diameter beyond which cord compression occurs is uncertain. In adults, cord compression has been reported when the canal diameter is less than 14 mm.

In children, cord compression may be inferred from the age-related diameter of the spinal canal. Morphologic investigations of the C1 vertebra in the growing spine, however, are limited. A prospective longitudinal study in 2001 attempted to provide more reliable reference values to objectively assess the developing cervical spine. The

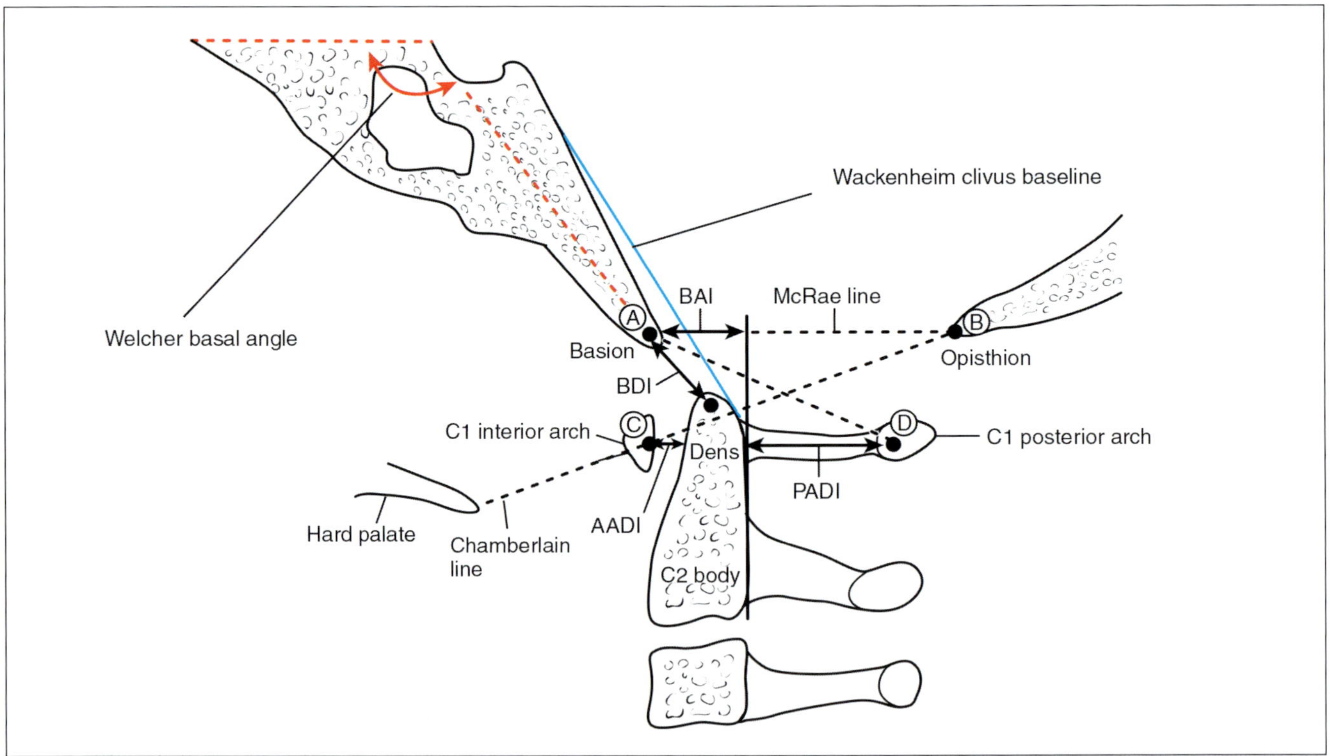

Figure 2 Schematic drawing of the upper cervical spine showing a lateral view of the common radiographic parameters. AADI = anterior atlantodens interval; BAI = basion-axial interval; BDI = basion-dens interval; PADI = posterior atlantodens interval; Powers ratio = AD/BC.

authors noted that cervical spine growth is most rapid in the first 3 years of life, by which time it has reached nearly 95% of its mature diameter. In males, the authors found the canal diameter of the upper cervical spine at C2 averaged 12.8 mm at 6 months of age, which increased to 16 mm in adolescence.[12] In a study using only lateral radiographs, the sagittal canal diameter at C1 in a developing spine was reported to increase from an average of 19.9 mm at age 3 to 6 years to 20.6 mm at age 7 to 10 years and 21.3 mm at age 11 to 14 years.[13] Another study described the average increase in the sagittal canal size at C1 from age 3 to 18 years to be 1.8 mm in boys and 2.9 mm in girls.[14] Most recently, researchers reported on the developmental morphology of the C1 vertebra using helical CT scans on 54 children and noted similar trends in the sagittal canal dimensions as those reported in earlier studies, with substantial increases in the canal area occurring up to 6 years of age and more gradual increase beyond this age.[4]

Morphologic studies of the cervical spinal cord are very limited. A review of 110 normal myelograms in children (age range, 1 month to 15 years) found that the ratio of the cord to subarachnoid space was independent of age and sex, with very little variability at different vertebral levels.[15] The spinal canal was found to be narrowest at C4 followed by C5, whereas the spinal cord was largest at C4-C5.[16] The area and circularity of the cervical spinal cord were not significantly correlated with any parameter of the spinal canal, and the spinal cord showed less individual variation than the bony canal.

The canal dimensions determine, in part, the space available for the cord and the susceptibility to spinal cord injury. In a study of adults, a comparison of CT parameters of normal control subjects with patients who sustained spinal cord injury found no substantial differences between the groups with regard to the cross-sectional area of the spinal canal; however, the sagittal diameters of the spinal canal of the control group were significantly larger than those of the spinal cord injury group. The study authors concluded that it is not the total volume of space within the spinal canal, but rather the shape that is the critical factor.[17]

CT and MRI have obvious noted advantages when assessing the pathology of the upper cervical spine, especially given the inherent limitations of plain radiographs of visualizing many of the osseous landmarks of the craniocervical junction. These studies, however, provide static information; for patients with dynamic instability, flexion-extension radiographs are still warranted. Dynamic CT as well as MRI have been shown to be of value in patients with neurologic symptoms but equivocal plain radiographs. Despite the added potential value of CT compared with plain radiography in assessing the pediatric cervical spine, the associated radiation dose and estimated increased cancer risk are important considerations. In 2013, researchers evaluated seven US healthcare systems and noted a sharp increase in pediatric CT use, with a fourfold to ninefold increase in spinal CTs from 1996 to 2010.[18] The authors noted that the projected lifetime attributable risks of solid cancer were higher in younger patients, in girls, and for abdomen/pelvic and spinal CTs. The risk for leukemia was highest for head CTs in children younger than 5 years.

Craniocervical and Upper Cervical Abnormalities

Atlantoaxial Rotatory Subluxation

Children with atlantoaxial rotatory subluxation (AARS) have a painful torticollis and limited neck motion. The head is rotated to one side and laterally flexed to the contralateral side. The associated muscle spasm is on the side of the long sternocleidomastoid muscle because the muscle is attempting to correct the deformity. This contrasts with congenital muscular torticollis, in which the muscle causes the deformity and is found to be tight on the opposite side of the deformity.

In normal rotation, C1 moves first; only after C1 rotates beyond 23° does C2 then begin to rotate. As C2 begins to rotate, C1 continues to move at a greater rate, such that the angular relationship between C1 and C2 continues to increase. The ligaments between C1 and C2 become taut after C1 has rotated approximately 65° from midline, at which point C1 and C2 rotate together until maximum head turn is achieved. It is important to note that the difference in rates of motion between the axis and the atlas produce a natural subluxation of the atlantoaxial facets during normal rotation. In AARS, the subluxation of the C1-C2 facets is prevented from returning to normal.[19]

Of the numerous causes of AARS, trauma and infection (Grisel syndrome) are the most common. The common denominator in AARS is a rotation of the atlantoaxial complex that is held in a fixed position and caused by either a muscle spasm or a mechanical block. Suspected pathophysiology after a retropharyngeal infection is believed to be involved because of a direct connection between the pharyngeal veins, the periodontal venous plexus, and the suboccipital epidural sinuses. This anatomic feature may facilitate the translocation of pharyngovertebral inflammatory products to the upper cervical spine, causing spastic contracture of the cervical muscles.[6] The presence of synovial folds in some atlantoaxial joints, which may be increased in children, have been reported. This abundance of soft-tissue structures adjacent to the mobile C1-C2 articulation may provide material that can become swollen or incarcerated during atlantoaxial motion, thus leading to AARS.

Although the Fielding and Hawkins classification is most widely used,[20] several authors have more recently proposed newer classification systems in an attempt to select the most appropriate treatment regimen. One group of authors established a classification system in 2005 by plotting C1-C2 motion curves generated from the dynamic CT scans of AARS patients.[21] In a subsequent study, these same authors found that patients in group 1 who had symptoms for more than 3 months' duration were more likely to have recurrent subluxation, undergo more prolonged treatment, and require more aggressive therapies.[22] A retrospective case study in 2012 used three-dimensional CT to classify AARS based on the lateral inclination of the atlas on the axis and the presence of C2 deformity. These authors described three types of AARS depending on the severity of the inclination, the degree of C2 deformity, and the duration of symptoms.[23]

Although in the past CT has been the most widely used imaging modality and is integral to several classification systems,[21,23] the value of diagnostic CT may be questioned because of more recent evidence. Because many patients with AARS do not have any intrinsic bony abnormality, and the subluxation noted on imaging is in the normal range, AARS is considered primarily a clinical diagnosis.[21,24] In 2002, researchers noted poor reliability and reproducibility of dynamic CT scanning and recommended against its routine use, especially in the acute setting.[25] Other authors found no important motion abnormalities on dynamic CT scanning and called into question its use in the acute setting.[24] In addition, all previous studies using CT scans for classification and treatment algorithms found that the more minor types of AARS were more likely to occur in patients with acute presentations.[22] These patients were more likely to have fewer observable abnormalities on CT and respond favorably to nonsurgical management. In chronic AARS, however, CT with three-dimensional reconstructions has a high accuracy of diagnosis and provides excellent anatomic detail of the abnormal C1-C2 relationship.

The treatment options for AARS continue to include cervical collars, halter or skeletal traction, halo immobilization, and surgery. The use of anti-inflammatory drugs and/or muscle relaxants also has shown benefit. The duration of symptoms prior to diagnosis remains the most important predictor of the type of treatment required.[21,22,26,27] No formal definition exists of when

AARS is considered acute, but most studies have reported on differences in the treatment required when AARS is diagnosed within 1 month from the onset of symptoms. Although earlier reports favor surgery for chronic AARS, recent literature reported treatment success by nonsurgical means in this setting with remodeling of the C2 facet deformity.[23] In a 2014 study, researchers reported successful outcomes at a mean follow-up of 10.3 months in 73% of the patients with chronic AARS who underwent reduction with traction and halo-thoracic vests.[28] The duration of treatment, in particular the time in an orthosis, remains variable, with ranges of 1 week to 6 months.[21,24,29] One group of researchers recommended an MRI protocol to determine the length of time in an orthosis. These researchers recommended immobilization in a cervical orthosis until repeat MRI shows resolution of hyperintensity in the transverse and alar ligaments.[29] A C1-C2 fusion is usually required for recurrent cases or those in whom nonsurgical treatment is unsuccessful. Rates of eventual fusion vary for chronic cases from 30% to 100%[21,27] (**Figure 3**).

Os Odontoideum

Os odontoideum is the most common anomaly of the dens and is seen as an oval-shaped, well-corticated bony ossicle positioned cephalad to the body of the axis. The cause of os odontoideum remains the subject of debate, but three general etiologies have been proposed: The os odontoideum represents (1) a fracture nonunion of the dens, (2) damage to the epiphyseal plate occurring in the first year of life, or (3) a congenital malformation of the dens itself. The congenital hypothesis has been challenged because the neurocentral synchondrosis is located below the level of the superior articular facet, whereas the gap in os odontoideum is frequently located above the plane of the superior articular facet. The most widely accepted etiology was proposed by a group of authors in 1980; these authors suggested that a fracture of the dens occurs in early childhood, and the alar ligaments attached to the apex gradually distract the fragment away from the base.[30] Subsequent case reports and series on the topic have highlighted the history of remote trauma in most patients, which has made the traumatic theory the most widely accepted theory.

The position of the os odontoideum can be either orthotopic or dystopic and should be carefully distinguished, especially if surgical stabilization is warranted. Orthotopic os odontoideum refers to an ossicle in anatomic position that moves in unison with the anterior arch of C1 and can be reducible to be normally aligned with the dens. In dystopic os odontoideum, it is abnormally positioned near the base of the clivus, where it may fuse with the basion and move functionally as an extension of the clivus, thus increasing the risk of neurologic injury. In orthotopic os odontoideum with instability, a C1-C2 arthrodesis can be considered; however, a dystopic os odontoideum with instability may require an occiput to C2 fusion (**Figure 4**).

In addition to cervical myelopathy, intracranial manifestations of vertebrobasilar ischemia, cerebral infarction, brain stem damage, and vertigo have been reported in patients with unstable os odontoideum.

Surgical intervention is warranted in patients with neurologic involvement, documented instability, or persistent cervical spine or neck symptoms. Patients with other risk factors for instability (for example, Down syndrome and skeletal dysplasias) also should be considered for surgical stabilization.

The natural history and risks associated with untreated os odontoideum are unclear, so prophylactic arthrodesis remains controversial. With advances in surgical techniques, more recent literature supports a consideration for surgical stabilization for patients with incidental os odontoideum because of the potential for sudden death and substantial morbidity highlighted from earlier reports.[31-33] A 2010 study reported on 10 patients with incidental os odontoideum who sustained an acute cervical spinal cord injury after minor trauma and recommended prophylactic fusion in patients with asymptomatic os odontoideum.[33] Although earlier studies advocate internal fixation using sublaminar wires, some authors caution against the use of posterior wiring techniques because the os odontoideum can be pulled back into the spinal canal.

Skeletal Dysplasias

Achondroplasia

Craniocervical manifestations in achondroplasia include foramen magnum stenosis and multisegmental spinal stenosis of the subaxial spine. Foramen magnum stenosis usually occurs within the first 2 years of life and is the direct result of defective enchondral bone growth and premature fusion of the two posterior basal synchondroses. The most common symptoms of this condition are excessive snoring and apnea; however, other signs and symptoms of chronic brainstem compression can manifest. These include lower cranial nerve dysfunction, hyperreflexia, hypotonia, weakness or paresis, clonus, swallowing difficulties, and developmental delay. Because foramen magnum stenosis can result in death, identification of the condition is critical. Polysomnography with or without other imaging studies may be used in making a diagnosis. Some authors recommend a screening MRI in all infants with achondroplasia to evaluate for foramen magnum stenosis.[34]

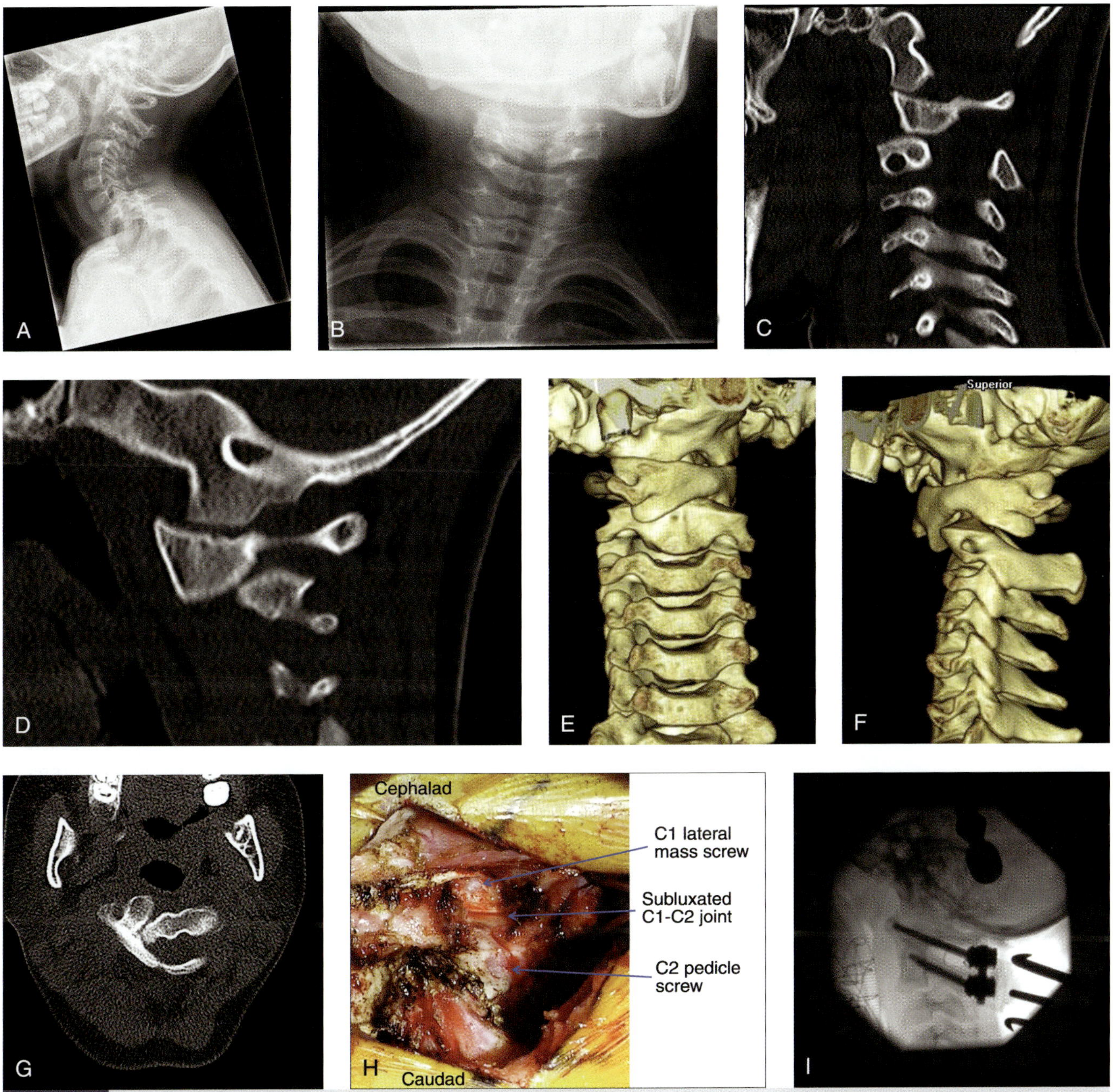

Figure 3 Images from a 9-year-old girl 6 months after torticollis secondary to Grisel syndrome. Lateral (**A**) and AP (**B**) radiographs show a decreased posterior atlantodens interval. **C,** Sagittal CT shows subluxated right C1-C2 joint. **D,** Sagittal CT shows subluxated left C1-C2 joint. AP (**E**) and lateral (**F**) three-dimensional CT reconstructions show gross subluxation of C1-C2. **G,** Axial CT shows gross subluxation of the C1-C2 facets. **H,** Intraoperative exposure of the right subluxated C1-C2 joint. **I,** Intraoperative lateral fluoroscopic image shows reduction and posterior segmental instrumented fusion of C1-C2.

Decompression of the foramen magnum generally is required in patients who are symptomatic within the first 2 years of life; however, symptoms may develop in older children and require treatment at that time. A 2006 study reported on the outcomes after cervicomedullary decompression and noted that although improvement of respiratory symptoms occurred soon after surgery, several complications also were encountered. Cerebrospinal fluid leaks, recurrent stenosis requiring revision surgery, and infection were the reported complications in 16 of 43 patients.[35]

Cervical stenosis results from several factors.

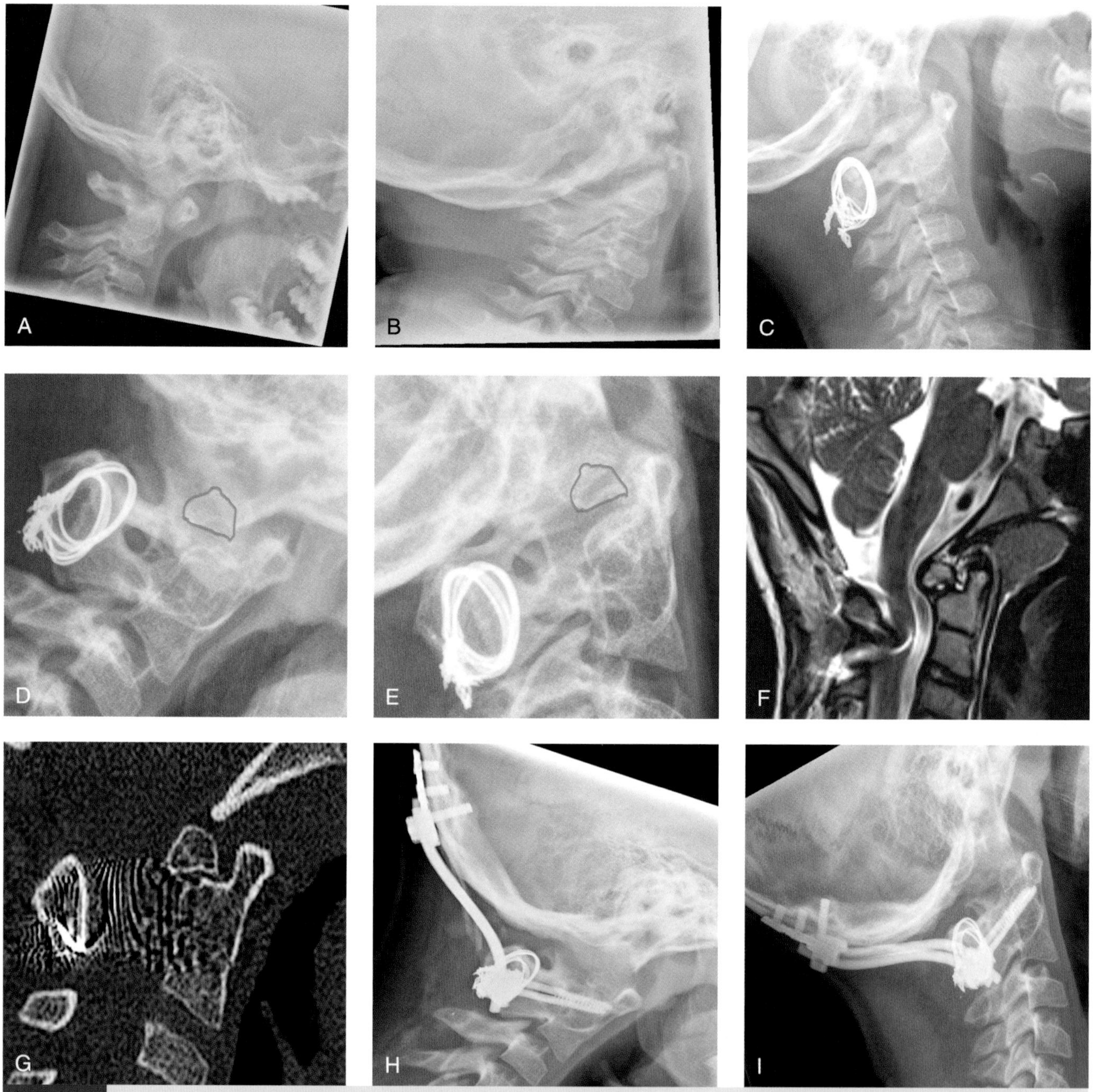

Figure 4 Images from an 8-year-old boy with os odontoideum diagnosed after a history of minor trauma. Lateral flexion (**A**) and lateral extension (**B**) cervical spine radiographs show unstable apparent orthotopic os odontoideum. **C,** Lateral cervical spine radiograph after the child was treated with C1-C2 fusion with a sublaminar wiring technique. Lateral flexion (**D**) and lateral extension (**E**) follow-up radiographs reveal os odontoideum behaving as the dystopic type. **F,** Sagittal midline MRI shows anterior compression of the spinal cord caused by the dystopic os odontoideum. **G,** Sagittal midline CT image shows posterior displacement of dystopic os odontoideum causing canal compression. Lateral flexion (**H**) and lateral extension (**I**) radiographs after revision fusion to the occiput show the os odontoideum and C1 move as a unit with no further instability.

Enchondral ossification defects shorten vertebral bodies and pedicles. The pedicles are thickened with a decrease in the interpedicular distance. The soft-tissue elements also are affected with hyperplasia of the intervertebral disks and the ligamentum flavum. Previous reports have noted a 40% reduction in sagittal and coronal diameters because of these abnormalities. Stenosis typically becomes symptomatic in the third and fourth decades of life but also can be seen in skeletally immature patients. The incidence of symptomatic stenosis is reported to be 10% in 10-year-old children.[36] Cervical stenosis can occur in skeletally immature individuals, whereas lumbar spinal stenosis is more commonly problematic in adults. Multilevel laminectomy can be considered in symptomatic patients, but in skeletally immature patients, a concurrent fusion should be performed to avoid postlaminectomy kyphosis.

Morquio Syndrome

In Morquio syndrome, the degradation of keratan sulfate and chondroitin sulfate is defective. The upper cervical manifestations of this autosomal recessive disease virtually always include atlantoaxial instability from odontoid hypoplasia as well the deposition of glycosaminoglycans posterior to the dens. The resultant cord compression causes substantial, progressive myelopathy in these patients. Prophylactic occipitocervical fusion has been advocated by some authors.[37,38] The anterior pannus at C1 typically resolves after posterior fusion, so anterior decompressive surgery usually is not warranted. Researchers in 2009 recommended that these patients should avoid contact sports and gymnastics and require cervical spine imaging before undergoing general anesthesia.[37]

Spondyloepiphyseal Dysplasia Congenita

Patients with spondyloepiphyseal dysplasia congenita (SEDC) are characterized by short-trunk disproportionate dwarfism. Atlantoaxial instability resulting from hypoplasia of the dens and/or lax ligaments can lead to myelopathy in up to 35% of patients. The sagittal atlas diameter also is reduced in most patients with SEDC, further compromising the spinal canal at C1. In a 2004 series, myelopathy developed in patients whose space available for the cord was less than 12 mm.[39] The authors also observed that a severe form of SEDC—with extreme short stature and coxa vara—was a risk factor for myelopathy. In their series, all patients with myelopathy were less than seven SDs below the mean. Spinal canal stenosis may not simply be addressed by reducing and stabilizing the atlantoaxial instability, and a concomitant C1 laminectomy may be required. The AADI in these patients increases with increasing age, so patients with SEDC should be followed into adulthood with regular cervical spine imaging.[40]

Syndrome-Related Abnormalities

Down Syndrome

Craniocervical instability has been reported in 8% to 63% of patients with Down syndrome, and atlantoaxial instability has been reported in 10% to 30% of these patients. Estimates of symptomatic disease, however, range from 1% to 2%. In addition to ligamentous laxity, patients with Down syndrome have a notably greater number of osseous anomalies of the upper cervical spine than do age- and sex-matched normal, healthy control subjects. Os odontoideum, persistent dentocentral synchondrosis of C2, spina bifida of C1, ossiculum terminale, and partial atlanto-occipital assimilation are the most frequently noted abnormalities. Patients with Down syndrome who have upper cervical instability are more likely to have bony anomalies than those without instability. Although no standard has been defined, occipitocervical subluxation of 7 to 10 mm is considered pathologic, and fusion is recommended. In 1996, some researchers noted difficulty with measuring occiput-C1 instability on plain radiographs and recommended confirmation with MRI;[41] other authors have suggested fusion for atlantoaxial instability in patients with an AADI greater than 10 mm or any symptomatic patients with cord changes on MRI.[42] Most studies indicate that ligamentous instability at the occipitocervical or atlantoaxial joint is unlikely to progress to clinically relevant subluxation; however, those children with bony anomalies are at higher risk of progression and should be followed closely.[43]

In 1983, the Special Olympics established radiographic screening guidelines,[44] which were endorsed in 1984 by the Committee on Sports Medicine of the American Academy of Pediatrics (AAP).[45] In 1995, the committee published a position paper questioning the value of lateral plain radiographs as a screening test in detecting patients with Down syndrome at risk for spinal cord injury and asserted that asymptomatic instability was not proven to be a risk factor for symptomatic instability.[46] Considerable debate exists regarding screening radiographs in the population with Down syndrome, and no consensus exists regarding the effectiveness of radiographs in preventing neurologic injury caused by upper cervical instability (**Figure 5**). The AAP published recommendations in 2001 and again in 2007 to screen all ambulatory children between the ages of 3 and 5 years, not just those participating in Special Olympics, using dynamic lateral cervical spine plain radiographs.[47,48] The need for subsequent serial radiographs in patients without instability on these index radiographs has not been agreed on, and it is important to note that instability may develop later in childhood in patients with Down syndrome despite normal screening radiographs at an early age (**Figure 5**). Therefore, more recently, the AAP changed its earlier 2001 and 2007 recommendations and now does not recommend routine radiologic evaluation of the cervical spine in asymptomatic patients. Pediatricians are advised by the AAP to rely on a careful history and

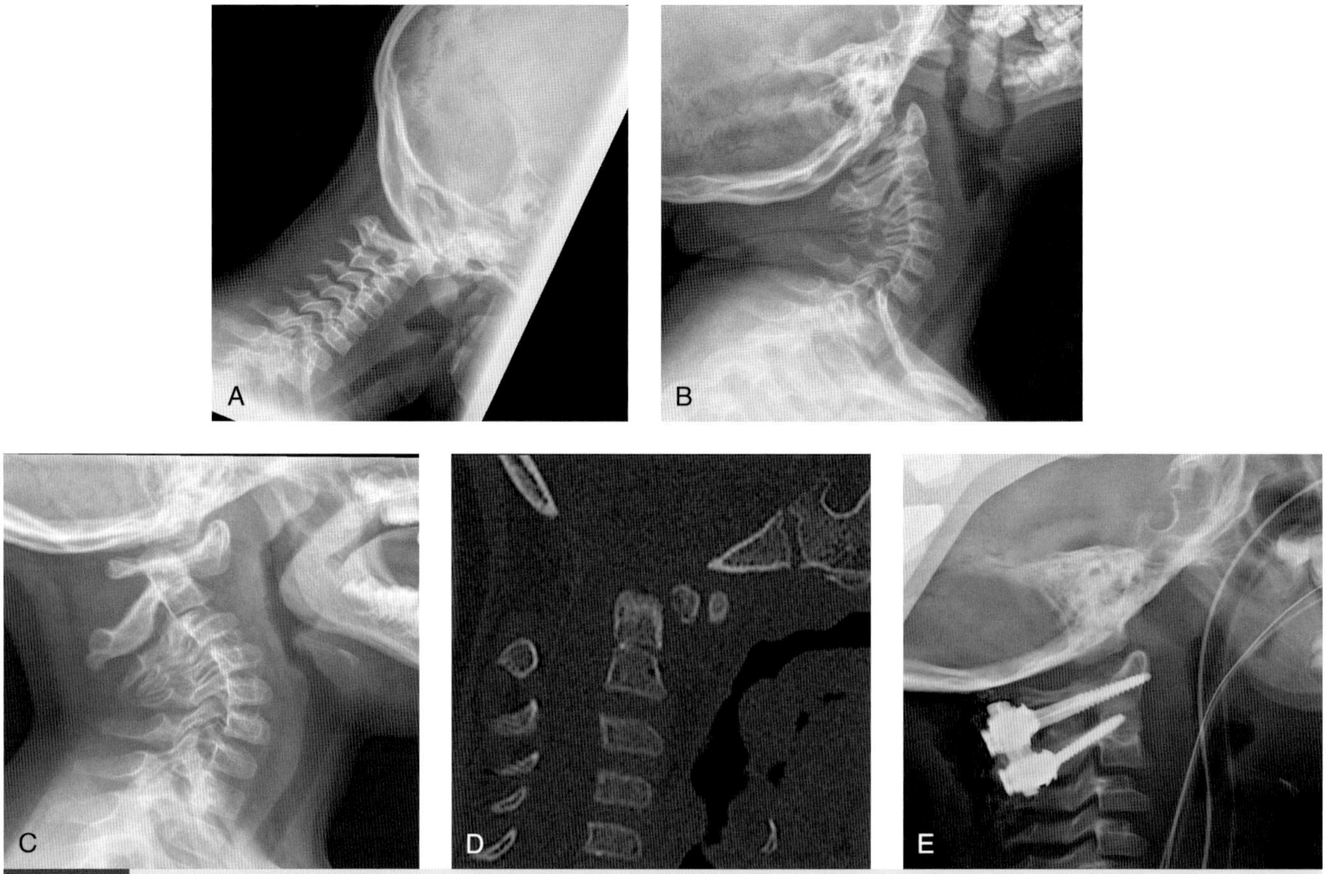

Figure 5 Images from a 9-year-old girl with trisomy 21. Screening lateral flexion (**A**) and extension (**B**) radiographs at age 5 years document no dynamic instability. **C,** Lateral radiograph obtained at age 9 years after the patient reported acute neck pain after going down a slide and dismounting uneventfully show gross C1-C2 subluxation. **D,** Sagittal midline CT shows os odontoideum. **E,** Lateral radiograph after urgent C1-C2 reduction and arthrodesis.

physical examination to identify myelopathic signs and symptoms and to discuss with parents the importance of universal precautions for protection of the cervical spine during anesthetic, surgical, or radiographic procedures. Participation in certain sports, including football, soccer, and gymnastics, as well as trampoline use, is discouraged by the AAP because of the increased risk of spinal cord injury.[49]

Klippel-Feil Syndrome

Klippel-Feil syndrome occurs in a heterogeneous group of patients, all of whom have two or more fused cervical vertebrae. The classic triad of a low posterior hairline, short neck, and decreased range of motion of the cervical spine occurs in less than 50% of patients. Associated cervical conditions include occipitocervical synostosis, basilar impression, and odontoid anomalies. Noncervical-associated conditions include congenital scoliosis, Sprengel deformity, synkinesia, genitourinary abnormalities, sensorineural hearing loss, and cardiac disease. A 2011 study reported that the prevalence of cervical scoliosis in patients with Klippel-Feil syndrome was 53.3%, with the presence of congenitally fused patterns and associated vertebral malformations indicating the greatest risk for the development of cervical scoliosis.[50] Interestingly, cervical scoliosis was not associated with cervical spine-related symptoms in this series.

Three common patterns of cervical instability have been described: C2-C3 fusion with occipitocervical synostosis; extensive fusion over several cervical levels with abnormal occipitocervical junction; and two fused segments separated by an open joint space. Abnormal biomechanics may cause neurologic symptoms in the second or third decades of life resulting from either stenosis or arthritic changes of the unfused segments.[51] Surgical intervention is warranted in patients with progressive neurologic compromise.

Although patients may have a decreased range of motion of the cervical spine, most patients with stable fusion patterns are usually asymptomatic. Those in whom instability develops may have central or peripheral neurologic sequelae. Pathologic changes within the spinal cord, instability and hypermobility at the motion segment adjacent to the fused vertebrae, and basilar invagination are reported mechanisms of neurologic sequelae in this population. Interestingly, some researchers assessed atlantoaxial segmental motion in patients with Klippel-Feil syndrome and noted an increased AADI on flexion-extension radiographs, most notably in patients with occipitalization and a fused C2-C3 segment; however, this hypermobility was not associated with symptoms or neurologic signs.[51] Early recommendations of prophylactic stabilization of patients with Klippel-Feil syndrome with hypermobility have therefore been challenged, and more recent studies do not advocate this approach.[51,52]

Subaxial Abnormalities

Cervical Kyphosis

Larsen Syndrome

Larsen syndrome is rare genetic disorder that may have an autosomal dominant or autosomal recessive inheritance. It is a connective tissue disorder caused by mutations of filamin B, whose clinical presentation typically includes multiple joint dislocations, distinct facial anomalies, clubfoot, heart defects, cleft palate, and neonatal tracheomalacia.

C1-C2 instability, lysis of the C2 pedicles, and substantial progressive cervical kyphosis are the cervical manifestations of Larsen syndrome. The risk of cord compression leading to paralysis and death because of progressive cervical kyphosis and instability warrants close surveillance of these patients, with at least serial plain radiography supplemented with CT and MRI when required. Surgical intervention depends on the age of the patient, the severity of the kyphosis, and the severity of the syndrome. In very young children, anterior arthrodesis alone is not recommended because of its high risk for spinal cord injury and arrest of anterior growth, thus eliminating the potential for kyphotic correction.[40] Posterior fusion alone in mild, flexible cases has been shown to produce good results. In patients with severe, rigid kyphosis with myelopathy, however, anterior decompression with circumferential fusion is warranted.[40,53]

Diastrophic Dysplasia

Diastrophic dysplasia is caused by mutations in the sulfate transporter gene, resulting in the production of abnormal cartilage that leads to many of the clinical manifestations associated with diastrophic dysplasia. Midcervical kyphosis with an apex at C3 or C4 present at birth typically occurs in up to one-third of this patient population. Kyphosis develops from ligamentous laxity and vertebral body wedging and hypoplasia. The natural history of cervical kyphosis in diastrophic dysplasia is favorable, with curves less than 60° typically resolving before age 6 years as the child holds up his or her head and strengthens the extensor muscles.[54] If the kyphosis exceeds 60° with an apical vertebra that is round or triangular and displaced posteriorly, then progression is likely.[54] Some authors advocate a Milwaukee brace in this setting to prevent progression; however, it remains unclear how effective nonsurgical treatment is in preventing the progression of kyphosis. Anterior decompression with posterior cervical arthrodesis has been shown to be the most effective method in preventing further progression and correcting the deformity.[40]

Neurofibromatosis

The most common cervical abnormality in patients with neurofibromatosis type 1 is kyphosis; this condition seldom requires surgery. Classic dystrophic changes of vertebral body scalloping, spinal canal widening, enlarged neural foramina, and defective pedicles may be present in cervical deformity. Severe progression of kyphosis and postoperative instability have been reported in 14% to 30% of patients after resection of intraspinal neurofibromas and spinal cord decompression[55,56] (**Figure 6**). Some authors advocate instrumented fusions as part of the decompressive laminectomy for patients with neurofibromatosis type 1 because of the frequency of severe postoperative kyphosis.[57] Hyperkyphosis that involves multiple vertebrae with dystrophic changes has been implicated as a predictor of curve progression.[58,59] More recently, strong consideration of instrumented fusion has been recommended in the management of patients with neurofibromatosis-1 who have cervical lesions, multiple levels of involvement, resection of lateral masses or facets, preexisting deformity, and involvement of either the occipitocervical or cervicothoracic junctions.[60] Despite the availability of more rigid modern instrumentation, many authors continue to favor preoperative traction with a combined circumferential fusion to optimize correction of the kyphosis and achieve a solid arthrodesis.[61]

Cervical Spondylolysis

Cervical spondylolysis is a rare condition with approximately 100 cases reported in the literature, of which only 25% have been noted in the pediatric population.[62] A diagnosis is made incidentally on routine radiographs or after minor trauma (**Figure 7**). It is characterized by a disruption of the articular mass at the junction of the superior and inferior facet joints, and it has been reported at all levels except C1 but is most commonly reported at C6.[63] Controversy exists regarding the etiology of cervical spondylolysis, with some authors favoring a congenital

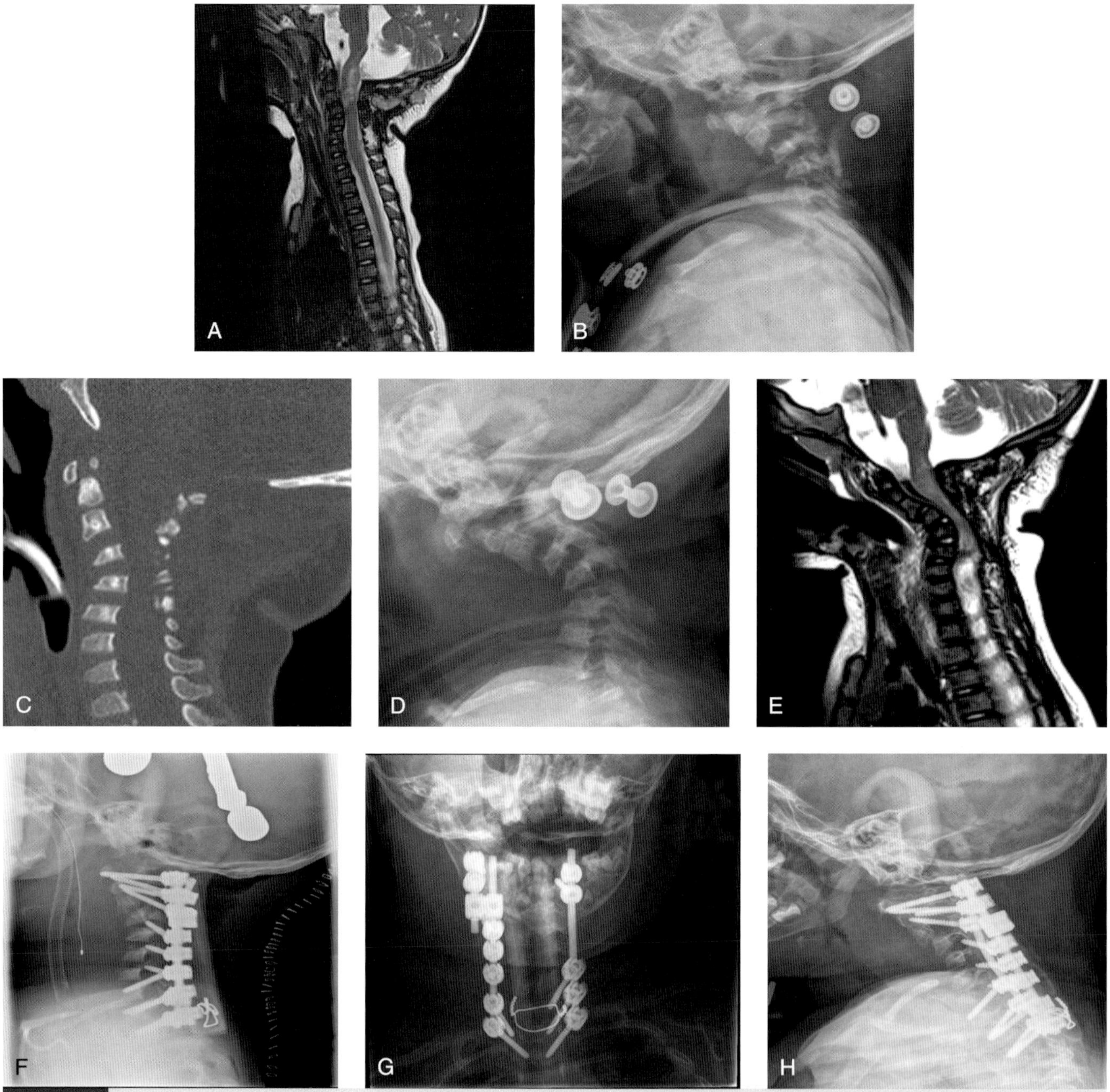

Figure 6 Images from a patient with neurofibromatosis type 1 at 3 months of age who underwent a C3-C5 laminectomy for debulking of an intraspinal tumor. MRI (**A**), lateral radiograph (**B**), and CT scan (**C**) at 10 months show postlaminectomy cervical kyphosis. Lateral cervical radiograph (**D**) and sagittal MRI (**E**) show the rapid progression of cervical kyphosis despite attempts at bracing with neurologic sequelae. **F,** Postoperative lateral cervical radiograph of the patient after undergoing C1-C7 posterior segmental instrumented fusion with tibial onlay allograft but no anterior procedure. AP (**G**) and lateral (**H**) radiographs show fusion with no recurrence of kyphosis at 4 years postoperatively.

cause and others reporting a traumatic etiology. Supporters for the traumatic theory base their argument on the fact that no cervical spondylolysis has been observed during autopsies of newborns, which implies that the disorder appears after birth. Repetitive trauma resulting in a stress fracture is now commonly accepted.[63] Rare reports of cord injury in cases of cervical spondylolysis have been noted. A 1999 study characterized cord compression in the presence of cervical spondylolysis.[64] Surgical management can be considered for pain, neurologic injury,

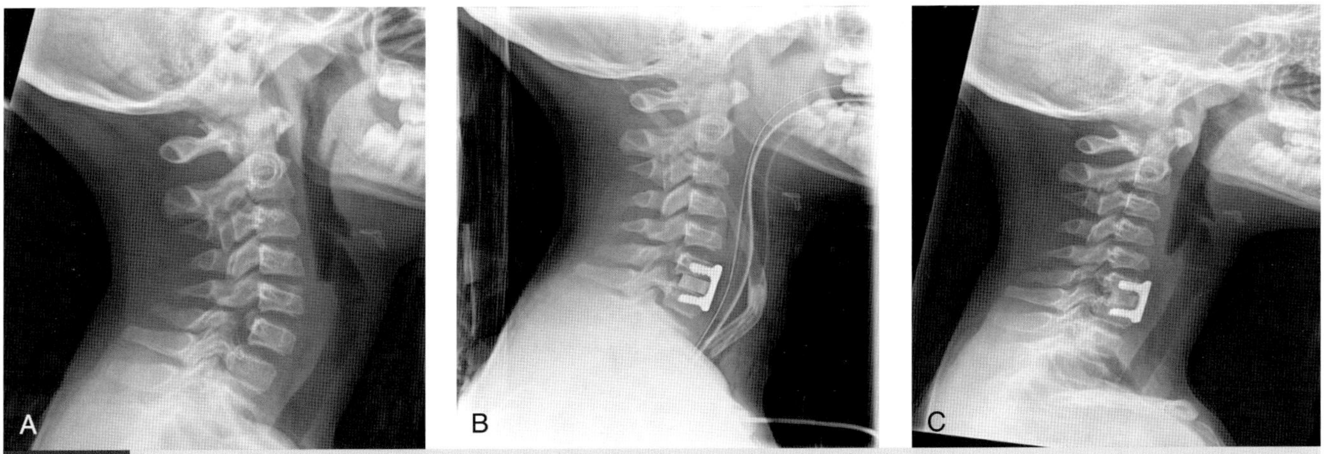

Figure 7 Images from an 8-year-old boy with a C6 pars defect and anterolisthesis after a minor fall. **A**, Lateral cervical spine radiograph shows C6 pars defect with anterolisthesis (C6 on C7). **B**, Immediate postoperative lateral cervical spine radiograph shows C6-C7 anterior cervical diskectomy and fusion. **C**, Lateral cervical spine radiograph at the 6-month follow-up shows graft incorporation.

instability on dynamic radiographs, or the presence of known risk factors for cervical spinal cord injury.[64] Optimal nonsurgical management in the absence of symptoms has yet to be fully defined.[62]

Trauma

Craniocervical and Upper Cervical Trauma

It is estimated that 1% of all pediatric injuries involve the cervical spine, with a male-to-female ratio of approximately 2:1.[65-68] The most common mechanism remains blunt trauma, with a fall from a height being the most common cause in patients younger than 8 years. Increased intrinsic elasticity with a large head-to-torso ratio results in a preponderance of upper cervical spine injuries in patients younger than 8 years.

Studies related to clinical decision making with regard to spinal imaging in pediatric cervical spine injuries are inconclusive. In adults, the National Emergency X-Radiography Utilization Study (NEXUS) criteria are well established. A 2001 study prospectively validated the NEXUS decision instrument in 3,065 pediatric patients and found a sensitivity of 100%, but the specificity was only 20%.[69] A major limitation of the NEXUS study was that only 2.8% of the included patients were younger than 2 years, which is the most crucial age group for the risk of ligamentous injury of the upper cervical spine. In 2008, two authors found a remarkably low sensitivity for the NEXUS criteria among children younger than 9 years.[70] This finding led the Congress of Neurologic Surgeons to recommend application of the NEXUS decision instrument only in children older than 9 years.[71] The Pediatric Emergency Care Applied Research Network conducted a large, multicenter case-control study to define the clinical clearance criteria specific to children; however, this study has not been validated prospectively.[72]

Most studies have historically described pediatric spine trauma in patients younger than 8 years compared with patients older than 8 years. In 2014, a group of researchers assessed differences in the epidemiology and characteristics of spine trauma in patients younger than 4 years with those between 4 and 9 years of age.[67] Important differences were identified. Upper cervical spine injuries and ligamentous injuries were more common in patients younger than 4 years. The younger group also had a higher rate of nonaccidental trauma causing spinal injury (19%) and a substantially higher mortality rate (25%).

Subaxial Cervical Trauma

Injuries of the subaxial cervical spine mainly occur after high-energy trauma in older children and adolescents in whom the cervical spine has matured. After age 8 years, the biomechanical properties of the cervical spine are more like those of adults, with injury patterns also similar to those in adults. The most common location of injury is between C5 and C7. Because this injury occurs predominantly in older children, some advocate the NEXUS criteria for decision making.[73] It has been suggested that more than 7° of kyphotic angulation between adjacent vertebral bodies implies ligamentous instability. Translation of more than 3.5 mm also should raise suspicion of injury.[74]

Because of the diagnostic limitations of plain radiographs, CT has emerged as the imaging modality of choice in the setting of acute trauma. However, with increasing concerns of radiation exposure in the pediatric

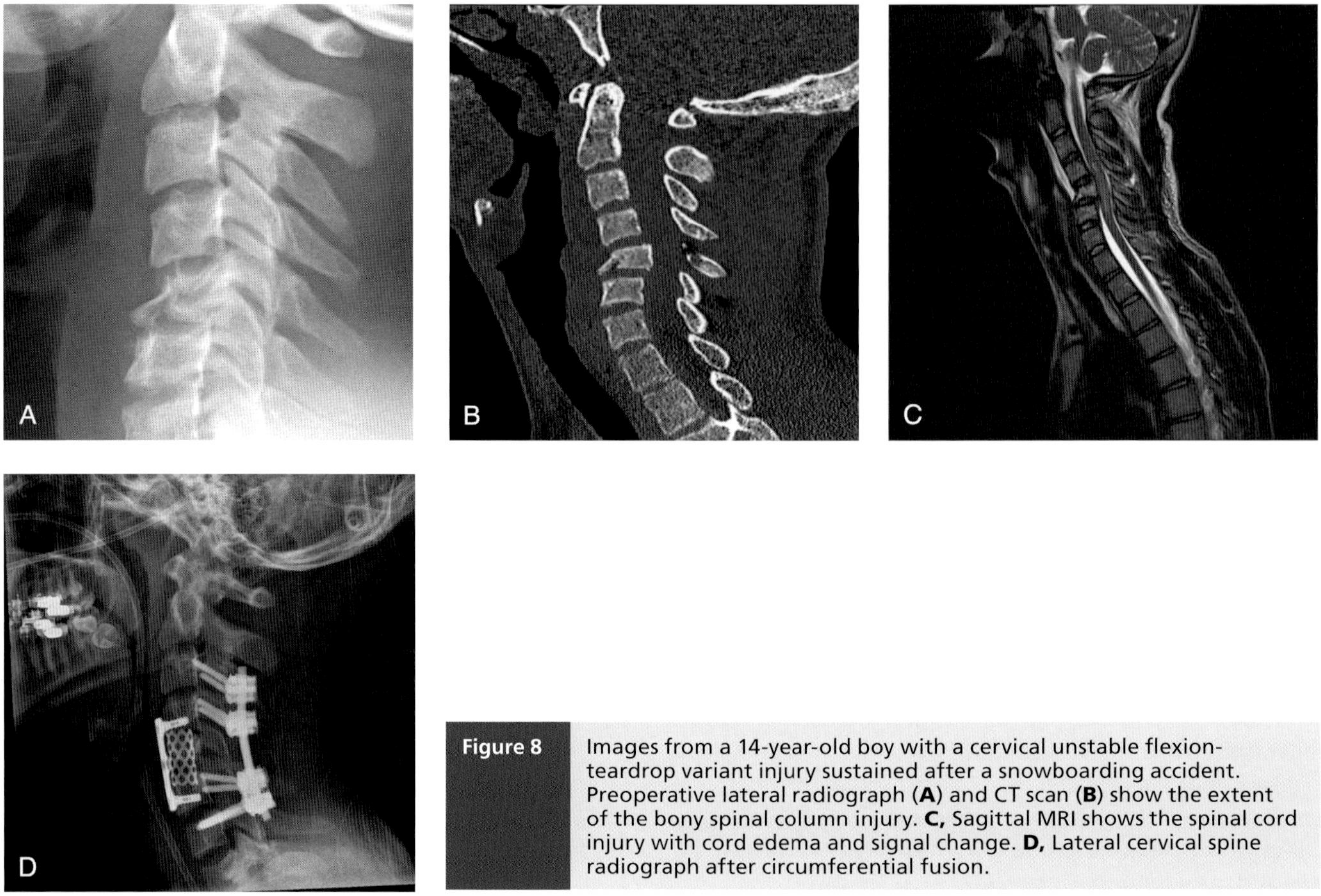

Figure 8 Images from a 14-year-old boy with a cervical unstable flexion-teardrop variant injury sustained after a snowboarding accident. Preoperative lateral radiograph (**A**) and CT scan (**B**) show the extent of the bony spinal column injury. **C**, Sagittal MRI shows the spinal cord injury with cord edema and signal change. **D**, Lateral cervical spine radiograph after circumferential fusion.

population,[18] MRI has recently been advocated as the study of choice in this setting.[75] One group of researchers found MRI to be 100% sensitive and 97% specific, with a negative predictive value of 75% and a positive predictive value of 100%, in detecting osseous injuries in the setting of pediatric cervical trauma.[75] Another group of researchers used clinical decision analysis to determine the optimal cervical spine evaluation strategy, balancing the risk of missed cervical spine injury with the risk of radiation-induced malignancy. Using literature-derived probabilities and clinical clearance, screening plain radiographs were preferred over CT for the evaluation of pediatric patients with blunt trauma.[68]

Despite advances in modern instrumentation techniques for pediatric cervical spine injuries, most injuries can be managed with external immobilization. When surgery is warranted, consideration must be given to the small size and growth potential of the pediatric spine.

Athletic Injuries

Athletic activities are one of the leading causes of cervical spine injuries in the pediatric population, accounting for the second most common cause of spinal cord injury in people younger than 30 years.[76] In children aged 10 to 14 years, sports participation is the most common cause of cervical spine injuries.[77] Football and ice hockey account for most of these injuries, followed by rugby, wrestling, diving, skiing, snowboarding, cheerleading, and equestrian sports (**Figure 8**). The mechanism of injury can be sport related, but it is more commonly independent of the sport. Although the mechanics of a cervical spine injury in athletes have been extensively studied, the true mechanism of injury remains controversial. Injury patterns include cervical sprain or strain, stingers and burners, cord neurapraxia and transient quadriplegia, discoligamentous injury, and fractures with and without dislocation.

The decision to allow an athlete to return to play after injury is complex and must be considered on an individual basis. Most published data offer expert opinion with limited objective data. In 1986, a point grading system was proposed to quantify a patient's clinical situation and offer an objective guideline for return to play.[78] In 2001, researchers attempted a questionnaire survey study to evaluate what factors, such as published guidelines, the type of sport of the patient, the physician's number of years in practice and subspecialty interests, and sport participation of the respondent, played a role in the return-to-play decision-making process.[79] The authors found that opinions vary regarding the decision to allow an athlete to return to play after a cervical spine injury. Most authors recommend that the decision be made on an individual basis. The literature remains inconclusive in providing firm, objective guidelines for sport participation after a cervical spine injury.

Summary

Recent morphologic studies have advanced the understanding of the growth and development of the upper cervical spine in the pediatric population, highlighting important variability in ossification patterns and the timing of synchondrosis fusion. Although CT has been the imaging modality of choice to quantify osseous anomalies, recent concerns of radiation-induced malignancy are making MRI a more favorable choice. Screening radiographs in patients at high risk continue to be controversial because the association between instability and neurologic sequelae remains poorly understood. Historically, pediatric cervical trauma had a clear delineation between those younger than 8 years and those older than 8 years; more recent literature further characterizes important differences in patients younger than 4 years and those older than 4 years. Modern surgical stabilization techniques may provide outcomes that are more favorable in patients at high risk, with recent literature favoring surgical intervention, even in incidental findings of osseoligamentous instability in the pediatric cervical spine.

Key Study Points

- The C1 posterior synchondrosis closure generally occurs by the age of 3 years, whereas the anterior C1 synchondrosis closure generally occurs at an older age.
- The duration of symptoms prior to the diagnosis of AARS is the most important predictor of the type of treatment required.
- The distinction between orthotopic and dystopic os odontoideum is critical in planning surgical stabilization.
- The AAP no longer recommends routine radiologic examinations in asymptomatic patients with Down syndrome to screen for upper cervical instability.
- The literature remains inconclusive in providing firm, objective guidelines for sport participation after a cervical spine injury.

Annotated References

1. Plaut HF: Fracture of the atlas or developmental abnormality. *Radiol* 1937;29(2):227-231.

2. Ogden JA: Radiology of postnatal skeletal development: XI. The first cervical vertebra. *Skeletal Radiol* 1984;12(1):12-20.

3. Piatt JH Jr, Grissom LE: Developmental anatomy of the atlas and axis in childhood by computed tomography. *J Neurosurg Pediatr* 2011;8(3):235-243.

   A convenience sample of CT scans from a single center was reviewed to recognize normal developmental anatomy from common variants in pediatric cervical spine fractures.

4. Rao RD, Tang S, Lim C, Yoganandan N: Developmental morphology and ossification patterns of the C1 vertebra. *J Bone Joint Surg Am* 2013;95(17):e1241-e1247.

   Data from this retrospective review of 54 CT scans of the cervical spine in young children quantified normative data as a function of age. The authors stated this should improve understanding of the developmental anatomy and biomechanical stability of the C1 vertebra. It also will help distinguish fractures of C1 from nonossified regions within vertebrae, congenital variations, and the effects of arthrodesis with or without internal fixation.

5. Junewick JJ, Chin MS, Meesa IR, Ghori S, Boynton SJ, Luttenton CR: Ossification patterns of the atlas vertebra. *AJR Am J Roentgenol* 2011;197(5):1229-1234.

   This review of CT scans characterized ossification patterns of the C1 (atlas) vertebra in children to better differentiate normal variants from traumatic injury. It found C1 ossification patterns and the timing of synchondrosis fusion to be variable between normal and traumatic injury.

6. Ghanem I, El Hage S, Rachkidi R, Kharrat K, Dagher F, Kreichati G: Pediatric cervical spine instability. *J Child Orthop* 2008;2(2):71-84.

7. Buhs C, Cullen M, Klein M, Farmer D: The pediatric trauma C-spine: Is the "odontoid" view necessary? *J Pediatr Surg* 2000;35(6):994-997.

8. Smoker WR: Craniovertebral junction: Normal anatomy, craniometry, and congenital anomalies. *Radiographics* 1994;14(2):255-277.

9. Harris JH Jr, Carson GC, Wagner LK, Kerr N: Radiologic diagnosis of traumatic occipitovertebral dissociation: 2. Comparison of three methods of detecting occipitovertebral relationships on lateral radiographs of supine subjects. *AJR Am J Roentgenol* 1994;162(4):887-892.

10. Dziurzynski K, Anderson PA, Bean DB, et al: A blinded assessment of radiographic criteria for atlanto-occipital dislocation. *Spine (Phila Pa 1976)* 2005;30(12):1427-1432.

11. Cattell HS, Filtzer DL: Pseudosubluxation and other normal variations in the cervical spine in children: A study of one hundred and sixty children. *J Bone Joint Surg Am* 1965;47(7):1295-1309.

12. Wang JC, Nuccion SL, Feighan JE, Cohen B, Dorey FJ, Scoles PV: Growth and development of the pediatric cervical spine documented radiographically. *J Bone Joint Surg Am* 2001;83(8):1212-1218.

13. Wills BP, Dormans JP: Nontraumatic upper cervical spine instability in children. *J Am Acad Orthop Surg* 2006;14(4):233-245.

14. Hinck VC, Hopkins CE, Savara BS: The size of the atlantal spinal canal: A sex difference. *Hum Biol* 1962;34:197-205.

15. Boltshauser E, Hoare RD: Radiographic measurements of the normal spinal cord in childhood. *Neuroradiology* 1976;10(5):235-237.

16. Inoue H, Ohmori K, Takatsu T, Teramoto T, Ishida Y, Suzuki K: Morphological analysis of the cervical spinal canal, dural tube and spinal cord in normal individuals using CT myelography. *Neuroradiology* 1996;38(2):148-151.

17. Matsuura P, Waters RL, Adkins RH, Rothman S, Gurbani N, Sie I: Comparison of computerized tomography parameters of the cervical spine in normal control subjects and spinal cord-injured patients. *J Bone Joint Surg Am* 1989;71(2):183-188.

18. Miglioretti DL, Johnson E, Williams A, et al: The use of computed tomography in pediatrics and the associated radiation exposure and estimated cancer risk. *JAMA Pediatr* 2013;167(8):700-707.

    Radiation doses from pediatric CT scans have increased and vary widely in clinical practice. The authors recommend reducing doses through standardized protocols and other methods.

19. Neal KM, Mohamed AS: Atlantoaxial rotatory subluxation in children. *J Am Acad Orthop Surg* 2015;23(6):382-392.

    This current review article on AARS in children discusses anatomy, etiology, classification, presentation, diagnostics, and treatment of AARS.

20. Fielding JW, Hawkins RJ: Atlanto-axial rotatory fixation. (Fixed rotatory subluxation of the atlanto-axial joint). *J Bone Joint Surg Am* 1977;59(1):37-44.

21. Pang D, Li V: Atlantoaxial rotatory fixation: Part 2. New diagnostic paradigm and a new classification based on motion analysis using computed tomographic imaging. *Neurosurgery* 2005;57(5):941-953.

22. Pang D, Li V: Atlantoaxial rotatory fixation: Part 3. A prospective study of the clinical manifestation, diagnosis, management, and outcome of children with atlantoaxial rotatory fixation. *Neurosurgery* 2005;57(5):954-972.

23. Ishii K, Toyama Y, Nakamura M, Chiba K, Matsumoto M: Management of chronic atlantoaxial rotatory fixation. *Spine (Phila Pa 1976)* 2012;37(5):E278-E285.

    A retrospective case series of chronic atlantoaxial rotatory fixation treated by a novel closed reduction method (remodeling therapy) was reviewed. The current study found no recurrence of symptoms or any observation of subluxation at a mean follow-up of 42 months.

24. Hicazi A, Acaroglu E, Alanay A, Yazici M, Surat A: Atlantoaxial rotatory fixation–subluxation revisited: A computed tomographic analysis of acute torticollis in pediatric patients. *Spine (Phila Pa 1976)* 2002;27(24):2771-2775.

25. Alanay A, Hicazi A, Acaroglu E, et al: Reliability and necessity of dynamic computerized tomography in diagnosis of atlantoaxial rotatory subluxation. *J Pediatr Orthop* 2002;22(6):763-765.

26. Tauchi R, Imagama S, Ito Z, et al: Surgical treatment for chronic atlantoaxial rotatory fixation in children. *J Pediatr Orthop B* 2013;22(5):404-408.

    The authors report on a case series of six patients who were treated with surgical fixation after unsuccessful nonsurgical management. The authors found that C1-C2 transarticular fixation, C1 lateral mass screw fixation, and C2 pedicle screw fixation were reliable methods for treating these patients.

27. Beier AD, Vachhrajani S, Bayerl SH, Aguilar CY, Lamberti-Pasculli M, Drake JM: Rotatory subluxation: Experience from the Hospital for Sick Children. *J Neurosurg Pediatr* 2012;9(2):144-148.

    The authors reviewed 40 patients in a 9-year series to explore the diagnosis and management of AARS at their center. They found that AARS management varies because of the spectrum of clinical presentations. Patients without neurologic deficits may be treated with collar therapy, whereas those in whom subluxation cannot be reduced or those who have a neurologic deficit may require traction and/or surgical fixation.

28. Glotzbecker MP, Wasser AM, Hresko MT, Karlin LI, Emans JB, Hedequist DJ: Efficacy of nonfusion treatment for subacute and chronic atlanto-axial rotatory fixation in children. *J Pediatr Orthop* 2014;34(5):490-495.

    A retrospective review of 14 patients with AARS and atlantoaxial rotatory fixation was conducted at a tertiary pediatric hospital. Recurrence may occur after a trial reduction and nonfusion treatment. In addition, patients with delayed presentation (>1 month) may be treated initially with a trial of nonsurgical treatment. Level of evidence: III.

29. Landi A, Pietrantonio A, Marotta N, Mancarella C, Delfini R: Atlantoaxial rotatory dislocation (AARD) in pediatric age: MRI study on conservative treatment with Philadelphia collar. Experience of nine consecutive cases. *Eur Spine J* 2012;21(suppl 1):S94-S99.

A case series of nine patients treated with a Philadelphia collar for atlantoaxial rotatory dislocation were evaluated with T2-weighted MRI and short tau inversion recovery (STIR) imaging. The authors found that MRI with STIR sequences was useful in addressing the duration of nonsurgical treatment.

30. Fielding JW, Hensinger RN, Hawkins RJ: Os odontoideum. *J Bone Joint Surg Am* 1980;62(3):376-383.

31. Klimo P Jr, Coon V, Brockmeyer D: Incidental os odontoideum: Current management strategies. *Neurosurg Focus* 2011;31(6):E10.

In this case report of a patient in whom an incidental discovery of os odontoideum was made, the authors reviewed embryologic aspects as well as upper cervical anatomy in context of the literature. The authors recommended surgical intervention for patients younger than 20 years who show evidence of radiographic instability at the atlantoaxial level and have bone anatomy favorable for screw fixation.

32. Arvin B, Fournier-Gosselin M-P, Fehlings MG: Os odontoideum: Etiology and surgical management. *Neurosurgery* 2010;66(3suppl):22-31.

A review of current literature found that nonsurgical treatment is successful in patients who are incidentally found to have radiologically stable and noncompressive os odontoideum. Surgical treatment (posterior decompression after reduction and fusion with C1 and C2 instrumentation) has a definite role in symptomatic patients.

33. Zhang Z, Zhou Y, Wang J, et al: Acute traumatic cervical cord injury in patients with os odontoideum. *J Clin Neurosci* 2010;17(10):1289-1293.

Ten patients with os odontoideum after acute cervical cord injury trauma were studied. The authors concluded that patients with asymptomatic or myelopathic atlantoaxial instability secondary to os odontoideum are at risk for spinal cord injury after a minor traumatic injury. Surgery is recommended for these patients.

34. White KK, Bompadre V, Goldberg MJ, et al: Best practices in the evaluation and treatment of foramen magnum stenosis in achondroplasia during infancy. *Am J Med Genet A* 2016;170(1):42-51.

The authors present a consensus-based best practice guideline with 22 recommendations for evaluating and treating foramen magnum stenosis in infants with achondroplasia.

35. Bagley CA, Pindrik JA, Bookland MJ, Camara-Quintana JQ, Carson BS: Cervicomedullary decompression for foramen magnum stenosis in achondroplasia. *J Neurosurg* 2006;104(3suppl):166-172.

36. Hunter AG, Bankier A, Rogers JG, Sillence D, Scott CI Jr: Medical complications of achondroplasia: A multicentre patient review. *J Med Genet* 1998;35(9):705-712.

37. White KK, Steinman S, Mubarak SJ: Cervical stenosis and spastic quadriparesis in Morquio disease (MPS IV): A case report with twenty-six-year follow-up. *J Bone Joint Surg Am* 2009;91(2):438-442.

38. Ransford AO, Crockard HA, Stevens JM, Modaghegh S: Occipito-atlanto-axial fusion in Morquio-Brailsford syndrome: A ten-year experience. *J Bone Joint Surg Br* 1996;78(2):307-313.

39. Miyoshi K, Nakamura K, Haga N, Mikami Y: Surgical treatment for atlantoaxial subluxation with myelopathy in spondyloepiphyseal dysplasia congenita. *Spine (Phila Pa 1976)* 2004;29(21):E488-E491.

40. McKay SD, Al-Omari A, Tomlinson LA, Dormans JP: Review of cervical spine anomalies in genetic syndromes. *Spine (Phila Pa 1976)* 2012;37(5):E269-E277.

A literature review of cervical spine anomalies in genetic syndromes concluded that it is important to be vigilant in the diagnosis and treatment of cervical spine anomalies.

41. Karol LA, Sheffield EG, Crawford K, Moody MK, Browne RH: Reproducibility in the measurement of atlanto-occipital instability in children with Down syndrome. *Spine (Phila Pa 1976)* 1996;21(21):2463-2467, discussion 2468.

42. Pizzutillo PD, Herman MJ: Cervical spine issues in Down syndrome. *J Pediatr Orthop* 2005;25(2):253-259.

43. Hankinson TC, Anderson RC: Craniovertebral junction abnormalities in Down syndrome. *Neurosurgery* 2010;66(3suppl):32-38.

44. Participation by individuals with Down syndrome who suffer from the atlantoaxial dislocation condition. Special Olympics Bulletin. March 31, 1983.

45. American Academy of Pediatrics, Committee on Sports Medicine: Atlantoaxial instability in Down syndrome. *Pediatrics* 1984;74(1):152-154.

46. American Academy of Pediatrics, Committee on Sports Medicine and Fitness: Atlantoaxial instability in Down syndrome: Subject review. *Pediatrics* 1995;96(1 pt 1):151-154.

47. American Academy of Pediatrics. Committee on Genetics: Health supervision for children with Down syndrome. *Pediatrics* 2001;107(2):442-449.

48. Policy statement: AAP publications reaffirmed and retired. *Pediatrics* 2007;120(3):683-684.

49. Bull MJ; Committee on Genetics: Health supervision for children with Down syndrome. *Pediatrics* 2011;128(2):393-406.

Guidelines for the care of children with Down syndrome are described.

50. Samartzis D, Kalluri P, Herman J, Lubicky JP, Shen FH: Cervical scoliosis in the Klippel–Feil patient. *Spine (Phila Pa 1976)* 2011;36(23):E1501-E1508.

This study found a high association of scoliosis in individuals with Klippel-Feil syndrome, and the presence of congenitally fused patterns and associated vertebral malformations leads to the greatest risk of the development of scoliosis.

51. Shen FH, Samartzis D, Herman J, Lubicky JP: Radiographic assessment of segmental motion at the atlantoaxial junction in the Klippel-Feil patient. *Spine (Phila Pa 1976)* 2006;31(2):171-177.

52. Nagashima H, Morio Y, Teshima R: No neurological involvement for more than 40 years in Klippel-Feil syndrome with severe hypermobility of the upper cervical spine. *Arch Orthop Trauma Surg* 2001;121(1-2):99-101.

53. Johnston CE II, Birch JG, Daniels JL: Cervical kyphosis in patients who have Larsen syndrome. *J Bone Joint Surg Am* 1996;78(4):538-545.

54. Remes V, Marttinen E, Poussa M, Kaitila I, Peltonen J: Cervical kyphosis in diastrophic dysplasia. *Spine (Phila Pa 1976)* 1999;24(19):1990-1995.

55. Isu T, Miyasaka K, Abe H, Ito T, Iwasaka Y, Tsuru M: Atlantoaxial dislocation associated with neurofibromatosis: Report of three cases. *J Neurosurg* 1983;58(3):451-453.

56. Yong-Hing K, Kalamchi A, MacEwen GD: Cervical spine abnormalities in neurofibromatosis. *J Bone Joint Surg Am* 1979;61(5):695-699.

57. Crawford AH: Pitfalls of spinal deformities associated with neurofibromatosis in children. *Clin Orthop Relat Res* 1989;245:29-42.

58. Funasaki H, Winter RB, Lonstein JB, Denis F: Pathophysiology of spinal deformities in neurofibromatosis: An analysis of seventy-one patients who had curves associated with dystrophic changes. *J Bone Joint Surg Am* 1994;76(5):692-700.

59. Wilde PH, Upadhyay SS, Leong JC: Deterioration of operative correction in dystrophic spinal neurofibromatosis. *Spine (Phila Pa 1976)* 1994;19(11):1264-1270.

60. Taleb FS, Guha A, Arnold PM, Fehlings MG, Massicotte EM: Surgical management of cervical spine manifestations of neurofibromatosis type 1: Long-term clinical and radiological follow-up in 22 cases. *J Neurosurg Spine* 2011;14(3):356-366.

This retrospective review of a heterogeneous group of 22 patients aged 8 to 74 years who have neurofibromatosis type 1 with symptomatic cervical spine neurofibromas underwent surgical decompression and tumor resection with or without instrumentation. The authors emphasized that early stabilization of the cervical spine prevents late deformity.

61. Kawabata S, Watanabe K, Hosogane N, et al: Surgical correction of severe cervical kyphosis in patients with neurofibromatosis type 1. *J Neurosurg Spine* 2013;18(3):274-279.

The authors reported on three cases of severe cervical kyphosis associated with neurofibromatosis type 1 that were successfully treated with combined anterior and posterior correction and fusion.

62. Alton TB, Patel AM, Lee MJ, Chapman JR: Pediatric cervical spondylolysis and American football. *Spine J* 2014;14(6):e1-e5.

This case report described C6 bilateral cervical spondylolysis with a bicuspid spinous process. The patient was asymptomatic and educated on ways to decrease the risk of spinal cord injury with contact sports, after which the patient was allowed to participate fully in sports without restriction.

63. Ahn PG, Yoon DH, Shin HC, et al: Cervical spondylolysis: Three cases and a review of the current literature. *Spine (Phila Pa 1976)* 2010;35(3):E80-E83.

64. Fessy MH, Durand JM, Gunepin FX, Chavane H, Béjui JB, Bouchet A: An unusual anomaly: Cervical spondylolysis in an adult [French]. *Rev Chir Orthop Reparatrice Appar Mot* 1999;85(2):174-177.

65. Firth GB, Kingwell SP, Moroz PJ: Pediatric noncontiguous spinal injuries: The 15-year experience at a level 1 trauma center. *Spine (Phila Pa 1976)* 2012;37(10):E599-E608.

This retrospective review of 211 pediatric patients determined the incidence of noncontiguous spinal injuries to be 11.8% over a 15-year period. The authors noted that 24% of the patients had a neurologic injury and recommended obtaining entire spine radiographs to exclude noncontiguous injuries for patients with a single-level spinal injury and a neurologic injury. Level of evidence: IV.

66. Schottler J, Vogel LC, Sturm P: Spinal cord injuries in young children: A review of children injured at 5 years of age and younger. *Dev Med Child Neurol* 2012;54(12):1138-1143.

One hundred fifty-nine children younger than 5 years with a spinal cord injury at a children's hospital were reviewed. The epidemiology, complications, and manifestations of spinal cord injuries in children are unique.

67. Knox JB, Schneider JE, Cage JM, Wimberly RL, Riccio AI: Spine trauma in very young children: A retrospective study of 206 patients presenting to a level 1 pediatric trauma center. *J Pediatr Orthop* 2014;34(7):698-702.

Many differences in characteristics are noted in spinal injuries of young children compared with older children. Cervical injuries are more common in young patients; they have more compression fractures and sustain more spinal cord injuries than older patients. Level of evidence: III.

68. Hannon M, Mannix R, Dorney K, Mooney D, Hennelly K: Pediatric cervical spine injury evaluation after blunt trauma: A clinical decision analysis. *Ann Emerg Med* 2015;65(3):239-247.

The authors presented a model to evaluate children with a cervical spine injury. The model highlighted the preferred strategies of clinical clearance and screening radiographs in a hypothetical trauma pediatric population. CT scanning is rarely the initial optimal evaluation.

69. Viccellio P, Simon H, Pressman BD, Shah MN, Mower WR, Hoffman JR; NEXUS Group: A prospective multicenter study of cervical spine injury in children. *Pediatrics* 2001;108(2):e20.

70. Garton HJ, Hammer MR: Detection of pediatric cervical spine injury. *Neurosurgery* 2008;62(3):700-708.

71. Management of pediatric cervical spine and spinal cord injuries. *Neurosurgery* 2002;50(3suppl):S85-S99.

72. Leonard JR, Jaffe DM, Kuppermann N, Olsen CS, Leonard JC; Pediatric Emergency Care Applied Research Network (PECARN) Cervical Spine Study Group: Cervical spine injury patterns in children. *Pediatrics* 2014;133(5):e1179-e1188.

This retrospective review describes cervical spine injuries in 540 children over a 5-year period. The authors explore the relationship between cervical spine injuries and age, mechanism of injury, comorbid injuries, surgical interventions, and neurologic outcomes.

73. Baumann F, Ernstberger T, Neumann C, et al: Pediatric cervical spine injuries: A rare but challenging entity. *J Spinal Disord Tech* 2015;28(7):E377-E384.

This review article used clinical cases as examples to demonstrate key points in the diagnosis and treatment of pediatric cervical spine injuries. The authors stated that knowledge of the biomechanical properties and radiographic presentation of the immature spine can improve the results with pediatric spinal cord injuries. Level of evidence: IV.

74. Mortazavi M, Gore PA, Chang S, Tubbs RS, Theodore N: Pediatric cervical spine injuries: A comprehensive review. *Childs Nerv Syst* 2011;27(5):705-717.

A review of the literature found that comprehensive knowledge of the special anatomy and biomechanics of the spine in children is essential in the diagnosis and treatment of spinal injuries.

75. Henry M, Riesenburger RI, Kryzanski J, Jea A, Hwang SW: A retrospective comparison of CT and MRI in detecting pediatric cervical spine injury. *Childs Nerv Syst* 2013;29(8):1333-1338.

In the setting of pediatric cervical spine trauma, using CT as the standard for osseous injury, MRI had a sensitivity of 100%, a specificity of 97%, a negative predictive value of 75%, and a positive predictive value of 100%. Using MRI as the standard for soft-tissue injury, CT had a sensitivity of 23%, a specificity of 100%, a negative predictive value of 88%, and a positive predictive value of 100%.

76. Bettencourt RB, Linder MM: Treatment of neck injuries. *Prim Care* 2013;40(2):259-269.

Spinal cord injuries are uncommon in sports; however, planning and practice for these types of injuries are important. Debate remains on sport participation after central cord neurapraxia in the setting of cervical spine stenosis, and these conflicts can present challenges to clinicians when forming a management plan and return-to-play recommendations.

77. Benjamin HJ, Lessman DS: Sports-related cervical spine injuries. *Clin Pediatr Emerg Med* 2013;14(4):255-266.

This review article described the evaluation of potential cervical spine injuries in an athlete. Prompt evaluation as well as knowledge and anatomic understanding are integral and necessary components in diagnosing such injuries. Clearance to play should be individually based and in conjunction with a specialist.

78. Watkins RG: Neck injuries in football players. *Clin Sports Med* 1986;5(2):215-246.

79. Morganti C, Sweeney CA, Albanese SA, Burak C, Hosea T, Connolly PJ: Return to play after cervical spine injury. *Spine (Phila Pa 1976)* 2001;26(10):1131-1136.

Chapter 33

Back Pain, Disk Disease, Spondylolysis, and Spondylolisthesis

A. Noelle Larson, MD

Abstract

Back pain is a common problem in children. Because many conditions can cause back pain, it is important to use appropriate physical examination and imaging methods to rule out specific conditions that are unique to children. Constant pain, abnormal findings on the physical examination, and progressive symptoms should prompt additional workups. Disk disease, spondylolysis, and spondylolisthesis are frequent causes of back pain in children. With the exception of high-grade spondylolisthesis, treatment is typically driven by symptomatology. Most patients respond to physical therapy, rest, and/or bracing. If nonsurgical measures are unsuccessful, surgical treatment may restore function.

Keywords: disk herniation; pars defect; pediatric back pain; spondylolisthesis; spondylolysis

Introduction

Historically, back pain in children was thought to indicate serious pathology and necessitated an extensive workup. However, back pain, particularly in adolescents, is quite common and has no identifiable underlying cause in up to 80% of patients. Intermittent back pain is experienced by 50% of adolescents.[1] An insurance registry evaluation of more than 200,000 adolescents with back pain reported that fewer than 20% had a specific associated diagnosis such as spondylolysis or disk disease given within 1 year.[2]

Dr. Larson or an immediate family member serves as a board member, owner, officer, or committee member of the Pediatric Orthopaedic Society of North America and the Scoliosis Research Society.

Conflicting evidence exists on whether back pain is more common in patients who are active and participate in sports.[3,4] Idiopathic back pain has been associated with older age, carrying heavy backpacks, an increased body mass index, and parental smoking.[5-7] A patient with idiopathic back pain may have detectable differences in his or her spine. A recent study using upright MRIs to analyze the response to backpack loads showed increased compression of the L5-S1 disks with backpack wear in children with idiopathic back pain compared with normal control subjects.[8] Effective management of back pain in adolescents is essential because back pain in children is associated with back pain later in life.[9,10]

It is important to identify the structural causes of back pain; however, these causes are present in only 20% to 30% of patients. Many diagnoses involving back pain are specific to the pediatric population, including tumor, infection, fracture, inflammatory arthritis, Scheuermann disease, spondylolysis, and spondylolisthesis. A diagnosis of idiopathic back pain can be made only after other important causes of back pain are ruled out by appropriate evaluations that are proportionate to the symptomatology.

Patient Evaluation

A thorough patient history, a physical examination, and, in many cases, standing PA and lateral radiographs make up the initial evaluation.[11,12]

History

Patients should be asked about the duration, characteristics, and onset of their pain, as well as any aggravating or alleviating factors. Night pain, progressive pain, or constant pain may indicate tumor or infection. Pain from osteoid osteoma is classically relieved by NSAIDs. Pain that results in a loss of function, missed participation in sports, or school absences is more concerning than activity-related back pain or mild symptoms at the end of the day. Extensive periods of missed school accompanied by chronic back pain may point to underlying psychosocial factors. Patients should be asked about constitutional symptoms, pertinent past medical history, and extracurricular activities that may put them at higher risk for spinal pathology. Patients who participate in hyperextension sports, such as gymnastics or diving, are at risk for spondylolysis. Weight lifting has been associated with lumbar Scheuermann disease and disk disease. A focused family history should be taken because disk disease may be a common condition in a patient's family. Careful questioning is needed regarding bowel and bladder function to elicit an accurate history because many patients and their families are reticent to volunteer this information. Tobacco use also should be verified.

Physical Examination

The physical examination should include inspection of the back for spinal deformity, including coronal balance and spinal asymmetry. The Adam forward bend test is used to assess for scoliosis and focal kyphosis. The skin should be examined for markings over the spine, such as a hairy patch or dimple, which may indicate spinal cord pathology. Findings such as multiple café au lait lesions or axillary freckling should prompt an evaluation for neurofibromatosis. Sagittal plane alignment should be noted as well as spinal range of motion. Restricted range of motion is concerning for any underlying pathologic process. Pain elicited from palpation or percussion also warrants evaluation. Excessive range of motion and generalized ligamentous laxity may be associated with idiopathic back pain. A complete neurologic examination is necessary, including motor strength, sensation, and reflexes. Gait should be assessed for asymmetry or limp. The feet should be examined for asymmetry or deformity, which could indicate a spinal cord tumor or a tethered cord.

Hip range of motion should be symmetric and pain free. Pain with provocative maneuvers, including pain with hip flexion and internal rotation or groin pain with resisted straight leg raises, may indicate hip pathology. Pain with the FABER (flexion/abduction/external rotation) maneuver or tenderness to palpation over the sacroiliac joints may indicate sacroiliac joint pathology, which may be attributable to degenerative causes, inflammatory arthritis, or infection (if unilateral). Hamstring tightness indicated by an increased popliteal angle is associated with spondylolysis, spondylolisthesis, kyphosis, and a tethered cord. Pain radiating below the knee with passive straight leg raises is indicative of nerve root tension. A positive, crossed straight leg raise is characterized by radicular pain in the opposite leg, which has even greater specificity. Radicular symptoms with palpation of the sciatic notch may indicate piriformis syndrome.

Imaging

Radiographs are the first imaging study to be considered and should be obtained prior to CT or MRI. Imaging studies should be performed based on clinical judgment and may be ordered selectively. Full-length standing two-view spine radiographs may show a spondylolytic defect, spondylolisthesis, scoliosis, diskitis (disk space narrowing), congenital segmentation anomalies, limb-length discrepancy, Scheuermann disease, or a compression fracture. A lumbar spine lateral view or L5-S1 spot lateral view may better show spondylolisthesis or spondylolysis because of parallax on a standard full-length lateral view unless low-dose biplanar slot scanning technology is used. Oblique views and flexion-extension views are not typically indicated in the pediatric population, particularly for the initial evaluation, because of the high radiation dose, particularly for the oblique views, which transmit as much radiation as a focal lumbar CT scan.

A variety of advanced imaging modalities are effective for evaluating severe or atypical back pain that has not responded to nonsurgical management. Advanced imaging is not warranted for every pediatric patient with back pain and should be used selectively. MRI can be useful for detecting disk or spinal cord pathology, lumbar Scheuermann disease, fracture, tumor, infection, or spondylolysis.[13] Evidence of diskitis can sometimes be seen on plain radiographs, although MRI is more sensitive. The hallmark of infection is a T2 signal change crossing a disk space and involving two adjacent levels. Inflammation of the lumbar apophyseal joints and interspinous ligament seen on MRI may be found in patients with enthesitis-related arthritis.[14] MRI is costly, may not be readily available, and requires sedation in younger children; however, it provides excellent visualization of soft tissues and does not expose the patient to radiation. Bone scintigraphy can be used to evaluate for spondylolysis, infection, tumor, and an apophyseal ring fracture, but it exposes the patient to deep ionizing radiation. Scintigraphy will not show spinal cord pathology.[15] A bone scan also is helpful in localizing the anatomic area of pain in a patient who is nonverbal and has back or leg pain. A normal bone scan can provide peace of mind for patients with severe, persistent generalized back pain that has not improved with nonsurgical management and has no other obvious diagnoses; however, bone scans should be used sparingly because of high radiation exposure.

Currently, CT provides the best three-dimensional visualization of bony structures. It is readily available at most centers, and images can be obtained quickly, so sedation in a younger child is less frequently needed. An apophyseal ring fracture may be better appreciated with CT than MRI. Also, CT allows for careful evaluation of the pars anatomy for spondylolytic defects and is more sensitive than radiography. Based on the injury mechanism, emergent CT of the spine may be warranted in an obtunded trauma patient or a patient with a distracting injury. CT entails greater ionizing radiation, although this modality typically has a lower dose than a bone scan.[16] Specific CT protocols should be adjusted based on the body weight and age of the child to limit radiation exposure. A recent high-quality population-based study from Australia with a mean 10-year follow-up showed one additional cancer for every 1,800 pediatric CT scans performed.[17] Therefore, CT should be reserved for patients with clear indications. CT myelography involves injection of dye into the dural sac and can be used to evaluate compression of the neural elements in patients who are unable to undergo MRI because of incompatible medical devices such as cochlear implants. The choice of imaging study should be tailored to the individual patient and the suspected diagnosis.

Laboratory Investigation

Certain signs and symptoms of back pain should prompt additional evaluation. For patients with constant pain, night pain, radicular pain, or an abnormal neurologic examination, further evaluation is indicated. Idiopathic back pain is more frequently seen in adolescents, so additional evaluation in a younger child may be warranted. A laboratory workup is indicated for patients with a history of fevers, weight loss, or fatigue. This evaluation should include a complete blood count with differential, C-reactive protein level, and erythrocyte sedimentation rate. A peripheral smear to evaluate cell morphology may identify early cases of leukemia. Routine screening for rheumatoid factor, antinuclear antibodies, and HLA-B27 is costly and not typically indicated unless other presenting features indicate a rheumatologic cause.

Common Categories of Back Pain and Treatment Options

Idiopathic Back Pain

If findings from radiography, the physical examination, and the patient history are all consistent with idiopathic back pain, a physical therapy program focused on core strengthening, hamstring stretches, and lumbar stabilization should be initiated. Treatment with physical therapy and strengthening exercises has been shown to improve idiopathic back pain in children.[18] Activity modification and a period of rest from sports may help relieve symptoms. Regular physical aerobic activity also may help improve back pain symptoms. In addition, smoking cessation and weight loss may be beneficial. The use of narcotic pain medications or muscle relaxants should be avoided. If the pain seems to warrant these types of prescriptions, further investigation is needed. Empiric spinal injections or oral corticosteroids are not warranted unless a discrete lesion is identified on imaging.

Disk Disease

Degenerative disk disease may be seen in adolescents and can result in back pain and, occasionally, radicular symptoms. Asymptomatic degenerative disk disease has been seen on MRIs of children without back pain,[19] although asymptomatic disk herniations are rare.[20] Imaging findings should be correlated with the physical examination findings. Degenerative disk disease may be familial in origin and has been associated with several genetic abnormalities. L4-L5 and L5-S1 are the most commonly affected levels.

Most patients younger than 21 years who have discogenic back pain can successfully be treated with nonsurgical measures,[21] including back and abdominal strengthening, weight loss, NSAIDs, activity restriction, low-impact aerobic conditioning, smoking cessation, and career counseling. Selective nerve root or epidural injections may be used as a second-line treatment and may achieve complete symptom relief.

Patients with congenital spinal stenosis (defined as less than 12 mm between the posterior wall of the vertebral body to the anterior margin of the lamina) may more frequently require surgical management.[21] Surgical management is indicated for cauda equina syndrome, neurologic deficit, or radicular symptoms refractory to 6 months of nonsurgical management (**Figure 1**). Although open diskectomy is the standard of care, successful microdiskectomy for symptomatic disk herniation in adolescents has been reported.[22,23] CT may be used to rule out an accompanying apophyseal ring fracture. Fusion is not indicated for discogenic back pain in children, and no studies on disk replacement have been done with children.

Surgeons should be aware of posterior spinal cord infarct, which is a rare condition associated with participation in high-intensity sports and degenerative disk changes in children and is thought to be caused by a fibrocartilaginous embolus.[24] Patients have acute back pain and neurologic deficit after a high-intensity activity. A spinal cord infarct can be detected on MRI with diffuse weighted imaging.

Apophyseal Ring Fracture

Apophyseal ring fractures (also known as limbus fractures) can occur in adolescents and young adults and have been reported in 28% to 38% of pediatric patients

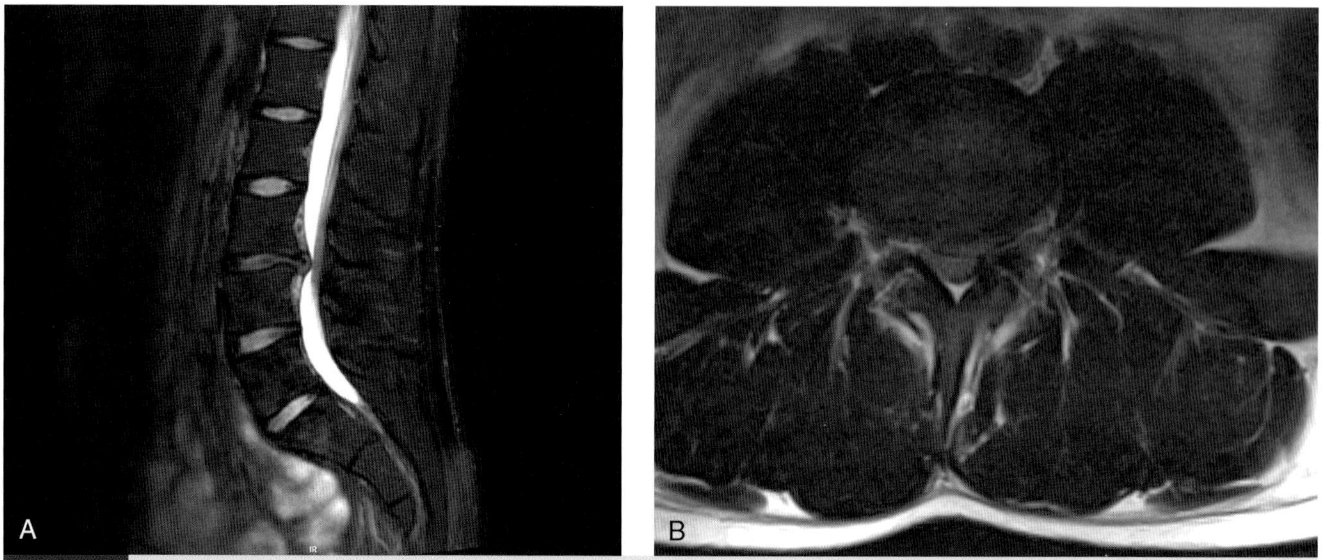

Figure 1 MRIs from a 17-year-old boy who presented with bilateral radicular pain and a positive straight leg raise test. He had increased knee and ankle jerk reflexes on the right side. **A,** Sagittal T2 MRI shows an L3 disk herniation. **B,** Axial T2 MRI shows pressure on the nerve roots. The patient was subsequently treated with microdiskectomy after 6 months of nonsurgical management with physical therapy, rest, and epidural steroid injections proved unsuccessful.

presenting with lumbar disk herniation.[25-27] Patients may have findings similar to a spondylolytic defect, with tight hamstrings, pain with hyperextension, possible radicular symptoms, a positive straight leg raise test, and/or neurologic findings.[25] The onset of symptoms may be insidious or acute after trauma. The lesion is best visualized on CT and may not be apparent on plain radiographs or MRI (**Figure 2**). On MRI, the disk herniation may be evident, but it can be difficult to appreciate the apophyseal fracture. Four types of apophyseal ring fractures have been described: (1) separation of the entire posterior vertebral margin; (2) an avulsion fracture, including a portion of the vertebral body; (3) a posterolateral fracture; and (4) a full-length fracture of the vertebral body between the end plates.

Compared with patients with disk herniation alone, patients with apophyseal ring fractures may be less likely to improve with nonsurgical management. Surgical treatment typically entails fragment excision, which is more complex than a simple diskectomy, requires wider exposure, and may require the use of a burr or an osteotome to remove the fragment. Patients with large apophyseal fragments treated nonsurgically are at risk for chronic back pain.[27] A 2012 study reported on 16 patients with apophyseal ring fractures treated nonsurgically and 8 patients treated surgically. At a mean follow-up of 13.8 years, no detectable difference in clinical outcomes occurred between the two groups.[28]

Lumbar Scheuermann Disease

Lumbar or atypical Scheuermann disease can be characterized on plain radiographs by Schmorl nodes, end plate irregularity, and loss of normal lumbar lordosis. MRI will show Schmorl nodes, degenerative disk disease, and narrowing of the disk space (**Figure 3**). The substantial kyphotic deformity and vertebral wedging seen in typical Scheuermann disease may not be present. Patients present with back pain and tend to be athletic male adolescents, sometimes with a history of weight lifting.[29,30] Treatment is nonsurgical. Interestingly, Schmorl nodes and end plate changes have been reported in up to 18% of the adult population and may be associated with chronic back pain.[31] Disk herniation in atypical Scheuermann disease can cause neurologic symptoms, but this is rare.[32]

Spondylolysis

Spondylolysis, a common cause of back pain in the pediatric population, is a defect of the lumbar pars interarticularis and can occur unilaterally or bilaterally. Patients may have acute or chronic low back pain in a band-like fashion across the lumbar spine. Hyperextension characteristically worsens the pain. Occasionally, patients may have radicular pain and/or a positive straight leg raise test.

Two recent structured literature reviews summarize the current state of knowledge on pediatric spondylolysis.[33,34] It is an acquired condition and more common in athletes, particularly those who participate in sports

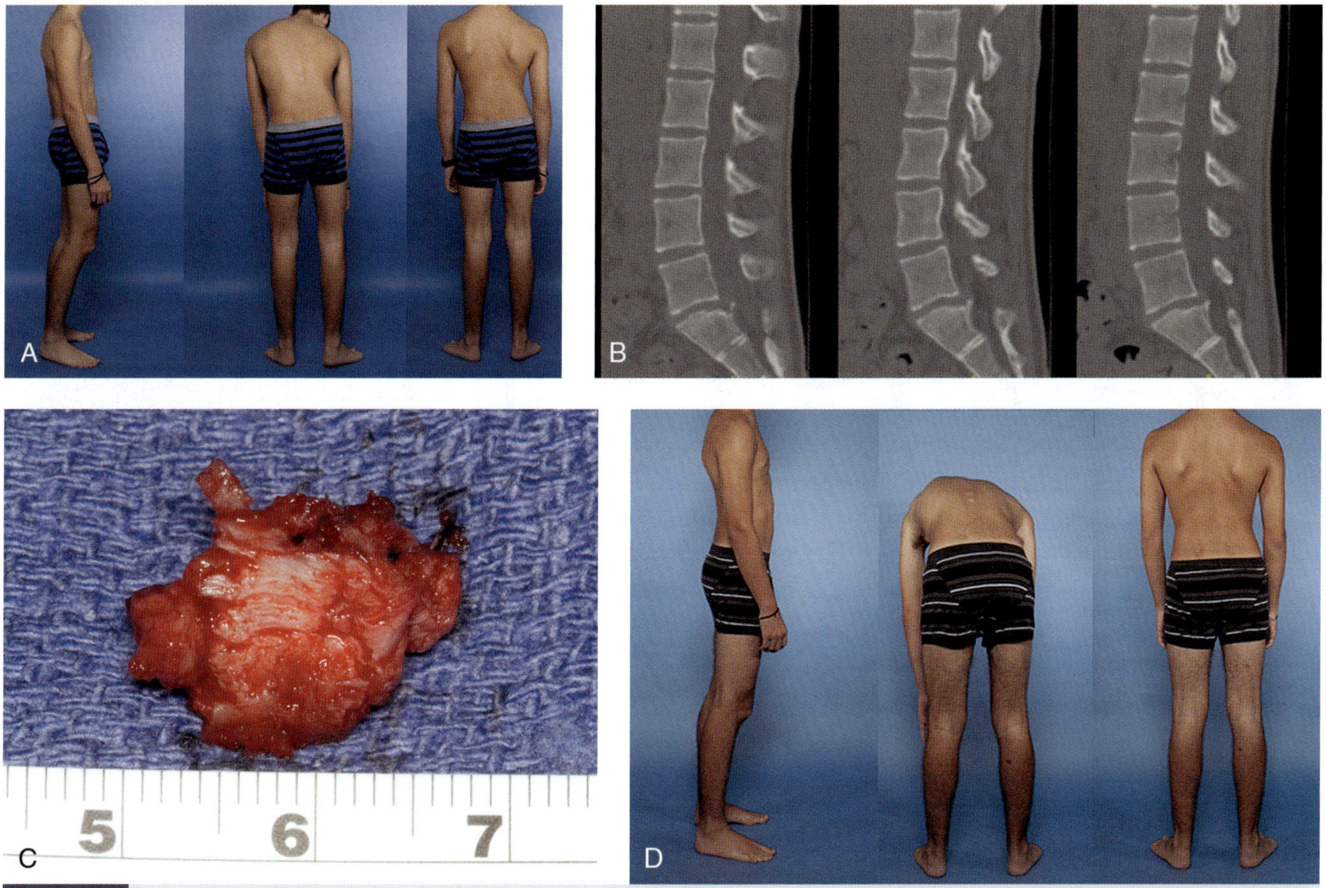

Figure 2 A 14-year-old boy presented with back pain, gait dysfunction, and bilateral radicular pain. **A,** Clinical photographs show olisthetic scoliosis, limited flexibility on forward bending (center panel), and loss of lumbar lordosis. **B,** Sagittal CT scans show an S1 apophyseal ring fracture associated with an L5-S1 disk herniation. **C,** Gross photograph of the resected lesion. **D,** Postoperative clinical photographs show resolution of scoliosis and improved forward bending (center panel).

requiring hyperextension, such as gymnastics. A unilateral defect can lead to a subsequent bilateral defect, which supports a mechanical etiology. L5 is the most commonly affected level. In the pediatric population, the prevalence of spondylolysis is 3% to 7%, although not all individuals are symptomatic.

Plain radiographs may show a defect up to 75% of the time, particularly when there is bilateral involvement.[16] Oblique radiographs do not add sensitivity or specificity in detecting spondylolysis and substantially increase radiation exposure.[35] Because limited CT through the pars interarticularis has a similar radiation dose as oblique lumbar spine radiographs and improved interrater reliability, oblique radiographs are not indicated in the pediatric population.[36] Standard CT also is an effective study and has a lower radiation dose than a bone scan (**Figure 4**). Skeletal single photon emission computed tomography (SPECT) is very sensitive for acute or subacute spondylolysis with increased uptake over the pars interarticularis. This imaging study results in substantial radiation exposure, with organ radiation doses up to 15 mSv, which is five times the annual background radiation and several times higher in radiation dose than a focal CT scan.[14,15,37,38] The incidence of cancer in individuals increases by 24% when these individuals had childhood exposure to a CT scan (mean estimated dose 4.5 mSv) compared with those without childhood exposure to CT.[17] Because first-line management for most cases of spondylolysis is physical therapy, the benefits of this type of imaging should be carefully weighed.[37]

MRI also can be used to evaluate T2 signal change over the pars interarticularis or visualize a fracture, and MRI is more sensitive than plain radiography. It is worthwhile to contact a musculoskeletal radiologist to develop a specific MRI protocol to best visualize the pars. In general, the MRI must be obtained with thin section images (3 mm) with both T1 and T2 fat suppression sequences in the axial and sagittal planes at high resolution. T2 edema

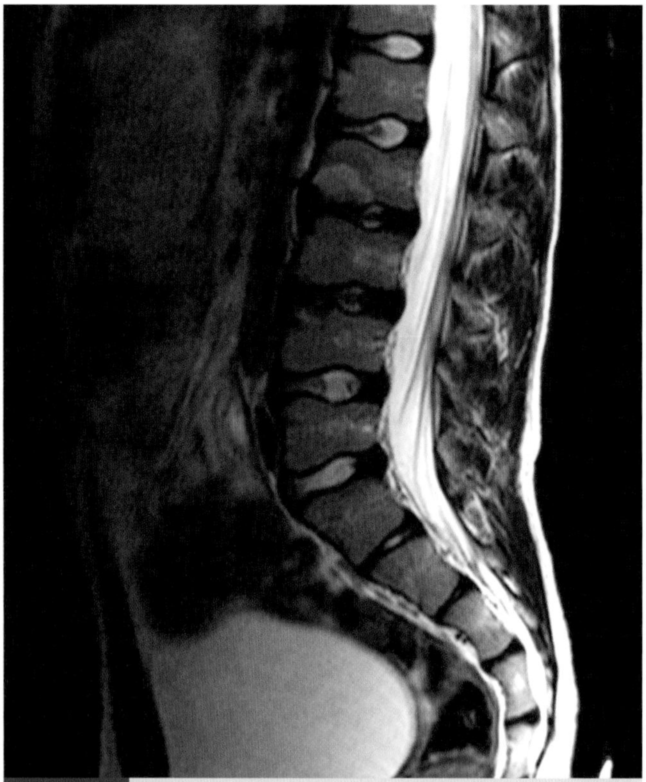

Figure 3 Sagittal MRI of the spine of a 14-year-old boy, who was active in multiple sports, including football, hockey, and snowmobiling, shows disk degeneration and Schmorl nodes.

in the pars corresponds to a subacute process. Specific sequences have been described in the literature.[39,40] Similar to SPECT or bone scans, MRI may identify prelytic lesions that may not be evident on CT.[38-40]

The preferred initial evaluation for spondylolysis is standing AP and L5-S1 spot lateral or low dose slot-scanner imaging without oblique views. For patients with chronic symptoms (>3 months), a trial of activity limitations and core strengthening physical therapy with scheduled follow-up is reasonable. Acute onset, severe pain, radicular symptoms, or the need for immediate return to sporting activities should prompt axial imaging with either selective CT of L4-S1 or MRI depending on imaging capabilities. Ongoing controversy exists whether CT, MRI, or SPECT is the best imaging study for the evaluation of spondylolysis. Specialized protocols can be used to lower the radiation dose of CT scans or provide effective imaging of the pars on MRI.

Nonsurgical treatment with rest has been shown to result in a good or excellent outcome in more than 80% of pediatric athletes.[41] Nonsurgical management consists of 2 to 6 months of activity restriction; physical therapy, with core strengthening and hamstring stretches; and/or bracing.[42] Cessation of sporting activities is more closely associated with a positive outcome than achieving bony union.[43] For active, early-stage unilateral lesions, healing occurs in 80% of patients with nonsurgical

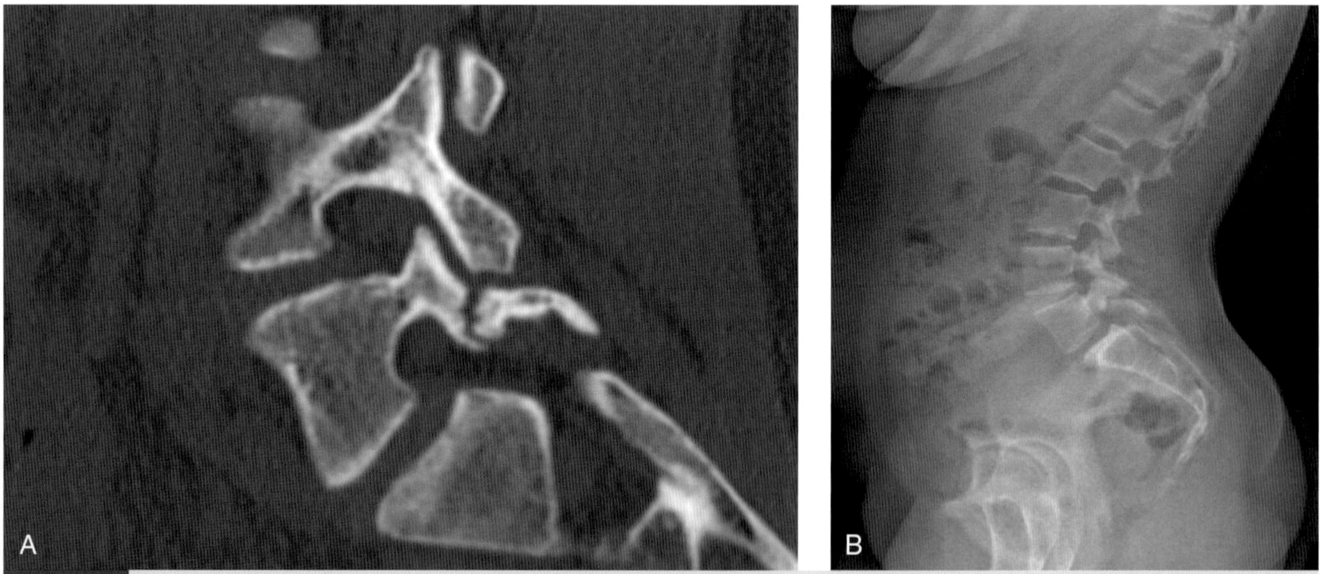

Figure 4 Images from a 13-year-old girl who presented with back pain. **A,** Sagittal CT shows a chronic-appearing L5 spondylolytic defect and increased sclerosis about the L4 pars interarticularis. After a period of rest followed by extensive core strengthening exercises, the patient successfully returned to all sports. **B,** Image obtained with biplane X-ray imaging (EOS Imaging) taken at 2-year follow-up shows bilateral L5 pars defects and grade 1 spondylolisthesis; however, the patient was asymptomatic.

management.[44] Immobilization in a thoracolumbosacral orthosis can be used in addition to rest and activity restriction to achieve bony union.[45] Healing is unlikely for patients with chronic-appearing unilateral lesions, bilateral disease, or spondylolisthesis. From 43% to 75% of patients with chronic bilateral pars defects will progress to low-grade spondylolisthesis.

Surgical treatment is indicated when 1 to 2 years of nonsurgical treatment are unsuccessful at achieving acceptable pain relief and the desired level of physical activity. Pars repair avoids fusion, and high success rates have been reported with methods such as intralaminar screw fixation, although revision for nonunion is reported at 15%.[46,47] Higher success rates are reported in L4 than L5 spondylolytic defects. Spondylolisthesis is a contraindication to pars repair. L5-S1 fusion also predictably relieves symptoms but may contribute to adjacent-segment disease later in life.

Spondylolisthesis

Spondylolisthesis refers to the forward translation of a vertebral body with respect to the vertebra beneath it. Isthmic spondylolisthesis and dysplastic spondylolisthesis are the most common types in children (**Table 1**). MRIs of children who are asymptomatic have shown spondylolisthesis in 2.3% of patients. Grade 1 and 2 spondylolisthesis (zero to 50% slip) is managed symptomatically. Nonsurgical treatment includes physical therapy, bracing, and activity modification. For a patient with persistent symptoms or neurologic deficit, in situ instrumented fusion is a treatment option. Six spinopelvic postures have been described for patients with spondylolisthesis, with types 1 through 3 slips being low grade and types 4 through 6 slips being high grade[48] (**Figure 5**). It is posited that increased pelvic incidence in a low-grade type 3 slip results in a higher risk of slip progression. Patients with types 3 and 4 slips have increased lumbar lordosis and are compensated in the sagittal plane. Types 5 and 6 slips are decompensated, and patients may have more symptoms and poorer patient-reported quality-of-life scores. If reduction is to be performed, types 5 and 6 slips may most benefit from correction of the slip angle. This classification has good reliability, but prospective long-term evidence to support these management recommendations is still needed.

Because of the high rate of progression and subsequent deformity, high-grade spondylolisthesis traditionally warrants surgical management, even in a patient who is asymptomatic. Although several studies reported successful nonsurgical management of even high-grade slips, the authors concluded that patients with symptoms benefit most from surgery.[49-51] An increased slip angle is associated with progression to surgical management. Decreased sacral slope is associated with more back pain.[52]

Table 1

The Wiltse-Neuman Classification of Spondylolisthesis

Type	Description
Dysplastic Congenital Developmental	Increased risk of slippage and incompetent L5-S1 articulation. The pars may be intact but elongated or fractured. The sacrum may be domed. L5 spina bifida occulta may be present.
Isthmic Spondylolytic	Secondary to bilateral stress fractures of the pars. Posterior elements are still in place.
Degenerative	Secondary to degenerative changes in adulthood.
Posttraumatic	Acute fracture and slippage.
Pathologic	Attenuation of the pars from bone pathology (such as osteogenesis imperfecta or Ehlers-Danlos syndrome).

Most patients with high-grade spondylolisthesis have back pain and/or radicular symptoms and merit surgical management. A variety of surgical strategies exists. Historically, in situ fusion was performed and achieved with postoperative immobilization in a pantaloon spica cast or a thoracolumbosacral orthosis with a thigh extension. Circumferential in situ fusion can be achieved using the Bohlman technique to place a fibular strut through the sacrum and into L5 to augment a standard posterolateral fusion. In situ fusion can result in progression of the slippage over time and may necessitate later reduction, particularly for patients with a high slip angle (**Figure 6**). Combined anteroposterior or all-posterior approaches can achieve reduction and circumferential fusion (**Figure 7**). The risk of neurologic deficit is substantially higher with reduction and can result in L5 nerve root irritation and foot drop. Performing a reduction to correct the slip angle is controversial because reduction is associated with a higher rate of neurologic compromise, although it is proposed to result in improved long-term durability compared with in situ fusion.

Bone morphogenetic protein is being used with increasing frequency for the surgical management of spondylolisthesis, although the indications and dosing are not clear and its use in children remains off-label.[53] Overall, there is an 11.5% rate of new neurologic defects after surgical treatment of spondylolisthesis.[54] Patients with

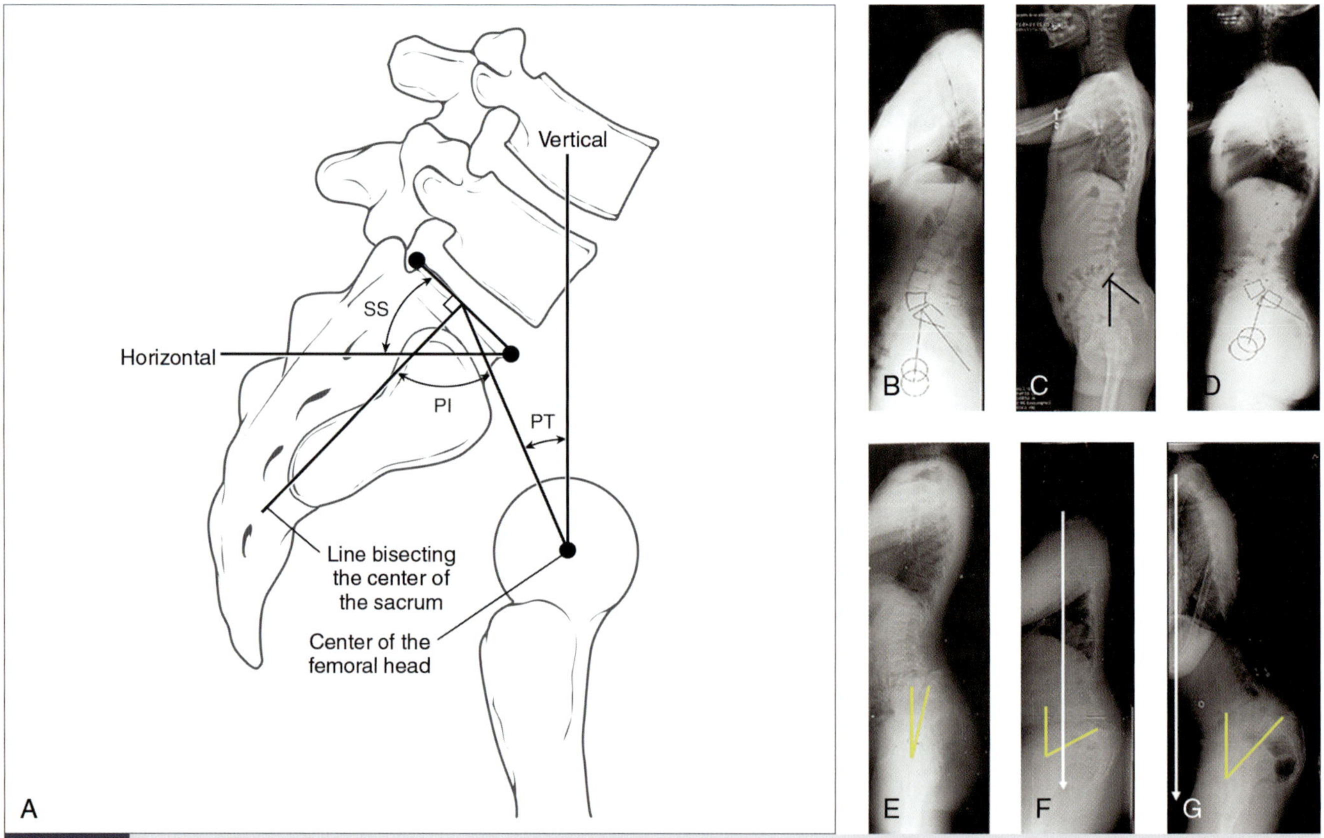

Figure 5 **A,** Schematic drawing shows a lateral view of the lumbosacral junction with standard parameters of pelvic morphology and spinopelvic balance in spondylolisthesis. In low-grade spondylolisthesis, the subtype depends on whether the pelvic incidence (PI) and the sacral slope (SS) are high or low. In high-grade spondylolisthesis, the subtype depends on whether the pelvic tilt (PT) and SS are high or low. **B** through **G,** Lateral radiographs demonstrate the six spinopelvic postures that have been described for patients with spondylolisthesis. **B,** Low-grade spondylolisthesis with low PI and low SS (nutcracker type). **C,** Low-grade spondylolisthesis with normal PI and SS. **D,** Low-grade spondylolisthesis with high PI and high SS (shear type). **E,** High-grade spondylolisthesis with a balanced pelvis, high SS, and low PT. **F,** High-grade spondylolisthesis with a retroverted pelvis, low SS, high PT, and a balanced spine. **G,** High-grade spondylolisthesis with an unbalanced spine. (Panel B through G reproduced with permission from Labelle H, Mac-Thiong JM, Roussouly P: Spino-pelvic sagittal balance of spondylolisthesis: A review and classification. *Eur Spine J* 2011;20[suppl 5]:641-646.)

neurologic symptoms should undergo either direct posterior or indirect anterior decompression as part of the surgical management process.

Other Causes of Back Pain in Children

Transitional anomalies at the lumbosacral junction are common and, occasionally, may generate back pain known as Bertolotti syndrome. Evaluation may include plain radiographs and MRI to evaluate radicular symptoms, if present. Bone scans or SPECT can be used to detect symptomatic articulations. Treatment begins with nonsurgical management. The injection of corticosteroid and local anesthetic at the site of a symptomatic articulation can temporarily improve symptoms and help target surgical management if nonsurgical measures are unsuccessful. The role of surgical treatment is unclear and entails fusion or resection of the symptomatic articulation.[55]

Diskitis and vertebral osteomyelitis can occur in children who are prone to hematogenous infections because of low-flow blood vessels and anastomoses to the disk and vertebral end plates. Young children may have a limp or refuse to walk, whereas adolescents typically have back or abdominal pain.[56] An altered gait pattern in an adolescent may indicate pelvic pyomyositis or psoas abscess. The patient also may have a fever. Elevation may be seen in the white blood cell count, the platelet count, the C-reactive protein level, and/or the erythrocyte sedimentation rate. The evaluation should include blood cultures; however, they are rarely positive.[56,57] End plate

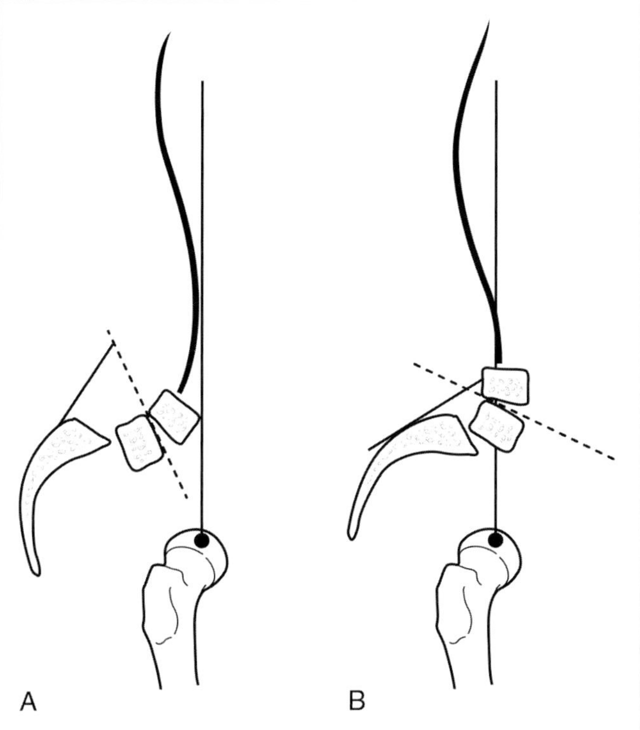

Figure 6 Illustrations of the slip angle, which can be used to describe the degree of spinal deformity. Surgical management of high-grade spondylolisthesis is focused on correcting the slip angle. **A,** Patients with a high slip angle, vertical sacrum, low sacral slope, and high pelvic tilt (a retroverted pelvis) may require correction of the deformity at the time of surgery. Patients with a retroverted pelvis may have a balanced spine or positive sagittal balance (as seen in Figure 5, G). **B,** Patients with a low slip angle may tolerate fusion in situ without reduction of the slip. These patients have neutral sagittal balance.

changes and disk space narrowing may be seen on plain radiographs. MRI will show changes earlier in the disease course and can rule out a paravertebral abscess or an epidural abscess (**Figure 8**). Biopsy is not indicated unless empiric treatment with anti-inflammatory drugs, rest, and oral or intravenous antibiotics fails. Bracing may be used for symptom management. Atypical organisms such as *Mycobacterium tuberculosis* should be suspected in multilevel disease, disease with an insidious onset, and in patients who are immunocompromised or have a history of exposure to such organisms. *Kingella kingae* infection can be considered in toddlers, but its role has not been established.[58] Generally, patients can be managed nonsurgically.

Tumor is a rare cause of back pain in children. Radiographs may show a vertebra plana lesion, which can be caused by eosinophilic granuloma (**Figure 9**). Osteoid osteoma and osteoblastoma classically affect the posterior vertebral elements. Twenty percent to 30% of patients with multiple hereditary exostosis may have an intracanal osteochondroma, which can cause progressive pain and/or neurologic deficit.[59,60] Patients with neurofibromatosis frequently have dural ectasia and plexiform neurofibromas involving the spine, which can result in chronic back pain. These lesions typically are not amenable to resection. Aneurysmal bone cysts can be locally aggressive and result in spinal instability. Preoperative embolization may reduce perioperative blood loss.[61,62] Malignant lesions, such as osteosarcoma, chondrosarcoma, lymphoma, leukemia, Ewing sarcoma, and metastatic disease, are rare. Spinal cord tumors include astrocytoma, ependymoma, and chordoma. CT or open biopsy may be necessary for making a diagnosis. A multidisciplinary team should treat malignant tumors. The management of nonmalignant tumors depends on the type and location of the tumor, spinal stability, and symptomatology.

Summary

Pediatric orthopaedic surgeons will frequently need to evaluate and treat back pain in their patients. It is essential to be aware of the features for common back pain diagnoses specific to children. Although most adolescents and school-age children have idiopathic back pain, severe pain or symptoms that do not respond to nonsurgical management warrant additional workup. Disk disease and spondylolytic conditions may occur in children but rarely require surgical management. High-grade spondylolisthesis typically requires surgical treatment and, although the need for reduction is controversial, correction of the slip angle will likely improve the long-term durability of the surgery by improving sagittal plane correction.

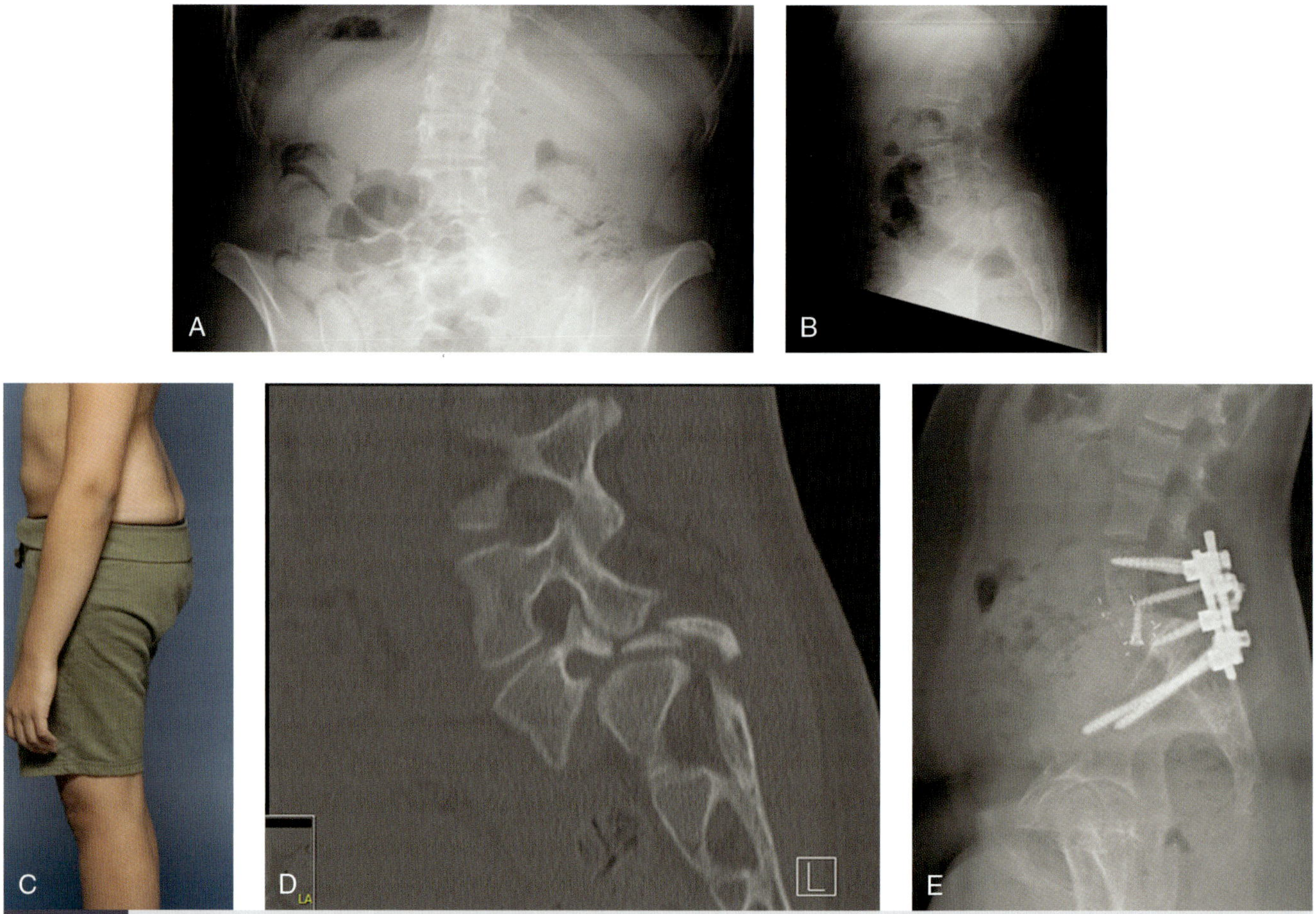

Figure 7 Images from a 13-year-old girl with back pain and deformity. **A,** PA standing radiograph shows apparent absence of the L5 vertebral body (the Napoleon hat sign). **B,** Lateral radiograph shows grade 4 spondylolisthesis and a retroverted pelvis. **C,** Clinical photograph shows a flattened sacrum. The L5 spinous process was not palpable. Lateral radiographs shows correction of the slip angle after anterior sacral dome osteotomy and fusion (**D**) and posterior instrumentation and fusion (**E**).

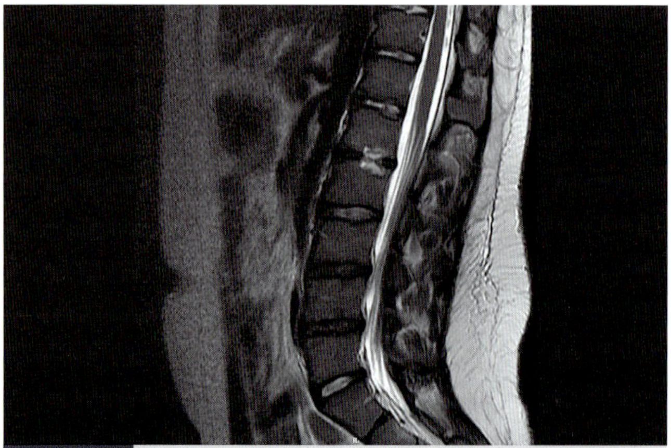

Figure 8 A 15-year-old boy presented with a 5-week history of acute severe back pain and elevated C-reactive protein level and erythrocyte sedimentation rate. MRI shows diskitis at L2-3 and vertebral osteomyelitis at L2 and L3. Symptoms resolved with oral antibiotics and anti-inflammatory medications.

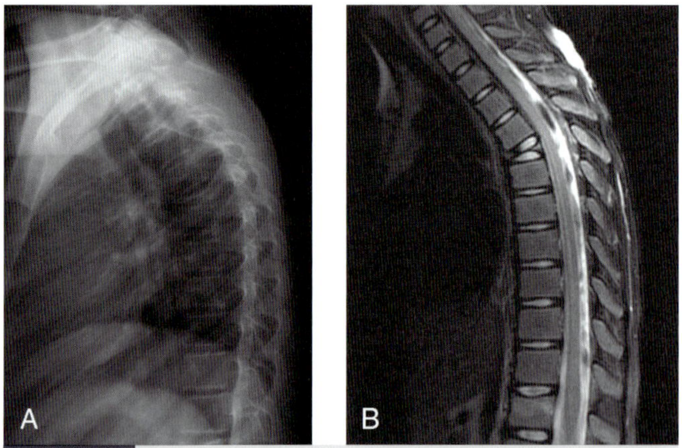

Figure 9 An 11-year-old girl had a 6-month history of severe back pain. **A,** Lateral radiograph shows vertebra plana secondary to eosinophilic granuloma. **B,** Sagittal MRI shows vertebra plana. The patient should be monitored in the future for progressive kyphosis with serial radiographs, but her current spinal alignment is satisfactory.

Key Study Points

- Patients younger than 18 years frequently have back pain, with 20% to 30% of patients having an underlying structural diagnosis.
- Further workup should be guided by the patient history and the findings of a careful neurologic examination and plain radiography. If the findings are benign, physical therapy and activity modification can be initiated without the need for advanced imaging.
- Symptoms from disk disease, spondylolysis, and low-grade spondylolisthesis are typically responsive to nonsurgical treatment. Surgery is indicated for patients with refractory symptoms.
- The treatment of high-grade spondylolisthesis is controversial, but surgery is typically recommended, particularly for patients who are symptomatic or those with documented progression.

Annotated References

1. Aartun E, Hartvigsen J, Wedderkopp N, Hestbaek L: Spinal pain in adolescents: Prevalence, incidence, and course: A school-based two-year prospective cohort study in 1,300 Danes aged 11-13. *BMC Musculoskelet Disord* 2014;15:187.

   The authors of this prospective cohort study evaluated adolescents with back pain to determine prevalence, severity, and progression over a 2-year period. Level of evidence: II.

2. Yang S, Werner BC, Singla A, Abel MF: Low back pain in adolescents: A 1-year analysis of eventual diagnoses. *J Pediatr Orthop* 2015; September 11 [Epub ahead of print].

   A review of the US national insurance registry between 2007 and 2010 identified 215,592 adolescents with back pain; less than 20% were given a secondary diagnosis within 1 year. Level of evidence: III.

3. Aartun E, Hartvigsen J, Boyle E, Hestbaek L: No associations between objectively measured physical activity and spinal pain in 11-15-year-old Danes. *Eur J Pain* 2016;20(3):447-457.

   Physical activity monitors revealed no association between physical activities and reported back pain in patients aged 11 to 15 years. Measurements were taken during a 2-year period. Level of evidence: III.

4. Sato T, Ito T, Hirano T, et al: Low back pain in childhood and adolescence: Assessment of sports activities. *Eur Spine J* 2011;20(1):94-99.

   In a cross-sectional study of Japanese school children, more hours of participation in sports were associated with increased lower back pain. The mean time of sporting activities was 9.8 hours per week. Level of evidence: III.

5. Sano A, Hirano T, Watanabe K, Endo N, Ito T, Tanabe N: Body mass index is associated with low back pain in childhood and adolescence: A birth cohort study with a 6-year follow-up in Niigata City, Japan. *Eur Spine J* 2015;24(3):474-481.

   This questionnaire-based study found that back pain was more frequently reported in older adolescents and those with an increased body mass index. Level of evidence: III.

6. Mwaka ES, Munabi IG, Buwembo W, Kukkiriza J, Ochieng J: Musculoskeletal pain and school bag use: A cross-sectional study among Ugandan pupils. *BMC Res Notes* 2014;7:222.

   A cross-sectional study of 532 students reported that 37% of the children reported low back pain. The increased weight of school bags was associated with reported back pain. Level of evidence: III.

7. Wirth B, Knecht C, Humphreys K: Spine Day 2012: Spinal pain in Swiss school children: Epidemiology and risk factors. *BMC Pediatr* 2013;13:159.

   Back pain in Swiss students was associated with older age and parental smoking as well as an increased body mass index. Level of evidence: III.

8. Shymon SJ, Yaszay B, Dwek JR, Proudfoot JA, Donohue M, Hargens AR: Altered disc compression in children with idiopathic low back pain: An upright magnetic resonance imaging backpack study. *Spine (Phila Pa 1976)* 2014;39(3):243-248.

   Standing MRIs were obtained in normal children and those with idiopathic back pain. While wearing a backpack, the children with back pain had increased compression at L5-S1 compared with normal children and also reported more pain with this activity. Level of evidence: III.

9. Brattberg G: Do pain problems in young school children persist into early adulthood? A 13-year follow-up. *Eur J Pain* 2004;8(3):187-199.

10. Harreby MS, Neergaard K, Hesselsøe G, Kjer J: Are low back pain and radiological changes during puberty risk factors for low back pain in adult age? A 25-year prospective cohort study of 640 school children [Danish]. *Ugeskr Laeger* 1997;159(2):171-174.

11. Bhatia NN, Chow G, Timon SJ, Watts HG: Diagnostic modalities for the evaluation of pediatric back pain: A prospective study. *J Pediatr Orthop* 2008;28(2):230-233.

12. Auerbach JD, Ahn J, Zgonis MH, Reddy SC, Ecker ML, Flynn JM: Streamlining the evaluation of low back pain in children. *Clin Orthop Relat Res* 2008;466(8):1971-1977.

13. Ramirez N, Flynn JM, Hill BW, et al: Evaluation of a systematic approach to pediatric back pain: The

6: Spine

utility of magnetic resonance imaging. *J Pediatr Orthop* 2015;35(1):28-32.

This prospective study evaluated the number of patients with back pain who had an identifiable pathology based on physical examination, radiographs, bone scans, and MRIs. Level of evidence: II.

14. Vendhan K, Sen D, Fisher C, Ioannou Y, Hall-Craggs MA: Inflammatory changes of the lumbar spine in children and adolescents with enthesitis-related arthritis: Magnetic resonance imaging findings. *Arthritis Care Res (Hoboken)* 2014;66(1):40-46.

A retrospective review compared MRI findings in pediatric patients with enthesitis-related arthritis with those of patients with mechanical back pain. Of those with enthesitis-related arthritis, 67% had abnormalities in the lumbar spine, and 78% had sacroiliitis visible on MRI. Level of evidence: III.

15. Alkhawaldeh K, Ghuweri AA, Kawar J, Jaafreh A: Back pain in children and diagnostic value of (99m)Tc MDP bone scintigraphy. *Acta Inform Med* 2014;22(5):297-301.

The authors reviewed the results of 68 patients undergoing bone scans for back pain. Technetium bone scintigraphy was found to have high sensitivity and specificity for detecting skeletal abnormalities that caused back pain. Level of evidence: IV.

16. Miller R, Beck NA, Sampson NR, Zhu X, Flynn JM, Drummond D: Imaging modalities for low back pain in children: A review of spondylolysis and undiagnosed mechanical back pain. *J Pediatr Orthop* 2013;33(3):282-288.

This retrospective cohort study of 2,846 patients who had back pain reported on the rates of spondylolysis found by each type of imaging modality. Level of evidence: IV.

17. Mathews JD, Forsythe AV, Brady Z, et al: Cancer risk in 680,000 people exposed to computed tomography scans in childhood or adolescence: Data linkage study of 11 million Australians. *BMJ* 2013;346:f2360.

A population-based study using Australian healthcare records found an increased cancer incidence in patients with a history of CT evaluation in childhood, with an overall incidence 24% greater in those with a previous CT scan. A dose-response relationship was found. Level of evidence: III.

18. Michaleff ZA, Kamper SJ, Maher CG, Evans R, Broderick C, Henschke N: Low back pain in children and adolescents: A systematic review and meta-analysis evaluating the effectiveness of conservative interventions. *Eur Spine J* 2014;23(10):2046-2058.

This systematic review evaluated the effects of physical therapy and exercise for treating back pain in children. Level of evidence: II.

19. Ramadorai U, Hire J, DeVine JG, Brodt ED, Dettori JR: Incidental findings on magnetic resonance imaging of the spine in the asymptomatic pediatric population: A systematic review. *Evid Based Spine Care J* 2014;5(2):95-100.

This systematic review evaluated the incidence of spine MRI findings in pediatric patients without back pain. Spondylolysis, spondylolisthesis, degenerative disk disease, and Scheuermann-type changes were found in patients who were asymptomatic. Level of evidence: II.

20. Urrutia J, Zamora T, Prada C: The prevalence of degenerative or incidental findings in the lumbar spine of pediatric patients: A study using magnetic resonance imaging as a screening tool. *Eur Spine J* 2015;25(2):596-601.

The spines of 103 patients who were undergoing studies for pelvic or abdominal complaints were reviewed. Degenerative disk disease was found in 10% of the patients; one patient had a disk bulge, but no patients had disk herniation. Level of evidence: IV.

21. Dimar JR II, Glassman SD, Carreon LY: Juvenile degenerative disc disease: A report of 76 cases identified by magnetic resonance imaging. *Spine J* 2007;7(3):332-337.

22. Thomas JG, Hwang SW, Whitehead WE, Curry DJ, Luerssen TG, Jea A: Minimally invasive lumbar microdiscectomy in pediatric patients: A series of 6 patients. *J Neurosurg Pediatr* 2011;7(6):616-619.

The results of six pediatric patients with radicular pain after microdiskectomy are described. Level of evidence: IV.

23. Çelik S, Göksu K, Çelik SE, Emir CB: Benign neurological recovery with low recurrence and low peridural fibrosis rate in pediatric disc herniations after lumbar microdiscectomy. *Pediatr Neurosurg* 2011;47(6):417-422.

The results of microdiskectomy for lumbar disk herniation are compared between adult and pediatric patients. Good results, excellent pain relief, and no recurrences were reported for 32 pediatric patients at a mean follow-up of 5 years. Level of evidence: III.

24. Bansal S, Brown W, Dayal A, Carpenter JL: Posterior spinal cord infarction due to fibrocartilaginous embolization in a 16-year-old athlete. *Pediatrics* 2014;134(1):e289-e292.

The authors present a case report of 16-year-old female athlete with acute myelopathy after exercise caused by a posterior spinal cord infarct from a fibrocartilaginous embolus. The patient's MRI showed degenerative disk disease and T2 signal change.

25. Bonic EE, Taylor JA, Knudsen JT: Posterior limbus fractures: Five case reports and a review of selected published cases. *J Manipulative Physiol Ther* 1998;21(4):281-287.

26. Singhal A, Mitra A, Cochrane D, Steinbok P: Ring apophysis fracture in pediatric lumbar disc herniation: A common entity. *Pediatr Neurosurg* 2013;49(1):16-20.

The authors report on 42 pediatric patients with a lumbar disk herniation. The authors concluded that a ring apophysis fracture is more frequently associated with lumbar disk herniation in children than in adults. Level of evidence: IV.

27. Chang CH, Lee ZL, Chen WJ, Tan CF, Chen LH: Clinical significance of ring apophysis fracture in adolescent lumbar disc herniation. *Spine (Phila Pa 1976)* 2008;33(16):1750-1754.

28. Higashino K, Sairyo K, Katoh S, Takao S, Kosaka H, Yasui N: Long-term outcomes of lumbar posterior apophyseal end-plate lesions in children and adolescents. *J Bone Joint Surg Am* 2012;94(11):e74.

The authors report on intermediate term retrospective follow-up of 24 patients with back and radicular pain with apophyseal end plate lesions.

29. Greene TL, Hensinger RN, Hunter LY: Back pain and vertebral changes simulating Scheuermann's disease. *J Pediatr Orthop* 1985;5(1):1-7.

30. Blumenthal SL, Roach J, Herring JA: Lumbar Scheuermann's: A clinical series and classification. *Spine (Phila Pa 1976)* 1987;12(9):929-932.

31. Liu N, Guo X, Chen Z, et al: Radiological signs of Scheuermann disease and low back pain: Retrospective categorization of 188 hospital staff members with 6-year follow-up. *Spine (Phila Pa 1976)* 2014;39(20):1666-1675.

MRIs were obtained for 188 hospital employees who were asymptomatic. The authors found that 18% had Scheuermann-like disk changes in the lumbar spine, and back pain more frequently developed in those individuals during a 2-year follow-up period. Level of evidence: III.

32. Song KS, Yang JJ: Acutely progressing paraplegia caused by traumatic disc herniation through posterior Schmorl's node opening into the spinal canal in lumbar Scheuermann's disease. *Spine (Phila Pa 1976)* 2011;36(24):E1588-E1591.

The authors present a case report of paraplegia after a fall following a herniated Schmorl node in a patient with Scheuermann changes to the lumbar spine. Level of evidence: IV.

33. Crawford CH III, Ledonio CG, Bess RS, et al: Current evidence regarding the etiology, prevalence, natural history, and prognosis of pediatric lumbar spondylolysis: A report from the Scoliosis Research Society Evidence-Based Medicine Committee. *Spine Deform* 2015;3(1):12-29.

An exhaustive, structured literature review evaluated multiple research questions regarding the diagnosis and natural history pediatric spondylolysis. Areas for further research were highlighted. Level of evidence: II.

34. Crawford CH III, Ledonio CG, Bess RS, et al: Current evidence regarding the surgical and nonsurgical treatment of pediatric lumbar spondylolysis: A report from the Scoliosis Research Society Evidence-Based Medicine Committee. *Spine Deform* 2015;3(1):30-44.

An exhaustive structured literature review evaluated multiple research questions regarding the treatment of pediatric spondylolysis. Areas for further research were highlighted. Level of evidence: II.

35. Beck NA, Miller R, Baldwin K, et al: Do oblique views add value in the diagnosis of spondylolysis in adolescents? *J Bone Joint Surg Am* 2013;95(10):e65.

Spine surgeons reviewed the radiographs of 50 patients with spondylolysis and 50 control subjects. Oblique views did not increase the sensitivity or specificity and imparted an additional radiation dose of 0.54 mSv. A four-view spine series imparted a 1.26 mSv dose, which was equivalent to one-third the annual background radiation dose. Level of evidence: III.

36. Fadell MF, Gralla J, Bercha I, et al: CT outperforms radiographs at a comparable radiation dose in the assessment for spondylolysis. *Pediatr Radiol* 2015;45(7):1026-1030.

CT had a much higher level of interobserver agreement compared with radiographs (kappa 0.88 versus 0.24-0.4). Oblique views did not improve the level of agreement. The effective radiation dose of the CT scans ranged from 0.15 to 1.04 mSv, depending on the CT settings and patient size. Level of evidence: III.

37. Spencer HT, Sokol LO, Glotzbecker MP, et al: Detection of pars injury by SPECT in patients younger than age 10 with low back pain. *J Pediatr Orthop* 2013;33(4):383-388.

A pars fracture was found in 18 of 72 patients younger than 10 years who were referred for a SPECT scan to evaluate back pain. There were two false negatives, with evidence of a pars defect found on CT or plain radiographs. Level of evidence: III.

38. Gum JL, Crawford CH III, Collis PC, Carreon LY: Characteristics associated with active defects in juvenile spondylolysis. *Am J Orthop (Belle Mead NJ)* 2015;44(10):E379-E383.

Pars defects in 57 patients were evaluated with MRI or CT. Males and patients without listhesis more frequently had early lesions, which may be amenable to attempts at osseous healing. Level of evidence: III.

39. Kobayashi A, Kobayashi T, Kato K, Higuchi H, Takagishi K: Diagnosis of radiographically occult lumbar spondylolysis in young athletes by magnetic resonance imaging. *Am J Sports Med* 2013;41(1):169-176.

The authors report on 200 pediatric athletes with back pain who underwent plain radiography and MRI of the lumbar spine. A pars fracture was diagnosed with MRI in 97 patients, and CT confirmed the pars defect in 92 patients. Level of evidence: III.

40. Rush JK, Astur N, Scott S, Kelly DM, Sawyer JR, Warner WC Jr: Use of magnetic resonance imaging in the evaluation of spondylolysis. *J Pediatr Orthop* 2015;35(3):271-275.

CT and MRI were obtained within 30 days of each other in 26 patients with pars lesions. In 9 patients, MRI identified 11 lesions that were not apparent on CT scans, which facilitated early treatment. Level of evidence: III.

41. Álvarez-Díaz P, Alentorn-Geli E, Steinbacher G, Rius M, Pellisé F, Cugat R: Conservative treatment of lumbar

spondylolysis in young soccer players. *Knee Surg Sports Traumatol Arthrosc* 2011;19(12):2111-2114.

A 2-year follow-up study reported that 28 of 35 soccer players with spondylolysis were able to return to sports after nonsurgical management. Level of evidence: IV.

42. Sairyo K, Sakai T, Amari R, Yasui N: Causes of radiculopathy in young athletes with spondylolysis. *Am J Sports Med* 2010;38(2):357-362.

43. El Rassi G, Takemitsu M, Glutting J, Shah SA: Effect of sports modification on clinical outcome in children and adolescent athletes with symptomatic lumbar spondylolysis. *Am J Phys Med Rehabil* 2013;92(12):1070-1074.

    More than 80% of patients with symptomatic spondylolysis had good or excellent results with nonsurgical treatment. Patients who stopped participating in their sport for 3 months were much more likely to have a satisfactory outcome. Level of evidence: IV.

44. Dunn AJ, Campbell RS, Mayor PE, Rees D: Radiological findings and healing patterns of incomplete stress fractures of the pars interarticularis. *Skeletal Radiol* 2008;37(5):443-450.

45. Sairyo K, Sakai T, Yasui N, Dezawa A: Conservative treatment for pediatric lumbar spondylolysis to achieve bone healing using a hard brace: What type and how long? Clinical article. *J Neurosurg Spine* 2012;16(6):610-614.

    Thoracolumbosacral bracing was used for 37 pediatric patients with 63 pars defects. Bony union rates were 94% for early-stage lesions (only hairline fracture on CT), 64% for lesions with high short tau inversion recovery signal on MRI, and 27% for lesions with normal appearance on MRI. No union was reported in those with chronic lesions. Level of evidence: III.

46. Menga EN, Kebaish KM, Jain A, Carrino JA, Sponseller PD: Clinical results and functional outcomes after direct intralaminar screw repair of spondylolysis. *Spine (Phila Pa 1976)* 2014;39(1):104-110.

    Thirty-one patients underwent direct pars repair with an intralaminar screw. Nonunion occurred in one patient, and fusion surgery was required. Level of evidence: IV.

47. Clegg T, Carreon L, Mutchnick I, Puno R: Clinical outcomes following repair of the pars interarticularis. *Am J Orthop (Belle Mead NJ)* 2013;42(2):72-76.

    Forty-nine patients with refractory spondylolysis underwent direct pars repair of 90 total pars defects. Seven patients required revision surgery. Level of evidence: IV.

48. Labelle H, Mac-Thiong JM, Roussouly P: Spino-pelvic sagittal balance of spondylolisthesis: A review and classification. *Eur Spine J* 2011;20(suppl 5):641-646.

    Work done by the Spinal Deformity Study Group led to the classification of spondylolisthesis into six types based on findings from sagittal spine and pelvic radiographs. Health-related quality-of-life measures differed substantially among patients with the six types of spondylolisthesis.

49. Lundine KM, Lewis SJ, Al-Aubaidi Z, Alman B, Howard AW: Patient outcomes in the operative and nonoperative management of high-grade spondylolisthesis in children. *J Pediatr Orthop* 2014;34(5):483-489.

    Twenty-four of 49 patients with high-grade spondylolisthesis were treated with surgery, and 25 patients were treated nonsurgically. Nonsurgical management failed in 10 of those patients, and they had subsequent surgical treatment. The failure of nonsurgical management was associated with an increased slip angle. Level of evidence: III.

50. Harris IE, Weinstein SL: Long-term follow-up of patients with grade-III and IV spondylolisthesis: Treatment with and without posterior fusion. *J Bone Joint Surg Am* 1987;69(7):960-969.

51. Bourassa-Moreau É, Mac-Thiong JM, Joncas J, Parent S, Labelle H: Quality of life of patients with high-grade spondylolisthesis: Minimum 2-year follow-up after surgical and nonsurgical treatments. *Spine J* 2013;13(7):770-774.

    Scoliosis Research Society-22 scores improved for 23 patients after surgery for high-grade spondylolisthesis. The five patients who were treated nonsurgically were stable and had no slip progression and no neurologic symptoms. Level of evidence: III.

52. Wang Z, Wang B, Yin B, Liu W, Yang F, Lv G: The relationship between spinopelvic parameters and clinical symptoms of severe isthmic spondylolisthesis: A prospective study of 64 patients. *Eur Spine J* 2014;23(3):560-568.

    Patients with high-grade spondylolisthesis with severe pain had an increased spondylolisthesis grade, sacral slope, and lumbar lordosis compared with those with only mild pain. Level of evidence: III.

53. Jain A, Kebaish KM, Sponseller PD: Factors associated with use of bone morphogenetic protein during pediatric spinal fusion surgery: An analysis of 4817 patients. *J Bone Joint Surg Am* 2013;95(14):1265-1270.

    Bone morphogenetic protein is frequently used in children for spondylolisthesis surgery according to the Nationwide Inpatient Sample database. Level of evidence: III.

54. Kasliwal MK, Smith JS, Shaffrey CI, et al: Short-term complications associated with surgery for high-grade spondylolisthesis in adults and pediatric patients: A report from the Scoliosis Research Society morbidity and mortality database. *Neurosurgery* 2012;71(1):109-116.

    A surgeon-reported complications registry reported that new neurologic deficits frequently occur after surgical treatment of high-grade spondylolisthesis. Level of evidence: III.

55. Li Y, Lubelski D, Abdullah KG, Mroz TE, Steinmetz MP: Minimally invasive tubular resection of the anomalous transverse process in patients with Bertolotti's syndrome:

Presented at the 2013 Joint Spine Section Meeting. Clinical article. *J Neurosurg Spine* 2014;20(3):283-290.

The authors report on a retrospective review of seven patients with chronic back pain treated with resection of the lumbosacral transition vertebra. Good pain relief occurred in five of the seven patients.

56. Spencer SJ, Wilson NI: Childhood discitis in a regional children's hospital. *J Pediatr Orthop B* 2012;21(3):264-268.

During an 18-year period, 12 cases of diskitis were reported at a tertiary referral center. Most of the patients were successfully treated with antibiotics, and no patients had symptom recurrence. Level of evidence: IV.

57. Brown R, Hussain M, McHugh K, Novelli V, Jones D: Discitis in young children. *J Bone Joint Surg Br* 2001;83(1):106-111.

58. Ceroni D, Belaieff W, Kanavaki A, et al: Possible association of Kingella kingae with infantile spondylodiscitis. *Pediatr Infect Dis J* 2013;32(11):1296-1298.

Ten patients younger than 4 years with diskitis were evaluated. Two had positive blood cultures for *K kingae*, and all 10 children had positive throat swabs. The authors proposed that this is a common organism causing diskitis in young children. Level of evidence: IV.

59. Roach JW, Klatt JW, Faulkner ND: Involvement of the spine in patients with multiple hereditary exostoses. *J Bone Joint Surg Am* 2009;91(8):1942-1948.

60. Ashraf A, Larson AN, Ferski G, Mielke CH, Wetjen NM, Guidera KJ: Spinal stenosis frequent in children with multiple hereditary exostoses. *J Child Orthop* 2013;7(3):183-194.

Two of nine patients with multiple hereditary exostoses undergoing spinal imaging had minimally symptomatic lesions compressing the spinal cord. The lesions were treated with decompression. Level of evidence: IV.

61. Zenonos G, Jamil O, Governale LS, Jernigan S, Hedequist D, Proctor MR: Surgical treatment for primary spinal aneurysmal bone cysts: Experience from Children's Hospital Boston. *J Neurosurg Pediatr* 2012;9(3):305-315.

The surgical treatment of 14 patients with spinal aneurysmal bone cysts was reviewed retrospectively. There was recurrence in two patients. Level of evidence: IV.

62. Novais EN, Rose PS, Yaszemski MJ, Sim FH: Aneurysmal bone cyst of the cervical spine in children. *J Bone Joint Surg Am* 2011;93(16):1534-1543.

The surgical treatment of seven patients with aneurysmal bone cysts in the cervical spine was reviewed retrospectively. One patient had local recurrence treated with additional surgery. Level of evidence: IV.

Section 7

Trauma

SECTION EDITOR:
Jeffrey E. Martus, MD, MS

Chapter 34

Pediatric Trauma Principles

Mauricio Silva, MD Anthony A. Scaduto, MD

Abstract

Fractures are common in children, with most caused by ground-level falls and sports activities. Certain fracture patterns, however, should raise concerns for an abusive etiology. The anatomy and physiology of children influence the types of fractures seen as well as their treatment options. By considering the effect of age and fracture location on the capacity for remodeling, most fractures in children can be safely managed nonsurgically. Ketamine and intravenous sedation are commonly used during closed manipulation, but local and regional drugs also can provide effective analgesia in the pediatric population. Effective casting is less dependent on the casting material than the technique used. Careful cast application and removal reduce the risk of complications such as thermal injuries and pressure sores that are associated with immobilization. Infections after an open fracture, compartment syndrome, and premature physeal arrest are some important complications of pediatric fractures. If intravenous antibiotics are administered soon after an open fracture, infections can be minimized with irrigation and débridement within 24 hours of the injury. An increasing need for pain medication can be the only sign of impending compartment syndrome in a child. Physeal fractures that have a high risk of growth arrest, such as distal femur and tibia fractures, require long-term surveillance to avoid angular deformities and limb-length discrepancies. The treatment of traumatic growth arrest includes bar resection, epiphysiodesis, osteotomy, or limb lengthening or shortening—depending on the extent of arrest and the amount of growth remaining.

Dr. Silva or an immediate family member serves as a board member, owner, officer, or committee member of the Pediatric Orthopaedic Society of North America and the World Federation of Hemophilia. Dr. Scaduto or an immediate family member serves as a board member, owner, officer, or committee member of the American Academy of Orthopaedic Surgeons, the Pediatric Orthopaedic Society of North America, and the Scoliosis Research Society.

Keywords: compartment syndrome; fracture; management; open fracture; physeal injury; polytrauma

Introduction

Each year, one of every four children in the United States requires urgent medical care for an accidental injury.[1] Although most of these injuries are sprains and contusions, nearly 50% of all boys and 25% of all girls sustain at least one fracture before reaching age 16 years,[2] with the incidence of fractures peaking in children aged 10 to 14 years. Pediatric fractures treated in the emergency department most commonly involve the forearm, hand, or wrist, and most (94%) are treated on an outpatient basis.[3] The most common pediatric fractures requiring hospitalization are fractures of the femur (20%) and humerus (18%).[4]

Although access to pediatric trauma care has diminished in many regions of the United States during the past decade,[5] orthopaedic surgeons continue to provide the bulk of fracture care to children. To optimize care, it is essential to understand the influence that growth can have on both fracture healing and remodeling as well as recognize complications unique to the growing skeleton.

Mechanisms of Injury

The rate and pattern of musculoskeletal injuries vary by age. Children younger than 5 years most commonly sustain low-energy fractures at home, whereas recreational and playground injuries are more common in school-aged children. Children who are obese may have an increased risk for fractures caused by ground-level falls.[6] Sleep deprivation also increases injury rates among middle school and high school athletes. One study found that adolescents who slept less than 8 hours per day were 1.7 times more likely to sustain an injury than students who slept more than 8 hours daily.[7]

Children older than 10 years are physically larger, stronger, and practice longer than younger children, all of which may contribute to a greater risk for sports-related injuries. Single-sport specialization has become more common in youth athletics. Even while accounting for more hours of physical activity, sports specialization is independently associated with higher injury rates.[8,9]

In 2000, the Centers for Disease Control and Prevention reported the top eight sport-related activities associated with injuries in children aged 5 to 14 years: baseball, basketball, bicycling, football, playground equipment, roller sports, soccer, and trampolining. One national database study found that sports-specific injury rates had substantially improved in the past decade for many sports, including bicycling (38%), roller sports (20%), and trampolining (17%). In contrast, football injuries, increased by 22% during the same period. Of concern to many, football-related concussions have more than doubled in the past decade.[10]

High-Energy Trauma

Severe and life-threatening musculoskeletal injuries in children are most commonly caused by falls from a height or motor vehicle crashes. Between 2007 and 2011, 2,238 pediatric traumatic amputations were reported in the national trauma databank. The most common injury mechanisms were being caught between two objects, machinery, powered lawnmowers, and motor vehicle collisions.[11] Motor vehicle collisions caused 8% of all amputations and were the leading cause of all amputations in adolescents. The increased use of child safety seats has reduced morbidity and mortality rates in children who are involved in motor vehicle crashes. Most children with motor vehicle–related injuries are pedestrians who were struck by a vehicle. All-terrain vehicles also remain a high-risk vehicle for children. Approximately 15% of all-terrain vehicle riders are children, but they account for 27% of all related injuries with such vehicles. Rollover is the most common mechanism of injury; however, children are substantially more likely than adults to be involved in collisions.[12,13]

Child Abuse

Fractures are a common finding in children who have sustained nonaccidental trauma. The orthopaedic surgeon plays a critical role in recognizing and treating child abuse. It is estimated that between one-third and one-half of all children who are abused are seen by an orthopaedic surgeon.[13] Certain fractures have a high likelihood of an abusive etiology, including posterior fractures of the ribs, metaphyseal corner fractures, long-bone fractures in nonambulatory children, or multiple fractures in different stages of healing. A spiral fracture of the femur in a young child has been thought to be possibly indicative of nonaccidental trauma; however, several studies have recently shown that transverse fractures of the femoral shaft rather than spiral fractures are better predictors of nonaccidental trauma.[14]

Pediatric Skeletal System and Fracture Patterns

Anatomy

Unlike adult bones, pediatric bones contain open growth plates and a thick periosteal layer. The presence of this thickened, highly osteogenic periosteum allows for faster fracture healing and the ability to remodel over time. With increasing age, the periosteum thins and its osteogenic capability decreases. Pediatric bones are less dense, are more porous, are penetrated by more vascular channels, and have a lower mineral content. Consequently, they have a lower modulus of elasticity and bending strength. The diaphysis, where the primary center of ossification is located during development, is highly vascular in a newborn. With age, vascularity decreases and the cortices thicken because of periosteum-induced bone formation. The metaphysis is wider than the diaphysis and has an increased amount of trabecular bone. After a fracture, much of the remodeling process occurs in the metaphysis. The physis is composed of an expandable matrix that allows long-bone growth through endochondral ossification. The epiphysis is completely cartilaginous at birth. It is rarely injured in its cartilaginous form. As the ossification of the epiphysis increases through the secondary center of ossification, so does the risk of injury.

Fracture Patterns

Pediatric bones are anatomically and mechanically different from adult bones. As such, many fracture patterns are unique to children. In general, pediatric fractures can be classified into five different types: plastic deformation, torus or buckle fractures, greenstick fractures, complete fractures, and physeal fractures. Plastic deformation is most commonly seen in the ulna and the fibula. Buckle fractures are mostly commonly seen in the metaphyseal portion of long bones where porosity is greatest. Greenstick fractures demonstrate a characteristic failure of the tension cortex, with a mirroring plastic deformity of the compression cortex. Complete fractures can be further subdivided into spiral, oblique, and transverse patterns. The thick periosteum tends to limit the amount of fracture displacement. An injury to the epiphysis frequently includes an associated injury to the growth plate. Conversely, not all growth plate injuries have an associated epiphyseal (or articular surface) injury. The physis and the epiphysis are firmly connected to the metaphysis by the periosteum. In children, most joint capsules and ligaments originate and insert on the epiphysis of a long bone. It has been generally accepted that such capsules and ligaments are stronger than the bones to which they attach; therefore, an injury that results in ligament stretching would result in a fracture in a child. (In an adult, however, ligament stretching results in a ligament strain.) This concept has been challenged with advanced imaging studies in pediatric patients with suspected nondisplaced physeal fractures of the distal fibula, suggesting that ligament sprains are actually quite common in this clinical scenario.[15] Injuries that involve the growth plate usually occur through the hypertrophic zone, although variability of the fracture plane within the physis has been suggested.[16]

Classification

Traditionally, fractures that involve the growth plate in a child have been classified using the Salter-Harris system (**Figure 1**). In general, a better prognosis is expected with lower-energy injuries not involving the epiphysis (types I and II); the prognosis is poorer for those that involve the epiphysis (types III and IV) or are associated with high energy (type V). Anatomic reduction is usually necessary to minimize growth arrest with types III and IV fractures. Although it has generally been accepted that anatomic reduction is not necessary for types I and II fractures, this might not be generalized to all anatomic locations. The risk of growth arrest is less reliably predicted by the Salter-Harris fracture type if the fracture is through a nonplanar physis.[17,18] It has been suggested that, when treating Salter-Harris types I and II fractures of the distal tibia, a residual physeal gap (>3 mm) may represent entrapped periosteum that could lead to a higher incidence of premature physeal closure if not removed surgically.[17] However, a recent study demonstrated that surgical management with removal of the interposed tissue and stable anatomic reduction improved joint alignment but did not reduce the incidence of premature physeal closure.[19] Although less commonly used, a comprehensive classification of long-bone fractures in children also has been described.[20]

Healing and Remodeling

Pediatric fractures heal faster and more predictably than adult fractures. Contributing factors include a thick and highly osteogenic periosteum, a more rapid initial inflammatory response because of higher bone vascularity (effectively shortening the early stages of fracture healing), and a lower likelihood of soft-tissue disruption. Pediatric bones have the ability to straighten residual deformities. The stresses and strains of the regular use of bone (Wolff law), as well as reorientation of the physis by asymmetric growth after a fracture (Hueter-Volkmann law), contribute to the remodeling capacity of pediatric bones (**Figure 2**). The ranges of acceptable fracture reduction parameters are, therefore, broader than those for adults. In general, the ability to remodel varies based on the bone involved, the patient's skeletal maturity, the location of the fracture and its proximity to the physis, the contribution of the closest physis to the overall growth of the affected bone, and the plane of deformity.[21] A 10-year-old boy with a sagittal malunion of the metaphysis of the distal radius will have a greater potential for remodeling than a 12-year-old girl with a sagittal malunion of the radial neck of the radius. In general, nonunion is uncommon in children. It appears that the risk of nonunion is highest with lateral condyle fractures of the humerus and open diaphyseal fractures of the tibia[22,23] (**Figure 3**).

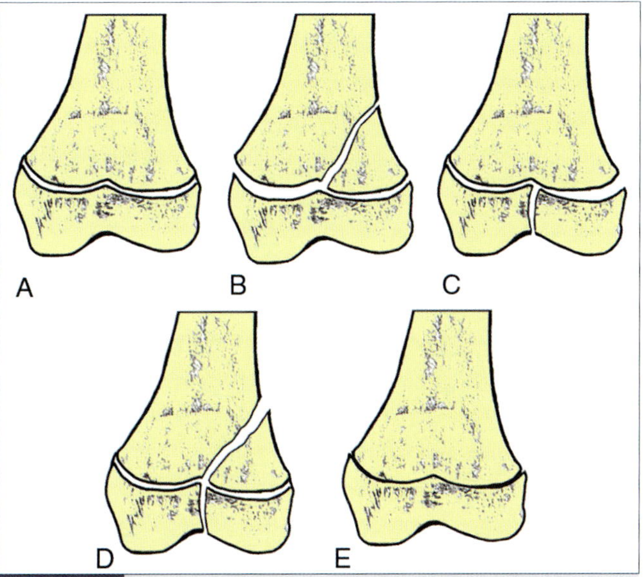

Figure 1 Illustration of the Salter-Harris classification for fractures. **A,** Type I. **B,** Type II. **C,** Type III. **D,** Type IV. **E,** Type V.

Fracture Management

History and Physical Examination

A complete patient history and a thorough physical examination are of primary importance when assessing a child with a possible fracture. It is crucial to determine the mechanism of injury. Although most fractures in children are isolated and the result of low-energy trauma, some are associated with high-energy mechanisms that often can involve multiple systems and result in life-threatening conditions. In such cases, coordinated management of all injuries by members of the trauma team is critical to minimize morbidity and mortality. In the event of an isolated, low-energy injury, the affected extremity is inspected for the presence of deformity, swelling, ecchymosis, skin breakdown, and the possibility of exposed bone.

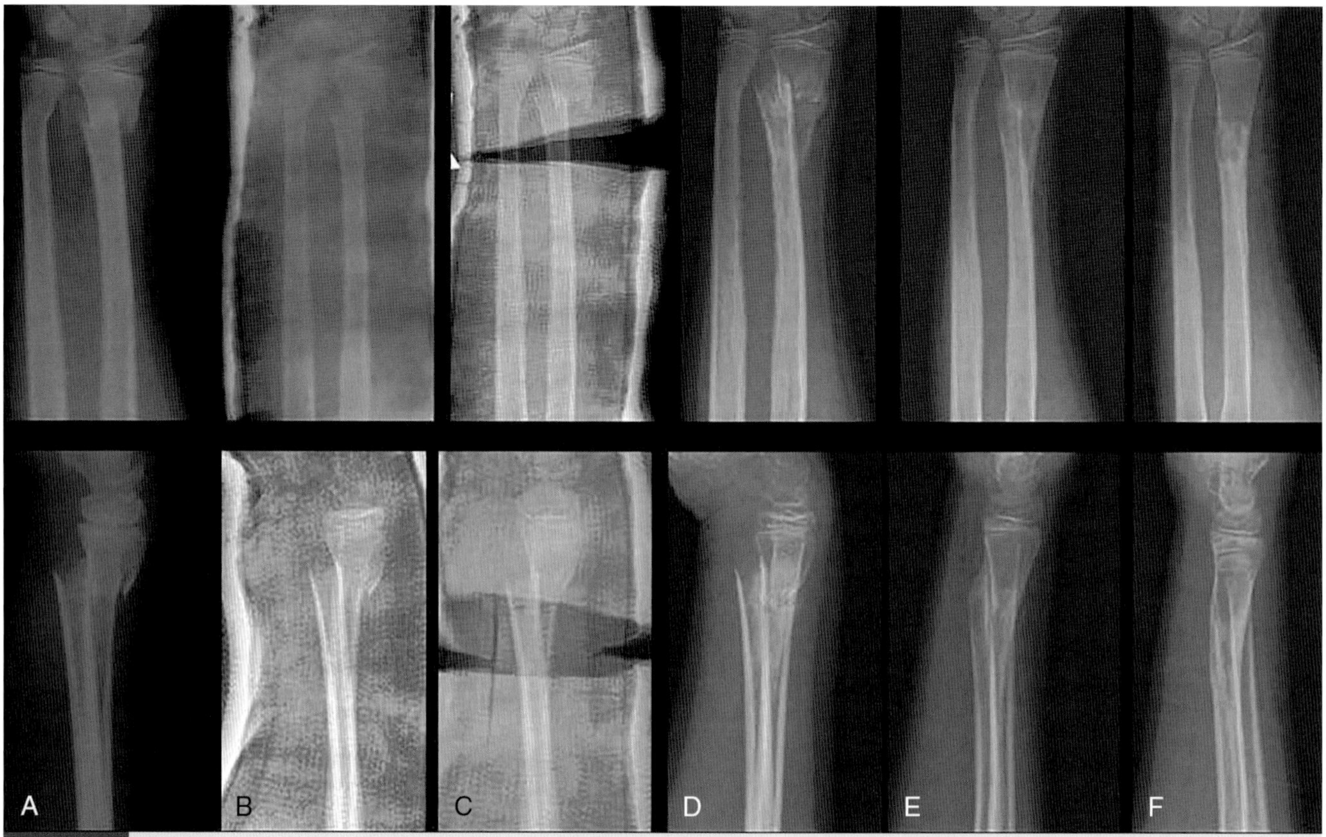

Figure 2 AP (top row) and lateral (bottom row) radiographs of remodeling after fracture of the distal radius and ulna. **A,** The initial injury. **B,** The fractures after reduction, **C,** The fractures after cast wedging at 1 week after injury. The fractures 1 month (**D**), 3 months (**E**), and 8 months (**F**) after injury.

All occluding dressings and splints should be removed to ensure a proper examination. Careful palpation of the entire affected extremity, with localization of the point of maximum tenderness, is helpful to determine the location of a possible fracture. Tenderness in more than one anatomic location should suggest the possibility of additional fractures. The compartments should be evaluated for the presence of excessive swelling and pain. A careful neurovascular examination should be performed, including motor and sensory examinations, the documentation of pulses, and assessment of capillary refill. After a focused examination of the affected extremity is performed, a rapid assessment of the remaining extremities should be completed to rule out the presence of additional injuries.

Imaging

Most fractures can be adequately evaluated with high-quality orthogonal radiographs of the affected area, including images of the joints above and below the suspected site of fracture. Oblique radiographs of the pediatric elbow and ankle are routinely obtained to facilitate the diagnosis of minimally displaced fractures (**Figure 4**). Special views could be helpful to determine displacement in specific anatomic areas. The routine use of comparison radiographs does not appear to increase diagnostic accuracy and is no longer favored. Although CT is useful for assessing pelvic, spinal, and intra-articular injuries, it is not routinely used for fracture assessment because it involves a large amount of ionizing radiation. Recently, ultrasonography has been used to detect minimally displaced fractures of the upper extremity in children.[24,25]

Pain Control

Local and Regional Drugs

Effective and safe levels of analgesia and sedation are desirable to minimize pain and apprehension during closed reduction and the immobilization of fractures in children. Several local and regional techniques have been described and are used in the pediatric population, including hematoma blocks, intravenous regional blocks, and regional nerve blocks. Infiltration of the fracture hematoma has commonly been used to reduce distal forearm and ankle fractures in children. It has been suggested that in the setting of a pediatric distal forearm fracture, local anesthesia

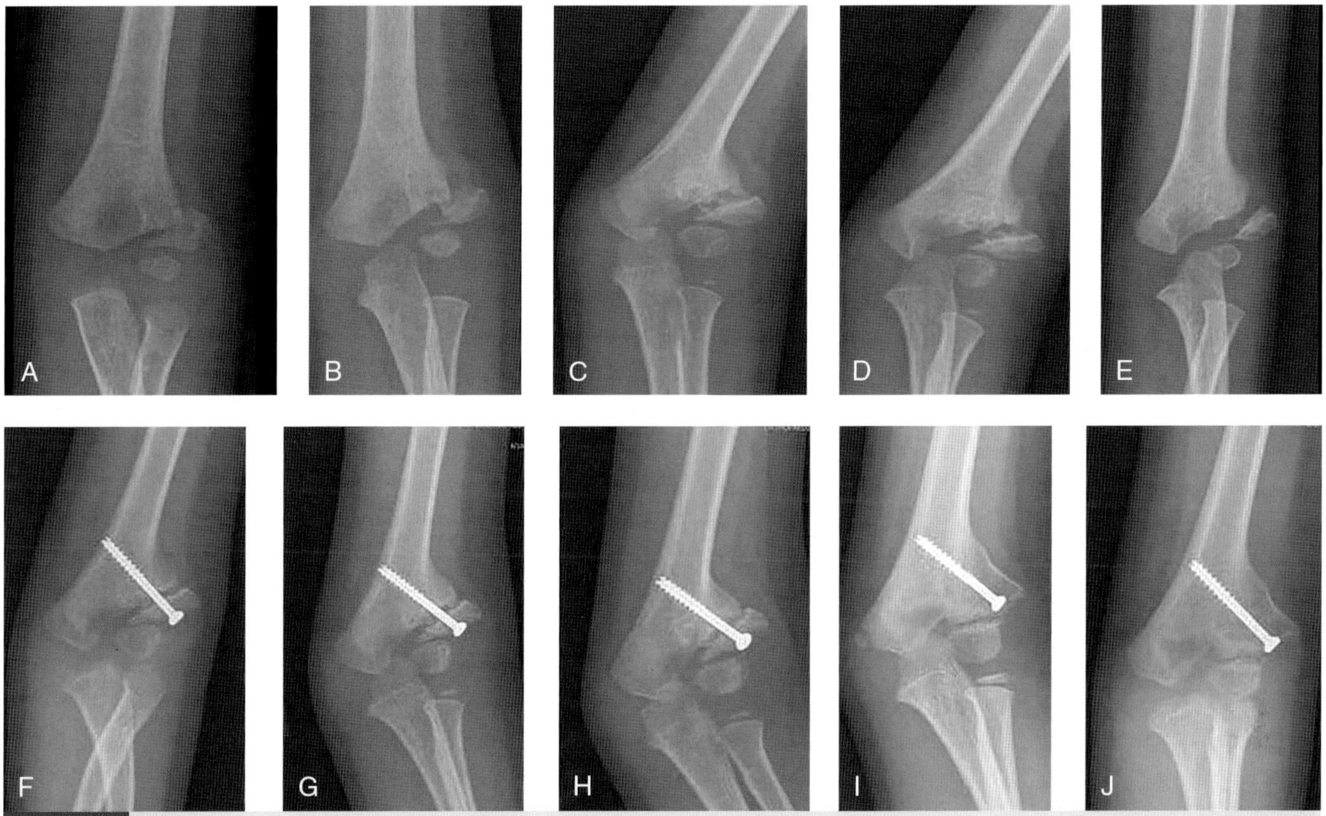

Figure 3 AP radiographs of fracture nonunion in a child, which is generally uncommon. The lateral condyle of the humerus is one of the few anatomic areas where nonunion can be observed. In this patient, a nonunion of the lateral condyle of the humerus was managed with percutaneous in situ screw fixation. **A,** The initial injury. The fracture at 2 months (**B**), 1 year (**C**), and 1.5 years (**D** and **E**) after injury. The fracture at 1 month (**F**), 2 months (**G**), 3 months (**H**), 1 year (**I**), and 2 years (**J**) after surgical fixation.

is less frequently used than sedation[26] and, as an adjunct to sedation, confers no additional benefits.[27] However, a 2015 report suggested that the use of a hematoma block in this setting provides similar clinical and radiographic outcomes (including pain and patient satisfaction) as those obtained with sedation, while substantially reducing the patient's time in the emergency department and the use of resources.[28] Intravenous regional anesthesia has been shown to be safe and cost-effective when reducing pediatric fractures, providing satisfactory analgesia in more than 90% of patients.[29,30] Although regional nerve blocks (brachial plexus) are more commonly used in surgical settings, their use in the emergency department has proved safe for pediatric forearm fracture manipulation and results in procedural distress and pain levels comparable with those obtained with deep sedation.[31]

Conscious Sedation and Dissociative Anesthesia

Conscious sedation, a state of depressed consciousness in which the patient maintains a patent airway and protective reflexes, is commonly used to achieve fracture reduction in the pediatric population. Sedation can be obtained by using either inhalational (nitrous oxide) or parenteral (opiate analgesics and benzodiazepines) agents. Pain relief and a safe level of sedation are usually obtained with these techniques. A combination of inhalational agents and a hematoma block also has been described.[32]

Dissociative anesthesia, a cataleptic, trancelike state induced by pharmacologic agents capable of causing dissociation of the thalamocortical and limbic areas of the brain, can impede the perception of noxious stimuli and provides a combination of sedation, analgesia, and amnesia.[30,33] Dissociative anesthesia is commonly used for fracture reduction in pediatric patients in emergency settings.[33-35] Ketamine, a dissociative anesthetic, is commonly combined with midazolam. When compared with other parenteral drug combinations, ketamine-midazolam therapy demonstrates fewer respiratory events and less need for supplemental oxygen and airway maneuvers.[34,35] Specific protocols to ensure the safety of the sedation procedure should be adopted.[36] The availability of personnel with up-to-date training and skills and appropriate equipment for airway management is essential.

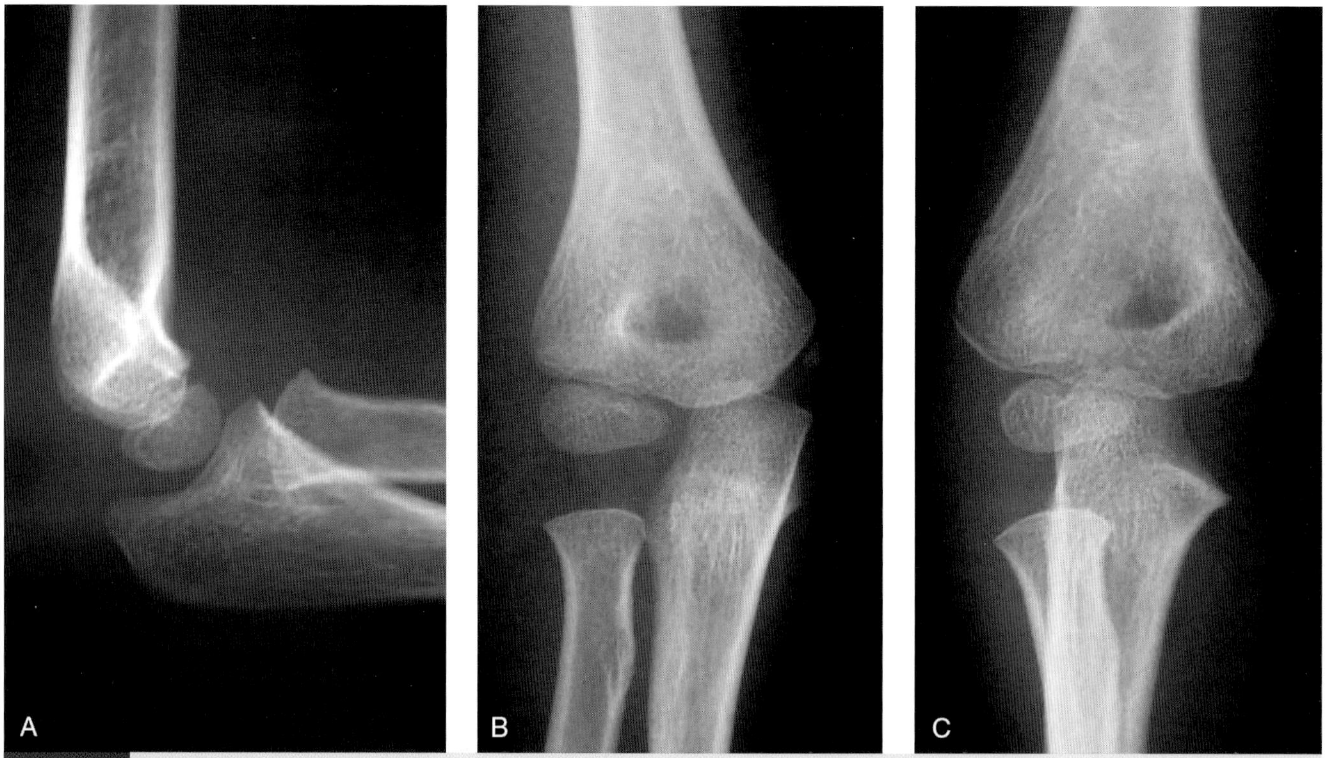

Figure 4 Lateral (**A**), AP (**B**), and internal oblique (**C**) radiographs of a minimally displaced fracture of the lateral condyle of the humerus in a child.

Splinting and Casting

Most pediatric fractures can be managed with immediate reduction and immobilization in a well-molded cast. Traditional splinting is usually preferred for patients if the injury is associated with severe swelling, in patients who are unable to communicate or insensate, or as a temporary measure in patients undergoing surgical treatment. It is generally accepted that a well-molded cast is more reliable than a traditional splint for maintaining fracture reduction. Removable splints have been shown to be advantageous for the treatment of some stable fractures.[37] Advocates of splint immobilization highlight the fact that splints can be taken off without exposing the child to the noise associated with a cast saw, a factor that has been identified as one of the most negative aspects of cast use from a child's perspective.[38-40]

No consensus is available on the optimal casting material for pediatric fractures. Plaster is more easily molded and is less expensive than fiberglass, but it is heavier and less resistant to water. Fiberglass is less malleable than plaster during the setting period and has a reduced capacity to create a good mold, but it is stronger, lighter, and water resistant.[41]

When applied by well-trained personnel, casting is usually safe. However, it is critical to be aware of potential complications associated with casting, including stiffness, thermal injuries, localized pressure, and compartment syndrome.[42] The setting of plaster involves an exothermic reaction that generates heat. Care must be taken to avoid using a dip-water temperature greater than 24°C, using excessively thick plaster, folding over the edges of splints (effectively increasing thickness), and placing the limb on a pillow during the curing process.[42,43] Although the risk of thermal injury is much lower with fiberglass, the risk of creating a constrictive bandage is greater. Proper application by stretching the material and allowing it to relax before rolling it on the affected extremity is critical to minimize this risk. Also, overwrapping of plaster in fiberglass should be delayed until the plaster is fully cured and cooled. The application of padding, including self-adhesive foam padding, over pressure-sensitive areas can minimize pressure sores.

The presence of increased pain and/or neurovascular change after cast application demands a careful evaluation and consideration of the possibility of compartment syndrome. Splitting or removing the cast might be necessary. Care must be taken to minimize the risk of cast-saw cuts and burns. Sliding the oscillating saw along the cast should be avoided. The risk of burns and cuts can be reduced by applying appropriate padding during casting, properly training personnel in the use of cast saws, frequently changing the saw blade (dull blades generate more heat), and cooling the blade periodically during cast removal.[44]

Special Situations

Polytrauma

Trauma is the leading cause of death in children aged 1 to 19 years in the United States.[45] Although extremity fractures are present in more than 60% of pediatric patients with polytrauma, approximately 80% of the deaths associated with high-energy trauma result from traumatic brain injury.[46] Compared with adult trauma centers, it has been reported that the treatment of a pediatric patient with multiple injuries at a pediatric trauma center results in a 20% lower rate of mortality.[47] The initial care of the pediatric patient with polytrauma should include a rapid assessment of any respiratory or circulatory compromise, with prompt management of any deficiency in oxygenation, ventilation, or perfusion. The assessment of life-threatening injuries is performed initially with radiographs of the chest, pelvis, and cervical spine. CT of the chest, abdomen, and pelvis provide a means of rapidly assessing multisystem organ failure. Unlike adult trauma patients, multisystem failure in children often occurs during resuscitation, affecting all organs almost simultaneously. However, reported rates of acute lung injury are nearly six times lower in children.[48,49] The lower rate of systemic damage is probably the result of an imbalanced inflammatory response to trauma in children, with a strong response at the tissue level but a diminished response at the systemic level.[50] Best outcomes are achieved with aggressive treatment of all musculoskeletal injuries and careful surveillance to detect any missed injuries.

Emergency Orthopaedic Management

The orthopaedic surgeon plays a critical role in the management of a child with polytrauma. A careful evaluation to identify potentially limb- or life-threatening injuries, including those to the spinal cord, the pelvic ring when associated with hemodynamic instability, fractures associated with vascular injury, and open fractures, is critical. When an injury to the cervical spine is suspected in a younger child, appropriate immobilization should be obtained using a backboard with an occipital recess. Using a standard trauma backboard will result in an unsafe position caused by neck flexion. Early stabilization with pelvic binders and external fixation may be beneficial in the presence of pelvic ring fractures associated with hemodynamic instability.[45] Temporary reduction and immobilization of pediatric fractures associated with vascular injuries can facilitate definitive vascular reconstruction and improve the overall outcome. Provisional splinting of affected extremities will increase patient comfort and minimize further tissue damage. Skeletal traction should be considered for patients with polytrauma if definitive treatment of femoral or unstable pelvic fractures is anticipated to be delayed by more than 24 hours.[45]

Damage Control

A traumatic event results in a sustained response of the immune system, with an early hyperinflammatory stage. In patients with polytrauma, lengthy initial surgery with substantial blood loss and hypothermia can result in an excessive inflammatory reaction (second hit), potentially triggering systemic inflammatory response syndrome, acute respiratory distress syndrome, and multiple organ failure. The concept of damage control orthopaedics in the trauma setting translates to performing only immediate lifesaving procedures aimed at stopping bleeding during the initial phase of care and achieving primary stabilization of major fractures by using external fixation.[51,52]

Recently, the preferential fixation of femoral fractures in the first 24 hours after injury, in contrast with other extremity fractures that could be splinted and fixed at a later date, has been described as early appropriate care.[53] Advocates of such care suggest that it represents a compromise between the earlier approach (wherein all fractures were treated immediately) and staged treatment, as long as an aggressive approach to resuscitation is used. In general, severely injured patients benefit from damage control orthopaedics, including those with an Injury Severity Score greater than 40, multiple injuries combined with thoracic trauma (an Injury Severity Score greater than 20), multiple injuries combined with severe abdominal or pelvic injuries and hemorrhagic shock, moderate or severe head trauma, radiographic evidence of a pulmonary contusion, bilateral femoral fractures, and those with a body temperature less than 35°C.[52] Although not specifically studied in children, damage control orthopaedics can be considered in the setting of children with severe head injuries who have an intracranial pressure greater than 30 mm Hg, those who are unstable and not easily controlled medically, those with profound hypothermia on admission, and those who are hypovolemic and hypotensive despite adequate ongoing resuscitation. Compared with adults, pediatric patients with polytrauma have a lower risk of sequential multiorgan failure in the first 48 hours after injury.[45] Early definitive orthopaedic stabilization after adequate resuscitation is critical to avoid complications associated with prolonged immobilization.

7: Trauma

Open Fractures

Although the principles of treating open fractures in children are similar to those in adults, the thicker and more active periosteum in children provides greater fracture stability. More rapid and reliable fracture healing also is usually achieved.

Open fractures typically result from high-energy or penetrating trauma. As with open fractures in adults, the Gustilo-Anderson system is used to classify open fractures in children. Open fractures represent approximately 2% of all pediatric fractures.[54,55] Careful evaluation of the patient in the emergency setting, after removing all dressings to allow for a complete skin assessment, is critical to diagnose smaller skin openings. The child's tetanus status should be confirmed. Little controversy exists with regard to the treatment of types II and III open fractures, including débridement of any devitalized tissue and abundant irrigation, in addition to the administration of intravenous antibiotics.[56] A first-generation cephalosporin is usually used in children with types II and III open fractures; an amino-glycoside and/or penicillin is added if the wound is severely contaminated or has been exposed to soil. The surgical treatment of type I open fractures has been questioned, with small studies suggesting that povidone-iodine and saline irrigation followed by closed reduction and cast immobilization in the emergency department (with either oral or intravenous antibiotics) have similar outcomes as those obtained with surgical treatment.[57-59] Prospective, randomized controlled trials are required to validate these findings.[56]

Timing of Irrigation and Débridement

In an effort to minimize the risk of infection, emergent surgical treatment was traditionally recommended for all open fractures. This recommendation was challenged by a large study in which the outcomes of 554 open fractures in children were analyzed. All patients received intravenous antibiotics at the time of admission to the emergency department, which were continued for 24 hours. Patients were retrospectively grouped based on whether they received surgical treatment before or after 6 hours from the time of injury. The infection rate was similar in both groups, regardless of the severity of the initial fracture.[60] Current recommendations suggest that emergent surgery is not required if intravenous antibiotics are administered soon after an injury.[56] Careful consideration of the vascular status of the limb and the severity of bone and soft-tissue injuries should help determine the need for immediate surgical treatment. All open fractures that require surgical treatment should receive it within 24 hours of the injury.

Surgical Considerations

The original wound should be extended as needed to gain adequate exposure to the bone ends. Muscle and other tissues should be inspected for signs of vitality. Any obviously devitalized tissue, including bone fragments completely stripped of periosteum, and other debris should be removed. If the vitality of any tissue is in question, it is best to preserve it and reevaluate it under general anesthesia 48 hours later.

Obtaining cultures before and after débridement appears to be of limited or no value in the treatment of open fractures.[56] A recent study in the adult population suggests that the use of very low pressure (1 to 2 psi) is an acceptable, low-cost alternative for the irrigation of open fractures, with rates of revision similar to those obtained with high (>20 psi) and low (5 to 10 psi) pressure.[61] Castile soap, as an additive in the irrigation fluid, has proved as effective as antibiotic (bacitracin) but has fewer wound healing problems.[62] However, castile soap appears to be associated with a higher revision rate compared with normal saline irrigation.[61]

Small, noncontaminated wounds can be closed over a drain. Negative pressure wound therapy with a vacuum-assisted closure system is helpful to reduce the need for free flaps and the risk of infection.[63-66] In general, stable fracture fixation is preferable to cast immobilization in patients with unstable fractures or a large soft-tissue injury. Sparse information is available regarding the length of antibiotic treatment after open fractures in children. In adults, the use of a first-generation cephalosporin for 24 to 48 hours after a type I open fracture and for 48 hours for types II and III open fractures, has been recommended.[67]

Outcomes

Compared with adults who have open fractures, children have better outcomes and a lower overall rate of infection. The rate of infection in children with open fractures is approximately 3%,[60] with an increasing rate as fracture severity increases (8% for type III fractures).[60] Although unlikely, delayed union and nonunion can occur, especially after a type III open fracture of the tibial shaft in an adolescent.

Compartment Syndrome

Compartment syndrome can be caused by a variety of factors, including fractures, crush injuries, vascular problems, burns, infections, casting complications, and intravenous infiltrations.[68] Regardless of the etiology, compartment syndrome occurs when an increase in intracompartmental pressure causes a decrease in perfusion pressure, which leads to hypoxemia of the tissues within the compartment. With hypoxemia, oxidant stress is increased. Because insufficient adenosine triphosphate is present, cell-membrane potential is lost and a resultant influx of chloride ions leads to cellular swelling and necrosis.[69]

Making a diagnosis of acute extremity compartment syndrome in a child can be challenging and often is delayed; the classic signs seen in adults are usually not helpful in children. The clinical diagnosis of acute extremity compartment syndrome in children should be based on the three A's: anxiety, agitation, and increasing analgesic requirement.[69] Although the most common scenarios for acute extremity compartment syndrome in a child include a tibial shaft fracture or a supracondylar humerus fracture, others include intravenous infiltrates, crush injuries, and thigh casts.[69]

For patients who are very young, are uncooperative, have altered mental status, or have unreliable or inconsistent clinical symptoms, the measurement of compartment pressures should be considered. The physiologic compartment pressures in children range from 10 to 15 mm Hg. An absolute pressure greater than 30 mm Hg is thought to indicate impaired tissue perfusion and the need for an emergency surgical fasciotomy; however, it is common practice now to use the differential pressure (Δp = diastolic blood pressure – intracompartmental pressure), with a proposed threshold of 30 mm Hg, as a more reliable indicator.[69] After fasciotomy, the skin edges should be approximated. Negative pressure wound therapy with a vacuum-assisted closure system can be helpful. Repeat evaluation and débridement often is needed after 48 to 72 hours, when delayed primary closure is sometimes possible. Split-thickness skin grafts are infrequently needed. In certain cases, passive stretching exercises and splinting might be helpful to minimize contractures. Timely diagnosis and prompt management with an appropriate fasciotomy can result in the recovery of function and favorable outcomes for children with acute compartment syndrome.

Growth Disturbance

The incidence of substantial disturbance of normal growth after a physeal injury is relatively low (<10%). Factors that can determine the extent of growth abnormality include the location and size of the physeal bar, the growth potential of the physis involved, and the age of the patient at the time of injury. Growth arrest can be complete or partial. With complete arrest, limb-length inequality will ensue. With a partial arrest, angular deformities or joint irregularities may be observed. The most common anatomic locations for growth arrest after a traumatic injury include the distal femur, the proximal tibia, and the distal tibia.[70,71]

Etiologies of Growth Arrest

In general, posttraumatic growth arrest usually is the result of partial or complete destruction of the physis at the time of injury, inadequate reduction of a physeal fracture, or tissue interposition at the fracture site.[70,71] A bridge of bone connecting the epiphysis and the metaphysis is responsible for growth arrest. Growth arrest can occur in the presence of an anatomic reduction.[70] Other causes of physeal bar formation include infection, tumors, irradiation, burns, vascular insufficiency, and metabolic disorders.[70] Crossing the physis with metal pins and drills, especially when threaded, and performing aggressive dissection of tissues, including the perichondrial ring, also can result in growth arrest.

Patterns of Bar Formation

Depending of the location of the bar within the physis, three common patterns are commonly seen: peripheral, central, or elongated (**Figure 5**). Peripheral bars are relatively common and can lead to angular deformities. Central bars are located away from the periphery and can tether growth, resulting in limb-length discrepancy or joint deformity. Elongated or linear bars run from one edge of the physis to the other (usually anterior to posterior) and can result in a combination of angular and joint deformities.

Treatment

One of the earliest signs of growth arrest is evidence of asymmetric growth recovery (Harris) lines. When growth is normal, growth recovery lines are parallel to the physis. With an arrest, the lines tend to converge toward the area of abnormal physis. Surveillance for growth arrest for at least 2 years is necessary after most physeal fractures. Particular attention should be paid to younger children with an injury known to have a high risk of growth disturbance such as a distal femoral fracture. Indistinct physeal margins and asymmetry or tilting at the joint are indirect radiologic signs that indicate the presence of a physeal bar.[72] Angular deformity and/or limb-length discrepancy are usually late radiographic manifestations. However, plain radiographs have limited ability to provide early identification and quantification of the extension of a physeal bar. Although CT has a better capacity to determine the size and location of physeal bars, it lacks the ability to detect early fibrous bars and is associated with high levels of radiation.[72] MRI is now widely accepted as the method of choice to provide early and complete evaluation of physeal bars, particularly when the three-dimensional gradient-recalled echo sequence is used.[72]

The precise location and size of the bar should be determined when surgical management is planned. Several

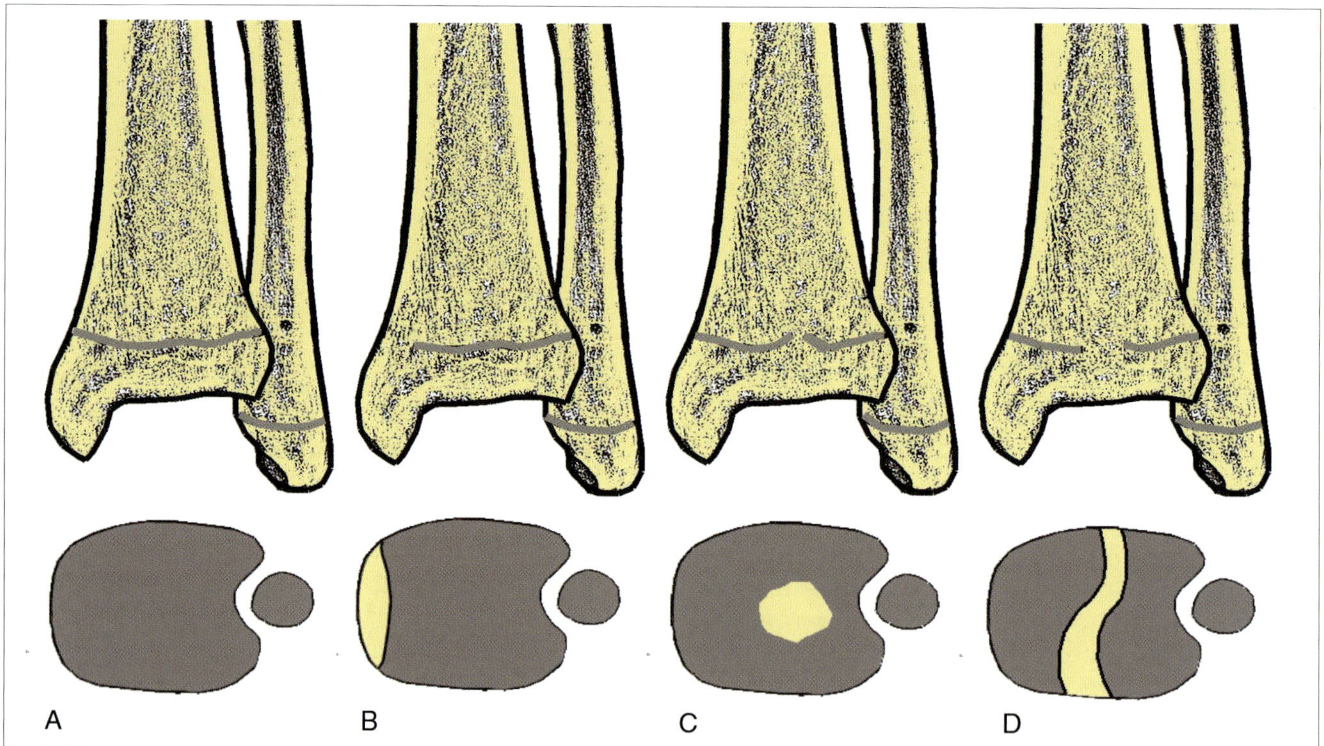

Figure 5 Illustrations of common patterns of physeal bar formation. **A,** Normal physis. **B,** Peripheral bars are relatively common and can lead to angular deformities. **C,** Central bars are located away from the periphery and can tether growth. **D,** Elongated or linear bars run from one edge of the physis to the other and can result in a combination of angular and joint deformities.

factors should be considered when planning surgical treatment after growth arrest, including the extent of the arrest, the anticipated discrepancy, and the age of the patient. In the presence of complete arrest, contralateral epiphysiodesis is chosen if the anticipated discrepancy is less than 5 cm. If the anticipated discrepancy is greater than 5 cm, lengthening of the short limb is performed. Partial arrest can be managed by resecting the physeal bar, completing the arrest through an epiphysiodesis (if no angular deformities have been noted), or combining epiphysiodesis and osteotomies and/or lengthening procedures if angular deformities and shortening are noted. Bar resection is indicated if the size of the bar represents less than 50% of the physis, the angular deformity is less than 20°, and at least 2 years of growth remain. Best results with resection are observed with traumatic bars that are located centrally and represent less than 25% of the entire size of the physis.

Summary

Most fractures in children result from falls from a low height or sports activities; however, certain fracture patterns should raise concerns for an abusive etiology. The anatomy and physiology of children influence the types of fractures and treatment options. The age of the child and the location of the fracture affect the capacity for remodeling. Most fractures in children can be managed nonsurgically. Ketamine and intravenous sedation are commonly used during closed manipulation, but local and regional drugs also can provide effective analgesia. Careful cast application and removal reduce the risk of complications such as thermal injuries and pressure sores associated with immobilization. Important complications after open fracture include compartment syndrome and premature physeal arrest. An increasing need for pain medication can be the only sign of an impending compartment syndrome in a child. Physeal fractures that have a high risk of growth arrest, such as distal femoral and tibial fractures, require long-term surveillance to avoid angular deformities and limb-length discrepancies. Depending on the extent of the arrest and the amount of growth remaining, the treatment of traumatic growth arrest can include physeal bar resection, epiphysiodesis, osteotomy, or limb lengthening or shortening.

Key Study Points

- By age 16 years, nearly 50% of all boys and 25% of all girls sustain at least one fracture.
- Posterior rib fractures, metaphyseal corner fractures, long-bone fractures in nonambulatory children, and multiple fractures in different stages of healing should raise concerns for nonaccidental trauma.
- Anatomic reduction is usually necessary to minimize growth arrest with Salter-Harris types III and IV physeal fractures.
- Effective and safe levels of analgesia and sedation are desirable to minimize pain and apprehension during closed reduction and the immobilization of fractures in children.
- The orthopaedic surgeon plays a critical role in the management of a child with polytrauma.
- The administration of intravenous antibiotics soon after the injury is a key step in the management of open fractures in children.
- Anxiety, agitation, and increasing analgesic requirement are common findings in a child with acute compartment syndrome.
- Physeal fractures of the distal femur and proximal tibia are associated with a high risk of growth arrest, requiring long-term surveillance to avoid angular deformities and limb-length discrepancies.

Annotated References

1. Danseco ER, Miller TR, Spicer RS: Incidence and costs of 1987-1994 childhood injuries: Demographic breakdowns. *Pediatrics* 2000;105(2):E27.

2. Landin LA: Epidemiology of children's fractures. *J Pediatr Orthop B* 1997;6(2):79-83.

3. Naranje SM, Erali RA, Warner WC Jr, Sawyer JR, Kelly DM: Epidemiology of pediatric fractures presenting to emergency departments in the United States. *J Pediatr Orthop* 2016;36(4):e45-e48.

   The authors report epidemiologic data for the most frequent pediatric fractures per 1,000 individuals using 2010 census data and a national injury database. Level of evidence: III.

4. Nakaniida A, Sakuraba K, Hurwitz EL: Pediatric orthopaedic injuries requiring hospitalization: Epidemiology and economics. *J Orthop Trauma* 2014;28(3):167-172.

   The authors identified the 10 most frequent pediatric orthopaedic injuries that required hospitalization and the most common causes of those injuries based on a longitudinal hospital care data set (the Kids' Inpatient Database).

5. Iobst C, Arango D, Segal D, Skaggs DL: National access to care for children with fractures. *J Pediatr Orthop* 2013;33(6):587-591.

   A survey of five general orthopaedic offices in every state showed decreasing access for pediatric fracture care. The ability to get an appointment for a simple pediatric fracture was lowest for mock patients with Medicaid (23%). Level of evidence: II.

6. Manning RL, Teach SJ, Searcy K, et al: The association between weight status and pediatric forearm fractures resulting from ground-level falls. *Pediatr Emerg Care* 2015;31(12):835-838.

   This retrospective case-control study found that children with fractures caused by ground-level falls had a 2.7 odds-adjusted risk of being at the 95th percentile or higher of weight compared with children with fractures that were the result of major trauma.

7. Milewski MD, Skaggs DL, Bishop GA, et al: Chronic lack of sleep is associated with increased sports injuries in adolescent athletes. *J Pediatr Orthop* 2014;34(2):129-133.

   A study of adolescent athletes correlated lower self-reported hours of sleep to higher rates of injuries recorded in a high school athletic department. Level of evidence: III.

8. Bell DR, Post EG, Trigsted SM, Hetzel S, McGuine TA, Brooks MA: Prevalence of sport specialization in high school athletics: A 1-year observational study. *Am J Sports Med* 2016;44(6):1469-1474.

   A cross-sectional study found that high school athletes who were highly specialized reported higher rates of overuse knee injuries compared with moderate or low-specialization athletes. Level of evidence: III.

9. Jayanthi NA, LaBella CR, Fischer D, Pasulka J, Dugas LR: Sports-specialized intensive training and the risk of injury in young athletes: A clinical case-control study. *Am J Sports Med* 2015;43(4):794-801.

   The odds of serious overuse injuries were increased in young athletes who participated in more hours of sports per week than their age in years or who participated in more organized sports than free play. Level of evidence: III.

10. Lykissas MG, Eismann EA, Parikh SN: Trends in pediatric sports-related and recreation-related injuries in the United States in the last decade. *J Pediatr Orthop* 2013;33(8):803-810.

    The authors reviewed sports-related injuries treated in emergency departments between 2000 and 2010. Football and soccer injuries increased by 22.8% and 10.8%, respectively. Injuries related to bicycling, roller sports, and trampolining decreased during the same period. Level of evidence: IV.

11. Borne A, Porter A, Recicar J, Maxson T, Montgomery C: Pediatric traumatic amputations in the United States: A 5-year review. *J Pediatr Orthop* 2015; Dec 2 [Epub ahead of print].

    All pediatric amputations in the United States from 2007 to 2011 are reviewed. Level of evidence: IV.

12. Su W, Hui T, Shaw K: All-terrain vehicle injury patterns: Are current regulations effective? *J Pediatr Surg* 2006;41(5):931-934.

13. Sink EL, Hyman JE, Matheny T, Georgopoulos G, Kleinman P: Child abuse: The role of the orthopaedic surgeon in nonaccidental trauma. *Clin Orthop Relat Res* 2011;469(3):790-797.

    The authors provide an extensive review of the literature on child abuse, with emphasis on the role of the orthopaedic surgeon. Level of evidence: IV.

14. Sawyer JR, Kelly DM, Kellum E, Warner WC Jr: Orthopaedic aspects of all-terrain vehicle-related injury. *J Am Acad Orthop Surg* 2011;19(4):219-225.

    An extensive review of the literature on injuries to children related to all-terrain vehicles is presented. Level of evidence: IV.

15. Boutis K, Narayanan UG, Dong FF, et al: Magnetic resonance imaging of clinically suspected Salter-Harris I fracture of the distal fibula. *Injury* 2010;41(8):852-856.

16. Wattenbarger JM, Gruber HE, Phieffer LS: Physeal fractures: Part I. Histologic features of bone, cartilage, and bar formation in a small animal model. *J Pediatr Orthop* 2002;22(6):703-709.

17. Barmada A, Gaynor T, Mubarak SJ: Premature physeal closure following distal tibia physeal fractures: A new radiographic predictor. *J Pediatr Orthop* 2003;23(6):733-739.

18. Arkader A, Warner WC Jr, Horn BD, Shaw RN, Wells L: Predicting the outcome of physeal fractures of the distal femur. *J Pediatr Orthop* 2007;27(6):703-708.

19. Russo F, Moor MA, Mubarak SJ, Pennock AT: Salter-Harris II fractures of the distal tibia: Does surgical management reduce the risk of premature physeal closure? *J Pediatr Orthop* 2013;33(5):524-529.

    Patients with displaced Salter-Harris type II distal tibial fractures were found to have a high rate of premature physeal closure. Surgical fixation with anatomic reduction and the removal of interposed tissue does not reduce the incidence of premature closure. Level of evidence: III.

20. Slongo T, Audigé L, Lutz N, et al: Documentation of fracture severity with the AO classification of pediatric long-bone fractures. *Acta Orthop* 2007;78(2):247-253.

21. Wilkins KE: Principles of fracture remodeling in children. *Injury* 2005;36(1):A3-A11.

22. Herman MJ, Martinek MA, Abzug JM: Complications of tibial eminence and diaphyseal fractures in children: Prevention and treatment. *Instr Course Lect* 2015;64:471-482.

    The authors present an extensive review of the literature regarding tibial fractures in children. Level of evidence: V.

23. Tejwani N, Phillips D, Goldstein RY: Management of lateral humeral condylar fracture in children. *J Am Acad Orthop Surg* 2011;19(6):350-358.

    The authors present an extensive review of the literature regarding lateral condyle fractures of the humerus in children. Level of evidence: V.

24. Supakul N, Hicks RA, Caltoum CB, Karmazyn B: Distal humeral epiphyseal separation in young children: An often-missed fracture-radiographic signs and ultrasound confirmatory diagnosis. *AJR Am J Roentgenol* 2015;204(2):W192-W1988.

    Often missed on radiographs, the diagnosis of distal humeral epiphyseal separation can be effectively confirmed with ultrasonography. Level of evidence: IV.

25. Neri E, Barbi E, Rabach I, et al: Diagnostic accuracy of ultrasonography for hand bony fractures in paediatric patients. *Arch Dis Child* 2014;99(12):1087-1090.

    Ultrasonographic imaging showed excellent sensitivity and specificity in the diagnosis of hand fractures in children when such imaging was performed by either a senior radiologist or a pediatric emergency physician. Level of evidence: III.

26. Constantine E, Steele DW, Eberson C, Boutis K, Amanullah S, Linakis JG: The use of local anesthetic techniques for closed forearm fracture reduction in children: A survey of academic pediatric emergency departments. *Pediatr Emerg Care* 2007;23(4):209-211.

27. Constantine E, Tsze DS, Machan JT, Eberson CP, Linakis JG, Steele DW: Evaluating the hematoma block as an adjunct to procedural sedation for closed reduction of distal forearm fractures. *Pediatr Emerg Care* 2014;30(7):474-478.

    This randomized, double-blind, placebo-controlled trial concluded that hematoma blocks, as an adjunct to procedural sedation with ketamine and midazolam for forearm fracture reduction in children, do not decrease pain scores, sedation time, or the total ketamine dose administered. Level of evidence: I.

28. Bear DM, Friel NA, Lupo CL, Pitetti R, Ward WT: Hematoma block versus sedation for the reduction of distal radius fractures in children. *J Hand Surg Am* 2015;40(1):57-61.

    In this prospective study of pediatric distal radius fractures, patients chose between hematoma blocks and procedural sedation before fracture reduction. Hematoma blocks provided radiographic alignment, patient satisfaction, and pain control comparable with that of procedural sedation. Level of evidence: III.

29. Aarons CE, Fernandez MD, Willsey M, Peterson B, Key C, Fabregas J: Bier block regional anesthesia and casting for forearm fractures: Safety in the pediatric emergency department setting. *J Pediatr Orthop* 2014;34(1):45-49.

A retrospective comparison of 600 patients who were treated with Bier block regional anesthesia and 645 patients who were treated with conscious sedation for displaced fractures of the forearm demonstrated comparable results regarding safety, time to discharge, and cost. Level of evidence: III.

30. McCarty EC, Mencio GA, Green NE: Anesthesia and analgesia for the ambulatory management of fractures in children. *J Am Acad Orthop Surg* 1999;7(2):81-91.

31. Kriwanek KL, Wan J, Beaty JH, Pershad J: Axillary block for analgesia during manipulation of forearm fractures in the pediatric emergency department: A prospective randomized comparative trial. *J Pediatr Orthop* 2006;26(6):737-740.

32. Luhmann JD, Schootman M, Luhmann SJ, Kennedy RM: A randomized comparison of nitrous oxide plus hematoma block versus ketamine plus midazolam for emergency department forearm fracture reduction in children. *Pediatrics* 2006;118(4):e1078-e1086.

33. McCarty EC, Mencio GA, Walker LA, Green NE: Ketamine sedation for the reduction of children's fractures in the emergency department. *J Bone Joint Surg Am* 2000;82(7):912-918.

34. Godambe SA, Elliot V, Matheny D, Pershad J: Comparison of propofol/fentanyl versus ketamine/midazolam for brief orthopedic procedural sedation in a pediatric emergency department. *Pediatrics* 2003;112(1):116-123.

35. Kennedy RM, Porter FL, Miller JP, Jaffe DM: Comparison of fentanyl/midazolam with ketamine/midazolam for pediatric orthopedic emergencies. *Pediatrics* 1998;102(4):956-963.

36. Coté CJ, Wilson S; American Academy of Pediatrics; American Academy of Pediatric Dentistry; Work Group on Sedation: Guidelines for monitoring and management of pediatric patients during and after sedation for diagnostic and therapeutic procedures: An update. *Pediatrics* 2006;118(6):2587-2602.

37. Boutis K, Willan A, Babyn P, Goeree R, Howard A: Cast versus splint in children with minimally angulated fractures of the distal radius: A randomized controlled trial. *CMAJ* 2010;182(14):1507-1512.

38. Carmichael KD, Westmoreland J: Effectiveness of ear protection in reducing anxiety during cast removal in children. *Am J Orthop (Belle Mead NJ)* 2005;34(1):43-46.

39. Katz K, Fogelman R, Attias J, Baron E, Soudry M: Anxiety reaction in children during removal of their plaster cast with a saw. *J Bone Joint Surg Br* 2001;83(3):388-390.

40. Liu RW, Mehta P, Fortuna S, et al: A randomized prospective study of music therapy for reducing anxiety during cast room procedures. *J Pediatr Orthop* 2007;27(7):831-833.

41. Inglis M, McClelland B, Sutherland LM, Cundy PJ: Synthetic versus plaster of Paris casts in the treatment of fractures of the forearm in children: A randomised trial of clinical outcomes and patient satisfaction. *Bone Joint J* 2013;95-B(9):1285-1289.

In this trial, children with forearm fractures were randomized to receive either a plaster-of-Paris cast or a synthetic cast. A higher complication rate was seen with plaster-of-Paris casts, including soft areas requiring revision and loss of reduction. Patient satisfaction was higher with synthetic casts. Level of evidence: II.

42. Halanski M, Noonan KJ: Cast and splint immobilization: Complications. *J Am Acad Orthop Surg* 2008;16(1):30-40.

43. Halanski MA, Halanski AD, Oza A, Vanderby R, Munoz A, Noonan KJ: Thermal injury with contemporary cast-application techniques and methods to circumvent morbidity. *J Bone Joint Surg Am* 2007;89(11):2369-2377.

44. Puddy AC, Sunkin JA, Aden JK, Walick KS, Hsu JR: Cast saw burns: Evaluation of simple techniques for reducing the risk of thermal injury. *J Pediatr Orthop* 2014;34(8):e63-e66.

This study suggested that, to reduce the temperature of the saw blade, the routine use of isopropyl alcohol or water on gauze, or running the saw and vacuum simultaneously, would substantially decrease the risk of discomfort and thermal injury during cast cutting. Level of evidence: III.

45. Pandya NK, Upasani VV, Kulkarni VA: The pediatric polytrauma patient: Current concepts. *J Am Acad Orthop Surg* 2013;21(3):170-179.

The authors present an extensive review of the literature regarding polytrauma in children. Level of evidence: V.

46. Jawadi AH, Letts M: Injuries associated with fracture of the femur secondary to motor vehicle accidents in children. *Am J Orthop (Belle Mead NJ)* 2003;32(9):459-462, discussion 462.

47. Oyetunji TA, Haider AH, Downing SR, et al: Treatment outcomes of injured children at adult level 1 trauma centers: Are there benefits from added specialized care? *Am J Surg* 2011;201(4):445-449.

A review of the data of 53,702 children included in the National Trauma Data Bank demonstrated that the adjusted odds of mortality were 20% lower for children seen at adult trauma centers with added qualifications in pediatrics. Level of evidence: II.

48. Zimmerman JJ, Akhtar SR, Caldwell E, Rubenfeld GD: Incidence and outcomes of pediatric acute lung injury. *Pediatrics* 2009;124(1):87-95.

49. Rubenfeld GD, Caldwell E, Peabody E, et al: Incidence and outcomes of acute lung injury. *N Engl J Med* 2005;353(16):1685-1693.

50. Wood JH, Partrick DA, Johnston RB Jr: The inflammatory response to injury in children. *Curr Opin Pediatr* 2010;22(3):315-320.

51. Lichte P, Kobbe P, Dombroski D, Pape HC: Damage control orthopedics: Current evidence. *Curr Opin Crit Care* 2012;18(6):647-650.

An extensive review of the literature regarding damage control orthopaedics is presented. Level of evidence: V.

52. Pape HC, Tornetta P III, Tarkin I, Tzioupis C, Sabeson V, Olson SA: Timing of fracture fixation in multitrauma patients: The role of early total care and damage control surgery. *J Am Acad Orthop Surg* 2009;17(9):541-549.

53. Nahm NJ, Como JJ, Wilber JH, Vallier HA: Early appropriate care: Definitive stabilization of femoral fractures within 24 hours of injury is safe in most patients with multiple injuries. *J Trauma* 2011;71(1):175-185.

This article reported that early definitive stabilization of femoral fractures is associated with low rates of complications. More complications and longer hospital stays were noted with delayed fixation. The presence of a severe abdominal injury was the greatest risk factor for complications. Level of evidence: III.

54. Cheng JC, Ng BK, Ying SY, Lam PK: A 10-year study of the changes in the pattern and treatment of 6,493 fractures. *J Pediatr Orthop* 1999;19(3):344-350.

55. Cheng JC, Shen WY: Limb fracture pattern in different pediatric age groups: A study of 3,350 children. *J Orthop Trauma* 1993;7(1):15-22.

56. Pace JL, Kocher MS, Skaggs DL: Evidence-based review: Management of open pediatric fractures. *J Pediatr Orthop* 2012;32(suppl 2):S123-S127.

The authors present an extensive review of the literature regarding the management of open pediatric fractures. Level of evidence: V.

57. Iobst CA, Spurdle C, Baitner AC, King WF, Tidwell M, Swirsky S: A protocol for the management of pediatric type I open fractures. *J Child Orthop* 2014;8(1):71-76.

The authors developed a protocol for the nonsurgical management of pediatric type I open forearm fractures that included antibiotics, local irrigation, and closed reduction. No infections were reported. The authors concluded that the protocol was safe and effective. Level of evidence: III.

58. Iobst CA, Tidwell MA, King WF: Nonoperative management of pediatric type I open fractures. *J Pediatr Orthop* 2005;25(4):513-517.

59. Doak J, Ferrick M: Nonoperative management of pediatric grade 1 open fractures with less than a 24-hour admission. *J Pediatr Orthop* 2009;29(1):49-51.

60. Skaggs DL, Friend L, Alman B, et al: The effect of surgical delay on acute infection following 554 open fractures in children. *J Bone Joint Surg Am* 2005;87(1):8-12.

61. Bhandari M, Jeray KJ, Petrisor BA, et al; FLOW Investigators: A trial of wound irrigation in the initial management of open fracture wounds. *N Engl J Med* 2015;373(27):2629-2641.

Patients with an open fracture were randomized to undergo irrigation with one of three irrigation pressures (high, low, or very low) and one of two solutions (castile soap or normal saline). Although the rates of reoperation were similar regardless of irrigation pressure, they were higher in the soap group. Level of evidence: I.

62. Anglen JO: Comparison of soap and antibiotic solutions for irrigation of lower-limb open fracture wounds: A prospective, randomized study. *J Bone Joint Surg Am* 2005;87(7):1415-1422.

63. Dedmond BT, Kortesis B, Punger K, et al: Subatmospheric pressure dressings in the temporary treatment of soft tissue injuries associated with type III open tibial shaft fractures in children. *J Pediatr Orthop* 2006;26(6):728-732.

64. Shilt JS, Yoder JS, Manuck TA, Jacks L, Rushing J, Smith BP: Role of vacuum-assisted closure in the treatment of pediatric lawnmower injuries. *J Pediatr Orthop* 2004;24(5):482-487.

65. Mooney JF III, Argenta LC, Marks MW, Morykwas MJ, DeFranzo AJ: Treatment of soft tissue defects in pediatric patients using the V.A.C. system. *Clin Orthop Relat Res* 2000;376:26-31.

66. Halvorson J, Jinnah R, Kulp B, Frino J: Use of vacuum-assisted closure in pediatric open fractures with a focus on the rate of infection. *Orthopedics* 2011;34(7):e256-e260.

Compared with historical control patients, this study showed that vacuum-assisted closure therapy for pediatric open fractures appears to be a safe and effective method for reducing infection rates. Level of evidence: IV.

67. Hauser CJ, Adams CA Jr, Eachempati SR; Council of the Surgical Infection Society: Surgical Infection Society guideline: Prophylactic antibiotic use in open fractures. An evidence-based guideline. *Surg Infect (Larchmt)* 2006;7(4):379-405.

68. Kanj WW, Gunderson MA, Carrigan RB, Sankar WN: Acute compartment syndrome of the upper extremity in children: Diagnosis, management, and outcomes. *J Child Orthop* 2013;7(3):225-233.

The authors presented a retrospective review of patients who underwent decompressive fasciotomy for an acute compartment syndrome of the upper extremity. The average time from injury to fasciotomy was more than

30 hours. Excellent long-term outcomes were observed in 74% of the patients. Level of evidence: IV.

69. von Keudell AG, Weaver MJ, Appleton PT, et al: Diagnosis and treatment of acute extremity compartment syndrome. *Lancet* 2015;386(10000):1299-1310.

The authors extensively reviewed the literature regarding acute compartment syndrome. Level of evidence: V.

70. Khoshhal KI, Kiefer GN: Physeal bridge resection. *J Am Acad Orthop Surg* 2005;13(1):47-58.

71. Wuerz TH, Gurd DP: Pediatric physeal ankle fracture. *J Am Acad Orthop Surg* 2013;21(4):234-244.

An extensive review of the literature regarding pediatric physeal ankle fractures is presented. Level of evidence: V.

72. Wang DC, Deeney V, Roach JW, Shah AJ: Imaging of physeal bars in children. *Pediatr Radiol* 2015;45(9):1403-1412.

The authors extensively reviewed the literature regarding the use of imaging modalities to diagnose physeal bars in children. Level of evidence: V.

Chapter 35

Child Abuse

Brian K. Brighton, MD, MPH Brian P. Scannell, MD

Abstract

Fractures are one of the most common injuries found in children who have been physically abused. The evaluation of such children, the identification of any associated injuries, and the creation of a management plan requires a multidisciplinary child maltreatment prevention team that includes communication and collaboration among pediatricians, orthopaedic surgeons, radiologists, nurses, and social workers.

Keywords: child abuse; nonaccidental trauma

Introduction

Child abuse remains a serious threat to the pediatric population. The incidence of nonaccidental trauma in the pediatric population is high, with reports ranging from 0.47 per 100,000 to 2,000 per 100,000.[1,2] Musculoskeletal injuries are one of the most common manifestations of physical abuse in children. Soft-tissue injuries are the most common injury, followed by fractures.[3,4] Many orthopaedic surgeons feel unprepared to manage these patients, and they may benefit from improved education and training related to nonaccidental trauma.[5]

Background

Numerous early reports of violence or abuse toward children have been published. In 1946, an association was highlighted between multiple fractures and subdural hematomas in a case series of six infants.[6] Although indications existed that the injuries were traumatic in etiology, no direct link could made to child abuse. It was not until 1962 that the medical profession fully recognized the reality of child abuse—when researchers published a landmark article describing battered child syndrome.[7] The journal article described the clinical profile of a child who has been abused and when physicians should have high levels of suspicion for abuse. This article resulted in increased public awareness to the societal and emotional trauma of child abuse.

Within a few years of this landmark article, nearly all states mandated the reporting of suspected abuse. In addition, the Child Abuse Prevention and Treatment Act of 1974 provided assistance to states to develop child abuse and neglect prevention and identification programs. This act was most recently amended in 2010, providing minimum standards to states for defining maltreatment; however, each state individually defines the parameters for the physical abuse of a child. The act defines child abuse as "any recent act or failure to act on the part of a parent or caretaker which results in death, serious physical or emotional harm, sexual abuse, or exploitation."[8]

Risk Factors for Abuse

Several child, parent, and environmental risk factors can indicate child abuse (**Table 1**). Very young children appear to be at the greatest risk.[9] Nearly 80% of all fractures caused by child abuse occur in children younger than 18 months.[10] In 2009, researchers found that the mean age of children with orthopaedic injuries resulting from nonaccidental trauma was 11.8 months.[11] In addition, children with disabilities are three times more likely to be maltreated than children without disabilities.[12]

Parental and environmental factors also may make children more vulnerable to physical abuse. Factors such as low parental self-esteem, substance abuse, and alcohol abuse may decrease a parent's ability to cope with the stresses of parenting, which may then be a predisposing factor in abuse.[13,14] Parents who were abused or neglected

Dr. Brighton or an immediate family member serves as a paid consultant to DePuy and serves as a board member, owner, officer, or committee member of the Pediatric Orthopaedic Society of North America and the American College of Surgeons. Neither Dr. Scannell nor any immediate family member has received anything of value from or has stock or stock options held in a commercial company or institution related directly or indirectly to the subject of this chapter.

Table 1

Child, Parental, and Environmental Risk Factors for Child Abuse

Child	Parental	Environment (Community and Society)
Emotional and/or behavioral difficulties	Low self-esteem	Social isolation
Chronic illness	Poor impulse control	Poverty
Physical disabilities	Substance and/or alcohol abuse	Unemployment
Developmental disabilities	Young maternal or paternal age	Low educational achievement
Premature birth	Parent abused as a child	Single parent
Unwanted child	Depression or other mental illness	Nonbiologically-related male living in the home
Unplanned pregnancy	Poor knowledge of child development or unrealistic expectations for child	Family or intimate partner violence
	Negative perception of normal child behavior	

Reproduced with permission from Flaherty EG, Stirling J Jr: Clinical report: The pediatrician's role in child maltreatment prevention. *Pediatrics* 2010;126(4):833-841.

as children are more likely to inflict abuse on their own children.[1,13] Socioeconomic status also appears to affect the incidence of abuse rates. Children from low socioeconomic households (annual income less than $15,000) are three times more likely to be abused.[15] Perpetrators of abuse often are known by the child and are more commonly male, with more than 50% of abusers being the child's father, the child's stepfather, or a male friend of the child's mother.[16] However, physical abuse can affect children of all ages, ethnicities, and socioeconomic groups.

Patient Evaluation

History and Physical Examination

A detailed history and physical examination are of utmost importance in children when abuse is suspected. History taking may vary based on the age and communication level of the child. When children are of school age and able to communicate, they should be interviewed apart from their caregivers. Parents or caregivers should be asked to describe events surrounding the reported injury. If more than one caregiver is present, it can be helpful to interview each caregiver separately.

The history should include details of the event, the developmental history of the child, and the family's social history to determine who lives in the house and who was present at the time of the injury.[17]A thorough family history is important to identify any bleeding, bone, and metabolic or genetic disorders.

Numerous key findings from the history should raise concern for abuse, including the following: (1) explicit denial of trauma in a child with obvious injury; (2) no explanation or only a vague explanation given for a substantial injury; (3) unexplained or notable delay in seeking medical care; (4) an injury explanation that is inconsistent with the child's physical and/or developmental capabilities; (5) an injury explanation that is inconsistent with the pattern, age, or severity of the injury; and (6) markedly different explanations for the injury between caregivers or the child and the caregiver.[17,18]

Each child requires a comprehensive head-to-toe physical examination, and it is of utmost importance that this examination be performed with the child undressed. The examination should include a thorough musculoskeletal and age-appropriate neurologic examination. In general, young children should be examined for signs of neglect, including malnutrition, dental issues, or neglected wound and/or skin issues, such as diaper dermatitis.[17] The head, eyes, ears, nose, and throat should be assessed, including the anterior fontanelle in infants; a detailed ophthalmology examination if abuse is suspected; and an evaluation for dental trauma and/or caries.

The skin examination may reveal bruises, lacerations, burns, or other injuries, and these should be documented in size, shape, and location.[17] Soft-tissue injuries are found in a high percentage (92%) of suspected child abuse cases.[4] Suspicion should be high for abuse for any soft-tissue injury in a child who is younger than 9 months or if multiple soft-tissue injuries are present in children ranging from 10 months to 2 years of age.[10] Certain sites of soft-tissue injury are more commonly associated with abuse, such as the face, back, buttocks, perineum, and genitalia; other

Table 2

Complete Skeletal Survey

Appendicular Skeleton	Imaging View
Humeri	AP
Forearms	AP
Hands	PA
Femurs	AP
Lower legs	AP
Feet	AP
Axial Skeleton	
Thorax	AP, lateral, right and left obliques, including ribs and thoracic and upper lumbar spine
Pelvis	AP, including midlumbar spine
Lumbosacral spine	Lateral
Cervical spine	Lateral
Skull	Frontal and lateral

locations, such as the anterior aspect of the lower leg, are more common with accidental injury.[19,20]

Imaging

In children undergoing an evaluation for both accidental and nonaccidental trauma, dedicated radiographs of the injured limb or joint should be obtained. In children younger than 2 years and select patients up to 5 years of age with injuries that are suspicious for physical abuse, a skeletal survey should be performed. A skeletal survey based on the parameters of the American College of Radiology and the Society for Pediatric Radiology includes images of the appendicular and axial skeleton[21] (**Table 2**). Using highly detailed skeletal surveys, additional unsuspected fractures may be present up to 20% of the time in cases of suspected abuse.[22] Repeating a skeletal survey 2 to 3 weeks after the initial evaluation of a child who has been abused improves the diagnostic accuracy of identifying skeletal injuries, including rib fractures and classic metaphyseal lesions.[23]

To document the level of suspicion for abuse in the presence of multiple fractures, surgeons must have a keen understanding of fracture healing in children. Typically, the resolution of soft-tissue swelling occurs in 4 to 10 days, and new periosteal reaction can be seen on radiographs in 10 to 14 days.[24]

In children with suspected head injuries and in infants younger than 1 year, CT is recommended to evaluate for a subdural hemorrhage or a brain injury. Brain MRI has become more frequently used for the diagnosis and prognostication of abusive head trauma.[25] Clinical signs of spinal cord injury may be masked by respiratory depression and impaired consciousness associated with the head injury.[26] Children who have abusive head trauma and are undergoing a brain MRI also should be considered for an MRI of the spine to assess for occult spinal cord injury, ligamentous disruption, or intrathecal blood.[27-29] In addition, spinal MRI may help differentiate between a traumatic and a nontraumatic intracranial subdural hemorrhage.[27] A chest CT can be used to identify rib fractures.[18] Bone scans may be used to detect rib fractures or other fractures when a skeletal survey is negative but when a high index of suspicion for abuse is present.[30,31] Whole-body MRI also may have a limited role in the evaluation of the child who is physically abused.[32]

Common Fractures

Fractures in children commonly occur as the result of accidental trauma. However, in young children and infants with skeletal trauma, the timely recognition of injuries associated with abuse can protect victims from further abuse.[33] In children with skeletal injuries, physical abuse should be included in the diagnosis if certain injury patterns are present. Several factors to consider are the patient age and history, the mechanism of injury, the fracture location and pattern, and associated injuries. It is important to correlate fracture findings with the history and physical examination because certain fractures should provoke a suspicion for abuse (**Table 3**). Although no absolutes exist, a high index of suspicion is appropriate in children who have a history of trauma that does not support the associated injury or certain fractures of the femur or tibia in children who are nonambulatory. If the presentation is delayed or multiple fractures in various states of healing are present, the concern for abuse increases. In addition, unusual fractures in infants and toddlers, such as rib fractures, sternal fractures, vertebral fractures, and classic metaphyseal lesions (metaphyseal corner fractures) without a history of trauma or known metabolic bone disorder should alert the physician to the high likelihood of abuse.[17] In a systematic review of the literature in 2008, researchers found that fractures resulting from abuse were most commonly found in infants younger than 1 year and toddlers (aged 1 to 3 years) and were located throughout the skeletal system.[34] Although any skeletal injury can be associated with physical abuse, rib fractures had the highest probability for abuse, followed by humeral, femoral, and skull fractures for a particular

Table 3

Specificity of Radiographic and Injury Findings

Specificity	Injury
High	Classic metaphyseal lesions Rib fractures, especially posterior Scapular process fractures Spinous process fractures Sternal fractures
Moderate	Multiple fractures, especially bilateral Fractures of different ages Epiphyseal separations Vertebral body fractures and subluxations Digital fractures Complex skull fractures Pelvic fractures
Low	Subperiosteal new bone formation Clavicular fractures Long-bone shaft fractures Linear skull fractures

Reproduced with permission from Kleinman PK, Rosenberg AE, Tsai A: Skeletal trauma: General considerations, in Kleinman PK, ed: *Diagnostic Imaging of Child Abuse*, ed 3. New York, NY, Cambridge University Press, 2015, pp 23-52.

developmental stage.[34]

Femoral Fractures

Fractures of the femur occur in association with both accidental and nonaccidental trauma. In general, a child younger than 18 months with a femoral fracture has a 1:3 to 1:4 chance of having been the victim of physical abuse. Femoral fractures in nonaccidental trauma occur more commonly in children who are nonambulatory.[34,35] In a single institution study in 2011, researchers found that among children with femoral fractures, evidence (physical and/or radiographic) of a prior injury, and being younger than 18 months were risk factors for abuse.[36]

Diaphyseal fractures of the femur can be nondisplaced, transverse, spiral, oblique, or comminuted, but no single fracture pattern is pathognomonic for abuse.[37] Using a fracture ratio, which is calculated by measuring the length of the fracture and dividing it by the diameter of the bone, researchers found that patients with nonaccidental trauma had femoral fractures with lower mean anteroposterior fracture ratios (that is, the fractures were more transverse).[38] As recommended in the American Academy of Orthopaedic Surgeons clinical practice guideline on the treatment of pediatric diaphyseal femur fractures, children younger than 3 years with a femoral fracture should be evaluated for the possibility of physical abuse.[39]

Humeral Fractures

In approximately 50% of children younger than 3 years who have a humeral fracture, the fracture is associated with physical abuse.[30] Fractures of the humeral shaft are more common in abuse, whereas supracondylar humerus fractures are more commonly seen with accidental trauma; however, supracondylar humerus and transphyseal distal humerus fractures also can occur in abuse situations.[40-42] In a single institution study in 2010, researchers found that a history suspicious for abuse, evidence (physical and/or radiographic) of a prior injury, and being younger than 18 months were the strongest predictors of child abuse in children with humeral fractures.[43]

Classic Metaphyseal Lesions

Classic metaphyseal lesions, also called corner fractures or bucket-handle fractures, were initially described by John Caffey but later explained in great detail by pediatric radiologist Paul Kleinman in his radiologic-histopathologic study in 1986.[6,23,44] These fractures carry a high specificity for abuse. The injury pattern is a transmetaphyseal fracture through the primary spongiosa and often is the result of a violent shake of the limbs or the trunk.[30] The resulting fractured disk of bone and calcified cartilage then appears as a corner fracture or a bucket-handle fracture based on the projection of the radiograph[45] (**Figures 1** and **2**).

Differential Diagnosis

In children with unexplained fractures, physical abuse remains a probable differential diagnosis; however, alternative diagnoses need to be considered. Osteogenesis imperfecta is the most commonly occurring diagnosis that is confused with nonaccidental trauma, especially in children with mild phenotypes and uncertain injury histories. Misdiagnosis can lead to unnecessary emotional, social, and financial distress for the families of such children.[46] Genetic bone disorders such as metaphyseal dysplasias, metabolic bone diseases such as vitamin D–deficient rickets, vitamin or mineral deficiencies such as scurvy or copper deficiency, disuse osteopenia, prematurity, osteomyelitis, and other systemic medical conditions also have been reported in children being evaluated for suspected abuse and can be further evaluated with laboratory or DNA analysis of a blood sample.[18,47]

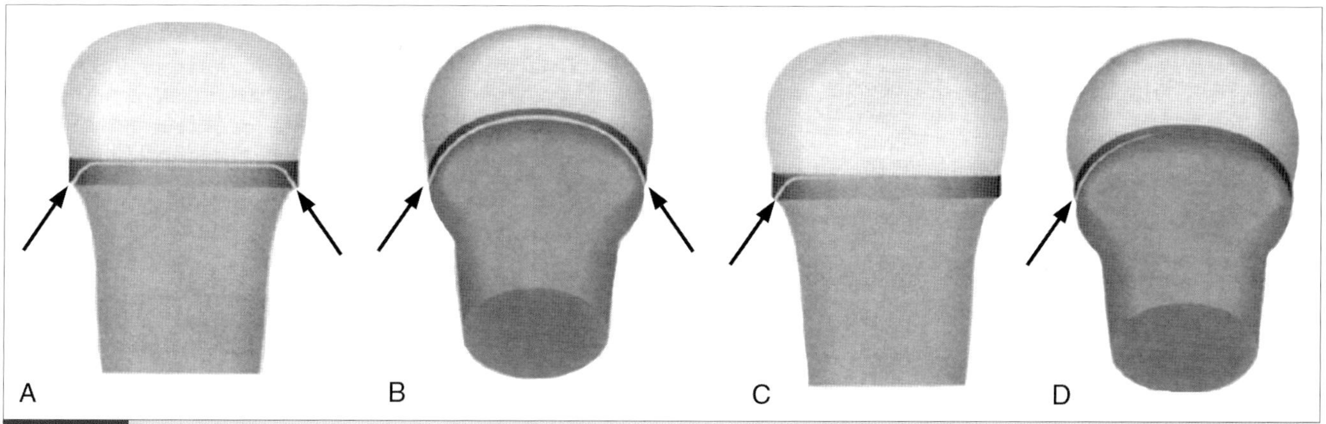

Figure 1 Diagrammatic representation of the relationship of the subperiosteal bone collar to a metaphyseal lesion. **A,** A tangential view of the metaphyseal margin shows a fracture line (arrows) that extends adjacent to the chondro-osseous junction centrally. Peripherally, the fracture line veers away from the growth plate to undermine a larger peripheral fragment incorporating the subperiosteal bone collar. **B,** When the fracture line (arrows) is projected obliquely, the thicker peripheral fragment, including the subperiosteal bone collar, is projected as a curvilinear fragment or a bucket-handle lesion. **C,** When the fracture line (arrow) is incomplete (it extends across only a portion of the metaphysis), the appearance suggests a focal, triangularly-shaped peripheral fragment encompassing the subperiosteal bone collar. **D,** When the fracture line (arrow) is tipped obliquely, the peripheral margin of the fragment is projected as a curvilinear density. (Reproduced with permission from Kleinman PK, Marks SC Jr: Relationship of the subperiosteal bone collar to metaphyseal lesions in abused infants. *J Bone Joint Surg Am* 1995;77[10]:1471-1476.)

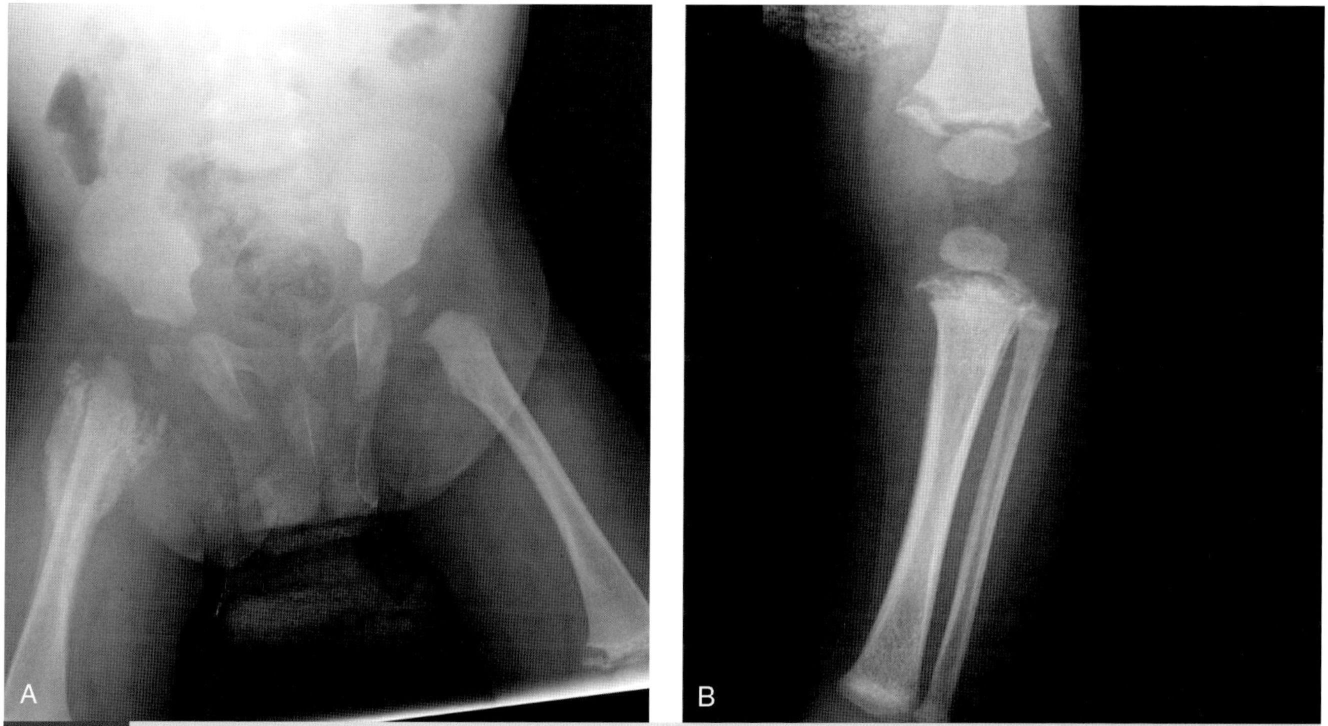

Figure 2 Radiographs from a 6-month-old male infant with multiple fractures caused by nonaccidental trauma. AP radiographs show a left proximal femoral fracture (**A**) and distal femoral and proximal tibial classic metaphyseal lesions (**B**). (Courtesy of Brian K. Brighton, MD, MPH, Charlotte, NC.)

7: Trauma

Management of Abuse

After a diagnosis of physical abuse has been made or if abuse is suspected, the orthopaedic surgeon must not only be involved with the management of the child's injuries but also must engage in ongoing evaluations with the multidisciplinary child maltreatment team. Orthopaedic management of many injuries associated with abuse is nonsurgical and includes splints or casts. Displaced fractures, such as displaced femoral fractures, may require closed reduction and casting.

Suspected cases of child abuse must be reported to the appropriate state or local child protective service agencies. The diagnosis of abuse often carries substantial social and legal implications in addition to the medical issues. Initiating a report of abuse must be nonjudgmental and presented as the standard of care. Clear and detailed documentation of the injuries and management within the medical record is extremely important in the event the surgeon is asked to participate in later legal proceedings.[48]

Summary

Orthopaedic surgeons play a critical role in the evaluation, management, and coordination of care of a child who is the victim of child abuse and suspected nonaccidental trauma. The physician must evaluate and treat the child's injuries in the context of the history and mechanism of injury and obtain additional imaging studies (such as a skeletal survey) if indicated. In addition, if abuse is suspected, involvement of a multidisciplinary child maltreatment prevention team is necessary.

Key Study Points

- Fractures are the second most common injury related to the physical abuse of children.
- Numerous risk factors exist for child abuse, including young age of the child, parental factors (such a single marital status and poor coping skills), and environmental factors (such as low socioeconomic status). However, physical abuse can affect children of all ages, ethnicities, and socioeconomic groups.
- Although any skeletal injury can be associated with physical abuse, certain fractures, such as rib and metaphyseal corner fractures, are highly specific for child abuse.
- Suspicion for physical abuse mandates physician reporting to the appropriate services and should initiate a multidisciplinary approach to the management of these patients.

Annotated References

1. Altemeier WA III, O'Connor S, Vietze PM, Sandler HM, Sherrod KB: Antecedents of child abuse. *J Pediatr* 1982;100(5):823-829.

2. Sibert JR, Payne EH, Kemp AM, et al: The incidence of severe physical child abuse in Wales. *Child Abuse Negl* 2002;26(3):267-276.

3. Loder RT, Feinberg JR: Orthopaedic injuries in children with nonaccidental trauma: Demographics and incidence from the 2000 kids' inpatient database. *J Pediatr Orthop* 2007;27(4):421-426.

4. McMahon P, Grossman W, Gaffney M, Stanitski C: Soft-tissue injury as an indication of child abuse. *J Bone Joint Surg Am* 1995;77(8):1179-1183.

5. Tenenbaum S, Thein R, Herman A, et al: Pediatric nonaccidental injury: Are orthopedic surgeons vigilant enough? *J Pediatr Orthop* 2013;33(2):145-151.

   Using a survey, the authors evaluated the level of knowledge that orthopaedic surgeons have regarding pediatric nonaccidental injury, including common practices and reporting attitudes. Only 35% of orthopaedic surgeons had specific and targeted training with respect to child abuse. More experienced physicians had lesser awareness but tended to further investigate cases with suspected nonaccidental injury. Level of evidence: III.

6. Caffey J: Multiple fractures in the long bones of infants suffering from chronic subdural hematoma. *Am J Roentgenol Radium Ther* 1946;56(2):163-173.

7. Kempe CH, Silverman FN, Steele BF, Droegemueller W, Silver HK: The battered-child syndrome. *JAMA* 1962;181(1):17-24.

8. The Child Abuse Prevention and Treatment Act (CAPTA) Reauthorization Act of 2010, P.L. 111-320 (42 USC and 5106a). Available at: http://www.acf.hhs.gov/programs/cb/laws_policies/cblaws/capta/capta2010.pdf. Accessed January 24, 2016.

9. Wu SS, Ma CX, Carter RL, et al: Risk factors for infant maltreatment: A population-based study. *Child Abuse Negl* 2004;28(12):1253-1264.

10. Coffey C, Haley K, Hayes J, Groner JI: The risk of child abuse in infants and toddlers with lower extremity injuries. *J Pediatr Surg* 2005;40(1):120-123.

11. Pandya NK, Baldwin K, Wolfgruber H, Christian CW, Drummond DS, Hosalkar HS: Child abuse and orthopaedic injury patterns: Analysis at a level I pediatric trauma center. *J Pediatr Orthop* 2009;29(6):618-625.

12. Sullivan PM, Knutson JF: Maltreatment and disabilities: A population-based epidemiological study. *Child Abuse Negl* 2000;24(10):1257-1273.

13. Oates RK, Davis AA, Ryan MG: Predictive factors for child abuse. *Aust Paediatr J* 1980;16(4):239-243.

14. Kelleher K, Chaffin M, Hollenberg J, Fischer E: Alcohol and drug disorders among physically abusive and neglectful parents in a community-based sample. *Am J Public Health* 1994;84(10):1586-1590.

15. Sedlak AJ, Mettenburg J, Basena M, et al: *Fourth National Incidence Study of Child Abuse and Neglect (NIS–4): Report to Congress.* Washington, DC, US Department of Health and Human Services, Administration for Children and Families, 2010.

16. Starling SP, Sirotnak AP, Heisler KW, Barnes-Eley ML: Inflicted skeletal trauma: The relationship of perpetrators to their victims. *Child Abuse Negl* 2007;31(9):993-999.

17. Christian CW; Committee on Child Abuse and Neglect, American Academy of Pediatrics: The evaluation of suspected child physical abuse. *Pediatrics* 2015;135(5):e1337-e1354.

    This clinical report provides guidance for the evaluation of suspected physical child abuse and discusses the role of the physician in diagnosing, reporting, and managing child abuse. Level of evidence: V.

18. Flaherty EG, Perez-Rossello JM, Levine MA, et al: Evaluating children with fractures for child physical abuse. *Pediatrics* 2014;133(2):e477-e489.

    This report is aimed at updating physicians in the appropriate evaluation and considerations when assessing a child with fractures from suspected abuse. Level of evidence: V.

19. Kemp AM, Maguire SA, Nuttall D, Collins P, Dunstan F: Bruising in children who are assessed for suspected physical abuse. *Arch Dis Child* 2014;99(2):108-113.

    Bruising of the buttocks, genitalia, face, trunk, upper arms, and front of the thighs was found to be more common in cases of suspected physical abuse. Petechia, or bruises with distinct patterns, and bruises in clusters were more likely in suspected abuse cases. Level of evidence: III.

20. Fassier A, Gaucherand P, Kohler R: Fractures in children younger than 18 months. *Orthop Traumatol Surg Res* 2013;99(1suppl):S160-S170.

    This review article discusses the circumstances that can cause fractures in infants and toddlers younger than 18 months as well as the management of these patients. Level of evidence: V.

21. American College of Radiology: ACR–SPR practice parameter for skeletal surveys in children. 2014. Available at: http://www.acr.org/~/media/ACR/Documents/PGTS/guidelines/Skeletal_Surveys.pdf. Accessed January 23, 2016.

    This updated practice parameter by the American College of Radiology and the Society for Pediatric Radiology outlines the goals, indications, and specifications for skeletal surveys of children and infants. Level of evidence: V.

22. Barber I, Perez-Rossello JM, Wilson CR, Kleinman PK: The yield of high-detail radiographic skeletal surveys in suspected infant abuse. *Pediatr Radiol* 2015;45(1):69-80.

    Using high-detail American College of Radiology standardized skeletal surveys that were performed for suspected abuse, 20% of the cases of suspected abuse were found to have unsuspected fractures on a skeletal survey. Level of evidence: III.

23. Kleinman PK, Nimkin K, Spevak MR, et al: Follow-up skeletal surveys in suspected child abuse. *AJR Am J Roentgenol* 1996;167(4):893-896.

24. Dwek JR: The radiographic approach to child abuse. *Clin Orthop Relat Res* 2011;469(3):776-789.

    Injuries have various specificities for abuse. A review of radiographic imaging of the more characteristic injuries related to abuse was performed. In addition, fracture healing and its correlation to radiographic findings was reviewed. Level of evidence: V.

25. Shaahinfar A, Whitelaw KD, Mansour KM: Update on abusive head trauma. *Curr Opin Pediatr* 2015;27(3):308-314.

    The authors present a review of clinical and imaging findings to aid in distinguishing accidental versus abusive head trauma. Level of evidence: V.

26. Kemp AM, Joshi AH, Mann M, et al: What are the clinical and radiological characteristics of spinal injuries from physical abuse: A systematic review. *Arch Dis Child* 2010;95(5):355-360.

27. Kadom N, Khademian Z, Vezina G, Shalaby-Rana E, Rice A, Hinds T: Usefulness of MRI detection of cervical spine and brain injuries in the evaluation of abusive head trauma. *Pediatr Radiol* 2014;44(7):839-848.

    This retrospective review of abusive head trauma demonstrated a 36% rate of associated cervical spine injuries and a high association with hypoxic-ischemic injuries. The authors suggest considering MRI of the brain and cervical spine in patients with suspected abusive head trauma. Level of evidence: IV.

28. Choudhary AK, Bradford RK, Dias MS, Moore GJ, Boal DK: Spinal subdural hemorrhage in abusive head trauma: A retrospective study. *Radiology* 2012;262(1):216-223.

    The authors describe a retrospective case-controlled study of patients with abusive head trauma and report an association with spinal subdural bleeding in the abusive head trauma cohort. Level of evidence: III.

29. Knox J, Schneider J, Wimberly RL, Riccio AI: Characteristics of spinal injuries secondary to nonaccidental trauma. *J Pediatr Orthop* 2014;34(4):376-381.

    This retrospective review identified nonaccidental trauma as a cause for spinal injuries in children, especially those younger than 2 years. The authors emphasize the importance of evaluating associated injuries outside the spine, multilevel injuries to the spine, and associated neurologic deficits. Level of evidence: IV.

30. Sink EL, Hyman JE, Matheny T, Georgopoulos G, Kleinman P: Child abuse: The role of the orthopaedic surgeon in nonaccidental trauma. *Clin Orthop Relat Res* 2011;469(3):790-797.

This article reviews the orthopaedic surgeon's role in recognizing and managing children who have been abused. Level of evidence: V.

31. Bainbridge JK, Huey BM, Harrison SK: Should bone scintigraphy be used as a routine adjunct to skeletal survey in the imaging of non-accidental injury? A 10 year review of reports in a single centre. *Clin Radiol* 2015;70(8):e83-e89.

In a 10-year period, 166 patients with both bone scans and skeletal surveys were reviewed. The addition of bone scans to the skeletal survey increased the confidence in radiographic findings. Occult injuries were identified with bone scans in 28 of 237 patients (12%) who were imaged. Level of evidence: III.

32. Perez-Rossello JM, Connolly SA, Newton AW, Zou KH, Kleinman PK: Whole-body MRI in suspected infant abuse. *AJR Am J Roentgenol* 2010;195(3):744-750.

33. Ravichandiran N, Schuh S, Bejuk M, et al: Delayed identification of pediatric abuse-related fractures. *Pediatrics* 2010;125(1):60-66.

34. Kemp AM, Dunstan F, Harrison S, et al: Patterns of skeletal fractures in child abuse: Systematic review. *BMJ* 2008;337:a1518.

35. Schwend RM, Werth C, Johnston A: Femur shaft fractures in toddlers and young children: Rarely from child abuse. *J Pediatr Orthop* 2000;20(4):475-481.

36. Baldwin K, Pandya NK, Wolfgruber H, Drummond DS, Hosalkar HS: Femur fractures in the pediatric population: Abuse or accidental trauma? *Clin Orthop Relat Res* 2011;469(3):798-804.

Seventy cases of femoral fractures resulting from abuse were compared with 139 patients with femoral fractures resulting from accidental trauma. Victims of abuse are generally younger than those with accidental trauma. Risk factors for femoral fracture from abuse were a history suspicious for abuse, prior physical or radiographic evidence of injury, and age younger than 18 months. Level of evidence: III.

37. Scherl SA, Miller L, Lively N, Russinoff S, Sullivan CM, Tornetta P III: Accidental and nonaccidental femur fractures in children. *Clin Orthop Relat Res* 2000;376:96-105.

38. Murphy R, Kelly DM, Moisan A, et al: Transverse fractures of the femoral shaft are a better predictor of nonaccidental trauma in young children than spiral fractures are. *J Bone Joint Surg Am* 2015;97(2):106-111.

The femur fracture ratio is an objective measure that can be used to evaluate children with femur fractures and suspected nonaccidental trauma. Level of evidence: III.

39. Kocher MS, Sink EL, Blasier RD, et al; American Academy of Orthopaedic Surgeons: American Academy of Orthopaedic Surgeons clinical practice guideline on treatment of pediatric diaphyseal femur fracture. *J Bone Joint Surg Am* 2010;92(8):1790-1792.

40. Gilbert SR, Conklin MJ: Presentation of distal humerus physeal separation. *Pediatr Emerg Care* 2007;23(11):816-819.

41. Strait RT, Siegel RM, Shapiro RA: Humeral fractures without obvious etiologies in children less than 3 years of age: When is it abuse? *Pediatrics* 1995;96(4 pt 1):667-671.

42. Shaw BA, Murphy KM, Shaw A, Oppenheim WL, Myracle MR: Humerus shaft fractures in young children: Accident or abuse? *J Pediatr Orthop* 1997;17(3):293-297.

43. Pandya NK, Baldwin KD, Wolfgruber H, Drummond DS, Hosalkar HS: Humerus fractures in the pediatric population: An algorithm to identify abuse. *J Pediatr Orthop B* 2010;19(6):535-541.

44. Caffey J: Some traumatic lesions in growing bones other than fractures and dislocations: Clinical and radiological features. The Mackenzie Davidson Memorial Lecture. *Br J Radiol* 1957;30(353):225-238.

45. Kleinman PK, Marks SC Jr: Relationship of the subperiosteal bone collar to metaphyseal lesions in abused infants. *J Bone Joint Surg Am* 1995;77(10):1471-1476.

46. Singh-Kocher M, Dichtel L: Osteogenesis imperfecta misdiagnosed as child abuse. *J Pediatr Orthop B* 2011;20(6):440-443.

The purpose of this study was to review the experience of families of 33 patients in which osteogenesis imperfecta was misdiagnosed as child abuse. The article highlights the clinical, radiographic, and family history features associated with this genetic disorder. Level of evidence: IV.

47. Pandya NK, Baldwin K, Kamath AF, Wenger DR, Hosalkar HS: Unexplained fractures: Child abuse or bone disease? A systematic review. *Clin Orthop Relat Res* 2011;469(3):805-812.

A systematic review of the literature found that injury caused by osteogenesis imperfecta is most frequently confused with nonaccidental trauma. Other genetic disorders, including metaphyseal dysplasia, disorders of phosphate metabolism, and temporary brittle bone disease, also have been reported as child abuse. Level of evidence: III.

48. Sullivan CM: Child abuse and the legal system: The orthopaedic surgeon's role in diagnosis. *Clin Orthop Relat Res* 2011;469(3):768-775.

The role of the orthopaedic surgeon often extends beyond the victim of child abuse and requires involvement with a multidisciplinary hospital-based team as well as coordination with social services and occasionally legal teams. Level of evidence: V.

Chapter 36

Shoulder, Humerus, and Elbow

David Lazarus, MD   Eric W. Edmonds, MD

Abstract

In the pediatric population, upper extremity trauma, particularly of the upper arm and elbow, is very common. Familiarity with specific injuries and a review of updates in the literature within the past 5 years pertaining to injuries about the clavicle, shoulder, humerus, and elbow will aid orthopaedic surgeons in caring for young patients with upper extremity traumatic injuries.

Keywords: clavicle dislocation; clavicle fracture; elbow fracture; shoulder management; shoulder trauma

Introduction

Pediatric injuries involving the shoulder and the elbow are common, with treatments that include both nonsurgical options and surgical interventions.[1] As with many childhood injuries, most can be managed without surgery or with minimally invasive procedures, such as closed reduction and percutaneous pinning. When planning the treatment program, it is critical to avoid complications such as deformity, physeal injury, and motion restriction. Despite the trend for referral of pediatric trauma to a children's hospital with specialized pediatric orthopaedic care, the general orthopaedic surgeon should be knowledgeable of pediatric injuries to decide on the appropriate management, whether primary treatment or referral.

Dr. Edmonds or an immediate family member serves as a board member, owner, officer, or committee member of the American Orthopaedic Society for Sports Medicine and the Pediatric Orthopaedic Society of North America. Neither Dr. Lazarus nor any immediate family member has received anything of value from or has stock or stock options held in a commercial company or institution related directly or indirectly to the subject of this chapter.

Shoulder

Sternoclavicular Dislocations

The sternoclavicular (SC) joint is unique in that the medial clavicle is the last long bone to ossify, and the epiphysis is the last to fuse. This makes a true SC dislocation difficult to differentiate from a medial physeal fracture in both children and adolescents, although the treatment may be similar for both injury patterns. Because of robust ligamentous support about the joint, SC dislocations are high-energy injuries. Much of the literature is focused on posterior dislocations because they place the mediastinal structures at risk, even though anterior SC dislocations are more common. A recent meta-analysis demonstrated that 71% of adolescent posterior SC dislocations occurred during sporting activities.[2] Serendipity radiographs or CT scans can help delineate the position of the medial clavicle. Unstable injuries with clavicular impingement on vital mediastinal structures should be reduced, with cardiothoracic surgery services aware and immediately available during the procedure. A 2014 retrospective review highlighted that only 8 of 22 posterior SC dislocations had successful closed reductions, and 86% of the unsuccessful cases were true dislocations versus medial clavicle physeal injuries. Moreover, all the successful closed reductions occurred within 24 hours of injury.[3] After open reduction, suture repair of capsular and ligamentous tissue may be necessary to maintain the clavicle in appropriate alignment during healing; however, reports of ligamentous reconstruction have appeared for patients with both acute and chronic injuries.

Clavicle Fractures

The spectrum of pediatric clavicle fractures ranges from the neonate with birth trauma to the adolescent with a sports injury, and these fractures carry different associated risks and treatment algorithms. Clavicle fractures secondary to birth trauma are associated with larger newborns, shoulder dystocia, and brachial plexus injuries. In an infant or a toddler with a suspected clavicle fracture, the differential diagnosis also includes osteomyelitis, septic shoulder, proximal humerus fracture, and, especially, brachial plexus injury if the child is unable to move his or her arm. Nonaccidental trauma must always be considered in the toddler with a clavicle fracture, especially when the lateral aspect is involved.[4] It may be difficult to determine the point of tenderness in young patients, even when it is evident that pain involving some aspect of the upper extremity is present. Radiographs or ultrasonography can be used to aid in the diagnosis. As with many other pediatric fractures, this injury will heal quickly. In infants, Velpeau splinting with an elastic bandage around the arm or pinning the sleeve at the wrist of the ipsilateral arm to the shirt can relieve pain and caretaker concern during the acute healing phase. Pseudarthrosis of the clavicle should be considered in a nontender presumed clavicle fracture if the radiographic appearance does not suggest an acute fracture with smooth bone ends. This diagnosis is most commonly seen in the diaphysis of the right clavicle.

In older cohorts, the diaphysis is the most common location for traumatic pediatric clavicle fractures. These fractures are classified based on location. Nonsurgical treatment continues to be the mainstay of treatment of all fractures, using a sling or figure-of-8 brace for 4 to 6 weeks. Although enthusiasm exists for the surgical treatment of displaced fractures based on adult biology and literature, increasing evidence supports historically validated nonsurgical management. A 2013 evaluation of nonsurgically treated, displaced clavicle fractures in adolescents demonstrated no differences in pain, strength, range of motion, or subjective function compared with the uninjured limb at 2 years after injury.[5]

A recent meta-analysis of randomized trials comparing surgery with no surgery showed that surgical treatment predictably led to a lower rate of nonunion and symptomatic malunion for adult clavicle fractures than nonsurgical management in patients 16 years and older. The study did show that the few existing randomized studies failed to demonstrate that long-term outcomes favored one method of treatment—either surgical or nonsurgical.[6] Regardless of these findings, increased numbers of pediatric clavicle fractures are being surgically treated, with one study of a public database showing an increase of nearly double from 2007 to 2011, mostly in the cohort aged 15 to 19 years.[7]

Because of the risk for symptomatic malunion, some surgeons prefer open reduction and internal fixation (ORIF) for displaced clavicle fractures in adolescents. A 2013 study that evaluated 16 clavicle fractures with more than 2 cm of displacement reported that those treated nonsurgically all went on to heal with radiographic malunion. Although the authors discovered that forward flexion and abduction were decreased compared with the contralateral side, they concurrently noted that no clinically significant differences in shoulder strength or functional outcomes were present.[8]

The midshaft, displaced, shortened clavicle fracture is the debated pattern discussed in the aforementioned studies. The current literature presents evidence to recommend either sling or surgery, unless absolute surgical indications are present, including open fracture or skin compromise. Surgical intervention may reduce the risk of union-related complications, but it is associated with other complications, including infection, implant complications, and neurovascular injury. Implant issues can and often require another surgical procedure for removal, which must be discussed in advance with the family.

ORIF with plates and screws, with or without a lag screw, is the most common form of surgical intervention, but intramedullary devices also can be considered. Precontoured plates are available to aid in decreasing the prominence of the plate on the curvy silhouette of the clavicle. Elastic intramedullary nails also can be successfully used in children and allow for earlier mobilization—similar to plates and screws.

Acromioclavicular Joint Injuries

The acromioclavicular (AC) joint has robust support with the AC ligaments and prevents anterior-posterior translation of the clavicle; the coracoclavicular ligament prevents superior migration of the lateral clavicle. The coracoclavicular ligamentous complex includes the conoid and the trapezoid ligament, from medial to lateral, respectively. Injury to the AC joint often occurs from a direct blow to the shoulder, resulting in either a true AC separation or a lateral clavicle physeal fracture. The lateral clavicle remains a cartilaginous structure until approximately age 20 years. AC injuries are seen more in contact athletes (and therefore are more common in males) and are more common at higher levels of play (more injuries occur in collegiate-level sports than intramural sports). Low-grade injuries have a mean loss of time from sports participation of approximately 10 days.[9] Radiographs are used for diagnosis, and contralateral AP radiographs are helpful when the diagnosis is questionable.

The Rockwood classification is widely used when discussing AC injuries (**Figure 1**). Classic teaching was that low-grade injuries (types I, II, and III) were treated nonsurgically, whereas high-grade injuries (types IV, V, and VI) were treated surgically. Currently, many type III injuries are considered for surgery, especially in the setting of failed nonsurgical management. A recent epidemiologic study demonstrated that 89% of AC injuries are low-grade types I and II. Rest and sling immobilization are the mainstays of treatment for low-grade AC injuries, with early rehabilitation including range-of-motion exercises

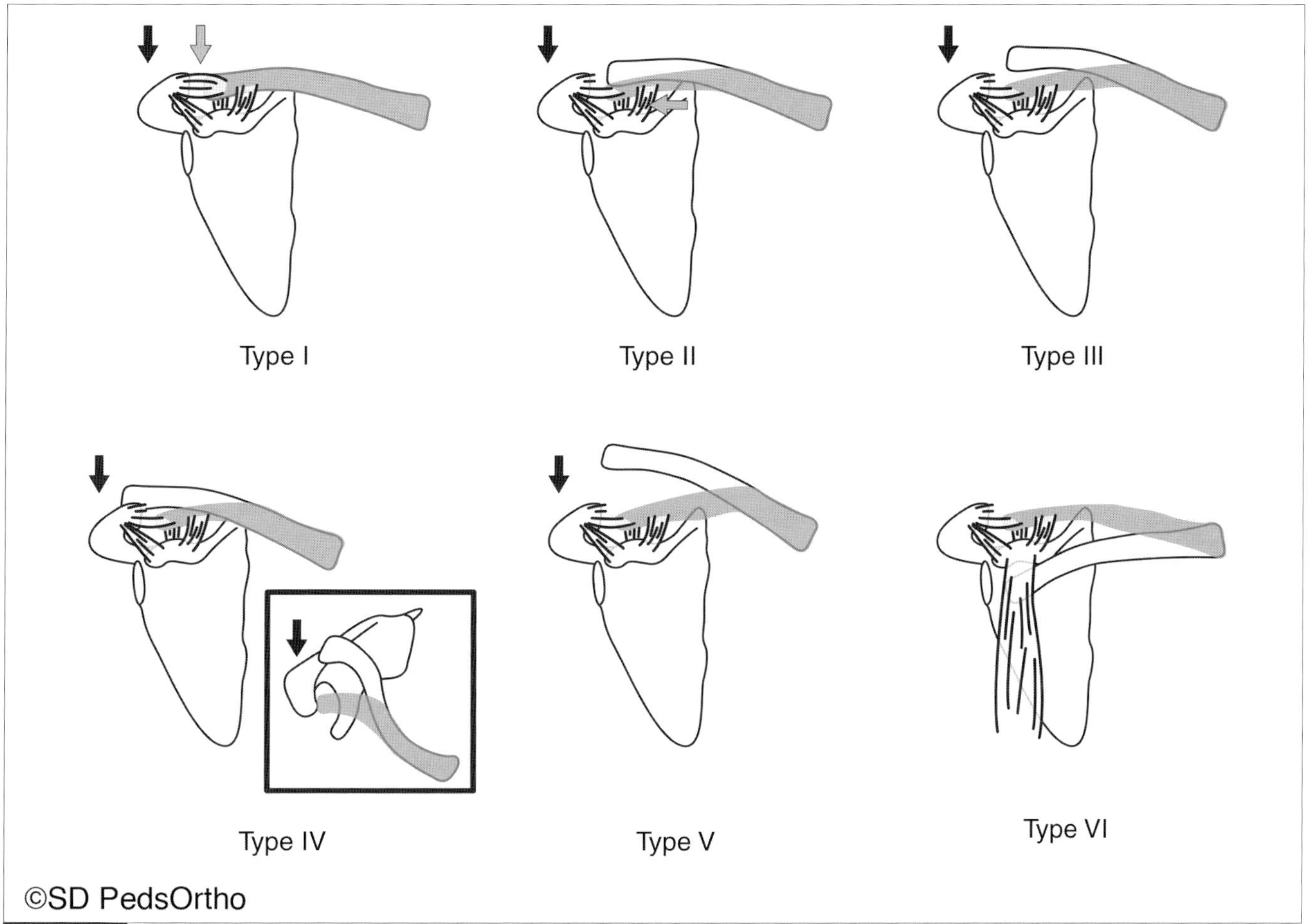

Figure 1 Illustration of the Rockwood classification of acromioclavicular (AC) joint injuries. **A,** Type I, AC ligament sprain. **B,** Type II, AC ligament tear. Coracoclavicular ligaments intact but stretched. **C,** Type III, AC and coracoclavicular ligament torn and displacement of the AC joint of 100% or less. **D,** Type IV, lateral clavicle displaced posteriorly, possibly through the trapezius muscle. **E,** Type V, more than 100% displacement superiorly, may rupture through the deltotrapezial fascia. **F,** Type VI, inferior displacement of the lateral clavicle. (Copyright James Bomar, San Diego Pediatric Orthopedics, San Diego, CA.)

and shoulder strengthening to maximize return to sports. For high-grade injuries, screw fixation from the clavicle to the coracoid, ligament reconstruction, or a hook plate construct are all options discussed in the literature. The hook plate requires a second surgical procedure for removal. A recent systematic review for AC injury treatment proved that no consensus exists on a specific surgical intervention, and no true agreed on treatment exists for the debated type III injury.[10] Individualization of treatment is recommended, with most patients receiving a trial of nonsurgical management before surgery is considered. AC joint injuries need high-quality research to help delineate the proper treatment of individual fracture types.

Shoulder Dislocations

The physis is a weak spot in the shoulder, thus making pediatric shoulder dislocations less common; however, pediatric shoulder dislocations do occur and can be recognized with proper imaging. Twenty percent of all shoulder dislocations occur in patients younger than 20 years, and they are more common in adolescents who participate in competitive contact sports, with most of the dislocations being anterior or anteroinferior. As expected, a prospective study demonstrated that the incidence is much higher in males (86.5%) than in females (13.5%).[11]

Radiographs are used for diagnosis and reduction confirmation. The AP, scapular Y, and axillary views are critical for evaluating the shoulder. Secondary to pain and the occasional difficulty of an adequate axillary view, a Velpeau radiograph can be taken with minimal shoulder manipulation to confirm proper reduction (**Figure 2**). To evaluate for any bony lesions, the Westpoint view allows glenoid examination, and the Stryker notch view helps identify a Hill-Sachs lesion. An MRI or a magnetic

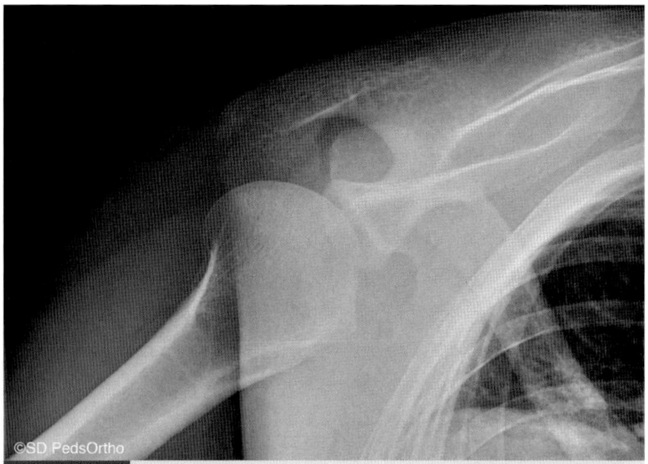

Figure 2 Lateral Velpeau radiographic view confirms a reduced glenohumeral joint. (Copyright James Bomar, San Diego Pediatric Orthopedics, San Diego, CA.)

resonance arthrogram is recommended for dislocations in younger patients to identify soft-tissue injuries that might make the shoulder prone to recurrent dislocations.

The natural history of shoulder dislocations has been well studied. The reported risk for recurrence in this younger cohort appears to be quite variable, yet previous studies have consistently demonstrated that young patients with shoulder dislocations have a higher chance of dislocating the shoulder again. Of 133 patients aged 13 to 18 years, the recurrence rate was 76.7%. In an evaluation of the survival of the shoulder reduction, 59% of reductions were intact at 1 year, but only 38% were without recurrence at 2 years, with decreasing numbers on the curve with time from the index event.[11] An epidemiologic study of shoulder dislocations in Canada in patients aged 10 to 16 years reported an overall recurrence rate of 38.2% at a mean of 10 months after the initial injury, although the authors of the study noted that the recurrence rate was lower in patients aged 10 to 13 years than in patients aged 14 to 16 years.[12]

After closed reduction, it is important to document a neurovascular examination because the axillary nerve is most commonly injured. Even if MRI shows mild pathology, nonsurgical treatment often is still recommended for the first traumatic shoulder dislocation, with a short period of sling immobilization followed by physical therapy. If a recurrent dislocation occurs, then the recommendations universally shift to surgical treatment, particularly if a large Hill-Sachs lesion, a Bankart tear, or a labral tear is present. The purpose of surgery is to prevent recurrence.

Arthroscopy is a good option if available and can be very successful in treating a traumatic shoulder dislocation in an adolescent with a minimal risk of complications.[13,14] At 27-month follow-up, the overall return to sports was 87% after arthroscopic labral repair for anterior instability and 69% for achieving a preinjury level of performance.[15] However, despite the ability to return to full activities, adolescents treated with either an arthroscopic or an open Bankart repair for instability had a 5-year shoulder survival rate of 49%.[16] Moreover, adolescent patients who later had revision surgery after failure of the primary repair demonstrated a rate of 33% repeat failure after the revision surgery.[17] This is clearly an age cohort and pathology that requires further investigation to optimize treatment outcomes.

Humerus

Proximal Humerus Fractures

Similar to clavicle fractures, proximal humerus fractures in children can range from birth trauma in the newborn to nonaccidental trauma in older children and sports injuries in adolescents. As with suspected clavicle injuries, surgeons must always be aware of differential diagnoses, including a septic joint. Because the proximal humeral physis contributes approximately 80% of the bone growth, the remodeling potential for fractures is excellent, but the risk for disruptive growth is greater with fractures that directly involve the physis. Fractures in newborns will heal quickly with a simple Velpeau splint applied for 2 weeks using an elastic wrap to secure the arm to the torso. In older children, a sling and swathe will suffice.

The Neer and Horowitz classification is commonly used for pediatric proximal humerus fractures. These fractures often involve the physis and can be classified with the Salter-Harris classification system, with types I and II being the most common. The capsule on the medial side attaches beyond the physis onto the metaphysis, which may lead to a Salter-Harris type II fracture pattern, which often is seen with the medial metaphysis still attached to the proximal piece.[18] Neer and Horowitz type I and II fractures can almost universally be treated nonsurgically, unless an open fracture or a neurovascular injury is present. Patient age and growth remaining are very important factors. In those with substantial growth remaining, larger deformities will have time for remodeling. The treatment of displaced fractures in older children and adolescents should be individualized, including surgical considerations. Although there is much literature focused on the proximal humerus, no evidence-based algorithm is available for treatment. Neer and Horowitz type III and IV fractures are commonly considered surgical fractures in children older than 10 years because displacement will have a low remodeling potential in this age group. A recent study comparing nonsurgical to surgical treatment of Neer and Horowitz type III and IV fractures in patients who are skeletally mature demonstrated no differences in complications, rate of return to full activity, or functional outcome.[19] However, the authors identified a trend for less desirable outcomes in children older than 12 years who were treated nonsurgically.

Multiple surgical options depend on proper reduction and maintenance of alignment. Whether closed or open reduction is obtained, stabilizing the fracture with either Kirschner wires (K-wires), cannulated screws, intramedullary nails, or plates and screws is necessary. K-wires are relatively easy to use when closed reduction is amenable, but there must be concern for the branches of the axillary nerve. K-wires may extend from the skin or be buried, although the complication rate of leaving them exposed is approximately 55%, whereas the treatment expense substantially increases when a second surgical procedure is required to remove buried pins.[20] Intramedullary nails can be used with a lower complication rate and achieve outcomes similar to those with percutaneous fixation but may involve a longer surgery time as well as a second surgical procedure for implant removal.[21]

As with any fracture, critical evaluation of the radiographic findings is important. Proximal humerus fractures often are associated with a pathologic lesion, most commonly unicameral bone cysts. Risks of fracture include greater than 85% involvement of the bone or a cyst wall less than 0.5 mm. In a study of 68 humeral unicameral bone cysts, 94% exhibited a fracture.[22] Overall, the goal is healing of the fracture followed by treatment of the cyst, as appropriate.

Elbow

Supracondylar Humerus Fractures

Supracondylar humerus fractures are the most common type of elbow fracture encountered in the pediatric patient. Most occur in children younger than 10 years who fall onto an outstretched hand. More than 90% of these fractures are the extension type commonly referred to in the Gartland classification. Flexion types are less common but are important to recognize because difficulty in closed reduction may require open exploration to confirm that the ulnar nerve is not entrapped. Extension-type fractures are classified based on their degree of posterior displacement, with partially and completely displaced accounting for type II and III fractures, respectively. Nondisplaced or minimally displaced type I fractures can be treated in a cast if the anterior humeral line intersects the capitellum and no coronal malalignment is present. On a lateral radiograph, the anterior humeral line should touch the capitellar ossific nucleus in patients of all ages. In patients age 5 years or older, the anterior humeral line should pass through the center third of the capitellum.[23] Percutaneous pin fixation is required for type II and III fractures to maintain anatomic alignment because the distal humerus has little inherent remodeling potential. This allows casting in less than 90° of flexion to reduce the risk of Volkmann ischemia.

With obesity becoming an epidemic in the United States, a recent study reported that children with supracondylar fractures who also are obese have injuries that are more complex, with more frequent perioperative nerve palsies and a greater number of surgical complications.[24] A study looking at nonsurgically treated, unreduced type II fractures at long-term follow-up demonstrated a mild cubitus varus deformity with increased extension of the injured arm and up to 37% unsatisfactory results in the nonreduced cohort.[25] Despite closed reduction, some type II fractures still lose reduction, often based on the amount of initial extension beyond the anterior humeral capitellar line. No specific criteria have been defined to delineate which type II fractures can be successfully treated with closed reduction.[26] However, the decision for nonsurgical treatment of these fractures can at least be influenced by finding minimal to no hyperextension at the contralateral elbow during a physical examination.

The extension-type injury is reduced with traction and the milking maneuver, if necessary, followed sequentially by flexion and then pronation to maintain the reduction. It is important to check AP, lateral, and oblique views to confirm proper reduction with alignment of the columns. Reducing radiation exposure in young children is important, and evidence suggests that postoperative radiographs are not necessary when fluoroscopic images are saved and adequate intraoperative stability of the fracture was obtained. Postoperative radiographs rarely change the treatment plan.[27]

Pin configuration can vary from all lateral pins to cross pins. Iatrogenic injury to the ulnar nerve is more common with medial pins,[28] but the superior biomechanical stability of crossed pins and certain fracture patterns (more proximal and oblique exiting distal lateral) maintains the relevance of this debate. Pin spread is important for stability and to decrease the risk of loss of reduction, with a goal of 13 mm at the level of the fracture.[29] A medial pin can be used to increase pin spread at the fracture site and can be done relatively safely to decrease the risk of iatrogenic ulnar nerve injury. The technique of extending the elbow to relax the ulnar nerve after lateral pin fixation to obtain further stability, and the surgeon using his or her thumb to press posteriorly from the medial epicondyle to hold the ulnar nerve in position while a medial pin

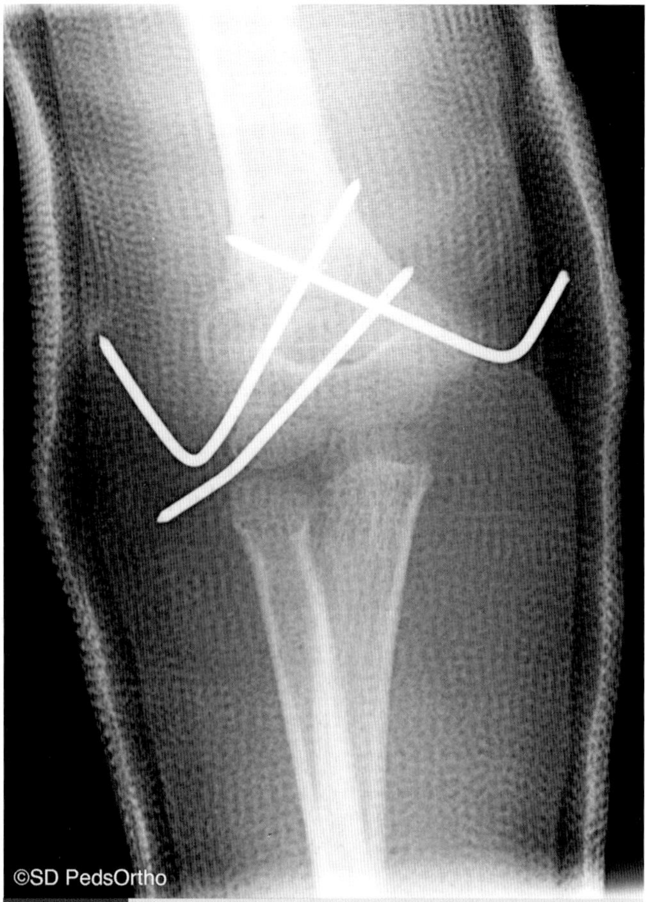

Figure 3 AP radiograph showing cross pinning of a supracondylar humerus fracture. (Copyright James Bomar, San Diego Pediatric Orthopedics, San Diego, CA.)

is placed, reduces the rate of ulnar nerve injury to 1%, even though historic literature states rates closer to 5%[30] (**Figure 3**). Alternatively, a small open approach to the medial epicondyle may be made with the elbow in relative extension, allowing the pin to be placed on the epicondyle under direct vision, avoiding ulnar nerve injury. If a patient has a new ulnar nerve deficit after the placement of cross pins, the medial pin should be removed, with maintenance of reduction in a cast or the placement of a third lateral pin. Pins should remain in place for 3 to 4 weeks, with further delay in pin removal increasing the infection risk. Pins are removed in the physician's office, but radiographs may not be indicated before pin removal.[31]

The displaced supracondylar humerus fracture has the potential for neurovascular injury. The physical examination is of extreme importance, even in a noncompliant young child, before and after surgery.

A pink or white pulseless hand is a cause for continued concern. A pulseless, poorly perfused hand requires emergent reduction and fixation, with the goal of restoring blood flow to the limb. The brachial artery may be draped over the fracture fragment and can be kinked, in spasm, or lacerated. If the hand is not perfused after pin fixation, exploration by a vascular surgeon should be performed. Vasodilating agents, thrombolytics, or grafting may be necessary and should be available. Concomitant median nerve deficits may be present and difficult to determine, depending on the child's cooperation with the physical examination. A study reviewing vascular deficiencies in type III supracondylar humerus fractures showed that 31% of type III fractures lacking a radial pulse also had a concomitant neurologic deficit.[32]

The management of a perfused but pulseless hand is controversial. Options include vascular exploration or close observation with serial examinations. If the artery has strong Doppler signals and the arm is neurologically intact, evidence indicates that observation in the hospital is a reasonable approach. Observation can help identify a child who may lose perfusion of the hand or require further intervention. In a study of 54 children without a palpable pulse before surgery, 20 continued to have a nonpalpable pulse, yet it was identifiable by Doppler after reduction and fixation of the fracture; only 1 child required vascular exploration 9 hours after the initial surgery that subsequently lost Doppler signals.[32] Any signs of worsening perfusion to the hand when all extraneous factors are resolved are reasons to consider vascular exploration. Patients managed expectantly with a pink pulseless hand usually do quite well; even with a risk of possible brachial artery occlusion, function often is not a problem.[33]

Extension-type fractures that injure the median nerve or the anterior interosseous nerve are important because an evolving compartment syndrome can be missed with a lack of sensation. A recent study evaluating isolated anterior interosseous nerve palsies showed no difference in outcome when comparing urgent surgery in the middle of the night versus the next day within 24 hours, with all patients having full return of function at an average of 49 days.[34] Because most neurologic deficits recover without complications, long-term follow-up for these patient is sparse. Ulnar nerve injuries are known to have less recovery potential, although with supracondylar fractures, the most common, long-term residual symptom of this palsy is referred paresthesias in the ulnar nerve distribution without a functional complaint.[35] With an ipsilateral both-bone forearm fracture, neurologic deficits are more common than in the isolated supracondylar fracture, with an association rate of up to 15%.[36]

Historically, type III fractures and fractures with any type of neurovascular compromise were treated with emergency surgical procedures, even in the middle of the night if required. New evidence has shown that few situations truly require emergency surgery. Type II fractures can be treated the next day or on an outpatient basis within a reasonable period without increased risk of complications.[37] Delaying surgery until the morning for a type III fracture without emergent indications (dysvascularity or impending compartment syndrome) does not increase the risk of the need for open reduction or increase the rate of complications.[38]

Lateral Condyle Fractures

Fractures of the lateral condyle are common and require anatomic restoration of the articular surface. Critical radiographic examination to determine the amount of displacement helps determine treatment, with the internal oblique view accepted as demonstrating true displacement. Arthrography can be beneficial in questionable cases to analyze the articular surface. The classic Milch classification type I and II fractures have a fracture line exiting the capitellum or the trochlea, respectively. The more clinically relevant Jakob classification is based on the maximal amount of lateral displacement and helps guide treatment based on the risk of articular displacement.[39] A Jakob type I fracture is less than 2 mm displaced, type II is more than 2 mm displaced without malrotation, and type III is more than 2 mm displaced with a rotational component. Type I fractures can be treated in a cast for 4 to 6 weeks but should have weekly radiographic follow-up (including lateral oblique views) for the first 2 weeks to confirm maintenance of reduction. Placement of the forearm in supination can help relax the extensor/supinator mass that originates from the lateral elbow and assist in reduction maintenance.

Jakob type II and III fractures require surgery to restore the joint. Closed reduction with percutaneous pinning is an attractive option for the fracture that can be manipulated closed into a reduced position, but an arthrogram to confirm joint congruity is required (**Figure 4**). Complication rates are relatively low with this method; one study showed a complication rate of 13% compared with 25% in the ORIF cohort.[40] The standard lateral open approach allows visualization of the fracture and the articular surface. Dissection along the posterior aspect of the lateral condyle should be avoided to preserve the blood supply and avoid osteonecrosis. Two or three divergent K-wires can be used for fixation, often with one parallel to the joint surface. Biomechanically, maximal divergence at the level of the fracture increases stability, as well as a third pin, if space is available. Open reduction with screw fixation also is described. Leaving the pins exposed and removing them at 4 weeks is recommended; however, burying the pins does not reduce the complication rate and increases cost.[41]

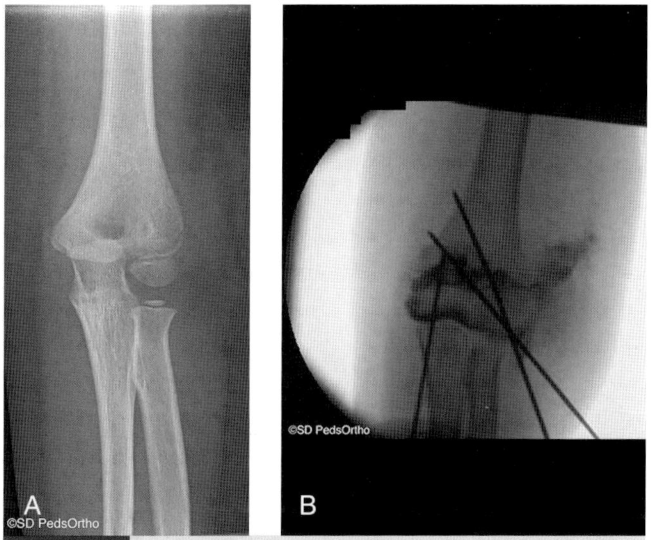

Figure 4 **A,** AP radiograph of an elbow with a lateral condyle fracture. **B,** Arthrogram confirming a congruent joint surface after closed reduction and percutaneous pinning. (Copyright James Bomar, San Diego Pediatric Orthopedics, San Diego, CA.)

Because of the articular nature of the fracture and exposure to synovial fluid, the lateral condyle fracture heals more slowly than other pediatric elbow fractures. Therefore, after pin removal, a cast often is reapplied for several weeks depending on the amount of callus formation seen on radiographs. An increased risk of delayed healing exists for fractures with residual displacement of the lateral cortex greater than 1 mm after fixation and in those who had a more difficult reduction at the time of surgery as indicated by increased fluoroscopic time and residual displacement of the fracture.[42] However, if the fracture is discovered later, a recent study demonstrated no differences in outcome or complications when surgery was performed within 14 days of injury.[43] Overall, the most common complication in the management of lateral condyle fractures is the development of a lateral spur, which occurs up to 73% of the time (**Figure 5**). This phenomenon correlates with the amount of initial displacement but, fortunately, does not affect outcome. However, families should be counseled preoperatively about the potential for lateral spur formation because it appears to be a cosmetic issue.[44]

Medial Epicondyle Fractures

The medial epicondyle ossifies at age 6 to 7 years, although the apophysis is the last to fuse around the elbow. A substantial force is needed to avulse the epicondyle,

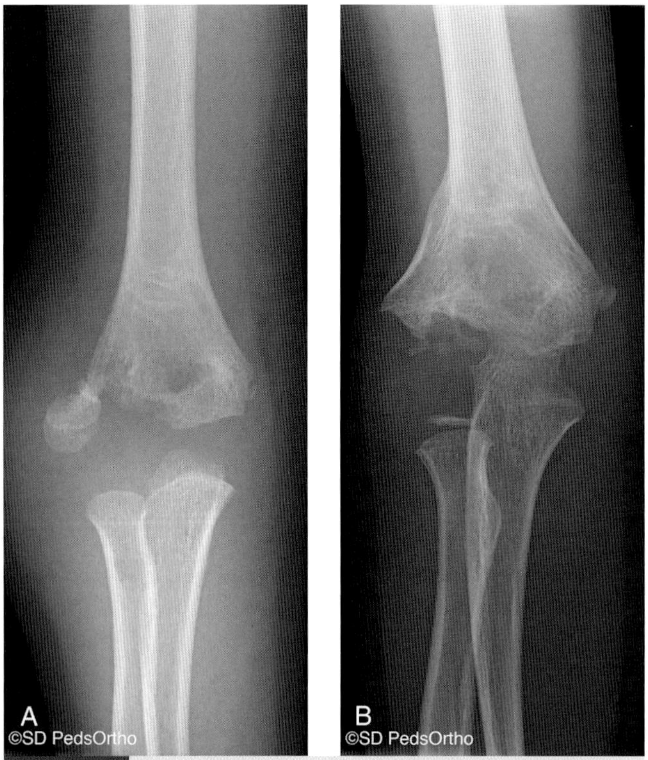

Figure 5 **A,** AP radiograph shows a severely displaced lateral condyle fracture. **B,** AP radiograph of a lateral spur after subsequent surgical treatment of the displaced lateral condyle fracture. Evidence of capitellar osteonecrosis is present. (Copyright James Bomar, San Diego Pediatric Orthopedics, San Diego, CA.)

such as the valgus force of a baseball pitcher or a fall during contact sports. Patients may report feeling a pop in the elbow with ulnar-sided elbow pain.

Plain radiographs often can be used to diagnose the medial epicondyle fracture, but it is debated whether plain radiographs can show the true amount of displacement to guide treatment. On a normal radiograph, the center of the medial epicondyle is 0.5 mm inferior to a line drawn horizontally through the bottom of the olecranon fossa on the AP view and 1.2 mm anterior to the posterior humeral line on the lateral view.[45] It is difficult to determine the amount of anterior displacement of the fracture even on the lateral view, which was shown in a CT study demonstrating that displacement may be greater than 1 cm even when plain radiographs suggest that the fracture is not displaced.[46] A newly described radiograph called the distal humeral axial view is performed with the humerus at 45° to the vertical, with the x-ray tube at the shoulder 25° anterior (**Figure 6**). With this radiographic technique, a cadaver study showed mean error in the measurement of displacement of only 1.5 mm in fractures displaced less than 10 mm and 0.8 mm in fractures displaced more than 10 mm[47] (**Figure 7**).

Medial epicondyle fractures are frequently associated with an elbow dislocation, and the dislocation should be reduced as soon as possible. Open fractures and fragments incarcerated in the joint are absolute indications for surgery (**Figure 8**). The presence of elbow instability also may influence the decision to use ORIF. In a young child, fixation choices include smooth K-wires or cannulated screws in the medial column, with or without a washer for additional strength; however, suture anchors can be used when the fragment is comminuted. At the time of surgery, the surgeon should be aware of the ulnar nerve and confirm that it is not being crushed or tethered when the fracture is reduced. The union rate will obviously be higher with surgical versus nonsurgical management, but debate is ongoing whether this is clinically relevant. A recent evaluation of return to sports after medial epicondyle fractures indicated that cast treatment is a good option for a low-energy injury with minimal displacement (5-8 mm), whereas ORIF is preferred for the high-energy, unstable, substantially displaced fracture.[48] In addition, the level of the patient's athletic participation may be considered when deciding on treatment; young athletes involved in sports requiring greater force from the flexor pronator mass may ultimately do better with surgery.

Elbow Dislocation

Elbow dislocations may occur in isolation but are commonly associated with fractures, most commonly of the medial epicondyle as previously discussed. In the young child, transphyseal supracondylar humerus fractures may be misdiagnosed as a dislocation, and child abuse also must be considered. A good neurovascular examination is important before and after reduction because the nerves and blood vessels are all in close proximity.

Carefully scrutiny of radiographs after closed reduction is necessary to assess the concentricity of reduction and recognize any fractures that may require surgery. Examination of the elbow after reduction is important to confirm stability and a smooth arc of motion. Two to 3 weeks of elbow immobilization before a range-of-motion program is initiated is adequate. Children and adolescents generally do well after elbow dislocations; however, fractures, surgery, and prolonged immobilization may lead to less-than-ideal outcomes.[49] Stiffness is the most common complication. An elbow that continues to be problematic with clinical instability that remains after initial treatment may warrant further study with MRI. Posterolateral instability may be present and masked by an elbow with a flexion contracture that can benefit from a lateral ulnar collateral ligament reconstruction.[50]

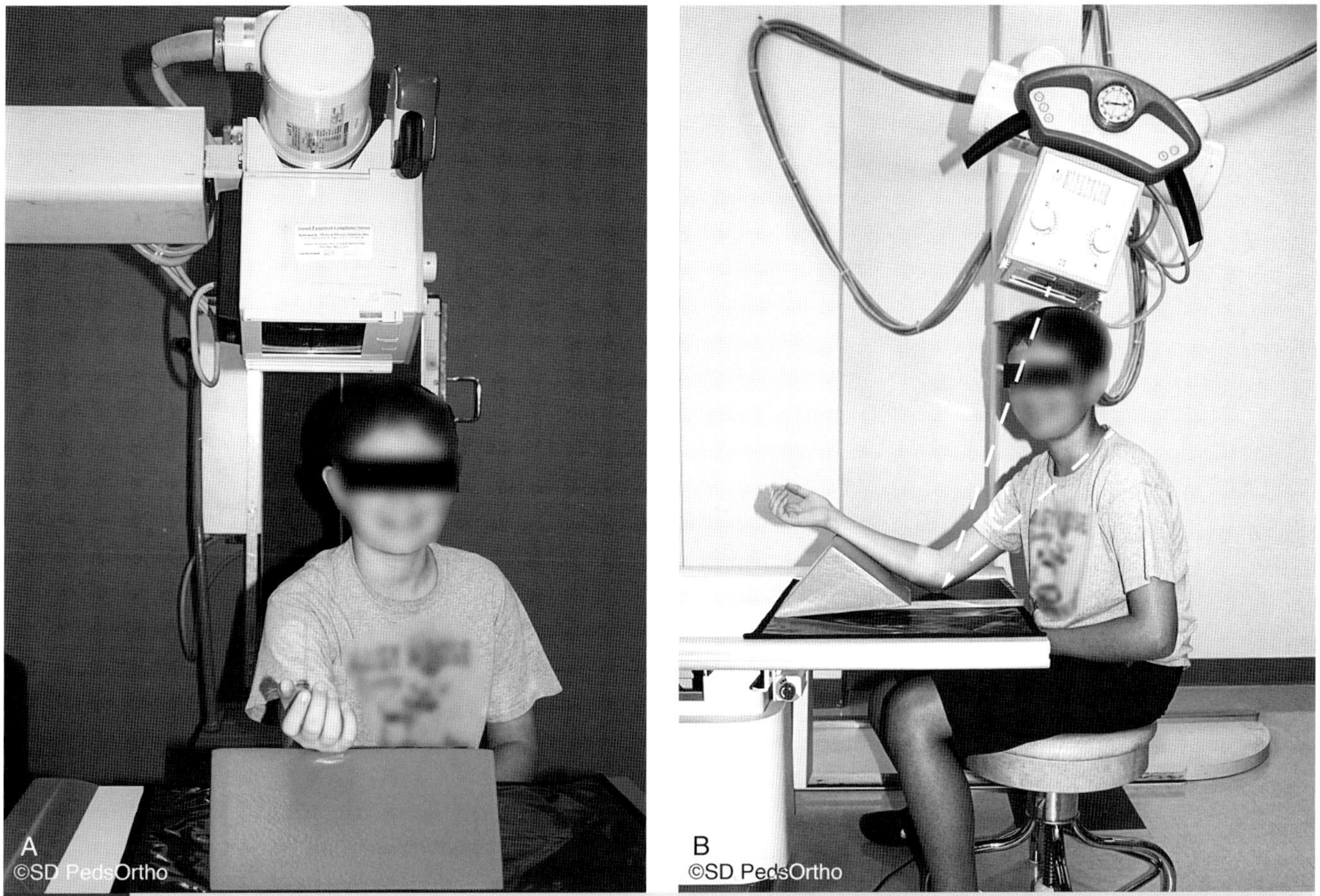

Figure 6 Clinical photographs show how to properly obtain a distal humeral axial view. **A,** The humerus should be angled 45° from vertical with the elbow resting at 90° on the table (a prop at the wrist may be helpful). The x-ray machine should be over the shoulder and shooting directly at the distal humerus at an angle 25° anterior to the humeral shaft. (Copyright James Bomar, San Diego Pediatric Orthopedics, San Diego, CA.)

Nursemaid's Elbow

In children younger than 5 years, pulling of the arm with the elbow in extension may cause subluxation of the radial head with displacement of the annular ligament, commonly referred to as nursemaid's elbow. The child often refuses to use his or her arm and holds the arm pronated and in slight flexion. Based on the classic history of these injuries, imaging is not routinely done in emergency departments. Radiographs can be used to rule out any other pathology, but radiographs in this situation are usually negative.[51] Flexion beyond 90° and supination with pressure on the radial head often will produce a click with immediate resolution of pain. The child may then use the arm, and no formal immobilization is necessary. Because this may recur with a similar mechanism, parents can learn the maneuver to perform at home, if necessary.

Olecranon Fractures

Olecranon fractures, a less common fracture sometimes seen in children, range from avulsion injuries in the athlete to comminuted traumatic fractures. The pull of the triceps on the proximal apophysis can displace the fracture. Minimally displaced fractures with an intact periosteum and a congruent articular surface can be treated closed in a cast. Extension relaxes the triceps and decreases the risk of displacement. Although routine radiographic follow-up is necessary for confirmation, the fracture will usually maintain the alignment set at casting. Displaced fractures require surgical fixation to restore the articular surface and maintain proper elbow mechanics. A tension band technique is attractive for transverse fracture patterns, which are most common. K-wires with a suture tension-band technique can be used, but the age of the patient and the fracture pattern must be considered. Comminuted fractures should be treated with open reduction and plate and screws fixation. Prominent implants often are symptomatic and may need to be removed after complete fracture healing.

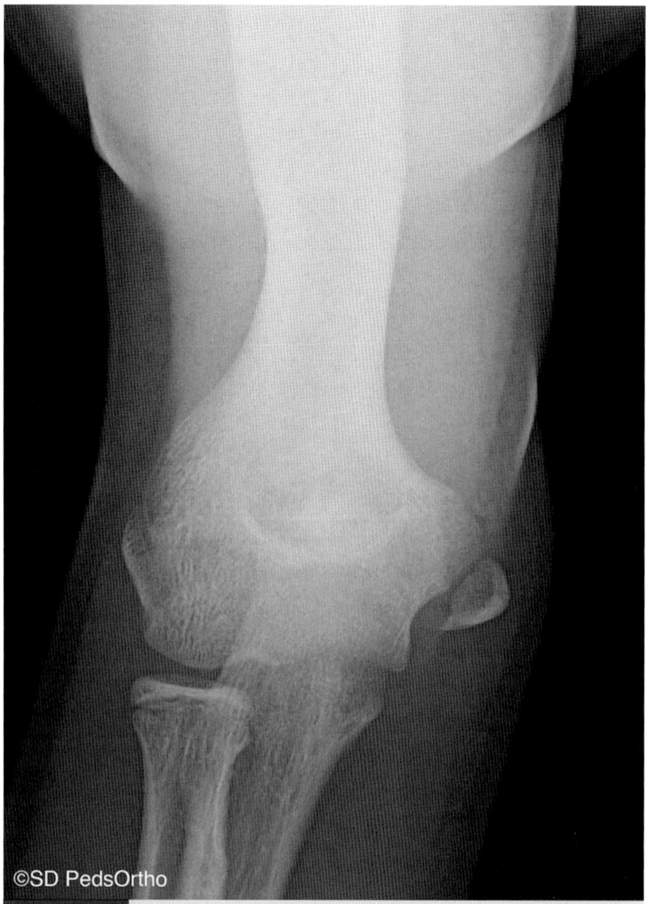

Figure 7 Distal humeral axial radiograph shows displacement of a medial epicondyle fracture. (Copyright James Bomar, San Diego Pediatric Orthopedics, San Diego, CA.)

Radial Head and Neck Fractures

Radial neck fractures are more common than radial head fractures in children. These often are Salter-Harris type II fractures resulting from a valgus force with a fall on an extended arm. Imaging to determine the true angulation of the fracture includes AP, lateral, and Greenspan views to show the radiocapitellar joint. The presence of the fat pad sign is suggestive of an occult fracture at the elbow, which is frequently a nondisplaced fracture of the radial neck.

Radial neck fractures angulated less than 30° often are well tolerated and can be treated in a cast in the skeletally immature child who has remodeling potential. Angulation greater than 30° and/or translation greater than 3 mm warrants a closed reduction attempt. Multiple closed reduction techniques have been described in the literature; some work better in certain settings, often depending on surgeon comfort with the technique. If closed reduction fails, percutaneous reduction can be obtained using a K-wire or a Steinmann pin as a joystick to lever the radial head or neck onto the shaft. If the radial shaft is translated ulnarly, then the Wallace technique can be used: a percutaneous joker elevator is placed medial to the radial shaft at the level of the biceps tuberosity to pull the radial shaft laterally while pressure is placed on the radial head to reduce the fragment[52] (**Figure 9**).

Older children are more likely to have displaced fractures that require open treatment, and open treatment is more likely to increase the complication rate seen with these fractures, particularly stiffness.[53] If entrapment of the annular ligament is preventing closed or percutaneous reduction, open reduction is indicated. Adequate treatment is K-wire stabilization of the radial head or neck (inserted proximally and avoiding the capitellum) for 3 to 4 weeks. Decreased satisfaction is more common with loss of supination-pronation, decreased flexion-extension, osteonecrosis of the radial head, premature physeal closure, and associated injuries.[54] A recent large series of surgically treated radial neck fractures showed that 31% of patients had suboptimal results, confirming the need to follow a protocol that at least attempts closed reduction before open treatment is undertaken.[55]

Radial head fractures are less common and may have displacement that requires ORIF, from an anterior or standard Kocher approach, depending on the fracture pattern. Plates at the bare spot or headless compression screws can be used for anatomic reduction. Although most radial head fractures have an extra-articular pattern, intra-articular fractures have worse outcomes and a substantially increased risk of complications.[56]

Summary

Fractures and dislocations of the upper extremity must receive a correct diagnosis and optimal treatment to prevent complications. A thorough physical examination and appropriate imaging studies are important in determining proper treatment.

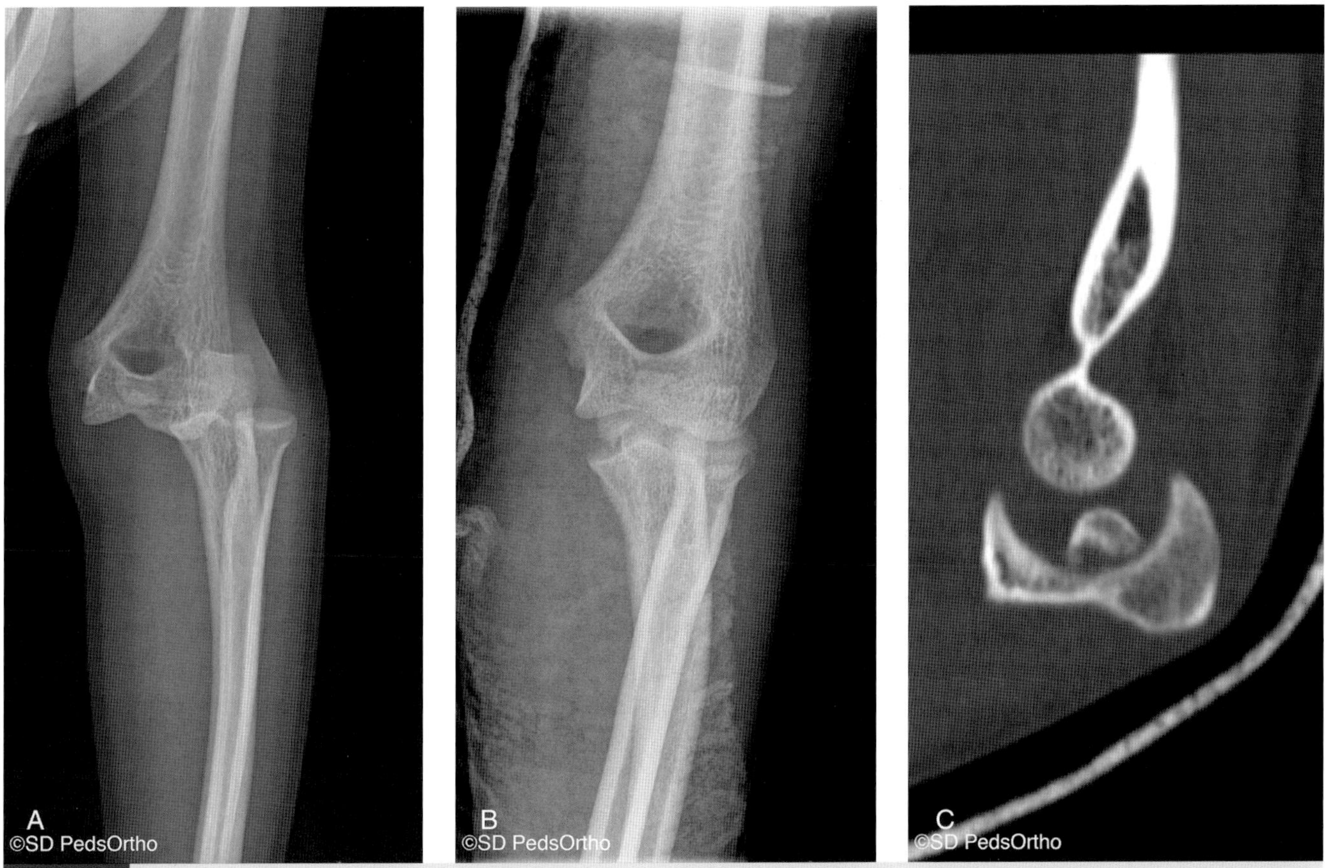

Figure 8 **A,** AP radiograph of a dislocated elbow. **B,** AP radiograph of the elbow after closed reduction showing a noncongruous reduction and a medial epicondyle fracture. **C,** CT scan of the elbow with the medial epicondyle fragment incarcerated in the joint. (Copyright James Bomar, San Diego Pediatric Orthopedics, San Diego, CA.)

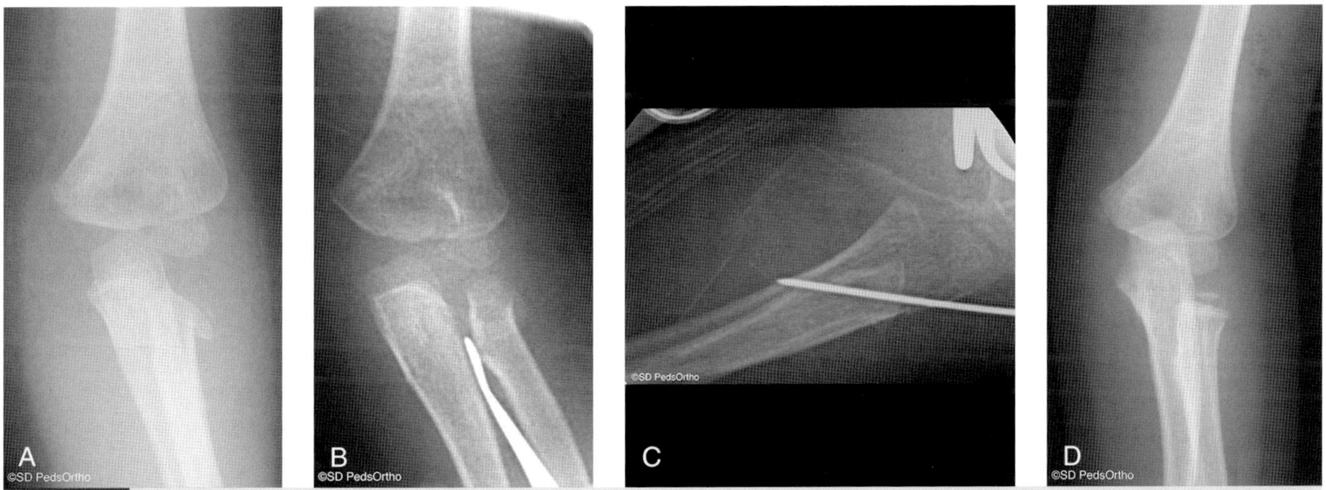

Figure 9 **A,** AP radiograph of a displaced, angulated radial neck fracture. **B,** AP radiograph shows a percutaneously inserted joker elevator on the medial side of the radial shaft, which is used to pull the shaft laterally to help reduce the radial head back onto the shaft. **C,** Radiograph shows Kirschner wire fixation to hold the fracture reduction. **D,** Postoperative radiograph after Kirschner wire removal shows the fracture healed. (Copyright James Bomar, San Diego Pediatric Orthopedics, San Diego, CA.)

Key Study Points

- The treatment of clavicle injuries (dislocations and fractures) remains controversial in pediatric and adolescent cohorts; recent literature suggests that children and adolescents have greater tolerance (acceptance) of deformity compared with adult cohorts with a similar pathology.
- Shoulder instability during adolescence can be treated surgically, as in adult patients; however, the outcomes are potentially worse with higher rates of recurrence.
- Although the recommendation for pin configuration in the treatment of supracondylar humerus fractures has not changed substantially in recent years, the attitude regarding the urgency of the intervention has shifted slightly toward delayed care being acceptable practice.
- Imaging of medial epicondyle fractures has evolved, shifting the assessment of the fracture displacement to be more axial in nature.
- The treatment of displaced lateral condyle fractures with closed or percutaneous reduction and percutaneous fixation has demonstrated promising results.

Annotated References

1. Dashe J, Roocroft JH, Bastrom TP, Edmonds EW: Spectrum of shoulder injuries in skeletally immature patients. *Orthop Clin North Am* 2013;44(4):541-551.

   This is a retrospective clinical and literature review on pediatric shoulder injuries, including epidemiology, treatment, and complications.

2. Tepolt F, Carry PM, Heyn PC, Miller NH: Posterior sternoclavicular joint injuries in the adolescent population: A meta-analysis. *Am J Sports Med* 2014;42(10):2517-2524.

   A meta-analysis on posterior SC joint injuries in the immature population reports that closed reduction is more successful within 48 hours of injury, and most patients do well whether closed or open reduction is required for treatment.

3. Lee JT, Nasreddine AY, Black EM, Bae DS, Kocher MS: Posterior sternoclavicular joint injuries in skeletally immature patients. *J Pediatr Orthop* 2014;34(4):369-375.

   This retrospective case series reported that when closed reduction fails, adolescents are more likely to have a posterior SC dislocation than a medial clavicle physeal fracture. Level of evidence: IV.

4. Jayakumar P, Barry M, Ramachandran M: Orthopaedic aspects of paediatric non-accidental injury. *J Bone Joint Surg Br* 2010;92(2):189-195.

5. Schulz J, Moor M, Roocroft J, Bastrom TP, Pennock AT: Functional and radiographic outcomes of nonoperative treatment of displaced adolescent clavicle fractures. *J Bone Joint Surg Am* 2013;95(13):1159-1165.

   In this case series of displaced pediatric clavicle fractures treated closed, no radiographic or functional outcome differences were found between the injured and uninjured shoulders.

6. McKee RC, Whelan DB, Schemitsch EH, McKee MD: Operative versus nonoperative care of displaced midshaft clavicular fractures: A meta-analysis of randomized clinical trials. *J Bone Joint Surg Am* 2012;94(8):675-684.

   A meta-analysis of randomized controlled trials showed a lower nonunion rate, less symptomatic malunion, and earlier functional return with surgical treatment compared with nonsurgical treatment for clavicle fractures in patients age 16 years and older.

7. Yang S, Werner BC, Gwathmey FW Jr: Treatment trends in adolescent clavicle fractures. *J Pediatr Orthop* 2015;35(3):229-233.

   This review reported increased surgical treatment of clavicle fractures in patients aged 15 to 19 years. Level of evidence: IV.

8. Bae DS, Shah AS, Kalish LA, Kwon JY, Waters PM: Shoulder motion, strength, and functional outcomes in children with established malunion of the clavicle. *J Pediatr Orthop* 2013;33(5):544-550.

   A case series concluded that clavicle malunions do not show clinically substantial loss of motion or strength in adolescents. Level of evidence: IV.

9. Pallis M, Cameron KL, Svoboda SJ, Owens BD: Epidemiology of acromioclavicular joint injury in young athletes. *Am J Sports Med* 2012;40(9):2072-2077.

   An epidemiologic study demonstrated that males, college athletes, and adolescents participating in contact sports are more likely to have low-grade AC injuries rather than high-grade injuries.

10. Beitzel K, Cote MP, Apostolakos J, et al: Current concepts in the treatment of acromioclavicular joint dislocations. *Arthroscopy* 2013;29(2):387-397.

    The authors present a systematic review of AC joint dislocations. Level of evidence: III.

11. Roberts SB, Beattie N, McNiven ND, Robinson CM: The natural history of primary anterior dislocation of the glenohumeral joint in adolescence. *Bone Joint J* 2015;97-B(4):520-526.

    Shoulder dislocations in adolescents have a high rate of recurrence, with most occurring within 2 years. The survival rate continues to decrease up to 5 years from the index event.

12. Leroux T, Ogilvie-Harris D, Veillette C, et al: The epidemiology of primary anterior shoulder dislocations in patients aged 10 to 16 years. *Am J Sports Med* 2015;43(9):2111-2117.

    The rate of recurrent shoulder dislocation is higher in adolescents aged 14 to 16 years than in children aged 10 to 13 years; the rate also is higher in males. Level of evidence: II.

13. Kraus R, Pavlidis T, Heiss C, Kilian O, Schnettler R: Arthroscopic treatment of post-traumatic shoulder instability in children and adolescents. *Knee Surg Sports Traumatol Arthrosc* 2010;18(12):1738-1741.

    A case series showed that a skilled arthroscopist can successfully treat pediatric shoulder instability pathology with arthroscopic techniques.

14. Edmonds EW, Lewallen LW, Murphy M, Dahm D, McIntosh AL: Peri-operative complications in pediatric and adolescent shoulder arthroscopy. *J Child Orthop* 2014;8(4):341-344.

    A retrospective review of arthroscopic complications in pediatric shoulders showed a 2.5% rate of complications that required physician intervention. No detrimental outcomes were reported.

15. Ozturk BY, Maak TG, Fabricant P, et al: Return to sports after arthroscopic anterior stabilization in patients aged younger than 25 years. *Arthroscopy* 2013;29(12):1922-1931.

    Ligamentous laxity, more than five dislocations, and a Hill-Sachs lesion are risk factors for recurrence of isolated anterior shoulder instability. The overall return-to-sports rate was 87%. Level of evidence: IV.

16. Shymon SJ, Roocroft J, Edmonds EW: Traumatic anterior instability of the pediatric shoulder: A comparison of arthroscopic and open Bankart repairs. *J Pediatr Orthop* 2015;35(1):1-6.

    A retrospective review showed no functional differences between arthroscopic and open Bankart repairs in children, although these techniques have higher failure rates in children than in adults. Level of evidence: III.

17. Blackman AJ, Krych AJ, Kuzma SA, Chow RM, Camp C, Dahm DL: Results of revision anterior shoulder stabilization surgery in adolescent athletes. *Arthroscopy* 2014;30(11):1400-1405.

    Revision surgery for anterior shoulder stabilization was unsuccessful in 5 of 15 adolescent patients at an average follow-up of 50 months. Level of evidence: IV.

18. Lefèvre Y, Journeau P, Angelliaume A, Bouty A, Dobremez E: Proximal humerus fractures in children and adolescents. *Orthop Traumatol Surg Res* 2014;100(1suppl):S149-S156.

    The authors present a review article on pediatric proximal humerus fractures, including epidemiology and anatomy.

19. Chaus GW, Carry PM, Pishkenari AK, Hadley-Miller N: Operative versus nonoperative treatment of displaced proximal humeral physeal fractures: A matched cohort. *J Pediatr Orthop* 2015;35(3):234-239.

    In matched cohorts, no significant differences were found for displaced proximal humerus fractures treated with or without surgery. Level of evidence: III.

20. Shore BJ, Hedequist DJ, Miller PE, Waters PM, Bae DS: Surgical management for displaced pediatric proximal humeral fractures: A cost analysis. *J Child Orthop* 2015;9(1):55-64.

    Leaving pins exposed outside the skin does not increase important complications and is less expensive than intramedullary fixation or burying pins.

21. Hutchinson PH, Bae DS, Waters PM: Intramedullary nailing versus percutaneous pin fixation of pediatric proximal humerus fractures: A comparison of complications and early radiographic results. *J Pediatr Orthop* 2011;31(6):617-622.

    Intramedullary nail fixation of pediatric proximal humerus fractures has a lower complication rate than percutaneous pins but requires more surgical time, has increased blood loss, and has increased cost because the hardware must be removed in the future. Level of evidence: III.

22. Kadhim M, Sethi S, Thacker MM: Unicameral bone cysts in the humerus: Treatment outcomes. *J Pediatr Orthop* 2015; May 8 [Epub ahead of print].

    This is a treatment review of humeral unicameral bone cysts. Level of evidence: III.

23. Ryan DD, Lightdale-Miric NR, Joiner ER, et al: Variability of the anterior humeral line in normal pediatric elbows. *J Pediatr Orthop* 2016;36(2):e14-e16.

    The authors reviewed normal pediatric elbow radiographs to determine the normal range of anterior humeral line intersection with the ossific nucleus of the capitellum. Level of evidence: III.

24. Seeley MA, Gagnier JJ, Srinivasan RC, et al: Obesity and its effects on pediatric supracondylar humeral fractures. *J Bone Joint Surg Am* 2014;96(3):e18.

    Obesity is associated with supracondylar humeral fracture patterns that are more complex and have additional complications. Level of evidence: III.

25. Moraleda L, Valencia M, Barco R, González-Moran G: Natural history of unreduced Gartland type-II supracondylar fractures of the humerus in children: A two to thirteen-year follow-up study. *J Bone Joint Surg Am* 2013;95(1):28-34.

    Functional outcomes are usually excellent despite slight increases in extension and a mild cubitus varus deformity

7: Trauma

in untreated Gartland type II supracondylar fractures. Level of evidence: IV.

26. Fitzgibbons PG, Bruce B, Got C, et al: Predictors of failure of nonoperative treatment for type-2 supracondylar humerus fractures. *J Pediatr Orthop* 2011;31(4):372-376.

    Evaluating the degree of extension of the distal fragment may help delineate fractures in which nonsurgical treatment will be unsuccessful. Level of evidence: III.

27. Karamitopoulos MS, Dean E, Littleton AG, Kruse R: Postoperative radiographs after pinning of supracondylar humerus fractures: Are they necessary? *J Pediatr Orthop* 2012;32(7):672-674.

    Early postoperative radiographs are not needed for supracondylar fractures because they do not change treatment or outcome. Level of evidence: IV.

28. Zhao J-G, Wang J, Zhang P: Is lateral pin fixation for displaced supracondylar fractures of the humerus better than crossed pins in children? *Clin Orthop Relat Res* 2013;471(9):2942-2953.

    A meta-analysis of randomized controlled trials showed that cross pins place the ulnar nerve at greater risk, so lateral pin fixation is recommended for supracondylar humerus fractures. Level of evidence: I.

29. Pennock AT, Charles M, Moor M, Bastrom TP, Newton PO: Potential causes of loss of reduction in supracondylar humerus fractures. *J Pediatr Orthop* 2014;34(7):691-697.

    Loss of reduction occurred in 4.2% of 192 fractures, with pin spread at the fracture site of less than 13 mm being the greatest predictor. Level of evidence: II.

30. Edmonds EW, Roocroft JH, Mubarak SJ: Treatment of displaced pediatric supracondylar humerus fracture patterns requiring medial fixation: A reliable and safer cross-pinning technique. *J Pediatr Orthop* 2012;32(4):346-351.

    Holding the ulnar nerve with a finger while the elbow is in extension allows for safe medial pin insertion for supracondylar humerus fractures. Level of evidence: III.

31. Schlechter JA, Dempewolf M: The utility of radiographs prior to pin removal after operative treatment of supracondylar humerus fractures in children. *J Child Orthop* 2015;9(4):303-306.

    Radiographs before pin removal are not needed and do not change the management plan for supracondylar humerus fractures in children. Level of evidence: III.

32. Weller A, Garg S, Larson AN, et al: Management of the pediatric pulseless supracondylar humeral fracture: Is vascular exploration necessary? *J Bone Joint Surg Am* 2013;95(21):1906-1912.

    Vascular exploration is not necessary for the perfused, pulseless supracondylar humerus fracture that has been treated with closed reduction and pinning, but it requires close observation in the hospital. Level of evidence: III.

33. Scannell BP, Jackson JB III, Bray C, Roush TS, Brighton BK, Frick SL: The perfused, pulseless supracondylar humeral fracture: Intermediate-term follow-up of vascular status and function. *J Bone Joint Surg Am* 2013;95(21):1913-1919.

    At latest follow-up, previously pink pulseless hands in patients with a supracondylar humerus fracture all had palpable radial pulses and good results, despite some having an occluded brachial artery. Level of evidence: IV.

34. Barrett KK, Skaggs DL, Sawyer JR, et al: Supracondylar humeral fractures with isolated anterior interosseous nerve injuries: Is urgent treatment necessary? *J Bone Joint Surg Am* 2014;96(21):1793-1797.

    Patients with isolated anterior interosseous nerve palsies from supracondylar humerus fractures do not require emergency treatment. A delay up to 24 hours did not change outcomes. Level of evidence: IV.

35. Valencia M, Moraleda L, Díez-Sebastián J: Long-term functional results of neurological complications of pediatric humeral supracondylar fractures. *J Pediatr Orthop* 2015;35(6):606-610.

    Supracondylar humerus fractures with nerve palsies largely have good outcomes, although the most common residual effect is a referred paresthesia in the ulnar nerve distribution. Level of evidence: IV.

36. Muchow RD, Riccio AI, Garg S, Ho CA, Wimberly RL: Neurological and vascular injury associated with supracondylar humerus fractures and ipsilateral forearm fractures in children. *J Pediatr Orthop* 2015;35(2):121-125.

    The rate of nerve injury is substantially higher in supracondylar humerus fractures with concomitant both-bone forearm fractures. Level of evidence: III.

37. Larson AN, Garg S, Weller A, et al: Operative treatment of type II supracondylar humerus fractures: Does time to surgery affect complications? *J Pediatr Orthop* 2014;34(4):382-387.

    Delaying the treatment of type II supracondylar humerus fractures more than 24 hours does not increase the complication rate of surgical treatment. Level of evidence: III.

38. Kronner JM Jr, Legakis JE, Kovacevic N, Thomas RL, Reynolds RA, Jones ET: An evaluation of supracondylar humerus fractures: Is there a correlation between postponing treatment and the need for open surgical intervention? *J Child Orthop* 2013;7(2):131-137.

    Delaying surgery for type III supracondylar humerus fractures beyond 12 hours after initial presentation did not increase the rate of open surgery.

39. Weiss JM, Graves S, Yang S, Mendelsohn E, Kay RM, Skaggs DL: A new classification system predictive of complications in surgically treated pediatric humeral lateral condyle fractures. *J Pediatr Orthop* 2009;29(6):602-605.

40. Pennock AT, Salgueiro L, Upasani VV, Bastrom TP, Newton PO, Yaszay B: Closed reduction and percutaneous pinning versus open reduction and internal fixation for type II lateral condyle humerus fractures in children displaced >2 mm. *J Pediatr Orthop* 2015; June 17 [Epub ahead of print].

Lateral condyle fractures displaced more than 2 mm but with a congruent joint surface can be treated open or percutaneously with no difference in outcomes. Level of evidence: III.

41. Das De S, Bae DS, Waters PM: Displaced humeral lateral condyle fractures in children: Should we bury the pins? *J Pediatr Orthop* 2012;32(6):573-578.

Leaving the pins exposed after open reduction percutaneous pinning is safe and cost-effective for treating lateral condyle fractures. Level of evidence: III.

42. Salgueiro L, Roocroft JH, Bastrom TP, et al: Rate and risk factors for delayed healing following surgical treatment of lateral condyle humerus fractures in children. *J Pediatr Orthop* 2015; June 3 [Epub ahead of print].

Delayed healing is seen more often with lateral condyle fractures that have residual displacement after surgery or if there was greater difficulty in obtaining reduction. Level of evidence: IV.

43. Silva M, Paredes A, Sadlik G: Outcomes of ORIF >7 days after injury in displaced pediatric lateral condyle fractures. *J Pediatr Orthop* 2015; August 28 [Epub ahead of print].

Open reduction of lateral condyle fractures up to 14 days after injury does not affect the outcome for such fractures. Level of evidence: II.

44. Pribaz JR, Bernthal NM, Wong TC, Silva M: Lateral spurring (overgrowth) after pediatric lateral condyle fractures. *J Pediatr Orthop* 2012;32(5):456-460.

The lateral spur is the most common complication seen with lateral condyle fractures, which is more evident with increased initial displacement and surgical treatment. Level of evidence: II.

45. Klatt JB, Aoki SK: The location of the medial humeral epicondyle in children: Position based on common radiographic landmarks. *J Pediatr Orthop* 2012;32(5):477-482.

This anatomic and radiographic study defined a reproducible radiographic position of the medial epicondyle.

46. Edmonds EW: How displaced are “nondisplaced” fractures of the medial humeral epicondyle in children? Results of a three-dimensional computed tomography analysis. *J Bone Joint Surg Am* 2010;92(17):2785-2791.

47. Souder CD, Farnsworth CL, McNeil NP, Bomar JD, Edmonds EW: The distal humerus axial view: Assessment of displacement in medial epicondyle fractures. *J Pediatr Orthop* 2015;35(5):449-454.

A cadaver study showed that the distal humeral axial radiograph allows estimations of displacement to be more accurate in medial epicondyle fractures.

48. Lawrence JT, Patel NM, Macknin J, et al: Return to competitive sports after medial epicondyle fractures in adolescent athletes: Results of operative and nonoperative treatment. *Am J Sports Med* 2013;41(5):1152-1157.

Patients who sustain low-energy injuries and have stable elbows with minimally displaced medial epicondyle fractures have a high rate of return to sports, whereas patients with more severe injuries are more likely to return to sports only after surgical management. Level of evidence: IV.

49. Murphy RF, Vuillermin C, Naqvi M, Miller PE, Bae DS, Shore B: Early outcomes of pediatric elbow dislocation: Risk factors associated with morbidity. *J Pediatr Orthop* 2015; Nov 3 [Epub ahead of print].

Most pediatric elbow dislocations do very well unless they have concomitant fractures, require prolonged immobilization, or undergo surgery. Level of evidence: IV.

50. Lattanza LL, Goldfarb CA, Smucny M, Hutchinson DT: Clinical presentation of posterolateral rotatory instability of the elbow in children. *J Bone Joint Surg Am* 2013;95(15):e105.

In this retrospective case series, the authors report on posterolateral instability of the elbow requiring lateral ulnar collateral ligament reconstruction. Level of evidence: IV.

51. Eismann EA, Cosco ED, Wall EJ: Absence of radiographic abnormalities in nursemaid’s elbows. *J Pediatr Orthop* 2014;34(4):426-431.

Radiographs from patients with nursemaid’s elbow do not show any acute findings and are used only to rule out other fractures before making the diagnosis of radial head subluxation. Level of evidence: III.

52. Pring M, Wenger DR, Rang M: Elbow, proximal radius, and ulna, in *Rang’s Children’s Fractures* ,ed 3. Philadelphia, PA, Lippincott Williams & Wilkins, 2005, pp 119-134.

53. De Mattos CB, Ramski DE, Kushare IV, Angsanuntsukh C, Flynn JM: Radial neck fractures in children and adolescents: An examination of operative and nonoperative treatment and outcomes. *J Pediatr Orthop* 2016;36(1):6-12.

This retrospective review compared outcomes of surgical and nonsurgical treatment and found an increased risk of worse outcomes and complications with the surgical management of more severely displaced fractures. Level of evidence: III.

54. Falciglia F, Giordano M, Aulisa AG, Di Lazzaro A, Guzzanti V: Radial neck fractures in children: Results when open reduction is indicated. *J Pediatr Orthop* 2014;34(8):756-762.

Outcomes are worse in elbows that required open reduction with residual radial head and/or neck deformity at

7-year follow-up and may be associated with functional losses, although 13 of 24 cases (55%) did well.

55. Zimmerman RM, Kalish LA, Hresko MT, Waters PM, Bae DS: Surgical management of pediatric radial neck fractures. *J Bone Joint Surg Am* 2013;95(20):1825-1832.

    Patients older than 10 years who had more severe displacement and underwent open reduction have an increased risk of suboptimal results for pediatric radial neck fractures. Level of evidence: IV.

56. Ackerson R, Nguyen A, Carry PM, Pritchard B, Hadley-Miller N, Scott F: Intra-articular radial head fractures in the skeletally immature patient: Complications and management. *J Pediatr Orthop* 2015;35(5):443-448.

    Intra-articular radial head fractures must be recognized because they have increased complication rates and need surgical management compared with extra-articular fractures. Level of evidence: III.

Chapter 37

Forearm, Wrist, and Hand

Joshua M. Abzug, MD   Theresa O. Wyrick, MD

Abstract

Pediatric forearm, wrist, and hand fractures are the most common fractures in children. Most of these fractures can be successfully treated with immobilization alone. If required, closed reduction maneuvers and casting with proper techniques can result in excellent outcomes for patients with these fractures. When surgery is necessary, successful outcomes can be expected along with low complication rates.

Keywords: distal radius fracture; forearm fracture; Galeazzi; Monteggia; pediatric; phalangeal neck; scaphoid fracture; Seymour fracture

Introduction

Forearm, wrist, and hand fractures are very common in the pediatric population. A recent study of the National Electronic Injury Surveillance System database assessed the epidemiology of pediatric fractures presenting to emergency departments in the United States and found that forearm fractures were the most common (17.8% of all fractures), followed by finger and wrist fractures, respectively.[1] This chapter focuses on recently published information regarding the epidemiology, treatment, and outcomes of these fractures in children and adolescents.

It is important to note that the reduction of displaced fractures in these anatomic locations was thought to involve less radiation when a mini C-arm was used; however, a recent study reported that radiation exposure during pediatric upper extremity fracture reduction was greater with the use of a mini C-arm than with the use of conventional radiography.[2] Less experienced orthopaedic residents had higher levels of radiation exposure than those with more experience. The authors recommended that formalized training and education be provided to residents about the use of a mini C-arm in fracture reduction.[2]

Both-Bone Forearm Shaft Fractures

Pediatric forearm fractures of the radius and ulna are classified by location, displacement, and fracture and deformity characteristics. The peak incidence of these fractures occurs between 12 and 14 years of age, and they usually result from a fall onto an outstretched hand.[3] In pediatric patients, most of these fractures can be managed nonsurgically with excellent outcomes, which is not the case in adult patients. The rapid healing and remodeling potential of children allow for a less than perfect reduction of these fractures in young patients.[4]

The determination of an acceptable reduction depends on many factors, but it is largely influenced by the remodeling potential of the individual patient. Because most of the longitudinal growth of the forearm bones comes from the distal physes of the radius (75%) and ulna (81%), distal forearm fractures have more remodeling potential than more proximal forearm fractures. Inadequate reduction or insufficient remodeling will result in malunion and contribute to loss of forearm rotation.[4] Remodeling of fractures of the forearm diaphysis cannot be expected in children who are within 1 to 2 years of skeletal maturity; therefore, these children should be treated in the same manner as adults are treated, with anatomic reduction and internal fixation.[5]

Plastic deformations, incomplete fractures (greenstick fractures), and complete fractures of the forearm are observed variations. Forearm fractures with an apex volar deformity occur when the outstretched arm is in supination during a fall. Conversely, a fall onto an outstretched pronated arm results in apex dorsal angulation of the

Dr. Abzug or an immediate family member is a member of a speakers' bureau or has made paid presentations on behalf of Checkpoint Surgical and serves as a paid consultant to Axogen. Neither Dr. Wyrick nor any immediate family member has received anything of value from or has stock or stock options held in a commercial company or institution related directly or indirectly to the subject of this chapter.

fracture. The closed reduction maneuver for a greenstick fracture includes rotation of the forearm in the opposite direction of that of the injuring force. In complete forearm fractures, a more complex maneuver may be needed to achieve adequate reduction.[4]

Current recommendations regarding what constitutes an acceptable deformity are based on the proximity of the fracture to the physis and the age of the patient. In children younger than 8 years, remodeling of up to 20° of angulation in diaphyseal fractures can be expected, whereas no more than 10° of diaphyseal angulation remodeling can be expected in children older than 10 years. Up to 1 cm of shortening is acceptable. Complete translation can remodel well in fractures located in the middle and distal forearm shaft in younger children, although translation in the radioulnar plane is less well tolerated and can lead to radioulnar impingement.[3] Malrotation of less than 45° is generally acceptable because functional motion is usually possible; however, remodeling will not occur. Bayonet apposition is acceptable in most instances except when the interosseous space is substantially narrowed because this leads to loss of motion secondary to radioulnar impingement with forearm rotation.[4,6]

Most pediatric forearm fractures can be treated with either immobilization alone or with closed reduction to achieve acceptable alignment, which is then followed by casting. Closed reduction is typically performed in the emergency department with the patient under conscious sedation or in the operating room. Most often, fluoroscopy is used in the reduction process; however, a recent study found that ultrasound can be used as well.[7] Close follow-up is warranted in patients with displaced or angulated forearm fractures, potentially unstable fractures, and reduced fractures. In those who have undergone fracture reduction, periodic radiographs should be obtained during the first 3 weeks after the injury to monitor for any loss of reduction. In patients with a greenstick fracture, however, a less stringent follow-up protocol may be indicated. A recent study reported that only two office visits and a total of three sets of radiographs provide adequate monitoring because only 1 of 109 study patients with greenstick fractures over a 10-year period required rereduction.[8] In contrast, loss of reduction occurs in 5% to 25% of patients with unstable forearm fractures of both bones. Many studies have been published on preventing loss of reduction.[3] Determination of the optimal type and position of immobilization (above- or below-elbow) as well as analyses of all of the factors contributing to loss of reduction are ongoing.

Malunion of forearm fractures results in loss of range of motion in as many as 60% of children but may not result in functional limitations. The risk of loss of range of motion is increased in older children and adolescents with fracture malunion because there is less remodeling potential; therefore, the need for surgical fixation of displaced forearm fractures is greater in these patients. To determine predictors of loss of reduction, a 2011 study evaluated 282 patients with complete both-bone forearm shaft fractures who were treated nonsurgically.[6] Loss of reduction that exceeded acceptable angulation criteria was found in 144 of the patients, with most of the reduction loss occurring in the first and second weeks after the initial closed reduction procedure. Risk factors for loss of reduction were patient age of 10 years or older, fracture of the proximal radius, and initial angulation of the ulna fracture of less than 15°. Another recent study in a similar patient population identified initial fracture displacement greater than 50% and an inability to achieve an anatomic initial reduction as major risk factors for redisplacement.[9]

Distal forearm fractures of both the radius and ulna and distal radius fractures can be successfully managed with a properly placed and molded below-elbow cast or splint. However, most displaced midshaft and proximal forearm fractures are better and more safely managed with an above-elbow cast. Careful attention to the casting technique is critical. The cast should be more narrow in the dorsal-ventral plane than in the radioulnar plane by a radiographic ratio of 0.7 (cast-index) while producing an adequate three-point mold around the fracture site (three-point index)[10] (**Figure 1**). If a long arm cast is needed because of the proximal nature of a fracture, it is critical that the cast does not migrate distally as swelling subsides so that late apex ulnar angulation is prevented. Careful attention to creating 90° of flexion at the elbow and a straight ulnar border on the cast can help prevent late angulation.

With the increase in obesity seen in the pediatric population, this comorbidity may be an additional risk factor contributing to the failure of nonsurgical treatment of forearm fractures. In a recent study of 157 pediatric patients with distal forearm fractures initially treated nonsurgically, 42% of the children were overweight and 29% of the children met the criteria for obesity (body mass index >95th percentile).[11] The children who were obese more often required a closed reduction in the operating room after initial closed treatment than children of normal weight. Children who were obese were significantly less likely to have an initial anatomic reduction in the emergency department ($P = 0.005$) and also had a significantly greater number of visits with radiographic follow-up ($P = 0.004$) than children who were not obese. Obesity is an important risk factor for failure of nonsurgical management of forearm fractures in the pediatric population.

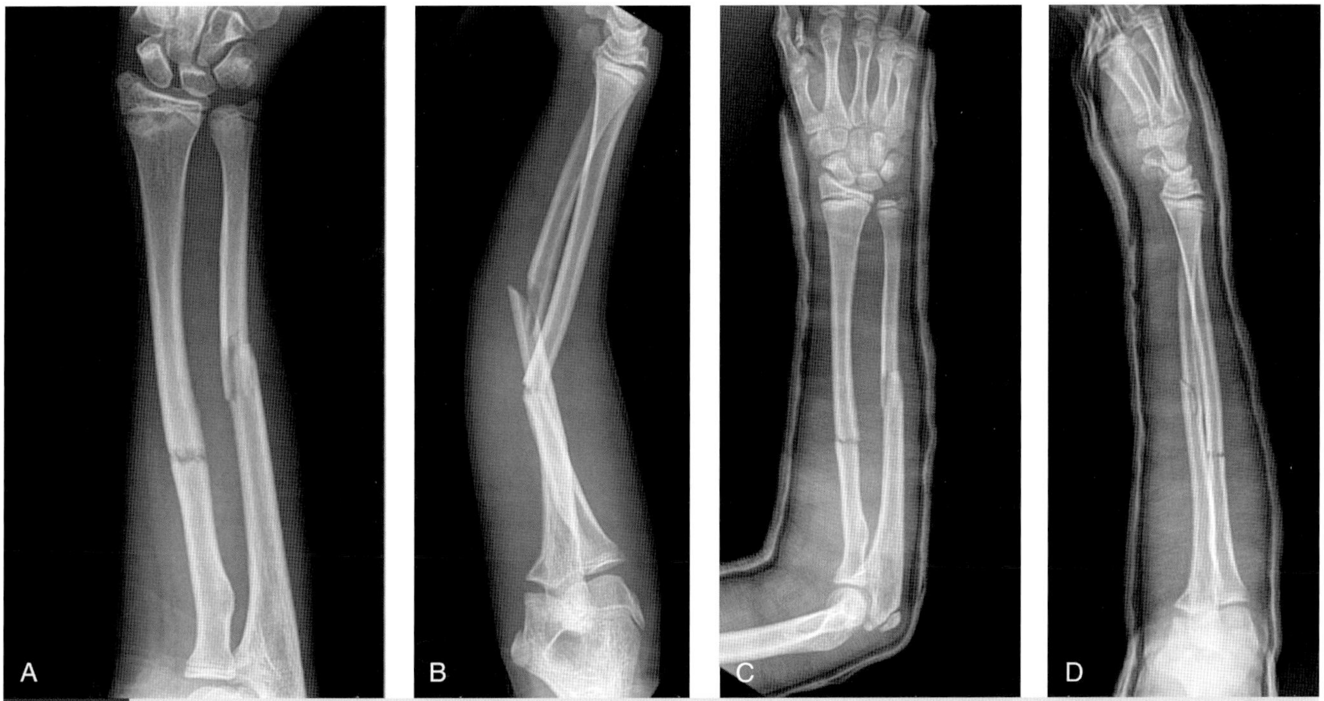

Figure 1 AP (**A**) and lateral radiographs (**B**) of the forearm of a 12-year-old girl who fell off of a trampoline sustaining a both-bone forearm fracture. AP (**C**) and lateral (**D**) radiographs of the forearm after closed reduction and the application of a long arm cast. Note that the cast applied is wider in the radioulnar plane compared with the dorsal-ventral plane, indicating a low cast index. (Copyright Joshua M. Abzug, MD, Timonium, MD.)

If nonsurgical treatment is unsuccessful, surgery is warranted in patients with open fractures, fractures with severe soft-tissue injury, displaced floating elbow injuries, irreducible fractures, and unstable fractures. A relative indication for surgery is a refracture of a previously nonsurgically treated forearm fracture. Older reports suggested a refracture rate of 5%; however, a recent large series reported a rate of 1.4%, with refractures most commonly occurring in the middle third of the forearm (72%) followed by the proximal third (24%).[12] Fractures with residual angulation of 15° or more refractured earlier than those with less angulation. Surgical treatment options include intramedullary fixation with Kirschner wires, Steinmann pins, elastic nails, or Rush rods; external fixation; and plate-and-screw fixation. Single-bone fixation is an option in some instances.[3]

Although most patients have excellent outcomes after surgical intervention, complications are relatively common, with reported complication rates of 14% to 21% for elastic nailing.[13,14] A recent study evaluating risk factors for tendon complications after intramedullary nailing of pediatric forearm fractures reported that 3 of 17 patients (18%) sustained extensor pollicis longus tendon ruptures.[15] No risk factors were identified, except all of the elastic nails had been placed using a dorsal approach to the radius, which suggested attritional tendon rupture secondary to implant prominence. Care should be taken to avoid tendon irritation when a dorsal entry elastic nail is used because of this possible associated complication. If tendon rupture occurs, it should be recognized and treated in a timely manner.

Monteggia Fracture-Dislocations

Monteggia injuries are most commonly seen in children between the ages of 6 and 10 years and are usually the result of a fall onto an outstretched arm. Although closed reduction and cast immobilization often provides sufficient treatment, close follow-up is warranted, with weekly radiographs for the first 3 weeks after injury to monitor for loss of fracture and radiocapitellar joint reduction. An algorithm to direct treatment strategies in patients with pediatric Monteggia fractures was described in 1998[16] and was expanded to a larger population of pediatric patients in 2015.[17] Using this algorithm, successful treatment of Monteggia fractures without subsequent loss of reduction of either the ulna or radiocapitellar joint at follow-up was reported.[16,17]

The treatment algorithm is directed by the ulna fracture pattern. In patients with plastic deformation or a greenstick fracture of the ulna, closed reduction with cast immobilization is recommended. For a complete

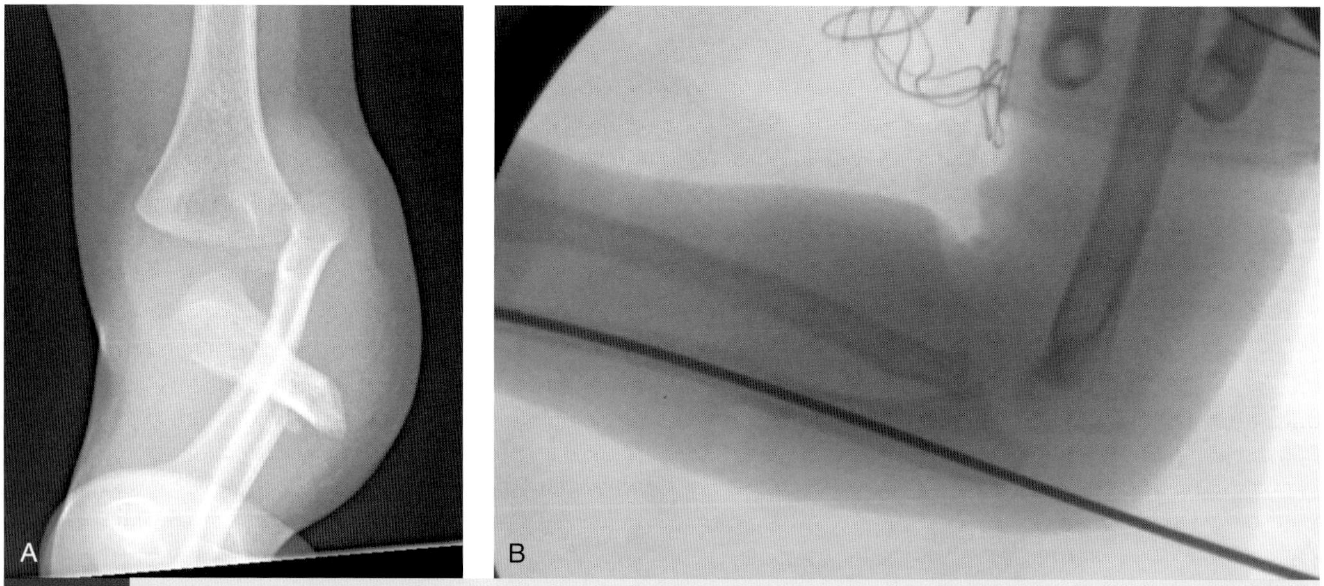

Figure 2 **A,** AP radiograph of the elbow of an 8-year-old girl with a Monteggia fracture-dislocation sustained in a fall from a bicycle. **B,** Intraoperative fluoroscopic lateral view of the elbow shows the reduction of the Monteggia fracture-dislocation and stabilization of the short oblique ulna fracture using intramedullary fixation. (Copyright Theresa O. Wyrick, MD, Little Rock, AR.)

fracture of the ulna that is length-stable (transverse or short oblique), intramedullary pin fixation of the ulna is recommended (**Figure 2**). In a complete fracture of the ulna that is length-unstable (long oblique or comminuted), open reduction with plate fixation is recommended. Complete fractures of the ulna, regardless of the fracture pattern, are at risk for treatment failure caused by loss of reduction of the ulna fracture and subsequent radial head subluxation or dislocation if surgical stabilization of the ulnar fracture is not undertaken initially.[16,17] It is rare for soft-tissue interposition to prevent reduction of the radial head dislocation after anatomic reduction of an ulnar shaft fracture. However, open reduction of the radiocapitellar joint is indicated in the setting of an irreducible radial head dislocation.

Complications associated with Monteggia fracture-dislocations in the pediatric population include loss of reduction; persistent pain; decreased motion; nonunion; compartment syndrome; and nerve palsies, which are usually transient. Loss of reduction can usually be prevented by treating complete fractures of the ulna with surgical stabilization, regardless of the amount of displacement. Close radiographic follow-up of patients with complete ulna fractures treated with closed reduction and cast immobilization is recommended, with early surgical intervention, including ulnar stabilization, if loss of anatomic radiocapitellar alignment is observed.[16,17]

Chronic Monteggia fracture-dislocations are occasionally seen in children and may result from a failure to recognize the initial radial head dislocation or because of subsequent loss of reduction during treatment. Initially, children often adapt well to a dislocated radial head, which usually causes little pain or functional deficit. However, over time, the radiocapitellar dislocation can cause valgus elbow instability, cubitus valgus, loss of motion, and pain.

Multiple techniques for corrective osteotomy of the ulna with subsequent closed or open reduction of the radiocapitellar joint have been described in the literature; results of these techniques have varied.[16] Soft-tissue reconstruction of the annular ligament also has been described using various methods. The age of the patient, the existing deformity of the radial head, and the length of time since the injury are all considerations when determining whether surgical treatment of a chronic Monteggia fracture-dislocation will be beneficial. Preferably, surgical treatment of this lesion should be undertaken within 1 year of the original injury for the best outcome. If little potential for remodeling exists and the radial head is radiographically deformed, the results of surgical treatment are less predictable.[16] No consensus exists on whether soft-tissue reconstruction of the annular ligament is warranted. In pediatric patients, overcorrection of an ulnar shaft deformity should be undertaken because of the extensive remodeling that occurs at the fracture site after the original injury. Fixation has been performed with various methods, including plate fixation, uniplane external fixation, intramedullary wire fixation, and ringed fixators; results have varied. Clearly, it is best to prevent the need for delayed treatment of this injury by pursuing diligent radiographic follow-up of the patient in the acute setting.

Galeazzi Fracture-Dislocations

A fracture of the shaft of the radius with an associated dislocation of the distal radioulnar joint is known as a Galeazzi fracture. This type of fracture was first described in 1934 by Riccardo Galeazzi of Milan.[18] It has also been called a reverse Monteggia fracture or a fracture of necessity. Galeazzi fractures are typically the result of a fall onto an outstretched arm. Good results are seen with nonsurgical treatment in children and adolescents after closed reduction and cast immobilization. In adults, open rigid internal fixation is necessary for the treatment of a Galeazzi fracture.[19]

The incidence of this relatively uncommon fracture-dislocation in children is reported to be between 0.3% and 2.8%, and it most commonly occurs in children between the ages of 9 and 13 years. A Galeazzi fracture must be considered with any isolated fracture of the radius and is more common in radius fractures at the junction of the middle and distal thirds of the diaphysis. Usually, the distal ulna is dislocated dorsally. Examination of the distal radioulnar joint should be performed after closed reduction of the radial shaft fracture to assess for instability when an anatomic reduction of the radius is achieved. If the radius or distal radioulnar joint is irreducible, soft-tissue interposition is likely, and an open approach to either the radius fracture, the distal radioulnar joint, or both is necessary to obtain an adequate reduction. Immobilization above the elbow is recommended after an anatomic reduction is achieved. Close follow-up is warranted to evaluate for loss of reduction of the radius and subsequent subluxation or dislocation at the distal radioulnar joint. Periodic radiographic assessments are recommended over the first 3 weeks after reduction to monitor for possible redisplacement. Fortunately, long-term instability of the distal radioulnar joint is not typical in pediatric patients with this injury pattern.[20]

Distal Both-Bone Forearm Fractures and Distal Radius Fractures

Distal radius fractures are common in the pediatric population and include metaphyseal and physeal injuries. Most wrist fractures result from a fall onto an outstretched hand. A recent study evaluating the epidemiology of pediatric wrist fractures found that the mean age of patients was 10.9 years, with approximately two-thirds of the fractures occurring in boys.[21] The top five activities associated with these fractures were bicycling, football, playground activities, basketball, and soccer. Subgroup classifications showed that, in patients from birth to 12 months of age, wrist fractures were most commonly associated with beds or bedframes, whereas in children aged 13 to 36 months, the fractures were most commonly associated with stairs, and in children aged 11 to 17 years, wrist fractures were associated with playing football.[21]

An increase in the incidence of pediatric distal radius fractures may also be associated with patient factors such as bone density, increased body mass index, participation in more intense or higher risk activities, and younger ages of participation in these activities. Multiple treatment options exist and many factors must be considered, including physeal involvement, articular displacement, remodeling potential, the risk of growth arrest, patient factors, and family expectations.[22]

A metaphyseal torus fracture of the distal radius is an incomplete or "buckle" fracture sustained as the result of an axial compression injury. Torus fractures do not require rigid immobilization or extended clinical follow-up and are expected to heal uneventfully within 3 weeks of injury. A removable splint provides sufficient immobilization. Splint removal at home 3 weeks after injury is acceptable and actually preferred by most families.[22] Similarly, minimally displaced and angulated metaphyseal fractures of the distal radius will typically remodel because of continued skeletal growth and the close proximity to the distal radial physis. Generally accepted radiographic parameters for this fracture pattern include 20° to 30° of sagittal plane angulation because sufficient remodeling will be possible.

Displaced fractures needing reduction require more discussion and consideration in decision-making. An initial closed reduction is recommended for displaced fractures that are not expected to sufficiently remodel based on established parameters. Factors to consider include patient age, skeletal immaturity, remaining growth, fracture pattern, and the presence of associated injuries. Closed reduction is most commonly performed with the patient sedated; however, this can lead to long times in the emergency department and high costs. A recent study comparing reductions performed under sedation versus reductions performed with only hematoma blocks found that there were no important differences in radiographic alignment, patient satisfaction, and pain control.[23] However, the use of a hematoma block alone substantially reduced the time spent in the emergency department (average, 2.2 fewer hours) as well as the resources required to perform the reduction.[23]

Displaced intra-articular fractures are rare in skeletally immature patients. Because these fractures will not remodel, surgical treatment is recommended. Other indications for surgical treatment include open fractures, displaced floating elbow injuries, and irreducible fractures. At the initial closed reduction procedure, either a cast or a splint can be used and both short- and long-arm immobilization are acceptable. Patients and families generally prefer short-arm immobilization. Careful attention to immobilization technique, whether a splint or cast is used, is important to prevent loss of reduction. It is essential to use a high-quality mold, as measured by the cast index and three-point index. Close radiographic follow-up is recommended, with weekly radiographic studies for the first 2 to 3 weeks after the reduction.[22]

Physeal arrest is a known sequela of distal radius fractures, with reported rates between 1% and 7%. Because of the increased risk of posttraumatic physeal arrest in the distal radius following late manipulations of displaced physeal fractures in pediatric patients, it is recommended that manipulations not be performed more than 10 days after the initial injury.[24] Because treatment of a subsequent malunion may be required if sufficient remodeling does not occur, the family should be informed of this possibility.

Multiple studies have shown that there is a substantial risk of pin site complications with the acute use of pin stabilization of displaced distal radius fractures to prevent loss of reduction. Outcomes in patients treated with reduction and pinning compared with those treated with reduction and cast immobilization are equivalent. Therefore, pinning of all displaced distal radius fractures is not indicated.[22]

Treatment variability exists among practitioners managing distal radius fractures in the pediatric population. A recent study of hand, pediatric, and general orthopaedic surgeons reported that hand surgeons and general orthopaedic surgeons were 2.9 and 1.6 times more likely, respectively, than pediatric orthopaedic surgeons to treat the same distal radius fracture surgically. In addition, orthopaedic surgeons in private practice were 1.5 times more likely to recommend surgery than surgeons with academic affiliations. This variation in treatment choices indicates that surgeons managing distal radius fractures in the pediatric population have varying criteria for acceptable alignment. Further investigation of the optimal treatment of these fractures is warranted.[25]

Scaphoid Fractures

Scaphoid fractures are relatively uncommon in children and adolescents; however, the incidence has increased as older children and adolescents are engaging in more intense sports participation and extreme sports.[26-28] Scaphoid fractures most commonly result from injuries sustained during participation in sports such as football, basketball, snowboarding, and skateboarding.[29]

Historically, scaphoid fractures were thought to more commonly involve the distal pole; however, recent studies have questioned the accuracy of this assumption. A retrospective analysis of 351 fractures seen over a 15-year period found that 71% of fractures occurred at the scaphoid waist, 23% at the distal pole, and 6% at the proximal pole.[29] The mean patient age in this series was 14.6 years.[29] In contrast, a smaller study that assessed 56 confirmed scaphoid fractures found that the most common fracture location was the distal pole (80%).[26] The mean patient age in that study was 12.2 years in boys and 10.3 years in girls, which may account for the differences in fracture patterns observed between the two studies. Both studies demonstrated that scaphoid fractures are more common in males. High-energy mechanisms, closed physes, and a high body mass index are associated with fractures of the scaphoid waist or proximal pole.[29]

Patient Evaluation

Patients with potential scaphoid fracture should be assessed with a thorough physical examination; the presence of tenderness to palpation in the snuffbox should be noted. Plain radiographs, including PA, lateral, and scaphoid views have been the mainstay of diagnostic imaging; however, a recent study showed that ultrasound can identify an acute scaphoid fracture, even if it is not visualized on plain radiographs.[30] MRI can be helpful in diagnosing an occult scaphoid fracture in the setting of normal findings on plain radiographs. CT can be helpful in determining the amount of displacement at the fracture site in subtle fractures in which the decision to proceed with surgical treatment is unclear based on plain radiographs. It is important to assess for associated injuries, including distal radius fractures, transscaphoid perilunate dislocations, ulnar styloid fractures, capitate fractures, and bilateral scaphoid fractures, which can be present in up to 10% of patients.[29]

Treatment

Cast immobilization is the mainstay of treatment of pediatric and adolescent scaphoid fractures. Healing in more than 90% of acute fractures was reported using cast immobilization alone.[29] Lower union rates are more likely in more proximal fractures, displaced fractures, and late-presenting fractures. In younger children who present acutely, union may occur as early as 4 to 6 weeks after injury, whereas longer times to union are more likely in older children and adolescents, older fractures, displaced

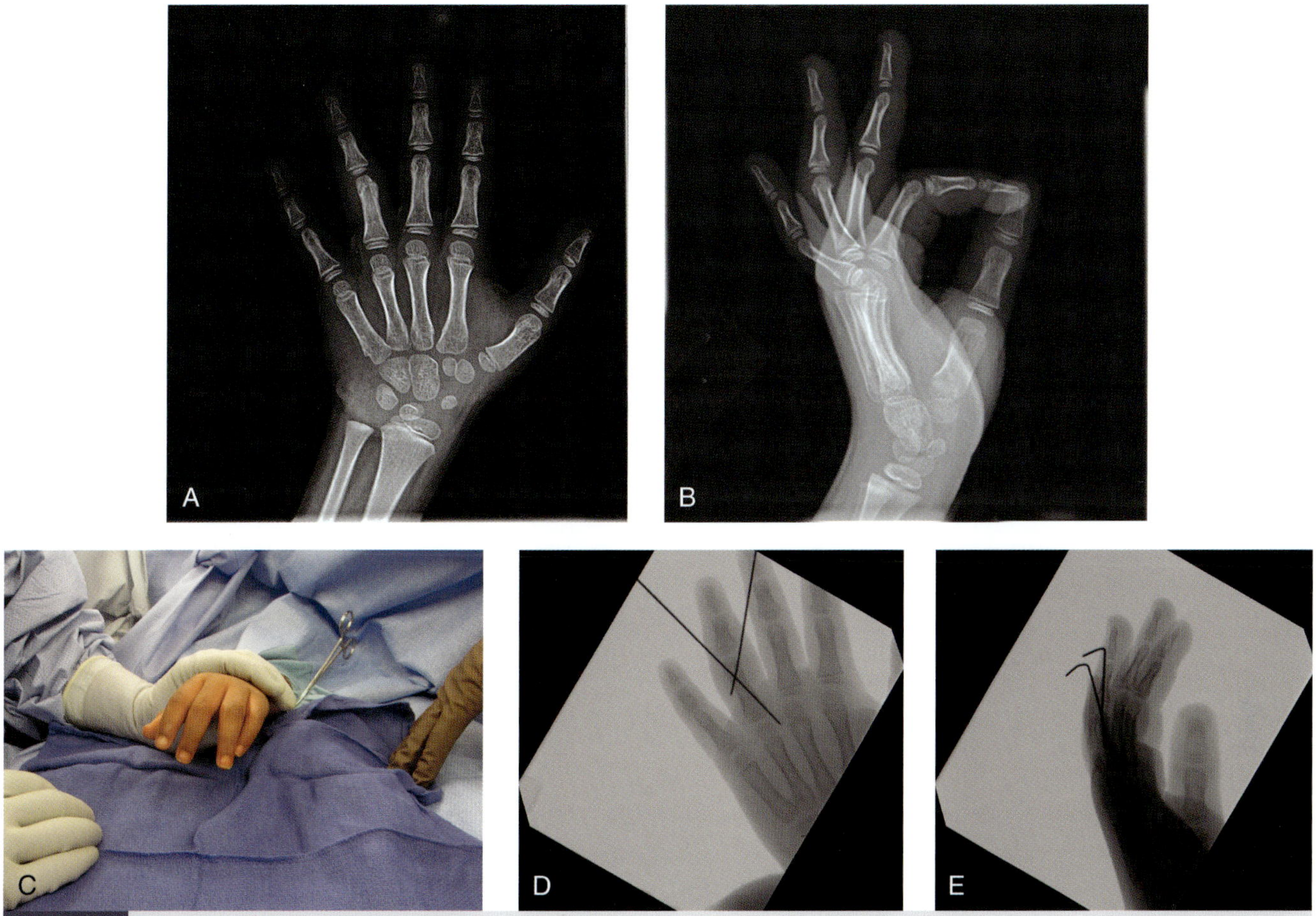

Figure 3 PA (**A**) and lateral (**B**) radiographs of a proximal phalanx phalangeal neck/subchondral fracture of the left ring finger of a 5-year-old boy sustained after his finger was caught in a door. Note the relatively benign appearance of the fracture. **C,** Intraoperative photograph shows the substantial deviation caused by the fracture. Intraoperative PA (**D**) and lateral (**E**) fluoroscopic images after closed reduction and percutaneous pinning of the fracture. (Copyright Joshua M. Abzug, MD, Timonium, MD.)

fractures, more proximal fractures, and fractures in patients with osteonecrosis.[29] CT is the most accurate and reliable modality to assess scaphoid fracture union. If a fracture does not unite with immobilization alone or in the case of displaced fractures or fractures with delayed presentations in which surgical treatment is indicated, surgical fixation is likely to be successful. One study reported a 98% union rate in pediatric patients treated with surgical fixation of scaphoid fractures for a variety of indications.[29]

Surgical fixation is warranted for acute displaced fractures (>1 mm), open fractures, and fractures with associated injuries such as transscaphoid perilunate fracture dislocations and displaced distal radius fractures requiring surgical treatment. A 2011 study reported a 96.5% union rate after surgical intervention.[29] Greater times to union after surgical intervention are associated with open physes, fracture displacement, more proximal fractures, the type of screw used for fixation, and bone grafting at the time of surgery.

Complications after nonsurgical and surgical treatment of pediatric and adolescent scaphoid fractures are relatively rare. However, late presentation of chronic fractures with nonunion is more common in this population. In one study, the use of immobilization only achieved union in 18 of 90 patients (20%) with chronic fractures.[29] A 2010 study reported successful treatment of scaphoid nonunion in 96% of the patients using bone grafting and internal fixation.[31] Union occurred at an average of 10.3 weeks (range, 8-14 weeks), with only 1 of 23 patients requiring a second bone grafting procedure to achieve union. Functional outcomes were excellent in approximately 75% of patients, with good outcomes in the remaining 25%.[31] These findings suggest that chronic scaphoid nonunions are optimally treated with surgical intervention.

Hand Fractures

Pediatric hand fractures are extremely common, with finger fractures representing the second most common pediatric fracture seen in emergency departments in the United States.[1] Most of these fractures can be treated nonsurgically with splint or cast immobilization followed by early active range of motion. Some fractures, including displaced fractures with malrotation or angulation, open fractures, displaced phalangeal neck fractures, and Seymour fractures are best treated surgically[32-34] (**Figure 3**). The complications and outcomes after surgical treatment of displaced pediatric proximal phalanx fractures have recently been reported.[32] The authors reported that most of the patients had excellent outcomes, with no pain, full function, and perfect aesthetics. However, 5% of the patients had complications, including infection, pin site complications, and malunions. Approximately 30% of the patients had stiffness and ultimately required a course of hand therapy to regain motion.[32]

Pediatric phalangeal neck or subchondral fractures deserve special mention because these fractures are often displaced and relatively unstable and require surgical treatment. A stepwise algorithm has been recommended to successfully treat these fractures.[34] The algorithm begins with an attempt at closed reduction. If this is successful, percutaneous pinning is performed. If closed reduction is not successful, a percutaneous reduction is recommended using a temporary intrafocal pin as a joystick for reduction and osteoclasis as needed. If these maneuvers fail, then open reduction with percutaneous pinning should be performed. Using this algorithm, the authors of a 2014 study reported that 80% of the fractures were treated with closed reduction and percutaneous pinning, and the remaining 20% were treated with percutaneous reduction and percutaneous pinning.[34] In all of the fractures that were treated more than 2 weeks after injury, percutaneous reduction and percutaneous pinning were required. Good or excellent outcomes were reported in 90% of the patients. Among those with fair or poor outcomes, four patients had complications, which included two patients with a flexion contracture, one patient with nonunion after a pin tract infection, and one patient with osteonecrosis after a crush injury.[34] A 2015 study that evaluated complications after surgical treatment of displaced proximal phalanx fractures reported that subcondylar fractures were associated with a greater likelihood of stiffness, angular deformity, and worse aesthetic outcomes.[32] In addition, a study assessing the sequelae of pediatric phalangeal fractures found that subcondylar fractures were associated with decreased range of motion, malunion, and osteonecrosis.[35]

Summary

Pediatric forearm, wrist, and hand trauma is extremely common. Most fractures can be treated nonsurgically with immobilization. When fracture alignment is unacceptable, closed reduction and casting performed using excellent techniques can achieve successful outcomes. Surgical intervention, when needed, typically achieves excellent outcomes with a low complication rate.

Key Study Points

- The casting technique plays an important role in the successful closed management of pediatric forearm fractures.
- Early recognition and treatment of Monteggia fracture-dislocations yields excellent outcomes, whereas a missed diagnosis may lead to permanent pain, instability, and decreased range of motion.
- Acute scaphoid fractures in children and adolescents can be successfully treated with immobilization alone in 90% of patients.
- Pediatric phalangeal neck and subchondral fractures are best managed surgically; however, even with optimal treatment these fractures are more likely to have a poor outcome compared with other pediatric phalangeal fractures.

Annotated References

1. Naranje SM, Erali RA, Warner WC Jr, Sawyer JR, Kelly DM: Epidemiology of pediatric fractures presenting to emergency departments in the United States. *J Pediatr Orthop* 2015.

   Using the National Electronic Injury Surveillance System database and 2010 US Census data, the occurrence rates of certain common pediatric fractures were extrapolated and analyzed. The peak age of fracture was between 10 and 14 years of age (15.23 per 1,000 children), with the annual occurrence rate in the entire pediatric population reported at 9.47 per 1,000 children. Fractures of the forearm were the most common (17.8%), and finger and wrist fractures were the second and third most common, respectively. Level of evidence: III.

2. Sumko MJ, Hennrikus W, Slough J, et al: Measurement of radiation exposure when using the mini C-arm to reduce pediatric upper extremity fractures. *J Pediatr Orthop* 2015.

   An evaluation of the amount of radiation exposure during the use of the mini C-arm by program year (PGY)2 and PGY3 residents when reducing upper extremity fractures was performed and compared with the amount of radiation that is typical in plain film radiography for two orthogonal wrist views. In the evaluation of 86 consecutive pediatric upper extremity fracture patients who underwent a reduction, it was found that PGY2 residents more often used fluoroscopy than PGY3 residents and more radiation exposure was seen with mini C-arm use in these reductions than with standard radiographic views.

3. Bae DS: Pediatric distal radius and forearm fractures. *J Hand Surg Am* 2008;33(10):1911-1923.

4. Noonan KJ, Price CT: Forearm and distal radius fractures in children. *J Am Acad Orthop Surg* 1998;6(3):146-156.

5. Zlotolow DA: Pediatric forearm fractures: Spotting and managing the bad actors. *J Hand Surg Am* 2012;37(2):363-366, quiz 366.

   A review article of treatment of pediatric forearm fractures is presented with a focus on so-called bad actors that have a higher chance of losing reduction and/or resulting in complications or poor outcomes. Highlighted fractures include the Monteggia variant with plastic deformation of the ulna; Monteggia and Galeazzi fractures and variants, including those with fractures of both bones and an associated distal radial ulnar joint or radiocapitellar joint disruption; forearm fractures of both bones with initial ulnar angulation of greater than 15° or with radius fractures located in the proximal third (prone to lose reduction with cast immobilization); and comminuted fractures with rotational malalignment caused by the difficulty in assessing the bony landmarks in children to properly determine appropriate rotation.

6. Bowman EN, Mehlman CT, Lindsell CJ, Tamai J: Nonoperative treatment of both-bone forearm shaft fractures in children: Predictors of early radiographic failure. *J Pediatr Orthop* 2011;31(1):23-32.

   Three hundred twenty-one pediatric patients with complete forearm fractures of both bones were retrospectively analyzed to assess the rates of loss of reduction and factors that might predict loss of reduction. Of those who lost reduction after initial closed reduction treatment, 55% of reductions failed by the end of the first week and 95% failed by 3 weeks. The odds of failure were greatest in patients 10 years or older, those with proximal radius fractures, and those with initial angulation of the ulna less than 15°. Level of evidence: II.

7. Wellsh BM, Kuzma JM: Ultrasound-guided pediatric forearm fracture reductions in a resource-limited ED. *Am J Emerg Med* 2016;34(1);40-44.

   The authors report on the treatment of 47 children with closed forearm fractures requiring reduction. Ultrasound was used to guide the reductions. There were 44 (94%) successful reductions, with only 3 patients (6%) requiring repeat reductions. No further adverse events were reported.

8. Ting BL, Kalish LA, Waters PM, Bae DS: Reducing cost and radiation exposure during the treatment of pediatric greenstick fractures of the forearm. *J Pediatr Orthop* 2015; June 5 [Epub ahead of print].

   The authors retrospectively analyzed 109 pediatric patients treated with closed reduction and cast immobilization for greenstick fractures of the forearm. With close radiographic and clinical follow-up, only one patient (0.9%) underwent repeat reduction because of loss of initial reduction and unacceptable radiographic alignment. On average, 3.5 sets of radiographs were obtained during the follow-up period. In this series of greenstick fractures, loss of reduction was rare and the number of follow-up radiographs could possibly be diminished by one radiograph leading to a 14.3% reduction in total cost of fracture care and a 41% reduction in radiation exposure. Level of evidence: IV.

9. McQuinn AG, Jaarsma RL: Risk factors for redisplacement of pediatric distal forearm and distal radius fractures. *J Pediatr Orthop* 2012;32(7):687-692.

   The authors present a review of 155 children with distal radius and forearm fractures treated with reduction and cast immobilization. Demographic factors, fracture characteristics, and initial reduction quality were assessed. Parameters regarding the cast quality also were measured on postreduction radiographs. Redisplacement was seen in 21% of the fractures. Factors associated with redisplacement included initial displacement of greater than 50% of the width of the radius and failure to achieve anatomic reduction and cast index greater than 0.7. Level of evidence: II.

10. Schreck MJ, Hammert WC: Comparison of above- and below-elbow casting for pediatric distal metaphyseal forearm fractures. *J Hand Surg Am* 2014;39(2):347-349.

   A case-based summary of the recent and current literature regarding above- and below-elbow casting in the treatment of pediatric distal metaphyseal forearm fractures is presented. A well-molded short arm cast offers adequate immobilization and protection against redisplacement after reduction compared with long arm casting. In addition, patient and family preference, decreased elbow stiffness, and decreased social burden relative to activities of daily living were reported with a short arm cast.

11. Auer RT, Mazzone P, Robinson L, Nyland J, Chan G: Childhood obesity increases the risk of failure in the treatment of distal forearm fractures. *J Pediatr Orthop* 2015.

   The authors retrospectively analyzed 157 consecutive patients with forearm fractures initially treated in a closed fashion with or without reduction. Sixty-six children (42%) were overweight and 46 children (29%) were obese. The children who were obese were significantly more likely to require a reduction in the operating room after initial treatment ($P = 0.02$), needed significantly more visits requiring radiography ($P = 0.004$), and were significantly less likely to have an initial perfect reduction in the emergency room ($P = 0.005$). Level of evidence: III.

12. Tisosky AJ, Werger MM, McPartland TG, Bowe JA: The factors influencing refracture of pediatric forearms. *J Pediatr Orthop* 2015;35(7):677-681.

A retrospective chart review of 2,590 pediatric patients who sustained a forearm fracture of both bones is presented. Thirty-seven patients sustained a refracture (1.4%), and the average time to refracture after healing of the original fracture was 128.7 days, with 36% of refractures occurring within 6 weeks of clinical clearance from the original fracture. Seventy-one percent of patients with refractures had more than 10° of residual angulation at the time of healing of the original fracture, and 72% of the refractures occurred in patients with fractures of the middle third of the forearm.

13. Flynn JM, Jones KJ, Garner MR, Goebel J: Eleven years experience in the operative management of pediatric forearm fractures. *J Pediatr Orthop* 2010;30(4):313-319.

14. Martus JE, Preston RK, Schoenecker JG, Lovejoy SA, Green NE, Mencio GA: Complications and outcomes of diaphyseal forearm fracture intramedullary nailing: A comparison of pediatric and adolescent age groups. *J Pediatr Orthop* 2013;33(6):598-607.

    The authors present a review of 4,161 pediatric forearm fractures treated at a single institution. Ninety-two percent of fractures were treated nonsurgically, and the remaining 8% of fractures (353 patients) were treated surgically with a variety of fixation methods. Those treated with intramedullary fixation (205 patients) were further studied. Outcomes were good or excellent in 91% of those patients. The rate of severe complications was found to be 17%, including three cases of compartment syndrome.

15. Lee AK, Beck JD, Mirenda WM, Klena JC: Incidence and risk factors for extensor pollicis longus rupture in elastic stable intramedullary nailing of pediatric forearm shaft fractures. *J Pediatr Orthop* 2015.

    Seventeen patients with pediatric forearm fractures treated surgically with flexible intramedullary nailing were analyzed retrospectively. The average follow-up was 5.5 years. All but one patient had their implants removed after fracture healing at an average of 21 weeks. Three patients sustained a rupture of the extensor pollicis longus tendon (18%). The authors found no independent risk factors or predictive factors for extensor pollicis longus rupture in this series of patients. Level of evidence: IV.

16. Ring D, Jupiter JB, Waters PM: Monteggia fractures in children and adults. *J Am Acad Orthop Surg* 1998;6(4):215-224.

17. Ramski DE, Hennrikus WP, Bae DS, et al: Pediatric Monteggia fractures: A multicenter examination of treatment strategy and early clinical and radiographic results. *J Pediatr Orthop* 2015;35(2):115-120.

    A retrospective analysis of 112 acute pediatric Monteggia fractures treated in a variety of ways is presented. Failure of treatment was defined as radiocapitellar subluxation or dislocation and/or loss of reduction of the ulna fracture. Monteggia fractures with a complete ulna fracture that were treated nonsurgically had a high failure rate of 33% (6 of 18) compared with no failures in the 52 fractures in this same group that were surgically treated. Other complications were similar among the treatment groups. Patients with comminuted fracture patterns in the ulna more frequently required open reduction of the radiocapitellar joint compared with other fracture patterns ($P < 0.001$). Level of evidence: III.

18. Sebastin SJ, Chung KC: A historical report on Riccardo Galeazzi and the management of Galeazzi fractures. *J Hand Surg Am* 2010;35(11):1870-1877.

19. Rettig ME, Raskin KB: Galeazzi fracture-dislocation: A new treatment-oriented classification. *J Hand Surg Am* 2001;26(2):228-235.

20. Eberl R, Singer G, Schalamon J, Petnehazy T, Hoellwarth ME: Galeazzi lesions in children and adolescents: Treatment and outcome. *Clin Orthop Relat Res* 2008;466(7):1705-1709.

21. Shah NS, Buzas D, Zinberg EM: Epidemiologic dynamics contributing to pediatric wrist fractures in the United States. *Hand (N Y)* 2015;10(2):266-271.

    An analysis of 53,265 patients with pediatric wrist fractures using the National Electronic Injury Surveillance System database was conducted to assess epidemiologic characteristics of the injuries and the patients. The most common locations of injuries were places of recreation/sports activities, home, and school. The top five consumer-product injuries were related to bicycles, football, playground activities, basketball, and soccer. Analysis of subgroups indicated the highest associations with beds (0 to 12 months of age), stairs (13 to 36 months of age), playgrounds (3 to 5 years and 6 to 10 years of age), and football (11 to 17 years of age).

22. Bae DS, Howard AW: Distal radius fractures: What is the evidence? *J Pediatr Orthop* 2012;32(suppl 2):S128-S130.

    An analysis of available randomized controlled trials looking at the treatment of undisplaced and displaced fractures of the pediatric distal radius is presented. Improved patient and family secondary outcomes were seen with equal radiographic alignment at healing in torus fractures and minimally displaced fractures treated with removable splints compared with cast immobilization. When comparing cast immobilization versus immediate pinning in displaced distal radius fractures in two small series, long-term outcomes were equivalent. However, more frequent loss of reduction was seen in the cast group and more pin complications were seen in the group treated with immediate pinning.

23. Bear DM, Friel NA, Lupo CL, Pitetti R, Ward WT: Hematoma block versus sedation for the reduction of distal radius fractures in children. *J Hand Surg Am* 2015;40(1):57-61.

    Fifty-two children with displaced distal radius fractures requiring reduction were prospectively offered either conscious sedation or hematoma block for analgesia for the reduction procedure. Factors, including family satisfaction, length of stay in the emergency department, patient discomfort during the reduction, and complications were assessed, as well as radiographic alignment after reduction. There were no important differences in any of the assessed factors between groups, with the exception of length of stay in the emergency department, which was substantially less in the hematoma block group (2.2 fewer hours).

24. Abzug JM, Little K, Kozin SH: Physeal arrest of the distal radius. *J Am Acad Orthop Surg* 2014;22(6):381-389.

A review of factors associated with physeal arrest after distal radius fractures is presented, including treatment options and recommendations. Factors associated with the increased incidence of physeal arrest after distal radius fracture include multiple attempts at fracture reduction and late reductions of physeal fractures performed after 12 days. Timely recognition of physeal arrest of the distal radius is important in helping to prevent more severe length discrepancies between the radius and ulna and more severe deformities of the radius. Surgical treatment options include physeal arrest of the ulna, resection of physeal bar of the radius with fat interposition, and radial lengthening versus ulnar shortening.

25. Bernthal NM, Mitchell S, Bales JG, Benhaim P, Silva M: Variation in practice habits in the treatment of pediatric distal radius fractures. *J Pediatr Orthop B* 2015;24(5):400-407.

An Internet-based survey was completed by 781 hand, pediatric, and general orthopaedic surgeons to assess variability in practice patterns in the management of 10 presented cases of pediatric distal radius fractures. Hand surgeons and general orthopaedic surgeons were 2.9 and 1.6 times more likely, respectively, to recommend surgical treatment in these cases than pediatric orthopaedic surgeons. Private practice surgeons were more likely to recommend surgical treatment than academic surgeons. Also noted was the discrepancy between surgeons' self-identified acceptable criteria and what they actually chose as treatment on these cases. Level of evidence: IV.

26. Ahmed I, Ashton F, Tay WK, Porter D: The pediatric fracture of the scaphoid in patients aged 13 years and under: An epidemiological study. *J Pediatr Orthop* 2014;34(2):150-154.

An epidemiologic study of 56 pediatric patients with scaphoid fractures is presented. The average annual incidence of the injury was found to be 11 per 100,000 individuals, with 70% of patients being male. The most common fracture location was the distal pole. The one patient who sustained a proximal fracture went on to have a nonunion. At a mean follow-up of 70 months, 60% of patients reported no limitations in daily activities and a mean Disabilities of the Arm, Shoulder and Hand score of 3. Level of evidence: IV.

27. Hayes JR, Groner JI: The increasing incidence of snowboard-related trauma. *J Pediatr Surg* 2008;43(5):928-930.

28. Larson AN, Stans AA, Shaughnessy WJ, Dekutoski MB, Quinn MJ, McIntosh AL: Motocross morbidity: Economic cost and injury distribution in children. *J Pediatr Orthop* 2009;29(8):847-850.

29. Gholson JJ, Bae DS, Zurakowski D, Waters PM: Scaphoid fractures in children and adolescents: Contemporary injury patterns and factors influencing time to union. *J Bone Joint Surg Am* 2011;93(13):1210-1219.

Three hundred fifty-one pediatric scaphoid fractures were retrospectively evaluated assessing fracture pattern and location, union rate, time to union, treatment, and clinical outcomes. Most of the fractures occurred at the scaphoid waist (71%), 23% occurred at the distal pole, and the remainder at the proximal pole. Treatment of acute fractures with cast immobilization alone resulted in a 90% union rate. Factors that resulted in a lower union rate and longer time to union with treatment included chronic fractures, displaced fractures, proximal pole fractures, and fractures in patients with osteonecrosis. A 96.5% union rate was reported in the 113 surgically treated patients.

30. Tessaro MO, McGovern TR, Dickman E, Haines LE: Point-of-care ultrasound detection of acute scaphoid fracture. *Pediatr Emerg Care* 2015;31(3):222-224.

Emergency department recognition and appropriate treatment with immobilization is important in minimizing nonunion in scaphoid fractures. Ultrasound performed by a skilled emergency department provider can be used to detect a scaphoid fracture in the setting of normal radiographs.

31. Masquijo JJ, Willis BR: Scaphoid nonunions in children and adolescents: Surgical treatment with bone grafting and internal fixation. *J Pediatr Orthop* 2010;30(2):119-124.

32. Boyer JS, London DA, Stepan JG, Goldfarb CA: Pediatric proximal phalanx fractures: Outcomes and complications after the surgical treatment of displaced fractures. *J Pediatr Orthop* 2015;35(3):219-223.

The authors report on 105 patients treated with closed reduction and percutaneous pinning of displaced proximal phalanx fractures. Thirty-one patients returned more than 1 year after surgery for further assessment. Complications included infection, pin site problems, and malunion. Thirty-one patients required hand therapy to address postoperative stiffness. Subcondylar fractures had a higher rate of stiffness. In the 31 patients assessed after 1 year, the visual analog scale scores were excellent, and clinical outcomes were equivalent to the contralateral side. Level of evidence: IV.

33. Abzug JM, Kozin SH: Seymour fractures. *J Hand Surg Am* 2013;38(11):2267-2270, quiz 2270.

A case report of a pediatric patient with a Seymour fracture is presented, and a review of the recent literature regarding the treatment for Seymour fractures is discussed. Surgical treatment of a Seymour fracture is indicated to extract soft-tissue interposition from the physeal fracture site. Pin fixation may be indicated if the fracture is unstable. The risk of osteomyelitis, nail dystrophy, and physeal disruption exists with this fracture pattern.

34. Matzon JL, Cornwall R: A stepwise algorithm for surgical treatment of type II displaced pediatric phalangeal neck fractures. *J Hand Surg Am* 2014;39(3):467-473.

The authors report on 61 children with displaced phalangeal neck fractures who were treated surgically based on a described algorithm. Using the algorithm, no fracture required open reduction. All patients treated surgically after 13 days following the injury required percutaneously placed pin-facilitated reduction. In the 53 patients followed for at least 1 year, 45 excellent, 4 good, 1 fair, and 3 poor results were reported. Fair and poor results were seen in four patients who had complications, which included flexion contracture (two patients), nonunion following pin tract infection (one patient), and osteonecrosis after a severe crush injury (one patient). Level of evidence: IV.

35. Huelsemann W, Singer G, Mann M, Winkler FJ, Habenicht R: Analysis of sequelae after pediatric phalangeal fractures. *Eur J Pediatr Surg* 2016;26(2):164-171.

A summary of the sequelae that developed after treatment of pediatric phalangeal fractures seen and treated in 40 patients is presented, including osteonecrosis, physeal arrest, malunion, and malposition. Transcondylar and subcondylar fractures resulted in sequelae in 10 patients, including limited motion and malposition. Fractures in the setting of severe soft-tissue damage resulted in sequelae seen in 10 patients. Most sequelae in this study could be related to the severity of the fracture and other fracture characteristics, although correct and timely treatment is important.

Chapter 38

Pelvis, Hip, Femur, and Knee

Gregory Hale, MD   Christopher Collins, MD   Jose Herrera-Soto, MD

Abstract

Trauma to the pelvis, hip, femur, and knee is mainly caused by high-energy trauma. However, because the immature hip has plasticity and elasticity, minor trauma can cause hip dislocation in a young patient that may go unnoticed. Femoral shaft fractures can be caused by simple falls and twisting injuries in young children, whereas these fractures in older children are more likely caused by sports injuries or high-energy trauma. The care of the fractured femur depends on the personality of the fracture and the age of the patient. Distal femoral injuries occur more commonly in the preadolescent and adolescent populations secondary to sports or high-energy injuries.

Keywords: femur; fracture; hip; knee; pelvis; physis; trauma

Pelvic Fractures

Pediatric pelvic fractures are relatively rare but can be the cause of substantial morbidity and mortality. These injuries can be described starting with the age of the patient. In the skeletally mature population consisting of adolescents with closed growth plates, fracture patterns more closely resemble those in the adult population. Younger patients with open growth plates can have similar patterns of pelvic ring disruption as adults, but such disruption requires higher forces because of the elasticity of the immature pelvis.[1] In general, the immature pelvis tends to deform under a load rather than fracture.[2] The immature pelvis can absorb more energy before fracturing because of the increased elasticity of the bone, stronger ligaments, thicker periosteum, and open growth plates.[2,3] When a fracture occurs, there is often less displacement because of the thicker periosteum of the immature pelvis.[2] In addition, the patient who is skeletally immature can sustain injuries to the growth centers themselves through apophyseal avulsions and triradiate fractures. Pelvic ring injuries account for only 0.3% to 4% of all pediatric injuries, and most of those injuries (83.3%) generally are caused by high-energy trauma.[2] Motor vehicle crashes and automobile versus pedestrian collisions account for most pelvic ring injuries in the pediatric population.[4]

The physical examination of a child with a suspected pelvic fracture should include inspection for pelvic asymmetry; limb-length discrepancy; vascular status; evidence of a hematoma or degloving around the pelvis, buttocks, and perineum; and sources of bleeding from the urethra or the vagina.[2] Radiographs of the pelvis remain the preferred method for determining the presence of a pelvic fracture, but in many orthopaedic centers, a shift toward routine CT for high-energy trauma is occurring. Obtaining CT studies also is important whenever evidence of hemodynamic instability exists. It is important to remember when examining radiographs of the pelvis that the width of the pubic symphysis is as wide as 10 to 12 mm in very young children, approximately 5.5 mm in adolescents, and 2 to 4 mm in adults.[2,3] The role of MRI in the diagnosis of these injuries is evolving but can be useful in young children when much of the pelvis is not fully ossified.[3]

Children who sustain a pelvic fracture can have several concomitant injuries, including bleeding (both retroperitoneal and intrapelvic) and injuries to the head,

Dr. Herrera-Soto or an immediate family member has received royalties from Biomet; is a member of a speakers' bureau or has made paid presentations on behalf of Biomet Spine and Biomet; serves as a paid consultant to Biomet Spine, Biomet, Orthopediatrics, Spine Form, and Spineguard; and serves as a board member, owner, officer, or committee member of the Pediatric Orthopaedic Society of North America and the Scoliosis Research Society. Neither of the following authors nor any immediate family member has received anything of value from or has stock or stock options held in a commercial company or institution related directly or indirectly to the subject of this chapter: Dr. Hale and Dr. Collins.

trunk, limbs, spine, thorax, abdomen, or genitourinary system.[2] When present, head injuries tend to be more severe than in adults and result in an increase in mortality from 3% to 30%.[5]

Numerous classification systems for pediatric pelvic fractures have been developed. The most widely used system was developed in 1985 by Torode and Zieg.[6] In this classification system, type I injuries are considered apophyseal avulsions, and type II injuries are iliac wing fractures. The classification system also described two types of pelvic ring fractures: type III, which are simple pelvic ring fractures (pubic rami fractures and stable symphyseal disruptions), and type IV ring disruptions, which are fractures with segmental instability, AP fractures, straddle fractures, and pelvic fractures with associated acetabular fractures. In 2012, the original classification system was modified to take into account CT data to incorporate a new division of type III injuries that show disruptions of both the anterior and posterior pelvic ring but remain stable with less than 2 mm of displacement. Such injuries are termed type IIIB injuries and are predictive of increased blood product usage and longer hospital stays. Type IIIB injuries are similar to type IV injuries but are adequately treated without surgery in most patients.[4]

The initial treatment of pelvic ring injuries depends largely on hemodynamic status. In the presence of a displaced, open book pelvic ring injury, any signs of shock will likely warrant the placement of a pelvic sheet or binder to decrease intrapelvic volume and bleeding. Although a true lateral compression fracture likely would not need a pelvic binder, most pelvic injuries result from a combination of more than one mechanism; therefore, the decision to use a pelvic sheet or binder should take into account more factors than just the radiographic appearance of the fracture. If hemodynamic status does not improve after this placement, then emergent angiography and embolization may be needed. Major venous bleeding may even necessitate surgical packing of the pelvis. Types II and III injuries can typically be treated nonsurgically with a short non–weight-bearing period. Instability (displacement of the pelvis with normal weight bearing) and displacement of greater than 1 cm are the main indications for surgical intervention.[3] Posterior sacroiliac screw fixation with concomitant anterior fixation of the pelvic ring, by either external fixation or anterior plating, is the preferred fixation method. In a skeletally immature patient, a plate placed over the symphysis must be removed after healing has occurred to allow for continued growth of the anterior pelvic ring.[3]

In a recent review of the literature, overall mortality results were reported to range from zero to 25% (averaging 6.4%).[2,4] In the same review, complex pelvic trauma or the presence of a crush injury was shown to have, on average, a mortality rate of 20%. However, the mortality rate is still less than that seen with adult pelvic fractures.[3] A recent review of the National Trauma Data Bank showed that children (younger than 13 years) had increased odds of death but decreased odds of severe complications compared with adults, whereas adolescents (aged 13 to 17 years) had decreased odds of both death and severe complications compared with adults.[7]

Long-term complications include delayed union and nonunion, sacroiliac joint subluxation, fusion of the sacroiliac joint, persistent symphysis, pubis diastasis, hemipelvic undergrowth, and lumbosacral scoliosis.[2] More than 30% of children who sustain unstable pelvic fractures can experience long-term sequelae, including pelvic and hip pain, a limp, scoliosis, low back pain, and a permanent neurologic deficit.[8]

Acetabular fractures are an even rarer occurrence in the pediatric population, representing 0.8% to 20% of pelvic injuries,[9,10] primarily because of the increased cartilage volume of the immature acetabulum compared with that of adults, which results in a greater ability to absorb energy from an impact before fracturing.[9] Injuries occurring in adolescents who are skeletally mature have largely been treated with surgical intervention, and similar results as those in adult acetabular fractures have been obtained. Complications include abductor weakness, heterotopic ossification, deep infection, and osteonecrosis of the femoral head when associated with a hip dislocation.[9]

Acetabular injuries in skeletally immature patients are sparsely reported in the literature and provide additional challenges when the triradiate cartilage is involved. A wide range, from 22% to 80%, of triradiate injuries can be missed on primary radiographs.[10] If suspicion exists for a triradiate injury, CT is recommended to fully evaluate the growth plate. MRI also can be useful for detecting an inverted labrum, loose osteochondral fragments, and triradiate injuries. In 1982, researchers proposed a classification for these injuries that is analogous to the Salter-Harris classification: type I, epiphysiolysis of one part of the triradiate cartilage; type II, epiphysiolysis with bony extension; and type V, crush injury to the growth plate.[11]

The mainstay of treatment of acetabular injuries remains nonsurgical, with surgical criteria limited to displacement of the weight-bearing surface, large posterior wall fragments, and incarcerated fragments. Patients with minimally displaced type I and II fractures typically fare well and have minimal long-term complications. However, late sequelae can include both posttraumatic femoral head necrosis and acetabular dysplasia (especially with type V injuries)—both of which can lead to arthrosis.

Other sequelae include limb-length discrepancy and, rarely, hip joint ankylosis. Routine surveillance radiographs until skeletal maturity are recommended so that any early signs of acetabular dysplasia can be detected.[10] Posttraumatic acetabular dysplasia is markedly different from other forms of hip dysplasia. In general, the femoral anatomy remains normal while the pelvis deforms, showing apparent lengthening compared with the other hemipelvis. However, the teardrop and inner wall have an increased size, which results in lateralization of the femoral head.[3]

Table 1

Delbet Classification of Pediatric Hip Fractures

Type	Description
I	Transepiphyseal fracture, with or without dislocation of the femoral head from the acetabulum
II	Transcervical fracture
III	Cervicotrochanteric fracture
IV	Intertrochanteric fracture

Hip Fractures

Hip fractures are uncommon in the pediatric population, accounting for less than 1% of all pediatric fractures. Most hip fractures in children are associated with high-energy trauma, such as a motor vehicle crash or a fall from a height. The exception to this would be pathologic fractures, such as those associated with bony lesions or metabolic conditions. Concomitant musculoskeletal and other injuries are common. The most popular classification system for hip fractures in children is the Delbet system, which is based on the location of the fracture (**Table 1**). The Delbet system has been shown to have prognostic value for osteonecrosis.[12-14] Displaced Delbet types I, II, and III fractures are considered orthopaedic emergencies because immediate treatment could potentially reverse injury to the blood supply of the femoral head.

Transepiphyseal Fractures

A Delbet type I fracture is the least common, accounting for 10% of all pediatric hip fractures, but it has the highest complication rate. These fractures tend to occur in younger children, often younger than 2 years. A type I fracture in a child younger than 2 years may be the result of child abuse. Fifty percent of the type I injuries encountered are accompanied by a dislocation of the capital femoral epiphysis, and the rate of osteonecrosis approaches 100% in such injuries. However, even in injuries not associated with dislocation, the rate of osteonecrosis has been reported to be as high as 100%.[14,15] A recent meta-analysis, however, showed a rate of osteonecrosis of only 38% with Delbet type I fractures.[12]

It has been reported that spontaneous remodeling can occur in children younger than 2 years who are treated with a hip spica cast without reduction. In most children, however, the treatment of a type I hip fracture starts with an attempt at closed reduction using traction, abduction, and internal rotation followed by pin fixation and spica casting. If closed reduction is unsuccessful, open reduction is indicated. Open reduction is performed with either an anterolateral or a direct anterior approach to the hip. However, if the dislocation is posterior, a posterior approach may be necessary. Fixation of the type I fracture necessitates crossing the physis. Fixation can be done with smooth pins in a child younger than 4 years or with screws in a child older than 4 years. The use of a spica cast is recommended for additional stability in children younger than 10 years.

Epiphyseal separation caused by birth trauma stemming from a breech delivery is a very rare Delbet type I fracture. The newborn infant usually has pseudoparalysis of the leg. Ultrasonography can help differentiate a fracture from an infection. Fortunately, epiphyseal separation in the newborn tends to remodel completely if the physis does not prematurely close. The recommended treatment is simple skin traction followed by casting and careful follow-up.

Transcervical and Cervicotrochanteric Fractures

Delbet type II transcervical hip fractures are the most common type of pediatric hip fracture, accounting for 45% of all pediatric hip fractures.[16] Osteonecrosis has been reported to be as high as 60% in such fractures. Cervicotrochanteric hip fractures (Delbet type III) are the second most common type of pediatric hip fracture, accounting for 30% of these fractures. Osteonecrosis has been reported to be approximately 30% for type III injuries.[16] Conversely, a meta-analysis showed that osteonecrosis develops in 28% of children with type II fractures and 18% of children with type III fractures.[12]

A nondisplaced type II or III fracture in a child younger than 6 years can be treated with spica casting and careful follow-up.[17] Percutaneous fixation and spica cast immobilization are recommended for most children with this injury to minimize the risk of secondary displacement and varus angulation.[18]

A displaced type II or III fracture is treated with anatomic reduction (either closed or open) and internal fixation.[19] Some authors have suggested that open reduction reduces the risk of osteonecrosis.[20] Alternatively, closed reduction with anterior capsulotomy to decompress the hip capsule and reduce the risk of osteonecrosis has been recommended.[21] Other authors recommend closed reduction with simple aspiration of the hip capsule. However, the quality and timing of the reduction may be the most important factors that influence the development of osteonecrosis rather than the use of capsular aspiration or decompression.[13] Patient age older than 11 years also may be an independent risk factor for the development of osteonecrosis.[22] After fracture fixation, a single-leg spica cast is used in children younger than 10 years to maximize fracture stability.[17,19]

In an adolescent, a type II or III injury often requires fixation across the proximal femoral physis to maximize stability. For these patients, achieving fracture stability is more important than preserving the proximal femoral physis. The resulting limb-length discrepancy is usually small, given the nearly 4 mm per year of remaining growth. Adolescents can use crutches and partial weight bearing on the injured leg; if needed, a hip-to-knee orthosis can add stability.

Intertrochanteric Fractures

Intertrochanteric fractures (Delbet type IV) account for approximately 15% of hip fractures in children and have the lowest incidence of osteonecrosis (5% to 10%).[12,14] In children younger than 8 years, these fractures can be treated with closed reduction or traction followed by hip spica casting. Because of remodeling, less than 10° of varus is considered acceptable.[17] Open reduction and internal fixation with a pediatric hip screw and side plate or a pediatric blade plate is recommended for an irreducible fracture in a child of any age, a fracture in a child with polytrauma, or a fracture in a child older than 10 years. In most type IV fractures, screw fixation can stop short of the physis; but in some fractures, fixation must cross the physis for fracture stability.

Hip Fracture Complications

Osteonecrosis of the femoral head is the most common complication resulting from a pediatric hip fracture.[12,14,17,21] The incidence of osteonecrosis after hip fracture varies in the literature (from zero to 100%)[22] and is dependent on multiple factors, including age, fracture location, and initial displacement.[13] Other factors, such as the timing of reduction (<12 hours after injury),[13] decompression of the hip capsule at the time of fixation,[21] and open versus closed reduction,[20] may contribute to the incidence of osteonecrosis. Injury to the vascular supply likely occurs at the time of actual hip fracture because of vessel kinking or laceration by the displaced fracture. Alternatively, femoral head ischemia may be provoked by tamponade of the epiphyseal vessels because of increased intracapsular pressure from the fracture hematoma.[12,16] Osteonecrosis may be recognized radiographically as late as 2 years after the injury.[17]

Other complications associated with pediatric hip fractures include varus angulation (25%), nonunion (5%), and limb-length discrepancy caused by premature physeal closure (2%).[12,16] Case reports and a small case series have suggested that delayed slipped capital femoral epiphysis is another potential complication that can occur after surgical fixation of a femoral neck fracture when the implants stop short of the physis.[23] Limb-length discrepancy can be treated based on the predicted magnitude at skeletal maturity.

Traumatic Hip Dislocation

Traumatic hip dislocation is an uncommon injury in children,[24-26] but because of ligamentous laxity, even minor trauma can cause a hip dislocation in children.[25] In children older than 10 years, a hip dislocation usually results from high-energy trauma, such as a motor vehicle crash. Approximately 90% of pediatric hip dislocations are posterior. A neurovascular examination should be performed, and radiographs should be obtained before reduction.[25] Closed reduction under conscious sedation or general anesthesia usually is successful. Epiphysiolysis of the femoral head during reduction of a traumatic hip dislocation can occur in children who have an open physis, and it also has been reported in adolescents.[27] Prior to reduction, if suspicion for a physeal injury exists on plain radiographs, or if physeal instability is observed under fluoroscopy, open reduction and internal fixation of the epiphysis is recommended to prevent inadvertent displacement of the epiphysis with closed reduction.[19,27] Hip stability after reduction should be assessed while the patient is still sedated.

Although reduction is usually easily achieved, careful attention should be paid to postreduction radiographs for nonconcentric reduction. As much as 3 mm of hip joint asymmetry may be caused by a hematoma or joint laxity.[28,29] If any concern exists for a hematoma or joint laxity, cross-sectional imaging with CT or MRI should be obtained. CT is preferable for detecting osteochondral lesions, and MRI is best for soft-tissue interposition. Labral, capsular, and osteochondral fragment interposition may prevent reduction, which usually requires surgery for anatomic reduction in as many as 15% of patients. In rare instances, the hip reduces spontaneously at the time of injury with interposition of bone or soft tissue with residual joint incongruity[29] (**Figure 1**). Open reduction is indicated for a patient with an intra-articular fragment,

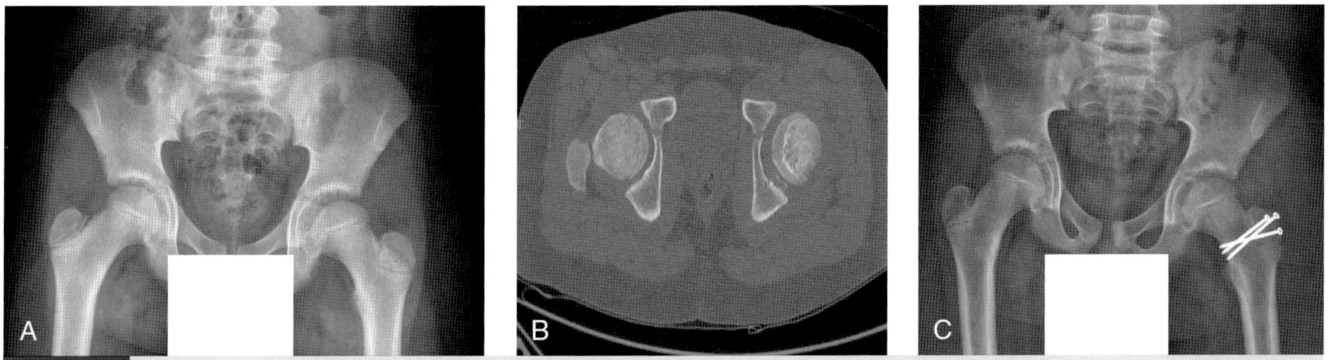

Figure 1 Images from a 13-year-old boy who had immediate left hip pain after a football tackle. **A,** AP radiograph shows widening in the medial joint space on the left side compared with the right side. **B,** Axial CT scan shows joint asymmetry and posterior bony interposition. **C,** Postoperative AP radiograph obtained 6 weeks after surgery shows a symmetric joint space. The patient was ambulatory and pain free.

a nonconcentric reduction, or an unstable acetabular rim fracture.[25]

Historically, the recommended surgical approach to the hip was from the direction of dislocation. Arthroscopic treatment of an interposed fragment also has been reported.[30,31] In addition, surgical hip dislocation has been introduced as a method for treating traumatic hip dislocations with interposed tissue.[32] To prevent redislocation in a child younger than 10 years, some authors recommend postreduction spica casting for 4 to 6 weeks.[25,33] An older child may benefit from a brace and protected weight bearing with crutches for 6 weeks.[25]

After a traumatic hip dislocation, osteonecrosis has been reported in 3% to 15% of patients.[28] Urgent reduction of the hip within 6 hours of the injury may decrease the risk of osteonecrosis.[25,28] In older children, a high-energy injury may be a risk factor for osteonecrosis.[26] Postreduction bone scanning or MRI does not appear to reliably predict the later development of osteonecrosis.[28,34] In the long term, asymptomatic coxa magna develops in approximately 20% of patients.[34] Prompt reduction of a hip dislocation can reduce the risk of sciatic or superior gluteal nerve palsy.[25]

In rare instances, a hip dislocation may be unrecognized for days or weeks in a pediatric patient with multiple trauma.[25] The rate of osteonecrosis in such patients is 100%.[35] Open reduction is recommended to position the femoral head into the acetabulum, stimulate growth of the femur and the pelvis, and minimize the deformity and limb-length inequality.[24]

Femoral Shaft Fractures

In the young child, femoral shaft fractures can be caused by simple falls and twisting injuries, whereas the cause among older children is more often a sports injury or high-energy trauma. There are many treatment options for femoral shaft fractures.[36,37] The type of treatment depends on the age and size of the patient, the type of fracture (transverse, oblique, comminuted), the social environment, and the surgeon's preference and expertise. The American Academy of Orthopaedic Surgeons has developed a clinical practice guideline to assist the treating physician in selecting the appropriate treatment option.[37]

Treatment Options by Age

During the first 6 months of life, most femoral shaft fractures can be safely treated in a Pavlik harness or a hip spica cast.[38] This allows relaxation of the deforming forces, decreases the chances of malunion, and allows space for diaper changes. Most of these fractures are healed and stable within 3 weeks.

Fracture manipulation, not reduction, and spica casting are the conventional methods of treatment for children aged 6 months to 6 years. However, some surgeons have elected to perform elastic nailing earlier in life.[39] The authors noted similar healing times, with earlier return to independent ambulation and full activities in the elastic nailing group. Spica casting can be done in either the surgical suite or the emergency department with similar results.[40]

Elastic nailing has been advocated for children aged 5 to 13 years. However, the size of the patient is an important factor. Poor outcomes are five times more frequent in patients who weigh more than 49 kg.[41] Most authors recommend filling approximately 80% of the shaft canal diameter with the nails. A biomechanical study evaluated adding a third nail, which demonstrated a substantial influence on stiffness in all four-point bendings as well as internal rotation compared with the classic two-nail configuration.[42] These researchers also reported that adding end caps did not improve stiffness in any direction.

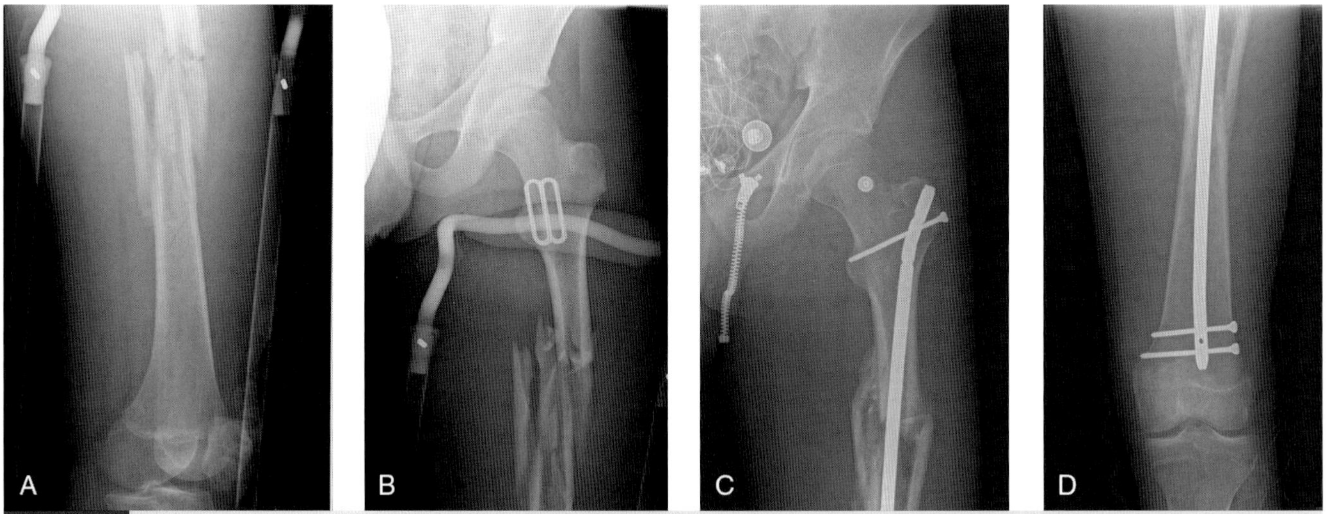

Figure 2 Images from a 14-year-old boy who sustained an injury to the left femur in a motor vehicle crash. Preoperative (**A**) and postoperative **(B)** AP radiographs after lateral trochanteric entry locked intramedullary nailing. Because of comminution, attention was given to restoring femoral length and rotation. **C** and **D,** AP radiographs obtained 6 weeks after surgery show abundant callus formation. The patient had started full weight bearing 5 weeks postoperatively without pain.

Another option is to use stainless steel elastic nails rather than titanium. Stainless steel has been shown to be stiffer in bending, torsion, and axial compression in an in vitro study.[43]

Studies have reported on malunion after elastic nailing of femoral shaft fractures.[44,45] In 2006, researchers noted that malangulation developed in 16 of 70 fractures, most often in the anteroposterior plane (11 of 16).[44] By studying their results, these researchers created a bone model for determining whether the direction of the nail shoe tip in the proximal fragment had any bearing on the radiographic outcome. They found that anterior bowing was the most common malangulation, and nail shoe tip direction influenced the likelihood of anterior bowing. They identified that having at least one of the tips pointing toward the anterior plane decreases the chances of malangulation. Other researchers reported a high rate of rotational malunion after elastic nailing, with 32 of 68 fractures (47%) healing with at least 15° of torsional malalignment, thus creating relative femoral retroversion in 31 of 32 fractures (97%).[45]

When considering older and heavier pediatric patients, the type of fixation can be modified to withstand mechanical stresses. Lateral trochanteric entry rigid nails have gained favor in such circumstances, particularly in patients older than 8 years with an intramedullary canal of ample size (**Figure 2**); however, the safe lower age limit of rigid intramedullary nailing is unclear. The advantages of locked nailing include stable fixation, small incisions, and early weight bearing. The disadvantages in a younger patient are concerns for proximal femoral growth disturbance and femoral head osteonecrosis. In 2011, researchers performed a systematic review of locked femoral nailing in patients who were skeletally immature and estimated the rates of femoral head osteonecrosis associated with piriformis entry (2%) and trochanteric tip entry (1.4%).[46] Osteonecrosis after lateral trochanteric entry locked nailing has not been reported in studies that describe the complications and outcomes of this technique.[47] A multicenter study compared elastic stable intramedullary nails with antegrade locking nails and found that patients who were older and heavier had shorter recovery times and a lower frequency of complications when they were treated with rigid nailing.[48] However, the outcomes for both groups were very similar. Other authors have biomechanically compared elastic nails and semirigid locking nails, demonstrating greater stability with the locking nails.[49]

Another option for unstable and comminuted fractures is submuscular plating, which is a relatively less invasive procedure compared with open plating because some of the screws can be placed in a percutaneous fashion, although a larger incision may be required if implant removal is necessary. A recent study reviewed 85 femoral shaft fractures treated with plate fixation and reported an overall complication rate of 12%.[50] One patient had a limb-length inequality that required epiphysiodesis. Valgus of 5° or more developed in 11% of femoral fractures treated with plating, and 30% of those fractures required an additional procedure to correct the deformity.[50] Patients with a plate-to-physis distance greater than or equal to 20 mm and a distal diaphyseal fracture were at a substantially higher risk for the development of a distal femoral valgus deformity. In 2012, researchers compared locked nailing and submuscular plating for adolescent femoral fractures and reported good results overall; however, they noted greater fluoroscopy time and a longer delay to full weight bearing in the submuscular plating group.[51]

Subtrochanteric Femoral Fractures

Subtrochanteric femoral fractures are more challenging to manage because varus malangulation is frequent when these fractures are treated with spica casting. At a younger age, these fractures will remodel. However, for the young adolescent and preadolescent years, either plating or nailing has been advocated.[47,52,53] In 2014, researchers evaluated the complication rate when using elastic nails for subtrochanteric fractures.[53] They reported a 22% complication rate, including revision of fixation in 11% and malunion in 6%. Excellent outcomes were found in 61% of the patients, and 33% of the patients had satisfactory outcomes at the latest follow-up. Other authors have identified plate fixation as having better outcomes than elastic nailing for the treatment of subtrochanteric femoral fractures.[52] In a report describing 10 patients, the use of statically locked intramedullary nailing was recommended.[47] Early ambulation was allowed, and no intraoperative complications were noted. In the postoperative period, the authors identified two patients with limb-length inequalities of less than 1 cm and two patients with grade 1 asymptomatic heterotopic ossification. For subtrochanteric fractures in preadolescents and young adolescents, the authors recommended locked nailing to minimize complications and maintain limb alignment.[47]

Knee (Distal Femur)

Supracondylar Metaphyseal Femoral Fractures

Supracondylar metaphyseal femoral fractures are uncommon in children. In nonambulatory infants, these fractures may be caused by child abuse,[54] but they also can be sustained during an accidental fall from a low height. These fractures, located proximal to the physis, usually occur just above the insertion of the gastrocnemius muscle on the distal femur.[55] The gastrocnemius and hip adductor muscles produce posterior and medial angulation of the distal fragment. With displaced fractures, the proximal fragment can buttonhole through the quadriceps and the extensor mechanism. Reduction can be difficult, but knee flexion may help reduce the pull of the gastrocnemius. Because it is difficult to obtain and maintain a reduction, the acceptable treatment options include closed or open reduction, crossed smooth-pin fixation with a cast, open reduction and internal fixation with a plate, and external fixation.[56] Traction and casting are acceptable for treating children younger than 10 years, although traction has largely been replaced by other treatment methods. Two-pin epiphyseal-metaphyseal traction has been suggested for controlled sagittal rotation.[56] In children aged 7 months to 5 years, acceptable angulation in a cast is less than 10° of varus or valgus, less than 10° of procurvatum, and less than 20° of recurvatum.

The use of plating and external fixation is limited by the size of the metaphyseal fragment.[56] The distal femoral physis should be avoided during plate fixation; a T-plate can be helpful. External fixation of a supracondylar femoral fracture can lead to knee joint sepsis (the knee joint capsule can be penetrated by the pins) or stiffness (caused by adhesions in the distal iliotibial band). Percutaneously placed pins can be buried under the skin to lessen the risk of sepsis; alternatively, they can be placed in antegrade fashion to avoid penetration of the joint capsule altogether.

Distal Femoral Physeal Fractures

Distal femoral physeal fractures are uncommon and most often result from a motor vehicle crash or a football injury.[57,58] Most distal femoral physeal fractures are Salter-Harris type II fractures.[58] Growth disturbance occurs after approximately 50% of these fractures and can lead to angular deformity and/or limb-length discrepancy; half of fractures that cause growth disturbance require later surgical intervention. Growth arrest is believed to result from bone bridge formation after direct physeal trauma or nonanatomic reduction.

Displaced Salter-Harris type II distal femoral fractures should undergo a gentle closed or open anatomic reduction while the patient is under general anesthesia, and fixation with smooth wires or screws should maintain the reduction (**Figure 3**). Threaded pins or screws should not be placed across the physis to avoid additional physeal injury. Pins used around the knee can be buried under the skin or placed in antegrade fashion to avoid an intra-articular pin infection, which can lead to septic arthritis. Fixation is recommended to prevent redisplacement, and usually it is supplemented with a cast or brace.[58] A postoperative long leg cast or a one leg spica cast is recommended depending on the age of the child. The pins can be removed and knee motion allowed approximately 6 weeks after fixation.

A nondisplaced distal femoral Salter-Harris type II fracture can initially be treated with a cast. Radiographic follow-up is recommended after 1 week; reduction and

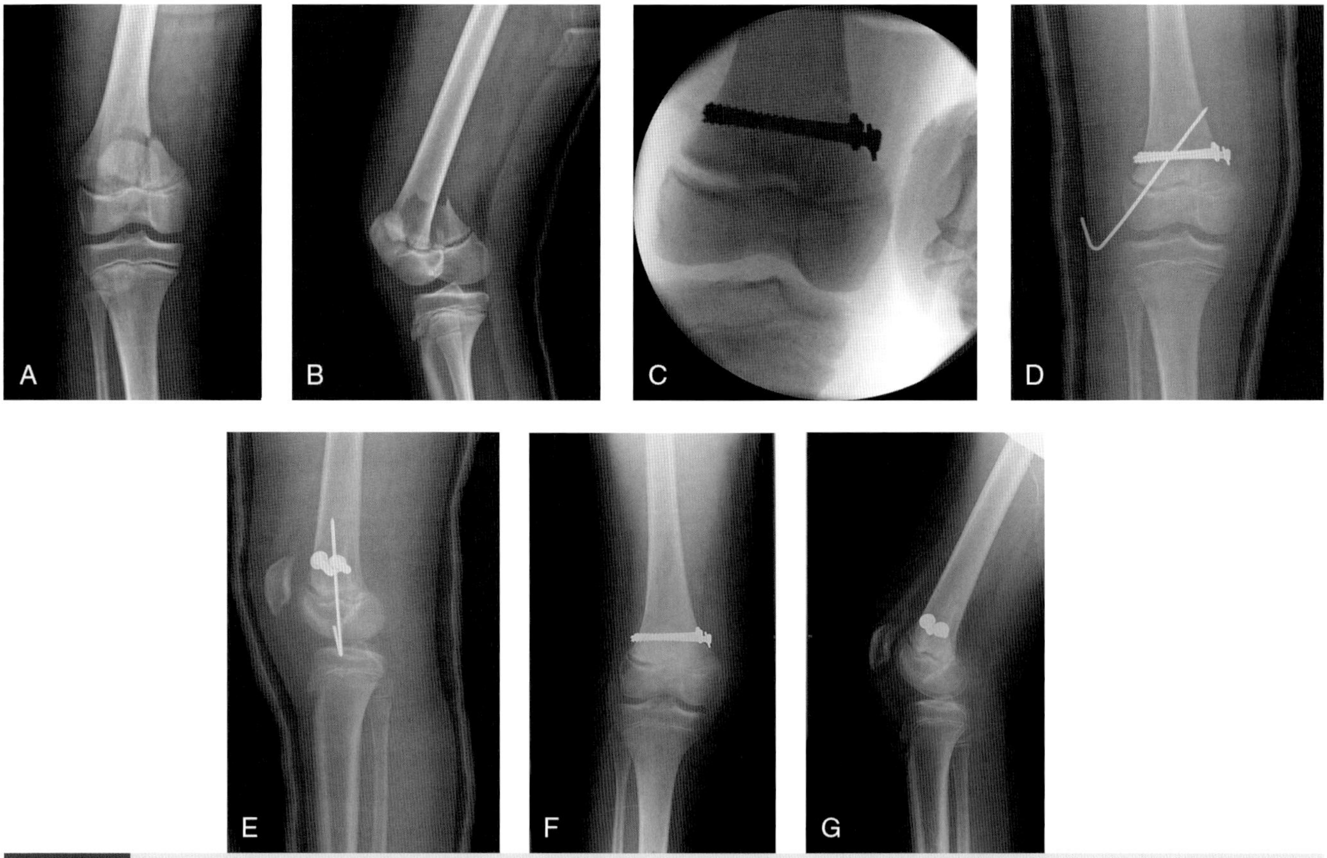

Figure 3 Images from a 12-year-old boy who sustained a distal femoral fracture after being tackled while playing football. Preoperative AP (**A**) and lateral (**B**) radiographs of the knee. The patient was treated with closed reduction and percutaneous fixation with cannulated screws and a washer in the Thurston Holland fragment. **C,** Intraoperative fluoroscopic radiograph after fixation. A varus load was applied, which showed physeal instability despite the screw fixation. AP (**D**) and lateral (**E**) radiographs after supplemental fixation with a Kirschner wire to provide stability. The wire was removed at 4 weeks postoperatively. AP (**F**) and lateral (**G**) radiographs 2 months after supplemental fixation show good alignment. The patient was able to ambulate freely and was scheduled for follow-up visits to monitor for potential growth arrest.

pinning can be done if displacement is detected at that time.[58]

A displaced Salter-Harris type III or IV fracture is more likely to require open reduction. Compression screws can be placed between the two epiphyseal fragments or between the metaphyseal spike and the femoral metaphysis. Casting for 6 weeks after the injury is recommended to provide additional stability.

Despite appropriate treatment, partial or complete growth arrest often leads to complications, including limb-length inequality and angulation.[58] Growth arrest is more common in a displaced fracture,[55,58] a Salter-Harris type III or IV fracture, or a fracture in which implants were placed across the physis. The patient should be followed for 2 years after the injury because of the risk of a physeal bar and growth disturbance.

Summary

The causes and treatment options for fractures of the pelvis, hip, knee, and femur vary depending on the age of the child. In younger children, trauma can be subtle. In adolescent and preadolescent patients, the modes of injury are more similar to those seen in adults. Care differs depending on the patient's age, from more conservative methods in younger patients to adult-type fixation methods in older patients. Growth disturbance is an important consideration and requires vigilance in young patients with distal femoral fractures.

Key Study Points

- Younger patients with open growth plates can have similar patterns of pelvic ring disruption as those of adults. In general, the immature pelvis tends to deform and can absorb more energy before fracturing because of the increased elasticity of the bone, stronger ligaments, thicker periosteum, and open growth plates.
- Epiphysiolysis of the femoral head during reduction of a traumatic hip dislocation can occur in adolescents with an open physis.
- Lateral trochanteric entry points decrease the incidence of osteonecrosis of the femoral head.
- Despite appropriate treatment of distal femoral physeal injuries, partial or complete growth arrest often leads to complications, including limb-length inequality and angulation.

Annotated References

1. Oransky M, Sanguinetti C: Surgical treatment of displaced acetabular fractures: Results of 50 consecutive cases. *J Orthop Trauma* 1993;7(1):28-32.

2. Gänsslen A, Heidari N, Weinberg AM: Fractures of the pelvis in children: A review of the literature. *Eur J Orthop Surg Traumatol* 2013;23(8):847-861.

   The authors present a comprehensive review of 27 articles on pelvic fractures in children and propose a new treatment protocol that focuses on fracture type and concomitant organ injuries.

3. Amorosa LF, Kloen P, Helfet DL: High-energy pediatric pelvic and acetabular fractures. *Orthop Clin North Am* 2014;45(4):483-500.

   A review of the literature on unstable pelvic fractures in children with special attention paid to acetabular and triradiate injuries is presented. The authors propose a novel diagnosis and treatment algorithm for pediatric acetabular fractures that takes into account the difficulty in imaging the immature pelvis.

4. Shore BJ, Palmer CS, Bevin C, Johnson MB, Torode IP: Pediatric pelvic fracture: A modification of a preexisting classification. *J Pediatr Orthop* 2012;32(2):162-168.

   The authors retrospectively reviewed 124 children with pelvic fractures. A modification to the traditional Torode classification was made based on the results identifying a subtype of pelvic ring injury that showed disruptions of both the anterior and posterior ring, but remained stable. Patients with this type of injury had substantially higher rates of blood transfusion and longer hospital stays than those with other types of stable pelvic ring disruptions. Level of evidence: III.

5. Snyder CL, Jain VN, Saltzman DA, Strate RG, Perry JF Jr, Leonard AS: Blunt trauma in adults and children: A comparative analysis. *J Trauma* 1990;30(10):1239-1245.

6. Torode I, Zieg D: Pelvic fractures in children. *J Pediatr Orthop* 1985;5(1):76-84.

7. Marmor M, Elson J, Mikhail C, Morshed S, Matityahu A: Short-term pelvic fracture outcomes in adolescents differ from children and adults in the National Trauma Data Bank. *J Child Orthop* 2015;9(1):65-75.

   The authors used the National Trauma Data Bank to evaluate 37,784 patients with pelvic fractures to determine the differences in complication and mortality rates between children, adolescents, and adults younger than 55 years. They found that children with pelvic fractures had an increased odds of death compared with adults, whereas adolescents with pelvic fractures had decreased odds of death and complications compared with adults.

8. Oransky M, Arduini M, Tortora M, Zoppi AR: Surgical treatment of unstable pelvic fracture in children: Long term results. *Injury* 2010;41(11):1140-1144.

9. Sen MK, Warner SJ, Sama N, et al: Treatment of acetabular fractures in adolescents. *Am J Orthop (Belle Mead NJ)* 2015;44(10):465-470.

   The authors present a retrospective study of 38 adolescents with acetabular fractures (mean follow-up, 3 years). Most of the patients required surgery. At follow-up, 29 patients had no pain and 34 had returned to full activity. Osteonecrosis of the femoral head was reported in two patients and was associated with concominant joint dislocation.

10. Gänsslen A, Hildebrand F, Heidari N, Weinberg AM: Acetabular fractures in children: A review of the literature. *Acta Chir Orthop Traumatol Cech* 2013;80(1):10-14.

    This literature review of acetabular fractures in skeletally inmature individuals documented succesful outcomes in many patients who were treated nonsurgically. However, surgical intervention was indicated when fractures showed more than 2 mm of displacement in the weight-bearing articular surface, instability of the hip, a posterior wall fracture of more than 50% of the articular surface, or the presence of incarcerated fragments.

11. Bucholz RW, Ezaki M, Ogden JA: Injury to the acetabular triradiate physeal cartilage. *J Bone Joint Surg Am* 1982;64(4):600-609.

12. Moon ES, Mehlman CT: Risk factors for avascular necrosis after femoral neck fractures in children: 25 Cincinnati cases and meta-analysis of 360 cases. *J Orthop Trauma* 2006;20(5):323-329.

13. Shrader MW, Jacofsky DJ, Stans AA, Shaughnessy WJ, Haidukewych GJ: Femoral neck fractures in pediatric

patients: 30 years experience at a level 1 trauma center. *Clin Orthop Relat Res* 2007;454:169-173.

14. Togrul E, Bayram H, Gulsen M, Kalaci A, Ozbarlas S: Fractures of the femoral neck in children: Long-term follow-up in 62 hip fractures. *Injury* 2005;36(1):123-130.

15. Canale ST, Tolo VT: Fractures of the femur in children. *Instr Course Lect* 1995;44:255-273.

16. Davison BL, Weinstein SL: Hip fractures in children: A long-term follow-up study. *J Pediatr Orthop* 1992;12(3):355-358.

17. Boardman MJ, Herman MJ, Buck B, Pizzutillo PD: Hip fractures in children. *J Am Acad Orthop Surg* 2009;17(3):162-173.

18. Forster NA, Ramseier LE, Exner GU: Undisplaced femoral neck fractures in children have a high risk of secondary displacement. *J Pediatr Orthop B* 2006;15(2):131-133.

19. Flynn JM, Wong KL, Yeh GL, Meyer JS, Davidson RS: Displaced fractures of the hip in children: Management by early operation and immobilisation in a hip spica cast. *J Bone Joint Surg Br* 2002;84(1):108-112.

20. Stone JD, Hill MK, Pan Z, Novais EN: Open reduction of pediatric femoral neck fractures reduces osteonecrosis risk. *Orthopedics* 2015;38(11):e983-e990.

    Of 22 patients who had 100% displaced femoral neck fractures, 6 were treated with open reduction and internal fixation with the Watson-Jones approach. Those six patients had no evidence of osteonecrosis, and all healed anatomically. Osteonecrosis was reported in 8 of the 16 patients treated with closed reduction and internal fixation, and only 7 of those patients healed anatomically. Level of evidence: III.

21. Swiontkowski MF, Winquist RA: Displaced hip fractures in children and adolescents. *J Trauma* 1986;26(4):384-388.

22. Riley PM Jr, Morscher MA, Gothard MD, Riley PM Sr: Earlier time to reduction did not reduce rates of femoral head osteonecrosis in pediatric hip fractures. *J Orthop Trauma* 2015;29(5):231-238.

    A literature review revealed osteonecrosis rates from zero to 100% in patients with pediatric hip fractures. In this study of 44 hip fractures, there was no osteonecrosis in patients younger than 11 years, and there was no association between osteonecrosis and time to reduction. Level of evidence: III.

23. Li H, Zhao L, Huang L, Kuo KN: Delayed slipped capital femoral epiphysis after treatment of femoral neck fracture in children. *Clin Orthop Relat Res* 2015;473(8):2712-2717.

    The authors report on a 12-year-old girl and a 6-year-old girl in whom slipped capital femoral epiphysis developed at 5 months and 9 months, respectively, after surgical fixation of a femoral neck fracture. A literature review found five additional similar cases. The authors note that physicians should be aware of this clinical scenario so it can be recognized promptly. Level of evidence: IV.

24. Kumar S, Jain AK: Neglected traumatic hip dislocation in children. *Clin Orthop Relat Res* 2005;431:9-13.

25. Herrera-Soto JA, Price CT: Traumatic hip dislocations in children and adolescents: Pitfalls and complications. *J Am Acad Orthop Surg* 2009;17(1):15-21.

26. Zrig M, Mnif H, Koubaa M, Abid A: Traumatic hip dislocation in children. *Acta Orthop Belg* 2009;75(3):328-333.

27. Herrera-Soto JA, Price CT, Reuss BL, Riley P, Kasser JR, Beaty JH: Proximal femoral epiphysiolysis during reduction of hip dislocation in adolescents. *J Pediatr Orthop* 2006;26(3):371-374.

28. Mehlman CT, Hubbard GW, Crawford AH, Roy DR, Wall EJ: Traumatic hip dislocation in children: Long-term followup of 42 patients. *Clin Orthop Relat Res* 2000;376:68-79.

29. Price CT, Pyevich MT, Knapp DR, Phillips JH, Hawker JJ: Traumatic hip dislocation with spontaneous incomplete reduction: A diagnostic trap. *J Orthop Trauma* 2002;16(10):730-735.

30. Kashiwagi N, Suzuki S, Seto Y: Arthroscopic treatment for traumatic hip dislocation with avulsion fracture of the ligamentum teres. *Arthroscopy* 2001;17(1):67-69.

31. Morris AC, Yu JC, Gilbert SR: Arthroscopic treatment of traumatic hip dislocations in children and adolescents: A preliminary study. *J Pediatr Orthop* 2015; October 30 [Epub ahead of print].

    The authors reports on seven patients between the ages of 8 and 17 years who had incongruent reduction of a traumatic hip dislocation. The patients were treated with hip arthroscopy and reduction and/or débridement of impediments to reduction without repair. Osteonecrosis or recurrent instability did not develop in any of the patients. Level of evidence: IV.

32. Podeszwa DA, De La Rocha A, Larson AN, Sucato DJ: Surgical hip dislocation is safe and effective following acute traumatic hip instability in the adolescent. *J Pediatr Orthop* 2015;35(5):435-442.

    Eleven patients with traumatic hip dislocations after incongruent closed reduction were treated with surgical hip dislocation as described by Ganz, with treatment of intra-articular pathology. Osteonecrosis did not develop in any of the patients. Level of evidence: IV.

33. Nirmal Kumar J, Hazra S, Yun HH: Redislocation after treatment of traumatic dislocation of hip in children: A report of two cases and literature review. *Arch Orthop Trauma Surg* 2009;129(6):823-826.

34. Vialle R, Odent T, Pannier S, Pauthier F, Laumonier F, Glorion C: Traumatic hip dislocation in childhood. *J Pediatr Orthop* 2005;25(2):138-144.

35. Banskota AK, Spiegel DA, Shrestha S, Shrestha OP, Rajbhandary T: Open reduction for neglected traumatic hip dislocation in children and adolescents. *J Pediatr Orthop* 2007;27(2):187-191.

36. Narayanan UG, Phillips JH: Flexibility in fixation: An update on femur fractures in children. *J Pediatr Orthop* 2012;32(suppl 1):S32-S39.

The authors discuss the surgical management of femoral fractures in children and emphasizes the many available treatment techniques.

37. Kocher MS, Sink EL, Blasier RD, et al: Treatment of pediatric diaphyseal femur fractures. *J Am Acad Orthop Surg* 2009;17(11):718-725.

38. Podeszwa DA, Mooney JF III, Cramer KE, Mendelow MJ: Comparison of Pavlik harness application and immediate spica casting for femur fractures in infants. *J Pediatr Orthop* 2004;24(5):460-462.

39. Heffernan MJ, Gordon JE, Sabatini CS, et al: Treatment of femur fractures in young children: A multicenter comparison of flexible intramedullary nails to spica casting in young children aged 2 to 6 years. *J Pediatr Orthop* 2015;35(2):126-129.

This study compares the results of immediate spica casting versus elastic nailing in patients 6 years of age or younger. The authors reported similar healing times, but earlier return to independent ambulation and full activities in the elastic nailing group.

40. Mansour AA III, Wilmoth JC, Mansour AS, Lovejoy SA, Mencio GA, Martus JE: Immediate spica casting of pediatric femoral fractures in the operating room versus the emergency department: Comparison of reduction, complications, and hospital charges. *J Pediatr Orthop* 2010;30(8):813-817.

41. Moroz LA, Launay F, Kocher MS, et al: Titanium elastic nailing of fractures of the femur in children: Predictors of complications and poor outcome. *J Bone Joint Surg Br* 2006;88(10):1361-1366.

42. Rapp M, Gros N, Zachert G, et al: Improving stability of elastic stable intramedullary nailing in a transverse midshaft femur fracture model: Biomechanical analysis of using end caps or a third nail. *J Orthop Surg Res* 2015;10:96.

The authors report that using a third elastic nail reduces axial deviation in transverse midshaft femoral fractures. The use of end caps did not improve stiffness in any direction.

43. Mahar AT, Lee SS, Lalonde FD, Impelluso T, Newton PO: Biomechanical comparison of stainless steel and titanium nails for fixation of simulated femoral fractures. J Pediatr Orthop 2004;24(6):638-641.

44. Sagan ML, Datta JC, Olney BW, Lansford TJ, McIff TE: Residual deformity after treatment of pediatric femur fractures with flexible titanium nails. *J Pediatr Orthop* 2010;30(7):638-643.

45. Salem KH, Keppler P: Limb geometry after elastic stable nailing for pediatric femoral fractures. *J Bone Joint Surg Am* 2010;92(6):1409-1417.

46. MacNeil JA, Francis A, El-Hawary R: A systematic review of rigid, locked, intramedullary nail insertion sites and avascular necrosis of the femoral head in the skeletally immature. *J Pediatr Orthop* 2011;31(4):377-380.

Based on a review of the literature, the authors reported that rigid intramedullary nail insertion into the lateral trochanter for femoral fracture fixation resulted in the lowest rate of osteonecrosis compared with insertion at other sites such as the tip of the greater trochanter.

47. Herrera-Soto JA, Meuret R, Phillips JH, Vogel DJ: The management of pediatric subtrochanteric femur fractures with a statically locked intramedullary nail. *J Orthop Trauma* 2015;29(1):e7-e11.

The use of a statically locked, lateral entry intramedullary nails for subtrochanteric femoral fracture fixation in children was evaluated in 10 patients. The authors found that it was a safe and efficacious method of treatment, with few complications and risks and satisfactory outcomes in the children older than 8 years. Level of evidence: IV.

48. Reynolds RA, Legakis JE, Thomas R, Slongo TF, Hunter JB, Clavert JM: Intramedullary nails for pediatric diaphyseal femur fractures in older, heavier children: Early results. *J Child Orthop* 2012;6(3):181-188.

The authors report that older, heavier pediatric patients who were treated for femoral fracture with lateral entry femoral nails had a shorter recovery time than similar patients treated with elastic, stable intramedullary nails.

49. Flinck M, von Heideken J, Janarv PM, Wåtz V, Riad J: Biomechanical comparison of semi-rigid pediatric locking nail versus titanium elastic nails in a femur fracture model. *J Child Orthop* 2015;9(1):77-84.

In biomechanical comparisons, semirigid pediatric locking nails provided the greatest stability in all planes compared with elastic nail models for femoral fracture fixation.

50. Heyworth BE, Hedequist DJ, Nasreddine AY, Stamoulis C, Hresko MT, Yen YM: Distal femoral valgus deformity following plate fixation of pediatric femoral shaft fractures. *J Bone Joint Surg Am* 2013;95(6):526-533.

In a review of 85 pediatric patients, distal femoral valgus was found to be a potential deformity after plate fixation of femoral shaft fractures. This deformity occurred in 30% of the patients with distal diaphyseal fractures and in 12% of the patients overall.

51. Park KC, Oh CW, Byun YS, et al: Intramedullary nailing versus submuscular plating in adolescent femoral fracture. *Injury* 2012;43(6):870-875.

    In this study, both intramedullary nailing and submuscular plating yielded good results and minimal complication in the fixation of femoral fractures in adolescent patients. However, intramedullary nailing may be advantageous because there is less need for fluoroscopy, greater technical ease in reduction, and early weight bearing for the patient.

52. Li Y, Heyworth BE, Glotzbecker M, et al: Comparison of titanium elastic nail and plate fixation of pediatric subtrochanteric femur fractures. *J Pediatr Orthop* 2013;33(3):232-238.

    The authors compared the use of plates versus elastic nails for the management of subtrochanteric femoral fractures. Patients with plate fixation had better outcome scores and a lower complication rate. Level of evidence: III.

53. Parikh SN, Nathan ST, Priola MJ, Eismann EA: Elastic nailing for pediatric subtrochanteric and supracondylar femur fractures. *Clin Orthop Relat Res* 2014;472(9):2735-2744.

    Elastic nailing represents an important option for femoral fractures that are difficult to manage. However, high complication rates were reported with elastic nailing of pediatric subtrochanteric and supracondylar femoral fractures (22% and 38%, respectively). Level of evidence: IV.

54. Arkader A, Friedman JE, Warner WC Jr, Wells L: Complete distal femoral metaphyseal fractures: A harbinger of child abuse before walking age. *J Pediatr Orthop* 2007;27(7):751-753.

55. Ilharreborde B, Raquillet C, Morel E, et al: Long-term prognosis of Salter-Harris type 2 injuries of the distal femoral physis. *J Pediatr Orthop B* 2006;15(6):433-438.

56. Butcher CC, Hoffman EB: Supracondylar fractures of the femur in children: Closed reduction and percutaneous pinning of displaced fractures. *J Pediatr Orthop* 2005;25(2):145-148.

57. Peterson HA, Madhok R, Benson JT, Ilstrup DM, Melton LJ III: Physeal fractures: Part 1. Epidemiology in Olmsted County, Minnesota, 1979-1988. *J Pediatr Orthop* 1994;14(4):423-430.

58. Arkader A, Warner WC Jr, Horn BD, Shaw RN, Wells L: Predicting the outcome of physeal fractures of the distal femur. *J Pediatr Orthop* 2007;27(6):703-708.

Chapter 39

Tibia, Ankle, and Foot

Ying Li, MD Mark A. Seeley, MD

Abstract

Fractures of the tibia, ankle, and foot are common in children. It is helpful to be familiar with the characteristics of the most frequent types of fractures, including epidemiology, mechanism of injury, diagnosis, classification, treatment options, and potential complications.

Keywords: foot fracture; proximal tibial fracture; tibial shaft fracture; Tillaux fracture; triplane fracture

Introduction

Fractures of the tibia, ankle, and foot are common in children. The incidence and pattern of each fracture type varies based on the age of the patient, the mechanism of injury, and the anatomic location. Nonsurgical treatment is successful for many of these fractures; surgical intervention is reserved for physeal malreductions, articular displacements, and unstable fractures. Long-term follow-up of physeal fractures in patients who are skeletally immature is required to monitor for growth arrest and resultant deformities.

Dr. Li or an immediate family member serves as a board member, owner, officer, or committee member of the Pediatric Orthopaedic Society of North America and the Scoliosis Research Society. Neither Dr. Seeley nor any immediate family member has received anything of value from or has stock or stock options held in a commercial company or institution related directly or indirectly to the subject of this chapter.

Proximal Tibial Fractures

Physeal Fractures

Proximal tibial physeal fractures comprise less than 1% of all physeal fractures.[1] These fractures result from substantial trauma, such as that sustained in a motor vehicle crash or from sports activity. The inciting mechanism is commonly a hyperextension force, which results in posterior displacement of the metaphysis. Vascular status must be carefully assessed because of tethering of the popliteal artery by the posterior tibia. A posteriorly displaced metaphyseal fragment may stretch or tear the artery[2,3] (**Figure 1**). Vascular surgical consultation is necessary if the limb is dysvascular after fracture reduction. Patients with proximal tibial physeal fractures should be closely monitored for the development of compartment syndrome.

Proximal tibial physeal fractures are classified according to the Salter-Harris system. Salter-Harris type I and II fractures are the most common.[3] Type I and II fractures can be treated with closed reduction and immobilization. Unstable fractures can be stabilized with smooth pins inserted percutaneously across the physis. Screw fixation also is an option for type II fractures with a large metaphyseal fragment. Irreducible type I and II fractures should undergo open reduction. The pes anserinus[4] and the periosteum[5] can block the reduction of type II fractures. Displaced type III and IV fractures should be treated with open reduction secondary to intra-articular involvement to ensure that articular congruity has been restored. Epiphyseal and metaphyseal screws are then inserted parallel to the physis. Proximal tibial physeal fractures can result in a growth disturbance and should be monitored for 1 to 2 years after injury for any development of shortening or angulation of the involved limb.

Tibial Tubercle Avulsion Fractures

Tibial tubercle avulsion fractures occur most commonly in male adolescents participating in jumping activities

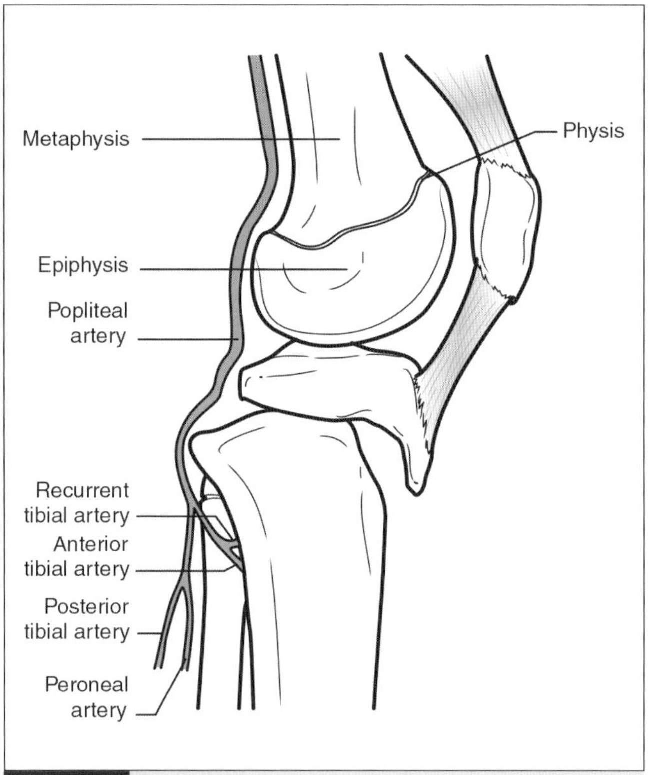

Figure 1 Illustration shows that posterior displacement of the metaphysis can lead to arterial injury secondary to close proximity and tethering of the popliteal artery near the proximal tibia.

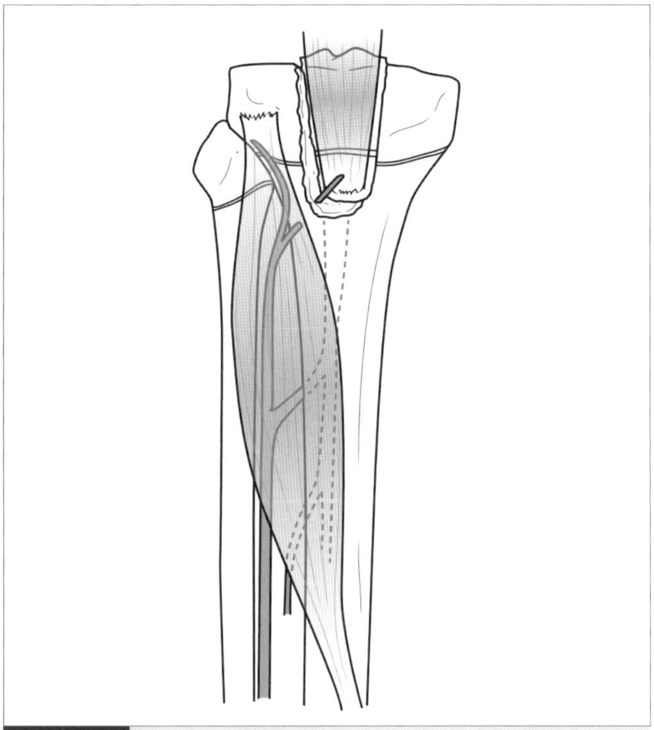

Figure 2 Illustration shows how the anterior tibial recurrent artery lies near the base of the tibial tubercle and can be torn with a tibial tubercle avulsion fracture. The artery retracts and bleeds into the anterior compartment, resulting in a possible compartment syndrome.

such as basketball.[6-13] These fractures occur through the apophysis at the posterior aspect of the tibial tubercle. Tibial tubercle avulsion fractures can be differentiated from Osgood-Schlatter disease based on the duration of symptoms.[7] Adolescents with Osgood-Schlatter disease will report a long history of symptoms but are able to continue with their athletic activities. In contrast, patients with tibial tubercle avulsion fractures report an acute injury and an inability to bear weight. Patients also will have difficulty extending their knees. Severely displaced fractures may tent the overlying skin. Patients with tibial tubercle avulsion fractures are at risk for the development of compartment syndrome secondary to avulsion of the anterior tibial recurrent artery near the base of the tibial tubercle[14] (**Figure 2**).

As modified in 1980, the Watson-Jones classification is used to describe tibial tubercle avulsion fractures[7] (**Figure 3**). Type I fractures occur distal to the junction between the apophysis and the proximal tibial physis. Type II fractures extend through the junction between the apophysis and the proximal tibial physis. Type III fractures propagate through the proximal tibial epiphysis and are intra-articular fractures (Salter-Harris type IV equivalent). Type IV fractures extend posteriorly through the proximal tibial physis. Type V injuries occur when the patellar tendon avulses with its large periosteal attachment off the tibial tubercle. Additional evaluation with CT or MRI may be necessary to assess intra-articular involvement.[12]

Nondisplaced type I fractures can be treated with immobilization with the knee in extension. However, even minimally displaced fractures may have a large flap of periosteum interposed in the fracture site.[8,9] Intra-articular fractures and fractures that are displaced more than 2 to 3 mm are treated with open reduction and internal fixation (ORIF).[9-12] Screws can be inserted in an anterior-to-posterior direction across the fracture (**Figure 4**). Tibial tubercle avulsion fractures usually occur in adolescents who are near skeletal maturity; however, in patients with more than 2 years of growth remaining, pins instead of screws can be used to avoid premature closure of the apophysis and the development of genu recurvatum. Tension-band wiring is also an option.[15] Intra-articular fractures may be associated with disruption of the meniscal-articular relationship. Repair of the coronary ligaments with suture anchors has been

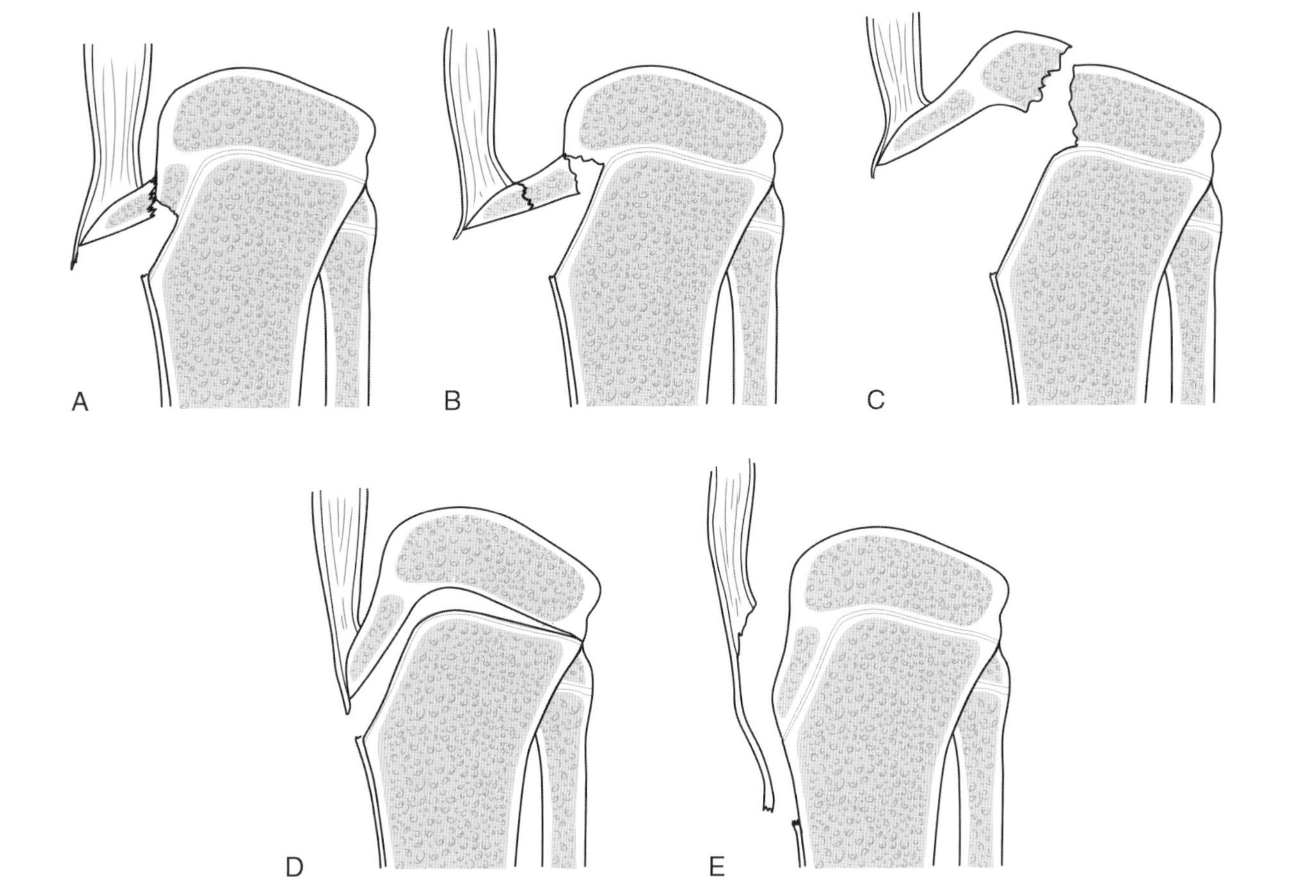

Figure 3 Illustrations of the Ogden modification of the Watson-Jones classification of tibial tubercle avulsion fractures. **A,** Type I fracture. **B,** Type II fracture. **C,** Type III fracture. **D,** Type IV fracture. **E,** Type V fracture.

described.[11] Prominent screw heads may necessitate implant removal after fracture healing.[13,16]

Proximal Tibial Metaphyseal Fractures

Proximal tibial metaphyseal fractures are most common in children aged 3 to 6 years.[17,18] These fractures usually result from a valgus force, wherein the fibula remains intact. Most patients can be treated nonsurgically with immobilization with the knee in slight flexion and application of a varus mold. The development of a late valgus deformity after these fractures was first described by Cozen.[17] This deformity can occur even after a nondisplaced fracture. One theory that has been proposed to explain the late valgus deformity is overgrowth secondary to increased vascularity to the medial proximal tibial physis after the fracture.[19,20] This uncommon deformity can develop up to 18 months after the fracture, and most patients will experience spontaneous improvement of the deformity with excellent long-term outcomes.[17,21] Persistent deformities can be corrected with medial proximal tibial hemiepiphysiodesis.[18]

Tibial Shaft Fractures

Tibial shaft fractures account for 15% of all pediatric long-bone fractures.[22] The most frequent mechanism of injury is indirect trauma, such as a twisting injury, and the most common resulting fracture pattern is spiral or oblique. Most of these fractures occur in the distal third of the tibia, followed by fractures in the middle third of the tibia.[22,23]

Most tibial shaft fractures can be treated with closed reduction and immobilization with the knee in 45° of flexion. Fracture alignment should be closely monitored during the first 3 weeks. Isolated tibial shaft fractures are at risk of varus angulation secondary to deforming forces from the anterior and deep posterior compartment musculature plus the tethering effect of the intact fibula.[23] In contrast, tibial shaft fractures with an associated fibula fracture result in valgus angulation secondary to forces from the anterior and lateral compartment musculature. Acceptable fracture alignment is controversial, but general principles are shown in **Table 1**. It is important to assess

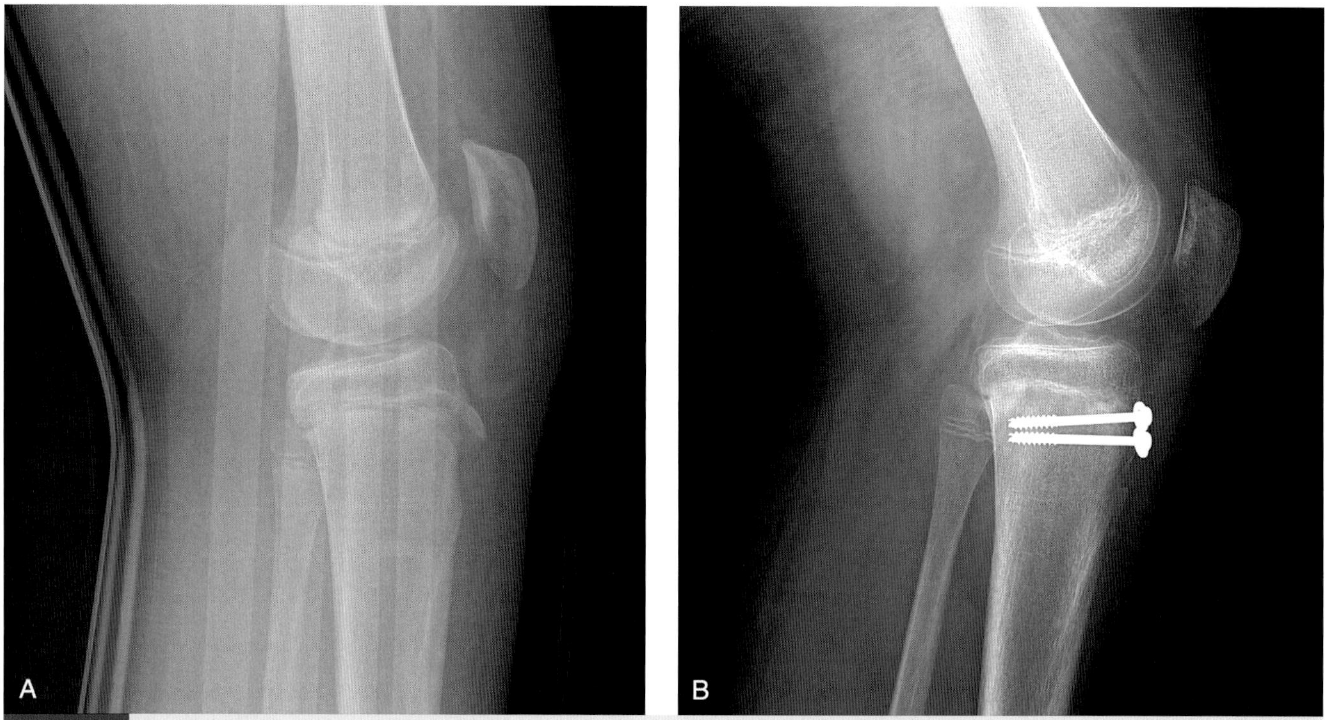

Figure 4 Lateral radiographs of a type II tibial tubercle avulsion fracture before (**A**) and after screw fixation (**B**).

for apex posterior angulation because this alignment will have the least remodeling of all the residual angular deformities.[24]

Although surgical treatment of pediatric tibial shaft fractures was rarely recommended in the past, fixation of these fractures became more popular over the past decade. Closed fractures that fail successful reduction, open fractures, fractures associated with a compartment syndrome, and polytrauma are now considered indications for surgical treatment. Flexible intramedullary nailing with titanium or stainless steel nails is most commonly performed. Two nails of the same diameter are inserted at the medial and lateral aspects of the proximal tibia, 2 cm distal to the physis (**Figure 5**). Flexible intramedullary nailing of tibial shaft fractures has been found to result in a substantially shorter time to union and better functional outcomes compared with external fixation.[25] Flexible intramedullary nailing of displaced tibial shaft fractures with an intact fibula can decrease the duration of immobilization compared with nonsurgical treatment.[26] After titanium elastic nailing of tibial shaft fractures, increased patient age and weight are associated with a higher risk of malunion or a longer time to healing.[27] Adolescents with a closed proximal tibial physis can be treated with a rigid intramedullary nail.

External fixation was previously considered the standard treatment of pediatric open tibial shaft fractures.

Table 1

Acceptable Alignment for Pediatric Tibial Shaft Fractures

	Age <8 years	Age ≥8 years
Valgus	5°	5°
Varus	10°	5°
Anterior angulation	10°	5°
Posterior angulation	5°	0°
Shortening	10 mm	5 mm
Rotation	5°	5°

Reproduced with permission from Heinrich SD, Mooney JF: Fractures of the shaft of the tibia and fibula, in Beaty JH, Kasser JR, eds: *Rockwood and Wilkins' Fractures in Children*, ed 7. Philadelphia, PA, Lippincott Williams and Wilkins, 2010, pp 930-966.

However, a high rate of complications with external fixation has been reported, including delayed union, malunion, limb-length discrepancy, and pin tract infections.[28] Although external fixation remains an option for unstable fractures and open fractures with extensive soft-tissue loss, immediate flexible intramedullary nailing of open tibial shaft fractures has not been found to result

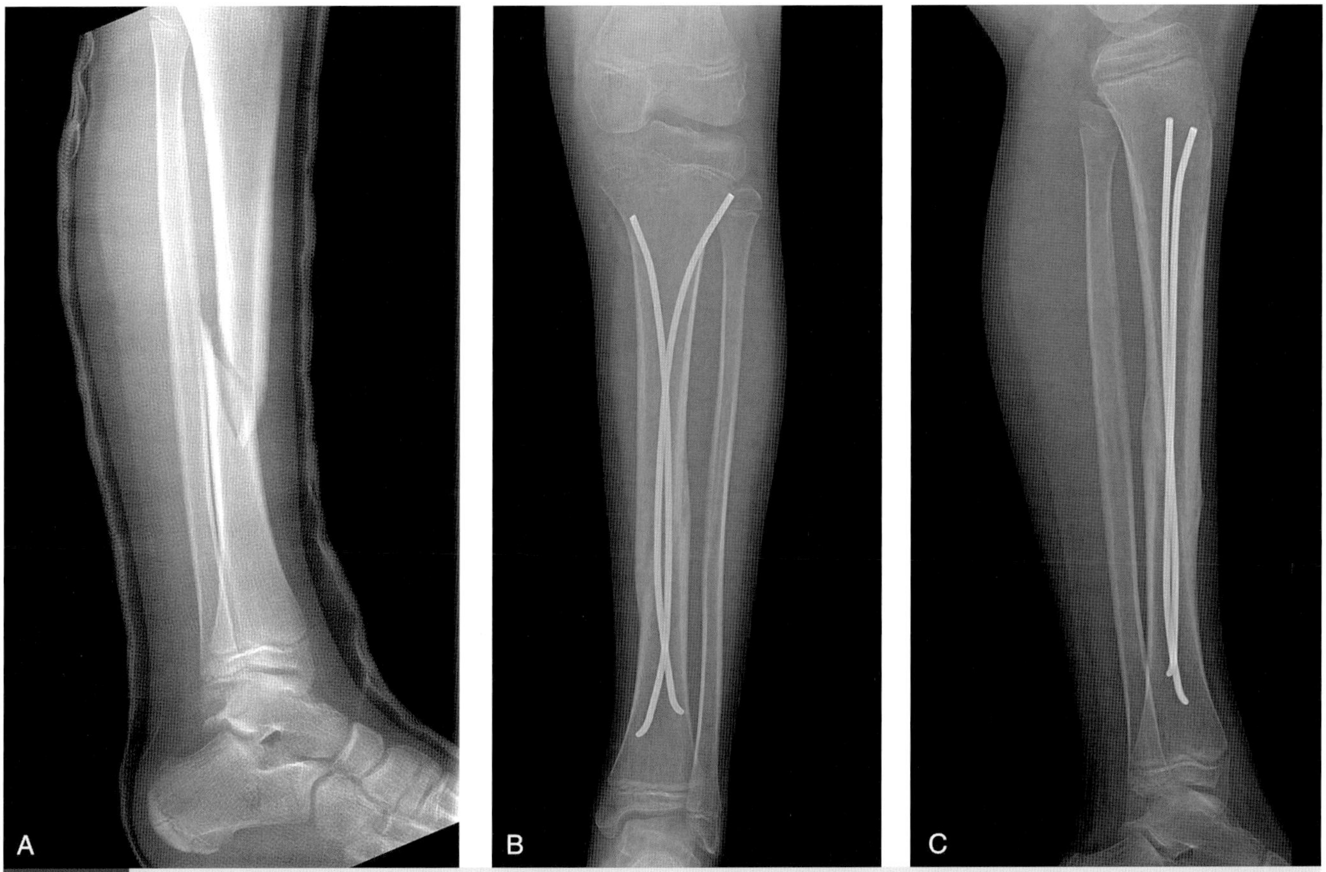

Figure 5 Lateral radiograph of a tibial shaft fracture in which apex posterior angulation persisted after attempted closed reduction (**A**). AP (**B**) and lateral (**C**) radiographs after titanium elastic nailing.

in increased rates of wound or infectious complications or compartment syndrome compared with closed fractures. Similar to external fixation, patients with Gustilo type II and III fractures treated with immediate flexible intramedullary nailing can experience substantially prolonged bone healing.[29]

Compartment syndrome has been reported in up to 12% of all pediatric tibial shaft fractures. Children at least age 14 years and those who are involved in a motor vehicle crash are at highest risk.[30] Compartment syndrome also has been reported in 20% of patients after flexible intramedullary nailing of tibial shaft fractures.[31] Close monitoring for compartment syndrome, both at the initial diagnosis and after nonsurgical or surgical intervention, is necessary.

Ankle Fractures

Distal Tibial Physeal Fractures

Ankle fractures account for 5% of all pediatric fractures.[32] The ankle ligaments are stronger than the distal tibial and fibular physes, making the physes susceptible to injury. Fracture morphology depends on the skeletal maturity of the patient and the mechanism of injury.[33] The central-medial portion of the distal tibial physis begins to close at approximately 12 to 15 years of age in girls and 13 to 17 years of age in boys. The central portion of the physis closes first, followed by the medial portion and then the lateral portion. Closure occurs over an 18-month period.[34]

The classification of distal tibial physeal fractures not only guides treatment but also provides prognostic implications. Most fractures can be classified with the Salter-Harris system. The Dias-Tachdjian classification is less commonly used because of its complexity, but this system is based on the position of the foot and the direction of force at the time of the injury.[35] Pronation injuries may have a higher rate of growth arrest than supination–external rotation injuries, thus requiring closer follow-up.[36-38] Abduction injuries have a relatively poor prognosis for premature physeal closure regardless of whether closed or open treatment is performed.[36-38] CT can be a valuable tool to evaluate intra-articular involvement and fracture displacement.[39]

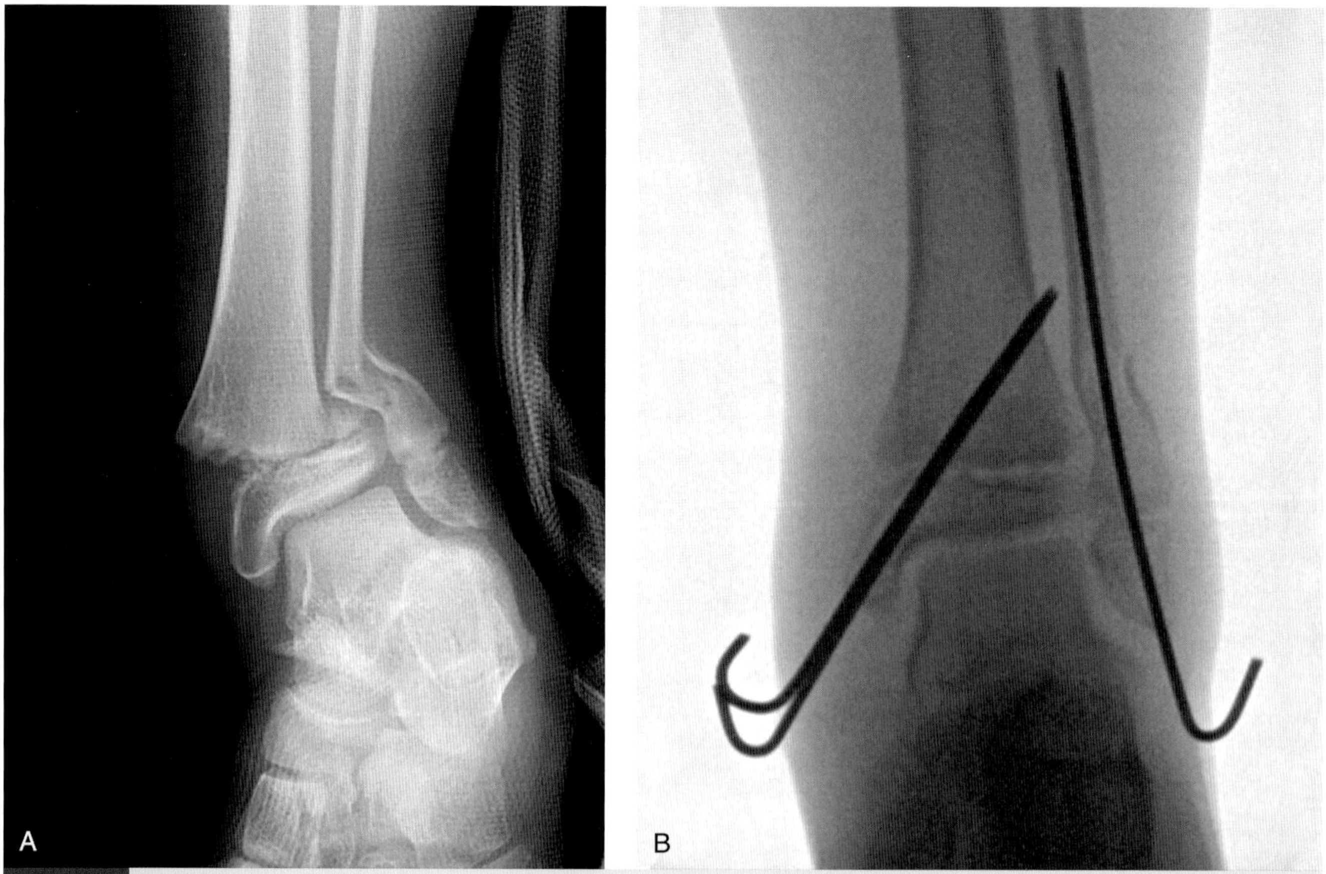

Figure 6 AP radiograph of a Salter-Harris type II distal tibia fracture and distal fibula fracture before (**A**) and after (**B**) open reduction and percutaneous pinning. A large flap of interposed periosteum was removed from the distal tibia fracture site.

Salter-Harris type I and II fractures can be treated with closed reduction and immobilization. In patients who are approaching skeletal maturity, mild residual displacement at the physis can be accepted if a large procurvatum deformity does not develop, which would hinder ankle dorsiflexion and predispose the patient to an Achilles contracture.[40] Surgical intervention is recommended for fractures with more than 2 mm of residual displacement, Salter-Harris type III and IV fractures with articular step-off, or external rotation deformity. Persistent gapping of greater than 3 mm suggests interposed periosteum, and premature physeal closure has been found to occur in 60% of these displaced fractures that are not treated with open reduction.[33,38] Fractures can be stabilized with the percutaneous insertion of smooth pins that cross the physis (**Figure 6**) or the placement of screws in the epiphysis and metaphysis parallel to the physis. Distal tibial physeal fractures should be followed for growth arrest for at least 1 year or until skeletal maturity.[41]

Tillaux Fractures

Tillaux fractures occur when an external rotational force leads to avulsion of the anterolateral distal tibial epiphysis by the anterior tibiofibular ligament. These injuries are Salter-Harris type III fractures, and the avulsed portion of the epiphysis is called the Tillaux fragment. These fractures are considered transitional fractures because they generally occur in adolescents who are within 1 year of closure of the distal tibial physis. As such, little risk exists for premature physeal closure resulting in growth arrest. The main goal in treatment is to restore articular congruity. CT scan is useful to assess fracture morphology[39] (**Figure 7**). Closed or open reduction plus fixation with pins or screws is recommended for fractures with more than 2 mm of displacement or articular step-off.[42]

Triplane Fractures

Triplane fractures are transitional fractures that occur earlier in adolescence than Tillaux fractures. Fracture morphology consists of two-, three-, or four-part fractures. A two-part triplane fracture is a Salter-Harris type

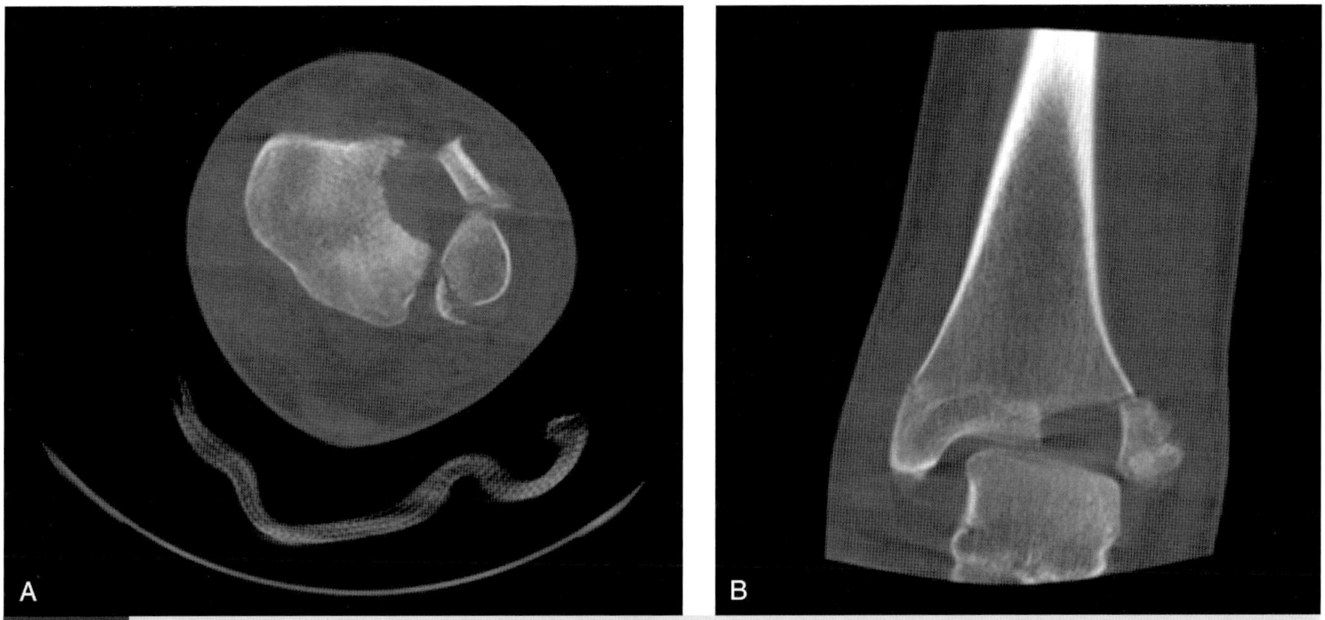

Figure 7 Axial (**A**) and coronal (**B**) CT scans show a Tillaux fracture.

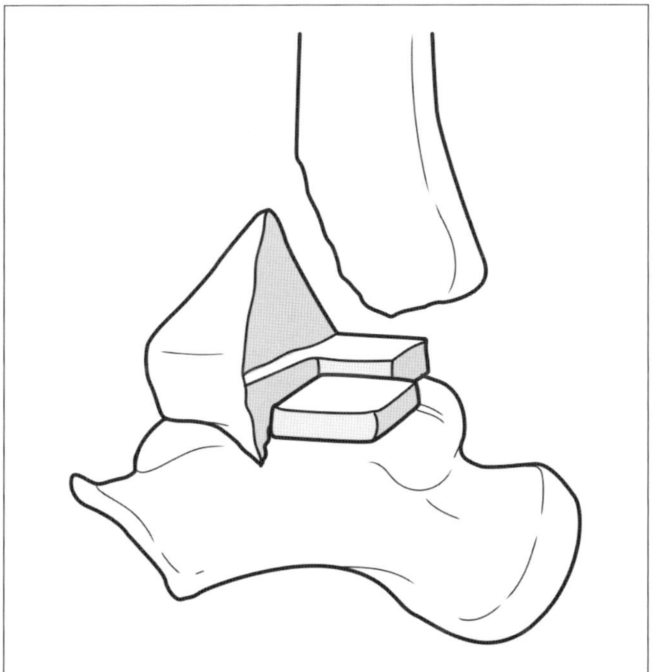

Figure 8 Schematic drawing of a three-part triplane fracture, which is a combined Salter-Harris type II and III fracture. The Salter-Harris type III fracture also is known as a Tillaux fragment.

IV fracture, whereas a three-part triplane fracture is a combined Salter-Harris type II and III fracture[43] (**Figure 8**). For intra-articular triplane fractures, treatment focuses on restoring articular congruity. Closed reduction by internally rotating the foot and immobilization in 30° of knee flexion can be performed. After closed reduction, a CT scan should be obtained to evaluate displacement of the fracture and the articular surface. If the reduction is unacceptable and surgical treatment is required, pins or screws are inserted across the metaphysis in an anterior-to-posterior direction and across the epiphysis in a lateral-to-medial or medial-to-lateral direction (**Figure 9**).

Foot Fractures

Calcaneus Fractures

Pediatric calcaneal fractures are uncommon and often are missed because of their subtle clinical and radiographic presentations.[44] A delay in diagnosis can occur in 30% to 50% of patients.[44,45] A CT scan should be considered in patients with pain if an appropriate mechanism of injury is involved. Extra-articular fractures are more common than intra-articular fractures, and most fractures can be treated nonsurgically with long-term satisfactory results.[45,46] In fractures with intra-articular extension, the posterior facet is usually intact, which likely explains why these fractures tend to do better in adolescents than in adults.[45,46] Substantially displaced fractures should be treated with ORIF.

Talus Fractures

Talar neck fractures are rare injuries that can occur from forced ankle dorsiflexion; however, 25% to 30% of fractures are associated with a medial malleolus fracture, suggesting a supination component.[47] Most of these fractures

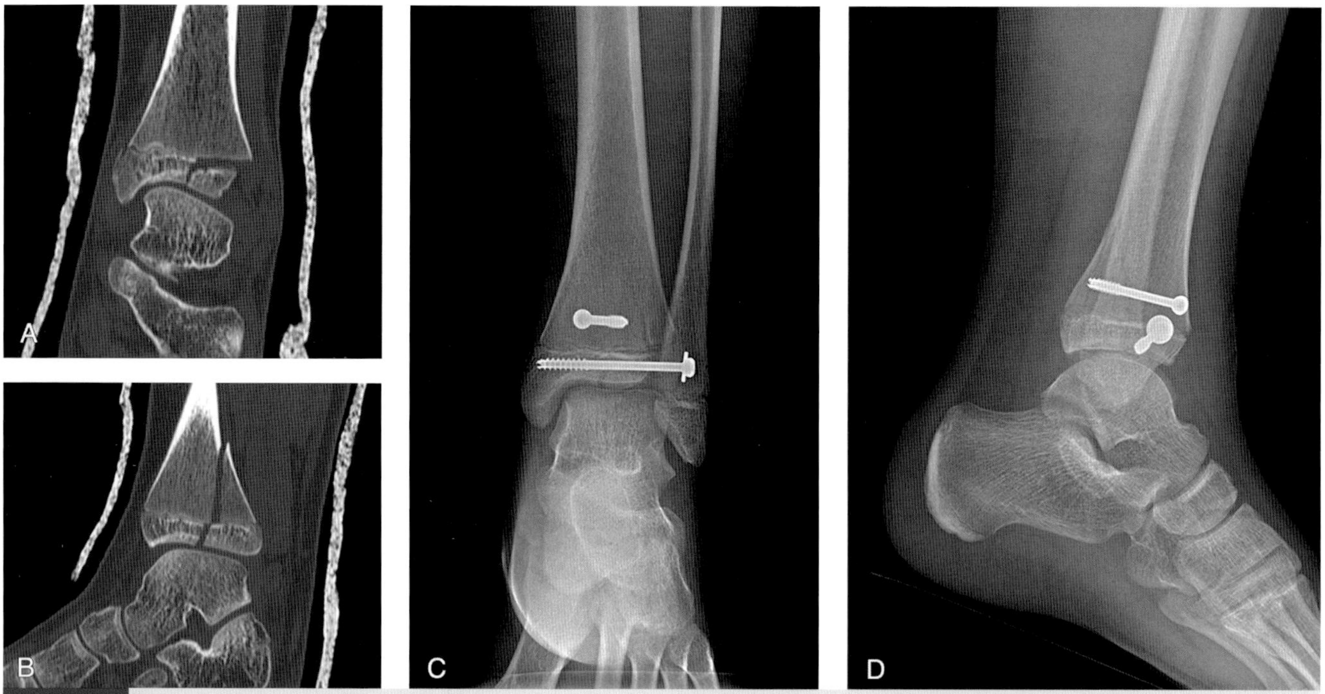

Figure 9 Coronal (**A**) and sagittal (**B**) CT scans demonstrating a triplane fracture. AP (**C**) and lateral (**D**) radiographs after screw fixation.

are nondisplaced and carry a lower risk of osteonecrosis than adult talar neck fractures. Nondisplaced fractures can be treated with immobilization for 6 to 8 weeks. Displaced fractures should be treated with screw fixation to avoid the displacement that could potentially occur with wire fixation. Patients are not allowed to bear weight until fracture union has been achieved.

Midfoot Fractures

Midfoot fractures are uncommon in children and often are misdiagnosed.[48] These fractures can occur from direct impact or from forced plantar flexion of the forefoot combined with a rotational force. Most of these fractures are avulsion injuries and can be managed conservatively. Although rare, Lisfranc injuries should be considered when a cuboid fracture is identified combined with a fracture at the base of the second metatarsal.[48] These injuries are usually associated with substantial soft-tissue swelling and ecchymosis. Nondisplaced fractures can be treated with immobilization for 4 weeks, whereas displaced fractures require closed versus open reduction plus fixation with pins or screws.

Metatarsal Fractures

Metatarsal fractures are the most common pediatric foot fracture, accounting for 5% to 7% of all pediatric fractures.[32] Children younger than 5 years are more susceptible to first metatarsal fractures, whereas children older than 10 years are more likely to sustain fractures at the base of the fifth metatarsal.[32] Midshaft fractures usually occur from direct trauma, whereas neck fractures result from indirect torsional forces. Patients who sustain a crush injury should be monitored for compartment syndrome. Growth arrest is rare but can cause shortening of the first ray, which has implications for the development of the longitudinal arch of the foot.[48]

The apophysis at the base of the fifth metatarsal should not be confused with an avulsion fracture. This secondary ossification center appears at approximately 8 years of age and fuses at age 12 years in girls and age 15 years in boys. Most metatarsal fractures can be treated nonsurgically. Surgical indications include open fractures, severely displaced metatarsal head fractures, and displaced intra-articular fractures. Smooth pins are most commonly used for fixation. Jones fractures, which occur at the metaphyseal-diaphyseal junction of the fifth metatarsal, also may benefit from surgical intervention. As in adults, a Jones fracture is at risk for delayed union or nonunion in an adolescent. The treatment of a Jones fracture can include a non–weight-bearing cast for 6 weeks for nondisplaced fractures and ORIF for displaced fractures.

Phalangeal Fractures

Most pediatric phalangeal fractures occur in the proximal phalanx and can be treated nonsurgically. A distal phalangeal fracture associated with an injury to the nail bed may result in an injury to the physis. These are open fractures and require irrigation, débridement, and the administration of antibiotics. Fractures that involve more than one-third of the joint surface may result in rotational deformities or joint instability and require stabilization with pins or a small screw.

Summary

Most fractures of the tibia, ankle, and foot in pediatric patients have good clinical and radiographic outcomes with nonsurgical treatment. Anatomic reduction and fixation of physeal fractures, intra-articular fractures, and unstable fractures is generally recommended. Complications, such as growth disturbances, can occur after certain fractures in patients who are skeletally immature and should be closely monitored over the long term.

Key Study Points

- Physeal fractures can lead to growth disturbance in patients who are skeletally immature.
- Compartment syndrome can result after proximal tibial physeal fractures, tibial tubercle avulsion fractures, and tibial shaft fractures. Careful initial assessment and monitoring are necessary.
- Closed tibial shaft fractures that fail reduction, open fractures, fractures associated with compartment syndrome, and polytrauma may be indications for surgical treatment.
- Distal tibial physeal fractures with persistent gapping of greater than 3 mm suggest interposed periosteum. These fractures have a high risk of premature physeal closure if open reduction is not performed.
- For Tillaux and intra-articular triplane fractures treatment focuses on restoring articular congruity.

Annotated References

1. Peterson HA, Madhok R, Benson JT, Ilstrup DM, Melton LJ III: Physeal fractures: Part 1. Epidemiology in Olmsted County, Minnesota, 1979-1988. *J Pediatr Orthop* 1994;14(4):423-430.

2. Burkhart SS, Peterson HA: Fractures of the proximal tibial epiphysis. *J Bone Joint Surg Am* 1979;61(7):996-1002.

3. Shelton WR, Canale ST: Fractures of the tibia through the proximal tibial epiphyseal cartilage. *J Bone Joint Surg Am* 1979;61(2):167-173.

4. Wood KB, Bradley JP, Ward WT: Pes anserinus interposition in a proximal tibial physeal fracture: A case report. *Clin Orthop Relat Res* 1991;264:239-242.

5. Ciszewski WA, Buschmann WR, Rudolph CN: Irreducible fracture of the proximal tibial physis in an adolescent. *Orthop Rev* 1989;18(8):891-893.

6. Mosier SM, Stanitski CL: Acute tibial tubercle avulsion fractures. *J Pediatr Orthop* 2004;24(2):181-184.

7. Ogden JA, Tross RB, Murphy MJ: Fractures of the tibial tuberosity in adolescents. *J Bone Joint Surg Am* 1980;62(2):205-215.

8. Christie MJ, Dvonch VM: Tibial tuberosity avulsion fracture in adolescents. *J Pediatr Orthop* 1981;1(4):391-394.

9. Hand WL, Hand CR, Dunn AW: Avulsion fractures of the tibial tubercle. *J Bone Joint Surg Am* 1971;53(8):1579-1583.

10. Bolesta MJ, Fitch RD: Tibial tubercle avulsions. *J Pediatr Orthop* 1986;6(2):186-192.

11. Howarth WR, Gottschalk HP, Hosalkar HS: Tibial tubercle fractures in children with intra-articular involvement: Surgical tips for technical ease. *J Child Orthop* 2011;5(6):465-470.

    Tibial tubercle avulsion fractures with intra-articular extension may be associated with intra-articular pathology such as capsular avulsion or coronary ligament disruption. This case series described using suture anchors to reestablish the meniscal-articular relationship. Level of evidence: IV.

12. Pandya NK, Edmonds EW, Roocroft JH, Mubarak SJ: Tibial tubercle fractures: Complications, classification, and the need for intra-articular assessment. *J Pediatr Orthop* 2012;32(8):749-759.

    This retrospective review found that intra-articular involvement in tibial tubercle avulsion fractures may be incompletely assessed on plain radiographs. Additional evaluation with CT or MRI should be considered. The authors also proposed a new fracture classification system. Level of evidence: III.

13. Pretell-Mazzini J, Kelly DM, Sawyer JR, et al: Outcomes and complications of tibial tubercle fractures in pediatric patients: A systematic review of the literature. *J Pediatr Orthop* 2015; Apr 10 [Epub ahead of print].

    This systematic review found that adolescents who underwent surgical fixation of tibial tubercle avulsion fractures had good clinical and radiographic outcomes. Intra-articular fractures can have associated injuries. Implant removal

7: Trauma

secondary to bursitis was the most common complication. Level of evidence: III.

14. Pape JM, Goulet JA, Hensinger RN: Compartment syndrome complicating tibial tubercle avulsion. *Clin Orthop Relat Res* 1993;295:201-204.

15. Nikiforidis PA, Babis GC, Triantafillopoulos IK, Themistocleous GS, Nikolopoulos K: Avulsion fractures of the tibial tuberosity in adolescent athletes treated by internal fixation and tension band wiring. *Knee Surg Sports Traumatol Arthrosc* 2004;12(4):271-276.

16. Wiss DA, Schilz JL, Zionts L: Type III fractures of the tibial tubercle in adolescents. *J Orthop Trauma* 1991;5(4):475-479.

17. Cozen L: Fracture of the proximal portion of the tibia in children followed by valgus deformity. *Surg Gynecol Obstet* 1953;97(2):183-188.

18. Jordan SE, Alonso JE, Cook FF: The etiology of valgus angulation after metaphyseal fractures of the tibia in children. *J Pediatr Orthop* 1987;7(4):450-457.

19. Zionts LE, MacEwen GD: Spontaneous improvement of post-traumatic tibia valga. *J Bone Joint Surg Am* 1986;68(5):680-687.

20. Tuten HR, Keeler KA, Gabos PG, Zionts LE, MacKenzie WG: Posttraumatic tibia valga in children: A long-term follow-up note. *J Bone Joint Surg Am* 1999;81(6):799-810.

21. Robert M, Khouri N, Carlioz H, Alain JL: Fractures of the proximal tibial metaphysis in children: Review of a series of 25 cases. *J Pediatr Orthop* 1987;7(4):444-449.

22. Yang JP, Letts RM: Isolated fractures of the tibia with intact fibula in children: A review of 95 patients. *J Pediatr Orthop* 1997;17(3):347-351.

23. Shannak AO: Tibial fractures in children: Follow-up study. *J Pediatr Orthop* 1988;8(3):306-310.

24. Dwyer AJ, John B, Krishen M, Hora R: Remodeling of tibial fractures in children younger than 12 years. *Orthopedics* 2007;30(5):393-396.

25. Kubiak EN, Egol KA, Scher D, Wasserman B, Feldman D, Koval KJ: Operative treatment of tibial fractures in children: Are elastic stable intramedullary nails an improvement over external fixation? *J Bone Joint Surg Am* 2005;87(8):1761-1768.

26. Canavese F, Botnari A, Andreacchio A, et al: Displaced tibial shaft fractures with intact fibula in children: Nonoperative management versus operative treatment with elastic stable intramedullary nailing. *J Pediatr Orthop* 2015; May 25 [Epub ahead of print].

    This retrospective study compared children with displaced tibial shaft fractures with an intact fibula treated with either closed reduction and casting or flexible intramedullary nailing. Both groups had similar clinical and radiographic outcomes. The surgical group had a substantially shorter period of immobilization. Level of evidence: III.

27. Goodbody CM, Lee RJ, Flynn JM, Sankar WN: Titanium elastic nailing for pediatric tibia fractures: Do older, heavier kids do worse? *J Pediatr Orthop* 2015; April 8 [Epub ahead of print].

    This retrospective review found that increased weight and age were not associated with a higher malunion rate or a longer time to healing after titanium elastic nailing of pediatric tibial fractures. Level of evidence: III.

28. Myers SH, Spiegel D, Flynn JM: External fixation of high-energy tibia fractures. *J Pediatr Orthop* 2007;27(5):537-539.

29. Pandya NK, Edmonds EW: Immediate intramedullary flexible nailing of open pediatric tibial shaft fractures. *J Pediatr Orthop* 2012;32(8):770-776.

    This retrospective study demonstrated that immediate flexible intramedullary nailing of open tibial shaft fractures was not associated with increased rates of wound or infectious complications compared with closed fractures. Gustilo type II or III fractures had more bone healing complications. Level of evidence: III.

30. Shore BJ, Glotzbecker MP, Zurakowski D, Gelbard E, Hedequist DJ, Matheney TH: Acute compartment syndrome in children and teenagers with tibial shaft fractures: Incidence and multivariable risk factors. *J Orthop Trauma* 2013;27(11):616-621.

    This retrospective study found an 11.6% rate of acute compartment syndrome in children with tibial shaft fractures. Risk factors were age at least 14 years and motor vehicle crashes. Level of evidence: III.

31. Pandya NK, Edmonds EW, Mubarak SJ: The incidence of compartment syndrome after flexible nailing of pediatric tibial shaft fractures. *J Child Orthop* 2011;5(6):439-447.

    This retrospective review demonstrated a 19.3% rate of compartment syndrome after flexible nailing of tibial shaft fractures. Risk factors were weight greater than 50 kg, complex or comminuted fractures, and neurologic deficit without compartmental swelling before surgical intervention. Level of evidence: III.

32. Landin LA: Epidemiology of children's fractures. *J Pediatr Orthop B* 1997;6(2):79-83.

33. Barmada A, Gaynor T, Mubarak SJ: Premature physeal closure following distal tibia physeal fractures: A new radiographic predictor. *J Pediatr Orthop* 2003;23(6):733-739.

34. Spiegel PG, Cooperman DR, Laros GS: Epiphyseal fractures of the distal ends of the tibia and fibula: A retrospective study of two hundred and thirty-seven cases in children. *J Bone Joint Surg Am* 1978;60(8):1046-1050.

35. Dias LS, Tachdjian MO: Physeal injuries of the ankle in children: Classification. *Clin Orthop Relat Res* 1978;136:230-233.

36. Russo F, Moor MA, Mubarak SJ, Pennock AT: Salter-Harris II fractures of the distal tibia: Does surgical management reduce the risk of premature physeal closure? *J Pediatr Orthop* 2013;33(5):524-529.

This retrospective study demonstrated that surgical fixation of displaced Salter-Harris type II distal tibia fractures with anatomic reduction and the removal of interposed tissue did not reduce the incidence of premature physeal closure. Level of evidence: III.

37. Rohmiller MT, Gaynor TP, Pawelek J, Mubarak SJ: Salter-Harris I and II fractures of the distal tibia: Does mechanism of injury relate to premature physeal closure? *J Pediatr Orthop* 2006;26(3):322-328.

38. Leary JT, Handling M, Talerico M, Yong L, Bowe JA: Physeal fractures of the distal tibia: Predictive factors of premature physeal closure and growth arrest. *J Pediatr Orthop* 2009;29(4):356-361.

39. Nenopoulos A, Beslikas T, Gigis I, Sayegh F, Christoforidis I, Hatzokos I: The role of CT in diagnosis and treatment of distal tibial fractures with intra-articular involvement in children. *Injury* 2015;46(11):2177-2180.

This retrospective review showed that CT evaluation led to changes in fracture classification and treatment decisions for distal tibial fractures with intra-articular involvement. The effect of the CT findings on treatment decision was particularly important for transitional fractures. Level of evidence: III.

40. Domzalski ME, Lipton GE, Lee D, Guille JT: Fractures of the distal tibial metaphysis in children: Patterns of injury and results of treatment. *J Pediatr Orthop* 2006;26(2):171-176.

41. Schurz M, Binder H, Platzer P, Schulz M, Hajdu S, Vécsei V: Physeal injuries of the distal tibia: Long-term results in 376 patients. *Int Orthop* 2010;34(4):547-552.

42. Choudhry IK, Wall EJ, Eismann EA, Crawford AH, Wilson L: Functional outcome analysis of triplane and Tillaux fractures after closed reduction and percutaneous fixation. *J Pediatr Orthop* 2014;34(2):139-143.

This retrospective study demonstrated that patients with residual displacement of less than 2.5 mm after closed reduction and percutaneous pinning of a transitional fracture had good medium-term outcomes. Level of evidence: III.

43. Cooperman DR, Spiegel PG, Laros GS: Tibial fractures involving the ankle in children: The so-called triplane epiphyseal fracture. *J Bone Joint Surg Am* 1978;60(8):1040-1046.

44. Inokuchi S, Usami N, Hiraishi E, Hashimoto T: Calcaneal fractures in children. *J Pediatr Orthop* 1998;18(4):469-474.

45. Brunet JA: Calcaneal fractures in children: Long-term results of treatment. *J Bone Joint Surg Br* 2000;82(2):211-216.

46. Petit CJ, Lee BM, Kasser JR, Kocher MS: Operative treatment of intraarticular calcaneal fractures in the pediatric population. *J Pediatr Orthop* 2007;27(8):856-862.

47. Jensen I, Wester JU, Rasmussen F, Lindequist S, Schantz K: Prognosis of fracture of the talus in children: 21 (7-34)-year follow-up of 14 cases. *Acta Orthop Scand* 1994;65(4):398-400.

48. Ribbans WJ, Natarajan R, Alavala S: Pediatric foot fractures. *Clin Orthop Relat Res* 2005;432:107-115.

Chapter 40

Spine

Daniel J. Hedequist, MD   Michael Glotzbecker, MD

7: Trauma

Abstract

Unique characteristics in children predispose them to spine injuries that differ from those in adults. The size of children, anatomic differences of the cervical spine, and normal radiographic variants all need to be considered during the initial evaluation of a spine injury. Routine plain radiographs are used in the primary setting of trauma, followed by MRI and CT when indicated. Younger children are predisposed to upper cervical spine injuries, the most common being odontoid fractures. Adolescents generally sustain subaxial cervical spine injuries as well as thoracic and lumbar injuries that are more consistent with adult spine trauma. Spinal cord injuries without radiographic abnormality, Chance fractures, and apophyseal ring injuries are unique to children, given their size and spinal plasticity. The treatment of individual injuries varies and may range from nonsurgical management with an orthosis to surgical management with instrumented stabilization and fusion.

Keywords: cervical spine; dentocentral synchondrosis; spinal cord injuries without radiographic abnormality (SCIWORA); spine trauma; thoracolumbar spine; vertebral fractures

Dr. Hedequist or an immediate family member serves as a board member, owner, officer, or committee member of the American Academy of Orthopaedic Surgeons and the Pediatric Orthopaedic Society of North America. Dr. Glotzbecker or an immediate family member serves as a paid consultant to DePuy and Medtronic, and has received research or institutional support from Synthes via the Chest Wall and the Spinal Deformity Study Group. This chapter is adapted from Hedequist D: Pediatric spine trauma, in Ricci WM, Ostrum RF, eds: Orthopaedic Knowledge Update: Trauma 5. *Rosemont, IL, American Academy of Orthopaedic Surgeons, 2016, pp 669-675.*

Introduction

Spine fractures represent approximately 1% of all fractures seen in level 1 pediatric trauma centers and are related to the patient's age and size. The anatomic differences in children vary and are deterministic of injury patterns. Younger children have a large head-to-body ratio and, consequently, sustain more upper cervical spine injuries, whereas adolescents sustain the most thoracolumbar injuries. For all children, the most common mechanism of fracture is a motor vehicle crash, with cervical trauma more common in younger children. The second most common cause of injury also is related to age, with falls more common in younger children and sports-related injuries more common in older children and adolescents. In up to 19% of patients, nonaccidental trauma is the cause of spine injuries in toddlers (children younger than 3 years), and it has a 25% mortality rate.[1] Spine trauma also is associated with nonspinal injuries, including head trauma, chest trauma, and abdominal injuries, as well as other noncontiguous spinal injuries.[2]

Anatomy

Anatomic differences in children predispose each pediatric age group to differing injury patterns. Children younger than 8 years have more horizontally aligned cervical facets, greater ligamentous laxity, and a larger head-to-body ratio, all of which predispose them to upper cervical spine injuries at the cranial-cervical junction and C1-C2. Children younger than 6 years also have open synchondroses (cartilaginous growth centers), the largest of which is at C2 (the dentocentral synchondrosis), which makes odontoid fractures through the physis much more common in younger children. The dentocentral synchondrosis fuses when a child is approximately 6 years of age; before that, younger children are at risk of sustaining an injury at the dens through this growth center (**Figure 1**). Subaxial spine fractures, thoracic burst or compression fractures, and lumbar spine injuries become more common as children develop (older than age 10 years) and their anatomy becomes more similar to that of an adult.

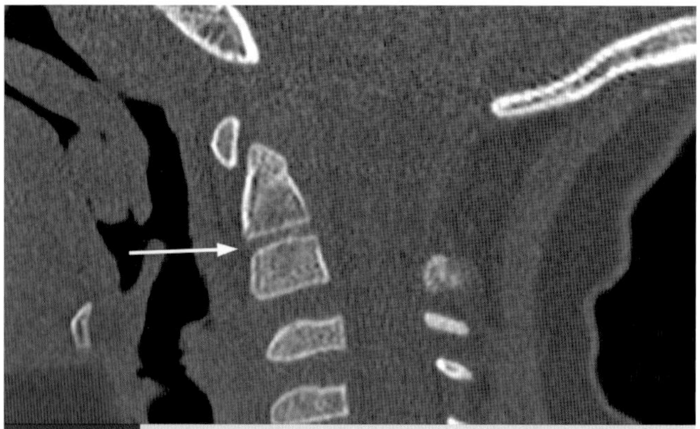

Figure 1 Sagittal CT scan of the spine of a 3-year-old patient. The arrow points to the dentocentral synchondrosis.

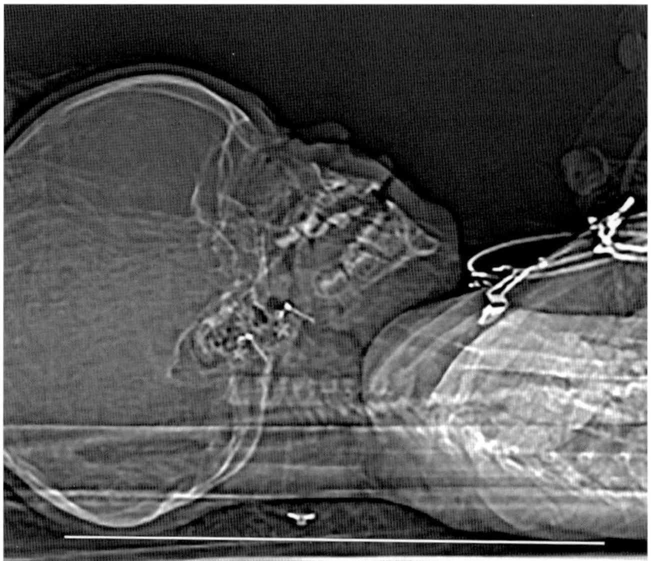

Figure 2 Lateral scout view in a CT scan of a 2-year-old patient being evaluated for neck trauma. Note the position of the child's neck in flexion; the white line extending from the back of the occiput to the shoulders at the bottom of the image indicates that no recess was applied to account for the large cranium because the occiput is in line with the thorax, not posterior.

Initial Evaluation

The initial evaluation of a child with suspected spine trauma begins in the field because children pose unique transport challenges related to their small size and anatomic differences. Children must be placed in cervical collars, with increased stability obtained by taping their heads to sandbags or intravenous fluid bags placed on either side of the head to further minimize cervical motion. Compared with adults, children have a larger cranium relative to their body size, and their occiput has a greater posterior offset that predisposes them to inadvertent cervical flexion when lying flat (**Figure 2**). This possible flexion must be counteracted by placing the child on a specialized pediatric backboard with an occipital recess cutout or elevating the child's body with blankets to allow the cranium to translate posteriorly. Generally, this is important in children younger than 8 years and can be assessed clinically by positioning the head so that the pinna is level with or posterior to the shoulder.

The initial physical examination should focus on all body systems. The evaluation of a child with suspected spine trauma should begin after a thorough primary survey because spine trauma often is associated with other injuries. The clinical evaluation of the back includes a standard inspection and palpation of the entire area, with care being taken to log roll the patient while using spinal precautions. A detailed neurologic examination should be performed because spine fractures and instability potentially can be associated with a spinal cord injury. Given the risk of lap-belt injuries in children, inspection and palpation of the anterior abdominal wall and the pelvic region are paramount in younger children who have been injured in a motor vehicle crash.

Radiographic Studies

At some medical centers, standard radiography remains the initial imaging modality of choice for pediatric trauma patients. At a minimum, radiographs should include a cross-table lateral view with an AP view of the cervical spine. Patients with substantial neck pain despite normal-appearing radiographs require further imaging (usually CT). Because of associated injuries, CT of the cervical spine should be considered for obtunded or uncooperative children with head injuries or facial trauma who will be undergoing CT. Plain radiographs of the thoracic and lumbar spine should be taken in cases of suspected injury indicated by the physical examination findings, associated injuries, or the patient's history. Normal anatomic variation exists for children younger than 8 years and may be mistaken for fractures or a ligamentous injury.[3] Ossification centers (most commonly the dens before age 5 years) can be mistaken for a fracture line. Vertebral height differences as well as differences in morphology may be mistaken for compression fractures. Cervical pseudosubluxation resulting from ligamentous laxity (most commonly C2 on C3), loss of normal cervical lordosis, and increased apparent anterior soft-tissue swelling caused by crying are all examples of normal variants in the pediatric cervical spine. Subtle wedging of thoracic and lumbar vertebra as well as apparent disk irregularities

(Schmorl nodes) must all be evaluated in context with the history and physical examination findings, and further imaging should be based on the complete evaluation.

CT is used to evaluate a suspected bony or ligamentous injury. Newer classification systems for spine trauma rely on CT for the anatomic classification of fractures. The increased use of CT for cervical screening has become more commonplace, especially in children who are more severely injured. In some centers, CT has been shown to be as efficacious as MRI in clearing the cervical spine in children who are severely injured to avoid the need for cervical collars and spinal precautions in patients who are obtunded.[4] However, the routine use of CT as a screening tool for cervical injuries is not appropriate because of the radiation dosing required and the ability to diagnose most suspected injuries with plain radiographs and a physical examination. Awake and alert patients with reliable examination findings do not require CT imaging based solely on the mechanism of injury. CT for thoracic and lumbar spine injuries should be limited to studying documented fractures. Prior to ordering CT, a discussion with the trauma team is warranted regarding the potential need for thoracic or abdominal CT for associated injuries. CT angiography should be considered in a patient with cervical facet fractures, upper cervical spine fractures, or fractures through the foramen because of the potential for vertebral artery injury with these fractures.[5]

In spinal trauma, MRI may be obtained for clearance and for the documentation of known injuries. MRI is an excellent cervical spine screening tool with high sensitivity and specificity when used within the first 48 hours of injury in children who are obtunded.[6] Children with a documented or suspected spine injury with a neurologic deficit should undergo MRI to determine the extent of neurologic injuries and/or compression, which may aid in treatment decisions. When surgical treatment of spine trauma is indicated, MRI and CT of the associated area should be obtained to clearly identify the extent of bony, ligamentous, and neural injuries.

Specific Injuries

Spinal Cord Injuries Without Radiographic Abnormality

Spinal cord injuries without radiographic abnormality (SCIWORA) describes a neurologic injury without apparent radiographic or CT evidence of a bony or ligamentous spinal column injury. The use of MRI has improved understanding of spinal column injuries in patients with apparently normal CT and radiographic findings. SCIWORA is thought to occur because of the plasticity of a child's spine, which allows stretch to occur without bony failure but causes damage to the neural elements that do not tolerate stretch as well. Most cases of SCIWORA occur in younger children secondary to motor vehicle and pedestrian-vehicle crashes. Infants and young children who have a SCIWORA should be screened for nonaccidental trauma. The degree of spinal cord injury ranges from mild and transient to severe and permanent, including profound quadriplegia. MRI evidence of facet and ligamentous injuries may be seen at the same level or even at levels away from the spinal cord injury. Spinal cord injuries seen on MRI range from mild cord contusions to complete disruptions. Treatment involves preventing further neurologic damage by stabilization with bracing and supportive care of the spinal cord injury. Bracing is worthwhile in patients with questionable ligamentous instability; however, if there is no evidence of injury other than neurologic injury, it is unclear if bracing plays any role.[7,8] Neurologic recovery is dependent on the initial degree of spinal cord injury, which was documented in a recent multicenter study in which 94% of the patients with SCIWORA and a normal MRI had full recovery compared with only 27% of patients with abnormal MRI findings having full recovery.[9]

Cranial-Cervical Junction Injuries

Injuries to the cranial-vertebral junction include ligament injuries, fractures, and combined injuries. Occipital condyle fractures are more common in the adolescent population and necessitate further evaluation of the supporting ligamentous structures to rule out more substantial injuries. Atlanto-occipital region injuries are high-energy injuries caused by sudden deceleration, with the head moving forward on the cervical spine. These injuries may be subtle and difficult to diagnose or highly unstable, such as atlanto-occipital dissociations. In the past, these injuries have universally been considered fatal injuries; however, improvements in modern emergency medical systems with rapid stabilization and transport have allowed some children to survive such injuries. Modern imaging techniques plus a high degree of suspicion have improved the accuracy of diagnosis, given the challenges in adequately assessing the craniovertebral junction with plain radiographs. Correlation of MRI findings with the degree of injury can be difficult; however, any radiographic evidence of distraction is highly suggestive of an unstable injury, and these patients have some degree of retroclival hematoma and posterior ligamentous signal on MRI. Patients have neck pain and frequently have complete or incomplete spinal cord injuries. Lateral gaze palsy secondary to injury to the sixth cranial nerve may be present. Multisystem injuries are common, including brain, chest, abdominal, and appendicular injuries. In

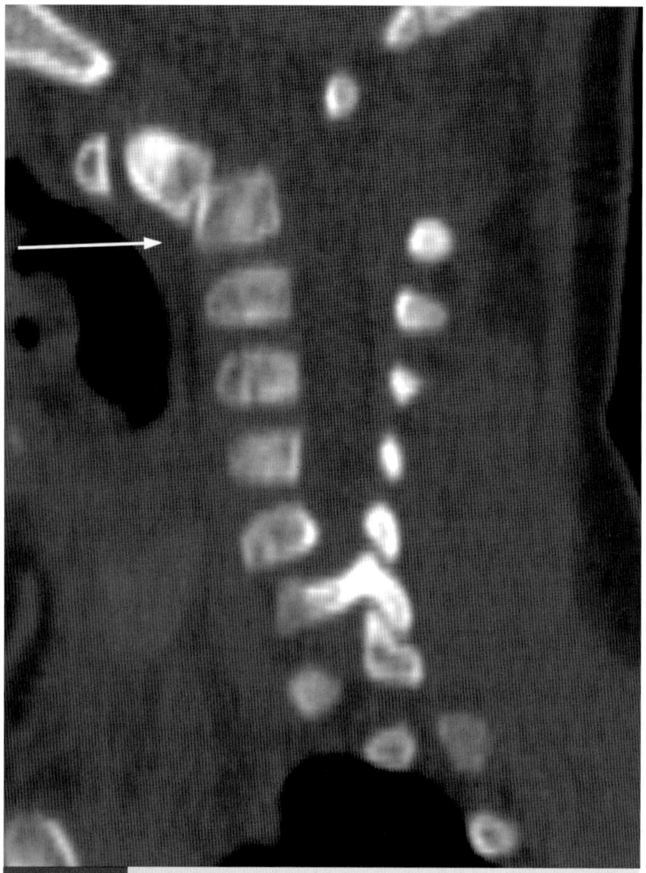

Figure 3 Sagittal CT scan of the spine of a 2-year-old child involved in a motor vehicle crash. The arrow points through the flexed odontoid fracture, which is a physeal fracture in a child of this age.

patients with true atlanto-occipital dissociations, an instrumented occiput to cervical fusion is required because halo immobilization is insufficient for these ligamentous injuries.[10] Among survivors of this injury, hydrocephalus and residual neurologic deficits are common.[10]

C1 Fractures

Fractures of the ring of C1 (also known as Jefferson fractures) in children may occur through the synchondroses of C1. These fractures are difficult to diagnose on plain radiographs and may be seen with CT or MRI in a child with a suspected fracture after the physical examination or by knowing the mechanism of injury.[11] The treatment of a Jefferson fracture is either with an orthosis or a halo vest. Stability of the fracture is determined by lateral overhang of the lateral mass of C1 on C2, which can best be appreciated with coronal CT reformatted images. Overlap of more than 5 mm on either side is indicative of a transverse atlantal ligament injury, which is best studied with MRI. Because of growth asymmetry, children younger than 7 years may have a pseudospread of the lateral masses in relationship to the dens. Edema seen on MRI or a definitive synchondrosis fracture in these children may help differentiate pseudospread from traumatic overhang. Injuries with greater severity ultimately need proof of ligamentous stability with flexion-extension radiographs after a period of treatment in a halo vest. Early stabilization and fusion are recommended only in cases of substantial displacement and evidence of complete ligamentous disruption.

Odontoid Fractures

Odontoid fractures are the most common pediatric cervical spine fracture. This fracture is commonly seen in children younger than 5 years through the dentocentral synchondrosis. Sudden deceleration with hyperflexion of the head is the mechanism most commonly seen in these patients, usually resulting from a motor vehicle crash. The child usually has substantial cervical apprehension and pain. Radiographs demonstrate the anterior and flexed position of the dens through the dentocentral synchondrosis. CT is usually sufficient to clarify the injury, although MRI also may be used (**Figure 3**). Neurologic function is usually intact, given the ample space available for the spinal cord at that level. Treatment is reduction under anesthesia with translation and hyperextension under fluoroscopy and immobilization in a halo vest for 6 to 8 weeks in a position of hyperextension. Nondisplaced fractures could potentially be treated in a noninvasive halo or a Minerva orthosis.

Hangman's Fractures

Hangman's fractures are rare in children and appear as defects in the pars of C2 with spondylolisthesis of C2 on C3. The mechanism of this fracture is thought to be related to forced hyperextension. Patients with acute injuries should be managed with a closed reduction and halo placement for 6 weeks. Occasionally, C2 pars defects may be seen on lateral radiographs in the workup of subacute neck pain. These defects may be differentiated from an acute injury by either the lack of edema on MRI or more sclerotic borders of the fracture edges on CT. Treatment options for subacute C2 pars defects include observation, Minerva-type bracing, and halo placement.[12] Attempts at closed treatment with immobilization are warranted and may result in complete healing of the defects. Persistent nonunions of the C2 pars region may result in instability. If worrisome amounts of translation are seen on flexion-extension radiographs, an instrumented fusion is warranted. Treatment should be individualized based on a variety of factors, including radiographic signs of instability and neurologic status.

Atlantoaxial Rotatory Subluxation

C1-C2 rotatory subluxation may result from an infection, head positioning during surgery, or trauma. Patients have neck pain and spasms, such as holding the head rotated to one side with the chin tilted, and resist attempts at movement secondary to pain. Confirmation of the subluxated C1-C2 complex is done with CT (**Figure 4**). The Fielding-Hawkins classification describes the severity of displacement; however, treatment is usually mandated depending on the physical presentation and the length of symptoms. High-energy mechanisms (such as those resulting from a motor vehicle crash) with acute torticollis deserve further workup with MRI to rule out a traumatic C1-C2 ligamentous injury. Low-energy mechanisms do not require additional imaging and can be managed with a soft collar, NSAIDs, and antispasmodics for the first week. Patients who do not have an initial response after 1 week may need to be admitted and placed in halter or halo traction. Reduction is usually seen with an improvement in pain and return to a normal clinical appearance. Failure of traction to reduce the subluxation then requires reduction by positioning the head in a neutral position under anesthesia with halo vest placement. If surgical repositioning does not reduce the subluxation, a period of halo traction may reduce it. If reduction can be obtained, treatment in a halo vest for 6 weeks will maintain reduction in more than 70% of patients.[13] Failure to obtain a reduction or recurrent subluxation after halo traction are treated with instrumented C1-C2 fusion. Traumatic torticollis with a ligamentous injury visible on MRI frequently requires C1-C2 fusion. However, a trial of halo-vest immobilization and subsequent assessment of stability with flexion-extension radiographs is reasonable before proceeding with arthrodesis.

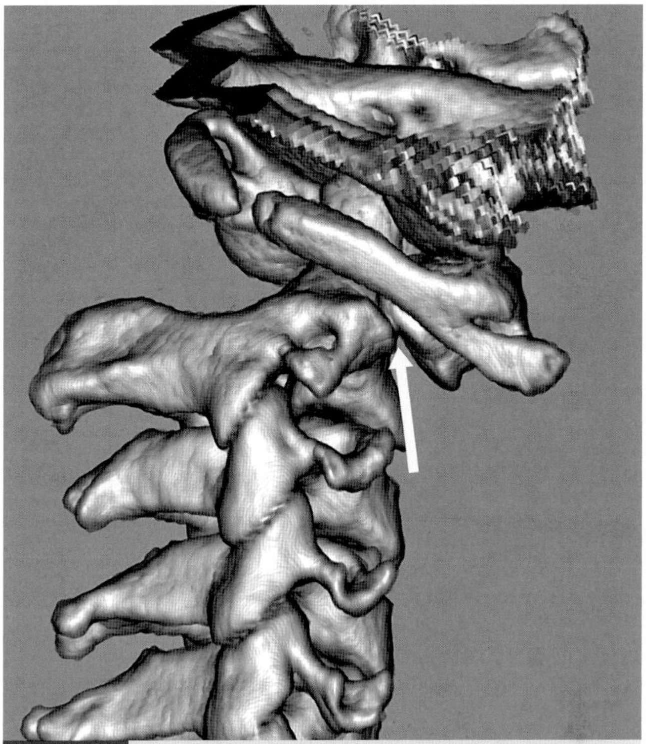

Figure 4 Reconstructed three-dimensional CT image from a 12-year-old child with fixed C1-C2 rotatory subluxation. The arrow points to the displacement of the C1 articular surface anteriorly and downward in relationship with the C2 joint surface.

Subaxial Cervical Injuries

Subaxial cervical spine injuries are more common in children older than 10 years and usually are the result of a motor vehicle crash or sport participation. Subaxial cervical injury patterns tend to resemble adult-type injuries because the anatomy of an adolescent has reached a mature state.[14] Injuries include spinous process avulsion fractures; ligamentous injuries, including facet subluxations and dislocations; facet fractures; compression fractures; and burst fractures with multicolumn involvement.

The AOSpine Group developed a working classification for cervical spine injuries in adults, which is transferrable to the adolescent population.[15] This classification describes fracture morphology, with more unstable injuries having posterior ligamentous injuries. Facet alignment, focal kyphosis, translation, and posterior spinous process distraction are factors in determining injury stability. CT as well as MRI are paramount for decision making. The classification system revolves around the CT findings, with MRI determining the degree of posterior ligamentous injury. Treatment is related to the injury pattern, the potential for stability, and the presence of neurologic deficit or cord compression. Stable injury patterns may be treated with cervical collars, whereas unstable injuries require stabilization and fusion with segmental rigid instrumentation. Facet subluxation or dislocations require MRI evaluation of the disk space before reduction to prevent exacerbation of a traumatic disk herniation. Some injuries, which are deemed stable, may subsequently demonstrate instability secondary to more severe ligamentous injury than was appreciated on imaging and will require stabilization. Flexion-extension radiographs in the nonacute setting ultimately determine cervical stability.

Thoracolumbar Spine Trauma

Multiple descriptive classifications for thoracolumbar spine trauma are primarily based on fracture morphology.

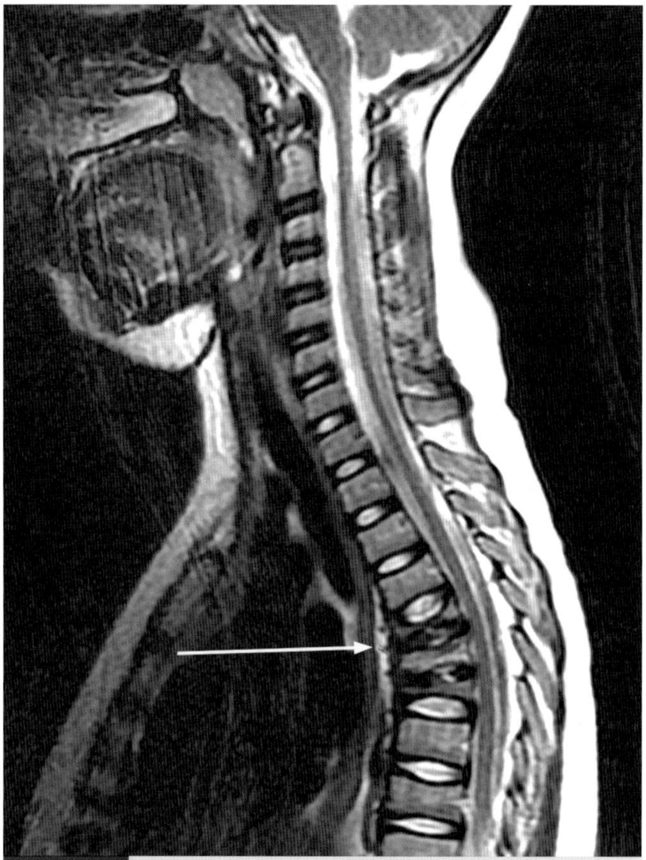

Figure 5 Sagittal T2-weighted MRI of the spine of a 7-year-old child with gradual onset of upper thoracic back pain. The arrow points to three continuous levels of compression fractures related to pathologic fractures resulting from leukemia.

In an effort to improve communication among treating physicians, provide standardization for research, and aid physicians in determining appropriate treatment, the AOSpine Group developed the thoracolumbar injury classification system. This system considers the bony and ligamentous aspects of injuries as well as the neurologic status of the patient in an attempt to guide treatment.[16] The thoracolumbar injury classification system has been applied to the pediatric population with relatively good specificity and sensitivity for morphology, but with poor reliability for predicting treatment.[17] The AOSpine classification currently is being studied in children. The following sections describe the classic fracture patterns according to relative severity.

Thoracic Compression Fractures

Compression fractures are commonly seen in children and usually occur in the thoracic spine and are contiguous over two or three levels. Frequently, compression fractures are related to a fall or athletic injury with a shock-wave effect through the spine, hence the multilevel nature of the injury. Radiographs will reveal a subtle loss of height over multiple levels, which should correspond to the region of back pain. Normal morphologic variations in children can resemble compression fractures; however, when associated with back pain and localized tenderness, radiographs should be interpreted as suggestive of fracture. If necessary, MRI may be helpful in differentiating true fractures from morphologic variations. Compression fractures are stable injuries, and a thoracic hyperextension-type brace is not required, although it may be useful for improving symptoms. Special mention should be made about patients with painful compression fractures in the absence of an injury. In this scenario, consideration should be given to an underlying bone density problem (such as juvenile osteoporosis) or the potential for malignancy, most notably leukemia, which may include malaise, atraumatic back pain, and compression fractures (**Figure 5**).

Burst Fractures

Burst fractures are high-energy injuries seen in older children and adolescents. The mechanisms of injury usually are motor vehicle trauma or high-velocity activities such as skiing, all-terrain vehicle use, or participation in motocross.[18] Although most patients are neurologically intact, some will have partial or incomplete spinal cord injuries. The risk of a spinal cord injury is higher in patients with thoracic burst fractures, and recovery is directly related to the severity of neurologic injury.[19] The degree of neurologic compression can be evaluated by MRI. Burst fractures may have extension to one or both end plates but classically involve the vertebral body, with the fracture extending through the posterior wall of the vertebral body. The presence of a posterior column injury may be difficult to define, but newer classification systems have focused on injuries to the posterior ligamentous complex. MRI evidence of a posterior ligamentous injury and CT scans showing interspinous widening or facet disruption signify a potentially unstable injury that may benefit from surgery. Treatment ranges from bracing with a thoracolumbar spinal orthosis to surgical stabilization and is based on a variety of factors, including canal compromise, loss of vertebral height, the location of the fracture, and the neurologic status of the patient. Most surgeons believe that an absolute indication for surgery is a burst fracture in the setting of an incomplete or a complete neurologic injury. Focal kyphosis with loss of height in the setting of an insufficient posterior ligamentous complex also is suggestive of the need for surgical stabilization. Surgical treatment varies and ranges from anterior decompression with structural support and instrumentation to

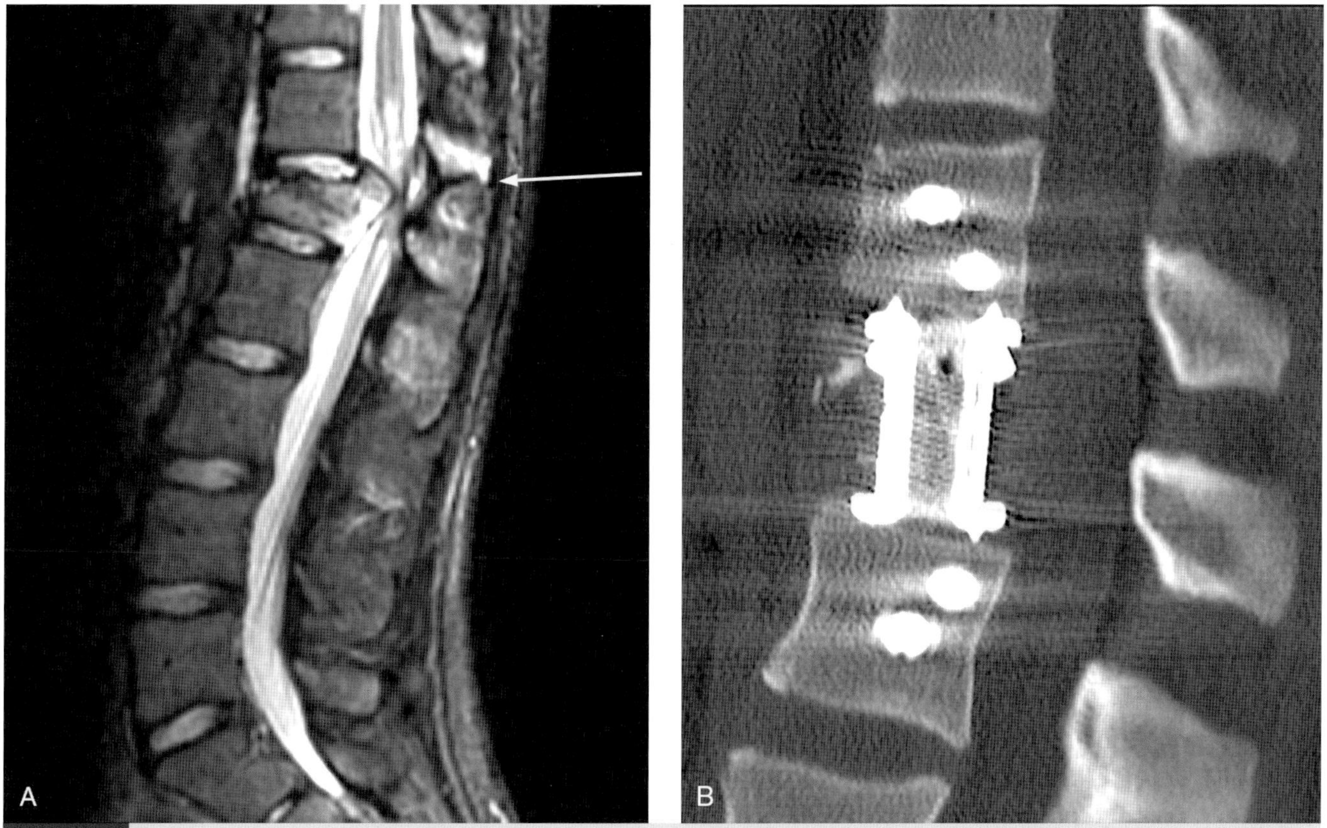

Figure 6 **A,** Sagittal T2-weighted MRI scan from a 14-year-old child involved in a high-speed motor vehicle crash. Note the fracture with retropulsion, cord compression, signal changes, and especially the signal change in the interspinous posterior ligamentous complex. All these variables signify a highly unstable fracture. **B,** Postoperative CT scan after corpectomy and anterior plating. Note the restoration of height and the decompressed canal.

posterior instrumentation with distraction and realignment (**Figure 6**). Nonsurgical treatment in patients who are neurologically intact is associated with good functional outcomes; however, care must be taken to monitor for progressive focal kyphosis, especially at the level of the thoracolumbar junction, where loss of alignment adversely affects overall sagittal alignment.

Flexion-Distraction Injuries (Chance Fractures)

Chance fractures are flexion-distraction injuries of the thoracolumbar spine and are commonly secondary to a sudden deceleration against a lap belt in a motor vehicle crash. Correct placement of a lap belt is dependent on the size of the child. Inherent to child safety is positioning the belt in contact with the pelvis, which is facilitated by using a booster seat for younger children. Chance fractures in children are a result of a sudden deceleration of the vehicle, with the momentum of a child going forward and flexing over an incorrectly applied lap belt, which is lying at the abdominal/umbilical level. This sudden deceleration results in a flexion injury to the anterior column and distraction of the posterior column. The resulting thoracolumbar injury may be ligamentous, bony, or mixed. Frequently, the diagnosis may be delayed because the association of this fracture with intra-abdominal injuries requiring laparotomy is high. In any patient with a Chance fracture, the trauma team must consider the possibility of intra-abdominal injuries. These injuries frequently occur in children younger than 10 years, with most cases occurring in the upper lumbar spine, These injuries are associated with neurologic deficit in more than 40% of patients.[20] Chance fractures may be treated nonsurgically with hyperextension casting or bracing if the injury is purely bony in nature without substantial kyphosis and in the absence of neurologic injury. A tendency exists for progressive kyphosis with nonsurgical management of this injury, so close follow-up is required. Patients with ligamentous injuries, greater deformity, and neurologic deficits are best treated with reduction and rigid posterior instrumentation and fusion (**Figure 7**).

Apophyseal Ring Injuries

In growing children, the disk attachment to the end plate is an apophysis, which may become avulsed during

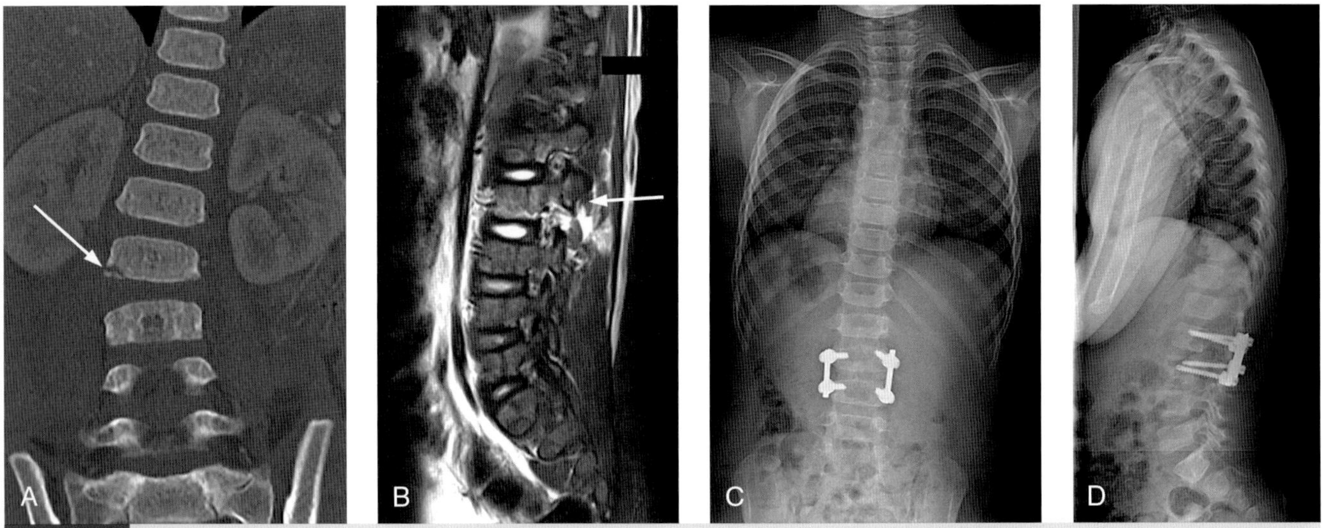

Figure 7 **A,** CT scan from a 3-year-old child with a suspected Chance fracture after a seat belt injury in a high-speed motor vehicle crash. The arrow points to the end plate fracture. Note the scoliosis present, which is indicative of a posterior ligament injury with facet subluxation. **B,** T2-weighted MRI scan from the same patient documents signal changes at the facet and posterior ligamentous complex indicative of a mixed bony-ligamentous Chance injury evident at the arrow. PA (**C**) and lateral (**D**) radiographs after reduction and instrumented fusion. At the time of the surgical procedure, the posterior ligaments were completely disrupted with a unilateral facet dislocation.

trauma. Frequently, apophyseal ring injuries occur in adolescents with trauma sustained during athletic events, and evidence of a previous apophysitis is usually present. Injuries are usually at the thoracolumbar junction and may include neurologic deficit if there is retropulsion into the canal. Lumbar apophyseal ring injuries frequently have radiculopathy. If no neurologic deficit is present, treatment usually involves bracing, which is followed by physical therapy. The presence of a motor deficit usually requires surgical treatment, which includes diskectomy and instrumented fusion. The described long-term outcomes after apophyseal ring injuries suggest that most patients do not have a permanent neurologic deficit and return to normal activities.[21] However, among patients managed nonsurgically, resorption of retropulsed bone did not occur, and those with large lesions had a higher frequency of chronic pain with limited activities.[21,22]

Summary

Successful management of pediatric spine trauma begins in the field with appropriate transport and is followed by a thorough assessment in the emergency department. Plain radiographs will document most injuries, with CT and MRI used as adjuncts to further classify injuries. Maintenance of a high degree of suspicion of injury is important in patients who are obtunded or younger children who may be uncooperative during the examination or are noncommunicative. Children younger than 8 years more commonly sustain upper cervical spine trauma, with odontoid fractures being more common in younger patients because of dentocentral synchondrosis. SCIWORA exists because of the plasticity of a young child's spinal column and should be suspected when the neurologic examination does not correlate with normal findings on plain radiographs and/or CT scans. Flexion-distraction injuries are caused by inappropriately applied lap belts, and evaluation of the spine is warranted in a child involved in a motor vehicle crash with a lap-belt sign and concern for an intra-abdominal injury. The treatment of all injuries should consider the age of the child, the alignment and stability of the fracture, and the presence of neurologic injury or compression.

Key Study Points

- Younger children have a larger head-to-body ratio than adults, thus predisposing them to upper cervical spine injuries.
- Chance fractures may be avoided by using booster seats for young children to ensure the correct placement of an automobile lap belt.
- SCIWORA exists in children because of the plasticity of the spine and should be suspected in a child with a neurologic deficit despite normal findings on plain radiographs.
- Normal radiographic variants exist in the pediatric cervical spine and must be considered when evaluating cervical spine imaging in the trauma setting.

Annotated References

1. Knox JB, Schneider JE, Cage JM, Wimberly RL, Riccio AI: Spine trauma in very young children: A retrospective study of 206 patients presenting to a level 1 pediatric trauma center. *J Pediatr Orthop* 2014;34(7):698-702.

   In this review of 206 patients younger than 10 years with spine fractures, upper cervical spine injuries were more frequent in younger children, and older children sustained more thoracic compression fractures. Nonaccidental trauma was the cause of 19% of the injuries. Level of evidence: III.

2. Hofbauer M, Jaindl M, Höchtl LL, Ostermann RC, Kdolsky R, Aldrian S: Spine injuries in polytraumatized pediatric patients: Characteristics and experience from a level I trauma center over two decades. *J Trauma Acute Care Surg* 2012;73(1):156-161.

   In this retrospective 20-year review of spinal trauma in children with multiple traumas who were stratified by age, younger children more commonly had cervical injuries, whereas lumbar injuries generally were seen only in adolescents. Level of evidence: III.

3. Lustrin ES, Karakas SP, Ortiz AO, et al: Pediatric cervical spine: Normal anatomy, variants, and trauma. *Radiographics* 2003;23(3):539-560.

4. Gargas J, Yaszay B, Kruk P, Bastrom T, Shellington D, Khanna S: An analysis of cervical spine magnetic resonance imaging findings after normal computed tomographic imaging findings in pediatric trauma patients: Ten-year experience of a level I pediatric trauma center. *J Trauma Acute Care Surg* 2013;74(4):1102-1107.

   This study evaluated the use of high-resolution CT as a screening modality for pediatric cervical spine clearance. The authors suggested using high-resolution CT for clearance when MRI is not readily available. Level of evidence: III.

5. Tolhurst SR, Vanderhave KL, Caird MS, et al: Cervical arterial injury after blunt trauma in children: Characterization and advanced imaging. *J Pediatr Orthop* 2013;33(1):37-42.

   This retrospective study evaluated the incidence of cervical vascular injuries associated with spinal trauma in children. Foraminal fractures, fracture-dislocations, and C1 through C3 injuries are at high risk for cervical vascular injuries. Level of evidence: IV.

6. Henry M, Scarlata K, Riesenburger RI, et al: Utility of STIR MRI in pediatric cervical spine clearance after trauma. *J Neurosurg Pediatr* 2013;12(1):30-36.

   The authors describe a level 1 trauma center's experience in using short tau inversion recovery MRI for cervical spine clearance in children. Short tau inversion recovery MRI was associated with a high specificity and sensitivity for clearance in trauma patients. Level of evidence: III.

7. Launay F, Leet AI, Sponseller PD: Pediatric spinal cord injury without radiographic abnormality: A meta-analysis. *Clin Orthop Relat Res* 2005;433:166-170.

8. Bosch PP, Vogt MT, Ward WT: Pediatric spinal cord injury without radiographic abnormality (SCIWORA): The absence of occult instability and lack of indication for bracing. *Spine (Phila Pa 1976)* 2002;27(24):2788-2800.

9. Mahajan P, Jaffe DM, Olsen CS, et al: Spinal cord injury without radiologic abnormality in children imaged with magnetic resonance imaging. *J Trauma Acute Care Surg* 2013;75(5):843-847.

   The authors of this study report that children younger than 16 years who were diagnosed with SCIWORA but had normal findings on MRI had a different presentation and better outcomes than those of children with MRI-detected cervical cord abnormalities.

10. Astur N, Klimo P Jr, Sawyer JR, Kelly DM, Muhlbauer MS, Warner WC Jr: Traumatic atlanto-occipital dislocation in children: Evaluation, treatment, and outcomes. *J Bone Joint Surg Am* 2013;95(24):e194(1-8).

    In a retrospective review of 14 pediatric patients with atlanto-occipital dislocation, the preferred management was occiput-to-cervical fusion. Level of evidence: IV.

11. AuYong N, Piatt J Jr: Jefferson fractures of the immature spine. Report of 3 cases. *J Neurosurg Pediatr* 2009;3(1):15-19.

12. Pizzutillo PD, Rocha EF, D'Astous J, Kling TF Jr, McCarthy RE: Bilateral fracture of the pedicle of the second cervical vertebra in the young child. *J Bone Joint Surg Am* 1986;68(6):892-896.

13. Glotzbecker MP, Wasser AM, Hresko MT, Karlin LI, Emans JB, Hedequist DJ: Efficacy of nonfusion treatment for subacute and chronic atlanto-axial rotatory fixation in children. *J Pediatr Orthop* 2014;34(5):490-495.

    In a retrospective review of a cohort of patients treated nonsurgically for chronic atlantoaxial rotatory subluxation, nonsurgical management with reduction and halo application was successful in more than 70% of the patients. Level of evidence: III.

14. Murphy RF, Davidson AR, Kelly DM, Warner WC Jr, Sawyer JR: Subaxial cervical spine injuries in children and adolescents. *J Pediatr Orthop* 2015;35(2):136-139.

    In a retrospective review of subaxial spine injuries at a level 1 pediatric trauma center, most of the injuries occurred in adolescents, were the result of motor vehicle crashes, and could be treated nonsurgically with a cervical collar. Level of evidence: IV.

15. Vaccaro AR, Koerner JD, Radcliff KE, et al: AOSpine subaxial cervical spine injury classification system. *Eur Spine J* 2015;25(7):2173-2184.

    This review article describes the AOSpine subaxial cervical spine injury classification.

16. Vaccaro AR, Oner C, Kepler CK, et al; AOSpine Spinal Cord Injury & Trauma Knowledge Forum: AOSpine thoracolumbar spine injury classification system: Fracture description, neurological status, and key modifiers. *Spine (Phila Pa 1976)* 2013;38(23):2028-2037.

This article describes the variables in the new AOSpine thoracolumbar injury classification system.

17. Savage JW, Moore TA, Arnold PM, et al: The reliability and validity of the thoracolumbar injury classification system in pediatric spine trauma. *Spine (Phila Pa 1976)* 2015;40(18):E1014-E1018.

A multisurgeon analysis evaluated the interobserver and intraobserver reliability of the thoracolumbar injury classification system when applied to pediatric spine trauma. Level of evidence: IV.

18. Sawyer JR, Beebe M, Creek AT, Yantis M, Kelly DM, Warner WC Jr: Age-related patterns of spine injury in children involved in all-terrain vehicle accidents. *J Pediatr Orthop* 2012;32(5):435-439.

In this retrospective database review of children who sustained spine injuries with all-terrain vehicle use, injuries also were associated with nonspine and noncontiguous spine injuries.

19. Vander Have KL, Caird MS, Gross S, et al: Burst fractures of the thoracic and lumbar spine in children and adolescents. *J Pediatr Orthop* 2009;29(7):713-719.

20. Arkader A, Warner WC Jr, Tolo VT, Sponseller PD, Skaggs DL: Pediatric Chance fractures: A multicenter perspective. *J Pediatr Orthop* 2011;31(7):741-744.

In a multicenter review of 35 patients younger than 18 years who had a Chance fracture, the fractures tended to be in the lumbar spine, frequently had associated neurologic deficit, and commonly required surgery. Level of evidence: III.

21. Higashino K, Sairyo K, Katoh S, Takao S, Kosaka H, Yasui N: Long-term outcomes of lumbar posterior apophyseal end-plate lesions in children and adolescents. *J Bone Joint Surg Am* 2012;94(11):e74.

The authors present a retrospective review of 24 patients (mean age, 14.5 years) treated for posterior apophyseal end plate lesions. At a mean follow-up of 13.8 years, outcomes were favorable for both the surgically and nonsurgically treated patients.

22. Chang CH, Lee ZL, Chen WJ, Tan CF, Chen LH: Clinical significance of ring apophysis fracture in adolescent lumbar disc herniation. *Spine (Phila Pa 1976)* 2008;33(16):1750-1754.

Section 8

Sports-Related Topics

SECTION EDITOR:

Jennifer M. Weiss, MD

Chapter 41

Ligamentous Knee Injuries

Cordelia W. Carter, MD   Melinda S. Sharkey, MD

Abstract

Sports-related injuries of the knee, including anterior cruciate ligament rupture and tibial spine fracture, have become increasingly common in skeletally immature patients. Mounting scientific evidence demonstrates that clinical and functional outcomes for patients with complete anterior cruciate ligament tears and displaced tibial spine fractures are generally better with acute surgery than with delayed or nonsurgical care. Careful preoperative evaluation of each patient's physiologic and skeletal maturity is necessary to determine the optimal surgical technique.

Keywords: anterior cruciate ligament (ACL) tear; knee ligament; pediatric sports; physeal injury; tibial eminence; tibial spine fracture

Introduction

Over the past 25 years, there has been a major shift in how children are coached and trained in youth sports programs. Currently, specialization in one sport is common from increasingly young ages. At the same time, young athletes are often asked to perform at increasingly higher levels. In parallel with this increase in intensity in youth sports, the incidence of sports-related injuries in the skeletally immature population has risen, with injury involving the anterior cruciate ligament (ACL) as one notable example.[1,2] This chapter reviews the clinical presentation, methods of evaluation, recommended treatments, functional outcomes, and common complications for young athletes who sustain injuries of the ACL and tibial spine.

ACL Injuries

Midsubstance ACL injuries were historically thought to be rare in the pediatric population; however, several recent studies have reported increasing rates of ACL injury and subsequent surgical ACL reconstruction for pediatric and adolescent patients.[2,3] A 2015 study reported that the nationwide increase in ACL injuries in children 10 to 14 years of age was 18.9% between the years 2007 and 2011; a concomitant increase in the rate of ACL reconstructions of 27.6% was reported for the years studied.[2] Proposed reasons for this increase include both enhanced awareness of the possibility of midsubstance ACL tears in the pediatric population and a true increase in the rate of ACL injuries as more children participate in sports in a systematic, specialized fashion.

Multiple risk factors for ACL injury in a pediatric athlete have been identified, including intrinsic anatomic factors such as increased posterior tibial slope,[4,5] increased quadriceps angle, and decreased width of the intercondylar notch.[6] Commonly identified mechanical and neuromuscular risk factors for ACL injury include reduced knee flexion angles, high quadriceps forces (increased quadriceps to hamstring strength ratio), and increased internal hip rotation and dynamic valgus landing postures.[7] A combination of these known risk factors has likely contributed to a higher incidence of ACL tears in young female athletes compared with their male peers. One recent study reported an adjusted relative risk for female athletes of 2.10, although the absolute number of ACL tears in young male athletes remains high.[8,9] Extrinsic risk factors that have been identified for ACL tears in the adolescent population include the level of competition and the sport played. Specifically, collegiate athletes have been shown to have higher rates of ACL tears than high school athletes.[8] In addition, athletes participating

Dr. Carter or an immediate family member serves as a board member, owner, officer, or committee member of the Pediatric Orthopaedic Society of North America and the American Academy of Orthopaedic Surgeons. Neither Dr. Sharkey nor any immediate family member has received anything of value from or has stock or stock options held in a commercial company or institution related directly or indirectly to the subject of this chapter.

in sports such as football, soccer, rugby, lacrosse, and basketball are at highest risk for ACL injury.[8,9]

Because ACL injuries are so common and devastating to a young athlete, various ACL injury prevention programs to screen at-risk athletes have been introduced and studied. In a recent systematic review of the literature on neuromuscular retraining intervention programs, the authors concluded that the Prevent Injury and Enhance Performance program, the Knee Injury Prevention Program, and the Sportsmetrics program each successfully reduced the rate of noncontact ACL injuries in adolescent female athletes. A range of 70 to 98 athletes needed to be trained to prevent one ACL injury.[7] A recently published cost-analysis of prevention and screening programs for ACL injuries in young athletes found that the introduction of neuromuscular prevention programs universally would be more cost-effective than screening for and training only at-risk athletes.[10]

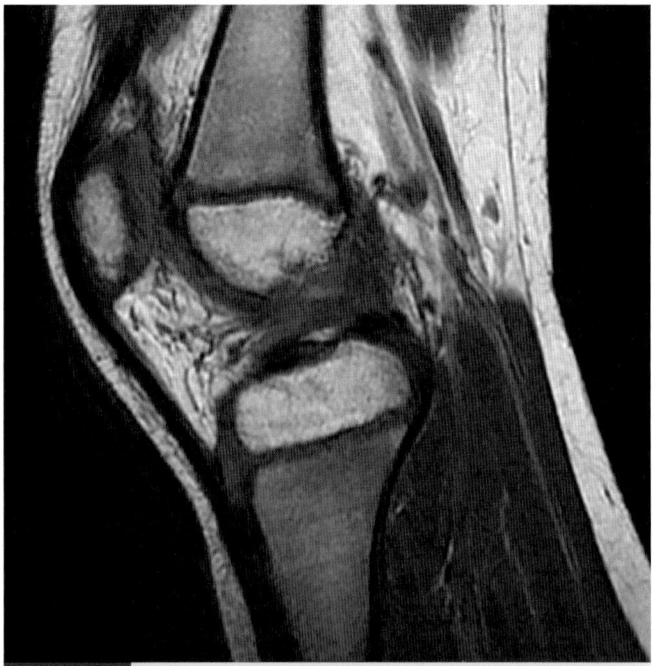

Figure 1 Sagittal T1-weighted MRI through the knee of a 9-year-old skeletally immature boy shows a complete midsubstance anterior cruciate ligament tear.

Evaluation

After a noncontact, twisting-type injury, young athletes with ACL tears frequently report the sudden onset of knee pain that is often accompanied by a popping sensation. Difficulty bearing weight and hemarthrosis are commonly present. The initial evaluation includes inspecting the soft tissues; performing passive motion of the ipsilateral hip, knee, and ankle; carefully palpating the entire affected limb; and assessing neurovascular status. Clinical tests for ACL deficiency include the Lachman, anterior drawer, and pivot shift tests. Because these tests may be difficult to perform and/or interpret in a young, anxious patient, results should be compared with similar tests performed on the contralateral, unaffected knee.

The presence of associated injuries of the menisci may be established by evaluating for tenderness of the joint line; decreased passive knee motion also may indicate a meniscal injury. Injuries of the collateral ligaments may be evaluated by varus and valgus stress testing of the knee performed at 0° and 30° of flexion. Specialized maneuvers such as the dial test and posterior drawer test also can be performed to evaluate other structures of the knee, including the posterolateral corner and posterior cruciate ligament. If ACL injury in a skeletally immature patient is suspected, limb alignment and lengths are assessed clinically. In addition, the patient's degree of physiologic maturity may be gauged by use of Tanner staging of sexual maturation.

Orthogonal radiographs of the affected knee should be obtained, with additional radiographs obtained as suggested by the physical examination findings. MRI of the knee is helpful for confirming an ACL tear (95% sensitivity and 88% specificity),[6] elucidating additional injuries, and assessing physeal patency (**Figure 1**). Before surgical treatment, a bone age study (for example, a PA radiograph of the left hand, which is then compared with the Greulich and Pyle atlas of normal standards) is generally done for skeletally immature patients to estimate the amount of remaining skeletal growth. Standing hip-to-ankle alignment radiographs may be obtained to evaluate for preexisting angular deformity or limb-length discrepancy of the lower limbs prior to surgical intervention.

Treatment

Partial tears of the ACL may occur in pediatric patients. The limited available data suggest that nonsurgical treatment may be successful in some patients with partial ACL tears.[11,12] In a prospective, cohort study of 45 skeletally immature patients with partial ACL tears, the authors reported that only one-third of the patients required surgical reconstruction for symptomatic instability. Tears involving more than 50% of the ACL fibers and predominantly the posterolateral bundle were more likely to require reconstruction. Similarly, nonsurgical treatment was more likely to be unsuccessful in patients older than 14 years and in those with objective signs of knee instability on clinical tests (such as the pivot shift test).[11]

Historically, full-thickness ACL tears in skeletally immature patients were treated with nonsurgical measures, including bracing, physical therapy, and activity modification until children reached skeletal maturity and a standard ACL reconstruction could be performed without risking injury to the physes. Although nonsurgical treatment should remain part of the discussion regarding the treatment of children with ACL injuries, there is mounting evidence that delayed surgical reconstruction is associated with worse outcomes in this population. A recent meta-analysis of studies examining nonsurgical versus surgical treatment of children and adolescents with ACL tears found that patients treated surgically had substantially less knee instability and pathologic laxity, substantially higher rates of return to activity, substantially lower rates of symptomatic posttreatment medial meniscus tears, and higher functional outcomes scores.[13]

Recent studies have attempted to clarify the relationship between delayed surgical reconstruction in this population and the presence of associated intra-articular injuries of cartilage and menisci.[14-17] One retrospective chart review evaluated 70 patients 14 years or younger who had undergone ACL reconstruction. The authors reported that increased time to surgery was independently associated with the presence of medial meniscal tears and chondral injuries of both medial and lateral compartments. In addition, patients who had undergone surgical stabilization more than 12 weeks after injury had substantially higher rates of severe or irreparable medial meniscal tears and lateral chondral injuries. Subjective knee instability was also associated with higher rates of meniscal tears in this study.[14] A second retrospective chart review of 370 pediatric patients who underwent ACL reconstruction found that patients treated more than 150 days after injury had substantially higher rates of medial meniscal tears than those treated sooner; when present, meniscal tears were significantly associated with chondral injury in the same compartment.[15] Two recent prospective cohort studies also examined this question. A substantial association was found between episodes of instability and the presence of medial meniscal tears and chondral injuries. Increased time to surgery also was associated with the increasing severity of concomitant injures.[16,17] Patients with ACL injury who undergo delayed reconstruction may have additional episodes of knee instability, especially if they return to sports and other physical activities; this in turn, puts them at risk for sustaining additional injuries of the meniscus and cartilage, which may be irreparable.

After the decision to proceed with surgical reconstruction of the ACL, the next step in the treatment algorithm is choosing an appropriate surgical technique. Traditional ACL reconstruction techniques involve the creation of tunnels in the distal femur and proximal tibia that would directly violate the open physes in a skeletally immature individual. Substantial work has been done to quantify the amount of physeal injury that reliably results in physeal arrest. Studies previously performed in animal models suggest that when less than 5% of the cross-sectional area of the physis is violated, growth arrest does not occur; however, when more than 7% to 9% of the physis is violated, growth disturbance—with resultant limb-length discrepancy and/or angular deformity—is possible. Growth disturbance also may result from placement of a bone block (for example, a bone-patellar tendon-bone graft) across an open physis and from peripheral physeal disruption, which is often attributed to overzealous dissection near the perichondrial ring of LaCroix and/or fixation devices placed in close proximity to the physes.[6,18]

Two studies have used computer modeling to generate three-dimensional MRI reconstructions of a skeletally immature knee and simulate transphyseal tunnels that would be made at the time of ACL reconstruction.[19,20] One study, using 8-mm tunnels and "optimal" trajectory angles for tunnel placement, determined that, in the 31 knees studied (patients age 10 to 15 years), 2.4% of the distal femoral physis and 2.5% of the proximal tibial physis were affected, on average, by tunnel drilling.[19] It was also determined that increasing the graft diameter by 1 mm resulted in an average 1.1% increase in the physeal volume affected. Changing the drill angle to achieve a more vertical tunnel had a much smaller effect, with a calculated decrease of 0.2% in the volume of injured physis for every 5° increase in the angle of the drill tunnel.

In a similar study performed in 2009, the volumetric injury produced by computer-generated creation of transphyseal tunnels in 10 children age 5 to 10 years was investigated.[20] The authors reported that drill holes measuring up to 9 mm in diameter resulted in an average physeal volume affected of less than 3.8% for the tibia and 5.4% for the femur, with the individual maximum percentage of volume removed remaining less than 9%, even with 9-mm drill holes placed across the physes of a 5-year-old child.

Physeal-Sparing ACL Reconstruction

Despite data supporting the use of transphyseal tunnels for ACL reconstruction in skeletally immature patients, physeal injury and subsequent growth disturbance remain important concerns. To address this issue, several physeal-sparing ACL reconstruction techniques have been developed. The two primary techniques are (1) the combined intra-articular and extra-articular extraphyseal technique in which no tunnels are drilled and fixation of the autograft iliotibial band (ITB) on both the femoral and tibial sides is achieved using sutures securing the graft

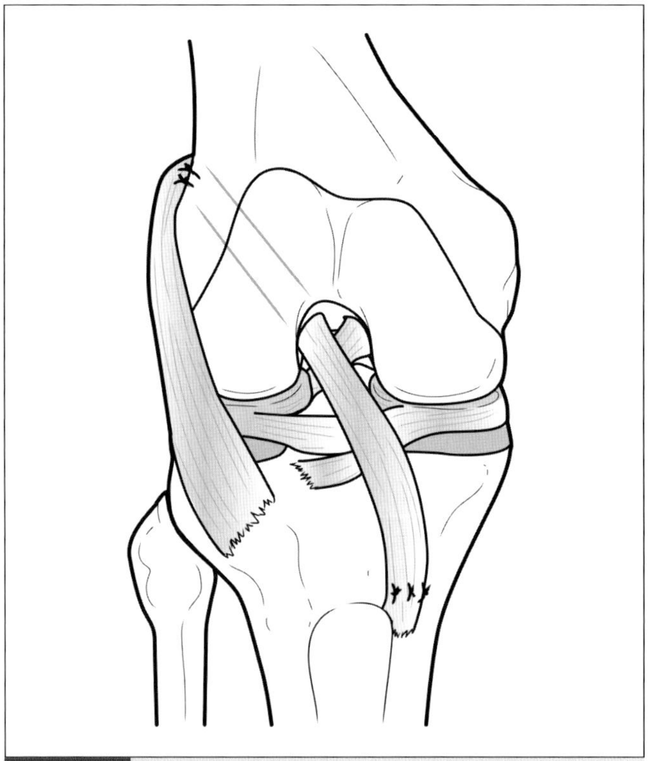

Figure 2 Illustration of a physeal-sparing anterior cruciate ligament reconstruction using iliotibial band autograft.

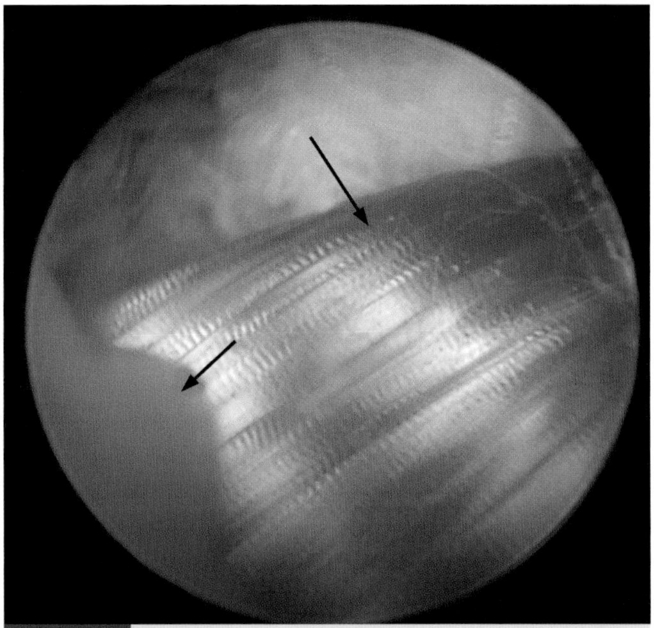

Figure 3 Arthroscopic image of the final intra-articular appearance of the anterior cruciate ligament in an 8-year-old girl after reconstruction using a physeal-sparing technique. Note the passage of the iliotibial band autograft (long arrow) anteriorly beneath the intermeniscal ligament (short arrow).

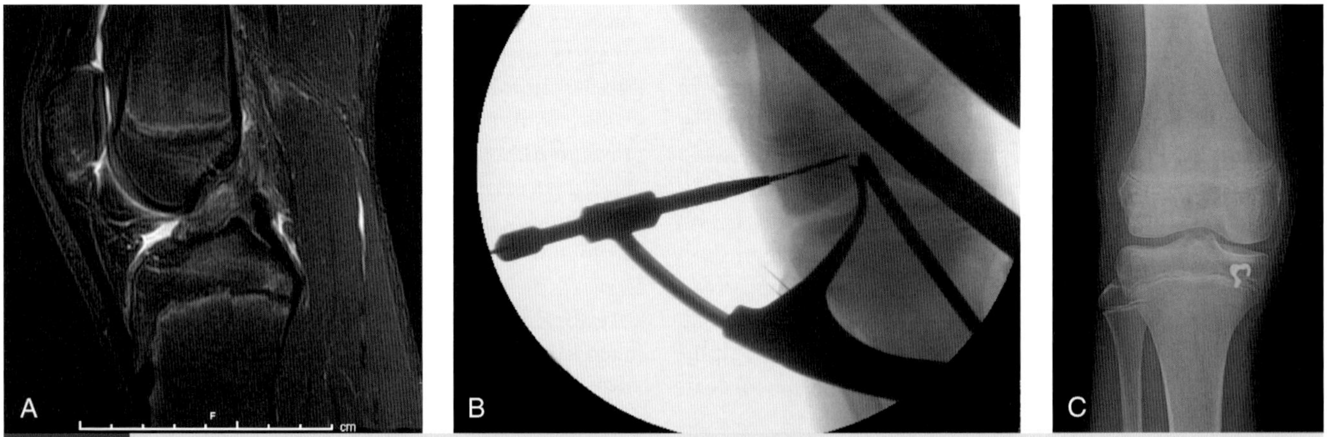

Figure 4 Images from a 12-year-old boy with an anterior cruciate ligament (ACL) injury and substantial remaining growth. **A,** Preoperative sagittal T2-weighted MRI through the knee shows a midsubstance ACL tear. **B,** Intraoperative image shows the drilling of an all-epiphyseal femoral tunnel. **C,** Postoperative AP radiograph shows the all-epiphyseal femoral and tibial tunnels.

to the periosteum[21,22] (**Figures 2** and **3**); and (2) the ACL reconstruction techniques in which tunnels are drilled in an all-epiphyseal fashion.[23] A variety of fixation methods for all-epiphyseal ACL reconstruction techniques exist, including suspensory fixation, epiphyseal interference screws, and/or a metaphyseal post[6] (**Figure 4**).

Recently, one group of authors evaluated the risk of MRI-documented physeal injury after ACL reconstruction using an all-epiphyseal technique performed in 15 skeletally immature patients.[24] The authors reported that, on average, 2.1% of the total tibial physeal area was compromised using this technique; however, no femoral

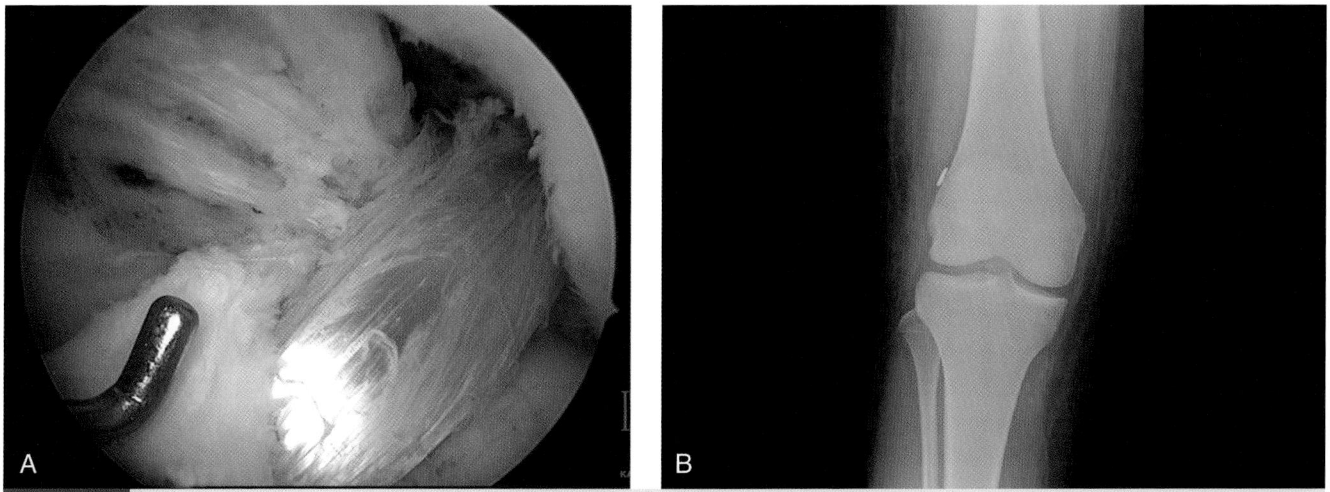

Figure 5 **A,** Arthroscopic image of the intra-articular appearance of the newly reconstructed anterior cruciate ligament (ACL) in a 14-year-old girl approaching skeletal maturity. ACL reconstruction was performed using a transphyseal technique. **B,** Postoperative AP radiograph shows placement of the transphyseal tunnel.

physeal disturbance was noted. At an average follow-up of 18 months after surgery, there were no cases of growth arrest or resultant limb deformity.

Considerable attention has been paid to evaluating the biomechanics of nontraditional ACL reconstruction techniques.[25-27] A 2011 study evaluated six adult cadaver knees in the intact state after ACL disruption and after ACL reconstruction using all-epiphyseal and ITB physeal-sparing techniques, and a hybrid method involving the creation of a transtibial tunnel coupled with an over-the-top (physeal-sparing) femoral technique. The authors reported that all three reconstruction techniques improved knee stability; the ITB method best restored both translational and rotational control, although it overconstrained the knee to rotational forces at some flexion angles.[25] In a follow-up study investigating pivot-shift kinematics, all three techniques improved knee stability. The ITB technique allowed for less translation and rotation than the normal ACL–intact state, and the all-epiphyseal technique was reported to achieve the best restoration of normal knee kinematics.[26]

Outcomes for patients undergoing physeal-sparing ACL reconstruction are generally good.[21,23,28,29] In a study in which the ITB physeal-sparing ACL reconstruction technique was used to treat 44 skeletally immature prepubescent patients (average age, 10.3 years), clinical (Lachman and pivot shift tests) and functional (International Knee Documentation Committee and Lysholm scores) outcome measures at the 5-year follow-up showed good results; only 2 patients required revision surgery. A clinically important growth disturbance did not develop in any of the patients, despite average patient growth of 21.5 cm.[21] A recent case series reported on 21 male patients (average age, 11.8 years) followed for 3 years after ACL reconstruction using the ITB technique. Similarly good results were reported. The authors reported a 14% rate of revision ACL surgery; for the patients not requiring revision, the clinical and functional outcomes were excellent, and no growth disturbances were detected.[28]

Reported outcomes in two studies of all-epiphyseal ACL reconstruction were generally good, although the number of patients studied in each series was small.[23,29] Patients undergoing all-epiphyseal ACL reconstruction usually have stable knees, high functional outcomes scores, no reported growth disturbance, and are able to return to sports activities after the surgical reconstruction.

Transphyseal ACL Reconstruction

Transphyseal ACL reconstruction is commonly performed in patients with a modest amount of growth remaining (**Figure 5**). Variations in transphyseal techniques have been described in the literature. In one hybrid technique, patients deemed at risk for growth disturbance from a transphyseal tunnel created in the femur undergo a physeal-sparing technique on the femoral side, with transphyseal tunnel drilling on the tibial side. (The distal femur is the fastest-growing physis in the body, and tunnel drilling for ACL reconstruction potentially affects the more vulnerable periphery of this physis.) This type of hybrid method is typically referred to as a partial transphyseal technique. In addition, physeal-respecting techniques may be used in children with modest amounts of remaining growth to minimize injury to the physis during a transphyseal ACL reconstruction. Physeal-respecting techniques can include the use of soft-tissue grafts and metaphyseal fixation, avoidance of dissection near the

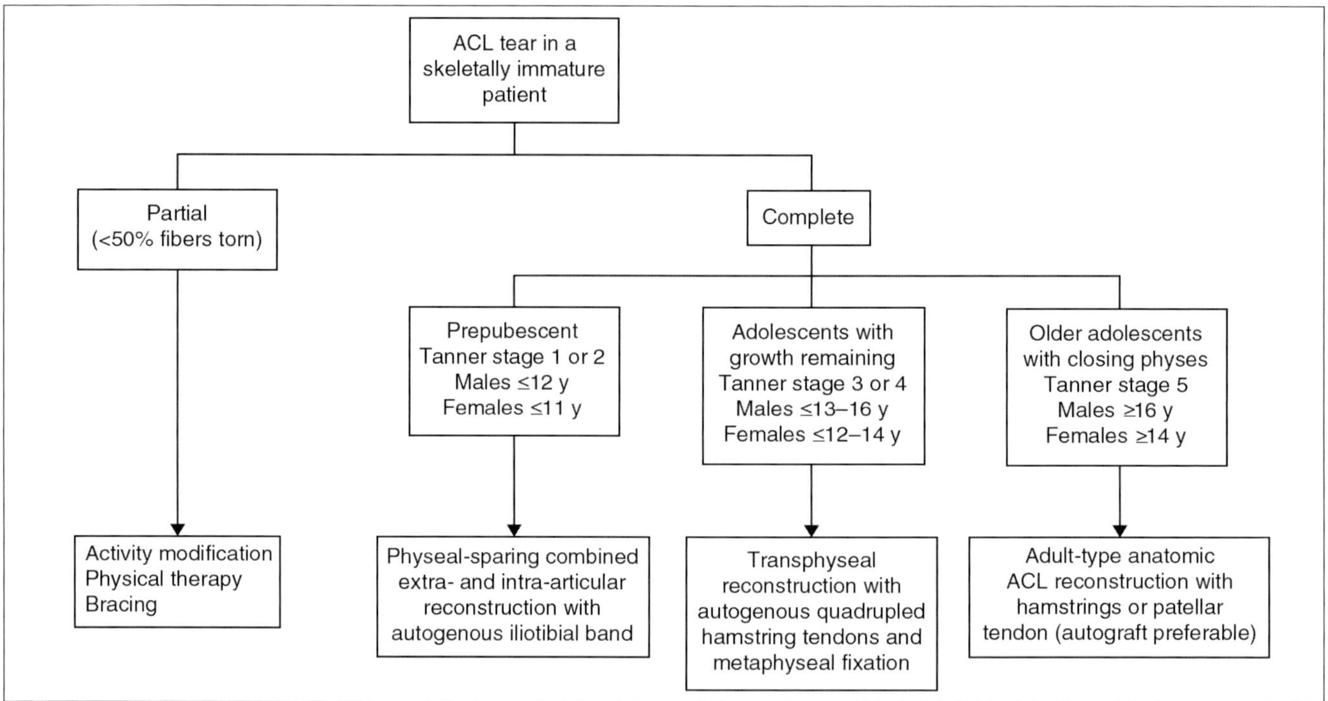

Figure 6 A treatment algorithm for the surgical management of complete anterior cruciate ligament (ACL) injuries in skeletally immature patients. (Reproduced from Frank JS, Gambacorta PL: ACL injuries in the skeletally immature athlete: Diagnosis and management. *J Am Acad Orthop Surg* 2013;21(2):78-87.)

perichondrial ring of LaCroix, optimization of tunnel size (as previously discussed, larger tunnels are associated with greater amounts of physeal disturbance), and the use of vertical tunnels. An algorithm for the surgical treatment of ACL injuries in skeletally immature patients is presented in **Figure 6**.

In terms of graft choice for ACL reconstruction, soft-tissue grafts such as quadrupled hamstring tendons are generally used in skeletally immature patients to minimize the risk of iatrogenic growth disturbance that accompanies placement of a bone plug across an open physis. In addition, data support the routine use of autograft tissue in this population. A recent case-control study of 73 pediatric patients (average age, 15 years) undergoing ACL reconstruction with either autograft or allograft tendon reported a more than fourfold greater risk of revision surgery for patients treated with allograft tendon.[30]

Outcomes of patients treated with transphyseal ACL reconstruction are generally good.[31-34] At an average follow-up of 3.6 years, a low rate of revision (3%), high functional outcomes scores, and no clinically detectable growth disturbance were reported in 59 patients (average age, 14.7 years) who had undergone transphyseal ACL reconstruction with soft-tissue autograft and metaphyseal fixation.[31] A 2013 study reported on the outcomes of 32 skeletally immature patients (average age, 11.3 years) treated with ACL reconstruction using a variation of the transphyseal technique in which the tibial and femoral tunnels were drilled comparatively vertical and a hamstring allograft was used for the reconstruction.[32] Fixation was kept far from the physes (screw and washer on the tibial side and an Endobutton [Smith & Nephew] on the femoral side). At a follow-up of 6 years, the functional outcomes measures of all of the patients had improved; one rerupture had occurred; and no limb-length discrepancy was noted, although valgus deformity occurred in one patient. A 2015 study described the outcomes of 27 skeletally immature patients (average age, 13 years) who had undergone transphyseal ACL reconstruction.[33] The authors reported that, at an average follow-up of 10.6 years, the patients had substantially improved functional outcomes scores and no detectable growth arrest; graft rerupture was reported in 3 of 27 patients (11%).

Postoperative Care, Rehabilitation, and Return to Play

No standardized guidelines exist for postoperative care, rehabilitation, and return to play for skeletally immature patients undergoing ACL reconstruction. As a result, recommendations vary based on the preference of the surgeon, patient factors, the reconstruction technique, the graft choice, and the need for associated procedures (such as meniscal repair). Despite considerable variability in postoperative regimens, the initiation of formal physical therapy usually occurs within the first several weeks after ACL reconstruction. Early goals include recovery of range of motion (ROM), particularly the achievement of terminal knee extension and patellar mobility, and isometric strengthening. Athletes are gradually advanced in weight bearing, ROM, strengthening, and endurance; sport-specific skills are introduced in a supervised setting after more basic skills have been mastered.

Numerous factors may contribute to the decision to allow an athlete to return to play, including recovery of quadriceps strength (as measured by muscle girth). Perhaps the most important indicator is the patient's ability to demonstrate functional readiness, which is typically assessed by performance on various testing measures (for example, the single-leg hop, triple-hop distance, crossover hop, and step-down tests). Although patients were traditionally cleared for return to play after a "safe" amount of time had elapsed (generally 6 to 9 months), a recent study found that even 9 months after ACL reconstruction, many adolescent patients do not demonstrate adequate functional movement patterns to allow safe return to sport.[35] It has been suggested that "maturity-specific" rehabilitation strategies may be needed to optimally prepare young athletes for return to play.

Complications

The most common complications occurring after ACL reconstruction in skeletally immature patients include secondary injury of the same or the contralateral knee requiring surgical intervention, arthrofibrosis, and growth disturbance. In a recent cohort study, the incidence of second ACL injury in young athletes (average age, 17 years) within 2 years of the index surgery was reported.[36] The authors found that the overall incidence of a second injury in this population of young patients who had returned to sports was more than five times greater than that of healthy control athletes. Nearly 30% of athletes sustained a second ACL injury within 24 months of return to sports, with approximately one-third of the injuries occurring in the ipsilateral knee and two-thirds in the contralateral knee. A 2014 case-control study found that patients younger than 20 years at the time of ACL reconstruction had a 29% chance of sustaining a second ACL injury (either knee) within 5 years of the index surgery; a return to cutting and pivoting sports increased the odds of injury.[37] A recent systematic review and meta-analysis of the existing literature confirmed that younger patients returning to high-level sporting activities were at greatest risk for subsequent knee injury.[38] The authors found that athletes younger than 25 years who return to sports had a secondary rate of ACL injury (ipsilateral or contralateral knee) of 23%.

Arthrofibrosis is a well-described complication after adult ACL reconstruction and has been shown to occur in children and adolescents. One recent retrospective case series described a single institution's experience with 902 young patients treated with ACL reconstruction.[39] An overall incidence of arthrofibrosis of 8.3% was reported in this population (average age, 15 years), with female sex, older age, the use of bone-patellar tendon-bone autograft, and concomitant meniscal repair being additional risk factors for arthrofibrosis.

Growth arrest sometimes occurs after ACL reconstruction in skeletally immature patients despite efforts to avoid this complication. One recent case series reported on four patients (average age, 14.2 years) in whom clinically important growth disturbances, including tibial recurvatum and genu valgum, developed after transphyseal ACL reconstruction using physeal-respecting techniques (for example, soft-tissue autograft, metaphyseal fixation on the femur).[40] Another group of researchers retrospectively reviewed the postoperative MRIs of 43 patients (average age, 14.8 years) who had undergone transphyseal ACL reconstruction using soft-tissue graft.[41] The authors found that the average bone tunnel to growth plate cross-sectional area ratios were 2.6% for the proximal tibia and 2.3% for the distal femur. Despite this, focal physeal bone bridges were noted in five knees, although no patient had resultant limb deformity.

Tibial Spine Fractures

Avulsion fractures of the tibial spine, also known as tibial eminence fractures, are uncommon injuries, with an annual incidence previously estimated to be 3 per 100,000 children and adolescents.[42] This injury is often referred to as the childhood equivalent of an ACL injury, with failure occurring through the bone-ligament interface rather than through the substance of the ligament itself. As tensile forces are initially applied to the knee, the ACL stretches, with resultant permanent plastic deformation of the ligament. Increased tensile load ultimately leads to failure of the incompletely ossified tibial plateau at the insertion of the ACL, resulting in a tibial spine avulsion fracture.[43]

Skeletally immature patients presenting with this injury are typically aged 8 to 14 years and commonly report a sports-related injury mechanism. Pedestrians struck by motor vehicles and bicyclists who sustain a fall also may have tibial spine fractures.[44]

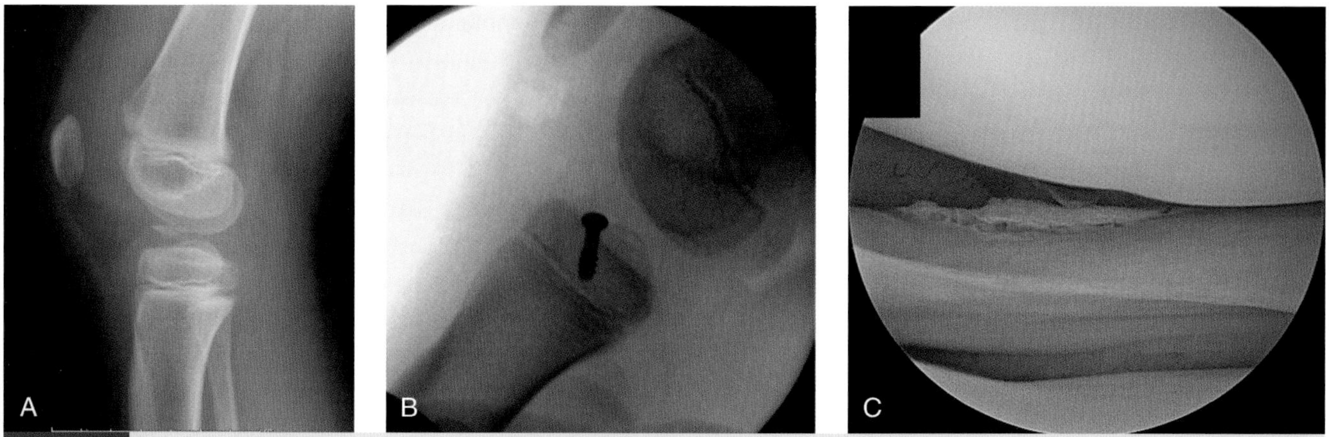

Figure 7 **A,** Preoperative lateral radiograph of the knee of a 7-year-old girl shows a type III tibial spine fracture. **B,** Intraoperative lateral fluoroscopic image of the knee of the patient in part A after arthroscopically assisted reduction and fixation using a cannulated, all-epiphyseal screw. **C,** Arthroscopic image shows a concomitant vertical tear of the posterior horn of the lateral meniscus.

Evaluation

Patients with tibial spine fractures report the acute onset of knee pain, which is often accompanied by swelling, decreased motion, and the inability to ambulate. The physical examination and the initial radiographic assessment are similar to those previously described for ACL tears.

The modified Myers and McKeever classification system is most commonly used to describe tibial spine fractures. Type I fractures are minimally displaced; type II are displaced anteriorly with an intact posterior bony hinge; type III fractures are completely displaced from the fracture bed (**Figure 7**); and type IV fractures are displaced and comminuted.[44]

Additional imaging studies such as CT and MRI may be useful for identifying associated intra-articular injuries of the meniscus and chondral surface that commonly occur in the setting of a tibial spine fracture. One recent retrospective evaluation of 20 patients with tibial eminence fractures who underwent preoperative MRI evaluation revealed that 90% of the patients had bone contusions similar to those seen in patients with midsubstance ACL tears; meniscal tears were present in 40% of these patients.[45]

Although a 2003 study demonstrated a 3.8% rate of associated meniscal tears,[46] more recent studies have shown the rate of concomitant intra-articular pathology to be as high as 30%.[42,47] In a retrospective review of 58 patients with anterior tibial spine fractures, the authors reported meniscal tears in 33% of the patients with type II fractures and 12% of those with type III fractures.[47] When present, meniscal tears most commonly affected the anterior horn of the medial meniscus and the posterior horn of the lateral meniscus (**Figure 7, C**). Chondral injury was identified in 7% of the patients.

Advanced imaging studies such as MRI may be useful for identifying potential blocks to fracture reduction. The anterior horn of the medial meniscus and the intermeniscal ligament are the two structures most frequently interposed in the fracture bed[46-48] (**Figure 8**). Soft-tissue impediments to fracture reduction are extremely common in the setting of displaced tibial spine fractures, with one study reporting a rate of soft-tissue entrapment to be as high as 65% for type III fractures.[46] A 2015 study reported a similarly high rate of meniscal entrapment, with 48% of the patients with type III fractures having entrapment of the meniscus within the fracture bed.[47]

Treatment

Patients with type I fractures are routinely treated with immobilization in a long leg cast. The position of the knee remains a subject of debate, with arguments made for placing the knee in either full extension (this theoretically allows the lateral femoral condyle to physically maintain fracture reduction) or in slight flexion (theoretically preventing elongation of the ACL during terminal extension).[49]

Closed reduction followed by radiographic confirmation of adequate alignment is the chosen treatment for most patients with type II fractures. One recent study suggested that less than 5 mm of displacement may be acceptable, with greater initial displacement correlating with a high rate of subsequent surgery to address late instability and impingement resulting from fracture malunion.[50] Type II fractures in which acceptable reduction cannot be achieved by closed means and fractures that are completely displaced (types III and IV) are candidates for surgical treatment.

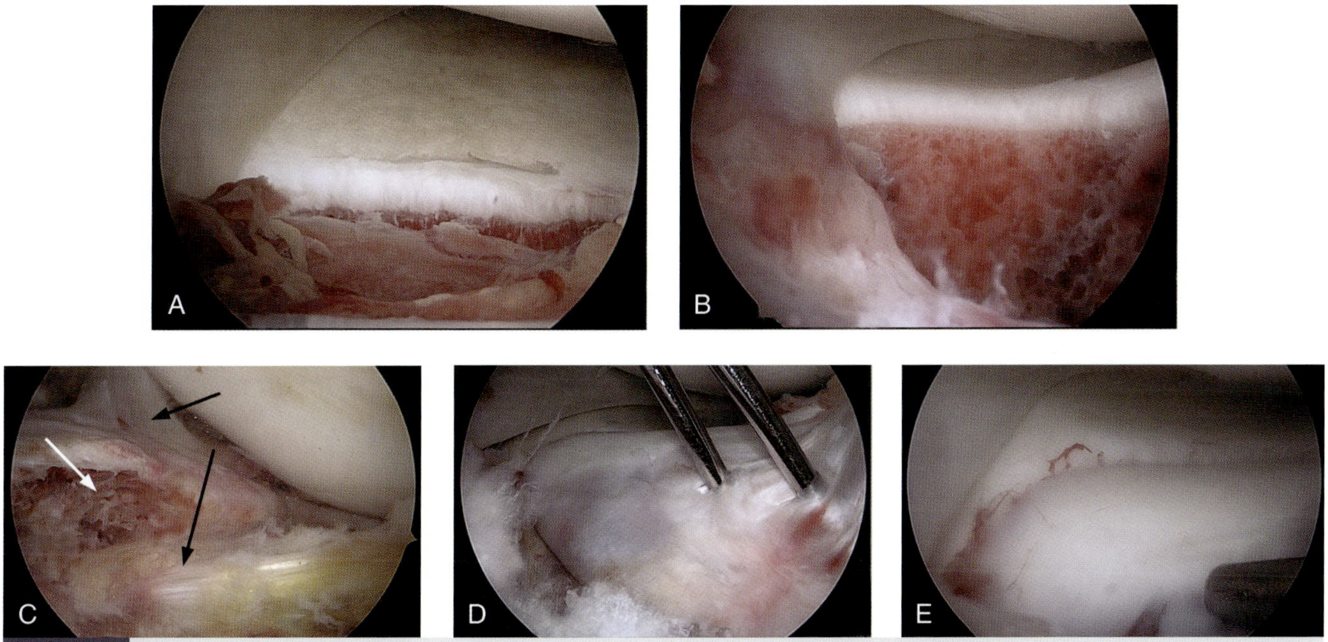

Figure 8 Arthroscopic images of the knee of a 13-year-old boy with a type III tibial spine fracture. **A,** Entrapment of the anterior horn of the medial meniscus in the fracture site. **B,** The fracture after removal of the entrapped meniscus. **C,** Residual interposition of the intermeniscal ligament (long black arrow) within the fracture bed (white arrow). The short black arrow points to the anterior cruciate ligament. **D,** The fracture after reduction and provisional fixation with Kirschner wires. **E,** Final alignment of the fracture after cannulated screw fixation.

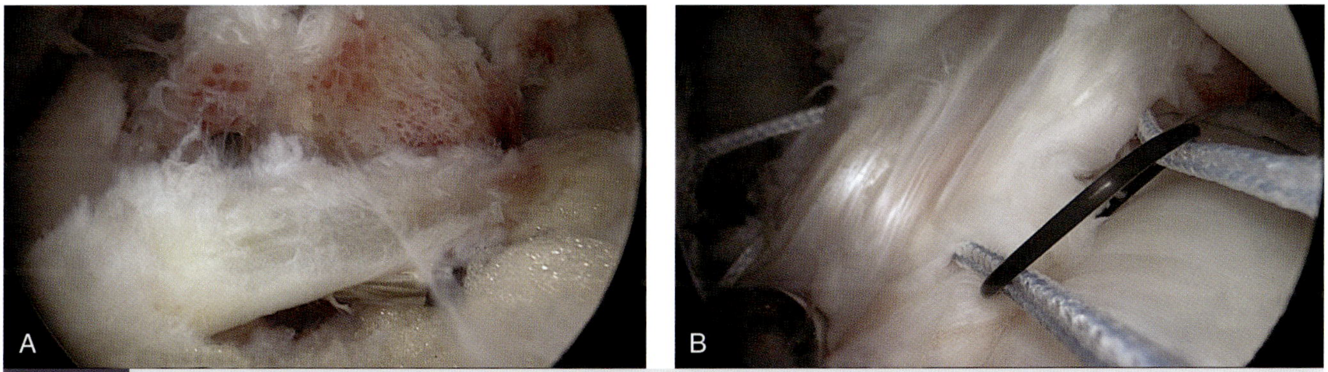

Figure 9 Arthroscopic images of a 13-year-old girl with a type IV tibial spine fracture treated with arthroscopically assisted reduction and suture fixation. **A,** The displaced fracture fragment, with the interposed intermeniscal ligament. **B,** Preparation for suture shuttling after fracture reduction.

Surgical treatment of displaced tibial spine fractures has traditionally consisted of open reduction and internal fixation via arthrotomy, although arthroscopically assisted reduction and internal fixation procedures have become increasingly commonplace. Concomitant intra-articular pathology, including meniscal tears and chondral injuries, is treated at the time of the index procedure. After surgical reduction and stabilization, patients are generally immobilized in a long leg cast or a hinged knee brace for a short period of time before knee range-of-motion exercises are begun.

Many methods of fixation have been described, with the two most common being (1) screw fixation, which typically involves the use of a self-tapping cannulated screw placed across the fracture fragments in an all-epiphyseal fashion, and (2) suture fixation, in which sutures are placed through the substance of the ACL, shuttled through small tunnels in the tibia, and tied over a bony bridge on the anterior tibial cortex[43] (**Figure 9**). A proposed advantage of screw fixation is the relative ease of the technique. Advantages of suture fixation include avoiding the possibility of subsequent hardware removal and the ability to fix comminuted fractures. Numerous variations of these techniques have been described, including the use of both absorbable and nonabsorbable suture materials, suture anchors, bioabsorbable implants (including nails and screws), and suture buttons.

Several attempts have been made to elucidate a difference in patient outcomes based on the surgical technique used. Two retrospective patient chart reviews have recently been published, each describing the authors' institutional experience in managing displaced tibial spine fractures.[50,51] In one study, the authors reviewed the charts of 31 patients, 13 of whom had been treated with open reduction and internal fixation and 18 of whom had undergone arthroscopically assisted reduction and internal fixation.[51] Patient sex, age, fracture type, fixation method (both screw and suture constructs were used), and length of postoperative immobilization were similar between the groups. The authors found that postoperative arthrofibrosis was more likely to develop in patients who waited longer for their surgery (>7-day delay from injury to surgery) and those who had longer surgical times (>120 minutes). They concluded that the method of surgery used should be the method that could be performed with the most efficiency.

The authors of a 2015 study reported on their institution's experience managing displaced tibial spine fractures using closed, open, and arthroscopic techniques.[50] In their review of 76 patients, it was found that open and arthroscopic methods of treatment achieved a similar amount of fracture reduction and comparable rates of complications, including arthrofibrosis (11% in the group treated with open reduction and internal fixation and 12.5% in the arthroscopic group). In addition, no substantial difference in functional outcomes as assessed by Lysholm scores was found between the two surgical groups. Although the closed management (casting) group had approximately 50% less initial displacement of the fracture than the surgically treated group, this group had higher rates of revision for symptomatic loose bodies, instability, and impingement. Because of this, the authors concluded that surgical management should be considered for tibial spine fractures with displacement greater than 5 mm. The study authors also suggest that surgeon comfort with the procedure should guide the choice between open and arthroscopic surgical techniques.

A recent systematic review of the literature regarding the treatment of tibial eminence fractures reported that the available level of evidence to support clinical decision-making in this setting is quite low (all studies were level III or IV).[52] The authors concluded that neither an open nor an arthroscopic method of fixation was demonstrated to be superior. They similarly noted that neither a screw nor a suture fixation technique demonstrated a clear superiority over the other, with appreciable healing noted in patients treated with each method. The need for higher-quality research in this area was recognized.

Mixed results have been reported from biomechanical studies performed to determine the optimal fixation techniques for patients with displaced tibial spine fractures. A 2007 study reported on 64 skeletally immature porcine knees in which tibial eminence fractures were created and then fixed with one screw, two screws, or nonabsorbable sutures.[53] In the laboratory, the construct using a commercially available ultra-high–molecular-weight polyethylene (UHMWPE) suture provided more fixation strength than a screw. It also was noted that the addition of a second screw did not enhance the construct strength. A 2005 study that used human cadaver knees reported similar findings, with UHMWPE suture fixation achieving greater ultimate strength than screw fixation.[54] However, the authors of a 2008 biomechanical study using immature bovine knees found no significant mechanical difference when comparing four methods of tibial spine fracture fixation (nonabsorbable suture, three bioabsorbable nails, one resorbable screw, and one metal screw).[55] The authors noted that the specimens repaired with a single metal screw demonstrated the greatest initial stiffness and failure force and the least amount of deformation. The suture and resorbable screw constructs demonstrated the highest levels of deformation at the fracture site during cyclic loading conditions.

Although suture and screw constructs have traditionally been used for fixation of tibial spine fractures, many other fixation methods exist. This heterogeneity is likely due, at least in part, to the fact that no single fixation method has been proved superior. Another recent cadaver biomechanical study compared four different methods of physeal-sparing fixation: (1) UHMWPE suture plus suture button, (2) suture anchors, (3) polydioxanone suture plus suture button, and (4) screw fixation.[56] After performing both load-to-failure and cyclic testing of the specimens in each group, the authors concluded that the UHMWPE suture plus button construct was biomechanically superior at the time of surgery. In addition, the suture anchor construct demonstrated the most variability in its ability to supply stable fixation for these fractures.

Complications

Residual laxity of the knee may be noted after treatment of a tibial spine fracture and usually is the result of plastic deformation of the ACL occurring at the time of initial injury. Although ACL laxity may be demonstrated objectively, clinical knee instability is rarely present after fracture fixation.[44] Common complications reported after treatment of tibial spine fractures include fracture malunion, fracture nonunion, hardware prominence, loss of fixation, and knee stiffness.

Arthrofibrosis is a well-documented complication of the surgical treatment of pediatric tibial spine fractures. In a study of 205 pediatric patients treated surgically for a displaced tibial spine fracture, arthrofibrosis (defined as 10° extension loss and/or less than 90° flexion at 3 months postoperatively) developed in 20 patients (10%).[57] The average time to surgery for these patients was 8.1 days, and postoperative immobilization was generally 4 to 6 weeks. The patients were treated with a second surgical procedure, which usually involved a combination of arthroscopic lysis of adhesions followed by manipulation under anesthesia. Of eight patients treated with manipulation under anesthesia alone, three sustained an intraoperative distal femoral physeal fracture. Isolated manipulation under anesthesia for postoperative arthrofibrosis in the skeletally immature knee, if performed, should be undertaken with extreme caution because of the documented risk of physeal injury.

In a 2012 study, the results of a retrospective chart review were reported for 40 patients treated surgically for a displaced tibial spine fracture. Arthrofibrosis developed in 7 of the 40 patients (17.5%), necessitating a second surgery.[58] Interestingly, the authors found that patients who had begun ROM therapy within 4 weeks of surgery had substantially faster return to full activity and were less likely to experience the development of arthrofibrosis than patients for whom ROM rehabilitation was initiated after 4 weeks. The goal of surgical treatment of these injuries is to achieve adequate fracture reduction in a timely fashion, with secure fracture fixation that will allow for early postoperative mobilization.

Summary

Sport-related injuries of the knee such as ACL rupture and tibial spine fracture have become increasingly common in skeletally immature patients. Clinical and functional outcomes for patients with complete ACL tears and displaced tibial spine fractures are generally better with early surgery than with delayed or nonsurgical care. Careful preoperative evaluation of the physes in these patients is important for determining the optimal surgical technique. Knowledge of potential complications after surgical treatment of these injuries (including physeal arrest) is crucial so that complications can be recognized and addressed in a timely manner.

Key Study Points

- Various physeal-sparing and physeal-respecting ACL reconstruction techniques have been developed for the skeletally immature knee.
- Growth disturbances related to physeal injury have been reported in a small number of skeletally immature patients after ACL reconstruction.
- Arthrofibrosis can commonly result after surgical fixation of tibial spine fractures, so secure fixation and early mobilization is paramount.

Annotated References

1. Carter CW, Micheli LJ: Training the child athlete for prevention, health promotion, and performance: How much is enough, how much is too much? *Clin Sports Med* 2011;30(4):679-690.

   The authors of this article review the existing literature on training young athletes, including the potential health benefits of physical activity and sport participation, as well as the potential negative consequences of overtraining such as injury and burnout.

2. Werner BC, Yang S, Looney AM, Gwathmey FW Jr: Trends in pediatric and adolescent anterior cruciate ligament injury and reconstruction. *J Pediatr Orthop* 2015.

   The authors of this retrospective cohort study evaluated the rates of ACL injury, ACL reconstruction, and associated surgical procedures in the pediatric population from 2007 to 2011 and found substantial increases in each rate compared with adult rates during the same period. Level of evidence: III.

3. Dodwell ER, Lamont LE, Green DW, Pan TJ, Marx RG, Lyman S: 20 years of pediatric anterior cruciate ligament reconstruction in New York State. *Am J Sports Med* 2014;42(3):675-680.

   The authors of this descriptive epidemiologic study used a New York State database to determine how the rates of pediatric ACL reconstruction had changed over a 20-year period ending in 2009. A steady rise in ACL reconstruction to 51 per 100,000 individuals aged 3 to 20 years was reported.

4. O'Malley MP, Milewski MD, Solomito MJ, Erwteman AS, Nissen CW: The association of tibial slope and anterior cruciate ligament rupture in skeletally immature patients. *Arthroscopy* 2015;31(1):77-82.

   The authors of this retrospective case-control study measured tibial slope using radiographs in 64 skeletally immature patients, 32 of whom had ACL deficiency. Increased posterior tibial slope was significantly associated with ACL injury in both males and females. Level of evidence: III.

5. Dare DM, Fabricant PD, McCarthy MM, et al: Increased lateral tibial slope is a risk factor for pediatric anterior cruciate ligament injury. *Am J Sports Med* 2015;43(7):1632-1639.

The authors of this case-control study measured lateral tibial slope using MRI in 152 skeletally immature patients, 76 of whom had ACL deficiency. Increased lateral tibial slope was significantly associated with ACL injury in both males and females. Level of evidence: III.

6. Fabricant PD, Jones KJ, Delos D, et al: Reconstruction of the anterior cruciate ligament in the skeletally immature athlete: A review of current concepts. AAOS exhibit selection. *J Bone Joint Surg Am* 2013;95(5):e28.

The authors of this current concepts review describe the clinical presentation, methods of evaluation, treatment options, surgical techniques, and functional outcomes for skeletally immature patients with an ACL tear.

7. Noyes FR, Barber-Westin SD: Neuromuscular retraining intervention programs: Do they reduce noncontact anterior cruciate ligament injury rates in adolescent female athletes? *Arthroscopy* 2014;30(2):245-255.

The authors of this systematic review of the existing literature regarding ACL prevention programs reported that three programs (Sportsmetrics, Prevent Injury and Enhance Performance, and Knee Injury Prevention) successfully reduced noncontact ACL injuries in female adolescent athletes. Level of evidence: II.

8. Beynnon BD, Vacek PM, Newell MK, et al: The effects of level of competition, sport, and sex on the incidence of first-time noncontact anterior cruciate ligament injury. *Am J Sports Med* 2014;42(8):1806-1812.

The authors of this cohort study of ACL injury in high school and college athletes reported that higher level of competition, female sex, and participation in certain sports (such as soccer) are risk factors for ACL injury. Level of evidence: II.

9. Gornitzky AL, Lott A, Yellin JL, Fabricant PD, Lawrence JT, Ganley TJ: Sport-specific yearly risk and incidence of anterior cruciate ligament tears in high school athletes. *Am J Sports Med* 2015; Dec 11 [Epub ahead of print].

The authors of this meta-analysis of the literature regarding ACL injury in high-school athletes concluded that females had a 1.57-fold greater rate of injury than males; female soccer players and male football players were at highest risk for ACL injury.

10. Swart E, Redler L, Fabricant PD, Mandelbaum BR, Ahmad CS, Wang YC: Prevention and screening programs for anterior cruciate ligament injuries in young athletes: A cost-effectiveness analysis. *J Bone Joint Surg Am* 2014;96(9):705-711.

A decision-analysis model was created to evaluate the cost-effectiveness of ACL injury prevention programs in young athletes. The authors found that universal training was the most cost-effective method compared with no screening and training or universal screening with training only for high-risk athletes.

11. Kocher MS, Micheli LJ, Zurakowski D, Luke A: Partial tears of the anterior cruciate ligament in children and adolescents. *Am J Sports Med* 2002;30(5):697-703.

12. Busch MT, Fernandez MD, Aarons C: Partial tears of the anterior cruciate ligament in children and adolescents. *Clin Sports Med* 2011;30(4):743-750.

The authors of this article review the clinical presentation, evaluation, treatment options, and existing literature for skeletally immature patients with a partial ACL tear.

13. Ramski DE, Kanj WW, Franklin CC, Baldwin KD, Ganley TJ: Anterior cruciate ligament tears in children and adolescents: A meta-analysis of nonoperative versus operative treatment. *Am J Sports Med* 2014;42(11):2769-2776.

This meta-analysis reported that pediatric patients with ACL injury treated with early stabilization have less instability and higher return-to-sport rates. The authors concluded that early surgical stabilization is favored over delayed or nonsurgical treatment, although the quality of the existing literature is low.

14. Lawrence JT, Argawal N, Ganley TJ: Degeneration of the knee joint in skeletally immature patients with a diagnosis of an anterior cruciate ligament tear: Is there harm in delay of treatment? *Am J Sports Med* 2011;39(12):2582-2587.

Seventy pediatric patients who had undergone ACL reconstruction were divided into two groups (based on surgical timing) and evaluated for associated injuries. Increased time to ACL reconstruction was associated with medial meniscal tears and chondral injuries as well as increased injury severity. Level of evidence: III.

15. Dumont GD, Hogue GD, Padalecki JR, Okoro N, Wilson PL: Meniscal and chondral injuries associated with pediatric anterior cruciate ligament tears: Relationship of treatment time and patient-specific factors. *Am J Sports Med* 2012;40(9):2128-2133.

In this retrospective chart review of 370 pediatric patients who had undergone ACL reconstruction, the patients were divided into two groups based on surgical timing. Patients with delayed surgery had more medial meniscus tears; chondral injuries were associated with same-compartment meniscal injuries. Level of evidence: III.

16. Anderson AF, Anderson CN: Correlation of meniscal and articular cartilage injuries in children and adolescents with timing of anterior cruciate ligament reconstruction. *Am J Sports Med* 2015;43(2):275-281.

In this cohort study, 130 pediatric patients were divided into three groups based on the timing of ACL reconstruction. Patients with delayed reconstruction had more chondral injuries, which were more severe. The severity of meniscal tears also correlated with surgical delay. Level of evidence: III.

17. Newman JT, Carry PM, Terhune EB, et al: Factors predictive of concomitant injuries among children and adolescents undergoing anterior cruciate ligament surgery. *Am J Sports Med* 2015;43(2):282-288.

In this retrospective cohort study, patients younger than 14 years and those 14 to 19 years were evaluated for injuries associated with ACL reconstruction. Delay to surgery was associated with injury severity in both groups. Concomitant injuries were correlated with surgical delay in the younger cohort. Level of evidence: III.

18. Frank JS, Gambacorta PL: Anterior cruciate ligament injuries in the skeletally immature athlete: Diagnosis and management. *J Am Acad Orthop Surg* 2013;21(2):78-87.

The authors of this article review the clinical presentation, evaluation, and treatment options for skeletally immature patients with an ACL tear.

19. Kercher J, Xerogeanes J, Tannenbaum A, Al-Hakim R, Black JC, Zhao J: Anterior cruciate ligament reconstruction in the skeletally immature: An anatomical study utilizing 3-dimensional magnetic resonance imaging reconstructions. *J Pediatr Orthop* 2009;29(2):124-129.

20. Shea KG, Belzer J, Apel PJ, Nilsson K, Grimm NL, Pfeiffer RP: Volumetric injury of the physis during single-bundle anterior cruciate ligament reconstruction in children: A 3-dimensional study using magnetic resonance imaging. *Arthroscopy* 2009;25(12):1415-1422.

21. Kocher MS, Garg S, Micheli LJ: Physeal sparing reconstruction of the anterior cruciate ligament in skeletally immature prepubescent children and adolescents. *J Bone Joint Surg Am* 2005;87(11):2371-2379.

22. Kocher MS, Garg S, Micheli LJ: Physeal sparing reconstruction of the anterior cruciate ligament in skeletally immature prepubescent children and adolescents: Surgical technique. *J Bone Joint Surg Am* 2006;88(suppl 1 pt 2):283-293.

23. Anderson AF: Transepiphyseal replacement of the anterior cruciate ligament using quadruple hamstring grafts in skeletally immature patients. *J Bone Joint Surg Am* 2004;86(pt 2suppl 1):201-209.

24. Nawabi DH, Jones KJ, Lurie B, Potter HG, Green DW, Cordasco FA: All-inside, physeal-sparing anterior cruciate ligament reconstruction does not significantly compromise the physis in skeletally immature athletes: A postoperative physeal magnetic resonance imaging analysis. *Am J Sports Med* 2014;42(12):2933-2940.

Authors of this series of 23 skeletally immature patients who underwent all-epiphyseal or partial transphyseal ACL reconstruction and follow-up MRI evaluation reported minimal femoral physeal disturbance in both groups. Tibial physeal disturbance was 2.1% and 5.4%, respectively. No growth arrest was reported. Level of evidence: IV.

25. Kennedy A, Coughlin DG, Metzger MF, et al: Biomechanical evaluation of pediatric anterior cruciate ligament reconstruction techniques. *Am J Sports Med* 2011;39(5):964-971.

This study used six adult cadaver knees to test knee kinematics after all-epiphyseal, over-the-top, and ITB ACL reconstruction. Each technique improved knee stability. ITB ACL reconstruction best restored stability and rotational control, although internal rotation was overconstrained.

26. Sena M, Chen J, Dellamaggioria R, Coughlin DG, Lotz JC, Feeley BT: Dynamic evaluation of pivot-shift kinematics in physeal-sparing pediatric anterior cruciate ligament reconstruction techniques. *Am J Sports Med* 2013;41(4):826-834.

This study used six adult cadaver knees to test pivot-shift kinematics after all-epiphyseal, over-the-top, and ITB ACL reconstruction. Each technique improved knee stability, although the ITB technique overconstrained the knee in adduction and internal rotation.

27. McCarthy MM, Tucker S, Nguyen JT, Green DW, Imhauser CW, Cordasco FA: Contact stress and kinematic analysis of all-epiphyseal and over-the-top pediatric reconstruction techniques for the anterior cruciate ligament. *Am J Sports Med* 2013;41(6):1330-1339.

This study used 10 human cadaver knees to test knee kinematics after physeal-sparing ACL reconstruction using all-epiphyseal and over-the-top techniques. The authors concluded that, although neither technique completely restored normal contact stresses and stability, both techniques resulted in improvements compared with the ACL-deficient state.

28. Willimon SC, Jones CR, Herzog MM, May KH, Leake MJ, Busch MT: Micheli anterior cruciate ligament reconstruction in skeletally immature youths: A retrospective case series with a mean 3-year follow up. *Am J Sports Med* 2015;43(12):2974-2981.

Authors of this retrospective case series of 21 skeletally immature males who underwent ITB ACL reconstruction reported a 14% revision rate at the 3-year follow-up. Patients not requiring revision had stable knees, excellent outcomes scores, and no growth disturbances. Level of evidence: IV.

29. Lawrence JT, Bowers AL, Belding J, Cody SR, Ganley TJ: All-epiphyseal anterior cruciate ligament reconstruction in skeletally immature patients. *Clin Orthop Relat Res* 2010;468(7):1971-1977.

30. Engelman GH, Carry PM, Hitt KG, Polousky JD, Vidal AF: Comparison of allograft versus autograft anterior cruciate ligament reconstruction graft survival in an active adolescent cohort. *Am J Sports Med* 2014;42(10):2311-2318.

This retrospective case-control study of 73 pediatric patients undergoing ACL reconstruction using either autograft or allograft tendon reported a significantly higher rate of graft failure in the allograft cohort (hazard ratio, 4.4). Level of evidence: III.

31. Kocher MS, Smith JT, Zoric BJ, Lee B, Micheli LJ: Transphyseal anterior cruciate ligament reconstruction

in skeletally immature pubescent adolescents. *J Bone Joint Surg Am* 2007;89(12):2632-2639.

32. Kumar S, Ahearne D, Hunt DM: Transphyseal anterior cruciate ligament reconstruction in the skeletally immature: Follow-up to a minimum of sixteen years of age. *J Bone Joint Surg Am* 2013;95(1e1):e1.

    The authors of this prospective case series of 32 skeletally immature patients treated with transphyseal ACL reconstruction and followed for 6 years postoperatively reported high functional outcomes scores, a low retear rate, and one case of valgus deformity. Level of evidence: IV.

33. Calvo R, Figueroa D, Gili F, et al: Transphyseal anterior cruciate ligament reconstruction in patients with open physes: 10-year follow-up study. *Am J Sports Med* 2015;43(2):289-294.

    The authors of this case series reported on the outcomes of 27 skeletally immature patients treated with transphyseal ACL reconstruction. Ten years postoperatively, functional outcomes were substantially improved. Five cases of recurrent instability and no physeal arrests were reported. Level of evidence: IV.

34. Hui C, Roe J, Ferguson D, Waller A, Salmon L, Pinczewski L: Outcome of anatomic transphyseal anterior cruciate ligament reconstruction in Tanner stage 1 and 2 patients with open physes. *Am J Sports Med* 2012;40(5):1093-1098.

    The authors of this case series report the results of transphyseal ACL reconstruction performed in 16 prepubescent patients (average age, 12 years). At the 2-year follow-up, all patients had returned to sports, International Knee Documentation Committee scores were high, and there was no case of clinical physeal arrest. Level of evidence: IV.

35. Boyle MJ, Butler RJ, Queen RM: Functional movement competency and dynamic balance after anterior cruciate ligament reconstruction in adolescent patients. *J Pediatr Orthop* 2016;36(1):36-41.

    This retrospective cohort study compared skeletally immature adolescents, skeletally mature adolescents, and adult patients who had undergone ACL reconstruction. At 9 months after surgery, all groups had deficits on functional movement screening, with unique deficits in the adolescent populations. Level of evidence: IV.

36. Paterno MV, Rauh MJ, Schmitt LC, Ford KR, Hewett TE: Incidence of second ACL injuries 2 years after primary ACL reconstruction and return to sport. *Am J Sports Med* 2014;42(7):1567-1573.

    Seventy-eight patients treated with ACL reconstruction who returned to sports were matched with 47 control subjects. At 24 months, the patients who underwent ACL reconstruction had a sixfold greater rate of subsequent ACL injury. The authors reported that 29.5% of the athletes had secondary ACL injuries (9% ipsilateral knee and 20.5% contralateral knee). Level of evidence: II.

37. Webster KE, Feller JA, Leigh WB, Richmond AK: Younger patients are at increased risk for graft rupture and contralateral injury after anterior cruciate ligament reconstruction. *Am J Sports Med* 2014;42(3):641-647.

    At 4.8 years after ACL reconstruction, 750 patients were evaluated. Patients younger than 20 years had the highest rate (29%) of subsequent ACL injury. Return to sports involving cutting and pivoting substantially increased the odds of reinjury. Level of evidence: III.

38. Wiggins AJ, Grandhi RK, Schneider DK, Stanfield D, Webster KE, Myer GD: Risk of secondary injury in younger athletes after anterior cruciate ligament reconstruction: A systematic review and meta-analysis. *Am J Sports Med* 2016;44(7):1861-1876.

    The authors of this systematic review found the rate of secondary ACL injury was 15% for patients who had undergone ACL reconstruction. Factors that increased the risk of reinjury included young age (<25 years) and return to sport (combined risk, 23%).

39. Nwachukwu BU, McFeely ED, Nasreddine A, et al: Arthrofibrosis after anterior cruciate ligament reconstruction in children and adolescents. *J Pediatr Orthop* 2011;31(8):811-817.

    The authors of this retrospective case series of 1,016 consecutive pediatric patients who underwent ACL reconstruction reported an overall incidence of postoperative arthrofibrosis of 8.3%. Female sex, older age, the use of patella tendon autograft, and concomitant meniscal repair increased the risk of arthrofibrosis. Level of evidence: IV.

40. Shifflett GD, Green DW, Widmann RF, Marx RG: Growth arrest following ACL reconstruction with hamstring autograft in skeletally immature patients: A review of 4 cases. *J Pediatr Orthop* 2015.

    The authors of this retrospective case series detailed the evaluation, treatment, and clinical outcomes of four skeletally immature patients (average age, 14.2 years) in whom growth disturbance occurred (recurvatum, genu valgum) after transphyseal ACL reconstruction. Level of evidence: IV.

41. Yoo WJ, Kocher MS, Micheli LJ: Growth plate disturbance after transphyseal reconstruction of the anterior cruciate ligament in skeletally immature adolescent patients: An MR imaging study. *J Pediatr Orthop* 2011;31(6):691-696.

    This retrospective review of MRI studies performed at approximately 16 months after transphyseal ACL reconstruction in 43 patients (average age, 14.8 years) demonstrated the presence of focal bone bridges in 5 patients and no evidence of a resultant growth disturbance. Level of evidence: IV.

42. Johnson AC, Wyatt JD, Treme G, Veitch AJ: Incidence of associated knee injury in pediatric tibial eminence fractures. *J Knee Surg* 2014;27(3):215-219.

    The authors of this retrospective chart review of 20 pediatric patients treated for tibial eminence fracture reported a 30% rate of associated meniscal injury, which was highest in patients with more displaced (type III) injuries. Concomitant chondral and ligamentous injuries rarely occurred. Level of evidence: IV.

43. Anderson CN, Anderson AF: Tibial eminence fractures. *Clin Sports Med* 2011;30(4):727-742.

    The authors of this article review the anatomy, clinical presentation, classification, and treatment of pediatric patients with tibial spine fractures and illustrate various surgical techniques for achieving fixation.

44. Herman MJ, Martinek MA, Abzug JM: Complications of tibial eminence and diaphyseal fractures in children: Prevention and treatment. *J Am Acad Orthop Surg* 2014;22(11):730-741.

    The authors review common complications of tibial eminence fractures in children, including fixation problems, ACL laxity, knee stiffness, and arthrofibrosis. Common complications of pediatric tibial shaft fractures, such as infection, bone healing, and compartment syndrome, are also reviewed.

45. Shea KG, Grimm NL, Laor T, Wall E: Bone bruises and meniscal tears on MRI in skeletally immature children with tibial eminence fractures. *J Pediatr Orthop* 2011;31(2):150-152.

    This retrospective MRI evaluation of 20 skeletally immature patients with tibial eminence fractures revealed meniscal tears in 40% of the patients. Subchondral bone contusions were present in 90% of the patients and closely approximated bruising patterns seen in adults with ACL injuries. Level of evidence: IV.

46. Kocher MS, Micheli LJ, Gerbino P, Hresko MT: Tibial eminence fractures in children: Prevalence of meniscal entrapment. *Am J Sports Med* 2003;31(3):404-407.

47. Mitchell JJ, Sjostrom R, Mansour AA, et al: Incidence of meniscal injury and chondral pathology in anterior tibial spine fractures of children. *J Pediatr Orthop* 2015;35(2):130-135.

    This retrospective review of 58 children treated for anterior tibial spine fractures reported that 59% of the patients had associated injury to the meniscus (including meniscal entrapment) and/or chondral surface; patients with displaced fractures had higher rates of associated injuries. Level of evidence: IV.

48. Archibald-Seiffer N, Jacobs J Jr, Zbojniewicz A, Shea K: Incarceration of the intermeniscal ligament in tibial eminence injury: A block to closed reduction identified using MRI. *Skeletal Radiol* 2015;44(5):717-721.

    This case report describes a 13-year-old male adolescent with a tibial spine fracture and an incarcerated intermeniscal ligament that was visible on preoperative MRI. The authors discuss the use of a preoperative diagnosis of entrapped soft tissues in preoperative planning and counseling patients.

49. Shin YW, Uppstrom TJ, Haskel JD, Green DW: The tibial eminence fracture in skeletally immature patients. *Curr Opin Pediatr* 2015;27(1):50-57.

    The authors review the existing literature on tibial eminence fractures in skeletally immature patients. They found that substantial heterogeneity exists in the literature, which makes it difficult to reach firm conclusions regarding preferred treatment. The authors conclude that displaced fractures should be treated surgically.

50. Edmonds EW, Fornari ED, Dashe J, Roocroft JH, King MM, Pennock AT: Results of displaced pediatric tibial spine fractures: A comparison between open, arthroscopic, and closed management. *J Pediatr Orthop* 2015;35(7):651-656.

    This retrospective chart review of 76 children treated for tibial eminence fracture concluded that closed management results in a higher rate of instability and the need for subsequent surgery, whereas fractures treated surgically had higher rates of arthrofibrosis, regardless of the fixation method used.

51. Watts CD, Larson AN, Milbrandt TA: Open versus arthroscopic reduction for tibial eminence fracture fixation in children. *J Pediatr Orthop* 2016;36(5):437-439.

    This retrospective chart review of 31 patients treated surgically for displaced tibial eminence fractures demonstrated that a delay in time to surgery (>7 days from injury) and longer surgical times (>120 minutes) were associated with higher rates of postoperative arthrofibrosis. Level of evidence: III.

52. Gans I, Baldwin KD, Ganley TJ: Treatment and management outcomes of tibial eminence fractures in pediatric patients. *Am J Sports Med* 2014;42(7):1743-1750.

    This systematic literature review of pediatric tibial eminence fractures reported that the existing data are of low quality and yield insufficient evidence to draw firm treatment conclusions regarding open versus arthroscopic surgical methods and screw versus suture fixation techniques. Level of evidence: IV.

53. Eggers AK, Becker C, Weimann A, et al: Biomechanical evaluation of different fixation methods for tibial eminence fractures. *Am J Sports Med* 2007;35(3):404-410.

54. Bong MR, Romero A, Kubiak E, et al: Suture versus screw fixation of displaced tibial eminence fractures: A biomechanical comparison. *Arthroscopy* 2005;21(10):1172-1176.

55. Mahar AT, Duncan D, Oka R, Lowry A, Gillingham B, Chambers H: Biomechanical comparison of four different fixation techniques for pediatric tibial eminence avulsion fractures. *J Pediatr Orthop* 2008;28(2):159-162.

56. Anderson CN, Nyman JS, McCullough KA, et al: Biomechanical evaluation of physeal-sparing fixation methods in tibial eminence fractures. *Am J Sports Med* 2013;41(7):1586-1594.

    The authors of this cadaver biomechanical study compared four methods of physeal-sparing fixation for tibial eminence fracture. They concluded that the UHMWPE suture plus suture button construct is biomechanically superior to suture anchor, screw, and polydioxanone suture plus suture button constructs.

57. Vander Have KL, Ganley TJ, Kocher MS, Price CT, Herrera-Soto JA: Arthrofibrosis after surgical fixation of tibial eminence fractures in children and adolescents. *Am J Sports Med* 2010;38(2):298-301.

58. Patel NM, Park MJ, Sampson NR, Ganley TJ: Tibial eminence fractures in children: Earlier posttreatment mobilization results in improved outcomes. *J Pediatr Orthop* 2012;32(2):139-144.

This retrospective chart review of 40 pediatric patients treated for tibial eminence fracture demonstrated that early initiation of ROM therapy (within 4 weeks of treatment) substantially decreased the rate of arthrofibrosis and hastened return to full activity. Level of evidence: III.

Chapter 42

Meniscal Tears in Children and Adolescents

Melinda S. Sharkey, MD   Cordelia W. Carter, MD

Abstract

The diagnosis and treatment of pediatric and adolescent meniscal injury is an evolving area of pediatric sports medicine practice. A growing body of literature is contributing to an evidence base for informing treatment decisions for different types of traumatic meniscal tears as well as the symptomatic discoid meniscus.

Keywords: discoid meniscus; meniscus injury; pediatric meniscus

Introduction

Meniscal tear rates are increasing in children and adolescents, partly because of increasing participation in organized sports and partly because of increased recognition of these injuries.[1,2] The menisci perform the critical functions of load distribution across the knee joint, shock absorption, and proprioception and also contribute to knee stability.[1-3] At birth, the menisci are completely vascularized and composed of cells with a large cytoplasm to nucleus ratio. By 10 years of age, the menisci have adult-like characteristics, with only the peripheral one-third of the meniscus having a direct blood supply and the tissue largely composed of collagen fibers arranged circumferentially.[1-3]

Dr. Carter or an immediate family member serves as a board member, owner, officer, or committee member of the Pediatric Orthopaedic Society of North America and the American Academy of Orthopaedic Surgeons. Neither Dr. Sharkey nor any immediate family member has received anything of value from or has stock or stock options held in a commercial company or institution related directly or indirectly to the subject of this chapter.

Evaluation

Most meniscal tears result from a noncontact, twisting injury that is frequently related to a sports activity. On presentation, patients generally report pain and may note mechanical symptoms such as locking, catching, and giving way. Physical examination may show knee effusion and joint line tenderness. If tolerated, meniscal compression tests may elicit pain. Because of the common association of meniscal tears with ligamentous injuries, an examination for knee stability is important. Plain radiographs of the knee should be obtained to evaluate for fractures, loose bodies, and osteochondritis dissecans lesions; however, results will often be negative in a patient with a meniscus injury. MRI is the study of choice (**Figure 1**). A 2015 study reported that MRI had high diagnostic accuracy for assessing knee disorders in children and adolescents, although lateral meniscus tears were one of the most frequently missed pathologies on MRI (18.8%) that were later identified at the time of arthroscopy.[4]

In addition to the known association between tears of the anterior cruciate ligament and the menisci, two recent reports have described a similarly high rate of meniscal injury in the setting of tibial eminence fractures in children.[5,6] The authors of one study found an overall 21% meniscal tear rate, with a 33% tear rate in children with type II tibial spine fractures.[5] The other study reported a 40% rate of meniscal tears in 20 children presenting with tibial spine fractures.[6]

Treatment

Some pediatric meniscal tears, such as partial thickness tears comprising less than 50% of the total meniscal thickness, may be suitable for nonsurgical treatment. An attempt at nonsurgical management also may be made for patients with small (<1 cm), stable, longitudinal tears in the peripheral red-red zone. These tears are generally found at the time of diagnostic arthroscopy in the setting of ligamentous injury. Most symptomatic meniscal tears

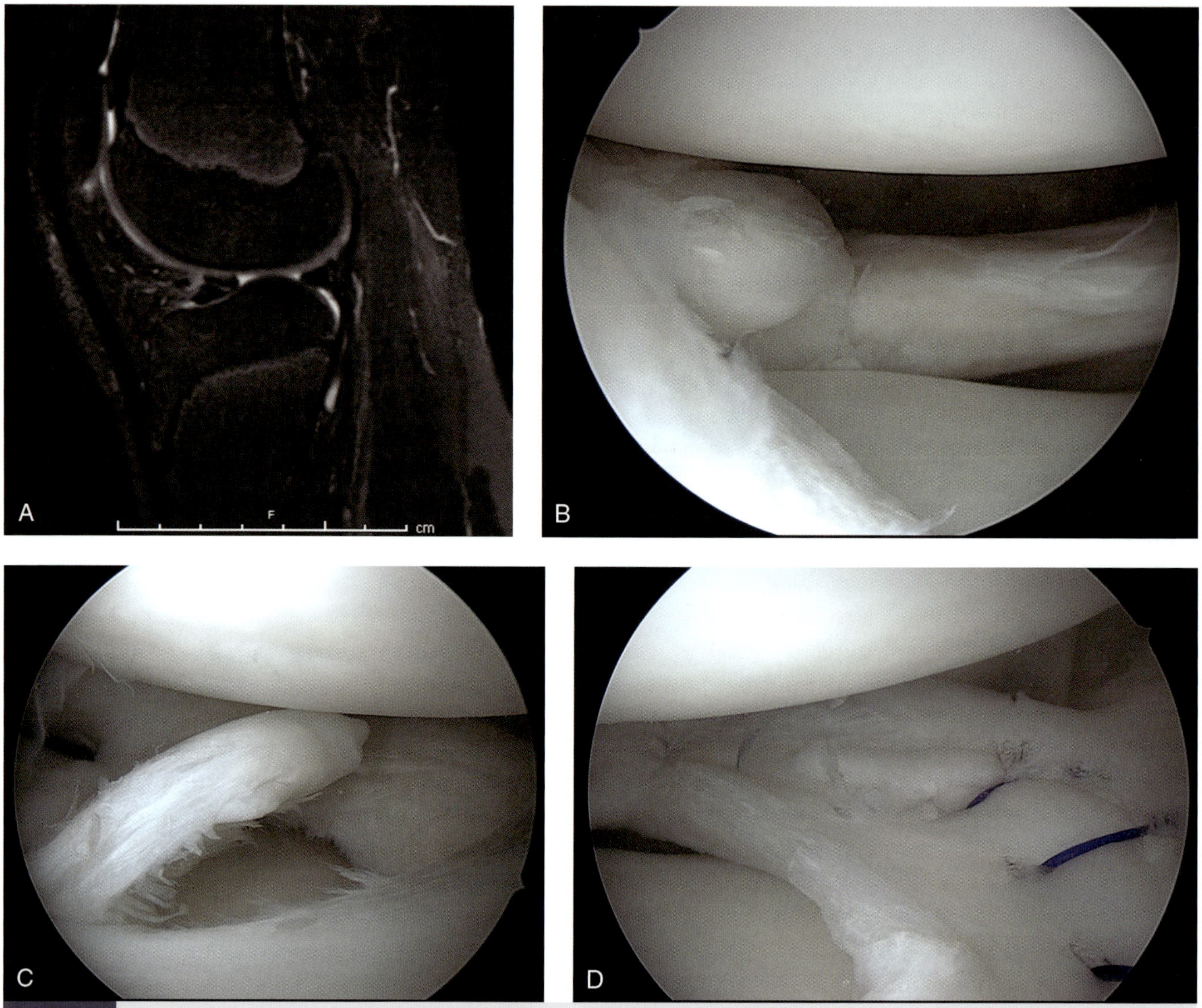

Figure 1 **A,** Sagittal T2-weighted MRI through the knee of a 13-year-old girl shows an anteriorly displaced bucket-handle tear of the posterior horn of the lateral meniscus. Arthroscopic images show the displaced tear (**B**), reduction of the tear (**C**), and final meniscal repair (**D**).

require surgical treatment (**Figure 1**). Treatment includes arthroscopic evaluation of the knee and débridement and/or repair of the meniscal tear(s).

If surgery is indicated, an attempt should be made to repair meniscal tears in pediatric patients whenever possible. Tear patterns that are generally considered amenable to repair are similar in children and adults and include longitudinal, vertical, and bucket-handle tear morphologies. Attempts are typically made to repair radial tears, especially if the tear extends to the periphery of the meniscus. Oblique and horizontal tear configurations are less amenable to repair. Meniscal tears that are complex in nature, with extensive tissue maceration or degeneration, may be irreparable.

As in adults, tears in the peripheral red-red zone in children are considered most likely to heal because of the robust blood supply. Surgical repair of tears in the more central zones of the meniscus, especially in younger children, may be attempted because of the perceived potential for healing in children and the known importance of an intact meniscus for long-term knee health.

Tears that are deemed irreparable by virtue of poor tissue quality, poor vascular supply, or some combination of factors, are best treated by partial meniscectomy, which may be performed using a combination of meniscal biters and/or punches and a small arthroscopic shaver. In this situation, the objective is to leave as much stable meniscal tissue as possible, with the goal of minimizing both the risk of recurrent meniscal tearing and that of future arthritic degeneration.

Viable methods of meniscal repair include all-inside, inside-out, and outside-in techniques, with the choice of technique depending on the location and morphology of the tear, the size of the patient, and the preference and comfort of the surgeon. Hybrid repairs, which include a combination of repair techniques, also may be performed. Typically, anterior horn tears are repaired in an outside-in fashion with monofilament suture. Tears of the body and posterior horn may be repaired with an all-inside fixation system or an inside-out technique with the sutures tied just outside the joint capsule. It is generally recommended to avoid an all-inside repair technique in younger children because the smaller distances from the meniscal anchors placed through the joint capsule and the popliteal neurovascular bundle may put the bundle at increased risk for direct injury.

Preparation of the meniscus and capsule by mechanically abrading the tissue on either side of the planned repair with a rasp or shaver is an important step in all meniscal repair procedures. In addition, young patients with isolated meniscal tears that are chronic in nature may benefit from techniques that are intended to optimize the vascularity of the repair. Trephination, injection of autologous blood clots, and microfracture of the notch at the level of the posterior cruciate ligament have all been described for this purpose.[1]

A recent study reported on the frequency of meniscal tear patterns in relation to skeletal maturity.[3] In 293 patients aged 10 to 19 years who underwent arthroscopy for a meniscal injury, 67% of the tears involved the lateral meniscus, 22% involved the medial meniscus, and 11% involved both menisci. The most frequent tear patterns were complex (28%), vertical (16%), discoid (14%), and bucket-handle (14%). The association with ligamentous injury varied based on the skeletal maturity of the patient. In patients who had open growth plates, 28% of the meniscal tears were associated with ligamentous injury compared with 51% in adolescents with closed growth plates. Skeletal maturity did not affect tear patterns, but male sex and obesity were associated with greater tear complexity, and discoid tears were more frequent in skeletally immature patients.

Although the outcomes literature for pediatric and adolescent meniscal surgery is still relatively sparse, more studies are being published. In one recent study, 49 knees in 45 patients 6 to 17 years of age were clinically evaluated at an average of 27 months after surgery (range, 17 to 52 months).[7] All of the repairs were performed in an inside-out fashion, and 31 of 49 knees (63%) had an associated anterior cruciate ligament tear that was reconstructed. Tears were repaired regardless of the meniscal zone (red-red, red-white, white-white). Excellent clinical outcomes were reported in 43 of 45 patients (96%). The two patients without excellent outcomes sustained reinjury of the knee; one at 15 months after the initial surgery and the other at 17 months after the initial surgery. The exceptionally low failure rates reported in this study may be the result of factors such as the short follow-up period, the young age of the patients, and the high rate of concomitant anterior cruciate ligament reconstruction. In addition, the study authors postulated that their remarkably high clinical success rate may be attributed, at least in part, to the repair technique used (an inside-out technique using permanent monofilament sutures placed in a vertical mattress fashion).[7]

In a recent single-center study of risk factors for failure of meniscal surgery in children and adolescents, 293 patients younger than 20 years with 324 meniscal surgeries (including 46 discoid meniscal surgeries) were evaluated at a mean follow-up of 40 months.[8] Surgical repair was performed in 47% of the cases. Most root detachments and vertical, bucket-handle, and horizontal tears were repaired, whereas few complex tears were repaired, and no radial, oblique, or fray tear patterns were repaired. Overall, 13% of the patients required revision surgery. The primary repair cohort had the highest rate of failure (18%), followed by the primary discoid saucerization cohort (15%) and the partial meniscectomy cohort (7%). Children with open physes and a bucket-handle tear had the highest rate of meniscal retear (46%). One weakness of this retrospective study is that there was no clear delineation of the criteria for performing a meniscal repair versus a partial meniscectomy at the time of the index procedure.[8]

Discoid Meniscus

The discoid meniscus is an uncommon meniscal variant that may present with symptomatic tearing and/or instability during childhood or adolescence. Discoid menisci are almost always lateral but, in rare instances, are found medially. The etiology of the discoid meniscus is not completely understood; however, it is considered a congenital anomaly with a possible genetic component. Studies have shown that the normal meniscus does not have a discoid precursor. Estimates of incidence vary, with a lower incidence (0.4% to 5.2%) in those of Western European decent and a much higher incidence (up to 17%) reported in Asian countries.[2,9,10]

The normal meniscus is wedge-shaped in the coronal plane and crescent-shaped in the axial plane. The central area of a discoid meniscus, however, is partially or

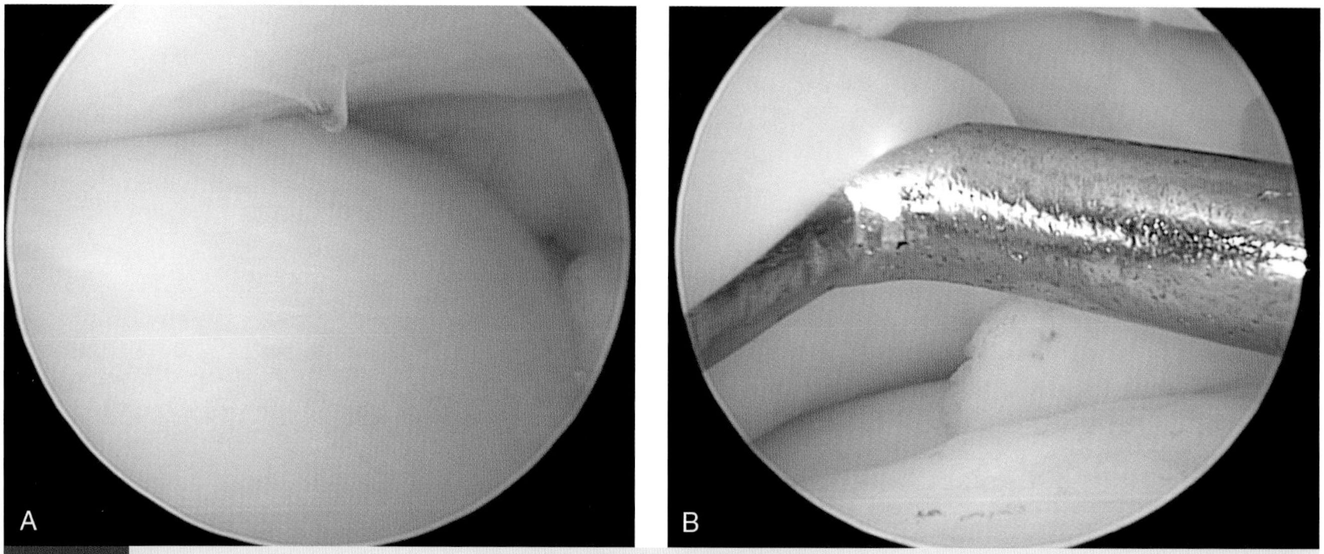

Figure 2 Arthroscopic images show a complete block-like discoid lateral meniscus in a 4-year-old boy. **A,** Native appearance of the discoid meniscus, with complete obstruction of the lateral tibial plateau. **B,** The arthroscopic probe is displacing the meniscus superiorly, revealing the tibial plateau beneath.

completely filled in and may lack normal attachments to the surrounding capsule, distal femur, and proximal tibia. In addition to an anomalous discoid shape, the thickness of the meniscus may be abnormally increased, resulting in a "block" of abnormal tissue (**Figure 2**). This variation may be responsible, at least in part, for the pathognomonic snapping of the knee as it is brought passively into flexion and extension. Increased meniscal thickness is one of the most difficult problems to correct surgically.[2,9-11]

Although the abnormal macromorphology of a discoid meniscus is generally the most striking feature, investigation into the histopathology of the discoid meniscus shows a disorganization of the circumferential collagen network at a molecular level. These structural abnormalities compromise the ability of the discoid meniscus to withstand normal stresses across the knee and predispose it to tears.

The traditional Watanabe classification system consists of three types of discoid meniscus variants: type I, complete discoid shape; type II, incomplete discoid shape; and type III, Wrisberg variant. The Wrisberg variant is described as a more normally shaped meniscus, but it lacks normal peripheral attachments (except the ligament of Wrisberg).[1,9,10] A contemporary classification system, which may be more clinically and surgically relevant, incorporates peripheral stability patterns.[9] Discoid menisci may be classified as complete or incomplete; stable or unstable, based on the presence or absence of peripheral attachments; and intact or torn, based on the presence or absence of a meniscal tear.[12] Peripheral instability may be present at any location along the meniscal margin and may be an important, although less obvious, contributing factor to symptomatology in the setting of a discoid meniscus.

Evaluation

Presenting symptoms in patients with a symptomatic discoid meniscus can include palpable and/or audible snapping, locking, pain, limited extension, quadriceps atrophy, giving way, effusion, and/or the inability to bear weight. Young children (5 to 10 years) tend to present with symptoms related to instability and abnormal shape (popping and snapping), whereas older children tend to present more acutely with symptoms related to an acute tear through the abnormal meniscal tissue.

The physical examination may demonstrate lateral joint line tenderness, possible snapping of the knee with flexion and extension, pain with meniscal compression tests (McMurray, Apley, and Thessaly tests), limited motion, and/or effusion. New or asymmetric flexion contracture of the knee in a young patient may indicate a torn and/or displaced discoid lateral meniscus.

Radiographs of the knee with a discoid lateral meniscus may show subtle differences compared with a nondiscoid knee. A recent comparison of radiographs of the knees of children with symptomatic discoid lateral menisci with those of age-matched control subjects found differences in the mean height of the lateral tibial spine, the lateral joint space distance, the height of the fibular head, and the obliquity of the lateral tibial plateau.[13]

MRI remains the modality of choice for making the diagnosis of a discoid meniscus (**Figure 3**). In a recent study, the performance of MRI and preoperative physical examination findings in the diagnosis of intra-articular pathology of the knee in children and adolescents was evaluated.[4] The overall diagnostic accuracy was 92.7% for MRI and 95.3% for preoperative clinical examination. Despite this accuracy, the most common pathology missed on MRI but found at the time of diagnostic arthroscopy was the presence of a discoid lateral meniscus (26.7% of cases). Because MRI criteria for discoid lateral meniscus have not been clearly defined in children, the adult diagnostic criteria (for example, three or more contiguous 5-mm sagittal cuts showing continuity between the anterior and posterior horns of the meniscus) are generally applied to children. For children, a ratio of meniscal coverage of the lateral tibiofemoral joint space also can be used to make the diagnosis. If greater than 50% of the lateral joint space is covered by meniscal tissue, the diagnosis of discoid lateral meniscus should be considered.[10]

Treatment

Surgical treatment may be beneficial for young patients with symptoms related to a discoid meniscus (pain, effusion, limited range of motion, mechanical symptoms, and associated activity restrictions). Surgical treatment of a symptomatic discoid meniscus has evolved over time. Previously, complete or subtotal meniscectomy was performed for a symptomatic discoid meniscus. Variable long-term outcomes have been reported for total meniscectomy, with some studies showing excellent results with no evidence of degenerative changes and other studies demonstrating poor function, osteoarthritis, pain, instability, and even the development of osteochondritis dissecans lesions associated with the discoid lateral meniscus.[9]

Currently, surgical treatment includes arthroscopic saucerization of the symptomatic discoid meniscus, with the goal of leaving a peripheral rim with a width of approximately 6 to 8 mm. Saucerization includes removal of abnormal, redundant central meniscal tissue, until "normal morphology" is achieved. Debulking an abnormally thick discoid lateral meniscus may be particularly difficult. After partial meniscectomy is completed, the remaining tissue is inspected for tearing and/or peripheral instability. Meniscal tears are repaired using the techniques described previously. Unstable menisci are stabilized by suturing them to the adjacent capsule (**Figure 4**). Menisci that have extensive complex tearing and tissue maceration may not be candidates for these techniques; patients with this type of unsalvageable meniscal tearing commonly undergo subtotal meniscectomy.

Few long-term outcome studies of arthroscopic saucerization exist, and the surgical treatment methods used are variable. One longer-term study, with an average follow-up of 8.5 years, reported on 104 knees.[14] The median age of patients at the time of surgery was 8 years. Treatment varied by age and discoid morphology. Patients aged

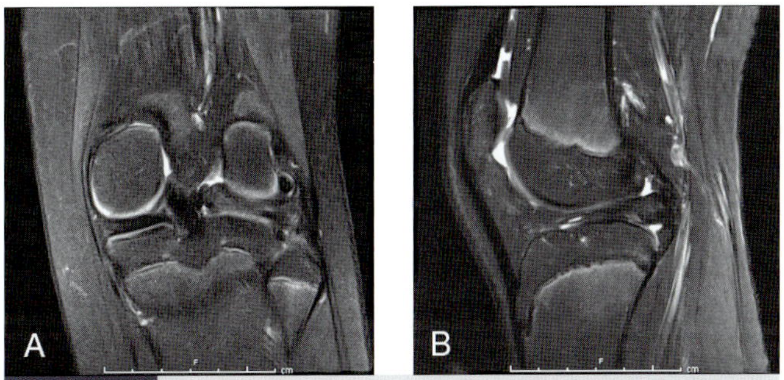

Figure 3 Coronal (**A**) and sagittal (**B**) MRIs show a torn, displaced discoid lateral meniscus in a symptomatic 12-year-old girl.

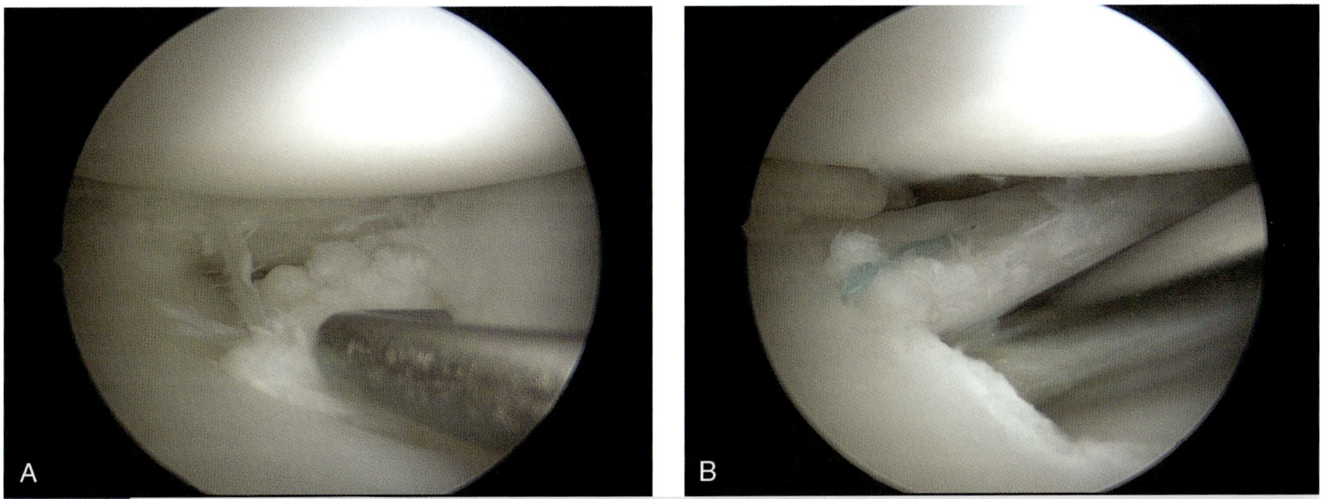

Figure 4 **A,** Arthroscopic image shows a complex tear of a discoid lateral meniscus. **B,** Arthroscopic image after saucerization and repair of the peripheral radial tear.

2 to 7 years underwent a subtotal meniscectomy, whereas those aged 8 to14 years underwent arthroscopic partial meniscectomy. Patients with Wrisberg type menisci underwent removal of the entire posterior horn (patients in this group who were older than 8 years were excluded from the analysis). Despite the variety of treatments and the exclusion of some patients from the final analysis, the authors concluded that patients in the younger group who underwent subtotal meniscectomy had the best outcomes based on clinical evaluation findings and questionnaire responses.

Another recent long-term outcome study (8- to 14-year follow-up) described patient-reported function and radiographic changes after arthroscopic reshaping of a discoid meniscus.[15] A total of 48 knees in 38 children (mean age, 9.9 years) were included. Patients were treated with arthroscopic partial meniscectomy (22 knees), partial meniscectomy with repair (18 knees), and subtotal meniscectomy (8 knees). In the 48 knees, the function of 45 knees (94%) was rated excellent or good at an average follow-up of 10 years. Follow-up radiographs demonstrated degenerative changes in 23% of knees in the partial meniscectomy group, 39% of knees in the partial meniscectomy with repair group, and 88% of knees in the subtotal meniscectomy group.

Short-term outcomes have been reported for contemporary treatment of the discoid meniscus, specifically in relation to peripheral rim stability. In a 2012 study, 57 knees underwent saucerization alone or saucerization and stabilization when the peripheral rim was unstable.[16] At an average follow-up of 15 months, outcomes were equivalent on self-reported outcomes measures and clinical examination findings. This led the authors to conclude that the need for peripheral stabilization does not negatively affect short-term clinical and functional outcomes if meniscal instability is recognized and appropriately treated at the time of surgery.

The authors of a 2015 study reported similarly good results at midterm follow-up.[17] In an evaluation of 100 knees in patients younger than 18 years (average follow-up, 4.7 years) equivalent results were found in the saucerization group, the saucerization and rim stabilization group, and the subtotal meniscectomy group. Subtotal meniscectomy (defined as <3 mm width of peripheral rim remaining) was performed when the remnant meniscal rim showed severe degeneration or complex tearing.

Summary

As increasing numbers of young children and adolescents participate in organized sports, meniscal injury rates have continued to increase. A growing body of literature is beginning to provide an evidence base for the evaluation and treatment of these injuries in children and adolescents. Short-term and midterm outcomes are generally quite good for young patients with meniscal pathology that is treated using contemporary surgical methods, although re-tearing of the meniscus requiring additional surgical procedures remains a concern. In addition, high-quality data on the long-term outcomes for pediatric patients with meniscus tears are lacking and should be a dedicated area of future research.

Key Study Points

- The lateral meniscus is most commonly injured in children and adolescents.
- Skeletally immature patients frequently present with an isolated meniscal injury; skeletally mature patients are more likely to sustain meniscal injury in the setting of a ligamentous injury of the knee.
- Children with open growth plates and bucket-handle meniscal tears have the highest rates of surgical revision after meniscal repair.
- In addition to anomalous macromorphology and microarchitecture, discoid lateral menisci commonly demonstrate peripheral instability.
- Arthroscopic saucerization, with repair and stabilization as necessary, is a procedure associated with good short-term and midterm clinical outcomes for patients with a symptomatic discoid lateral meniscus.

Annotated References

1. Carter CW, Kocher MS: Meniscus repair in children. *Clin Sports Med* 2012;31(1):135-154.

   The authors present a comprehensive review article on meniscal injury and treatments, including a discussion of the discoid meniscus.

2. Francavilla ML, Restrepo R, Zamora KW, Sarode V, Swirsky SM, Mintz D: Meniscal pathology in children: Differences and similarities with the adult meniscus. *Pediatr Radiol* 2014;44(8):910-925, quiz 907-909.

   This comprehensive review article discusses meniscal injury, with a focus on radiologic evaluation of meniscal tears.

3. Shieh A, Bastrom T, Roocroft J, Edmonds EW, Pennock AT: Meniscus tear patterns in relation to skeletal immaturity: Children versus adolescents. *Am J Sports Med* 2013;41(12):2779-2783.

This study reports on 293 patients 10 to 19 years of age who underwent surgery for meniscal injuries. The authors documented tear patterns and association with ligamentous injury in relation to patient age. Lateral meniscus tears were most common, and older children were more likely to have an associated ligamentous injury. Level of evidence: III.

4. Gans I, Bedoya MA, Ho-Fung V, Ganley TJ: Diagnostic performance of magnetic resonance imaging and pre-surgical evaluation in the assessment of traumatic intra-articular knee disorders in children and adolescents: What conditions still pose diagnostic challenges? *Pediatr Radiol* 2015;45(2):194-202.

   The authors found that preoperative MRI and preoperative clinical examination were quite accurate in assessing intra-articular knee disorders in children. Overall, the diagnostic accuracy of MRI and clinical examination were 92.7% and 95.3%, respectively. The most common diagnosis missed on MRI but found at arthroscopy was discoid meniscus (26.7% of cases). Level of evidence: III.

5. Mitchell JJ, Sjostrom R, Mansour AA, et al: Incidence of meniscal injury and chondral pathology in anterior tibial spine fractures of children. *J Pediatr Orthop* 2015;35(2):130-135.

   Of 58 patients with tibial spine fractures, 7% had cartilage injury, 21% had meniscus injury, and 4% had loose bodies. Level of evidence: IV.

6. Shea KG, Grimm NL, Laor T, Wall E: Bone bruises and meniscal tears on MRI in skeletally immature children with tibial eminence fractures. *J Pediatr Orthop* 2011;31(2):150-152.

   Of 20 skeletally immature children with tibial eminence fractures, 90% had subchondral bone contusions and 40% had meniscal tears. Level of evidence: IV.

7. Vanderhave KL, Moravek JE, Sekiya JK, Wojtys EM: Meniscus tears in the young athlete: Results of arthroscopic repair. *J Pediatr Orthop* 2011;31(5):496-500.

   At an average 27-month follow-up, excellent clinical outcomes were seen after arthroscopic meniscal repair in 43 of 45 patients. Two patients sustained knee reinjury. Level of evidence: III.

8. Shieh AK, Edmonds EW, Pennock AT: Revision meniscal surgery in children and adolescents: Risk factors and mechanisms for failure and subsequent management. *Am J Sports Med* 2016;44(4):838-843.

   At a single center, 293 patients younger than 20 years with 324 meniscal surgeries (including 46 discoid meniscus surgeries) were evaluated at a mean follow-up of 40 months. Overall, 13% of the patients required revision surgery. Level of evidence: III.

9. Kushare I, Klingele K, Samora W: Discoid meniscus: Diagnosis and management. *Orthop Clin North Am* 2015;46(4):533-540.

   The authors present a comprehensive review of discoid meniscus pathology, evaluation, and treatment.

10. McKay S, Chen C, Rosenfeld S: Orthopedic perspective on selected pediatric and adolescent knee conditions. *Pediatr Radiol* 2013;43(suppl 1):S99-S106.

    A comprehensive review of pediatric knee conditions, including discoid meniscus with a focus on radiographic evaluation, is presented.

11. Flouzat-Lachaniette CH, Pujol N, Boisrenoult P, Beaufils P: Discoid medial meniscus: Report of four cases and literature review. *Orthop Traumatol Surg Res* 2011;97(8):826-832.

    In this case series, four medial discoid menisci are described. Level of evidence: IV.

12. Klingele KE, Kocher MS, Hresko MT, Gerbino P, Micheli LJ: Discoid lateral meniscus: Prevalence of peripheral rim instability. *J Pediatr Orthop* 2004;24(1):79-82.

13. Choi SH, Ahn JH, Kim KI, et al: Do the radiographic findings of symptomatic discoid lateral meniscus in children differ from normal control subjects? *Knee Surg Sports Traumatol Arthrosc* 2015;23(4):1128-1134.

    A study of the radiographic findings in 91 discoid knees compared with the normal knees of 91 age- and sex-matched control subjects found that there were important differences in mean height of the lateral tibial spine, the lateral joint space, the height of fibular head, and the obliquity of the lateral tibial plateau. Level of evidence: II.

14. Stilli S, Marchesini Reggiani L, Marcheggiani Muccioli GM, Cappella M, Donzelli O: Arthroscopic treatment for symptomatic discoid lateral meniscus during childhood. *Knee Surg Sports Traumatol Arthrosc* 2011;19(8):1337-1342.

    A retrospective review with a mean follow-up of 8.5 years after surgery assessed outcomes after arthroscopic surgery for the treatment of symptomatic discoid lateral meniscus. Surgery (subtotal meniscectomy versus partial meniscectomy) varied based on patient age. Better clinic results were described in the group treated with subtotal meniscectomy; these patients were younger at the time of surgery. Level of evidence: IV.

15. Ahn JH, Kim KI, Wang JH, Jeon JW, Cho YC, Lee SH: Long-term results of arthroscopic reshaping for symptomatic discoid lateral meniscus in children. *Arthroscopy* 2015;31(5):867-873.

    A retrospective study of 38 children (48 knees) who underwent arthroscopic surgery for a symptomatic discoid lateral meniscus is presented. Satisfactory clinical outcomes were recorded at mean follow-up of 10 years. However, progressive degenerative changes appeared in 40% of the patients. The subtotal meniscectomy group had a substantially increased progression of degenerative changes compared with the partial meniscectomy group. Level of evidence: IV.

16. Carter CW, Hoellwarth J, Weiss JM: Clinical outcomes as a function of meniscal stability in the discoid meniscus: A preliminary report. *J Pediatr Orthop* 2012;32(1):9-14.

A retrospective chart review of 57 knees with symptomatic discoid meniscus was done to compare outcomes in those requiring peripheral rim stabilization and those who did not require stabilization. No significant difference was found between the groups at an average follow-up of 15 months. Level of evidence: III.

17. Yoo WJ, Jang WY, Park MS, et al: Arthroscopic treatment for symptomatic discoid meniscus in children: Midterm outcomes and prognostic factors. *Arthroscopy* 2015;31(12):2327-2334.

The results of a study of 100 knees in patients younger than 18 years who underwent surgery for a symptomatic discoid meniscus is presented. At an average follow-up of 4.7 years, the authors reported good and equivalent results in the saucerization group, saucerization and rim stabilization group, and the subtotal meniscectomy group. Level of evidence: IV.

Chapter 43

Patellar Instability

Corinna CD Franklin, MD

Abstract

Patellar instability refers to subluxation or dislocation of the patella out of the trochlear groove, usually laterally. This condition is thought to be more common in adolescent girls. The medial patellofemoral ligament is the key medial structure resisting lateral subluxation of the patella dynamically, and the vastus medialis obliquus is the main muscular contributor to patellar stability. Important radiographic measurements are patellar height, patellar tilt, sulcus angle, and the tibial tubercle-trochlear groove distance. No preferred method exists for the management of patellar instability. Patients with a first-time patellar dislocation may be treated with measures such as physical therapy to strengthen the vastus medialis obliquus, core, and gluteal musculature. Current surgical management typically involves reconstruction of the medial patellofemoral ligament, with correction of underlying anatomic factors if necessary.

Keywords: patellar instability; patellofemoral instability; pediatric knee; pediatric sports

Introduction

Patellar instability refers to subluxation or dislocation of the patella out of the trochlear groove of the femur, usually laterally. Acute, traumatic patellar dislocations are the most common acute knee disorder in adolescent athletes.[1] Atraumatic patellar instability is also possible, particularly in patients with ligamentous laxity.

Dr. Franklin or an immediate family member serves as a board member, owner, officer, or committee member of the American Academy of Orthopaedic Surgeons and the Pediatric Orthopaedic Society of North America.

Epidemiology

An often-cited 1994 study from Finland reported the incidence of acute patellar dislocation in children younger than 16 years to be 0.04% (43 per 100,000 children).[2] A 2004 study reported the highest incidence of patellar instability in girls between the ages of 10 and 17 years.[3] More recently, a longitudinal epidemiologic study of emergency department visits for patellar dislocation reported the annual overall rate to be 2.29 per 100,000 individuals.[4] The highest incidence occurred in individuals between the ages of 15 and 19 years; sex was not an important differentiating factor. Half of patellar dislocations occurred during sports participation. The estimates for recurrence rates have ranged from 15% to 44%.[1]

A recent study specifically evaluating patellofemoral instability in high school athletes found that, for comparable sports, girls had higher rates of patellar instability than boys.[5] Injury rates were higher in competition than in practice, and physical contact was a common injury mechanism.

Reported risk factors for patellar instability include female sex, race (black or white being at higher risk than Hispanic individuals), sports participation, anatomic factors, and a personal or family history of patellar instability.[3,4,6] Ligamentous laxity may also play a role; patients should be examined for generalized laxity or hypermobility, with referral to a geneticist if Ehlers-Danlos syndrome is suspected.[7] A recent study found trochlear dysplasia to be an important risk factor for recurrent patellar instability, particularly in skeletally immature patients.[6]

The natural history of patellar instability has not been fully characterized. Limited high-level data exist, and comparing studies is difficult, in part because of the wide variety of reconstruction procedures and treatment options.

Anatomy and Pathoanatomy

The medial patellofemoral ligament (MPFL) is thought to be the most important restraint in preventing lateral subluxation and dislocation of the patella, particularly from full extension to 30° of flexion, and it is most taut

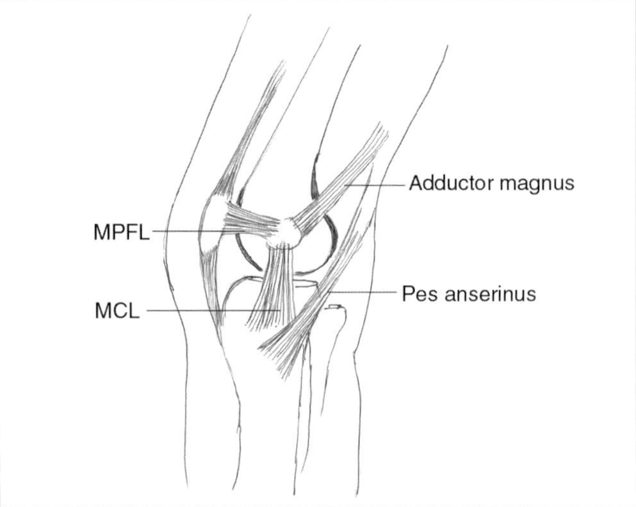

Figure 1 Illustration of the anatomy of the lateral aspect of the knee showing the insertion of the medial patellofemoral ligament (MPFL) on the patella. MCL = medial collateral ligament. (Reproduced from Hennrikus W, Pylawka T: Patellofemoral instability in skeletally immature athletes. *Instr Course Lect* 2013;62:445-453.)

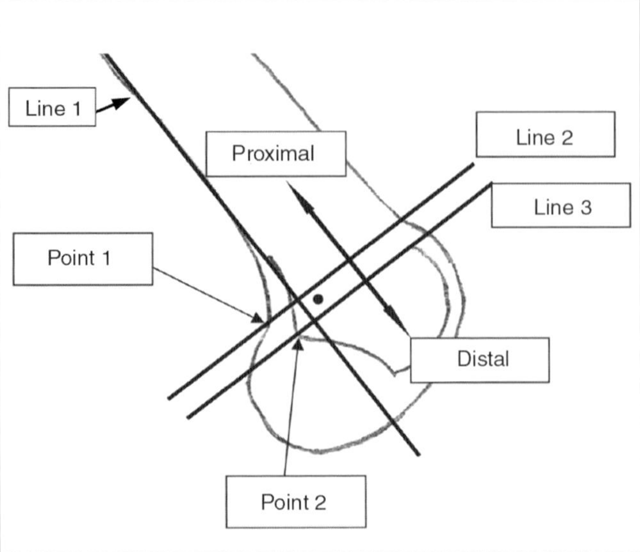

Figure 2 Illustration showing the femoral origin of the medial patellofemoral ligament, which is just anterior (1.3 mm) to the posterior cortex extension (line 1), just distal (2.5 mm) to the posterior origin of the medial femoral condyle (point 1/line 2), and just proximal to the level of the posterior point of the Blumensaat line on a lateral radiograph (point 2/line 3). (Adapted with permission from Schöttle PB, Schmeling A, Rosenstiel N, Weiler A: Radiographic landmarks for femoral tunnel placement in medial patellofemoral ligament reconstruction. *Am J Sports Med* 2007;3[5]:801-804.)

at full extension.[1,8] The MPFL is approximately 55 mm long and variably thick (ranging in thickness from 3 to 30 mm).[8] Studies seem to agree that its insertion is along the superomedial aspect of the patella,[8,9] although the MPFL insertion is more variable in skeletally immature patients[10] (**Figure 1**). The origin of the MPFL is more controversial. Using a radiographic method, authors found the MPFL origin to be just proximal to the femoral physis.[11] However, a later anatomic study reported that the MPFL originates at or below the physis in children.[12] A radiographic method has been described for placing the origin of the MPFL. On a lateral radiograph of the knee, with the posterior condylar margin overlapped, the origin should be 1.3 mm anterior to the posterior cortex extension and 2.5 mm distal to the posterior origin of the medial femoral condyle, just proximal to the level of the posterior point of Blumensaat line[13] (**Figure 2**). In agreement with these findings, the authors of a 2011 study used a radiographic method to determine that the MPFL originates just distal to the femoral physis.[14]

After the patella is engaged, at approximately 20° of flexion, the trochlear groove provides stability. As a result, trochlear dysplasia can contribute to patellar instability. A 2011 study described the relationship between trochlear dysplasia (a morphologically abnormal and/or shallow trochlear) and recurrent patellar dislocations. However, it is unknown whether the dysplasia is congenital or a result of recurrent dislocations.[15] Data from a 2010 case-controlled study found trochlear dysplasia to be more common in women with patellar dislocations.[16]

The main contributor to dynamic stability of the patella is the vastus medialis obliquus, which exerts a medial and posterior force that opposes lateral patellar instability.[17] Alignment of the lower limb is also an important factor. A higher quadriceps (Q) angle indicates a more lateral pull of the quadriceps on the patella, potentially increasing the risk of subluxation or dislocation.[17] Internal femoral rotation and/or external tibial rotation also may be predisposing factors to patellar instability; these factors may be dynamically worsened by hip or core weakness.[17]

The position of the patella also contributes to its stability. In patella alta, the knee must flex further for the patella to engage with the trochlea, allowing a greater range for instability before attaining the bony stability of the trochlea.

Imaging

When evaluating patients with patellar instability, plain radiographs of the knee (AP, lateral, and Merchant views) should be obtained. MRI is also often helpful. Relevant

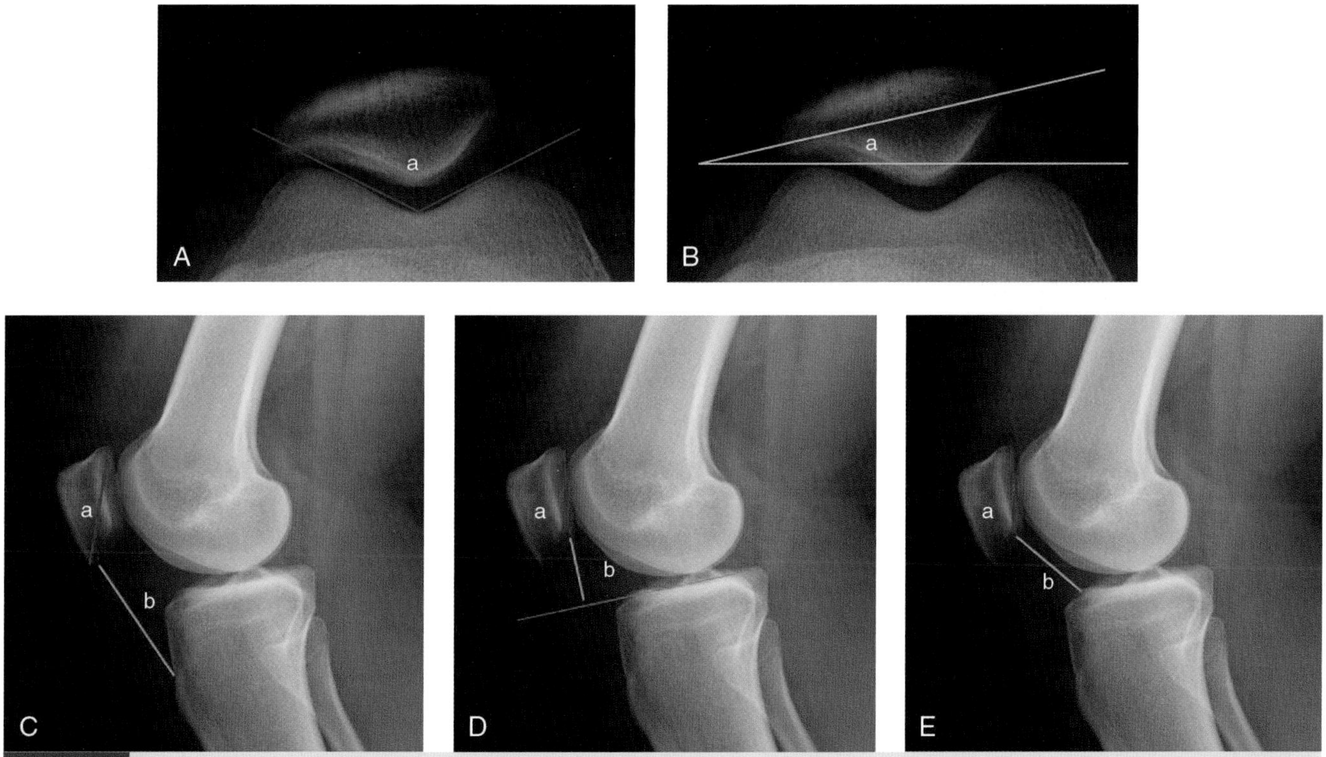

Figure 3 Measurements on plain radiographs can be used to evaluate patellar instability. **A,** A normal sulcus angle (a) is 138° with 6° SD. **B,** Patellar tilt (a) greater than 5° is abnormal. **C,** The Insall-Salvati ratio (b/a) is the ratio of the length of the patellar tendon (blue line) to the diagonal length of the patella (red line); normal is 0.8-1.2. **D,** The Blackburne-Peel ratio (b/a) is the height of the articular surface of the patella from the plateau (blue line) to the length of the articular surface of the patella (red line); greater than 1 suggests patella alta. **E,** The Caton-Deschamps index (b/a) is the distance between the articular facet of the patella and the anterior corner of the superior tibial epiphysis (blue line) and the articular facet length of the patella (red line); normal is 0.6-1.3.

measurements on plain radiographs are the sulcus angle (normal = 138°, with 6° SD)[18] (**Figure 3, A**); patellar tilt (>5° is abnormal)[19](**Figure 3, B**); and patellar height. Several indices can be used to determine patella height, including the Insall-Salvati ratio, which is the ratio of the diagonal length of the patella to the length of the patellar tendon (normal is 0.8-1.2)[20](**Figure 3, C**); the Blackburne-Peel ratio, which is the ratio of the height of the articular surface of the patella from the plateau to the length of the articular surface of the patella (>1 suggests patella alta)[21] (**Figure 3, D**); and the Caton-Deschamps index, which is the ratio between the articular facet length of the patella and the distance between the articular facet of the patella and the anterior corner of the superior tibial epiphysis (normal = 0.6-1.3)[22](**Figure 3, E**). A recent study found the Caton-Deschamps index to be a useful measurement in children and adolescents.[23]

Rupture of the MPFL may be seen on MRI, and it is best seen on T2-weighted images. In addition, osteochondral damage may be noted, and the patella may remain tilted or subluxated[24] (**Figure 4**). Importantly, MRI allows for the measurement of the distance between the tibial tubercle and the trochlear groove, known as the TT-TG distance. If the tibial tubercle is positioned directly under the trochlear groove, there will be a direct line of pull keeping the patella aligned; however, if the tibial tubercle is lateral to the trochlea, the resultant force will tend to pull the patella laterally, which can contribute to instability. This can be assessed by measuring the medial/lateral distance between the tibial tubercle and trochlear grove on successive MRIs or CTs. A TT-TG distance less than 15 mm is normal, whereas a TT-TG distance greater than 20 mm is excessive.[24] A recent comparison study reported that MRI may underestimate the TT-TG distance compared with measurements determined with CT; this should be considered in surgical planning.[25]

Loose bodies may be appreciated on either plain radiographs or MRIs. The use of MRI may help to better localize the location of the loose body and determine its origin; this may help in surgical planning.

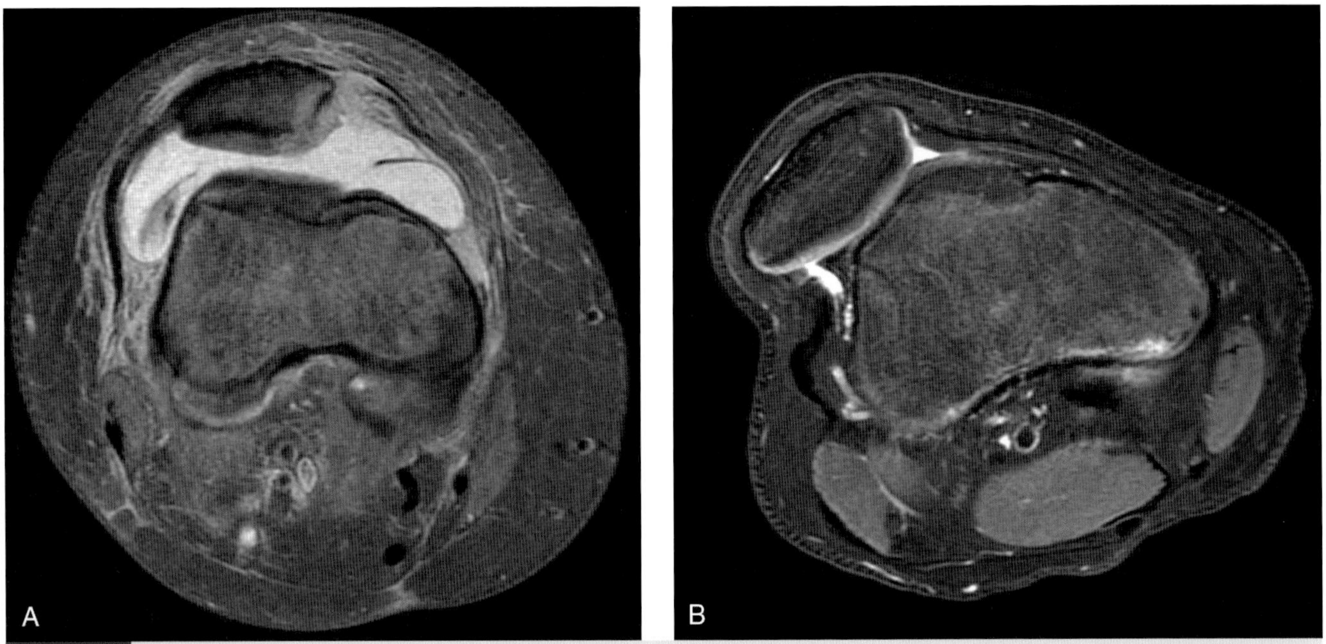

Figure 4 **A,** MRI shows rupture of the medial patellofemoral ligament and osteochondral damage to the patella with a loose body. **B,** MRI shows a patellar dislocation.

Management

There is currently no preferred method for the treatment of patellar instability and only limited high-level data are available to guide treatment decisions. The authors of a recent systematic review were unable to determine whether surgical management of primary patellar dislocation was indicated because of insufficient data.[26] Nonsurgical measures are often used, particularly in patients with first-time dislocations or those with instability without frank dislocation.

Physical Therapy

Physical therapy for patellar instability generally focuses on strengthening the vastus medialis obliquus and the gluteal and core musculature.[1] Weak gluteal muscles can cause adduction and internal rotation of the femur, which exacerbates patellar instability.[27] Closed kinetic chain exercises are likely a more effective therapy for patellar instability.[28,29] Bracing or taping to assist with patellar tracking and prevent lateral subluxation may also be helpful.[27,30]

Surgical Care

More than 100 procedures have been described for the surgical management of patellar instability. Relevant criteria to consider when deciding on a particular procedure should include the age and skeletal maturity of the patient, the underlying pathoanatomy (patella alta, femoral and tibial rotation, patellar tilt, and Q angle), the condition of the cartilage, and associated injuries.

Lateral Release

Isolated lateral release is no longer recommended for the treatment of patellar instability.[1] It may be appropriate in combination with other procedures, particularly in the setting of patellar tilt, but should be used judiciously because, if excessive or not indicated, lateral release can lead to medial instability.[31]

Primary Repair and Medial Reefing

A recent randomized controlled trial examined whether primary repair of the medial structures in patients with acute patellar dislocation improved outcomes compared with nonsurgical management.[32] The authors reported that the rate of recurrent dislocation and long-term outcomes did not differ substantially, and they did not advocate primary repair. In patients with recurrent patellar instability and normal anatomy, medial reefing without lateral release was shown to be an effective treatment in a recent case series.[33]

Proximal Realignment

In 1979 Insall described a proximal realignment involving a lateral release and a long, open medial tightening.[34] However, this procedure has been reported to exacerbate patellofemoral arthritis.[35]

Distal Realignment

For patients with an increased TT-TG distance, the tibial tubercle may be osteotomized and moved anteromedially to correct misalignment of the extensor mechanism. In patients with patella alta, some distalization also can be performed. A recent cadaver study demonstrated that lateralizing the tibial tubercle increased patellar tilt and decreased patellar stability, whereas the reverse was the case for medializing the tibial tubercle.[36] Another recent cadaver study found that 3.5-mm screws were adequate for fixation of the tibial tubercle, and their use may reduce screw irritation.[37] Tibial tubercle transfer may be combined with other reconstruction procedures; a recent case series reported good results when combining MPFL reconstruction with tibial tubercle transfer.[38] This procedure has limited application in skeletally immature patients because of the open tibial apophysis.

Several additional distal soft-tissue procedures have been described, including transfer of the patellar tendon medially (whole or in part) or transfer of the semitendinosus muscle to the patella.[1] A modification of the Roux-Goldthwait technique has been described in which the patellar tendon is split and the lateral half is detached distally and then passed under the medial half and sewn to the insertion of the sartorius.[39] A lateral release also is performed with this modified technique.

MPFL Reconstruction

Most recently, the main focus of surgical management of patellar instability has been reconstruction of the MPFL using tendon graft to restore medial resistance to lateral subluxation and dislocation. Many different options have been described for graft choice, the fixation method, the location of fixation, the appropriate position for fixation, and graft tension. A 2016 systematic review reported no difference in recurrent instability with the use of allografts versus autografts; however, this study included only level IV evidence.[40]

A 2012 case series described a representative technique using ipsilateral semitendinosus autograft. This is looped and fixed through a patellar tunnel with a cortical suspensory system, and a femoral tunnel with an interference screw. Placement of the femoral tunnel is based both on radiographic landmarks and checking the isometry of the graft in tension between 0° and 30° of knee flexion.[41]

A 2013 study described a technique for MPFL reconstruction in patients with open growth plates using gracilis autograft.[42] Two tunnels are made in the proximal two-thirds of the patella, and both ends of the whipstitched graft are fixed into the patella. Using the method described by Schottle et al,[13] a guide pin is placed at the MPFL origin and drilled across to the lateral side, using fluoroscopy to avoid the physis. This is overdrilled to produce a tunnel, and the looped graft is inserted with a suture and fixed with an interference screw at 30° of knee flexion (**Figures 5** and **6**). The vastus medialis obliquus aponeurosis is sutured back over to the patella.

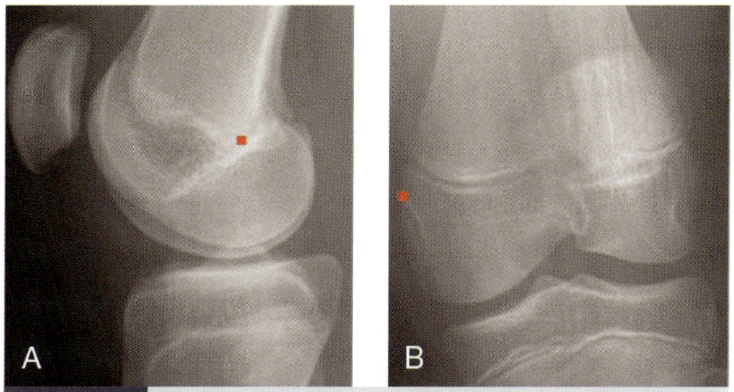

Figure 5 Cross-reference of the physis on a lateral radiographic view is made onto an AP radiographic view. This technique was used to demonstrate that the same point (dot) that is projected on or proximal to the physis on the lateral radiographic view is distal to the physis on the AP view. (Reproduced with permission from Nelitz M, Dreyhaupt J, Reichel H, Woelfle J, Lippacher S: Anatomic reconstruction of the medial patellofemoral ligament in children and adolescents with open growth plates: Surgical technique and outcome. *Am J Sports Med* 2013;41[1]:58-63.)

A method of MPFL reconstruction using the medial portion of the quadriceps tendon has been described.[43] This portion of the quadriceps tendon is amputated proximally (but remains attached at the patella) and is turned down and oversewn. The free portion is sewn under the medial retinaculum to the medial intermuscular septum. This technique is particularly useful in very young patients because there is no drilling near the physis.

A recent systematic review analyzed the existing literature to report on complications and determine the use of various methods. Notably, the authors found a dearth of high-level studies, with no level I studies and only two level II studies. Among the studies included in the analysis, the overall complication rate was 26.1%. Complications included continued apprehension, persistent instability, stiffness, patellar fracture, and pain. Clear conclusions about the superiority of one procedure over the others were not possible.[44]

Guided Growth

A 2015 study described hemiepiphysiodesis to correct genu valgum in patients with patellar instability.[45] Improvements in the anatomic lateral distal femoral angle and symptoms were reported. Hemiepiphysiodesis may be

8: Sports-Related Topics

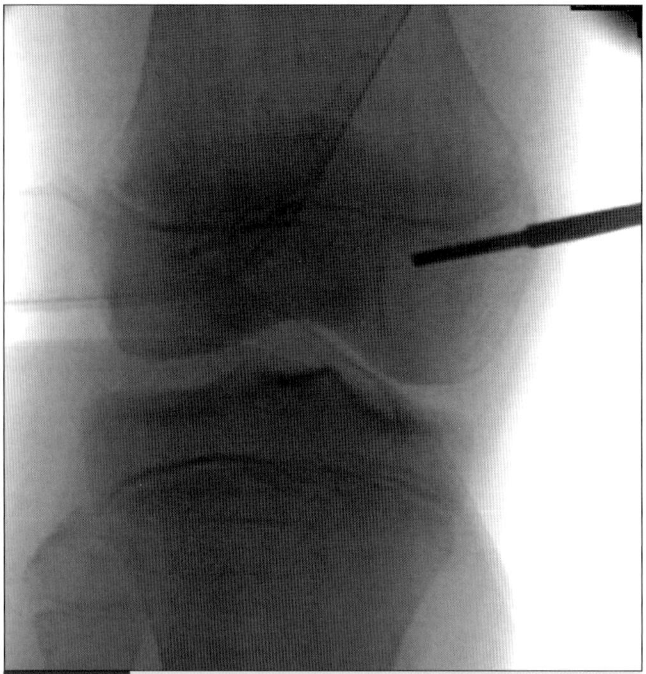

Figure 6 Radiograph shows a bioresorbable interference screw used to secure the graft, with the medial condyle tunnel distal to the physis. Graft placement distal to the physis is demonstrated. (Reproduced with permission from Nelitz M, Dreyhaupt J, Reichel H, Woelfle J, Lippacher S: Anatomic reconstruction of the medial patellofemoral ligament in children and adolescents with open growth plates: Surgical technique and outcome. *Am J Sports Med* 2013;41[1]:58-63.)

considered for skeletally immature patients with patellar instability and genu valgum.

Trochleoplasty

There has been a recent increase in interest in trochleoplasty as an adjunct to surgical procedures for patellar instability. Several recent case series have reported good midterm results with trochleoplasty for patients with severe trochlear dysplasia.[46-48] Trochleoplasty is often combined with other procedures such as MPFL reconstruction. This procedure has had limited application in the United States. The authors of a 2010 review of complications in patellar stabilization surgery urge caution because of concerns about irreversible articular and subchondral injury.[49]

Return to Sports

Limited data exist on return to sports after surgical management of patellar instability. A 2010 systematic review was unable to draw conclusions on return to sports efficacy after MPFL reconstruction because of the quality of the reviewed studies.[50] However, a 2014 case series reported that 100% of patients returned to sports after MPFL reconstruction, but only approximately 50% were able to participate at their prior level or a higher level.[51] A 2013 study suggested that skeletally immature athletes may return to sports participation 4 to 6 months after surgery for patellofemoral instability.[1]

Summary

No preferred method exists for the treatment of patellar instability; additional high-level studies are needed to better clarify appropriate treatment strategies. Current treatment generally involves nonsurgical management for primary dislocations and subluxation in the absence of a loose fragment in the joint. Physical therapy is used to strengthen the vastus medialis obliquus, core, and gluteal musculature. Current surgical management typically involves reconstruction of the MPFL, with correction of underlying anatomic factors if necessary.

Key Study Points

- The MPFL is the primary restraint to lateral subluxation of the patella from 0° to 30° of knee flexion.
- Patella alta, femoral anteversion, and external tibial torsion can contribute to patellar instability.
- An abnormal TT-TG distance (>20 mm) can predispose an individual to patellar instability.
- Physical therapy for patellar instability includes strengthening of the vastus medialis obliquus, core, and gluteal musculature.
- Lateral release in isolation is not recommended for treatment of patellar instability.
- Current surgical management of patellar instability often includes MPFL reconstruction with correction of anatomic parameters if indicated.

Annotated References

1. Hennrikus W, Pylawka T: Patellofemoral instability in skeletally immature athletes. *Instr Course Lect* 2013;62(2):445-453.

The authors review patellofemoral instability in skeletally immature athletes and discuss pathoanatomy and management.

2. Nietosvaara Y, Aalto K, Kallio PE: Acute patellar dislocation in children: Incidence and associated osteochondral fractures. *J Pediatr Orthop* 1994;14(4):513-515.

3. Fithian DC, Paxton EW, Stone ML, et al: Epidemiology and natural history of acute patellar dislocation. *Am J Sports Med* 2004;32(5):1114-1121.

4. Waterman BR, Belmont PJ Jr, Owens BD: Patellar dislocation in the United States: Role of sex, age, race, and athletic participation. *J Knee Surg* 2012;25(1):51-57.

   A longitudinal, prospective epidemiologic database was used to determine the incidence and demographic risk factors for patellar dislocations in patients presenting to emergency departments in the United States. Level of evidence: II.

5. Mitchell J, Magnussen RA, Collins CL, et al: Epidemiology of patellofemoral instability injuries among high school athletes in the United States. *Am J Sports Med* 2015;43(7):1676-1682.

   This cross-sectional study of patellofemoral instability in high school athletes used an online sports injury surveillance system. Level of evidence: III.

6. Lewallen LW, McIntosh AL, Dahm DL: Predictors of recurrent instability after acute patellofemoral dislocation in pediatric and adolescent patients. *Am J Sports Med* 2013;41(3):575-581.

   The authors of this case-controlled study describe patient demographics for first-time patellar dislocations and determine predictors of recurrent instability. Level of evidence: III.

7. Hinton RY, Sharma KM: Acute and recurrent patellar instability in the young athlete. *Orthop Clin North Am* 2003;34(3):385-396.

8. Amis AA, Firer P, Mountney J, Senavongse W, Thomas NP: Anatomy and biomechanics of the medial patellofemoral ligament. *Knee* 2003;10(3):215-220.

9. Smirk C, Morris H: The anatomy and reconstruction of the medial patellofemoral ligament. *Knee* 2003;10(3):221-227.

10. Shea KG, Polousky JD, Jacobs JC Jr, et al: The patellar insertion of the medial patellofemoral ligament in children: A cadaveric study. *J Pediatr Orthop* 2015;35(4):e31-e35.

    This cadaver study examined nine pediatric knees to determine the patellar insertion of the MPFL.

11. Shea KG, Grimm NL, Belzer J, Burks RT, Pfeiffer R: The relation of the femoral physis and the medial patellofemoral ligament. *Arthroscopy* 2010;26(8):1083-1087.

12. Shea KG, Polousky JD, Jacobs JC Jr, et al: The relationship of the femoral physis and the medial patellofemoral ligament in children: A cadaveric study. *J Pediatr Orthop* 2014;34(8):808-813.

    The authors of this cadaver study examined six skeletally immature knees to determine the relationship between the MPFL and the distal femoral physis.

13. Schöttle PB, Schmeling A, Rosenstiel N, Weiler A: Radiographic landmarks for femoral tunnel placement in medial patellofemoral ligament reconstruction. *Am J Sports Med* 2007;35(5):801-804.

14. Nelitz M, Dornacher D, Dreyhaupt J, Reichel H, Lippacher S: The relation of the distal femoral physis and the medial patellofemoral ligament. *Knee Surg Sports Traumatol Arthrosc* 2011;19(12):2067-2071.

    True lateral radiographs were used to determine the relationship between the MPFL and the distal femoral physis in children and adolescents.

15. Bollier M, Fulkerson JP: The role of trochlear dysplasia in patellofemoral instability. *J Am Acad Orthop Surg* 2011;19(1):8-16.

    The authors present a review article on trochlear dysplasia as related to patellar instability.

16. Balcarek P, Jung K, Ammon J, et al: Anatomy of lateral patellar instability: Trochlear dysplasia and tibial tubercle-trochlear groove distance is more pronounced in women who dislocate the patella. *Am J Sports Med* 2010;38(11):2320-2327.

17. Greiwe RM, Saifi C, Ahmad CS, Gardner TR: Anatomy and biomechanics of patellar instability. *Oper Tech Sports Med* 2010;18(2):62-67.

18. Merchant AC, Mercer RL, Jacobsen RH, Cool CR: Roentgenographic analysis of patellofemoral congruence. *J Bone Joint Surg Am* 1974;56(7):1391-1396.

19. Grelsamer RP, Bazos AN, Proctor CS: Radiographic analysis of patellar tilt. *J Bone Joint Surg Br* 1993;75(5):822-824.

20. Insall J, Salvati E: Patella position in the normal knee joint. *Radiology* 1971;101(1):101-104.

21. Blackburne JS, Peel TE: A new method of measuring patellar height. *J Bone Joint Surg Br* 1977;59(2):241-242.

22. Phillips CL, Silver DA, Schranz PJ, Mandalia V: The measurement of patellar height: A review of the methods of imaging. *J Bone Joint Surg Br* 2010;92(8):1045-1053.

23. Thévenin-Lemoine C, Ferrand M, Courvoisier A, Damsin J-P, Ducou le Pointe H, Vialle R: Is the Caton-Deschamps index a valuable ratio to investigate patellar height in children? *J Bone Joint Surg Am* 2011;93(8):e35.

    This study used lateral radiographs of the knees of 300 healthy pediatric patients taken after minor trauma to demonstrate that the Caton-Deschamps index is useful in children.

8: Sports-Related Topics

24. Diederichs G, Issever AS, Scheffler S: MR imaging of patellar instability: Injury patterns and assessment of risk factors. *Radiographics* 2010;30(4):961-981.

25. Camp CL, Stuart MJ, Krych AJ, et al: CT and MRI measurements of tibial tubercle-trochlear groove distances are not equivalent in patients with patellar instability. *Am J Sports Med* 2013;41(8):1835-1840.

This diagnostic cohort study demonstrated that CT and MRI measurements for TT-TG distance are not interchangeable. Level of evidence: II.

26. Magnussen RA, Duffee AR, Kalu D, Flanigan DC: Does early operative treatment improve outcomes of primary patellar dislocation? A systematic review. *Curr Orthop Pract* 2015;26(3):281-286.

The authors of this systematic review examined early surgical intervention for patellar dislocation but were unable to draw conclusions because of insufficient data.

27. Colvin AC, West RV: Patellar instability. *J Bone Joint Surg Am* 2008;90(12):2751-2762.

28. Stensdotter AK, Hodges PW, Mellor R, Sundelin G, Häger-Ross C: Quadriceps activation in closed and in open kinetic chain exercise. *Med Sci Sports Exerc* 2003;35(12):2043-2047.

29. Escamilla RF, Fleisig GS, Zheng N, Barrentine SW, Wilk KE, Andrews JR: Biomechanics of the knee during closed kinetic chain and open kinetic chain exercises. *Med Sci Sports Exerc* 1998;30(4):556-569.

30. Cowan SM, Bennell KL, Hodges PW: Therapeutic patellar taping changes the timing of vasti muscle activation in people with patellofemoral pain syndrome. *Clin J Sport Med* 2002;12(6):339-347.

31. Song G-Y, Hong L, Zhang H, Zhang J, Li Y, Feng H: Iatrogenic medial patellar instability following lateral retinacular release of the knee joint. *Knee Surg Sports Traumatol Arthrosc* 2015.

A review of multiple existing studies concluded that aggressive or inappropriate lateral retinacular release of the knee joint leads to medial instability. Level of evidence: IV.

32. Palmu S, Kallio PE, Donell ST, Helenius I, Nietosvaara Y: Acute patellar dislocation in children and adolescents: A randomized clinical trial. *J Bone Joint Surg Am* 2008;90(3):463-470.

33. Boddula MR, Adamson GJ, Pink MM: Medial reefing without lateral release for recurrent patellar instability: Midterm and long-term outcomes. *Am J Sports Med* 2014;42(1):216-224.

The authors of this case series found that arthroscopically assisted medial reefing without lateral release is an effective long-term treatment for patients with recurrent patellar instability and normal bony anatomy. Level of evidence: IV.

34. Insall J, Bullough PG, Burstein AH: Proximal "tube" realignment of the patella for chondromalacia patellae. *Clin Orthop Relat Res* 1979;144:63-69.

35. Schüttler KF, Struewer J, Roessler PP, et al: Patellofemoral osteoarthritis after Insall's proximal realignment for recurrent patellar dislocation. *Knee Surg Sports Traumatol Arthrosc* 2014;22(11):2623-2628.

This case series demonstrated that patellofemoral osteoarthritis progressed after proximal realignment. Level of evidence: IV.

36. Stephen JM, Lumpaopong P, Dodds AL, Williams A, Amis AA: The effect of tibial tuberosity medialization and lateralization on patellofemoral joint kinematics, contact mechanics, and stability. *Am J Sports Med* 2015;43(1):186-194.

This controlled laboratory study evaluated the effects of medialization and lateralization of the tibial tubercle on patellofemoral joint kinematics, contact pressure, and stability.

37. Warner BT, Kamath GV, Spang JT, Weinhold PS, Creighton RA: Comparison of fixation methods after anteromedialization osteotomy of the tibial tubercle for patellar instability. *Arthroscopy* 2013;29(10):1628-1634.

The authors of this cadaver study examined the biomechanical strength of two screw configurations for tibial tubercle fixation after osteotomy.

38. Ahmad R, Calciu M, Jayasekera N, Schranz P, Mandalia V: Combined medial patellofemoral ligament reconstruction and tibial tubercle osteotomy: Results at a mean follow-up of two years. *Bone Joint J* 2015;97-B(suppl 10):8.

This study described good results in a series of patients treated with MPFL reconstruction and tibial tubercle osteotomy.

39. Marsh JS, Daigneault JP, Sethi P, Polzhofer GK: Treatment of recurrent patellar instability with a modification of the Roux-Goldthwait technique. *J Pediatr Orthop* 2006;26(4):461-465.

40. Weinberger JM, Fabricant PD, Taylor SA, Mei JY, Jones KJ: Influence of graft source and configuration on revision rate and patient-reported outcomes after MPFL reconstruction: A systematic review and meta-analysis. *Knee Surg Sports Traumatol Arthrosc* 2016;Feb 6 [Epub ahead of print].

The authors of this systematic review examined the influence of the graft source (allograft versus autograft) and the configuration (single- versus double-limbed) on the failure rate and outcomes of MPFL reconstruction. No difference was found between graft sources with regard to revision rates; however, it was concluded that a double-limbed configuration should be used. Level of evidence: IV.

41. Howells NR, Barnett AJ, Ahearn N, Ansari A, Eldridge JD: Medial patellofemoral ligament reconstruction: A

prospective outcome assessment of a large single centre series. *J Bone Joint Surg Br* 2012;94(9):1202-1208.

This prospective case series examined outcomes after MPFL reconstruction.

42. Nelitz M, Dreyhaupt J, Reichel H, Woelfle J, Lippacher S: Anatomic reconstruction of the medial patellofemoral ligament in children and adolescents with open growth plates: Surgical technique and clinical outcome. *Am J Sports Med* 2013;41(1):58-63.

    A technique for physis-respecting MPFL reconstruction in skeletally immature patients is described. Level of evidence: IV.

43. Noyes FR, Albright JC: Reconstruction of the medial patellofemoral ligament with autologous quadriceps tendon. *Arthroscopy* 2006;22(8):904.e1-904.e7, 904.e7.

44. Shah JN, Howard JS, Flanigan DC, Brophy RH, Carey JL, Lattermann C: A systematic review of complications and failures associated with medial patellofemoral ligament reconstruction for recurrent patellar dislocation. *Am J Sports Med* 2012;40(8):1916-1923.

    A meta-analysis of MPFL reconstructions reported an overall complication rate of 26.1%.

45. Kearney SP, Mosca VS: Selective hemiepiphyseodesis for patellar instability with associated genu valgum. *J Orthop* 2015;12(1):17-22.

    A case series review of 26 knees with patellar instability and genu valgum treated with hemiepiphysiodesis is presented.

46. McNamara I, Bua N, Smith TO, Ali K, Donell ST: Deepening trochleoplasty with a thick osteochondral flap for patellar instability: Clinical and functional outcomes at a mean 6-year follow-up. *Am J Sports Med* 2015;43(11):2706-2713.

    Good results after trochleoplasty for patients with patellar instability and trochlear dysplasia were reported in this case series. Level of evidence: IV.

47. Ntagiopoulos PG, Byn P, Dejour D: Midterm results of comprehensive surgical reconstruction including sulcus-deepening trochleoplasty in recurrent patellar dislocations with high-grade trochlear dysplasia. *Am J Sports Med* 2013;41(5):998-1004.

    Good midterm results after trochleoplasty for patients with patellar instability and trochlear dysplasia were reported in this case series. Level of evidence: IV.

48. Nelitz M, Dreyhaupt J, Lippacher S: Combined trochleoplasty and medial patellofemoral ligament reconstruction for recurrent patellar dislocations in severe trochlear dysplasia: A minimum 2-year follow-up study. *Am J Sports Med* 2013;41(5):1005-1012.

    The authors report good results after MPFL reconstruction and trochleoplasty for patients with patellar instability and trochlear dysplasia. Level of evidence: III.

49. Bowers AL, Shubin Stein BE: Complications of patellar stabilization surgery. *Oper Tech Sports Med* 2010;18(2):123-128.

50. Fisher B, Nyland J, Brand E, Curtin B: Medial patellofemoral ligament reconstruction for recurrent patellar dislocation: A systematic review including rehabilitation and return-to-sports efficacy. *Arthroscopy* 2010;26(10):1384-1394.

51. Lippacher S, Dreyhaupt J, Williams SR, Reichel H, Nelitz M: Reconstruction of the medial patellofemoral ligament: Clinical outcomes and return to sports. *Am J Sports Med* 2014;42(7):1661-1668.

    Two years after MPFL reconstruction most patients were able to return to sports participation, at least at a recreational level. Level of evidence: IV.

Chapter 44

Osteochondritis Dissecans of the Knee and Elbow

Matthew D. Milewski, MD Marc A. Tompkins, MD Kevin G. Shea, MD Theodore J. Ganley, MD

Abstract

Osteochondritis dissecans commonly affects the knee and elbow, particularly in young, athletic individuals. An understanding of the epidemiology, pathophysiology, clinical presentation, diagnostic imaging characteristics, and nonsurgical and surgical treatment options is important to optimize patient outcomes.

Keywords: capitellum; cartilage repair; elbow; knee; OCD; osteochondritis dissecans; osteoarthritis; osteochondrosis

Introduction

Osteochondritis dissecans (OCD) is a disease that continues to challenge surgeons, medical providers, and patients and their families. A current working definition of OCD states it is a focal, idiopathic alteration of subchondral bone with risk for instability and disruption of adjacent articular cartilage that may result in premature osteoarthritis.[1] Despite the relatively low incidence of OCD in the general population, this condition is encountered in most orthopaedic and sports medicine clinics, and the American Academy of Orthopaedic Surgeons has produced a clinical practice guideline for the diagnosis and treatment of OCD of the knee.[2,3] Although many of the AAOS recommendations lack strong evidence from the literature, they have helped guide future research efforts for this vexing condition.

Osteochondritis Dissecans of the Knee

Epidemiology

Recent data from a large US managed healthcare system has estimated the incidence of OCD of the knee in patients between age 6 and 19 years as 9.5 per 100,000 individuals overall.[4] In that population, patients aged 12 to 19 years had a 3.3 times greater risk of OCD compared with patients aged 6 to 11 years, with males having a 3.8 times greater risk of OCD compared with females. This study suggested a rate of bilaterality of 7%, but another recent study suggested the rate of bilaterality was as high as 29%.[5] In patients presenting for treatment of an OCD lesion, 40% of contralateral OCD lesions were asymptomatic. The authors of a 2014 study found the incidence of knee lesions to be 64% in the medial femoral condyle, 32% in the lateral femoral condyle, and less than 4% in the patella, trochlear groove, and tibial plateau.[4] Although lesions of the trochlea and patella are rare, recent reports suggest that 38% of trochlear lesions are unstable, and there is another type of coexistent OCD lesion in 24% of knees with a trochlear lesion.[6,7] Another recent report found that in patients with multifocal lesions within the knee, 74% of the lesions required surgical treatment.[8]

Pathophysiology

Historically, OCD was thought to be caused by inflammation, but this theory has since been refuted. The potential etiologies of OCD lesions include trauma, repetitive

Dr. Milewski or an immediate family member serves as a board member, owner, officer, or committee member of the Pediatric Orthopaedic Society of North America. Dr. Shea or an immediate family member serves as an unpaid consultant to Clinical Data Solutions and SourceTrust and serves as a board member, owner, officer, or committee member of the Pediatric Orthopaedic Society of North America; Pediatric Research in Sport Medicine Society; and Research for OsteoChondritis Dissecans of the Knee Study Group. Neither of the following authors nor any immediate family member has received anything of value from or has stock or stock options held in a commercial company or institution related directly or indirectly to the subject of this chapter: Dr. Tompkins and Dr. Ganley.

injury, overload resulting from malalignment, and genetic predisposition. A recent study examining potential genetic links for OCD found potential loci suggesting association with OCD.[9,10] Some authors have recently proposed genetic links to vitamin D insufficiency and fluoroquinolone use.[11,12]

OCD is referred to as osteochondrosis in the veterinary literature and has caprine, porcine, bovine, and equine models.[13-15] Osteochondrosis is the leading cause of lameness in horses and leg weakness in pigs, and parathyroid hormone receptor has been identified as a strong candidate gene in equine and bovine models.[9] These animal models also have been used to reexamine the potential vascular etiology of OCD lesions. CT and MRI coupled with histologic sectioning have confirmed an area of subchondral vascular failure in a porcine model.[14,16] It is hoped that additional animal studies will aid in determining potential vascular etiologies and genetic predispositions for OCD in humans.

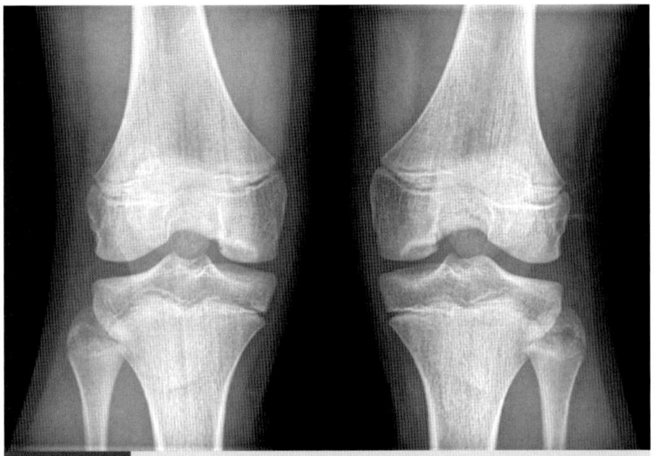

Figure 1 Notch radiograph of the knees of a 13-year-old-boy with bilateral knee pain shows evidence of bilateral lesions of the medial femoral condyle. (Reproduced with permission from St. Luke's Clinic, Intermountain Orthopaedics, Boise, ID).

History and Physical Examination

Patients with OCD of the knee can have a wide range of symptoms that may be benign for an extended period. Occasional, activity-related pain without swelling is noted in patients with stable lesions and often only progresses to limping, swelling, and mechanical symptoms in patients with advanced lesions.

Physical examination findings are typically subtle unless unstable, advanced lesions are present. Mild effusion or tenderness to palpation over the lesion site may be noted. The Wilson sign may elicit pain with internal tibial rotation as the knee is extended, particularly in patients with lesions of the medial femoral condyle. However, the Wilson sign is positive in only 25% of patients with a known OCD lesion.[17] Physical examination results in some patients with OCD lesions may be entirely normal. Occasionally, these lesions are found during the workup for unrelated trauma.

Radiographic Evaluation

Radiographic evaluation of children and adolescents with knee pain is essential when making a diagnosis of OCD because the physical examination findings are often nonspecific. Radiographic studies should include AP, lateral, sunrise, and notch views. Some OCD lesions may be missed if sunrise and notch views are not obtained. The authors of a 2015 study advocated obtaining bilateral radiographs because of the reported high rate (29%) of bilateral lesions[5] (**Figure 1**). Weight-bearing radiographs or radiographs of the left hand and wrist can help determine bone age and may be necessary if surgical intervention is being considered.[18]

Recently, a multicenter research group identified specific radiographic features of OCD lesions, including location, epiphyseal plate maturity, size, fragmentation, displacement, boundary, central radiodensity, and contour.[19] These features have been found to correlate with stability and therefore have prognostic value. The authors of a 2015 study found that a smaller intercondylar notch width index was associated with OCD of the medial femoral condyle.[20] This anatomic risk factor could contribute to impingement of the tibial eminence. Greater medial and posterior tibial slope has been reported in knees with lesions of the medial femoral condyle.[21] A 2010 study found an association between OCD lesions of the medial femoral condyle and varus alignment and between OCD lesions of the lateral femoral condyle and valgus alignment.[18] Further studies are needed to define the most reliable specific radiographic features that correlate with prognosis and healing.

Three-phase bone scans and CT have been replaced to a substantial extent by MRI as the imaging modality of choice for the initial assessment of articular cartilage integrity, subchondral bone status, and OCD lesion instability. In adult patients, MRI criteria for the assessment of unstable lesions include a hyperintense signal seen on T2-weighted MRI sequences at the fragment-femur interface, an adjacent cystic area (high-signal intensity line), a focal defect in the articular cartilage (>5 mm), and a hyperintense signal line equal to fluid that traverses both the articular cartilage and subchondral bone.[22] The presence of all of the criteria is not needed to make the diagnosis of an unstable OCD lesion. The authors of a 2008 study described MRI criteria for juvenile patients as follows: a

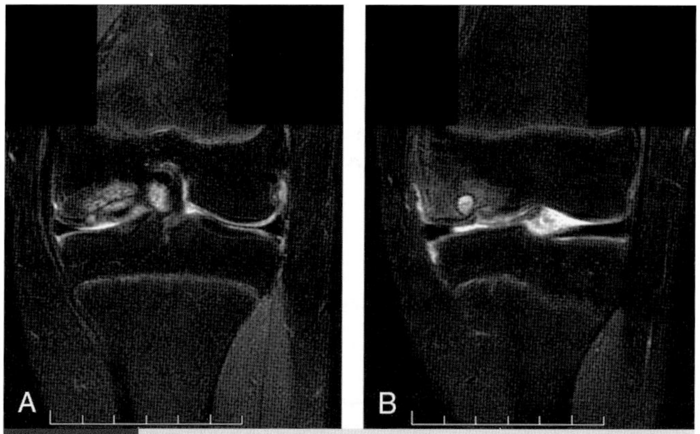

Figure 2 MRIs of the knees of a 13-year-old girl with an osteochondritis dissecans lesion of the medial femoral condyle **(A)**; note the cyst-like structure (**B**). (Reproduced with permission from Milewski MD, Nissen CW, Shea K: Treatment of juvenile osteochondritis dissecans of the knee, in Diduch D, Bedi A: *Insall and Scott: Surgery of the Knee*, ed 6. Philadelphia, PA, Elsevier, in press.)

rim-like, hyperintense signal equal to joint fluid, plus a second, deeper linear margin of low signal, plus multiple sites of discontinuity of subchondral bone.[23] These MRI criteria were 100% sensitive and specific for instability in this younger population. (**Figure 2**) The authors also found that multiple cyst-like foci or a single cyst-like focus greater than 5 mm in size was highly specific for instability (100%) but had low sensitivity (25% to 38%). A 2013 study, which assessed the diagnostic performance of three-dimensional gradient-recalled echo sequence T1-weighted MRIs combined with routine sequences, also showed exceptional sensitivity, specificity, and accuracy in the detection of unstable OCD lesions in juveniles.[24]

Treatment

Treatment of OCD lesions of the knee in young patients can vary depending on the age of the patient and the location, size, and stability of the lesion. Goals of treatment, especially in young patients, include saving the native fragment if possible and preventing osteoarthritis through early detection and prompt treatment.

Nonsurgical

Nonsurgical treatment may achieve successful healing of OCD lesions in younger patients, particularly those with open physes. Nonsurgical treatment is recommended in patients with open physes, minimal symptoms, and stable lesions on initial imaging. The age of the patient, size of the lesion, and presence or absence of mechanical symptoms each play a role in the predictability of healing.[25] To predict healing, the authors of a 2013 study developed a nomogram that included the age of the patient, the size of the normalized region, and the size of cyst-like lesions as demonstrated on MRI.[26] Healing may take 6 to 12 months with activity restrictions, bracing, and/or casting. No consensus exists on the exact methods that should be used in nonsurgical treatment.

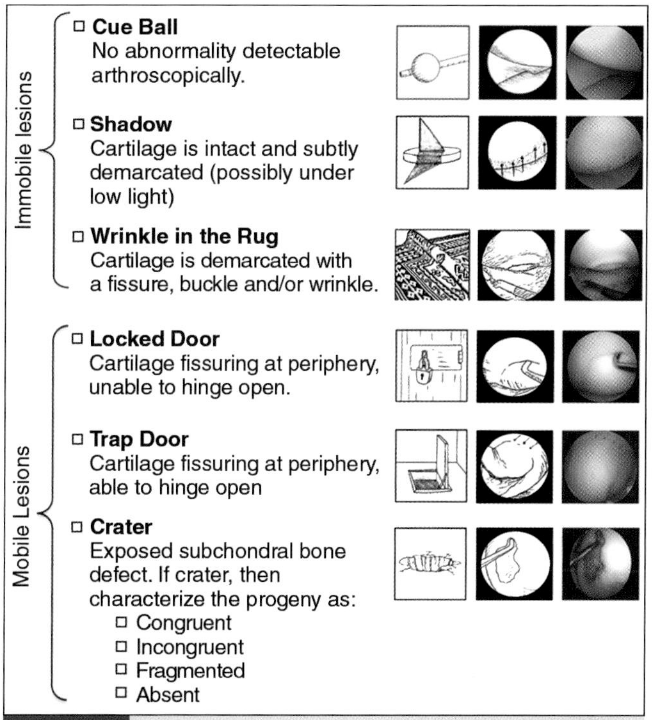

Figure 3 Image depicts the Research on OsteoChondritis Dissecans of the Knee Arthroscopy Classification System to better assess the stability of osteochondritis dissecans lesions. (Reproduced with permission from Milewski MD, Nissen CW, Shea K: Treatment of juvenile osteochondritis dissecans of the knee, in Diduch D, Bedi A: *Insall and Scott: Surgery of the Knee*, ed 6. Philadelphia, PA, Elsevier, in press.)

Surgical

If nonsurgical treatment is unsuccessful or the OCD lesions are interpreted to be unstable at the time of initial diagnosis, surgical treatment is an option. A variety of surgical options are available depending on the size and stability of the lesion, age of the patient, and the need for salvage treatment because of a nonviable native fragment. In general, surgical treatment begins with arthroscopic assessment of the lesion's stability. Multiple prior classifications have been described but lack rigorous assessment of interrater and intrarater reliability.[27] A multicenter OCD research group has developed and validated a new arthroscopic classification system to help better assess lesion stability (**Figure 3**).

Many surgical techniques and implants are available for lesion stabilization. The goals of OCD treatment

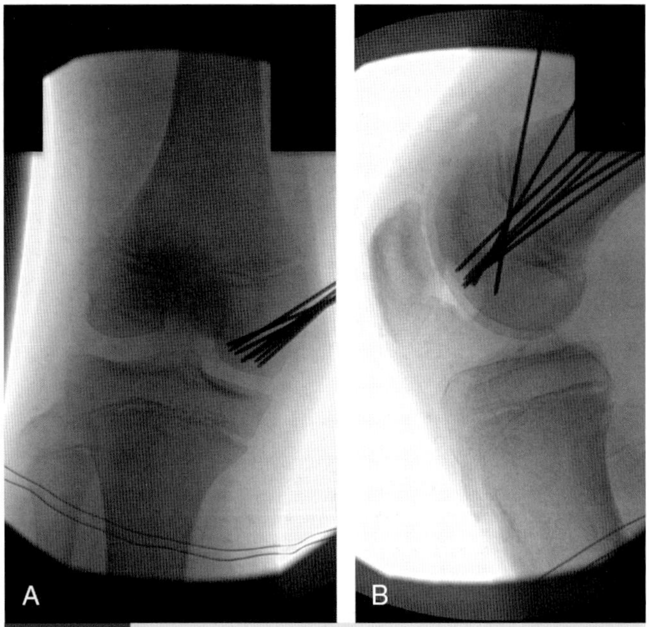

Figure 4 AP (**A**) and lateral (**B**) fluoroscopic images of the knee of a 12-year-old girl with an osteochondritis dissecans lesion of the medial femoral condyle. After nonsurgical treatment failed, the patient underwent arthroscopy. The lesion was found to be stable and the lesion was treated with retroarticular drilling of the subchondral bone. (Reproduced with permission from Milewski MD, Nissen CW, Shea K: Treatment of juvenile osteochondritis dissecans of the knee, in Diduch D, Bedi A: *Insall and Scott: Surgery of the Knee*, ed 6. Philadelphia, PA, Elsevier, in press.)

include drilling to stimulate or incite a vascular healing response to the avascular subchondral bone; fixation to stabilize loose subchondral bone and articular cartilage; bone grafting when needed to support contour, stability, and vascularity of articular cartilage; and, when needed, salvage of articular cartilage and subchondral bone with biologic replacements. A recent review of the literature found surgical excision of the OCD lesion without a salvage procedure to be the only surgical treatment with clear evidence for inferior results.[28]

Drilling of the subchondral bone adjacent to an OCD lesion is performed to stimulate a vascular healing response by disrupting the sclerotic margin and introducing biologic factors from adjacent, healthier cancellous bone.[29] A variety of drilling techniques have been described. The two main techniques can be divided into transarticular drilling (through the articular cartilage into the subchondral bone) and retroarticular drilling (from behind the lesion through the subchondral bone into the lesion but not through the articular cartilage)[29-31] (**Figure 4**). Intercondylar notch drilling along with retroarticular drilling with bone grafting also have been described.[32,33] No studies have shown superiority of one drilling technique over another, and reported outcomes for properly chosen younger patients with fairly stable lesions have been good.[29]

Fixation of unstable OCD lesions as demonstrated on preoperative imaging and/or confirmed at the time of arthroscopy can be performed with a variety of fixation devices.[34] Fixation with metal screws (headed or headless), bioabsorbable screws or implants, and biologic fixation have been described.[35] Metal screws offer the advantage of rigid fixation without a potential synovitic response to a bioabsorbable device but may require hardware removal. In addition, metal screws can complicate follow-up MRIs. Bioabsorbable screws and implants do not require hardware removal and do not impede postoperative MRI but have the potential for hardware failure and synovitis-type reactions.[36-38] Biologic fixation with small osteochondral autograft transplantation (OAT) plugs has also been described along with a hybrid technique combining biologic fixation using an OAT plug with metal screw fixation.[39] Future prospective studies are needed to determine whether an advantage exists for the use of specific fixation devices (**Table 1**).

Salvage procedures should be considered when fixation or previous excision procedures have been unsuccessful. Marrow stimulation procedures have been used in the treatment of OCD lesions but the additional subchondral bone loss associated with OCD lesions makes marrow stimulation techniques challenging in these patients. Microfracture has been shown to produce results inferior to those of other techniques such as OAT in adult populations with chondral defects of varying etiologies.[40] Biologic restoration of both the subchondral bone and the articular cartilage surface is an advantage of OAT both in terms of lesion fixation and salvage.[39,41] Limitations to OAT include lesion size and donor site morbidity; however, donor knee function was not adversely affected in younger patients after osteochondral autograft harvesting.[42]

Fresh frozen osteochondral allografts can address some of the limitations associated with OAT and have been used to treat large OCD lesions in two studies.[43,44] No donor site morbidity exists with fresh frozen osteochondral allografts, and they can be used to address much larger defects. Disadvantages of fresh frozen osteochondral allografts include concerns about lack of bone integration between the graft and the host, host immune response, and chondrocyte viability after transplantation. A 2007 study showed the 5-year survivorship rate to be 91%.[43] Further studies are needed to address the long-term viability of these allografts as salvage for large OCD lesions in a young patient population.

Table 1

Bioabsorbable Versus Metal Implants for Osteochondritis Dissecans Fixation

Implant	Advantages	Disadvantages
Bioabsorbable	Removal may not be necessary Does not produce substantial artifact with MRI	Concerns about strength and implant failure Incomplete absorption Backing out from bone May result in substantial cyst formation around implants
Metal	Does not leave cystic lesions during screw absorption Titanium screws may induce less MRI artifact	May produce substantial artifact on MRI studies Removal may be necessary if close to cartilage surface and not recessed within stable bone Backing out from bone

Autologous chondrocyte implantation (ACI) is another technique that can be used to salvage knees with OCD. Long-term results of ACI show good survivorship rates and clinical outcomes for osteochondral defect treatment, and ACI provides the advantage of using the patient's own chondrocytes. One disadvantage of treatment of OCD of the knee with ACI is the cost of a second procedure. In addition, ACI does not necessarily address the subchondral bone deficiency associated with OCD lesions unless concomitant bone grafting is done. Midterm results have been promising for the use of ACI with bone grafting in the treatment of OCD of the knee.[45] Long-term studies are needed to confirm these results and examine other newer-generation cartilage regeneration options such as minced juvenile cartilage in the treatment and salvage of knees with OCD.

Osteochondritis Dissecans of the Elbow

Epidemiology and Pathophysiology

The exact incidence of OCD of the elbow is unknown. Although the condition is rare, a prevalence as high as 3% and possibly higher has been documented in young athletes in certain sports.[46,47] Participants in baseball, gymnastics, and other overhead sports are at relatively high risk for this condition.[46,47] Those who begin play at a young age, play for longer periods, or experience elbow pain have a higher risk for OCD.[46] In many athletes, the cause of OCD is thought to be related to overload of the lateral compartment of the elbow[48] and perhaps limitations in elbow vascularity. The possible vascular etiology for elbow OCD is thought to be caused by a vascular watershed area in the location of an OCD lesion.[49] Secondary overload in these areas may also enhance the risk of development and/or progression of the condition.[49]

OCD of the elbow and Panner disease may represent different stages of a related condition. Historically, Panner disease has been described in patients younger than 10 years; in many patients, the condition will resolve with time.[50] OCD of the elbow is thought to arise in older patients and, in many patients, these lesions do not heal.[51]

History and Physical Examination

Many young patients with OCD of the elbow have relatively minor symptoms, including occasional mechanical symptoms, minimal loss of motion, and occasional effusion.[52] In some patients, the only notable physical examination finding may be a 5° to 10° loss of full extension compared with the contralateral elbow.

Radiographic Evaluation

Most OCD lesions of the elbow can be seen on plain radiographs. However, certain aspects of the lesions may be better seen with MRI, such as surrounding bone edema, cystic change, loose bodies, or more subtle lesions not fully appreciated on radiographs[53] (**Figures 5** and **6**). Some of these findings can affect clinical decision-making for specific treatments. Newer techniques of cartilage evaluation, including those with ultrasound, may complement other forms of advanced imaging in the future.[54]

Treatment

Nonsurgical

Younger patients with substantial growth remaining may respond well to activity modifications. In some patients, both rest and short periods of immobilization may be beneficial. For throwing athletes, switching to another position may be valuable, such as having a pitcher play as a first baseman.

Surgical

For patients who do not respond to activity modifications and/or restrictions, surgical intervention may be necessary.[55-57] Larger lesions, including those that expand to involve the lateral wall and those with intra-articular loose bodies, may progress to surgery more frequently

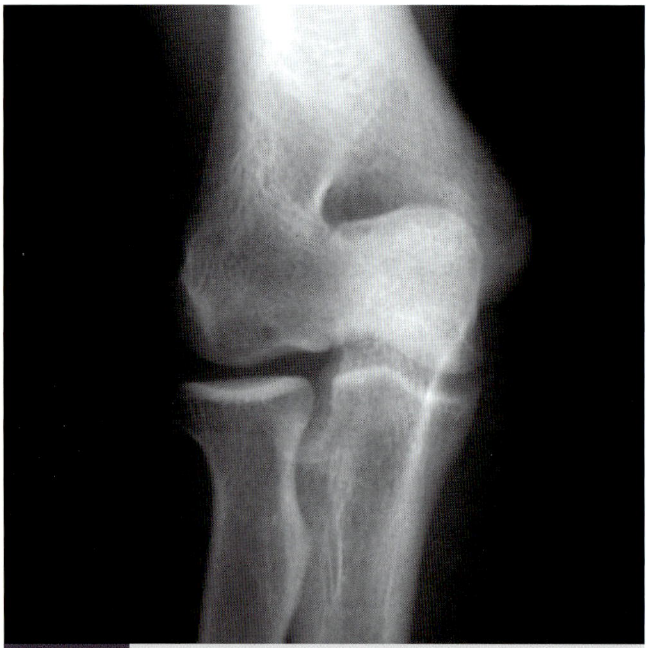

Figure 5 AP radiograph shows an osteochondritis dissecans lesion of the elbow. (Reproduced with permission from St. Luke's Clinic, Intermountain Orthopaedics, Boise, ID.)

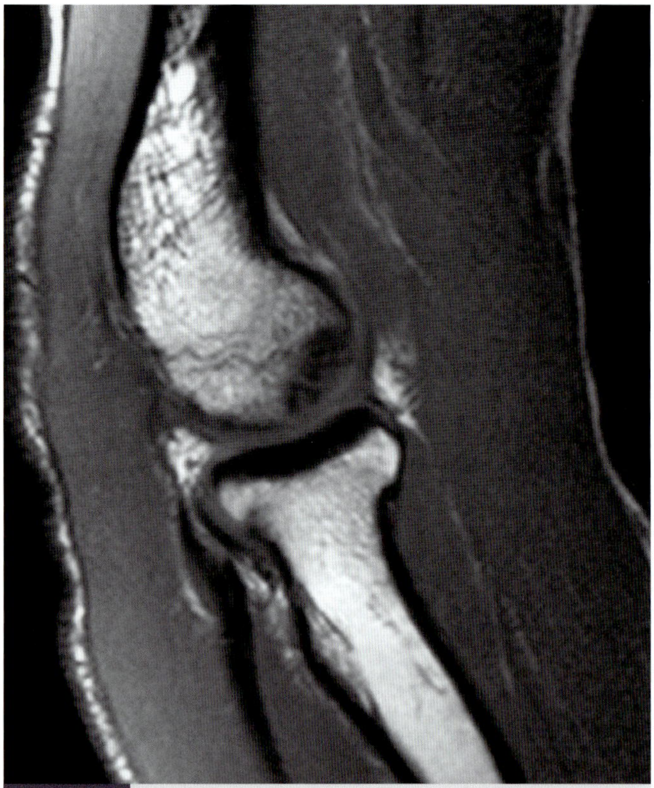

Figure 6 Sagittal MRI shows osteochondritis dissecans of the elbow. (Reproduced with permission from St. Luke's Clinic, Intermountain Orthopaedics, Boise, ID.)

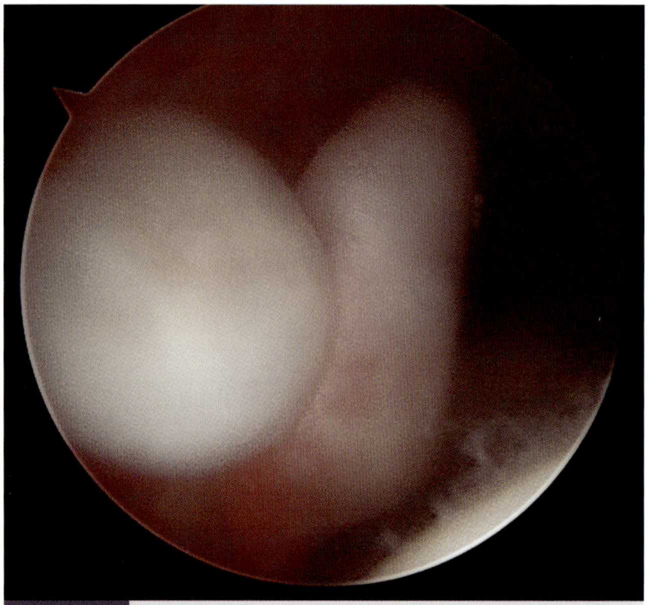

Figure 7 Arthroscopic view depicts osteochondritis dissecans of the elbow with intra-articular free bodies. (Reproduced with permission from St. Luke's Clinic, Intermountain Orthopaedics, Boise, ID.)

than small lesions (**Figure 7**). The authors of a 2011 study developed a staging system that may be helpful for the evaluation and management of this condition.[58] Most of the published series on OCD of the elbow represent level IV evidence, so surgical treatment recommendations must be understood in that context.[55,59]

Arthroscopic débridement with and without drilling has shown reasonable outcomes in shorter-term follow-ups, although outcomes are limited in longer-term follow-ups for those that participate in throwing sports; gymnastics; and other high-demand, upper extremity athletic activities.[56,60,61] Larger or uncontained lesions may have a worse prognosis than contained lesions.[52] To address these larger or uncontained lesions, the harvest of osteochondral autografts from the knee and mosaicplasty procedures have been reported.[62-64]Accessing the joint to treat certain size lesions at some locations can be technically challenging, so novel techniques, including the use of oblique grafts, have been developed to address challenges with joint access.[65]

Summary

OCD of the knee and elbow continue to be a challenging disease process in regard to diagnosis, prognosis, and treatment. The goals of treatment, whether surgical or nonsurgical, are to resolve symptoms and retain as much normal bone and cartilage as possible at the lesion site. Multicenter prospective studies are needed to assess optimal outcomes and refine treatment algorithms.

Key Study Points

- Radiographic evaluations are essential when diagnosing an OCD lesion of the knee and elbow; however, important aspects of the OCD lesions may be better seen with MRI. Diagnostic imaging modalities continue to evolve.
- Assessing the potential instability of an OCD lesion is key to early treatment.
- Surgical intervention should be considered for patients that have unstable OCD lesions of the knee and elbow and/or OCD lesions that do not heal with nonsurgical treatment such as activity modification.
- Surgical treatment of OCD of the knee and elbow can involve drilling, fixation, or salvage techniques depending on the stability of the native fragment.

Annotated References

1. Edmonds EW, Shea KG: Osteochondritis dissecans: Editorial comment. *Clin Orthop Relat Res* 2013;471(4):1105-1106.

   In this symposium, the histology, natural history, outcomes, and treatment of OCD were reviewed, and a working definition of OCD was developed.

2. Chambers HG, Shea KG, Anderson AF, et al; American Academy of Orthopedic Surgeons: Diagnosis and treatment of osteochondritis dissecans. *J Am Acad Orthop Surg* 2011;19(5):297-306.

   Clinical questions regarding the evaluation and treatment of OCD of the knee are presented.

3. Chambers HG, Shea KG, Anderson AF, et al; American Academy of Orthopaedic Surgeons: American Academy of Orthopaedic Surgeons clinical practice guideline on: The diagnosis and treatment of osteochondritis dissecans. *J Bone Joint Surg Am* 2012;94(14):1322-1324.

   Sixteen clinical practice recommendations for the diagnosis and treatment of OCD of the knee are presented. This consensus statement will guide current practice and future research endeavors.

4. Kessler JI, Nikizad H, Shea KG, Jacobs JC Jr, Bebchuk JD, Weiss JM: The demographics and epidemiology of osteochondritis dissecans of the knee in children and adolescents. *Am J Sports Med* 2014;42(2):320-326.

   This study evaluated the demographics and epidemiology of OCD of the knee in children and adolescents. Patients aged 12 to 19 years had three times the risk of OCD of the knee compared with patients aged 6 to 11 years, and males had a greater incidence of OCD and almost four times the risk of OCD compared with females. Level of evidence: IV.

5. Cooper T, Boyles A, Samora WP, Klingele KE: Prevalence of bilateral JOCD of the knee and associated risk factors. *J Pediatr Orthop* 2015;35(5):507-510.

   The authors evaluated 108 juvenile patients with OCD of the knee. A 29% incidence of bilateral disease was found, and 40% of the contralateral lesions were found to be asymptomatic. Bilateral radiographic evaluation was recommended for all patients with juvenile OCD. Level of evidence: IV.

6. Kramer DE, Yen YM, Simoni MK, et al: Surgical management of osteochondritis dissecans lesions of the patella and trochlea in the pediatric and adolescent population. *Am J Sports Med* 2015;43(3):654-662.

   This study assessed the outcomes of surgical treatment of patellofemoral OCD in children and adolescents. The authors found that surgical treatment resulted in a high rate of satisfaction and return to sports. Risk factors associated with worse outcomes included female sex, a prolonged duration of symptoms, and internal fixation. Level of evidence: IV.

7. Wall EJ, Heyworth BE, Shea KG, et al: Trochlear groove osteochondritis dissecans of the knee patellofemoral joint. *J Pediatr Orthop* 2014;34(6):625-630.

   The authors found that MRI effectively aids in the diagnosis and staging of OCD of the trochlear groove. Level of evidence: IV.

8. Backes JR, Durbin TC, Bentley JC, Klingele KE: Multifocal juvenile osteochondritis dissecans of the knee: A case series. *J Pediatr Orthop* 2014;34(4):453-458.

   In this study of 28 patients with multifocal juvenile OCD, the authors found that lesions located on the medial femoral condyle healed at a statistically significant greater rate than other locations within the knee. The prognosis was not affected by sex, age, or associated discoid menisci. Level of evidence: IV.

9. Bates JT, Jacobs JC Jr, Shea KG, Oxford JT: Emerging genetic basis of osteochondritis dissecans. *Clin Sports Med* 2014;33(2):199-220.

   A review of the currently available literature supporting a genetic basis for OCD is presented. Parathyroid hormone receptor was found to have a strong link to OCD and was identified in both horses and pigs.

10. Yellin JL, Trocle A, Grant SF, Hakonarson H, Shea KG, Ganley TJ: Candidate loci are revealed by an initial genome-wide association study of juvenile osteochondritis dissecans. *J Pediatr Orthop* 2015.

In this study, the authors found that multiple single-nucleotide polymorphisms may be associated with a genetic basis for OCD.

11. Bruns J, Werner M, Soyka M: Is vitamin D insufficiency or deficiency related to the development of osteochondritis dissecans? *Knee Surg Sports Traumatol Arthrosc* 2014.

    In this review of mostly an adult population with OCD lesions, vitamin D_3 deficiency was associated with high-grade OCD lesions. Level of evidence: IV.

12. Jacobs JC Jr, Shea KG, Oxford JT, Carey JL: Fluoroquinolone use in a child associated with development of osteochondritis dissecans. *BMJ Case Rep* 2014;2014.

    The authors present a case report of a 10-year-old child who underwent a prolonged course of fluoroquinolone therapy for recurrent urinary tract infections. An OCD lesion of the medial femoral condyle subsequently developed. An association between fluoroquinolone use and OCD is described.

13. McCoy AM, Toth F, Dolvik NI, et al: Articular osteochondrosis: A comparison of naturally-occurring human and animal disease. *Osteoarthritis Cartilage* 2013;21(11):1638-1647.

    Links between osteochondrosis in animal models and OCD in humans were examined. Naturally occurring and surgically induced animal models may be useful for testing treatment options to improve treatment of OCD lesions in humans.

14. Olstad K, Ekman S, Carlson CS: An Update on the Pathogenesis of Osteochondrosis. *Vet Pathol* 2015;52(5):785-802.

    The origin of osteochondrosis in animals, particularly pigs and horses, was examined along with the link to OCD in humans. A vascular origin with ischemic chondronecrosis was examined and radiographic and histologic data were reviewed.

15. Tóth F, Nissi MJ, Wang L, Ellermann JM, Carlson CS: Surgical induction, histological evaluation, and MRI identification of cartilage necrosis in the distal femur in goats to model early lesions of osteochondrosis. *Osteoarthritis Cartilage* 2015;23(2):300-307.

    A goat model was used to induce cartilage necrosis similar to osteochondrosis and then examined with histologic confirmation and MRI examination using the adiabatic $T1\varrho$ sequence. The authors concluded that this technique may aid in the early diagnosis of osteochondrosis in the future.

16. Tóth F, Nissi MJ, Ellermann JM, et al: Novel application of magnetic resonance imaging demonstrates characteristic differences in vasculature at predilection sites of osteochondritis dissecans. *Am J Sports Med* 2015;43(10):2522-2527.

    A 9.4 Tesla MRI scanner was used to examine cadaver femurs from juvenile humans, pigs, and goats and delineate the epiphyseal vasculature. Humans and pigs were found to have similar distal predilection sites for OCD lesions and osteochondrosis.

17. Conrad JM, Stanitski CL: Osteochondritis dissecans: Wilson's sign revisited. *Am J Sports Med* 2003;31(5):777-778.

18. Jacobi M, Wahl P, Bouaicha S, Jakob RP, Gautier E: Association between mechanical axis of the leg and osteochondritis dissecans of the knee: Radiographic study on 103 knees. *Am J Sports Med* 2010;38(7):1425-1428.

19. Wall EJ, Polousky JD, Shea KG, et al; Research on OsteoChondritis Dissecans of the Knee (ROCK) Study Group: Novel radiographic feature classification of knee osteochondritis dissecans: A multicenter reliability study. *Am J Sports Med* 2015;43(2):303-309.

    The Research on OsteoChondritis Dissecans of the Knee group reviewed the radiographs of 45 knees with OCD lesions and reported excellent reliability for measuring sizes and growth plate maturity. In the subset of knees with visible bone in the lesion, the fragmentation, displacement, boundary, central radiodensity, and contour (concave/nonconcave) of the lesion bone were classified with moderate to substantial reliability. Level of evidence: III.

20. Chow RM, Guzman MS, Dao Q: Intercondylar notch width as a risk factor for medial femoral condyle osteochondritis dissecans in skeletally immature patients. *J Pediatr Orthop* 2015.

    Thirty-five patients with medial femoral condyle OCD lesions were compared with matched control subjects. The authors found a substantially smaller notch width index in patients with OCD lesions. Level of evidence: III.

21. Wechter JF, Sikka RS, Alwan M, Nelson BJ, Tompkins M: Proximal tibial morphology and its correlation with osteochondritis dissecans of the knee. *Knee Surg Sports Traumatol Arthrosc* 2015;23(12):3717-3722.

    Proximal tibial slope measurements were performed in 72 patients with OCD lesions and compared with normal control subjects. Knees with medial femoral condyle OCD lesions had greater medial tibial slope and posterior tibial slope when compared with the control subjects. Level of evidence: III.

22. De Smet AA, Ilahi OA, Graf BK: Reassessment of the MR criteria for stability of osteochondritis dissecans in the knee and ankle. *Skeletal Radiol* 1996;25(2):159-163.

23. Kijowski R, Blankenbaker DG, Shinki K, Fine JP, Graf BK, De Smet AA: Juvenile versus adult osteochondritis dissecans of the knee: Appropriate MR imaging criteria for instability. *Radiology* 2008;248(2):571-578.

24. Chen CH, Liu YS, Chou PH, Hsieh CC, Wang CK: MR grading system of osteochondritis dissecans lesions: Comparison with arthroscopy. *Eur J Radiol* 2013;82(3):518-525.

    This study evaluated the combined diagnostic performance of three-dimensional gradient-recalled echo T1-weighted MRIs and routine sequence MRIs for the evaluation of OCD as confirmed by arthroscopy. The sensitivity, specificity, and accuracy for detection of unstable OCD lesions were 100%, 100%, and 100% in juvenile lesions, respectively, and 93%, 100%, and 96% in adult lesions, respectively.

25. Wall EJ, Vourazeris J, Myer GD, et al: The healing potential of stable juvenile osteochondritis dissecans knee lesions. *J Bone Joint Surg Am* 2008;90(12):2655-2664.

26. Krause M, Hapfelmeier A, Möller M, Amling M, Bohndorf K, Meenen NM: Healing predictors of stable juvenile osteochondritis dissecans knee lesions after 6 and 12 months of nonoperative treatment. *Am J Sports Med* 2013;41(10):2384-2391.

    This study used a predictive model for healing potential of stable OCD lesions based on MRI findings. Age, size of cyst-like lesions, and normalized lesion width were most predictive of healing after 6 months. Cyst-like lesion size was most predictive of healing. Level of evidence: II.

27. Jacobs JC Jr, Archibald-Seiffer N, Grimm NL, Carey JL, Shea KG: A review of arthroscopic classification systems for osteochondritis dissecans of the knee. *Orthop Clin North Am* 2015;46(1):133-139.

    In this review of arthroscopic classification systems for OCD of the knee, the authors found no consensus regarding a universal system. The need to establish a clear, consistent, and reliable method for classifying OCD lesions of the knee during arthroscopy was described. Level of evidence: IV.

28. Trinh TQ, Harris JD, Flanigan DC: Surgical management of juvenile osteochondritis dissecans of the knee. *Knee Surg Sports Traumatol Arthrosc* 2012;20(12):2419-2429.

    This study evaluated clinical and radiographic outcomes at short-term, midterm, and long-term follow-ups and demonstrated that surgical treatment of juvenile OCD substantially improved clinical and radiographic outcomes after unsuccessful nonsurgical treatment. Level of evidence: IV.

29. Heyworth BE, Edmonds EW, Murnaghan ML, Kocher MS: Drilling techniques for osteochondritis dissecans. *Clin Sports Med* 2014;33(2):305-312.

    The authors reviewed the currently available indications and techniques for drilling in the treatment of OCD of the knee.

30. Boughanem J, Riaz R, Patel RM, Sarwark JF: Functional and radiographic outcomes of juvenile osteochondritis dissecans of the knee treated with extra-articular retrograde drilling. *Am J Sports Med* 2011;39(10):2212-2217.

    This study examined the outcomes of retrograde extra-articular drilling in juveniles with OCD of the knee. In most juveniles with OCD lesions in whom nonsurgical treatment had failed, the authors found that retrograde extra-articular drilling resulted in clinical and radiographic improvement. Level of evidence: IV.

31. Gunton MJ, Carey JL, Shaw CR, Murnaghan ML: Drilling juvenile osteochondritis dissecans: Retro- or transarticular? *Clin Orthop Relat Res* 2013;471(4):1144-1151.

    This systematic review of the literature in regards to transarticular versus retroarticular drilling modalities for OCD lesions demonstrated excellent healing rates for both techniques (91% versus 86%, respectively) with no complications reported.

32. Kawasaki K, Uchio Y, Adachi N, Iwasa J, Ochi M: Drilling from the intercondylar area for treatment of osteochondritis dissecans of the knee joint. *Knee* 2003;10(3):257-263.

33. Lykissas MG, Wall EJ, Nathan S: Retro-articular drilling and bone grafting of juvenile knee osteochondritis dissecans: A technical description. *Knee Surg Sports Traumatol Arthrosc* 2014;22(2):274-278.

    A technique for retroarticular drilling for the management of stable juvenile OCD lesions of the knee was described. The authors concluded that the use of a bone marrow biopsy needle could facilitate bone grafting when compared with previously described techniques. Level of evidence: V.

34. Grimm NL, Ewing CK, Ganley TJ: The knee: Internal fixation techniques for osteochondritis dissecans. *Clin Sports Med* 2014;33(2):313-319.

    After a diagnosis of OCD is made in an athlete, the stability of the lesion should be determined. The athlete's level of play, type of sport, and overall goals should be considered when choosing the fixation method. Level of evidence: IV.

35. Webb JE, Lewallen LW, Christophersen C, Krych AJ, McIntosh AL: Clinical outcome of internal fixation of unstable juvenile osteochondritis dissecans lesions of the knee. *Orthopedics* 2013;36(11):e1444-e1449.

    This retrospective study evaluated the use of bioabsorbable versus metal screw fixation for OCD lesions of the knee. The authors found that osseous integration was evident in 15 of 20 knees (75%) at final follow-up. Bioabsorbable fixation for symptomatic stable lesions and metal compression screws with staged removal for unstable lesions was recommended.

36. Adachi N, Deie M, Nakamae A, Okuhara A, Kamei G, Ochi M: Functional and radiographic outcomes of unstable juvenile osteochondritis dissecans of the knee treated with lesion fixation using bioabsorbable pins. *J Pediatr Orthop* 2015;35(1):82-88.

    In this study, the functional and radiographic outcomes of fixation of unstable juvenile OCD of the knee were evaluated. The use of bioabsorbable pins resulted in improved clinical outcomes and high healing rates at a mean follow-up of 3.3 years. The authors recommended this procedure for patients with unstable juvenile OCD lesions of sufficient quality to enable fixation. Level of evidence: IV.

37. Camathias C, Festring JD, Gaston MS: Bioabsorbable lag screw fixation of knee osteochondritis dissecans in the skeletally immature. *J Pediatr Orthop B* 2011;20(2):74-80.

    The authors found that simple arthroscopic fixation of OCD with biodegradable lag screws resulted in substantial improvement in function in pediatric patients. Level of evidence: IV.

8: Sports-Related Topics

38. Camathias C, Gögüs U, Hirschmann MT, et al: Implant failure after biodegradable screw fixation in osteochondritis dissecans of the knee in skeletally immature patients. *Arthroscopy* 2015;31(3):410-415.

This series reported a 23% rate of failure of bioabsorbable screws associated with OCD lesion fixation. Level of evidence: IV.

39. Lintz F, Pujol N, Pandeirada C, Boisrenoult P, Beaufils P: Hybrid fixation: Evaluation of a novel technique in adult osteochondritis dissecans of the knee. *Knee Surg Sports Traumatol Arthrosc* 2011;19(4):568-571.

A promising technique that combines biologic fixation using an autograft osteochondral plug with metallic screw fixation is described. Level of evidence: IV.

40. Gudas R, Kalesinskas RJ, Kimtys V, et al: A prospective randomized clinical study of mosaic osteochondral autologous transplantation versus microfracture for the treatment of osteochondral defects in the knee joint in young athletes. *Arthroscopy* 2005;21(9):1066-1075.

41. Miura K, Ishibashi Y, Tsuda E, Sato H, Toh S: Results of arthroscopic fixation of osteochondritis dissecans lesion of the knee with cylindrical autogenous osteochondral plugs. *Am J Sports Med* 2007;35(2):216-222.

42. Nishimura A, Morita A, Fukuda A, Kato K, Sudo A: Functional recovery of the donor knee after autologous osteochondral transplantation for capitellar osteochondritis dissecans. *Am J Sports Med* 2011;39(4):838-842.

This study of 12 patients with severe capitellar OCD demonstrated a time lag in recovery between postoperative symptoms and muscle power at 3 months. The authors found that harvesting osteochondral grafts had no adverse effects on function of the donor knee in young athletes at 2 years following OAT for capitellar OCD. Level of evidence: IV.

43. Emmerson BC, Görtz S, Jamali AA, Chung C, Amiel D, Bugbee WD: Fresh osteochondral allografting in the treatment of osteochondritis dissecans of the femoral condyle. *Am J Sports Med* 2007;35(6):907-914.

44. Lyon R, Nissen C, Liu XC, Curtin B: Can fresh osteochondral allografts restore function in juveniles with osteochondritis dissecans of the knee? *Clin Orthop Relat Res* 2013;471(4):1166-1173.

The authors suggested that fresh osteochondral allografts restored short-term function in juvenile patients whose juvenile OCD did not respond to standard treatments. Level of evidence: IV.

45. Filardo G, Kon E, Berruto M, et al: Arthroscopic second generation autologous chondrocytes implantation associated with bone grafting for the treatment of knee osteochondritis dissecans: Results at 6 years. *Knee* 2012;19(5):658-663.

The authors found that second-generation ACI associated with bone grafting was a valid treatment option for OCD of the knee and resulted in a statistically significant improvement in all test scores at a mean follow-up of 6 years postoperatively. Level of evidence: IV.

46. Kida Y, Morihara T, Kotoura Y, et al: Prevalence and clinical characteristics of osteochondritis dissecans of the humeral capitellum among adolescent baseball players. *Am J Sports Med* 2014;42(8):1963-1971.

In a study of adolescent baseball players in Japan, an incidence of OCD of the elbow of 3.4% was noted. Risk factors included beginning play at earlier ages, playing for longer periods, and experiencing more elbow pain. Level of evidence: III.

47. Dexel J, Marschner K, Beck H, et al: Comparative study of elbow disorders in young high-performance gymnasts. *Int J Sports Med* 2014;35(11):960-965.

The authors report on 30 young, high-performance gymnasts who were evaluated with MRIs of the elbow; 7 of the athletes were found to have OCD of the capitellum. The control group of athletes who did not participate in sports with high upper limb demands had only two cases of asymptomatic OCD. Level of evidence: II.

48. van den Ende KI, McIntosh AL, Adams JE, Steinmann SP: Osteochondritis dissecans of the capitellum: A review of the literature and a distal ulnar portal. *Arthroscopy* 2011;27(1):122-128.

In this literature review, the authors discuss the likely role of capitellar overload in the etiology of OCD of the elbow.

49. Nissen CW: Osteochondritis dissecans of the elbow. *Clin Sports Med* 2014;33(2):251-265.

In this study, the authors found that patients who are involved in overhead-dominant sports and sports that require the arm to be a weight-bearing limb are predisposed to OCD of the elbow. Level of evidence: IV.

50. Claessen FM, Louwerens JK, Doornberg JN, van Dijk CN, Eygendaal D, van den Bekerom MP: Panner's disease: Literature review and treatment recommendations. *J Child Orthop* 2015;9(1):9-17.

In this literature review, the notion that Panner disease is typically seen in patients younger than those experiencing OCD of the elbow is supported.

51. Ruchelsman DE, Hall MP, Youm T: Osteochondritis dissecans of the capitellum: Current concepts. *J Am Acad Orthop Surg* 2010;18(9):557-567.

52. Shi LL, Bae DS, Kocher MS, Micheli LJ, Waters PM: Contained versus uncontained lesions in juvenile elbow osteochondritis dissecans. *J Pediatr Orthop* 2012;32(3):221-225.

The authors found that uncontained OCD lesions of the elbow had greater flexion contracture, higher rates of joint effusion, and a broader and shallower presentation when compared with contained lesions. Level of evidence: IV.

53. Zbojniewicz AM, Laor T: Imaging of osteochondritis dissecans. *Clin Sports Med* 2014;33(2):221-250.

The authors describe the advantages of MRI over plain radiography in the diagnosis of OCD and discuss important MRI findings that can have an effect on clinical decision-making.

54. Nishitani K, Nakagawa Y, Gotoh T, Kobayashi M, Nakamura T: Intraoperative acoustic evaluation of living human cartilage of the elbow and knee during mosaicplasty for osteochondritis dissecans of the elbow: An in vivo study. *Am J Sports Med* 2008;36(12):2345-2353.

55. de Graaff F, Krijnen MR, Poolman RW, Willems WJ: Arthroscopic surgery in athletes with osteochondritis dissecans of the elbow. *Arthroscopy* 2011;27(7):986-993.

In this review, the results of arthroscopic surgery for the treatment of athletes with OCD were assessed. The authors suggested that surgical treatment be considered for athletes with OCD after a period of unsuccessful nonsurgical therapy. Level of evidence: III.

56. Lewine EB, Miller PE, Micheli LJ, Waters PM, Bae DS: Early Results of Drilling and/or Microfracture for Grade IV Osteochondritis Dissecans of the Capitellum. *J Pediatr Orthop* 2015.

At a minimum follow-up of 2 years, approximately 70% of patients who underwent fragment removal and microfracture for grade IV capitellar OCD lesions demonstrated improvement, which was identified as no further tenderness in the joint or resolution of bony edema on MRI. Level of evidence: IV.

57. Uchida S, Utsunomiya H, Taketa T, et al: Arthroscopic fragment fixation using hydroxyapatite/poly-L-lactate acid thread pins for treating elbow osteochondritis dissecans. *Am J Sports Med* 2015;43(5):1057-1065.

Eighteen adolescent baseball players underwent fragment fixation using hydroxyapatite/poly-lactate acid pins for primarily grade 2 and 3 capitellar OCD lesions. At 3 years postoperatively, an improvement in outcomes scores and range of motion was noted, and nearly all patients had returned to the same or higher level of play. Level of evidence: IV.

58. Ahmad CS, Vitale MA, ElAttrache NS: Elbow arthroscopy: Capitellar osteochondritis dissecans and radiocapitellar plica. *Instr Course Lect* 2011;60:181-190.

Radiocapitellar plica was found to cause chondromalacic changes on the radial head and capitellum, with symptoms including painful clicking and effusions. The authors concluded that arthroscopic plica resection is indicated when nonsurgical treatment fails. Level of evidence: IV.

59. Chen NC: Osteochondritis dissecans of the elbow. *J Hand Surg Am* 2010;35(7):1188-1189.

Both reconstruction and arthroscopic débridement were found to yield notable improvement after surgery for OCD of the elbow. Some evidence exists that reconstruction yielded better results than débridement for larger defects at midterm follow-up. Level of evidence: IV.

60. Arai Y, Hara K, Fujiwara H, Minami G, Nakagawa S, Kubo T: A new arthroscopic-assisted drilling method through the radius in a distal-to-proximal direction for osteochondritis dissecans of the elbow. *Arthroscopy* 2008;24(2):237.e1-237.e4.

61. Rahusen FT, Brinkman JM, Eygendaal D: Results of arthroscopic debridement for osteochondritis dissecans of the elbow. *Br J Sports Med* 2006;40(12):966-969.

62. Yamamoto Y, Ishibashi Y, Tsuda E, Sato H, Toh S: Osteochondral autograft transplantation for osteochondritis dissecans of the elbow in juvenile baseball players: Minimum 2-year follow-up. *Am J Sports Med* 2006;34(5):714-720.

63. Iwasaki N, Kato H, Ishikawa J, Masuko T, Funakoshi T, Minami A: Autologous osteochondral mosaicplasty for osteochondritis dissecans of the elbow in teenage athletes. *J Bone Joint Surg Am* 2009;91(10):2359-2366.

64. Lyons ML, Werner BC, Gluck JS, et al: Osteochondral autograft plug transfer for treatment of osteochondritis dissecans of the capitellum in adolescent athletes. *J Shoulder Elbow Surg* 2015;24(7):1098-1105.

Eleven adolescent patients with capitellar OCD lesions larger than 1 cm underwent an OAT procedure with a donor site from the knee. All patients returned at least to their original level of play, and improved results from the Disabilities of the Arm, Shoulder and Hand test and range of motion were reported. Level of evidence: IV.

65. Miyamoto W, Yamamoto S, Kii R, Uchio Y: Oblique osteochondral plugs transplantation technique for osteochondritis dissecans of the elbow joint. *Knee Surg Sports Traumatol Arthrosc* 2009;17(2):204-208.

Chapter 45

Shoulder Injuries

Natasha Trentacosta, MD J. Lee Pace, MD

Abstract

With increasing participation of children and adolescents in organized sports and early specialization in a single sport, the risk of shoulder injuries in young athletes will continue to increase. Children and adolescents experience acute traumatic injuries to the shoulder during both practice and competition, and chronic overuse injuries occur secondary to the repetitive shoulder motions required in sports such as baseball, swimming, and racquet sports. The unique nature of the pediatric shoulder requires a different diagnostic, prognostic, and treatment approach to shoulder injuries than that needed in adult patients.

Keywords: overuse injuries; shoulder injuries; shoulder trauma; sports injuries

Introduction

Shoulder injury in athletic children and adolescents is likely to continue to increase as this population increases its participation in organized sports, focuses on a single sport throughout the year without cross training, and achieves higher levels of competitive play. Although lower extremity injuries are seen more commonly in athletes, children involved in sports such as baseball, judo, gymnastics, and snowboarding are more likely to sustain upper extremity injuries.[1] A recent study found 2.15 shoulder injuries per 10,000 athlete exposures in high school students, with the highest rates seen in football, wrestling, and baseball.[2] The shoulders of children and adolescents are subject to acute traumatic athletic injuries as well as chronic overuse injuries resulting from participation in overhead sports. The pattern of these injuries often is different than that seen in their adult counterparts. Early recognition of these injuries and proper management may help avoid long-term disability.

Dr. Pace or an immediate family member serves as a paid consultant to Arthrex and Ceterix and serves as a board member, owner, officer, or committee member of the Pediatric Orthopaedic Society of North America. Neither Dr. Trentacosta nor any immediate family member has received anything of value from or has stock or stock options held in a commercial company or institution related directly or indirectly to the subject of this chapter.

Shoulder Anatomy

The shoulder complex encompasses a group of joints that acts in concert to provide mobility and function to the upper extremity. The four joints that work in a coordinated manner are the glenohumeral, sternoclavicular (SC), acromioclavicular (AC), and scapulothoracic joints. Although not a true joint, the scapulothoracic articulation results from the concave nature of the anterior scapular gliding over the convex posterior thorax to provide stability and motion to the shoulder complex. This articulation is an important component in propagating the kinetic chain of energy.

The presence of epiphyseal plates and the altered collagen composition of the shoulder ligaments and tendons define the pediatric shoulder and predispose it to injury patterns dissimilar to those seen in adults. The three main ossification centers in the proximal humeral epiphysis are the humeral head, the greater tubercle, and the lesser tubercle (**Figure 1**). The tubercles fuse at approximately age 15 years, whereas the humeral epiphysis fuses to the diaphysis near age 20 years. The three ossification centers of the clavicle are the lateral epiphysis, the medial epiphysis, and the diaphysis. The clavicle is unique in that the epiphyses both ossify and fuse very late in adolescence. The lateral epiphysis often appears at approximately age 18 years and rapidly fuses within 1 year. The medial epiphysis also appears near age 18 years, but it may not completely fuse until age 25 years. The cartilage of the physis represents a weak link that makes it susceptible to injury, particularly just before skeletal maturity.

Much of the stability of the shoulder complex arises from the soft-tissue structures. The glenohumeral joint has both static and dynamic stabilizers. The static stabilizers include the glenohumeral capsule, the labrum, and the glenohumeral ligaments. The dynamic stabilizers include

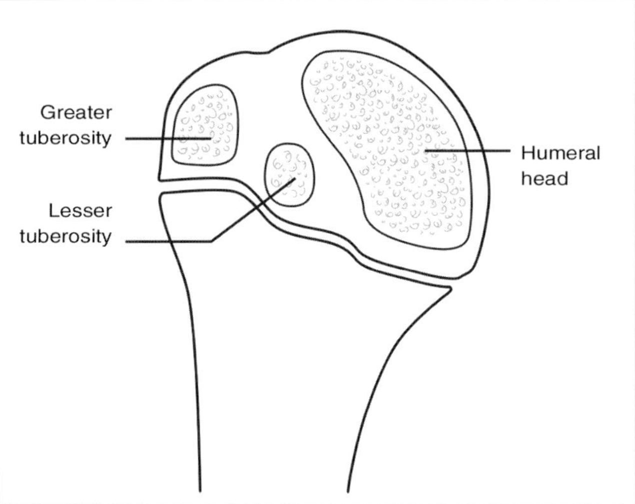

Figure 1 Illustration shows the centers of ossification in the proximal humerus. The ossification center of the humeral head is typically identified after age 6 months. The ossification center of the greater tuberosity is identified by age 7 months to 3 years and that of the lesser tuberosity by age 2 to 5 years.

the rotator cuff muscles, the long head of the biceps, the deltoid muscle, and the other scapulothoracic muscles. The SC joint is stabilized by the anterior and posterior SC ligaments, the costoclavicular ligament, and the interclavicular ligament. The AC joint is predominantly stabilized by the coracoclavicular ligaments, with contributions from the joint capsule and the AC ligament.

Kinetic Chain Mechanics

Overhead sports, including baseball, swimming, racquet sports, and volleyball, rely on the coordinated generation and transfer of energy from the lower extremities through the hips, torso, and upper extremities. The kinetic chain is a sophisticated chain of muscle contractions that allows for efficient energy transfer and prepares the body to withstand the muscle imbalances generated by the act of overhead motion. The kinetic chain generates tremendous force and control during various athletic overhead motions. The disruption of any part of this mechanism can lead to poor performance and may ultimately predispose the athlete to injury. Knowledge and evaluation of the kinetic chain in the overhead athlete will aid in the diagnosis and treatment of many shoulder injuries. Typically, an abnormality in the chain results in either a slower velocity at the distal end of the mechanism or an overcompensation of the distal segment in an attempt to maintain a certain velocity despite a disruption earlier in the chain. The area that overcompensates often is the area that becomes injured because excessive forces are concentrated in that area.

Patient Evaluation

History

As with any injury, a thorough history and physical examination are imperative to the diagnosis and treatment of shoulder injuries in a young athlete. The athlete's sport and position as well as the mechanism of injury are important considerations. Most injuries sustained to the shoulder during football are a result of direct trauma. Because spearing has been banned in football, more shoulder injuries are possible because more focus has been placed on shoulder-body contact for tackling. Judo has a substantially higher proportion of shoulder injuries caused by throwing, flipping, and falling compared with other disciplines, such as karate and tae kwon do.[3] Higher injury rates are seen with higher levels of contact and, interestingly, in the amount of protective equipment worn by male athletes playing hockey and lacrosse.[4] Among high school baseball players, especially pitchers, the shoulder is the most common site of injury, with muscle strains the most predominant injury.[5]

Knowledge of an athlete's training is helpful because unsound practices and abrupt changes may lead to overuse injuries. For throwing athletes, knowledge of the number and types of pitches per week is critically important. The patient's growth history should be assessed because peak growth velocity is a risk factor for injury. The passive elongation of soft tissues over actively elongating bone leads to temporary inflexibility, muscle imbalance, and an increased risk of injury. A history of joint laxity should be ascertained in patients with instability symptoms.

Physical Examination

A focused musculoskeletal examination can provide objective measures to aid in making a diagnosis of shoulder pain. The range of motion should be assessed in overhead athletes, with a comparison to the contralateral side to check for differences. Stability should be assessed in both traumatic and atraumatic situations. Muscle atrophy may be a sign of nerve impingement disorders. Provocative impingement tests are important to assess for subacromial bursitis and impingement as well as rotator cuff strength. Biceps strength and irritability could indicate superior labral pathology. Dynamic examination of the scapula also is imperative when evaluating scapular dyskinesis or winging.

Given the proximity of neurovascular structures to many of the bony structures of the shoulder girdle, a careful examination of neurovascular status is warranted in all patients with suspected fractures and brachial plexus injuries. Traction to the brachial plexus can produce radicular pain into the arm and hand after a shoulder tackle in football. Open fractures and those that could cause neurovascular injury should be attended to immediately.

Imaging

Appropriate imaging is undertaken after the history is obtained and the physical examination is completed. When dealing with traumatic injuries to the shoulder, radiography often reveals the pathology. Pathologic bone lesions may be found incidentally in patients who have a fracture through a weak bone lesion. Advanced imaging is usually needed only if nonsurgical measures are unsuccessful or for those who have an abnormal physical examination or radiographic findings suggestive of internal derangement in the shoulder. A CT scan of the SC joint is important when a posterior dislocation of the SC joint is suspected.

Traumatic Shoulder Injuries

Patients with a traumatic shoulder injury often report a single event or an acute event superimposed on a history of overuse. These injuries often occur in contact sports such as football, basketball, hockey, and wrestling.

Sprains and Strains

Sprains and strains account for approximately 38% of all shoulder injuries seen in high school athletes.[2] Injuries may occur to the AC joint, the SC joint, or about the glenohumeral joint as a result of direct trauma or a fall onto an outstretched arm, which often leads to bony injuries in younger adolescent athletes and sprains in older adolescent athletes.

Injuries to the AC joint may involve a sprain to the supporting ligaments or result in a distal clavicle fracture. For making a diagnosis and treatment, radiographic evaluation, including standard shoulder views, as well as Zanca views, are needed. Most AC injuries are successfully managed with nonsurgical methods, with the arm placed in a sling followed by physical therapy. Surgical intervention is reserved for patients with advanced injuries.

Similarly, trauma to the SC joint can cause ligamentous injury; in severe cases, the medial clavicular physis may dislocate or fracture. Dislocations can be either anterior or posterior, depending on the mechanism of injury. These injuries should be suspected in children with trauma to the chest region so that a posterior dislocation or physeal injury is not missed; a serendipity radiographic view (40° cephalic tilt view of the SC joint) or CT often is required to make the diagnosis. Closed treatment of anterior dislocations often can lead to successful outcomes without complications. Historically, posterior SC dislocations have been thought to be stable after closed reduction, with surgical intervention required only for recurrent or symptomatic dislocations. However, the authors of a 2014 study reported more failed closed reductions with SC joint dislocation versus physeal fractures.[6] They also found that posterior SC joint dislocation and medial clavicular physeal fractures occur with nearly equivalent frequency in patients with open medial physes, although the differentiation of such often is unreliable based on radiography and CT because of the late ossification and fusion of the medial clavicle epiphysis. Open stabilization procedures with the consultation of a thoracic surgeon are currently being advocated because of this increased recognition of recurrent instability, difficulty of differentiation from physeal fractures, increased reports of mediastinal complications, and consistently good surgical outcomes.

Fractures

Acute fractures to the shoulder are uncommon in the pediatric and adolescent populations, with the exception of midshaft clavicle fractures. Participation in certain sports predisposed participants to fractures of the shoulder. A large number of fractures occur in children who are horseback riders, with nearly two-thirds of these fractures occurring in the upper extremity (particularly the proximal humerus).[7] In martial arts, nearly 50% of the injuries seen in the shoulder region are fractures.[3]

The management of proximal humerus fractures is largely nonsurgical in pediatric athletes because 80% of humeral growth occurs at this physis, which allows for substantial remodeling potential. In children older than 12 years, remodeling capacity decreases to approximately 40° angulation and 50% displacement; surgical correction may be considered in these patients.[8] As adolescents age, their remodeling capacity decreases, and the ability for the shoulder to compensate for deformity in adolescent athletes is compromised. The fracture often falls into varus, with the pectoralis major muscle pulling the distal fragment medially while the rotator cuff and deltoid muscles pull the proximal fragment upward. This deformity also can arise from partial growth plate arrest, which leads to angular growth. If not corrected, this residual deformity will lead to limitations in forward flexion and abduction with greater tuberosity-acromial impingement, making overhead sporting activities difficult. Recently, the literature has shifted from nonsurgical management to surgical treatment of older pediatric patients and those with greater displacement. Surgical stabilization may be achieved with percutaneous pinning or retrograde elastic stable intramedullary nailing, which has gained popularity in recent years.

In pediatric athletes, the location and thin nature of the clavicular bone makes it susceptible to fracture, with approximately 15% of all fractures in this population involving the clavicle. The acts of blocking, tackling, and using the shoulder as a battering ram in football, hockey, and rugby place the clavicle at risk for injury. When a cyclist is thrown over the handlebars and lands directly on his or her shoulder, a distal clavicle fracture (known as bicycle shoulder) often occurs.

Nonsurgical management with a sling or figure-of-8 bracing is the preferred treatment for a nondisplaced or minimally displaced clavicular fracture. In patients younger than 15 years, regardless of displacement, excellent healing and remodeling potential allows for the successful use of nonsurgical measures. In patients older than 15 years, longitudinal growth and remodeling potential is minimal, and the risk of nonunion increases to more than 15%.[9] Although not the standard of care, many physicians recommend surgical intervention to allow for a more rapid union and a decreased incidence of symptomatic nonunion in older adolescents with substantially shortened or displaced clavicular fractures.[10] Return to contact sports should be delayed until radiographically confirmed bony union is achieved, usually at 2 to 4 months after injury.

An increasing number of insertional injuries and avulsion fractures are occurring as the result of poor training techniques. During puberty, the development of muscle mass increases in adolescents while tendon and bony insertions remain weak and unable to absorb generated loads. Avulsion injuries can result from this developmental imbalance.

Avulsion of the lesser tuberosity is an uncommon injury; however, several reports of acute and missed chronic cases exist in the literature.[11,12] The diagnosis of an avulsion of the lesser tuberosity often may be delayed because symptoms overlap those of other shoulder injuries, such as instability, physeal injury, or muscle strain. Clinical awareness of this condition will help ensure that (1) a proper physical examination is performed and (2) radiographs are carefully evaluated to avoid missing an avulsion of the lesser tuberosity and prevent its potential sequelae of malunion, nonunion, impingement, instability, pain, or weakness. Although the size of a bony avulsion may vary, this injury is treated with surgical repair of the fragment to the humerus.

Similarly, the coracoid is vulnerable to avulsion in adolescents before fusion of the physis. This injury often results from collisions in football. Given the amount of force required to sustain this type of injury, concurrent injuries may be seen. Treatment often is successful with nonsurgical measures.

Glenohumeral Dislocations

The prevalence of glenohumeral dislocations in patients younger than 18 years is 31.0 per 100,000 person-years for males and 8.2 per 100,000 person-years for females.[13] These dislocations account for approximately 0.01% of all injuries in children, with most occurring in patients 10 years and older.[14,15] Similar to their adult counterparts, approximately 90% of shoulder dislocations are anterior traumatic dislocations that result from a fall onto an abducted, externally rotated arm.[16] Nearly 30% of upper extremity injuries involving the shoulder, mostly consisting of shoulder dislocations or sprains, result from skiing injuries.

Accurate diagnosis and prompt treatment are necessary to identify any bony or labral pathology requiring surgical management and allow a quick return to play. Magnetic resonance arthrography is the preferred modality for identifying the hallmark imaging findings of a Hill-Sachs humeral impaction fracture or a Bankart lesion of the anterior inferior glenoid rim. Initial management of acute shoulder dislocations includes closed reduction under conscious sedation followed by postreduction immobilization.

The natural history of traumatic shoulder dislocation in patients younger than 20 years follows a course of recurrent instability and dislocation. Recurrent instability produces persistent symptoms that can interfere with sports participation and activities of daily living and may damage the articular cartilage of the glenoid fossa and humeral head. The rate of recurrent dislocation in patients with open physes varies widely in the literature, with reported rates ranging from 40% to 100%.[17-20]

A recent study examined a focused cohort of 10- to 16-year-old patients with shoulder dislocations and found that recurrent dislocation was substantially greater in those aged 14 to 16 years than in those 13 years or younger.[13] Similar results of lower dislocations rates in patients younger than 13 years were reported in an earlier study.[17] It has been hypothesized that the inherent laxity of the shoulder in children imparts more resiliency to structural damage than that seen in the shoulders of adolescents and adults.[17] The difference in recurrence rates also may be a reflection of the variation in the type of sport played and lower participation rates of children in contact sports. Those at risk for subsequent dislocations include adolescent boys and those participating in contact sports.[13,21]

Definitive management for pediatric shoulder dislocations is controversial. Although many physicians choose definitive treatment with immobilization and physical therapy for adolescents older than 13 years with first-time dislocations, the higher rates of recurrent shoulder dislocations in this population warrants consideration of early stabilization.[13,22] In a comparison of early arthroscopic intervention with nonsurgical treatment followed by delayed arthroscopic treatment in a pediatric population, the authors found that early surgical intervention was beneficial.[23] In clinical studies looking at shoulder dislocations in pediatric patients, up to 44% of the patients required surgical intervention.[14,24]

When surgery is necessary, arthroscopic treatment with no modification from adult techniques has become the standard treatment. In a study of anterior surgical shoulder stabilization in high school and collegiate athletes, the authors reported an 11% dislocation rate in patients younger than 20 years.[25] In a 2010 study, no recurrences were reported in five of six patients aged 11 to 15 years who underwent surgical stabilization for posttraumatic shoulder instability.[26] A 2012 study of adolescents who underwent arthroscopic shoulder stabilization found that 81% of the patients returned to their preinjury sport; however, a 21% dislocation recurrence rate was reported, with higher rates seen in water polo and rugby players.[27]

Multidirectional Instability

Multidirectional instability of the shoulder, which is characterized by involuntary subluxation in any combination of anterior, inferior, and posterior directions, is a complex entity seen in overhead athletes and often is characterized by pain. This pathologic laxity may result from repetitive microtrauma to the static stabilizers of the shoulder that create a large patulous inferior capsular pouch with a widened rotator interval, usually in conjunction with some predisposing laxity. The quality and quantity of collagen in patients with multidirectional instability has been shown to be reduced compared with those without the syndrome.[28] This condition is commonly seen in throwing athletes, swimmers, and gymnasts who experience episodes of subluxation with spontaneous reductions. The physical examination may reveal hyperlaxity in other joints of the body and scapulothoracic dyskinesis.

A regimented rehabilitation program that focuses on strengthening the dynamic stabilizers of the shoulder is successful in more than 80% of these patients.[29] If pain and instability persist after a least 6 months of regimented rehabilitation, arthroscopic management with capsulolabral shift with or without rotator interval closure may lead to improved outcomes.[30-32]

Chronic Overuse Injuries

Overhead athletes involved in throwing, swimming, volleyball, gymnastics, and racquet sports often have chronic shoulder pain secondary to repetitive microtrauma, which is generally referred to as an overuse injury. These injuries occur when training demands exceed the physiologic ability of an individual's body to compensate because submaximal forces are repetitively loaded on tissue, causing microscopic tissue damage.[33] Children are at particular risk for overuse injuries because of their weaker physes and muscle imbalance. The adolescent growth spurt is a unique time in development that can make pediatric patients more susceptible to such injury. During the growth spurt, bone tends to be weaker because of slower bone mineralization compared with the rate of linear bone growth, the physeal cartilage tends to be weaker in general, the musculotendinous junction tightens as lengthening bones impart more tension, and coordination is lacking.[34-36]

Throwing athletes produce high levels of force throughout the upper extremity that lead to overuse of the stabilizing structures in an attempt to create a stable shoulder joint during the arc of motion. This force increases during the midteen to late teen years because of the increase in muscle development. Poor biomechanics and scapular dyskinesis along with excessive throwing contribute to the development of these common conditions.

Proper biomechanics, particularly core activation in the initiation of kinetic chain events, is important in preventing overuse injuries. A coordinated approach is needed among trainers, therapists, and physicians in assessing pitching mechanics in pediatric athletes. Since the mid 1990s, efforts have been undertaken to decrease the number of overuse injuries in pediatric throwing athletes by limiting pitch counts and mandating rest days between pitching appearances. Muscle fatigue from overuse can lead to poor dynamic stability and subsequent injury. Cross training in different seasons also is encouraged because it allows the body time to recover, which is not possible if a single sport is played throughout the year. A recent study found that youth league baseball coaches had poor knowledge of the current recommendations to prevent overuse injuries in pediatric pitchers.[37]

Little Leaguer's Shoulder

Commonly seen in pediatric baseball pitchers, Little Leaguer's shoulder is considered a chronic stress form of a nondisplaced Salter-Harris type I fracture of the proximal humerus. This condition typically manifests as insidious shoulder pain (particularly in the follow-through phase of throwing) and limited range of motion. It often is seen in male pitchers aged 11 to 13 years because this is the period of maximal physeal growth resulting in relatively weak physes. Those who throw curve balls, continue throwing through fatigue, are overweight, lift weights, and play on multiple teams are at increased risk for this overuse condition.[38] The repetitive stress of throwing produces radiographic physeal widening of the proximal humeral physis compared with the contralateral side. In patients with severe overuse injuries, premature closure of the growth plate may occur and can lead to angular deformity. The diagnosis of this condition relies mainly on clinical assessment and can be supported by radiographic widening (**Figure 2**). MRI, although rarely needed to make the diagnosis, may show widening and edema within the proximal humeral physis.

The rehabilitation regimen for Little Leaguer's shoulder is cessation of throwing activities for 8 to 12 weeks, followed by gradual rehabilitation of the shoulder and return to play. A graduated program progresses from range of motion through strengthening, endurance, and speed and stresses the importance of control and proper biomechanics. Prevention of injury is paramount and requires adherence to recommendations on pitch counts and rest days as well as maintenance of proper pitching biomechanics. An undiagnosed overuse injury can lead to chronic pain with throwing, shoulder instability, and degenerative arthritis.[39]

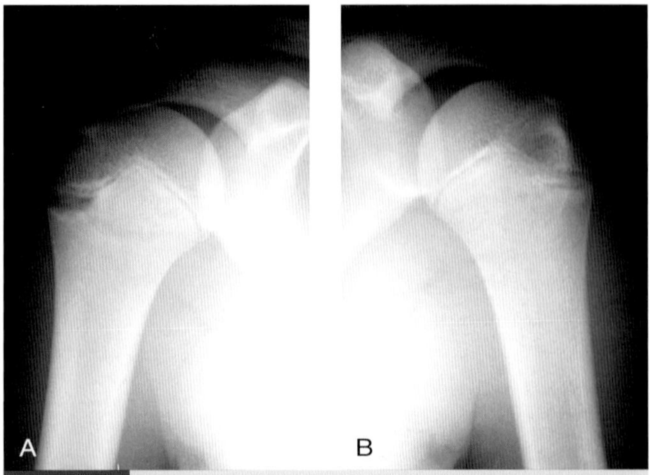

Figure 2 External rotation AP comparison radiographs of the proximal humerus from a patient with Little Leaguer's shoulder show the affected shoulder (**A**) and the contralateral normal shoulder (**B**). Note widening of the proximal humeral physis. (Reproduced with permission from Carson WG, Gasser SI: Little leaguer's shoulder: A report of 23 cases. *Am J Sports Med* 1998;26[4]:575-580.)

Glenohumeral Internal Rotation Deficit

Glenohumeral internal rotation deficit (GIRD) is a shoulder syndrome commonly seen in pitchers and other overhead athletes such as swimmers and tennis players. It is defined by the objective loss of internal rotation compared with the contralateral side and results from derangements of the dynamic shoulder restraints. The posteroinferior capsule becomes contracted with corresponding stretching of the anterior capsular structures, resulting in a posterosuperior translation of the humeral head on the glenoid with combined external rotation and abduction of the shoulder. This can result in structural injury to the labrum or rotator cuff tendons. The changes in range of motion and resulting torsional stresses of overhead activities can lead to bony adaptations in the humerus, such as increased humeral head retroversion and, ultimately, alteration of the normal scapular and shoulder biomechanics.

Posterior capsule stretching to decrease pain and the adaptive changes seen in throwing are integral to the treatment and prevention of GIRD. A strengthening program that focuses on strengthening the posterior shoulder muscles to counterbalance the stronger internal rotators of the shoulder helps treat and prevent shoulder pain in throwing athletes with GIRD.

Internal Impingement and Rotator Cuff Injury

In children and adolescents, rotator cuff injury tends to be rare when compared with such injuries in adults, but rotator cuff tendinitis has been increasingly described in the adolescent population, particularly in swimmers, throwers, and racquetball and tennis players, and it often occurs with other intra-articular pathology, especially labral tears.[16,40-42] Rotator cuff tendinitis is believed to result from internal impingement and instability. With internal impingement, the rotator cuff, the labrum, and the joint capsule are repetitively pinched between the greater tuberosity and the superior glenoid rim at the extremes of abduction and external rotation, which occurs multiple times in overhead sports. Recently, it has been reported that frank tears of the rotator cuff, which were thought to occur only in adults, also exist in the pediatric population[43,44] (**Figure 3**).

High-performance swimmers experience high repetitive forces across the shoulder caused by multiple shoulder revolutions needed to propel their bodies long distances in the water. An increase in overuse shoulder injuries occurs in these swimmers, usually after age 10 years. A condition called swimmer's shoulder often develops in these athletes. This condition is an ill-defined overuse injury of the shoulder synonymous with rotator cuff tendinitis and impingement syndrome. It results in pain from impingement of the humeral head and rotator cuff on the coracoacromial ligament. Gymnasts also experience rotator cuff tendinitis, predominantly in the supraspinatus tendons.[45]

The treatment options for rotator cuff pathology tend to involve nonsurgical modalities, relying on a course of physical therapy. Surgical intervention may be considered

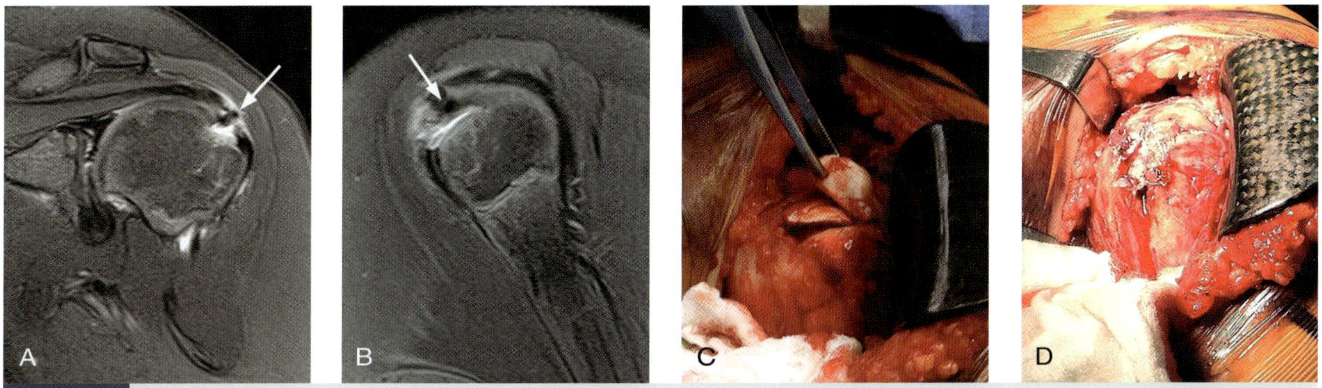

Figure 3 Images from a 12-year-old boy with a rotator cuff tear. Four weeks after falling off a cargo net in gym class, the child was unable to lift his left arm. With normal radiographic findings, an MRI of the left shoulder was obtained. Coronal T2-weighted (**A**) and sagittal T2-weighted (**B**) MRIs show a periosteal avulsion of the supraspinatus footprint (arrows) in a patient with open growth plates. **C,** Intraoperative photograph of the deltopectoral approach, wherein the avulsion of the supraspinatus footprint was identified with no bony component. **D,** Intraoperative photograph of an open rotator cuff repair with medial row fixation using suture anchors and lateral row soft-tissue fixation. (Courtesy of Micah Lissy, MD; UHS Sports Medicine, Binghamton, NY.)

if nonsurgical management is unsuccessful and symptoms and some degree of rotator cuff tearing and/or persistent impingement exist; however, the results of surgical treatment are largely undetermined in the pediatric population.[41,46]

Superior Labrum Anterior to Posterior Tears

Although uncommon, superior labrum anterior to posterior (SLAP) tears can occur in the pediatric overhead athlete and cause insidious nonspecific shoulder pain during overhead activities.[47] The etiology is believed to be the peel-back phenomenon that results in a more vertical and posterior force vector on the biceps tendon in the abducted and externally rotated position. There should be a high suspicion for SLAP tears in throwing athletes who have refractory pain; MRI may be needed in making the diagnosis.

Initial management should consist of nonsurgical measures, including rest and physical therapy. The role for surgical treatment of SLAP tears remains controversial. Arthroscopic treatment of SLAP tears has been suggested if no improvement occurs after rest, NSAID administration, and physical therapy.[48]

Gymnast Shoulder

Gymnasts tend to experience sustained forces rather than the repetitive motions seen in other overhead athletes. This type of stress produces a benign cortical hypertrophy (known as a ringman's shoulder lesion) at the insertion of the pectoralis major muscle at the anterolateral aspect of the proximal humerus.[49] The lesion, which is asymptomatic, is thought to occur exclusively in gymnasts and does not warrant intervention. Awareness of the imaging findings in these athletes may allow for accurate diagnosis and avoid unnecessary imaging studies and biopsy.

Snapping Scapula Syndrome

Snapping scapula syndrome is an uncommon condition associated with a painful shoulder in an overhead athlete. Because a sport injury is associated with this condition in most pediatric patients, an overuse injury is believed to be the most likely factor contributing to snapping scapula syndrome in this population. The authors of a 2015 study reported that 75% of the patients with this syndrome were able to return to sports after treatment with nonsurgical measures that focused on physical therapy, which included strengthening of the rhomboids and trapezius muscles and stretching of the pectoralis muscles.[50] If nonsurgical measures are unsuccessful in relieving symptoms, further workup is indicated, including CT to assess for structural causes such as osteochondromas or anatomic anomalies in angulation of the scapula. This information will aid in surgical planning if a structural lesion, a hooked superomedial border, or anterior angulation is found that requires mass excision or superomedial border excision.

Scapular Dyskinesis

An increased incidence of scapular dyskinesis and shoulder injury was found in adolescents who participate in throwing sports compared with preadolescent overhead throwing athletes. In these patients, the dyskinesis often is secondary to another problem, such as glenohumeral instability, impingement syndrome, rotator cuff weakness, or labral injury. Management consists of scapular stabilization rehabilitation focusing on strengthening and stretching of the scapular muscles to regain control of scapular protraction, retraction, depression, elevation, and rotation, along with treatment of any underlying pathology.

Osteolysis of the Distal Clavicle

Stress osteolysis of the distal clavicle is rare in adolescent athletes but can be seen in those who participate in overhead weight lifting. This condition results in a decrease in mineralization of the distal clavicle and causes resorption of the distal tip of the clavicle.[51] Although most patients improve within 3 to 6 months with nonsurgical measures, including modification of weight-training techniques, NSAIDs, and ice application, a small percentage of patients may require distal clavicle excision to continue overhead and weight-lifting activities.

Other Causes of Shoulder Pain

Less common causes of shoulder pain include quadrilateral space syndrome, suprascapular nerve entrapment, axillary artery occlusion, axillary vein thrombosis, posterior capsule laxity, and glenoid spurs. These alternative diagnoses should be considered when evaluating pediatric patients with shoulder pain.

Summary

The participation of children and adolescents in organized sports and the early specialization of these individuals in a single sport has led to an increasing rate of injuries in pediatric shoulders. Acute traumatic injuries to the shoulder can result in sprains, strains, fractures, and dislocations. Chronic overuse injuries also occur in pediatric patients. The presence of open physes and differences in collagen composition in pediatric shoulder tissue compared with the adult shoulder create a unique environment for injury and require special treatment considerations.

Key Study Points

- Shoulder injuries in pediatric athletes continue to rise with increasing sports participation and specialization.
- The adolescent growth spurt is a unique time in development and can make older children more susceptible to shoulder injury.
- Knowledge of the kinetic chain of energy generation in the overhead athlete is important for understanding injury treatment and prevention.
- Acute traumatic events during practice or, more likely, competition can lead to sprains, strains, dislocations, or fractures of the structures that encompass the shoulder region.
- Overhead athletes are susceptible to overuse injuries in the shoulder because of repetitive motions across the joint.

Annotated References

1. Caine D, Caine C, Maffulli N: Incidence and distribution of pediatric sport-related injuries. *Clin J Sport Med* 2006;16(6):500-513.

2. Robinson TW, Corlette J, Collins CL, Comstock RD: Shoulder injuries among US high school athletes, 2005/2006-2011/2012. *Pediatrics* 2014;133(2):272-279.

   In high school athletes, a rate of 2.15 shoulder injuries per 10,000 athlete exposures was reported. Injury rates were highest in football players, with 4.86 shoulder injuries per 10,000 athlete exposures. Thirty-seven percent of the injuries were strains and sprains, and 29.2% were dislocations and separations of the shoulder. Level of evidence: IV.

3. Yard EE, Knox CL, Smith GA, Comstock RD: Pediatric martial arts injuries presenting to emergency departments, United States 1990-2003. *J Sci Med Sport* 2007;10(4):219-226.

4. Yard EE, Comstock RD: Injuries sustained by pediatric ice hockey, lacrosse, and field hockey athletes presenting to United States emergency departments, 1990-2003. *J Athl Train* 2006;41(4):441-449.

5. Krajnik S, Fogarty KJ, Yard EE, Comstock RD: Shoulder injuries in US high school baseball and softball athletes, 2005-2008. *Pediatrics* 2010;125(3):497-501.

6. Lee JT, Nasreddine AY, Black EM, Bae DS, Kocher MS: Posterior sternoclavicular joint injuries in skeletally immature patients. *J Pediatr Orthop* 2014;34(4):369-375.

Of 48 patients treated for posterior SC joint injuries, 50% had a true SC joint dislocation, and 50% had a medial clavicle physeal fracture. The authors found that an attempted closed reduction may be more successful if performed within 24 hours after injury. Failure of closed reduction is more likely to occur in posterior SC joint dislocations than in physeal fractures. Level of evidence: IV.

7. Landin LA: Fracture patterns in children: Analysis of 8,682 fractures with special reference to incidence, etiology and secular changes in a Swedish urban population 1950-1979. *Acta Orthop Scand Suppl* 1983;202:1-109.

8. Bishop JY, Flatow EL: Pediatric shoulder trauma. *Clin Orthop Relat Res* 2005;432:41-48.

9. Zlowodzki M, Zelle BA, Cole PA, Jeray K, McKee MD; Evidence-Based Orthopaedic Trauma Working Group: Treatment of acute midshaft clavicle fractures: Systematic review of 2144 fractures. On behalf of the Evidence-Based Orthopaedic Trauma Working Group. *J Orthop Trauma* 2005;19(7):504-507.

10. Sarwark J, King E, Luhmann S: Proximal humerus, scapula and clavicle, in Beaty J, Kasser J, eds: *Rockwood and Wilkin's Fractures in Children* , ed 6. Philadelphia, PA, Lippincott-Raven, 2006, pp 704-771.

11. Garrigues GE, Warnick DE, Busch MT: Subscapularis avulsion of the lesser tuberosity in adolescents. *J Pediatr Orthop* 2013;33(1):8-13.

    The authors reported that six cases of lesser tuberosity avulsion fractures in adolescents treated with diagnostic arthroscopy and open fixation of the avulsion fracture resulted in good outcomes despite diagnosis delays. Level of evidence: IV.

12. LaMont LE, Green DW, Altchek DW, Warren RF, Wickiewicz TL: Subscapularis tears and lesser tuberosity avulsion fractures in the pediatric patient. *Sports Health* 2015;7(2):110-114.

    A series of five cases of lesser tuberosity avulsion fractures in pediatric patients resulted in good outcomes with arthroscopic repair. A high index of suspicion should be maintained for lesser tuberosity avulsion fractures in adolescent boys with chronic shoulder pain without instability to avoid missed injuries. Level of evidence: V.

13. Leroux T, Ogilvie-Harris D, Veillette C, et al: The epidemiology of primary anterior shoulder dislocations in patients aged 10 to 16 years. *Am J Sports Med* 2015;43(9):2111-2117.

    In patients aged 10 to 16 years, the incidence of anterior shoulder dislocation among boys was 164.4 per 100,000 person-years. In patients aged 10 to 12 years, the incidence of primary shoulder dislocation was rare. The recurrent dislocation rate was 38.2%; the rate was higher among patients aged 14 to 16 years but substantially lower in younger patients. Level of evidence: II.

14. Lawton RL, Choudhury S, Mansat P, Cofield RH, Stans AA: Pediatric shoulder instability: Presentation, findings, treatment, and outcomes. *J Pediatr Orthop* 2002;22(1):52-61.

15. Zacchilli MA, Owens BD: Epidemiology of shoulder dislocations presenting to emergency departments in the United States. *J Bone Joint Surg Am* 2010;92(3):542-549.

16. Edmonds EW, Roocroft JH, Parikh SN: Spectrum of operative childhood intra-articular shoulder pathology. *J Child Orthop* 2014;8(4):337-340.

    In children aged 8 to 16 years undergoing shoulder arthroscopy, labral pathology was seen as the primary pathology in 93% of the patients. Twenty-three percent of the patients had pathology involving only the posterior or posterosuperior labrum, and 25% of the patients had pathologies associated with rotator cuff tendon injuries. Level of evidence: IV.

17. Postacchini F, Gumina S, Cinotti G: Anterior shoulder dislocation in adolescents. *J Shoulder Elbow Surg* 2000;9(6):470-474.

18. Hovelius L: Anterior dislocation of the shoulder in teenagers and young adults: Five-year prognosis. *J Bone Joint Surg Am* 1987;69(3):393-399.

19. Marans HJ, Angel KR, Schemitsch EH, Wedge JH: The fate of traumatic anterior dislocation of the shoulder in children. *J Bone Joint Surg Am* 1992;74(8):1242-1244.

20. Robinson CM, Howes J, Murdoch H, Will E, Graham C: Functional outcome and risk of recurrent instability after primary traumatic anterior shoulder dislocation in young patients. *J Bone Joint Surg Am* 2006;88(11):2326-2336.

21. Leroux T, Wasserstein D, Veillette C, et al: Epidemiology of primary anterior shoulder dislocation requiring closed reduction in Ontario, Canada. *Am J Sports Med* 2014;42(2):442-450.

    The incidence of shoulder dislocations in Ontario, Canada was 23.1 per 100,000 person-years, with the highest rate seen in males younger than 20 years (98.3 per 100,000 person-years). The rate of recurrent dislocation was 19%. Level of evidence: II.

22. Li X, Ma R, Nielsen NM, Gulotta LV, Dines JS, Owens BD: Management of shoulder instability in the skeletally immature patient. *J Am Acad Orthop Surg* 2013;21(9):529-537.

    The management of shoulder instability in skeletally immature patients requires prompt reduction and sling immobilization. Athletic patients older than 14 years involved in high-risk sports or those with intra-articular pathology may be at increased risk of recurrent dislocation, so surgical intervention should be considered.

23. Jones KJ, Wiesel B, Ganley TJ, Wells L: Functional outcomes of early arthroscopic Bankart repair in adolescents aged 11 to 18 years. *J Pediatr Orthop* 2007;27(2):209-213.

24. Simonet WT, Cofield RH: Prognosis in anterior shoulder dislocation. *Am J Sports Med* 1984;12(1):19-24.

25. Mazzocca AD, Brown FM Jr, Carreira DS, Hayden J, Romeo AA: Arthroscopic anterior shoulder stabilization of collision and contact athletes. *Am J Sports Med* 2005;33(1):52-60.

26. Kraus R, Pavlidis T, Heiss C, Kilian O, Schnettler R: Arthroscopic treatment of post-traumatic shoulder instability in children and adolescents. *Knee Surg Sports Traumatol Arthrosc* 2010;18(12):1738-1741.

27. Castagna A, Delle Rose G, Borroni M, et al: Arthroscopic stabilization of the shoulder in adolescent athletes participating in overhead or contact sports. *Arthroscopy* 2012;28(3):309-315.

    Arthroscopic stabilization of the shoulder improved the functional outcomes in patients aged 13 to 18 years who sustained traumatic shoulder instability. A 21% failure rate was reported. Higher rates of recurrence were correlated with participation in high-energy contact sports. Level of evidence: IV.

28. Rodeo SA, Suzuki K, Yamauchi M, Bhargava M, Warren RF: Analysis of collagen and elastic fibers in shoulder capsule in patients with shoulder instability. *Am J Sports Med* 1998;26(5):634-643.

29. Burkhead WZ Jr, Rockwood CA Jr: Treatment of instability of the shoulder with an exercise program. *J Bone Joint Surg Am* 1992;74(6):890-896.

30. Kim SH, Kim HK, Sun JI, Park JS, Oh I: Arthroscopic capsulolabroplasty for posteroinferior multidirectional instability of the shoulder. *Am J Sports Med* 2004;32(3):594-607.

31. Gartsman GM, Roddey TS, Hammerman SM: Arthroscopic treatment of multidirectional glenohumeral instability: 2- to 5-year follow-up. *Arthroscopy* 2001;17(3):236-243.

32. Baker CL III, Mascarenhas R, Kline AJ, Chhabra A, Pombo MW, Bradley JP: Arthroscopic treatment of multidirectional shoulder instability in athletes: A retrospective analysis of 2- to 5-year clinical outcomes. *Am J Sports Med* 2009;37(9):1712-1720.

33. Lord J, Winell JJ: Overuse injuries in pediatric athletes. *Curr Opin Pediatr* 2004;16(1):47-50.

34. Micheli LJ: Overuse injuries in children's sports: The growth factor. *Orthop Clin North Am* 1983;14(2):337-360.

35. Caine D, Maffulli N, Caine C: Epidemiology of injury in child and adolescent sports: Injury rates, risk factors, and prevention. *Clin Sports Med* 2008;27(1):19-50, vii.

36. Bright RW, Burstein AH, Elmore SM: Epiphyseal-plate cartilage: A biomechanical and histological analysis of failure modes. *J Bone Joint Surg Am* 1974;56(4):688-703.

37. Fazarale JJ, Magnussen RA, Pedroza AD, Kaeding CC, Best TM, Classie J: Knowledge of and compliance with pitch count recommendations: A survey of youth baseball coaches. *Sports Health* 2012;4(3):202-204.

    In a survey of youth baseball coaches, only 43% of the respondents were able to correctly answer questions regarding pitch counts and rest periods, although 73% believed they were following recommendations. Thirty-five percent of the coaches reported that their pitchers reported shoulder or elbow pain during the season, and 19% reported that one of their players pitched a game with a sore arm during the season. Level of evidence: IV.

38. Lyman S, Fleisig GS, Waterbor JW, et al: Longitudinal study of elbow and shoulder pain in youth baseball pitchers. *Med Sci Sports Exerc* 2001;33(11):1803-1810.

39. Sabick MB, Kim YK, Torry MR, Keirns MA, Hawkins RJ: Biomechanics of the shoulder in youth baseball pitchers: Implications for the development of proximal humeral epiphysiolysis and humeral retrotorsion. *Am J Sports Med* 2005;33(11):1716-1722.

40. Drakos MC, Rudzki JR, Allen AA, Potter HG, Altchek DW: Internal impingement of the shoulder in the overhead athlete. *J Bone Joint Surg Am* 2009;91(11):2719-2728.

41. Kibler WB, Dome D: Internal impingement: Concurrent superior labral and rotator cuff injuries. *Sports Med Arthrosc* 2012;20(1):30-33.

    Internal impingement refers to the pathologic combination of a SLAP injury and a partial-thickness rotator cuff injury in throwing shoulders. Treatment should address all existing pathologies.

42. Eisner EA, Roocroft JH, Edmonds EW: Underestimation of labral pathology in adolescents with anterior shoulder instability. *J Pediatr Orthop* 2012;32(1):42-47.

    Clinical history and physical examination have 59% accuracy and 79% positive predictive values for detecting labral pathology in adolescent patients, whereas magnetic resonance arthrography has 86% accuracy and 95% positive predictive values. Level of evidence: III.

43. Ryu RK, Fan RS: Adolescent and pediatric sports injuries. *Pediatr Clin North Am* 1998;45(6):1601-1635, x.

44. Ireland ML, Andrews JR: Shoulder and elbow injuries in the young athlete. *Clin Sports Med* 1988;7(3):473-494.

45. Snook GA: A review of women's collegiate gymnastics. *Clin Sports Med* 1985;4(1):31-37.

46. Kibler WB: Rehabilitation of rotator cuff tendinopathy. *Clin Sports Med* 2003;22(4):837-847.

47. Bedi A, Dodson C, Altchek DW: Symptomatic SLAP tear and paralabral cyst in a pediatric athlete: A case report. *J Bone Joint Surg Am* 2010;92(3):721-725.

48. Kocher MS, Waters PM, Micheli LJ: Upper extremity injuries in the paediatric athlete. *Sports Med* 2000;30(2):117-135.

49. Fulton MN, Albright JP, El-Khoury GY: Cortical desmoid-like lesion of the proximal humerus and its occurrence in gymnasts (ringman's shoulder lesion). *Am J Sports Med* 1979;7(1):57-61.

50. Haus B, Nasreddine AY, Suppan C, Kocher MS: Treatment of snapping scapula syndrome in children and adolescents. *J Pediatr Orthop* 2015; Apr 9 [Epub ahead of print].

Although most patients with snapping scapula syndrome can be treated successfully with nonsurgical measures, those who do not respond well require a further workup to look for possible structural components to the syndrome. These patients often obtain relief from surgical intervention. Level of evidence: IV.

51. Auringer ST, Anthony EY: Common pediatric sports injuries. *Semin Musculoskelet Radiol* 1999;3(3):247-256.

Chapter 46

Ankle Injuries

Joel Kolmodin, MD   Paul M. Saluan, MD

Abstract

Ankle injuries are exceedingly common in pediatric athletes and represent a leading cause of missed athletic participation. The incidence of acute ankle injuries may be increased in patients with underlying abnormalities, such as tarsal coalition or Achilles tendon contracture. Acute ankle injuries, such as ankle sprains and peroneal tendon injuries, generally can be treated nonsurgically with a short period of immobilization and limited weight bearing followed by focused rehabilitation. Chronic ankle pain, often the result of repetitive ankle trauma, is typically caused by abnormalities such as talar osteochondral lesions, ankle tendon instability, and peroneal tendon pathology. Surgical management is sometimes indicated for the treatment of chronic ankle pathologies.

Keywords: peroneal tendon; sprain; syndesmosis; talus; talar osteochondritis dissecans (OCD)

Introduction

Ankle injuries are exceedingly common in pediatric athletes and are a leading cause of missed athletic participation. Such injuries are expected to increase as the rate of athletic participation increases and sports participation begins at younger ages. A thorough understanding of ankle anatomy and pathology is needed to accurately diagnose and treat pediatric patients who have ankle pain. Athletic injuries, such as a distal fibular physeal fracture, a lateral process talus fracture, peroneal tendon injuries, osteochondral defects of the talus, and sequelae of tarsal coalition, can be very subtle on imaging and at the physical examination and often are misdiagnosed. This chapter will highlight diagnostic and treatment considerations when treating commonly encountered ankle injuries in pediatric athletes.

Low Ankle Sprain

Ankle sprains—90% of which are low ankle sprains—represent the most common reason for missed athletic participation in adolescent athletes, and they may result in long-term dysfunction if not treated appropriately. The classic low ankle sprain is defined as a sprain that results in an injury to the lateral ligamentous structures of the ankle, which occur below the level of the distal tibiofibular syndesmosis. These sprains are typically inversion injuries, and the position of the foot during inversion determines the location of the lateral ankle ligamentous injury. Excessive inversion of the plantarflexed foot leads to injury to the anterior talofibular ligament (ATFL), the most common ligament injured by an ankle sprain. Excessive inversion of the dorsiflexed foot causes injury to the calcaneofibular ligament and, less commonly, the posterior talofibular ligament. An increased propensity for these inversion injuries is known to occur in conjunction with obvious cavovarus foot deformity as well as in conjunction with subtle cavovarus foot deformity.[1]

Acute low ankle sprains are typically manifest by a large amount of lateral ankle swelling, pain with weight bearing, and pain in the lateral ankle. The physical examination characteristically shows focal tenderness to palpation over the involved lateral ankle ligamentous structures. The patient may have pain with resisted eversion of the foot, a sign of peroneal tendon injury during the inversion episode. In patients with a history of numerous ankle sprains, the anterior drawer test may be

Dr. Saluan or an immediate family member is a member of a speakers' bureau or has made paid presentations on behalf of Arthrex; serves as a paid consultant to DJ Orthopaedics; serves as an unpaid consultant to Middle Path Innovations and Triatrix; has stock or stock options held in Middle Path Innovations; and has received research or institutional support from Zimmer. Neither Dr. Kolmodin nor any immediate family member has received anything of value from or has stock or stock options held in a commercial company or institution related directly or indirectly to the subject of this chapter.

positive. This test involves anterior translation of the slightly plantarflexed foot; excessive anterior translation represents chronic laxity of the injured ATFL. In addition, inversion stress testing of the neutral foot may demonstrate increased laxity, such as in the setting of an attritional calcaneofibular ligament.

The Ottawa Ankle Rules have been proven as a reliable tool for determining when radiography is necessary in the evaluation of an acute ankle sprain.[2,3] In this case, a fracture is suspected when there is (1) difficulty with weight bearing, (2) tenderness to palpation over the medial or lateral malleolus, (3) tenderness over the navicular, or (4) tenderness over the base of the fifth metatarsal. A lower threshold for obtaining radiographs exists after a patient referral in the outpatient setting, because referrals are often made in situations of more severe injury or chronic symptoms. When radiographs are necessary, weight-bearing AP, lateral, and mortise views are recommended. Varus stress views can be used to evaluate for excessive talar tilt in the setting of ATFL laxity. External rotation stress views should be obtained to rule out a syndesmotic injury, which is characteristic of a high ankle sprain. MRI is rarely warranted, except in the setting of prolonged pain or instability. In this case, MRI is performed to evaluate for associated injuries such as peroneal tendon pathology, talar osteochondral lesions, fractures of the anterior calcaneal process, or fractures of the lateral talar process. Lateral process talar fractures are especially important to consider in the differential diagnosis; a recent study demonstrated that as many as 42% of these injuries are initially misdiagnosed as ankle sprains.[4]

The treatment of an acute low ankle sprain includes rest, ice, compression, and elevation. After the acute phase of injury has resolved, physical therapy is recommended, focusing on peroneal strength and proprioceptive training.[5] Return to play is most efficient when early functional rehabilitation occurs.[6] Bracing also is used to prevent recurrent ligament sprains, and bracing has proved to be a far more reliable method for ankle stabilization during athletic participation than rehabilitation alone.[7]

Surgical management is recommended when patients demonstrate persistent pain and instability despite aggressive nonsurgical treatment. The most common surgical technique is the anatomic technique developed by Broström[8] and later modified by Gould et al.[9] This technique involves shortening and reattaching the ATFL and the calcaneofibular ligament to the distal fibula followed by reinforcement with the extensor retinaculum. Various studies have demonstrated good to excellent results in 90% of patients using this technique.[10,11] Alternative reconstruction methods exist, such as peroneal tenodesis to augment the lax lateral ligaments, but these are not typically used in the pediatric population because of their nonanatomic nature and propensity to produce subtalar stiffness.

High Ankle Sprain

The classic high ankle sprain is an injury to the distal tibiofibular syndesmosis. A much less common variant than a low ankle sprain, high ankle sprains represent less than 10% of all ankle sprains, although this incidence is higher in collision sports. These injuries are invariably rotational injuries, usually caused by external rotation of the foot relative to the leg. Such excessive external rotation causes the talus to drive the distal tibia and fibula apart, leading to a failure of the ligaments that normally maintain their position relative to one another. Associated injuries are quite common, including Weber type B and C ankle fractures, osteochondral defects, and peroneal tendon injuries.

The distal tibiofibular syndesmosis is a complex arrangement of ligaments whose purpose is to maintain the relationship between the distal tibia and the fibula. The ligamentous complex primarily acts to control translational and rotational forces, while allowing small amounts of physiologic motion. The most important ligaments of the syndesmosis include the anterior-inferior tibiofibular ligament, the posterior-inferior tibiofibular ligament, the transverse tibiofibular ligament, and the interosseous ligament. The deltoid ligament also contributes to syndesmotic stability; it prevents lateral translation of the talus. The anterior-inferior tibiofibular ligament originates from the anterior distal tibia (Chaput tubercle) and inserts into the anterior aspect of the distal fibula (Wagstaffe tubercle). The posterior-inferior tibiofibular ligament, which originates from the posterior distal tibia (Volkmann tubercle) and inserts into the posterior aspect of the lateral malleolus, is the strongest component of the syndesmosis. The interosseous ligament represents a distal thickening of the interosseous membrane, transversely connecting the tibia and the fibula.

Patients with high ankle sprains often report pain slightly above the ankle joint. They are frequently unable to bear weight on the injured limb, a factor that distinguishes the high ankle sprain from the classic low ankle sprain. Patients typically demonstrate tenderness to palpation over the distal tibial syndesmosis anterolaterally, which can extend up the leg. In fact, the level of the proximal tenderness (the tenderness length) has been shown to correlate with return-to-play time. Patients also may demonstrate medial ankle pain in situations in which the deltoid ligament is injured; deltoid injury signifies increased instability of the ankle joint.

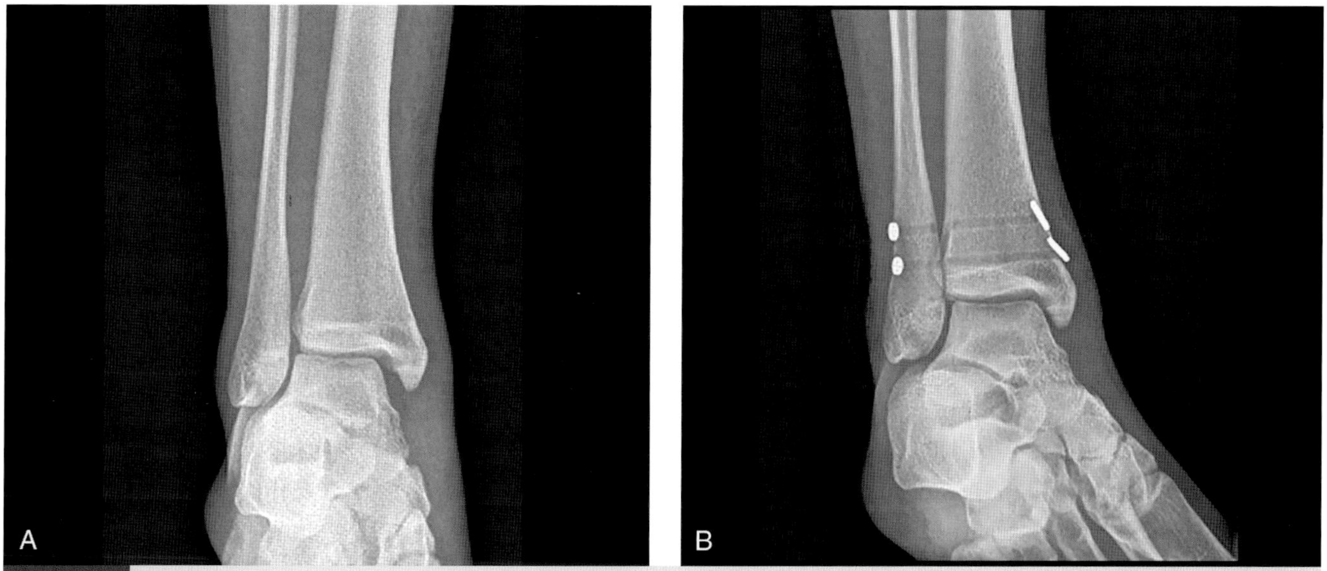

Figure 1 **A,** AP stress radiograph of the ankle of an adolescent athlete shows an isolated syndesmotic sprain. **B,** Mortise radiograph after fixation of the syndesmosis with a suture-button.

Various provocative tests are used to diagnose a high ankle sprain. The Hopkin squeeze test is performed by applying compressive pressure to the mid-calf level; the response is considered positive if pain is elicited during the maneuver. The external rotation test is performed by dorsiflexing and externally rotating the foot—essentially re-creating the forces that caused the injury. The test is positive if pain is elicited.

As with low ankle sprains, radiographic evaluation of suspected high ankle sprains includes AP, lateral, and mortise views of the ankle (**Figure 1**). Decreased tibiofibular overlap on the AP view and increased tibiofibular clear space on the mortise view are suggestive of a syndesmotic injury, which can be confirmed with external rotation stress and gravity stress views. Because Tillaux fractures can be misdiagnosed by those who have limited knowledge of the distal tibial physeal closure pattern, careful attention must be paid to ankle radiographs of skeletally immature patients. Advanced imaging is rarely indicated, although MRI can be used when there is a high suspicion of injury in a patient with negative radiographic findings. MRI is highly sensitive and specific for syndesmotic injury.[12]

The management of distal tibiofibular syndesmotic injuries varies depending on the nature and the severity of the injury. Syndesmotic sprains with no evidence of tibiofibular diastasis can be treated with a short non–weight-bearing period. Weight bearing is then gradually reinstituted, and bracing with a rigid orthosis is used to prevent external rotation forces at the ankle. Patients should be counseled regarding the prolonged recovery time after a high ankle sprain. Patients also should be observed closely after nonsurgical treatment because a known complication of a high ankle sprain is distal tibiofibular synostosis, which is rarely symptomatic but can require surgical excision if it is excessively painful.

Surgical indications for syndesmotic injuries include failed nonsurgical treatment, evidence of instability on stress radiographs, and an associated fracture. The surgical treatment of these injuries has evolved. Traditional management included reduction and screw fixation of the syndesmosis, and screw fixation was attained by capturing either three or four cortices. Excellent results have been reported when the syndesmosis was accurately reduced.[13] However, the use of a syndesmotic screw requires eventual screw removal and adds risk for screw breakage and other complications if it is left in place too long.[14] To address these shortcomings, suture-button fixation recently has been advocated. Theoretically, suture-button fixation allows a small amount of physiologic motion at the syndesmosis, which may prevent subtle, inaccurate reduction.[15] In addition, the suture-button device does not require removal. Early results using the suture-button technique have been very encouraging, showing comparable outcomes and a faster return to activity.[14,15]

Ankle Sprain Equivalent Fractures

Ankle injuries can vary greatly depending on the skeletal status of the patient. For the patient who is skeletally immature, ankle fractures are more common than ankle sprains. In fact, fractures of the distal tibia and fibula are second only to fractures of the distal radius as the most common physeal fractures in children. Classically, the distal fibular physeal fracture has been considered the equivalent injury to the low ankle sprain in the athlete who is skeletally immature. Thus, a patient with normal radiographs and symptoms of an ankle sprain with focal tenderness over the distal fibular physis is presumed to have a physeal fracture because the cartilage of the growth plate is biomechanically weaker than the neighboring lateral ankle ligaments. However, subsequent studies have demonstrated that this is not always the case. Two recent studies found that the incidence of a distal fibular physeal fracture in a patient who is skeletally immature and has lateral ankle pain and negative radiographs is rather low, ranging from 14% to 18%.[16,17] Further, a recent study found that unrecognized ATFL avulsion fractures occur in up to 26% of skeletally immature patients with a presumed ankle sprain.[18] These three studies demonstrate that ligamentous injuries of the ankle do occur in patients who are skeletally immature, despite the presence of open physes. Thus, the accurate diagnosis of ankle injuries can be challenging in the pediatric population.

Equivalent injuries to the high ankle sprain in the patient who is skeletally immature are the Tillaux fracture (**Figure 2**) and the triplane fracture. It has been established that distal tibial physeal closure occurs in a characteristic central-to-medial-to-lateral fashion, which means that the anterolateral portion of the physis is the last to close. This process occurs during an 18-month window for adolescents aged 13 to 16 years, during which time "transitional" fractures such as these occur.[19] Because the anterolateral tibial epiphysis is the site of distal tibiofibular ligament attachment, this area is the most susceptible to fracture during rotational ankle injuries. The Tillaux fracture is a Salter-Harris type III fracture that involves fracture in the sagittal and axial planes within the epiphysis only. The triplane fracture is a Salter-Harris type IV fracture that includes a coronal fracture that extends into the distal tibial metaphysis.

For the patient with a Tillaux or triplane fracture, closed reduction with or without fixation is the standard treatment. An internal rotation reduction maneuver is used to achieve reduction (**Figure 3**); if the fracture is displaced, fixation is typically performed with cannulated screws in the epiphysis and/or the metaphysis, depending on the nature of the fracture. Postreduction CT scans are recommended in cases when a nonanatomic reduction is obtained. A recent study demonstrated that good long-term outcomes could be achieved with residual fracture displacement up to 2.5 mm after reduction.[20] Larger amounts of displacement necessitate open, anatomic reduction and internal fixation. Reduction often can be obtained in a closed manner, and internal fixation is typically accomplished with two anterior-to-posterior screws through the epiphysis (Tillaux fracture) or metaphysis (triplane fracture). Because the fracture is transitional in nature, expeditious physeal closure is expected, and angular deformity is rarely a concern.

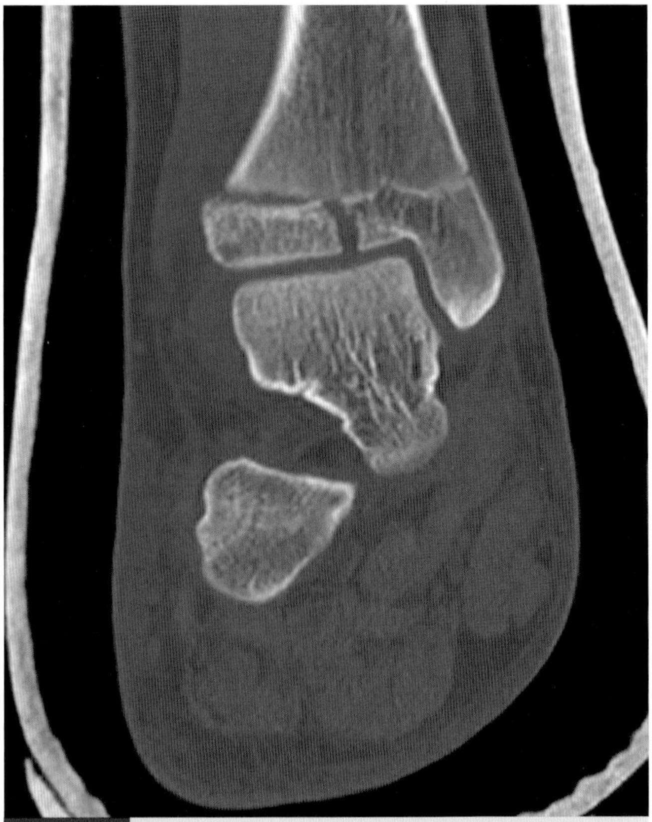

Figure 2 Coronal slice CT image from an adolescent athlete shows a Tillaux fracture with 4 mm of displacement at the articular surface.

Peroneal Tendon Injuries

Peroneal tendon injuries—both acute and chronic—are uncommon in the young, athletic population, although they remain an overlooked cause of lateral ankle pain. Peroneal tendon pathology takes many forms, including tenosynovitis, a tendon tear, and tendon instability. These injuries often are observed in the setting of lateral ankle ligamentous instability. Anatomic studies have demonstrated that the tendons are perched along the distal fibula at 15° to 25° of plantar flexion, making them susceptible to inversion injury at this position. Thus, peroneal tendon injury occurs when there is rapid dorsiflexion of the inverted foot. This rapid movement causes reflexive contraction of the peroneus brevis and longus, which

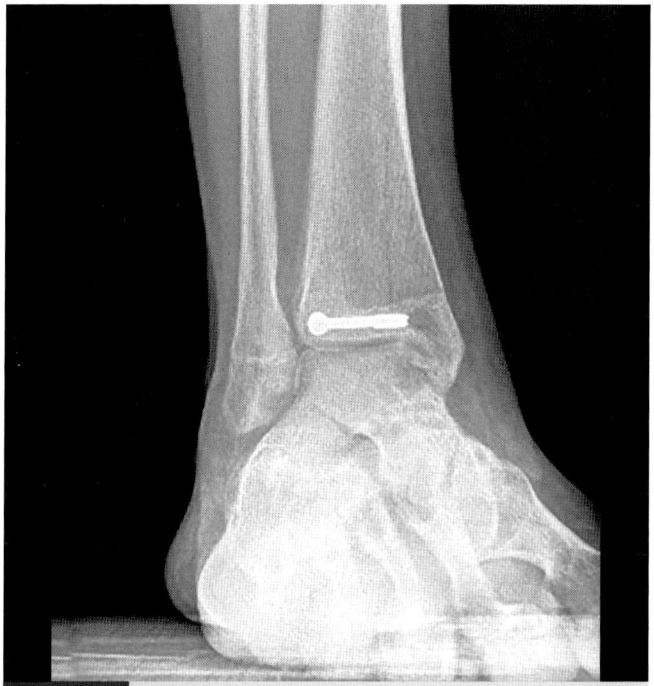

Figure 3 Mortise radiograph of the ankle of the patient shown in Figure 2 after open reduction and internal fixation through the distal tibial epiphysis.

can lead to frank tendon injury or injury to the superior peroneal retinaculum (SPR).[21] Chronic symptoms can develop when the tendons are not anatomically located in their retromalleolar position and subsequently subluxate abnormally with ankle motion. In cases in which the SPR is disrupted, the peroneal tendons will subluxate repeatedly, which often leads to longitudinal tears, most frequently in the peroneus brevis where it runs within the fibular groove. Peroneal tendon injuries at the level of the ankle should be differentiated from Iselin disease, which is a traction apophysitis seen in the pediatric population and results from repetitive traction of the peroneus brevis at its attachment at the base of the fifth metatarsal.

The peroneal tendons include the peroneus brevis and peroneus longus. The peroneus brevis originates from the distal half of the lateral fibula and inserts into the base of the fifth metatarsal, making it a strong evertor and plantar flexor of the foot. The peroneus longus originates more proximally on the lateral fibula and inserts into the medial cuneiform and the first metatarsal base, thus allowing it to assist in foot eversion and plantar flexion. Together, the peroneal tendons provide supplemental lateral ankle stability. Both the peroneus brevis and peroneus longus run posterior to the lateral malleolus in the retromalleolar sulcus. This sulcus is deepened by a fibrocartilaginous rim, which provides moderate inherent stability to the tendons as they course through the region. Within the sulcus, the peroneus longus is found posterior to the peroneus brevis; the brevis can be easily identified further by its low-lying muscle belly, which typically terminates approximately 3 cm from the tip of the fibula. The SPR, which runs from the posterolateral ridge of the fibula to the lateral calcaneus, is essential to the proper function of the peroneal tendon complex. This retinacular structure functions as the primary restraint to peroneal tendon subluxation within the retromalleolar sulcus.

Young patients with peroneal tendon pathology often report an acute injury, usually accompanied by a popping sound or sensation. They typically experience localized pain posterior to the lateral malleolus, with symptoms of clicking and popping with ankle motion, signifying either peroneal tendon instability or tendinopathy. The physical examination will exhibit tenderness to palpation in this region, as well as pain elicited with dorsiflexion and eversion against resistance. In some instances, patients may be able to voluntarily subluxate the tendons with eversion of the foot.

Plain radiographs are used in the initial evaluation of suspected peroneal tendon injuries, including weight-bearing foot and ankle radiographs. Occasionally, a cortical avulsion of the SPR can be seen, which is classically termed a rim fracture. It can be seen on a mortise view of the ankle, which brings the distal fibula into profile as the leg is internally rotated. CT can be used to assess the osseous anatomy of the lateral ankle, specifically the convexity of the retromalleolar sulcus. MRI often is useful in identifying specific peroneal tendon pathology, such as an SPR tear, a pathologic low-lying peroneus brevis muscle belly, the presence of an anomalous peroneus quartus muscle, and tendon tears.

SPR injuries are characterized according to the Ogden classification.[21] Grade I injuries are characterized by partial avulsion of the SPR from the distal fibula, allowing subluxation of the tendons. Grade II injuries involve separation of the SPR from the distal fibrocartilaginous rim; in this case, the tendons pass between the SPR and the rim. In grade III injuries, there is a frank cortical avulsion of the SPR from the distal fibula, forming the classic rim fracture. Grade IV injuries are characterized by SPR failure at the calcaneus instead of the fibula.

Acute peroneal tendon injuries in the pediatric population should initially be treated nonsurgically with rest, ice, and NSAIDs. Physical therapy and ankle bracing can be effective in preventing further ankle instability episodes. In more severe cases where SPR injury and peroneal tendon subluxation are suspected, immobilization in a short-leg cast and protected weight bearing for 4 to 6 weeks is advocated. Care should be taken to make sure that the peroneal tendons are appropriately reduced in the retromalleolar sulcus during casting; slight ankle plantar flexion during casting is sometimes necessary and is well tolerated in the pediatric population.

Acute repair of the SPR is rarely indicated, except in a serious athlete. With acute repair, the torn retinaculum or the cortical avulsion can be directly repaired to its fibular origin with excellent success and quick return to function. Chronic peroneal tendon injuries, such as a chronically lax SPR or a peroneal tendon tear, frequently require surgical management; prior studies have demonstrated success rates of less than 50% with the nonsurgical treatment of chronic disorders.[21]

The management of chronic peroneal subluxation or dislocation focuses on reestablishing a competent SPR and retromalleolar sulcus. SPR repair is typically performed by detaching and reattaching the retinacular tissue in a pants-over-vest manner, allowing the redundant SPR tissue to reinforce the repair. This construct can be augmented by local tissue, such as local Achilles tendon tissue or the plantaris tendon. In cases of a dysplastic, shallow retromalleolar sulcus, a groove-deepening procedure may be indicated to enhance the stability of the tendons.[22] Current techniques involve removal of the subcortical bone of the posterior lateral malleolus and subsequent impaction of the thin cortical rim of bone that remains. These techniques produce a deepened sulcus that is characterized by a smooth remaining floor.

Peroneal tendon tears are uncommon in the pediatric athlete, although they can occur as the result of repetitive tendon subluxation. When present, tears are usually longitudinal and involve the peroneus brevis. This tendon is prone to injury from the sharp posterolateral ridge of the distal fibula.

Tears of the peroneus longus are far less common. When present, these tears are frequently seen in conjunction with peroneus brevis tears and occur distal to the tip of the fibula. Nonsurgical treatment of peroneal tendon tears has poor outcomes, so surgical management often is indicated. The standard repair of longitudinal tears involves débridement, repair, and tubularization of the tendon using a small monofilament suture.[23] Peroneus brevis tenodesis is a reliable method to manage chronic tears,[24] but this procedure is not routinely performed in the pediatric population.

Talar Osteochondritis Dissecans

In the pediatric population, talar osteochondritis dissecans (OCD) occurs infrequently. Originally thought to be the result of an avascular process, OCD is now thought to be caused by acute or repetitive microtrauma. The talus is the third most common joint at which to find evidence of OCD, behind only the knee and the capitellum. OCD is 1.5 times more frequent in females than males, and it is 7 times more likely to occur in adolescents than in younger children.[25] Talar OCD occurs almost exclusively in the talar dome, although it has been reported in the talar head.[26] For OCD involving the talar dome, lesions on the medial and lateral aspects of the talar dome occur at approximately equal rates, although a slight trend is toward an increased prevalence of medial lesions.[27] Numerous studies have demonstrated distinct differences between medial and lateral talar OCD lesions. Lateral lesions are invariably associated with a history of trauma, and they tend to be smaller and more superficial. Medial lesions are less frequently associated with trauma (64% to 82%) but tend to be larger and deeper.[28,29]

The talus articulates with the tibia, the fibula, the navicular, and the calcaneus. The talar dome, which articulates with the tibial plafond, is trapezoidal in shape—narrower posteriorly than anteriorly. The talus has no tendinous attachments and is mostly covered by cartilage. Thus, its blood supply is provided by a limited number of small branches of the dorsalis pedis, peroneal, and posterior tibial arteries. Blood supply to the talar dome occurs in a retrograde fashion. Because of the relatively limited vascularity of the talar dome and the inherent avascularity of its articular cartilage, talar OCD lesions have limited capacity for spontaneous healing. In addition, talar OCD lesion healing is inhibited by the fact that the tibiotalar joint is subjected to a tremendous amount of force—more per unit area than any other joint in the body.

Patients with talar OCD report a history of prolonged ankle pain, usually following a traumatic episode or a series of traumatic episodes. They often experience mechanical symptoms, such as catching and grinding, which may signal the presence of a loose body or an unstable cartilage flap. Because it is an intra-articular process, most patients also report swelling and ankle stiffness. These patients may be referred to an orthopaedic surgeon after a prolonged period of unsuccessful nonsurgical management. Evaluation often demonstrates swelling and diffuse ankle pain, with restricted range of motion. Because these lesions are associated with recurrent trauma, instability testing is vital in patients with suspected talar OCD, including anterior drawer and inversion/eversion testing.

Radiographic evaluation begins with standard ankle radiographs, including weight-bearing AP, lateral, and mortise views. However, many talar OCD lesions, particularly low-grade lesions, are not visible on plain radiographs. CT can be used for evaluation (**Figure 4**), but it is successful only in evaluating the integrity of subchondral bone; it is not effective in the diagnosis and characterization of lesions that are purely cartilaginous. Thus, MRI is recommended for further evaluation of all known or suspected talar OCD lesions. MRI also is useful for evaluating the integrity of articular cartilage, bone edema, and surrounding soft-tissue pathology.

Various classifications exist for talar OCD lesions. The best-recognized system is the Berndt and Harty classification,[27] which characterizes lesions based on plain radiography. Stage I lesions are those with an area of subchondral compression; stage II lesions are those with a partially detached osteochondral fragment; stage III lesions are those with a fully detached osteochondral fragment; and stage IV lesions are those with a visible loose body. A second frequently used classification system is the Hepple staging system, which is based on MRI findings.[30] This staging system is very useful for surgical planning because MRI has been found to correlate closely with arthroscopic findings.[31]

Nonsurgical management typically involves immobilization and strict adherence to a non–weight-bearing period for 6 to 9 weeks, which is followed by gradual transition to full weight bearing and physical therapy. This treatment is routinely recommended for Berndt and Harty grade I and II lesions, although the original article (1959) reported overall poor outcomes in 75% of the talar OCD lesions treated nonsurgically.[27] A more recent systematic review in 2003 supported these findings, demonstrating a success rate of only 45% with nonsurgical management based on radiographic and clinical outcomes.[32] The treating surgeon should be aware, however, that the patient who responds well to nonsurgical management may demonstrate persistent radiographic evidence of disease despite having no symptoms.[26]

Surgery is generally indicated for patients with symptomatic OCD lesions if radiographs do not demonstrate radiographic healing or if there is no improvement in symptoms despite nonsurgical management. In contrast with OCD lesions of the knee and elbow in which skeletal maturity and larger lesion size clearly have a negative effect on healing potential and outcomes with nonsurgical management, outcomes of nonsurgical and surgical treatment of OCD lesions of the talus do not appear to be directly related to lesion size or skeletal status.[33] This finding may suggest that there is less overall functional healing capacity for OCD lesions in the ankle compared with those of the knee and elbow, even in skeletally immature patients with small lesions. Thus, prolonged nonsurgical management of small lesions in skeletally immature patients may not be beneficial, and surgical intervention may be indicated in these patients.

Numerous surgical strategies for the management of talar OCD lesions are available. Regardless of the treatment, the goal is to restore the anatomy of the talar dome, thus reestablishing normal joint reactive forces within the ankle joint. The broad categories of surgical management are as follows: repair of the lesion, débridement and stimulation of the lesion, and transplantation to fill the lesion.[34] Current trends favor arthroscopic management over open treatment, although open measures in the form of an arthrotomy and a medial malleolar osteotomy may be needed for surgical therapies that are more aggressive[35] (**Figure 5**).

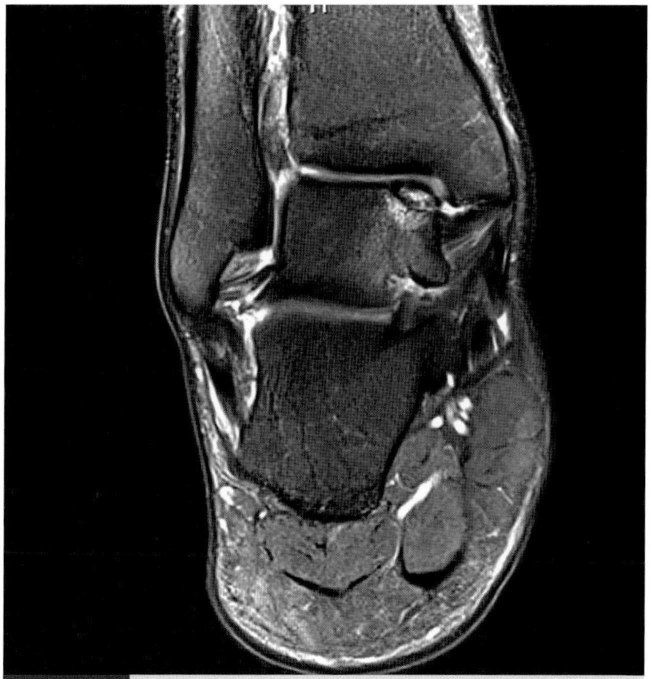

Figure 4 Coronal slice CT of the ankle of an adolescent athlete shows a posteromedial talar osteochondritis dissecans lesion.

In patients in whom the cartilage surface is intact and stable, as with grade I lesions, antegrade or retrograde drilling may be used. This drilling stimulates healing by opening the sclerotic subchondral bone and allowing bleeding into the defect. Antegrade drilling occurs through the intact cartilage of the OCD lesion. It is accomplished arthroscopically and is the most accurate way to confirm penetration of the subchondral bone. Retrograde drilling is accomplished by inserting 0.062-inch Kirschner wires into the defect through the tarsal sinus laterally or the talar body medially; image guidance is used to triangulate the defect. Prior studies have shown up to 91% fair or good outcomes with antegrade and retrograde techniques.[36]

In cases of grade II lesions with relatively normal cartilage and adequate attached subchondral bone, simple fragment fixation is recommended. Fixation can occur

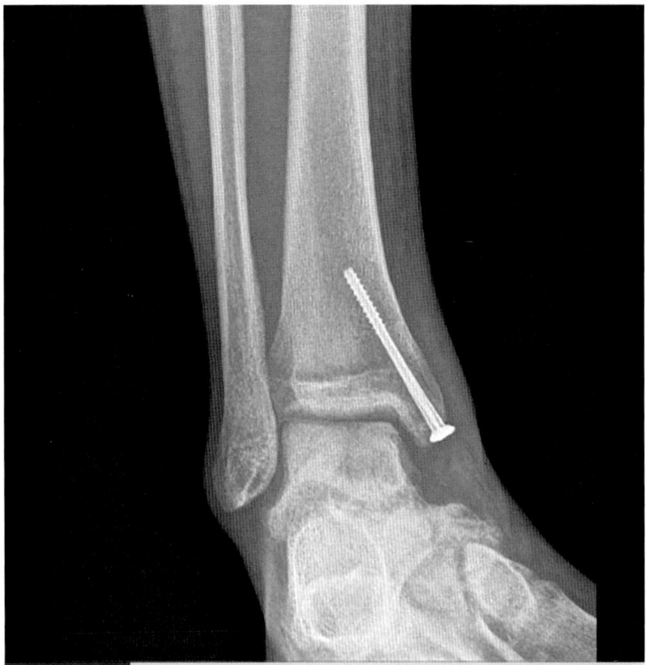

Figure 5 Mortise radiograph of the patient shown in Figure 4 after medial malleolar osteotomy and osteochondral autograft from the ipsilateral knee.

with either screws or bioabsorbable devices. It is important to débride the back side of the fragment and remove any loose tissue before fixation of the fragment. Lesions that are located anteriorly may be amenable to arthroscopic fixation. However, lesions that are focused on the posterior talar dome are difficult to access with appropriate instrumentation. In these cases, a medial malleolar osteotomy (for medial lesions) or an anterolateral tibial osteotomy (for lesions located further laterally) may be indicated. Recently, some authors have advocated lesion salvage procedures, such as drilling or fixation, whenever possible, because they yield reliable results in most patients. Lesion salvage procedures have been shown, however, to have slightly higher revision rates compared with techniques that are more aggressive, such as microfracture or osteochondral transfer techniques.[33]

The most common surgical intervention for grade III and IV lesions involves the removal of loose bodies, aggressive débridement, and drilling of the subchondral bone (microfracture). This process allows for the release of marrow elements into the defect, resulting in the formation of fibrocartilage in the cartilage gap. Débridement and microfracture have produced reliable results in recent studies.[33,35,37] In the largest systematic review to date, a group of researchers found good or excellent results in 85% of patients who were treated with débridement and microfracture; most of these patients had lesions of grade III or higher.[38]

Débridement and microfracture have produced reliable results, although these techniques are limited by their inability to address large defects and provide hyaline cartilage within the defect. It also is unclear how well these techniques can address an uncontained OCD lesion, a lesion that includes the lateral or medial shoulder of the talus. A recent large study of talar OCD in the adolescent population found a high revision rate of 27% for patients who had undergone drilling, fragment fixation, or microfracture.[33] Thus, recent research has sought to determine the optimal surgical strategy based on the characteristics of a given lesion. Newer strategies have been developed to address situations in which drilling, fragment fixation, or microfracture may not be effective options and include osteochondral transfer (autograft or allograft) and autologous chondrocyte implantation.

Within the pediatric population, the most frequently used technique is osteochondral autograft transfer. This procedure involves the harvest of circular osteochondral plugs from a patient donor site (typically the ipsilateral knee) and insertion into the talar defect in a side-by-side manner, frequently through a tibial osteotomy. The largest series using this technique was published in 2008 and reported good to excellent results in 93% of the patients, with only 3% of the patients exhibiting donor site knee pain.[39] Subsequent studies have shown high rates of return to sport, although many patients modify their sporting activities.[40] For uncontained defects, small, circular osteochondral plugs may not be able to effectively re-create the shoulder of the talus, leading to excessive shear forces at the site and premature graft failure. Thus, some authors advocate using large (partial talar body) allograft transfer in this case. This is an area of active research, however, because outcomes studies in this particular clinical situation are lacking.

Summary

Ankle injuries are commonly seen in the pediatric population and often are the cause of missed athletic participation. Subtle pediatric ankle injuries, such as physeal fractures, peroneal tendon injuries, and osteochondral injuries, commonly go unnoticed at the initial evaluation by primary care providers. Accurate diagnosis by the orthopaedic provider requires knowledge of pediatric ankle anatomy and injury patterns, which are different from those in the adult athlete. Indications for the nonsurgical management of ankle injuries are expanded in the pediatric athlete compared with their adult counterparts.

Surgical intervention for various pathologies can be effective when used for the correct indication.

Key Study Points

- Ankle injuries can vary depending on the skeletal status of a patient. Distal fibula fractures are common in patients who are skeletally immature, although purely ligamentous injuries and ATFL avulsion fractures occur regularly.
- Syndesmotic reduction with screw or suture-button fixation yields reliable results. Suture-button fixation, however, has been shown to produce a lower rate of malreduction and rarely requires a second surgery for removal.
- Poor outcomes are seen with nonsurgical management of talar OCD lesions. Surgical options vary depending on lesion characteristics. In the pediatric population, first-line management typically entails osteochondral fragment salvage procedures, such as drilling or fragment fixation whenever possible.

Annotated References

1. Fortin PT, Guettler J, Manoli A II: Idiopathic cavovarus and lateral ankle instability: Recognition and treatment implications relating to ankle arthritis. *Foot Ankle Int* 2002;23(11):1031-1037.

2. David S, Gray K, Russell JA, Starkey C: Validation of the Ottawa Ankle Rules for acute foot and ankle injuries. *J Sport Rehabil* 2016;25(1):48-51.

   This review of strictly applying the Ottawa Ankle Rules in 124 consecutive high school and college athletes within 1 hour after injury resulted in no missed fractures but overestimated the need for radiographs.

3. Plint AC, Bulloch B, Osmond MH, et al: Validation of the Ottawa Ankle Rules in children with ankle injuries. *Acad Emerg Med* 1999;6(10):1005-1009.

4. Wu Y, Jiang H, Wang B, Miao W: Fracture of the lateral process of the talus in children: A kind of ankle injury with frequently missed diagnosis. *J Pediatr Orthop* 2016;36(3):289-293.

   A review of 12 consecutive children who had treatment of a lateral process talus fracture at one institution demonstrated that 5 fractures (42%) were missed at the initial visit to the emergency department. Nonetheless, outcomes were good or excellent in 11 of the 12 patients.

5. Hupperets MD, Verhagen EA, van Mechelen W: Effect of unsupervised home based proprioceptive training on recurrences of ankle sprain: Randomised controlled trial. *BMJ* 2009;339:b2684.

6. Maffulli N, Ferran NA: Management of acute and chronic ankle instability. *J Am Acad Orthop Surg* 2008;16(10):608-615.

7. Janssen KW, van Mechelen W, Verhagen EA: Bracing superior to neuromuscular training for the prevention of self-reported recurrent ankle sprains: A three-arm randomised controlled trial. *Br J Sports Med* 2014;48(16):1235-1239.

   A randomized controlled trial showed that bracing is superior to neuromuscular training in preventing recurrent ankle sprains at 1-year follow-up.

8. Broström L: Sprained ankles. VI. Surgical treatment of "chronic" ligament ruptures. *Acta Chir Scand* 1966;132(5):551-565.

9. Gould N, Seligson D, Gassman J: Early and late repair of lateral ligament of the ankle. *Foot Ankle* 1980;1(2):84-89.

10. Cho BK, Kim YM, Kim DS, Choi ES, Shon HC, Park KJ: Outcomes of the modified Brostrom procedure using suture anchors for chronic lateral ankle instability: A prospective, randomized comparison between single and double suture anchors. *J Foot Ankle Surg* 2013;52(1):9-15.

    A randomized controlled trial compared outcomes for single- versus double-suture anchor Broström repair at greater than 2-year follow-up. Comparable improvement in outcomes scores was seen between the two groups, and satisfactory results were seen in 90% of the cases.

11. Petrera M, Dwyer T, Theodoropoulos JS, Ogilvie-Harris DJ: Short- to medium-term outcomes after a modified Broström repair for lateral ankle instability with immediate postoperative weightbearing. *Am J Sports Med* 2014;42(7):1542-1548.

    A case series of 55 patients underwent modified Broström repair. At an average follow-up of 42 months, the return-to-sport rate was 94%, and only 6% of the patients reported residual instability. Level of evidence: IV.

12. Sikka RS, Fetzer GB, Sugarman E, et al: Correlating MRI findings with disability in syndesmotic sprains of NFL players. *Foot Ankle Int* 2012;33(5):371-378.

    A study of 36 National Football League players who sustained syndesmotic injures showed that a positive squeeze test and increased injury severity on MRI correlated with an increase in the number of games missed.

13. Schepers T: Acute distal tibiofibular syndesmosis injury: A systematic review of suture-button versus syndesmotic screw repair. *Int Orthop* 2012;36(6):1199-1206.

    In this systematic review of syndesmotic screw versus suture-button repair of isolated syndesmotic disruptions, similar outcomes between the methods were observed, and implant removal was lower for the suture-button technique (10% versus 52%).

14. Schepers T, Van Lieshout EM, de Vries MR, Van der Elst M: Complications of syndesmotic screw removal. *Foot Ankle Int* 2011;32(11):1040-1044.

In this retrospective review of 76 consecutive patients who underwent syndesmotic screw removal at a level II trauma center, the overall complication rate was 22.4%, including infection in 9.2% and screw breakage in 6.6%.

15. Naqvi GA, Cunningham P, Lynch B, Galvin R, Awan N: Fixation of ankle syndesmotic injuries: Comparison of tightrope fixation and syndesmotic screw fixation for accuracy of syndesmotic reduction. *Am J Sports Med* 2012;40(12):2828-2835.

This cohort study of 46 patients compared suture-button fixation to screw fixation. The outcomes scores were similar between the groups, although malreduction was seen in 21.7% of patients treated with a syndesmotic screw. Malreduction was not found in the patients treated with suture-button fixation. Level of evidence: II.

16. Sankar WN, Chen J, Kay RM, Skaggs DL: Incidence of occult fracture in children with acute ankle injuries. *J Pediatr Orthop* 2008;28(5):500-501.

17. Farley FA, Kuhns L, Jacobson JA, DiPietro M: Ultrasound examination of ankle injuries in children. *J Pediatr Orthop* 2001;21(5):604-607.

18. Kwak YH, Lim JY, Oh MK, Kim WJ, Park KB: Radiographic diagnosis of occult distal fibular avulsion fracture in children with acute lateral ankle sprain. *J Pediatr Orthop* 2015;35(4):352-357.

This diagnostic study found a 26% incidence of ATFL avulsion fractures in patients who were skeletally immature with an ankle sprain and negative initial radiographs. Level of evidence: IV.

19. Kleiger B, Mankin HJ: Fracture of the lateral portion of the distal tibial epiphysis. *J Bone Joint Surg Am* 1964;46:25-32.

20. Choudhry IK, Wall EJ, Eismann EA, Crawford AH, Wilson L: Functional outcome analysis of triplane and tillaux fractures after closed reduction and percutaneous fixation. *J Pediatr Orthop* 2014;34(2):139-143.

In a review of 78 patients with a Tillaux or triplane fracture, closed reduction and percutaneous fixation yielded good results at long-term follow-up as long as residual articular displacement was less than 2.5 mm. Level of evidence: III.

21. Philbin TM, Landis GS, Smith B: Peroneal tendon injuries. *J Am Acad Orthop Surg* 2009;17(5):306-317.

22. Walther M, Morrison R, Mayer B: Retromalleolar groove impaction for the treatment of unstable peroneal tendons. *Am J Sports Med* 2009;37(1):191-194.

23. Steel MW, DeOrio JK: Peroneal tendon tears: Return to sports after operative treatment. *Foot Ankle Int* 2007;28(1):49-54.

24. Heckman DS, Reddy S, Pedowitz D, Wapner KL, Parekh SG: Operative treatment for peroneal tendon disorders. *J Bone Joint Surg Am* 2008;90(2):404-418.

25. Kessler JI, Weiss JM, Nikizad H, et al: Osteochondritis dissecans of the ankle in children and adolescents: Demographics and epidemiology. *Am J Sports Med* 2014;42(9):2165-2171.

In this retrospective epidemiologic review of 85 pediatric (mostly adolescent) patients with talar OCD lesions, the lesions were 1.5 times more likely to occur in females than males.

26. Thacker MM, Dabney KW, Mackenzie WG: Osteochondritis dissecans of the talar head: Natural history and review of literature. *J Pediatr Orthop B* 2012;21(4):373-376.

This is case report of two patients with OCD of the talar head. The natural history and course of the disorder to skeletal maturity are described.

27. Berndt AL, Harty M: Transchondral fractures (osteochondritis dissecans) of the talus. *J Bone Joint Surg Am* 1959;41:988-1020.

28. Canale ST, Belding RH: Osteochondral lesions of the talus. *J Bone Joint Surg Am* 1980;62(1):97-102.

29. Flick AB, Gould N: Osteochondritis dissecans of the talus (transchondral fractures of the talus): Review of the literature and new surgical approach for medial dome lesions. *Foot Ankle* 1985;5(4):165-185.

30. Hepple S, Winson IG, Glew D: Osteochondral lesions of the talus: A revised classification. *Foot Ankle Int* 1999;20(12):789-793.

31. Mintz DN, Tashjian GS, Connell DA, Deland JT, O'Malley M, Potter HG: Osteochondral lesions of the talus: A new magnetic resonance grading system with arthroscopic correlation. *Arthroscopy* 2003;19(4):353-359.

32. Verhagen RA, Struijs PA, Bossuyt PM, van Dijk CN: Systematic review of treatment strategies for osteochondral defects of the talar dome. *Foot Ankle Clin* 2003;8(2):233-242, viii-ix.

33. Kramer DE, Glotzbecker MP, Shore BJ, et al: Results of surgical management of osteochondritis dissecans of the ankle in the pediatric and adolescent population. *J Pediatr Orthop* 2015;35(7):725-733.

In a retrospective review of 109 consecutive cases of talar OCD treated with fragment fixation, transarticular drilling, or microfracture at one institution, 82% of the patients were satisfied, and 84% of the patients returned to sport, although the revision rate was high at 27%.

34. Murawski CD, Kennedy JG: Operative treatment of osteochondral lesions of the talus. *J Bone Joint Surg Am* 2013;95(11):1045-1054.

    This review article highlights current concepts and surgical techniques for addressing OCD lesions of the talus.

35. Goh GS, Bin Abd Razak HR, Mitra AK: Outcomes are favorable after arthroscopic treatment of osteochondritis dissecans of the talus. *J Foot Ankle Surg* 2015;54(1):57-60.

    In a prospective study of 61 consecutive patients who underwent microfracture of talar OCD lesions, 74% of the patients were satisfied with their outcomes at greater than 1-year follow-up, although 41% of the patients had fair or poor outcomes.

36. Kumai T, Takakura Y, Higashiyama I, Tamai S: Arthroscopic drilling for the treatment of osteochondral lesions of the talus. *J Bone Joint Surg Am* 1999;81(9):1229-1235.

37. Barnes CJ, Ferkel RD: Arthroscopic debridement and drilling of osteochondral lesions of the talus. *Foot Ankle Clin* 2003;8(2):243-257.

38. Zengerink M, Struijs PA, Tol JL, van Dijk CN: Treatment of osteochondral lesions of the talus: A systematic review. *Knee Surg Sports Traumatol Arthrosc* 2010;18(2):238-246.

39. Hangody L, Vásárhelyi G, Hangody LR, et al: Autologous osteochondral grafting: Technique and long-term results. *Injury* 2008;39(suppl 1):S32-S39.

40. Paul J, Sagstetter M, Lämmle L, et al: Sports activity after osteochondral transplantation of the talus. *Am J Sports Med* 2012;40(4):870-874.

    In a case series of 131 patients who underwent osteochondral autograft transplantation to address talar OCD lesions, the return-to-sport rate was high (97%), although sport modification was necessary for many patients involved in high-impact sports. Level of evidence: IV.

Chapter 47

Overuse Conditions

Jennifer J. Beck, MD Pamela Lang, MD Richard E. Bowen, MD

Abstract

Promoting safe, well-rounded participation in youth athletics can help develop a lifetime of physical activity and healthy habits while decreasing the risk of injuries. It has become clear that current training regimens of early sport specialization, year-round activity participation, and training of increasing intensity are leading to an increase in overtraining and burnout in young athletes. Although the medical community has a clear understanding of the problem of overuse and burnout, further research is needed on the efficacy of prevention programs, the treatment of overuse injuries, and the appropriate timing of return to sports after an injury.

Keywords: burnout; chronic pain; overtraining; overuse; young athletes

Introduction

According to the National Federation of State High School Associations, participation in high school athletics has increased dramatically from approximately 4 million participants in 1971 to approximately 8 million participants in 2014.[1] Along with this increase in sports participation, the intensity and time requirements of competition and training have amplified. With an increase in the popularity of club sports participation, many children are now playing a single sport throughout the year, without periods of rest and recovery. Consequently, there are increasing numbers of overuse conditions being diagnosed in children. Currently, approximately 50% of childhood sports-related injuries are attributed to overuse.[2-8]

Overuse injuries are caused by repetitive submaximal loading with inadequate rest, resulting in the inability for structural repair and adaptation.[2,3,9] For the purpose of research, an overuse injury has been defined as "a condition to which no identifiable single external transfer of energy could be associated but that led to the athlete being unable to take full part in athletics training."[10] The four stages of overuse are (1) pain after activity, (2) pain during activity but without hindering performance, (3) pain during activity leading to detrimental effects on performance, and (4) unrelenting pain, even at rest.[11] The loss of practice and competition time would be expected for injuries that progress to stages three or four.

Recent research has focused on understanding the etiology and epidemiology of pediatric overuse injuries, describing overuse injuries in pediatric-specific subpopulations and sports, determining risk factors associated with pediatric overuse injuries, and defining prevention strategies for coaches, parents, and medical providers.[2-4,12-15] The treatment of pediatric overuse injuries has received little attention because the traditional treatment modalities of rest, anti-inflammatory medications, physical therapy, and bracing still apply for most patients. For example, a 12-year-old runner with heel pain secondary to Sever disease can be successfully managed with activity modification and stretching.

Epidemiology and Risk Factors

Overuse injuries make up at least 50% of the sports-related injuries that occur during childhood.[2-8,14] Approximately 50% of overuse injuries in high school athletes result in loss of play time or sports participation of more than 1 week.[3] A 2015 study reported that 7.7% of chronic or overuse injuries in high school athletes resulted in more than 21 days of lost competition time, and 2.5% of the athletes required surgical intervention to treat cartilage and disk injuries, tendinosis, tendinitis, or

Dr. Beck or an immediate family member serves as a board member, owner, officer, or committee member of the Pediatric Orthopaedic Society of North America. Neither of the following authors nor any immediate family member has received anything of value from or has stock or stock options held in a commercial company or institution related directly or indirectly to the subject of this chapter: Dr. Lang and Dr. Bowen.

muscle strain.[2] Stress fractures were the most common season-ending overuse injury.[2] Two recent studies found that the most common site of an overuse injury is the lower leg, with approximately 70% of overuse injuries in high school athletes involving the leg.[2,3]

Girls have a higher rate of overuse injuries than boys (13.3% versus 5.5%, respectively) and these injuries occur early during the high school years (30.7% of overuse injuries occurred during the ninth grade).[3] The same sex prevalence was found in high school and collegiate athletes.[2] The lower leg, knee, and ankle, in particular, are the areas that are more commonly affected in girls compared with boys. In a report on high school distance runners, tibial stress injuries were found in 41% of the girls and 34% of the boys, and patellofemoral pain occurred in 21% of the girls and 16% of the boys.[5] The authors of a 2015 study reported that the variability in body mass index (BMI) and sport characteristics between sexes is responsible for approximately 50% of the increased risks of overuse injuries in girls, with the other 50% attributable to biologic differences.[16]

Risk factors for overuse injury can be categorized as either intrinsic or extrinsic.[13,17] Intrinsic risk factors are those that are unique to an individual. Some intrinsic risk factors are not modifiable, including sex and maturation status. Factors such as BMI, biomechanical movement patterns, and anatomic alignment are potentially modifiable intrinsic risk factors.[17] Skeletally immature athletes with joint hypermobility, muscle weakness, and muscle tightness are at increased risk for overuse injury.[9]

Extrinsic risk factors include environment, equipment, and (probably most importantly) training regimens.[17] The authors of an investigation of extrinsic risk factors involved in overuse injury described three scenarios in which these factors play a role in the development of overuse injury.[18] These scenarios involved (1) a rapid increase in training load after a period of decreased activity, (2) participation at an athletic level that exceeds an individual's skill or fitness level, and (3) continuous participation at a high level of athletics or in a single activity or sport.[18]

Physiologic Considerations in the Growing Athlete

Skeletally immature athletes have areas of rapidly growing cartilage, physes, and apophyses, with decreased tensile strength compared with that of surrounding bone and up to five times less tensile strength than surrounding ligaments and tendons.[9,19] The hypertrophic zone, including the zone of provisional calcification, is the weakest portion of the physis; this increases its propensity to injury during phases of rapid growth.[9,20] In addition, muscle and tendon adaptations lag behind longitudinal bone growth, which results in the need for a greater percentage of muscle force to perform the same movements.[19] This increased relative muscle contraction force leads to increased forces transferred to the apophysis and makes the physis and apophysis more vulnerable to injury.[19]

Repetitive stress on the physis may lead to widening, early calcification, and physeal bar formation, which ultimately lead to growth disturbances such as premature distal radius physeal closure in the wrists of gymnasts.[20-24] Growth disturbances related to physeal stress injury also have been documented in the proximal humerus, distal femur, and proximal tibia.[13,21,25,26] One theory is that repetitive stress leads to a disruption of the metaphyseal blood supply, altered endochondral ossification of the physis, and physeal widening caused by chondrocyte accumulation in the proliferative zone.[20]

Not only is there greater stress on the physis and apophysis of bone during periods of growth, but also the mechanical structure of the bone itself may not be able to withstand the demands of high-level, continuous competition. Muscle adaptation and bone mineralization in skeletally immature individuals lags behind linear bone growth.[21,27] Measurements of bone mineral density in a group of boys and girls during the adolescent growth period found that bone mass decreased relative to bone size just before the time of peak height velocity.[28] Following this drop in bone mineral density, a continuous increase occurred until approximately 4 years after peak height velocity.[28] These findings imply that the risk of osseous overuse injury may be highest during the period just before peak height velocity growth.

Specialization, Overtraining, and Burnout

Burnout, which also is known as overtraining syndrome or nonfunctional overreaching, is a maladaptive process resulting from excessive exercise and inadequate rest.[9] It may be caused by an increased training load with inadequate recovery, monotony of training, or overscheduling. Ultimately, burnout increases an athlete's risk for an overuse injury.[9] A 2011 study surveyed 360 pediatric athletes aged 6 to 18 years presenting to sports medicine clinics for injury evaluation. The authors found a substantial association between an athlete's or his or her parent's perception of too much training or competitive play without enough rest between scheduled activities and the time immediately leading up to the onset of symptoms.[15]

The pathophysiology behind burnout is a systemic inflammatory response, affecting the neurohormonal axis (hypothalamus, pituitary, and end organs such as the thyroid, the gonad, and the adrenal glands).[9] As a result, there are detrimental effects on immunity and mood in addition to a decreased level of athletic performance.[9] A survey of 376 English athletes found a lack of confidence and bad feelings in athletes with burnout when their level of performance did not meet their expectations.[29] Diagnostic criteria of burnout include a persistent decrease in performance even after weeks to months of rest, along with mood disturbances that cannot be attributed to other causes.[30] Burnout in a child has been described as decreased enthusiasm to participate in practices or games, chronic muscle or joint pain, an elevated resting heart rate, personality changes, and difficulty in successfully completing familiar routines.[11]

Overtraining and burnout in athletes are becoming more common or, at least, are more widely recognized. At least one occurrence of overtraining was reported by 110 of the 376 athletes (29%) in a survey of English athletes.[29] Women, elite athletes, and participants in sports with low physical demands were more likely to report overtraining.[29] In this group, athletes with overtraining syndrome were more likely to rate their sport as their most important activity, and they spent a limited amount of time engaged in other hobbies.[29] This survey suggests that specialization in a single sport may increase the risk of burnout by allowing an individual to focus all of his or her energy on one sport. A 2015 study attempted to find a relationship between sport specialization and injury in skeletally immature athletes.[12] This study defined specialization as "year-round intensive training in a single sport at the exclusion of other sports."[12] Sport specialization was found to be an independent risk factor for overuse and serious overuse injuries, even when accounting for patient age and hours spent participating in that sport.[12] In addition, a dose-response relationship between the degree of specialization and the severity of the overuse injury was found, with a serious overuse injury more likely to develop in the youth athletes who were the most specialized.[12]

Prevention

In response to the rising concern about overuse injuries in youth athletes, the "STOP Sports Injuries" campaign was initiated in 2007 by the American Orthopaedic Society for Sports Medicine. It is estimated that approximately 50% of overuse injuries in children and adolescents may be preventable.[23] It is believed that prevention of overuse injuries during childhood may be important in preventing chronic overuse conditions later in life and promoting lifelong activity and sports participation.[2,7,13,31] The prevention of overuse injury is a multidisciplinary undertaking and involves improved injury surveillance, identification of risk factors, thorough preparticipation physical examinations, proper supervision and education of coaches and medical staff, improved training and conditioning, sport alterations, and delayed specialization.[13,23,32]

A detailed patient history is important in screening for overuse injury or burnout. The history should include assessment of the athlete's attitude and level of fatigue, parental pressure, and coach involvement. To determine an athlete's training workload, an assessment should be made regarding the number of hours per week of participation in a structured sport along with sport-specific measures such as pitch counts, miles run per week, and the number of team memberships, conditioning or strength training sessions, and days off per week.[9,13] The physical examination should include methods to screen for joint hypermobility (such as the Beighton and Horan Joint Mobility Index) and muscle tightness or imbalances (such as the Ober test, the Thomas test, and evaluation of the popliteal angle, the degree of ankle dorsiflexion, and the glenohumeral internal rotation deficit).[9]

Prevention programs should be aimed at encouraging an appropriate training progression. Training and prevention programs should ultimately strive to help young athletes improve their ability to dampen forces applied to their body.[17] The American Academy of Pediatrics Council on Sports Medicine and Fitness released recommendations aimed at reducing overuse injuries and overtraining in skeletally immature individuals.[11,33] It was suggested that the amount of time in any single sporting activity be limited to a maximum of 5 days per week, with at least 1 day off from any organized physical activity each week.[11,33] The recommendations also include allowing 2 to 3 months away from any particular sport each year.[11,33] In addition, children and adolescents should get at least 7 hours of sleep per night to decrease chronic fatigue and reduce the injury rate.[15,34] In 2015, the International Olympic Committee published their consensus statement on youth athletic development[35] (**Table 1**).

Update on Common Overuse Injuries

Common pediatric overuse injuries of the upper extremity, lower extremity, and spine are listed in **Table 2**.

Elbow Injuries in Young Throwers

With more than 5 million children participating in baseball, rates of elbow injuries seem to be increasing in throwing athletes despite regulations and safety measures implemented by organizational leagues.[36,37] The diagnosis and treatment of pediatric elbow overuse injuries warrants attention.

Table 1

International Olympic Committee Consensus Statement on Youth Athletic Development

General Principles	Conditioning for Injury Prevention	Coaching	Nutrition, Hydration, Heat	Sports Medicine Governing Bodies
Allow for a wider definition of sport success Commit to psychological development of resilient and adaptable athletes Use an evidence-based framework for athlete development and coaching Encourage unstructured play Promote safety, health, and respect for rules, athletes, and the game Assist athletes with sport-life balance	Encourage varied strength and conditioning programs Develop programs with diversity and variability of athletic exposure Promote injury prevention programs, protective equipment legislation, and rule changes No youth athlete should compete, train, or practice in a way that loads the affected injured area or interferes with or delays recovery when in pain or not completely rehabilitated and recovered from an illness or injury	Provide a challenging and enjoyable environment Use research-based techniques that promote innovation and proper technique Encourage athlete intrapersonal and interpersonal skill development Seek interdisciplinary support and guidance	Provide dietary education on a healthy, balanced diet Provide education on risks associated with dietary supplements and energy drinks Mitigate risks of energy deficiency in athletes Educate and train on heat-related illness Create a written emergency plan for treating medical emergencies	Protect the health and well-being of youth in sports with education and safeguards Diversification and variability of athletic exposure should be encouraged Competitions should be age and skill appropriate, with sufficient rest and recovery

In the past, elbow pain was described by the general term Little Leaguer's elbow; however, it is now understood that multiple etiologies contribute to elbow pain in young, throwing athletes. Ulnar collateral ligament injuries, olecranon stress fractures, capitellar osteochondritis dissecans, medial epicondyle apophysitis, and fractures commonly occur in throwing athletes. An increased risk of pitching-related arm pain has been shown in young athletes who pitch on consecutive days, pitch on multiple teams with overlapping seasons, and pitch multiple games per day.[36,38] Throwing curveballs is associated with a 1.66 increased risk of pitching-related injuries in athletes aged 9 to 18 years, whereas those who pitch with arm tiredness and pain have more than a sevenfold greater risk of pitching-related injury.[38]

In response to the increasing incidence of pediatric elbow injuries in throwing athletes, a set of guidelines for youth pitchers based on established guidelines and clinical experience was proposed in 2012[37] (**Table 3**); however, despite these guidelines, elbow injuries continue to occur. The treatment of these elbow injuries often includes temporary cessation of pitching and overhead activities, the administration of anti-inflammatory medications, icing of the elbow, and the implementation of physical therapy that focuses on core strengthening along with shoulder and elbow flexibility and strengthening. Instructions for performing the "sleeper stretch" for the shoulder is an important part of the physical therapy program. Young athletes with elbow injuries may require individual coaching or performance evaluations to improve their technique and decrease the risk for future injury. Surgical intervention is rarely required, and it is typically reserved for patients in whom an extensive period of nonsurgical management has been unsuccessful.

Anterior Knee Pain

Patellofemoral pain or patellofemoral stress syndrome is the most common overuse injury in runners and those

Table 2

Common Overuse Injuries in Pediatric Patients

Location	Conditions
Upper extremity	Distal clavicle osteolysis
	Proximal humeral physeal separation
	Rotator cuff tendinitis
	Olecranon stress fractures
	Capitellum osteochondritis dissecans
	Ulnar collateral ligament strain/tear
	Medial epicondyle apophysitis/fracture
	Chronic exertional compartment syndrome
	Gymnast wrist
Lower extremity	Femoral/tibial/metatarsal stress fracture
	Femoroacetabular impingement
	Medial tibial stress syndrome
	Chronic exertional compartment syndrome
	Patellofemoral syndrome
	Iliotibial band friction syndrome
	Osteochondritis dissecans
	Osgood-Schlatter disease
	Sinding-Larsen-Johansson disease
	Patellar tendinitis
	Symptomatic plica
	Hoffa fat pad syndrome
	Sever disease
	Symptomatic accessory navicular bone
	Symptomatic os trigonum
Spine	Posture-related back pain
	Spondylolysis and spondylolisthesis

Table 3

Guidelines for Young Throwing Athletes

- Watch and respond to signs of fatigue; rest for any symptoms
- Minimum 2 to 3 months of rest per year, with 4 months preferred
- Do not pitch >100 game innings in any calendar year
- Follow limits for pitch counts and days of rest
- Avoid pitching on multiple teams with overlapping seasons
- Learn proper throwing mechanics with gradual progression
- Avoid using radar guns
- A pitcher should not also be a catcher
- Any elbow or shoulder pain should initiate a sports medicine referral
- Encourage athletes' involvement in various activities in which they show interest and enthusiasm

who participate in running sports such as basketball and soccer. This syndrome has been termed runner's knee and is described as peripatellar knee pain that increases with activities such as running, jumping, stair climbing, squatting, and sitting with the knees flexed for a prolonged time.[17] Specialization in a single sport incurs a 1.5-fold increased relative risk of anterior knee pain in adolescent female athletes and a fourfold increase in Sinding-Larsen-Johansson disease, patellar tendopathy, and Osgood-Schlatter disease.[39]

Recently, biomechanical etiologies for the development of patellofemoral stress syndrome have gained attention.[17,40-42] Proximal muscle weakness (specifically, decreased hip strength and activation) has been targeted as a risk factor for patellofemoral stress because increasing loads across the patellofemoral joint increase the functional quadriceps angle.[40-42] Rehabilitation protocols have focused on core and hip strengthening.[40] In addition to proximal stability, excessive or mistimed pronation is thought to alter transverse and frontal plane mechanics at the patellofemoral joint, thereby increasing patellofemoral joint compression forces.[40,41] Proper shoes, the addition of foot orthoses, or gait training may improve foot biomechanics while running. Surgical interventions, such as diagnostic arthroscopy, isolated lateral release, and/or plica excision, have been performed with inconsistent results, with less than 40% of patients reporting pain-free outcomes after surgery.[43] These poor surgical results reinforce the importance of multimodal nonsurgical management for anterior knee pain, including multiple pain management strategies, bracing, physical therapy, coaching on proper techniques, and performance evaluations.

Tibial Stress Injury

Tibial stress injury represents a spectrum of overuse injuries ranging from medial tibial stress syndrome (MTSS), also known as shin splints, to a radiographically evident stress fracture. Leg pain caused by tibial stress injury is common in runners and athletes who participate in running sports. In a survey of high school cross-country runners, 68% of the girls and 59% of the boys had some lower extremity overuse injury or chronic injury in their lifetimes.[5] In an investigation of risk factors associated with chronic exercise-related leg pain in a group of high school cross-country athletes, it was found that 82.4% of athletes had experienced exercise-related leg pain at some time, with 48% experiencing pain during the current season.[7] More than 50% of the athletes who participated in cross-country running experienced leg pain related to running, and 58.4% reported that the pain had interfered with participation in their sport.[7] Most (97.8%) of those who experienced pain during the current season also had similar symptoms in the past.[7] This finding suggests that a history of running-related leg pain is a risk factor for recurrence of symptoms. In high school athletes, a higher weekly mileage total is associated with overuse injury in boys but not in girls. This finding suggests that other factors, such as mechanical alignment or biomechanics may play a role in the development of overuse injuries.[5] No associations between running-related leg pain and training distance, sex, BMI, foot type, years of running, or age were found.[7]

MTSS is defined as an exercise-induced, localized pain along the distal two-thirds of the posteromedial tibia.[17,44] MTSS is more common in girls than in boys. Risk factors include a lack of running experience, a history of MTSS, and an increased BMI. It is unclear whether overpronation is associated with MTSS.[17,44] A retrospective study of adults showed decreased plantar flexor strength in runners with MTSS, which suggests that decreased plantar flexor muscle endurance may also be a risk for MTSS in younger athletes.[45] The treatment of MTSS is nonsurgical and includes foot orthoses, leg taping and bracing, anti-inflammatory medications, icing, physical therapy to address muscle imbalance and weakness, and running analyses to improve foot strike forces and body position.

Tibial stress fractures occur in healthy bone when repetitive loading surpasses the bone's ability to remodel, resulting in the accumulation of microdamage within the bone.[17,46] Fatigue stress fractures are the more common type of stress fracture in pediatric athletes. In contrast, insufficiency stress fractures occur under normal loading conditions in the setting of pathologic bone.[17]

A stress fracture in a juvenile or an adolescent girl should raise suspicion that the patient may be affected by the female athlete triad. These patients should be assessed for amenorrhea and decreased bone mineral density. More recently, the female athlete triad has been renamed relative energy deficiency in sport (RED-S) to address the increasing rate of male patients with this metabolic abnormality.[47] The definition has been broadened to include dysfunction of metabolism, menses, bone health, immunity, protein synthesis, and cardiovascular health. Because pain associated with an osseous injury is often the presenting symptom, orthopaedic surgeons should be aware of the proper workup and referral for these patients. Confirmation of the diagnosis may include laboratory blood tests, bone mineralization tests, and nutritional and psychological evaluations. Although the multidisciplinary treatment plan is often best coordinated by a primary care physician who is knowledgeable about RED-S, it is often initiated by an orthopaedic surgeon.

Summary

Promoting safe, well-rounded participation in youth athletics can help develop a lifetime of physical activity and healthy habits while decreasing the risk for injuries. It has become increasingly clear that current training regimens of early sport specialization, year-round activity participation, and increasingly intense training are leading to the increase in overtraining and burnout in youth athletes. Although the medical community has a clear understanding of the problems of overuse injuries and burnout, further research is needed on the efficacy of prevention programs, the treatment of overuse injuries, and the appropriate amount of time needed before return to sports after an injury.

Key Study Points

- Approximately 50% of sports-related injuries in pediatric patients are overuse injuries.
- The education of parents, coaches, and medical providers can help prevent overuse injuries.
- Early specialization in a single sport increases the risk of overuse injuries in pediatric patients.
- Evaluation for the female athlete triad, now known as RED-S, should be considered in any female athlete with a stress fracture.

Annotated References

1. National Federation of State High School Associations: Participation statistics: 2013-14 high school athletics participation survey. Available at: http://www.nfhs.org/ParticipationStatistics/PDF/2013-14_Participation_Survey_PDF.pdf. Accessed January 22, 2016.

   Data are available on high school athletic participation in the United States during the 2013 to 2014 academic year.

2. Roos KG, Marshall SW, Kerr ZY, et al: Epidemiology of overuse injuries in collegiate and high school athletics in the United States. *Am J Sports Med* 2015;43(7):1790-1797.

This descriptive epidemiologic study reports on overuse injury rates for college and high school athletes using surveillance data for 16 sports from the National Collegiate Athletic Association Injury Surveillance System (2004-2009) and 14 sports from High School Reporting Information Online (2006-2013). Level of evidence: III.

3. Schroeder AN, Comstock RD, Collins CL, Everhart J, Flanigan D, Best TM: Epidemiology of overuse injuries among high-school athletes in the United States. *J Pediatr* 2015;166(3):600-606.

   This descriptive epidemiologic study uses the High School Reporting Information Online study data from 2006 to 2012 to examine high school overuse injury rates and patterns based on sex and sport. A better understanding of overuse injury patterns may help direct preventive measures. Level of evidence: III.

4. Hoang QB, Mortazavi M: Pediatric overuse injuries in sports. *Adv Pediatr* 2012;59(1):359-383.

   The authors provide a review of the epidemiology, risk factors, diagnosis, treatment, and prevention of overuse injuries in the pediatric and adolescent populations. Level of evidence: V.

5. Tenforde AS, Sayres LC, McCurdy ML, Collado H, Sainani KL, Fredericson M: Overuse injuries in high school runners: Lifetime prevalence and prevention strategies. *PM R* 2011;3(2):125-131, quiz 131.

   This retrospective review of high school distance runners at 28 high schools in the San Francisco Bay Area used online survey data to describe overuse injury patterns in this population. Level of evidence: III.

6. Hjelm N, Werner S, Renstrom P: Injury profile in junior tennis players: A prospective two year study. *Knee Surg Sports Traumatol Arthrosc* 2010;18(6):845-850.

7. Reinking MF, Austin TM, Hayes AM: Risk factors for self-reported exercise-related leg pain in high school cross-country athletes. *J Athl Train* 2010;45(1):51-57.

8. Bonza JE, Fields SK, Yard EE, Dawn Comstock R: Shoulder injuries among United States high school athletes during the 2005-2006 and 2006-2007 school years. *J Athl Train* 2009;44(1):76-83.

9. Smucny M, Parikh SN, Pandya NK: Consequences of single sport specialization in the pediatric and adolescent athlete. *Orthop Clin North Am* 2015;46(2):249-258.

   The authors provide data to support the argument that early specialization in a single sport may increase the risk of overuse injuries in skeletally immature individuals. Level of evidence: V.

10. Timpka T, Jacobsson J, Dahlström Ö, et al: The psychological factor 'self-blame' predicts overuse injury among top-level Swedish track and field athletes: A 12-month cohort study. *Br J Sports Med* 2015;49(22):1472-1477.

    The authors report on 278 Swedish track and field athletes who participated in an injury surveillance program and were surveyed to examine psychological factors associated with injury among these athletes. Level of evidence: IV.

11. Brenner JS; American Academy of Pediatrics Council on Sports Medicine and Fitness: Overuse injuries, overtraining, and burnout in child and adolescent athletes. *Pediatrics* 2007;119(6):1242-1245.

12. Jayanthi NA, LaBella CR, Fischer D, Pasulka J, Dugas LR: Sports-specialized intensive training and the risk of injury in young athletes: A clinical case-control study. *Am J Sports Med* 2015;43(4):794-801.

    This case-control study surveyed 1,214 young athletes to identify risk factors for injury in pediatric and adolescent athletes. Specialization in a single sport was found to be an independent risk factor for injury. Level of evidence: III.

13. DiFiori JP, Benjamin HJ, Brenner J, et al: Overuse injuries and burnout in youth sports: A position statement from the American Medical Society for Sports Medicine. *Clin J Sport Med* 2014;24(1):3-20.

    The authors of this systematic, evidenced-based review provide recommendations for the prevention of overuse injuries in young athletes. The authors also discuss the presentation of overuse conditions, risk factors for injury, and specific injuries that are unique to pediatric athletes. Level of evidence: III.

14. Franklin CC, Weiss JM: Stopping sports injuries in kids: An overview of the last year in publications. *Curr Opin Pediatr* 2012;24(1):64-67.

    This review of the current literature provides an update on pediatric and adolescent sports injuries. Overuse injuries highlighted include elbow injuries in throwing athletes and knee injuries in young girls. Level of evidence: IV.

15. Luke A, Lazaro RM, Bergeron MF, et al: Sports-related injuries in youth athletes: Is overscheduling a risk factor? *Clin J Sport Med* 2011;21(4):307-314.

    Athletes 6 to 18 years of age at six university-based sports medicine clinics in North America were surveyed over a 3-month period. Clinical and survey data were analyzed for correlations between participation hours and injury. Level of evidence: IV.

16. Stracciolini A, Casciano R, Friedman HL, Meehan WP III, Micheli LJ: A closer look at overuse injuries in the pediatric athlete. *Clin J Sport Med* 2015;25(1):30-35.

    This cross-sectional epidemiologic study analyzed sex differences in overuse injuries over a 10-year period. Other factors evaluated included age, BMI, history of injury, and activity type. Level of evidence: III.

17. Paterno MV, Taylor-Haas JA, Myer GD, Hewett TE: Prevention of overuse sports injuries in the young athlete. *Orthop Clin North Am* 2013;44(4):553-564.

    The authors review the literature regarding the etiology of overuse injuries in children and adolescent athletes and suggest strategies to prevent overuse injuries in young athletes. Level of evidence: V.

18. Hogan KA, Gross RH: Overuse injuries in pediatric athletes. *Orthop Clin North Am* 2003;34(3):405-415.

19. Hawkins D, Metheny J: Overuse injuries in youth sports: Biomechanical considerations. *Med Sci Sports Exerc* 2001;33(10):1701-1707.

20. Paz DA, Chang GH, Yetto JM Jr, Dwek JR, Chung CB: Upper extremity overuse injuries in pediatric athletes: Clinical presentation, imaging findings, and treatment. *Clin Imaging* 2015;39(6):954-964.

    The authors describe upper extremity overuse injuries in pediatric athletes. Imaging findings associated with these injuries are reported. Level of evidence: V.

21. Caine D, Purcell L, Maffulli N: The child and adolescent athlete: A review of three potentially serious injuries. *BMC Sports Sci Med Rehabil* 2014;6(1):22.

    An overview of three injuries seen in pediatric athletes—anterior cruciate ligament injury, concussion, and physeal injury—is presented. These injuries are considered potentially serious because of their frequency, potential for adverse long-term health outcomes, and escalating healthcare costs. Level of evidence: V.

22. De Smet L, Claessens A, Lefevre J, Beunen G: Gymnast wrist: An epidemiologic survey of ulnar variance and stress changes of the radial physis in elite female gymnasts. *Am J Sports Med* 1994;22(6):846-850.

23. Valovich McLeod TC, Decoster LC, Loud KJ, et al: National Athletic Trainers' Association position statement: Prevention of pediatric overuse injuries. *J Athl Train* 2011;46(2):206-220.

    This article provides a review of the epidemiology and risk factors associated with overuse sports injuries in pediatric athletes and provides evidence-based recommendations on best practices for the prevention of those injuries. Level of evidence: V.

24. DiFiori JP: Overuse injury and the young athlete: The case of chronic wrist pain in gymnasts. *Curr Sports Med Rep* 2006;5(4):165-167.

25. Blatnik TR, Briskin S: Bilateral knee pain in a high-level gymnast. *Clin J Sport Med* 2013;23(1):77-79.

    This is a case report of the presentation, diagnosis, and treatment of a skeletally immature gymnast with bilateral distal femoral physeal stress injuries. Level of evidence: IV.

26. Laor T, Wall EJ, Vu LP: Physeal widening in the knee due to stress injury in child athletes. *AJR Am J Roentgenol* 2006;186(5):1260-1264.

27. Cuff S, Loud K, O'Riordan MA: Overuse injuries in high school athletes. *Clin Pediatr (Phila)* 2010;49(8):731-736.

28. Faulkner RA, Davison KS, Bailey DA, Mirwald RL, Baxter-Jones AD: Size-corrected BMD decreases during peak linear growth: Implications for fracture incidence during adolescence. *J Bone Miner Res* 2006;21(12):1864-1870.

29. Matos NF, Winsley RJ, Williams CA: Prevalence of nonfunctional overreaching/overtraining in young English athletes. *Med Sci Sports Exerc* 2011;43(7):1287-1294.

    This study evaluated the incidence of overtraining in a cohort of young English athletes and described their signs and symptoms when they presented for treatment. Level of evidence: IV.

30. Kreher JB, Schwartz JB: Overtraining syndrome: A practical guide. *Sports Health* 2012;4(2):128-138.

    A review of overtraining syndrome is presented, and recommendations for workup and management of the condition are provided. Level of evidence: V.

31. Maffulli N, Longo UG, Gougoulias N, Loppini M, Denaro V: Long-term health outcomes of youth sports injuries. *Br J Sports Med* 2010;44(1):21-25.

32. Hill DE, Andrews JR: Stopping sports injuries in young athletes. *Clin Sports Med* 2011;30(4):841-849.

    The authors review the epidemiology of overuse injuries in young athletes and identify risk factors for injury. Methods for prevention of overuse injuries in pediatric and adolescent athletes are suggested. Level of evidence: V.

33. Intensive training and sports specialization in young athletes: American Academy of Pediatrics. Committee on Sports Medicine and Fitness. *Pediatrics* 2000; 106(1 pt 1):154-157.

34. Milewski MD, Skaggs DL, Bishop GA, et al: Chronic lack of sleep is associated with increased sports injuries in adolescent athletes. *J Pediatr Orthop* 2014;34(2):129-133..

    This study reports the results of an online survey of 112 adolescents at a single school, along with a retrospective review of injury records from the school's athletic department. The goal of the study was to investigate the relationship between injuries and sleep practices of the cohort. Level of evidence: III.

35. Bergeron MF, Mountjoy M, Armstrong N, et al: International Olympic Committee consensus statement on youth athletic development. *Br J Sports Med* 2015;49(13):843-851.

    The authors provide evidence-based recommendations regarding youth sports participation and strategies to prevent and treat overuse injuries in pediatric and adolescent athletes. Level of evidence: V.

36. Popchak A, Burnett T, Weber N, Boninger M: Factors related to injury in youth and adolescent baseball pitching, with an eye toward prevention. *Am J Phys Med Rehabil* 2015;94(5):395-409.

This article provides a summary of risk factors for pitching injuries in adolescent throwers. The development and use of pitching guidelines in youth baseball as a strategy to decrease the incidence of overuse injuries in young throwers is discussed. Level of evidence: V.

37. Fleisig GS, Andrews JR: Prevention of elbow injuries in youth baseball pitchers. *Sports Health* 2012;4(5):419-424.

    The authors describe the risk factors for elbow injury and the need for elbow surgery in young baseball pitchers and present strategies to prevent injuries in these athletes. Level of evidence: V.

38. Yang J, Mann BJ, Guettler JH, et al: Risk-prone pitching activities and injuries in youth baseball: Findings from a national sample. *Am J Sports Med* 2014;42(6):1456-1463.

    This study reports the results of a national survey of 754 youth pitchers. Self-reported risk-prone pitching activities were identified and compared with recommendations by the American Sports Medicine Institute to determine relationships between pitching activities and injury. Level of evidence: III.

39. Hall R, Barber Foss K, Hewett TE, Myer GD: Sport specialization's association with an increased risk of developing anterior knee pain in adolescent female athletes. *J Sport Rehabil* 2015;24(1):31-35.

    This retrospective cohort study compared the incidence of patellofemoral pain in female athletes who participated in multiple sports and those who competed in a single sport to determine whether there was a difference in incidence of anterior knee pain between the athletes. The authors concluded that early specialization was associated with an increased risk of anterior knee pain. Level of evidence: III.

40. Earl JE, Hoch AZ: A proximal strengthening program improves pain, function, and biomechanics in women with patellofemoral pain syndrome. *Am J Sports Med* 2011;39(1):154-163.

    This study evaluated the effect of an 8-week program to strengthen the hip and core muscles and improve dynamic lower extremity alignment associated with patellofemoral pain in a cohort of 19 college-aged women. Level of evidence: IV.

41. Powers CM: The influence of altered lower-extremity kinematics on patellofemoral joint dysfunction: A theoretical perspective. *J Orthop Sports Phys Ther* 2003;33(11):639-646.

42. Zazulak BT, Hewett TE, Reeves NP, Goldberg B, Cholewicki J: Deficits in neuromuscular control of the trunk predict knee injury risk: A prospective biomechanical-epidemiologic study. *Am J Sports Med* 2007;35(7):1123-1130.

43. Kramer DE, Kalish LA, Abola MV, et al: The effects of medial synovial plica excision with and without lateral retinacular release on adolescents with anterior knee pain. *J Child Orthop* 2016;10(2):155-162.

    Although most adolescent patients with knee pain are satisfied with the results of plica excision with or without lateral release, residual symptoms are common. Level of evidence: IV.

44. Hubbard TJ, Carpenter EM, Cordova ML: Contributing factors to medial tibial stress syndrome: A prospective investigation. *Med Sci Sports Exerc* 2009;41(3):490-496.

45. Madeley LT, Munteanu SE, Bonanno DR: Endurance of the ankle joint plantar flexor muscles in athletes with medial tibial stress syndrome: A case-control study. *J Sci Med Sport* 2007;10(6):356-362.

46. Pepper M, Akuthota V, McCarty EC: The pathophysiology of stress fractures. *Clin Sports Med* 2006;25(1):1-16, vii.

47. Mountjoy M, Sundgot-Borgen J, Burke L, et al: The ICO consensus statement: Beyond the female triad. Relative energy deficiency in sports (RED-S). *Br J Sports Med* 2014;48(7):491-497.

    Replacement of the term female athlete triad with RED-S addresses the involvement of both sexes and the multiple physiologic systems that extend beyond the classic three systems of the female athlete triad. Level of evidence: V.

Chapter 48

Pediatric and Adolescent Athletes: Special Considerations

Andrew J.M. Gregory, MD, FAAP, FACSM

Abstract

The care of young athletes involves special considerations. Those caring for these young patients should be aware of sport-related concussion, exertional heat illness, the female athlete triad, sudden cardiac arrest, and other medical conditions affecting sports participation. Familiarity with preparticipation screening, the benefits of strength training, and the potential harm of performance-enhancing supplements will assist caregivers in preventing injuries and providing the best possible care when injury occurs.

Keywords: female athlete triad; heat-related illness; medical conditions affecting sports participation; performance-enhancing supplements; preparticipation screening; sport-related concussion; strength training

Introduction

Children are participating in organized sports at younger ages than in past decades. Physicians who care for young athletes should be aware of considerations that are unique to patients in this age group. Although young athletes generally heal faster from injury than older athletes, certain conditions such as concussion may take longer to heal. Congenital conditions such as Marfan syndrome or hypertrophic cardiomyopathy that preclude sports participation may occur in childhood and should be recognized early to prevent poor outcomes. Other conditions such as heat illness may be more common in children because young athletes may not recognize early symptoms. Many infections that commonly occur in children also can affect sports participation.

Sport-Related Concussion

Young athletes are at increased risk for concussion sustained during sports participation.[1] The incidence of concussion varies widely across different sporting disciplines. For athletes younger than 18 years, the sports with the highest incidence rates of concussion per athletic exposure are rugby, hockey, and American football at 4.18 per 1,000, 1.20 per 1,000, and 0.53 per 1,000, respectively. The sports with the lowest incidence rates of concussion are volleyball, baseball, and cheerleading at 0.03 per 1,000, 0.06 per 1,000, and 0.07 per 1,000, respectively.[2] Because athletes may not report symptoms of concussion, a high index of suspicion must be maintained when any young athlete sustains a blow to the head or chest. A child-specific symptom checklist for athletes, parents, and teachers is recommended for use in children younger than 12 years. Although not yet validated, the Child-SCAT3, introduced in 2013 by the Concussion in Sport Consensus Group, is a standardized concussion assessment tool for use in children aged 5 to 12 years.[3] A helpful checklist of concussion symptoms is available from the Centers for Disease Control and Prevention.[4]

Based on comparative studies, it appears that recovery from concussion is somewhat slower (a few days) in adolescent athletes than in their adult counterparts.[5] Data are not available for young athletes for comparison with data from high school and college athletes. Although management of concussion in younger athletes is similar to that of adults, a more conservative approach is warranted regarding return to play for younger athletes with sport-related concussion. Management of concussion includes rest from activity, avoidance of any triggers that

Dr. Gregory or an immediate family member serves as a paid consultant to DJ Orthopaedics and serves as a board member, owner, officer, or committee member of the American College of Sports Medicine.

worsen symptoms, treatment of headache, rehabilitation for neck pain, and cognitive or vestibular therapy if indicated. Complete brain rest is not recommended because this has been shown to extend the duration of symptoms. Return to play should be considered only when the athlete is symptom free at rest. The return-to-play protocol includes graded increases in exertion before return to full activity. A minimum of 24 hours is recommended between each stage, and progression to the next stage is allowed only if no symptoms are present at the previous stage. The stages are (1) light activity such as jogging or biking, (2) moderate activity such as sprinting or jumping, (3) intense activity such as sports-specific activity or ball kicking or shooting baskets, (4) sports practice without contact, and (5) sports practice with full contact.

Strength Training in Children

Although participation in strength training historically has been considered unsafe for children, it has since proven to be a safe activity for young athletes when simple guidelines are followed. The guidelines of the American Academy of Pediatrics for strength training in children include recommendations to avoid power lifting, bodybuilding, and maximal lifts until physical and skeletal maturity is reached. Adequate fluid and nutritional intake, inclusion of aerobic conditioning, warm-up and cool-down periods, the initial learning of exercises with no weights, the gradual increase in weight if proper form is maintained, and addressing all major muscle groups also are recommended. The guidelines also include recommendations for a preparticipation physical examination, evaluation of any illness or injury before resumption of strength training, and appropriate adult supervision.[6]

In addition to being a safe activity for children, strength training may prevent injury during sports participation as well as improve overall body composition. Injury prevention programs have been shown to substantially reduce injury rates in adolescent athletes.[7] The specific reason for their efficacy is unknown; however, it may be related to program content and improvements in muscle strength, proprioceptive balance, and flexibility. Strength training can make positive alterations in overall body composition while reducing body fat, improving insulin sensitivity in adolescents who are overweight, and enhancing cardiac function in children who are obese.[8]

Performance-Enhancing Supplements

Performance-enhancing supplements are used by young athletes beginning as early as middle school. Most young athletes do not have the ideal diet and hydration for sports performance and do not understand the potential harm that these supplements can cause. Supplements by their definition are not drugs and do not have to undergo the same rigorous testing and regulation as drugs. Consequently, supplements may not contain ingredients shown on their labels and may contain undesirable impurities. Common supplements used by young athletes include creatine, anabolic steroids, human growth hormone, stimulants, and amino acids and other proteins. Few studies exist on the safety of supplement use in adults, and no studies exist regarding the safety of supplements for children.

Creatine is used by young athletes trying to gain muscle, usually in the setting of strength training. Studies of creatine use in adults have demonstrated a positive effect in repeated short bouts of intense activity, but no effects in single sprints or endurance activities. These results have not been replicated in children, and no studies exist on competitive benefits. Weight gain is the most common side effect of creatine use. Athletes who consume meat as a regular part of their diet are unlikely to require a creatine supplement. The intake of creatine and other protein should be limited in any athlete with kidney disease.

Anabolic steroids have been shown to have ergogenic effects in adult athletes, but they also cause serious adverse side effects in various body systems. Of chief concern in young athletes is the effect that anabolic steroids have on early closure of the physes of the long bones. In addition, there appears to be a clear relationship between steroid use and abuse of illegal substances and other risk-taking behaviors in adolescents. Anabolic steroids should only be prescribed for children by endocrinologists in the setting of a growth hormone deficiency. Little information is available about human growth hormone use in young athletes.

Stimulants are commonly used by athletes to maintain a high level of alertness during a sports activity and for performance enhancement. Common stimulants include caffeine, ephedrine, synephrine, and amphetamine. Stimulants have been extensively studied for treatment of attention deficit hyperactivity disorder in children but not for effects on sports performance. Commonly reported adverse side effects include increased pulse rate and palpitations, restlessness, and difficulty sleeping.[9] Potential other adverse effects include addiction, hypertension, arrhythmia, and increased susceptibility to heat-related illness.

Because new supplements are continually introduced in the marketplace, it is difficult for efficacy studies to keep pace. Many new products contain either anabolic steroids or stimulants in different or undetectable forms. Some recently introduced supplements such as products containing beet juice have a high nitrate content. Recent studies of nitrate supplementation revealed either a minor positive effect or no systematic effect on exercise performance. The sugar content of whole beetroot juice might have a slightly more pronounced effect on athletic performance. Although reasonable intake of nitrate supplements (<1g/d) has no detrimental effect on kidney function, the risk and benefit of higher nitrate intake is unknown.[10]

The continued use of performance-enhancing supplements by young athletes is concerning. Education of athletes by their coaches may reduce the intention to use supplements. Efforts should concentrate on the education of coaches regarding performance-enhancing supplements.

Female Athlete Triad

In 1992, the female athlete triad was defined as having the following components: an eating disorder, amenorrhea, and osteoporosis. Over time, it was realized that athletes who did not meet the strict definition of the female athlete triad were still experiencing higher rates of sports injuries. In 2007, the American College of Sports Medicine updated the diagnostic guidelines, and the female athlete triad was redefined as a spectrum of abnormalities in energy availability, menstrual function, and bone mineral density.[11] The new definition is less restrictive and allows for the presence of only one or two components to make a diagnosis; therefore, this condition also can apply to male athletes.

Low energy availability is defined as a body mass index less than 17.5 kg/m^2 or less than 85% of expected body weight in adolescents.[12] Other methods for assessing energy availability, dietary intake, and energy expenditure are imprecise. An experienced sports dietitian or an exercise physiologist can provide assistance with these assessments. Athletes with primary or secondary amenorrhea (<6 menses over 12 months) should be evaluated to rule out pregnancy, systemic diseases, and endocrinopathies. The diagnosis of functional hypothalamic amenorrhea in athletes secondary to low energy availability is a diagnosis of exclusion. Screening for low bone mineral density should be done if an athlete has at least one high risk factor or at least two moderate risk factors as defined by the Female Athlete Triad Coalition Consensus Statement[12] (**Table 1**).

All adolescent female athletes should be screened for symptoms of the female athlete triad during a preparticipation physical examination. Particular attention should be given to athletes participating in high-risk sports such as gymnastics, cheerleading, dancing, ice skating, cross-country running, and wrestling. An athlete with an abnormality in any of the three components should be educated on injury risks (particularly stress fractures) and the importance of proper nutrition and exercise modifications. The use of oral contraceptives for return of menses without proper nutrition and exercise modification is less desirable. Increased energy availability should allow for return of normal menses and improved bone health. For athletes who do not respond to education alone, treatment by a multidisciplinary team, including a physician, a mental health counselor, and a sports nutritionist, is recommended.

Table 1

Risk Factors for Low Bone Mineral Density

High Risk Factors
History of a DSM-V diagnosed eating disorder
BMI <17.5 kg/m^2, <85% expected body weight, or recent weight loss of ≥10% in 1 month
Menarche at 16 years of age or older
Currently experiencing or has a history of <6 menses over 12 months
Two prior stress reactions or stress fractures, one high-risk stress reaction or stress fracture, or one low-energy nontraumatic fracture
Prior Z-score of less than −2.0 SD (after at least 1 year from baseline DEXA)
Moderate Risk Factors
Currently experiencing or has a history of disordered eating for 6 months or more
BMI between 17.5 kg/m^2 and 18.5 kg/m^2, 85% to 90% expected body weight, or recent weight loss of 5% to 10% in 1 month
Menarche between 15 and 16 years of age
Currently experiencing or has a history of six to eight menses over 12 months
One prior stress reaction or stress fracture
Prior Z-score between −1.0 and −2.0 SD (after at least a 1-year interval from baseline DEXA)

DSM-V = *Diagnostic and Statistical Manual of Mental Disorders*, Fifth Edition; BMI = body mass index; DEXA = dual-energy x-ray absorptiometry.

Adapted with permission from De Souza MJ, Nattiv A, Joy E, et al: 2014 Female Athlete Triad Coalition Consensus Statement on treatment and return to play of the female athlete triad: 1st international conference held in San Francisco, California, May 2012 and 2nd international conference held in Indianapolis, Indiana, May 2013. *Br J Sports Med* 2014;48:289.

Exertional Heat Illness

Exertional heat illness occurs in children and adolescents just as it does in adults. It is no longer believed that children are at greater risk than adults; however, heat-related deaths occur almost yearly in children who play high school football.[13] With appropriate preparation, activity modifications, and monitoring, most healthy children and adolescents can safely participate in outdoor sports and other physical activities in warm to hot climatic conditions.[14] Personnel capable of treating all forms of heat illness, especially exertional heat stroke, by rapidly lowering core body temperature, should be on-site during youth athletic events and community programs involving vigorous physical activity in warm or hot weather conditions. Children and adolescents should be educated on the importance of proper preparation, hydration, reporting of symptoms, and effectively managing recovery and rest, which directly affect exercise heat tolerance and safety.

A core body temperature measurement should be obtained for a young athlete who exhibits signs or symptoms of exertional heat illness, which include fatigue, weakness, lightheadedness, and muscle cramps. The most accurate measurement of core body temperature is with a rectal, not an oral, thermometer.[15] An athlete with acute mental status change and core body temperature greater than 104°F should undergo rapid cooling treatment. Ice water or cold water immersion provides the most efficient cooling treatment for exercise-induced hyperthermia and is recommended as the definitive treatment of exertional heat stroke.[16] Heat stroke can be distinguished from heat exhaustion by the presence of an altered mental status (such as hysteria or delirium), syncope, paralysis, ataxia, seizure, and coma. If immersion treatment is not available, immediate and continual dousing of the patient with water, combined with fanning and continually rotating cold, wet towels, is an alternative. Because morbidity is directly related to the duration of the high body temperature, it is import to cool first and transport second.

Sudden Cardiac Death and Preparticipation Screening

There is general agreement that young athletes should undergo preparticipation screening before participation in athletic events. Controversy exists regarding when to begin screening, how often to screen, and the best screening methods. The American Heart Association recommends screening that includes a targeted personal history, a family history, and a physical examination. Some key elements of screening are a history of elevated systemic blood pressure, knowledge of certain cardiac conditions in family members, and the presence of a heart murmur. The identification of these elements is designed to identify or at least raise suspicion of cardiovascular diseases. Athletes with positive findings of cardiovascular disease should be referred for further evaluation and testing.[17] Recent studies have supported the use of electrocardiography for screening for potentially lethal cardiac disorders in athletes. Electrocardiography is 5 times more sensitive than a patient history and 10 times more sensitive than a physical examination in detecting cardiac disorders and has a higher positive likelihood ratio, a lower negative likelihood ratio, and a lower false-positive rate than a history or examination.[18] Electrocardiographic screening is currently being used by many major sporting organizations, but it is not widely used in most youth sports organizations.

Every organization that sponsors athletic activities should have a written, structured emergency action plan that includes instructions, preparations, and expectations for the athletes, parents or guardians, coaches, strength and conditioning trainers, athletic directors, and health-care professionals who provide medical care during practices and games. Precise injury prevention, recognition, treatment, and return-to-play policies for the common causes of sudden death in athletes also are needed. The emergency action plan should be developed and coordinated with local emergency medical services staff, school public safety officials, on-site first responders, school medical staff, and school administrators. The plan should be specific to each athletic venue and should be practiced at least annually with all involved personnel.[19]

General Medical Conditions

Certain medical conditions can affect a child's ability to participate in sports. The American Academy of Pediatrics Council of Sports Medicine Fitness has prepared a list of medical conditions that affect sports participation.[20] These conditions range from congenital absence of organs to infections and illnesses. It is recommended that children born with a single eye, kidney, or testicle protect the solitary organ with approved polycarbonate eyewear, a flak jacket, or an athletic cup, respectively, as required. Children with a transplanted kidney may require a specially made abdominal pad for protection. Children with medical illnesses such as diabetes mellitus and epilepsy can participate safely in sports with proper medication and monitoring.

In general, if an illness keeps a child from attending school, he or she should not participate in sports activities. Athletes with a fever (temperature > 101°F) should avoid participation in hot and humid environments because an increased body temperature is a predisposing factor for heat illness. Athletes with diarrhea or nausea should avoid participation because of the risk for dehydration and the possibility of infecting other athletes. Skin rashes should be evaluated by a physician before allowing athletic participation because several skin infections can be transmitted via skin-to-skin contact. Athletes with herpes, staphylococcal, streptococcal, tinea, or molluscum skin infections should not participate until the infection is treated and the lesions are healed. Covering skin lesions is no longer considered sufficient to prevent transmission. Universal precautions should be used when handling blood or body fluids in the athletic environment in the same manner as in a hospital or clinic.

Infectious mononucleosis from an Epstein-Barr viral infection is a unique situation because the spleen may be enlarged and consequently at risk for rupture. Although rupture is quite rare, death may occur. Most documented spleen ruptures have occurred within the first 3 weeks of the illness and were atraumatic, so a minimum of 3 weeks of rest from all physical activities starting from the first day of onset of illness is recommended.[21] Manual palpation of the spleen is known to be unreliable, and imaging of the spleen is challenging to interpret because the baseline size differs in individuals.

Summary

Young athletes are unique and should be treated differently than adults. Because an increasing number of children are participating in organized sports at younger ages, care providers should be aware of sports-related health concerns, including concussion, the use of performance-enhancing supplements, the female athlete triad, exertional heat illness, and sudden cardiac death. Care providers should keep their Basic Life Support training current if providing sideline coverage for sporting events. Strength training programs; early recognition of factors that predispose a young athlete to injury; the development of a written emergency action plan that is practiced yearly with staff at each specific venue; and the education of athletes, parents, and coaches will aid in ensuring the safety of young athletes and encouraging a lifetime of sports participation.

Key Study Points

- Although management of concussion in young athletes is similar to that of adults, a more conservative approach is warranted regarding return to play for younger athletes.
- In addition to being a safe activity for children, strength training may actually prevent injury during sports participation and improve overall body composition.
- Continued use of performance-enhancing supplements by young athletes is a cause for concern. Education of athletes by their coaches reduces the intention to use supplements.
- Adolescent female athletes should be screened for symptoms of the female athlete triad during the preparticipation physical examination. Those with abnormalities in any of the three components should be educated on injury risks, proper nutrition, and exercise modifications.
- A core body temperature measurement with a rectal thermometer should be obtained for a young athlete who exhibits signs or symptoms of exertional heat illness. An athlete with an acute mental status change and core body temperature greater than 104°F should undergo a rapid cooling treatment with ice water or cold water immersion.
- Every organization that sponsors athletic activities should have a written, structured emergency action plan that includes instruction, preparation, and expectations for those who provide medical care during practices and games. In addition, precise prevention, recognition, treatment, and return-to play policies for the common causes of sudden death in athletes are needed.

Annotated References

1. Halstead ME, Walter KD; Council on Sports Medicine and Fitness: American Academy of Pediatrics: Clinical report. Sport-related concussion in children and adolescents. *Pediatrics* 2010;126(3):597-615.

2. Pfister T, Pfister K, Hagel B, Ghali WA, Ronksley PE: The incidence of concussion in youth sports: A systematic review and meta-analysis. *Br J Sports Med* 2016;50(5):292-297.

   Sports with a high degree of physical contact had the highest estimated incidence of concussion, including rugby, American football, and hockey. Level of evidence: II.

3. McCrory P, Meeuwisse WH, Aubry M, et al: Consensus statement on concussion in sport: The 4th International Conference on Concussion in Sport held in Zurich, November 2012. *Br J Sports Med* 2013;47(5):250-258.

   The authors described the consensus-based recommendations for clinicians caring for athletes with concussions. Management and return-to-play decisions should be based on clinical judgment and on an individualized basis. Level of evidence: V.

4. Heads up to clinicians: Addressing concussion in sports among kids and teens. Concussion Symptom Checklist. Centers for Disease Control and Prevention. Available at: http://www.cdc.gov/concussion/headsup/clinicians/resource_center/pdfs/Concussion_Symptoms_Checklist.pdf. Accessed June 27, 2016.

   The somatic, cognitive, affective, and sleep symptoms of concussion are presented.

5. Foley C, Gregory A, Solomon G: Young age as a modifying factor in sports concussion management: What is the evidence? *Curr Sports Med Rep* 2014;13(6):390-394.

   Recovery from sports-related concussion is somewhat slower (a few days) in adolescent athletes than in adults. Level of evidence: III.

6. McCambridge TM, Stricker PR; American Academy of Pediatrics Council on Sports Medicine and Fitness: Strength training by children and adolescents. *Pediatrics* 2008;121(4):835-840.

7. Soomro N, Sanders R, Hackett D, et al: The Efficacy of Injury Prevention Programs in Adolescent Team Sports: A Meta-analysis. *Am J Sports Med* 2015;0363546515618372.

   Injury prevention programs resulted in a total injury risk reduction of approximately 40% in adolescents participating in team sports. Level of evidence: I.

8. Lloyd RS, Faigenbaum AD, Stone MH, et al: Position statement on youth resistance training: The 2014 International Consensus. *Br J Sports Med* 2014;48(7):498-505 .

   The focus of youth resistance training should be on developing the technical skill and competency to perform a variety of resistance training exercises at the appropriate intensity and volume, while providing an opportunity to participate in programs that are safe, effective, and enjoyable. Level of evidence: V.

9. Stephens MB, Attipoe S, Jones D, Ledford CJ, Deuster PA: Energy drink and energy shot use in the military. *Nutr Rev* 2014;72(suppl 1):72-77.

   The use of energy drinks (53%) and energy shots (19%) is prevalent in the military, particularly in younger soldiers. Side effects are common (65%). Level of evidence: III.

10. Poortmans JR, Gualano B, Carpentier A: Nitrate supplementation and human exercise performance: Too much of a good thing? *Curr Opin Clin Nutr Metab Care* 2015;18(6):599-604.

    Use of -arginine, beetroot juice, or nitrate supplements revealed either a minor positive effect or no effect on exercise performance in trained athletes. Level of evidence: IV.

11. Matzkin E, Curry EJ, Whitlock K: Female athlete triad: Past, present, and future. *J Am Acad Orthop Surg* 2015;23(7):424-432 .

    A thorough history and physical examination by a healthcare provider is prudent in discovering if a female athlete is at risk for the development of any of the pathologic entities of the triad. Treating this cohort of athletes is a multidisciplinary effort. Level of evidence: V.

12. Joy E, De Souza MJ, Nattiv A, et al: 2014 Female Athlete Triad Coalition Consensus Statement on treatment and return to play of the female athlete triad. *Curr Sports Med Rep* 2014;13(4):219-232 .

    An evidenced-based, risk stratification point system for the female athlete triad is provided to assist the physician regarding sport participation, clearance, and return to play. Level of evidence: V.

13. Kucera KL, Klossner D, Colgate B, Cantu RC: *Annual Survey of Football Injury Research. March, 2015.* Available at: https://nccsir.unc.edu/files/2013/10/Annual-Football-2014-Fatalities-Final.pdf. Accessed June 9, 2016.

    Sixteen direct and indirect fatalities were recorded for the 2014 football season. Even though the rate of direct fatal injuries was low (0.14 per 100,000 football participants), most occurred during competition situations.

14. Bergeron MF, Devore C, Rice SG; Council on Sports Medicine and Fitness and Council on School Health; American Academy of Pediatrics: Policy statement: Climatic heat stress and exercising children and adolescents. *Pediatrics* 2011;128(3):e741-e747.

    Trained personnel and facilities capable of effectively treating all forms of heat illness, especially exertional heat stroke, by rapidly lowering core body temperature should be readily available on-site during all youth athletic activities and community programs that involve vigorous physical activity and are held in the hot weather. Level of evidence: V.

15. Mazerolle SM, Ganio MS, Casa DJ, Vingren J, Klau J: Is oral temperature an accurate measurement of deep body temperature? A systematic review. *J Athl Train* 2011;46(5):566-573.

    Oral body temperature does not accurately reflect core body temperature, and reliance on oral temperature in an emergency, such as exertional heat stroke, might grossly underestimate temperature and delay making a proper diagnosis and starting treatment. Level of evidence: III.

16. McDermott BP, Casa DJ, Ganio MS, et al: Acute whole-body cooling for exercise-induced hyperthermia: A systematic review. *J Athl Train* 2009;44(1):84-93.

17. American Heart Association/American Stroke Association: Preparticipation *Cardiovascular Screening of Young Competitive Athletes: Policy Guidance.* Available at: https://www.heart.org/idc/groups/ahaecc-public/@wcm/@adv/documents/downloadable/ucm_443945.pdf. Accessed June 9, 2016.

    Preparticipation sports screening should consist of a targeted personal history; a family history, including the 12 key elements; and a physical examination. The use of tests such as a 12-lead electrocardiogram or echocardiogram in mandatory preparticipation screening programs was not recommended. Level of evidence: V.

18. Harmon KG, Zigman M, Drezner JA: The effectiveness of screening history, physical exam, and ECG to detect potentially lethal cardiac disorders in athletes: A systematic review/meta-analysis. *J Electrocardiol* 2015;48(3):329-338.

    The most effective strategy for screening for cardiovascular disease in athletes is electrocardiography. It is 5 times more sensitive than a patient history and 10 times more sensitive than a physical examination; it has a higher positive likelihood ratio, a lower negative likelihood ratio, and a lower false-positive rate. Level of evidence: II.

19. Casa DJ, Guskiewicz KM, Anderson SA, et al: National athletic trainers' association position statement: Preventing sudden death in sports. *J Athl Train* 2012;47(1):96-118.

    Every organization that sponsors athletic activities should have a written, structured, emergency action plan that is developed and coordinated with local emergency medical services, staff, school public safety officials, on-site first responders, school medical staff, and school administrators. The plan should be specific to each athletic venue and practiced at least annually with all those involved. Level of evidence: IV.

20. Rice SG; American Academy of Pediatrics Council on Sports Medicine and Fitness: Medical conditions affecting sports participation. *Pediatrics* 2008;121(4):841-848.

21. Putukian M, O'Connor FG, Stricker P, et al: Mononucleosis and athletic participation: An evidence-based subject review. *Clin J Sport Med* 2008;18(4):309-315.

Index

Page numbers with *f* indicate figures.
Page numbers with *t* indicate tables.

A

Abatacept, 207, 208
Abdominal strengthening, 417
Acanthosis nigricans, 87
Accessory navicular, 309
Acetabular dysplasia, 129
Acetabular osteotomy, 275–276
Acetabulum
  dysmorphology, 261
  injuries to, 486–487
Acetaminophen, intravenous, 29
Achilles tendon
  contractures, 131–132, 181, 303
  lengthening, 132, 305
  stretching program, 305–306
  tightness, 182
Achilles tenotomy, 147, 182
Achondroplasia, 87–88, 102, 400–403
  kyphosis and, 390–391, 392*f*
Acoustic neuromas, 101
Acromioclavicular (AC) joint
  anatomy of, 567
  injuries to, 458–459, 459*f*
Acrosyndactyly, 222
Active Movement Scale (AMS), 228
Acute compartment syndrome, 28, 30*t*. *See also* Compartment syndrome
Acute hematogenous osteomyelitis, 113–114
Acute lymphoblastic leukemia, 166
Acute rheumatic fever, 209*f*
Adalimumab, 207
Adam forward bend test, 355, 355*f*, 416
Adams-Oliver syndrome, 236
Adaptive equipment, in spinal muscular atrophy, 189–191
Adductor canal block, 28, 29*f*
Adolescent idiopathic scoliosis (AIS), 76–77, 341–342, 351–363, 352*f*, 355*f*, 358*f*, 389
Adolescents
  ACL injuries in, 522
  athletes, 581*f*, 601–607
  back pain in, 415
  FAI in, 264
  growth spurts, 385
  kyphosis in, 388
  meniscal tears, 537–544
  neuromuscular diseases, 177–201
  Osgood-Schlatter disease in, 498
  patellofemoral instability in, 545
  posterior sternoclavicular dislocations in, 457
  syndesmotic sprain in, 581*f*
  thoracolumbar injuries, 509
  Tillaux fractures, 582*f*
Aerobic conditioning, 417
African Americans, Ewing sarcoma risk in, 74–75
Age/aging, mutations during, 72
Aggrecan, 85
AKT1 gene, 75
Alagille syndrome, 343
Alanine transaminase, 181
Alpha (α)-angle, 231, 248, 248*f*
Alveolar soft-part sarcomas, 54*t*
Amenorrhea, female athlete triad, 603
American Academy of Orthopaedic Surgeons (AAOS)
  AUC for supracondylar humerus fractures, 19*f*
  Clinical Practice Guidelines, 14–15, 15*t*, 16*t*
  Committee on Evidence-Based Quality and Value, 14
  Department of Research and Scientific Affairs, 14
  evidence-based medicine, 14
  systematic review process, 14–15
American Academy of Pediatrics (AAP)
  on Down syndrome screening, 403
  on strength training, 602
American College of Medical Genetics, 73
American College of Radiology skeletal surveys, 451
American football, concussion in, 601
American Heart Association, on sports screening, 604
American Society of Anesthesiologists, 108–109
Amniotic band syndrome (ABS), 222, 222*f*, 236
Amphetamines, performance and, 602
Amputations, in limb deficiencies, 330–332
Amyoplasia, 154, 156*f*, 159–161
Anabolic steroids, 602
Analgesia, 107–109
  postoperative, 28–30
Anderson-Green-Messner growth remaining charts, 62, 65
Anencephaly, folate deficiency and, 137–138
Anesthesia
  dissociative, 437
  intravenous regional, 437
  neurotoxicity, 25–33
  pediatric, 25–33
  regional, 25–33
Anesthesia-induced rhabdomyolysis, 184
Aneurysmal bone cysts, 423
Angelman syndrome, 103
Angle of Lequesne, 250
Angular correction, 64–65
Angular limb deformities, 319–320, 319*t*
  eight-Plate for, 291
Anhidrosis, 228
Ankle-foot orthoses, 141
Ankle sprain equivalent fractures, 581–582
Ankles
  after ORIF, 583*f*
  fractures, 501–503
  high sprains, 580–581
  injuries, 579–589
  low sprains, 579–580
Anterior atlantodens intervals (AADIs), 397, 398*f*
Anterior capsule release, 127
Anterior cruciate ligament (ACL)
  in congenital knee dislocation, 284
  evaluation of, 522
  full-thickness tears, 522–523
  midsubstance injuries, 521, 524*f*
  partial tears, 522
  postoperative care, 526–527
  reconstruction, 28, 523–525, 525*f*, 527
  rehabilitation after injury, 526–527
  return to play after injury, 526–527
  risk factors for injury to, 521
  tears, 522*f*, 539
  transphyseal reconstruction, 525–526
  treatment of injuries, 522–523, 526*f*
Anterior drawer test, 522, 579–580, 584
Anterior interosseous nerve injury, 463
Anterior talofibular ligament (ATFL), 579, 580, 582
Anterolateral tibial osteotomy, 586
Anterolisthesis, 407*f*
Anti-tumor necrosis factor (TNF), 204–205, 207
Antibiotics
  classes of, 113*f*
  mechanisms of action, 113*f*
  in musculoskeletal infections, 37–39
  oral, 37
  in pediatric orthopaedics, 112–113
Anticonvulsant medications, 369
Antifibrinolytics, 25–33, 26–27
Antinuclear antibodies, 417
Antisclerostin antibodies, 168
Antistreptolysin O titer, 204
Antoni A areas, 54
Antoni B areas, 54
Aortic root dilatation, 165
AOSpine Group, 513
Apert syndrome, 306
Apical ectodermal ridge (AER), 235
Apical epithelial caps, 239
Apley tests, 540
Apophyseal ring fractures, 416–418
Apophyseal ring injuries, 515–516
Apophysis, 310
Apparent diffusion coefficient (ADC), 272

Appropriate use criteria (AUC), 13, 15–17, 16*t*, 18*t*, 19*f*
Aprotinin, 26
Arnold-Chiari malformations, 103, 137
Arthritis, 203–213
enthesitis-related, 205–206, 416
immune-mediated, 203
juvenile, 203–208
juvenile idiopathic, 205–208
Lyme-type, 41, 209, 209*t*
osteoarthritis, 86, 246
poststreptococcal, 209
proximal interphalangeal, 204
reactive, 208–210
septic, 36, 40–41, 113–114
systemic, 205–206
ultrasonography in, 204
undifferentiated, 205
Arthrodesis, for scoliosis, 61
Arthrofibrosis, 527, 530, 531
Arthrogryposis, 153–164, 370
congenital dislocation of the knee and, 283
general management, 157
patellar dislocation and, 285
Ponseti method in, 305
syndromes, 153–164
types of, 154–157
Arthrogryposis multiplex congenita, 153
Asfotase-α therapy, 100
Aspirin, for arthritis, 206
Assisting Hand Assessment, 127, 229
Astrocytomas, 101, 423
Ataluren, 186
Ataxias, 124, 130, 367
Athetosis, in cerebral palsy, 124
Athletes. *See also* Overuse conditions
ACL injuries, 521–522
adolescent, 581*f*, 601–607
cam lesions, 263
cervical spine injuries, 408–409
female athlete triad, 596, 603
femoroacetabular impingement and, 263
injury prevention programs, 602
patellofemoral instability in, 545
pediatric, 601–607
preparticipation screening, 604
skeletally immature, 592
syndesmotic sprain, 581*f*
traumatic injuries in, 433–434
Atlanto-occipital joint space, 397, 511–512
Atlantoaxial instability, Down syndrome and, 403
Atlantoaxial rotatory subluxation (AARS), 399–400, 513, 513*f*
Atlas method, 63
Atrial septal defects, 344
Attention-deficit hyperactivity disorder, 602
Atypical cleft hand, 220
Autologous chondrocyte implantation (ACI), 559
Avulsion fractures, 166, 497–499, 527–531, 582
Avulsion injuries, brachial plexus palsy and, 227
Axillary freckling, 416
Axillary nerve injuries, 460
Axonotmesis, 228*t*
Azathioprine, 207

B

Bacitracin, 440
Back pain
in children, 415–429
imaging in, 416–417
laboratory investigation of, 417
patient history, 415–418
physical examination in, 416
thoracic, 514*f*
Back strengthening, 417
Backboards, pediatric, 510
Baclofen, for cerebral palsy, 126
Bacteremia, osteomyelitis and, 36
Baker techniques, 130
Bankart lesions, 570
Bankart repairs, 460
Barlow maneuver, 246
Barlow provocative test, 248
Barlow sign, 189, 250
Barrel chest, 86
Baseball injuries, 568, 601
Basic Life Support training, 605
Basion-axial interval (BAI), 397, 398*f*
Basion-dens interval (BDI), 397, 398*f*
Basketball injuries, 497–499
Beals syndrome, 283
Bebax orthoses, 308
Becker muscular dystrophy, 178, 179, 181, 184, 186
Beckwith-Wiedemann syndrome, 45–46, 101
Beetroot juice, in performance enhancement, 603
Benzodiazepines, 30, 437
Berndt and Harty classification, 585
Bertolotti syndrome, 422
Beta (β)-angle, 248, 248*f*
Biceps tendon lengthening, 127
Bilevel positive airway pressure ventilation, 181
Biopsies, 48, 48*f*
Bipolar radiofrequency hemostatic sealers, 373
Birch classification, 328*f*
Birth brachial plexus palsy (BBPP), 227–234
Birth trauma
brachial plexus palsy and, 227–234, 457–458
clavicular fractures, 457–458
humeral fractures, 460
Birth weights
brachial plexus palsy and, 227
cerebral palsy risk and, 123
Bisphosphonates, 109, 111–112, 112*f*, 370. *See also* Diphosphonates
in DMD, 185
fracture healing and, 167
mineralization and, 112*f*
in osteogenesis imperfecta, 168
side effects of, 168
Blackburne-Peel ratio, 547
Blastemal cell formation, 239
Blauth classification system, 220
Blood loss, in polytrauma, 439
Blount disease, 65, 289. *See also* Tibia vara
infantile, 320
Blount staples, 291
Blue-gray sclera, 165
Blumensaat line, 546
Body mass index (BMI), 60. *See also* Obesity
SCFE and, 259
tibia vara and, 289–290
Bohlman technique, 421
Bone age, 59–68
Bone anchor fixation, 369–370
Bone blocks, 523
Bone cysts, 49–50, 50*f*
Bone density, fractures and, 141
Bone islands, differential diagnoses, 47*t*
Bone lesions, differential diagnoses, 47*t*
Bone mass
factors affecting, 169*t*
low, 166–167
Bone mineral density (BMD), 141
bisphosphonate therapy in, 168
low, 166–167
in neuromuscular diseases, 369–370
risk factors, 603*t*
spinal, 171
Bone morphogenetic protein (BMP), 100, 293, 421–422
Bone scans, 47, 416, 451
Bone tumors, 48–51, 49*t*. *See also* *specific* tumors
Bones. *See also specific* bones
elasticity of, 485
fracture patterns, 434–435
hypertrophic zones, 592
longitudinal growth, 592
plastic deformation, 434–435
pseudoarthrosis, 100
remodeling of, 487
resorption of, 171
transport, 292
Both-bone forearm fractures, 473–475
Botulinum toxin, 126, 229, 284
Bowel incontinence, 370
Boyd amputation, 330

Braces
in AIS, 354–357
compliance with wear of, 304
in Legg-Calvé-Perthes disease, 275
in spinal deformity, 367–368
Brachial artery injuries, 463
Brachial plexus injuries, 227–234, 457–458, 569
Brachial plexus palsy, 227–234
Brachialis tendon lengthening, 127
BRAF enzyme inhibitors, 51
BRAF V600E mutations, 51
Brain-machine interfaces, 238
Brainstem, chronic compression, 400
BRCA1 genes, 73
BRCA2 genes, 73
British Medical Research Council scale, 230
Brodie abscess, 47*t*
Brown tumors, 47*t*
Bruck syndrome, 157, 157*f*
Bucket-handle fractures, 452
Buckle fractures, 434–435, 477
Bupivacaine, 30, 30*t*
Burnout, in sports training, 592–593
Burst fractures, 514–515

C

C-natriuretic protein, 102
C-reactive protein levels, 417
Café au lait lesions, 416
Caffeine, athletic performance and, 602
Calcaneal apophysitis, 310. *See also* Sever disease
Calcaneofibular ligament, 579, 580
Calcaneonavicular coalition, 306*f*
Calcaneus fractures, 503–504
Calcipenic rickets, 165, 169
Calcitriol therapy, 170
Calcium
dietary allowance, 111
homeostasis, 109, 110*f*
insufficiency, 111
supplementation, 109, 168
Calf enlargement, 179, 179*f*
Camptomelic dysplasia, 89, 102
Canakinumab, 208
Candida albicans, 40
Candida parapsilosis, 40
Capsulorrhaphy, posterior, 231
Carcinogenesis, Knudson two-hit theory, 93
Cardiac function, in DMD, 182
Cardiomyopathies, muscular dystrophies and, 369
Cardiopulmonary compromise, 365
Caregiver Priorities and Child Health Index of Life With Disabilities (CPCHILD), 377
Carpal hypoplasia, 220
Cartilage oligomeric matrix protein (COMP), 84
Castile soap, in wound irrigation, 440
Castle procedure, 129
Casts
in clubfoot, 304–305
in fractures, 438–439
in rigid flatfoot, 306
CAT-1004 (Catabasis), 186
Cataracts, 193
Caton-Deschamps index, 547
Catterall classification system, 271
Cauda equina syndrome, 417
Caudal anesthetics, 108
Cavovarus foot deformity, 579
Cavus deformity, imaging of, 194–195
CBFA1 gene, 89
Center-edge angle of Wiber, 250
Centers for Disease Control and Prevention
growth charts, 65
on sports-related injuries, 434
Cephalosporins, 113
Cerebral palsy (CP), 123–136
classification, 124
diagnosis, 124
epidemiology of, 123
etiology, 123–124
goal setting, 124–126
nonorthopaedic treatment, 126–127
orthopaedic treatment, 127–128
outtoeing in, 318
physical therapy, 126
scoliosis and, 366*t*
selective dorsal rhizotomy, 126–127
spinal deformity and, 367
Cerebral Palsy Computer-Adapted Testing Battery, 20
Cervical collars, 510
Cervical kyphosis, 92, 405–406
Cervical pseudosubluxation, 510
Cervical spine
development of, 396*f*
growth of, 61
imaging, 397–399
injuries, 408–409, 509, 512
lower vertebrae, 397
ossification centers, 61
pediatric disorders, 395–413
Cervical spondylosis, 406–407
Cervical stenosis, 402
Cervical trauma, 407–408, 408*f*
Cervicotrochanteric fractures, 487–488
Chamberlain line, 397, 398*f*
Chance fractures, 515, 516, 516*f*
Change, after treatment intervention, responsiveness to, 18
Chaput tubercle, 580
Charcot-Marie-Tooth (CMT) disease, 177, 194–198, 196*f*, 197*f*, 198*f*, 366*t*
CHARGE syndrome, 76
Charleston nighttime braces, 356
CHD7 gene, 76
CHEK2 suppressor gene, 45
Chiari iliac osteotomy, 370
Chiari osteotomy, 86, 276
Child abuse, 449–456
background, 449
elbow dislocation in, 464
fractures in, 451–452, 491
imaging in, 451
misdiagnosis, 452–453
patient evaluation, 450–451
radiographic findings, 452*t*
risk factors for, 449–450, 450*t*
traumatic injuries in, 434
Child Abuse Prevention and Treatment Act of 1974, 449–450
Child-SCAT3, 601
Childhood Arthritis and Rheumatology Research Alliance, 206–208
CHL1 gene, 353
Chondroblastoma, 47*t*, 49–51
Chondroid lesions, 50
Chondroitin sulfate, 85, 403
Chondrosarcomas, 46, 423
Chordomas, back pain and, 423
Choreiform movements, 124
CHRNG gene, 156
Chronic osteomyelitis, 114–115
Chronic recurrent multifocal osteomyelitis (CRMO), 39–40, 203, 209
Chronologic growth, 60
Cisplatinum, 51
Classic test theory, 18
Classification of Early-Onset Scoliosis (C-EOS), 340, 340*f*
Clavicle
fractures of, 457–458
impingement, 457
ossification centers, 567
osteolysis of, 574
pseudoarthrosis, 458
Clear cell chondrosarcoma, 47*t*
Cleft-type symbrachydactyly, 220
Cleidocranial dysplasia, 89, 102
Clinical practice guidelines (CPG)
AAOS, 14–15, 15*t*, 16*t*
description of, 13–15
Institute of Medicine, standards for, 13–15, 14*t*
musculoskeletal infections, 36–37
Clonidine, 108
Clostridium botulinum, 126
CLOVES syndrome, 75
Clubfoot, 303–305, 344
arthrogryposis and, 153
comorbidities in, 75–76
congenital, 304*f*
imaging, 304*f*
myelomeningocele and, 137, 146–147
recurrence, 305
CNTNAP2 gene, 353

Coagulopathies, 372
Cobb angles, 100, 368
 diurnal variations, 356
 spinal growth and, 340
Cobb elevator, 195
Codeine, 30, 73
Coenzyme Q, 186
Cognitive function
 in congenital myotonic dystrophy, 193
 in Duchenne muscular dystrophy, 183
Cohen kappa, 18
COL2A1 gene, 86
COL9A genes, 84
COL1A1 mutations, 165
COL1A2 mutations, 165
Coleman block test, 195
Collagen, type 1, 165
Collagen, type II, 86
Collagen type IX, 84, 85
Collagenopathies, 86
Committee on Evidence-Based Quality and Value (AAOS), 14
COMP gene, 85
Compartment syndrome, 440–441. *See also* Acute compartment syndrome
 diagnosis, 108
 pressure, 441
 in pyomyositis, 41
 risk for, 31*t*
 in supracondylar humerus fractures, 463
Competition, healthcare, 6
Complex genetic disease, 72*t*
Compression fractures, thoracic, 514
Compressive wrapping, 92
Computed tomography (CT)
 in evaluation of back pain, 416–417
 radiation doses, 399
Computerized adaptive testing, 13, 18–20
Computerized gait analysis (CGA), 137, 143*f*
Concussion, sports-related, 601–602
Concussion in Sport Consensus Group, 601
Congenital dislocations, 283–287
Congenital disorders, spinal, 339–349
Congenital hand deficiencies, 235–241
Congenital kyphosis, 389–390
Congenital myotonic dystrophy, 177, 191–193, 192*f*
Congenital posteromedial bowing of the tibia (CPMBT), 294–295, 295*f*
Congenital pseudoarthrosis of the tibia (CPT), 292–294, 294*f*, 295*f*
Congenital scoliosis, 343–346
Congenital talipes equinovarus. *See* Clubfoot
Congenital vertical talus, 159, 307–308, 307*f*
Connective tissue disorders, inherited, 165
Conoid ligaments, 458
Conscious sedation, 25, 437
Consensus guidelines, 5, 13–14
Constipation, opioids and, 30
Construct validity, 18
Content validity, 17
Continuous peripheral nerve blocks, 28
Continuum of disease, 36
Contraceptives, oral, 603
Cookie test, 228
Coracoid, avulsion injuries, 570
Cord compression, 397–398
Core body temperatures, 604
Cornelia de Lange syndrome, 89–90
Corpectomy, partial, 375
Corticosteroids, 184–185, 185*t*
Cost shifting, in healthcare expenditures, 6
Costs, measures of, 7–8
CoughAssist device, 181, 191
Coxa vara, 84
Cranial-cervical junction injuries, 511–512
Craniocervical abnormalities, 399–405
Craniocervical trauma, 407
Craniometry, 397–399
Craniosynostosis, 87
Craniovertebral angle, 397
Crankshaft phenomenon, 61
Creatine supplements, 602
Creatinine kinase levels, 180–181
Criterion validity, 18
Crossover hop, 527
Crouch gait, 130*f*, 131
Crouzon syndrome, 87
Crush injuries, 480, 486
CTNNB1 mutations, 53
Cubitus valgus, 89
Cutaneous syndactyly, 221
Cyclooxygense-2 inhibitors, 206
Cyclosporine, 207
CYP2D6 enzyme polymorphisms, 73
Cystic ear swelling, 92
Cytochrome P450 metabolism, 30
Cytotoxic T cell lymphocyte antigen-4, 208

D

D10 gene, 307
De novo, definition of, 72*t*
De novo variants, 72
Deceleration injuries, 511–512
Deflazacort, 184–185
Delbet system, 487–488, 487*f*, 487*t*
Denis Browne bar orthosis, 304, 318
Denosumab, 168
Dentocentral synchondrosis, 509, 510*f*, 512
Department of Research and Scientific Affairs (AAOS), 14
Derotational femoral osteotomy, 253
Desmoid tumors, 53–54
Developmental dysplasia of the hip (DDH), 245–257
 complications of, 251, 253–254
 etiology, 245–246
 imaging, 246–250
 older children, 251–254
 pathologic anatomy of, 246, 246*f*
 radiography, 249–250
 screening for, 246, 247*f*
 young infants, 250–251
Devices, fatigue fractures, 374
Dexmedetomidine, 27, 108
Diarrhea, sports participation and, 604
Diastematomyelia, 89, 102, 137
Diastrophic dysplasia, 92, 285, 405
Diazepam, 126
Differential diagnoses, of bone lesions, 47*t*
Diphosphonates, 51, 109, 370. *See also* Bisphosphonates
Diplegia, 124
Disabilities of the Arm, Shoulder and Hand score, 20
Discoid meniscus, 539–542, 540*f*
Disease-modifying antirheumatic drugs (DMARDS), 207
Disk disease, weight lifting and, 416
Disk diseases, degenerative, 417
Disk pathology, imaging in, 416
Diskitis, infections and, 422, 424*f*
Distal arthrogryposis, 154–155, 155*f*, 161–162, 162*f*
Distal femoral extension osteotomy, 193
Distal tibial corrective osteotomies, 318
Distal tibial syndesmosis, 580
Distal tibiofibular syndesmosis, 579, 581
DMD. *See* Duchenne muscular dystrophy (DMD)
DMIAC (define, measure, analyze, improve, and control), 4
DNA variants, definition of, 72*t*
Documentation of injuries, in child abuse, 450–451
Dorsal carpal wedge osteotomy, 161
Down syndrome (trisomy 21), 102, 285, 403–404, 404*f*
Doxorubicin, 51
Drowsiness, opioids and, 30
Drug resistance, 115
DSCAM gene, 353
Dual growing rod technique, 342
Duchenne muscular dystrophy (DMD), 177
 anesthesia-induced rhabdomyolysis in, 184
 back pain in, 185*f*
 bone health in, 184
 clinical symptoms, 179*t*
 clinical trials, 185–186
 cognitive function in, 183

diagnosis, 179–181
genetics of, 178–179
historical findings, 179*t*
medical treatment, 184–185
natural history of, 181–182
novel therapies for, 185–187
occupational therapy, 182–183
orthopaedic treatment, 182
pathophysiology, 178
physical therapy, 182–183
progressive scoliosis in, 183–184
rehabilitation treatment, 182
scoliosis and, 366*t*
screening for, 181
somatosensory-evoked potentials in, 371
spinal deformity and, 367
Dunn lateral views, radiation doses in, 263
Dunn-McCarthy S-hooks, 373–374
Dunn procedure, modified, 260
Dupuytren fibromatosis, 53
Dwarfism, 219, 403
Dynamic Standard Minimum Examination, 247
Dyskinesia, in cerebral palsy, 124
Dysplasia, myelomeningocele and, 137
Dysplasia epiphysealis hemimelica, 47*t*
Dystonia, in cerebral palsy, 124
Dystrophic scoliosis, 100
Dystrophin, 178, 185–186

E

Early-onset idiopathic scoliosis (EOIS), 342–346
Early-onset scoliosis, classification of, 340*f*
Early-Onset Scoliosis Questionnaire (EOSQ), 340
Ears, cystic swelling of, 92
Eating disorders, female athlete triad, 603
Effect sizes, 18
EGR2 gene, 74
Ehlers-Danlos syndrome, 283, 308, 545
Elbow
contractures, 127, 160
dislocations, 464, 467*f*
injuries in young throwers, 593–594
osteochondritis dissecans, 555–565
pediatric injuries to, 461–466
Electrocardiography (ECG), presports participation, 604
Electrocautery, 373
Electromyographic (EMG) signals, 238
Electrooculography, 238
Ellis-van Creveld syndrome, 285
Embryonal rhabdomyosarcoma, 54*t*
Emergency orthopaedic management, 439
Enabling the Future organization, 238
Endobutton, 526
Enthesitis-related arthritis, 205–206, 416
Environmental factors, child abuse risk and, 449–450, 450*t*
Eosinophilia with polyangiitis, 210
Eosinophilic granuloma, 423, 424*f*
Ependymomas, back pain and, 423
Ephedrine, athletic performance and, 602
Epidural anesthetics, 108
Epilepsy, neuromuscular scoliosis and, 369
Epinephrine, injection, 373
Epiphyseal ossification, 85
Epiphyseal plates, shoulder, 567
Epiphyseal separation, 487
Epiphysiodesis
contralateral, 442
in limb-length discrepancies, 324–325
reversible, 66
Epiphysiolysis, 259
Epithelioid sarcoma-proximal, 54*t*
Epsilon-amino-caproic acid (EACA), 26–27
Epstein-Barr virus infection, 605
Equinocavovarus deformity, 132
Equinoplanovalgus deformity, 132
Equinus contractures, 130
Equinus gait, 130–131, 130*f*
Errors of commission, 5
Errors of omission, 5
Escobar syndrome, 156
Ethnicity
CYP2D6 polymorphisms and, 73
SCFE and, 259
vitamin D deficiency and, 169
ETS family transcription factors, 74
Evans procedure, modified, 132
Evidence-based guidelines, 5
Evidence-based medicine, 14
Ewing sarcoma, 52–53, 52*f*, 73–75, 423
EWS-FLO 1 gene, 52
Exertional heat illness, 603–604
Exome sequencing, 72
Exostoses, 103
Exostosin *(EXT)* genes, 46, 50, 93, 103, 223
Expenditures in healthcare, value and, 6–8
Extensor carpi radialis brevis, 161
Extensor digitorum communis, 196
External rotation test, 581
External tibial torsion, 318
EXTL genes, 93
Extraskeletal Ewing sarcoma, 54*t*
Extraskeletal myxoid chondrosarcoma, 54*t*

F

FABER (flexion/abduction/external rotation) maneuver, 416
Face validity, 17
Facet alignment, 513
Facial asymmetry, 76*f*
Factor XIII, 372
FAI. *See* Femoroacetabular impingement (FAI)
Falls, musculoskeletal injuries in, 434
Fanconi anemia, 218
Farnesyl transferase inhibitors, 100
Fassier-Duval telescopic rods, 292
FBFR3 mutations, 87
FBN genes, 76
Female athlete triad, 596, 603
Femoral anteversion, 131, 315–318
Femoral condyle dysplasia, 89
Femoral deficiency, 328–329
Femoral derotation osteotomy, 131
Femoral head, 85, 488
Femoral nerve block, 28, 284
Femoral osteotomy, 275–276
Femoral shaft fractures, 489–491
Femoral shortening, 284
Femoral shortening osteotomy, 253
Femoroacetabular impingement (FAI), 259–268
Femur
development of, 315–316
fractures, 439, 490*f*
child abuse and, 452
diaphyseal, 452
in osteogenesis imperfecta, 166*f*
subtrochanteric, 491
supracondylar metaphyseal, 491–492
rotation of, 316*f*
subtrochanteric fractures, 491
transverse fractures, 434
Femur, distal aspect
fractures, 491
growth arrest, 441
physeal fractures, 491–492
Femur, proximal aspect
development of, 270*f*
dysplasias, 84
fractures, nonaccidental, 453*f*
Fentanyl, 108
Fever, sports participation and, 604
FGF10 gene, 327
Fibroadipose tissue, 178
Fibroblast growth factor (FGF) antibodies, 170
Fibroblast growth factor receptor-3 *(FGFR3)* gene, 102, 390
Fibroblast growth factor receptors (FGFR), 87–88
Fibromatosis, 53–54, 53*f*
Fibrosarcomas, 46
Fibrous dysplasia, 50–51
Fibular deficiencies, 327–328, 328*f*

Fibular graft, free vascularized, 293
Fibular osteotomy, 295*f*
Fielding and Hawkins classification, 399
Filamin B, 405
Fingers, thumb-in-palm deformity, 161
Finite element modeling, fracture risk, 167
Flatfoot, 305–307
Flatt type thumbs, 220–221, 221*f*
Fleiss criteria, 20*t*
Flexor carpi ulnaris transfer, 127
Flexor digitorum superficialis (FDS) opponensplasty, 220
FLNB gene, 155–156
Folate deficiency, 137
Foot. *See also* Clubfoot; Flatfoot
  congenital disorders of, 303–313
  deformities, 147
  fractures, 503–505
  planovalgus, 131
Foot and ankle surgery, 131–132
Foot-progression angle, 316
Foramen magnum, 400–402
  stenosis, 87–88
Forced vital capacity (FVC), in neuromuscular diseases, 181
Forearm
  fractures, 25–26, 473–475
  pronation, 127
Fractures
  ankle sprain equivalent, 581–582
  avulsion-type, 166
  bone density and, 141
  casting, 438–439
  causes in older children, 166
  child abuse and, 451–452
  classification of, 435
  displaced, 438*f*
  fragility-related, 369–370
  healing, 435
  imaging of, 436
  malunion, 458, 474, 490
  manipulation of, 25–26
  morphology of, 501
  multiple, 451
  in neuromuscular diseases, 369–370
  nonaccidental, 453*f*
  nonunion, 437*f*, 458, 488
  open, 440
  in osteogenesis imperfecta, 166
  pain management in, 25–26, 107–108, 436–437
  pathologic, 36
  patient history, 435–436
  patterns in osteogenesis imperfecta, 168
  physical examination, 435–436
  remodeling, 435, 436*f*
  splinting, 438–439
Freeman-Sheldon syndrome, 154, 159
Freiberg disease, 309–310
Friedrich ataxia, 366*t*, 367, 377
Functional Assessment Questionnaire, 20
Functional Mobility Scale, 139, 140*f*

G

Gabapentin, 27
Gait analyses, 130, 130*f*
Galeazzi fracture-dislocations, 477–478
Galeazzi sign, 246
Galveston construct, 375
Gartland classification, 461–463
Gastric motility, 369
Gastrocnemius contractures, 305–306
Gastrocnemius recession procedure, 130–131
Gastrocnemius-soleus complex lengthening, 131
General Anesthesia Compared to Spinal Anesthesia trial, 26
Generalized arterial calcification in infancy, 109
Genetic associations, definition of, 72*t*
Genetic profiling, 71–73
Genetics, personalized medicine and, 71–80
Genome-wide association studies (GWAS), 71
Genu recurvatum, 499
Genu valgum, 89, 101
Genu varum, 87
Germline mutations, 72, 72*t*
Giant cell tendon sheath tumors, 54
Giant cell tumors, 47*t*
Glenohumeral dysplasia, 227–234, 232*f*
Glenohumeral internal rotation deficit (GIRD), 572
Glenohumeral joint, 567, 570–571
Glenohumeral subluxation, 230
Glucocorticoids, 109, 367
Gluteus maximus release, 189, 193
GNAS gene, 46
GNAS1 mutation, 50
Gowers maneuver, 179, 180*f*
GPR126 gene, 76, 353
Granulomatosis, 209–210
Greater tubercle, ossification centers, 567
Greenstick fractures, 434–435, 473–474
Greulich and Pyle method, 63
Grisel syndrome, 399, 401*f*
Gross Motor Function Classification System, 18, 124, 125*f*, 366–367, 367*f*
Gross Motor Function Measures, 20
Growing rod breakage, 343
Growth, 59–68
  amount remaining, 62–66
  areas of, 59
  arrest of, 65–66, 527
  chronologic, 60
  disturbances, 441–442
  guided, 170
  lower limbs, 59
  normal, 59–60
  peak height velocity, 353
  spinal, 60–61
  trunk, 59
Growth hormone supplements, 602
Growth velocity curves, 60
Gustilo-Anderson system, 440
Gymnasts, rotator cuff tendinitis, 572
Gymnast shoulder, 573

H

Hallux valgus, 308
Halo-gravity traction, preoperative, 371
Halo placement, 512
Halo vests, 512
Hamartomas, 100
Hamstring tightness, 416
Hand fractures, 480
Hand plate only symbrachydactyly, 220–222
Hand transplants, 238
Hangman's fractures, 512
Harris hip scores, 261, 263
Harris lines, 441
Head trauma, MRIs in, 451
Health-related quality of life (HRQoL) scores, 236
Healthcare expenditures, 6–8
Hearing loss, in osteogenesis imperfecta, 165
Heart defects, in congenital scoliosis, 344
Heart disease, skeletal dysplasia and, 82
Heat illness, exertional, 603–604
Heat stroke, 604
Heel-bisector line, 316, 317, 317*f*
Height, documentation of, 59
Hemangiomas, midline, 156*f*
Hematoma blocks, 436–437, 477
Hemiepiphysiodesis, 65, 345, 549–550
Hemihypertrophy, 93, 101
Hemimegalencephaly, 76*f*
Hemiplegia, 124
Hemivertebra excision, 345
Hemophagocytic lymphohistiocytosis, 206
Henoch-Schönlein purpura, 209–210
Hepatosplenomegaly, 90
Hepple staging system, 585
Hereditary motor neuropathies, 177, 366*t*
Hereditary multiple exostosis (HME), 93
Hereditary retinoblastomas, 46
Herpes infection, 605
Herring lateral pillar systems, 271, 272, 274*f*
Hibb technique, 373
High ankle sprains, 580–581

Hill-Sachs humeral impaction fractures, 570
Hill-Sachs lesions, identification of, 459–460
Hindfoot equinus, 303
Hindfoot varus, 303
Hip
  cervicotrochanteric fractures, 487–488
  clicks, 84*f*
  contractures, 158, 189
  developmental dysplasia of, 245–257
  dislocations, 158, 259–268, 488–489
  fractures, 487–489, 487*t*, 489*f*
  instability, 365
  neuromuscular subluxation, 128
  premature osteoarthritis, 86
  subluxation, 84–85
Hip dysplasia, 198, 198*f*, 344
Hip-knee-ankle-foot orthoses, 140–141, 143*f*
Hip spica cast, 489
HLA-B27, 417
Holt-Oram syndrome, 218
Hopkin squeeze test, 581
Horner syndrome, 228
HOX genes, 75–76, 343
Huber opponensplasty, 220
Hueter-Volkman law, 435
Human leukocyte antigen B27, 204
Humeral head displacement, 231, 231*f*
Humeral shaft fractures, 452
Humerus
  displaced fracture, 438*f*
  fractures, child abuse and, 452
  supracondylar fractures, 461–463, 463*f*
Humerus, distal aspect, 465*f*
Humerus, proximal aspect
  fractures, 460–461, 569
  ossification centers, 567, 568*f*
  pediatric injuries, 460–461
Hunter syndrome, 90, 91–92
Hurler syndrome, 90
Hydrocephalus, 137, 138, 141
Hydrocodone, 30
Hydromyelia, 89, 102
Hydrotherapy, in osteogenesis imperfecta, 168
Hydroxyapatite, in osteoporosis, 109
Hydroxychloroquine, 207
1,25-hydroxyvitamin D, 168, 170. *See also* Vitamin D
Hyperalimentation, parental, 377
Hypercalcemia, 165
Hyperkyphosis, 387, 405
Hypersomnolence, 193
Hypertelorism, 86
Hyperthermia, exercise-induced, 604
Hypertrophic cardiomyopathy, 193
Hypocalcemia, 110, 168
Hypochondroplasia, 88
Hypofibrinogenemia, 372
Hypoglycemia, neonatal, 101
Hypothermia, 439
Hypovolemia, 372
Hypoxemia, 440–441

I

Ibuprofen, 107–108, 206
Idebenone, 187
Idiopathic back pain, 415, 417
Idiopathic scoliosis, 27, 89, 339–340
  adolescent, 341–342
  early-onset, 341–343
Ifosfamide, 51
Ileus, opioids and, 30
Iliac apophysis, ossification of, 353
Iliotibial band (ITB) autograft, 523, 524*f*, 525*f*
Ilizarov bone transport, 292
Ilizarov external fixation, 293
Ilizarov technique, 325
Immobilization of fractures, 438
Immune system, overtraining and, 593
Immunodeficiency, primary, 37
Immunosuppression therapy, 238
Impaired consciousness, 451
Impaired sitting balance, 365
Incentives, volume-based, in healthcare delivery, 6
Infantile fibrosarcoma, 54*t*
Infantile myofibromatosis, 47
Infantile scoliosis, 341
Infants, fractures in, 451
Infections
  back pain in, 415
  continuum of disease, 36
  indications of, 422–423
  MRI hallmarks, 416
  musculoskeletal, 35–44
  sports participation and, 604
  superficial, 35
Infectious mononucleosis, 605
Inflammation
  burnout and, 592–593
  in traumatic injuries, 439
Infliximab, 207
Infraspinatus muscles, 230
Injury prevention programs, 602
Injury Severity Score, 439
INK4A tumor suppressor gene, 74
Innominate osteotomy, 253
Insall-Salvati ratio, 547, 547*f*
Institute of Medicine (IOM), 13–15, 14*t*
Institutional guidelines, 5
Insulin-like growth factor, 101
Insulin resistance, 193
Interleukin-1 (IL-1), 208
Interleukin-6 (IL-6), 271
Interleukin-1 (IL-1) inhibitors, 207
Internal tibial torsion, 131, 317–318
International Classification of Functioning, Disability, and Health (ICF), 236
International Hip Outcome Tool, 264
International Olympic Committee, statement on youth athletic development, 593, 594*t*
Intervertebral disks, 402
Intoeing, 317
Intraclass correlation coefficient (ICC), 18, 20*t*
Intramedullary nailing, 490*f*, 501
Intramedullary Skeletal Kinetic Distractor (ISKD), 326
Intrarater reliability, 18
Intravenous regional blocks, 436–437
Iselin disease, 310, 583

J

Jacob classification, 463
Jagged1 gene, 179
Janus-kinase inhibitors, 208
Jefferson fractures, 512
Joint Commission for the Accreditation of Healthcare Organizations, 13
Joints, hypermobility, 593
Jones classification, 329*f*, 330*f*
Jones criteria, acute rheumatic fever, 209*f*
Jones fractures, 504
Jones transfer, 196
Jump gait, 130*f*, 131
Jumping activities, 497–499
Junctional kyphosis, 343
Juvenile arthritis, 203–208
Juvenile dermatomyositis, 209–210
Juvenile hallux valgus, 308
Juvenile idiopathic arthritis (JIA), 205–208

K

Kappa coefficient, 18
Kawasaki disease, 209–210
Keratan sulfate, 90, 91*t*, 92, 403
Ketamine, 26, 108, 437
Ketorolac, postoperative, 30
Kidney transplants, sports participation and, 604–605
KIDSCREEN, 20
Kinetic chain mechanics, overhead sports, 568
Kingella kingae, 37, 40, 423*f*
Klinefelter syndrome, 76
Klippel-Feil syndrome, 235, 344, 370, 404–405
Knee
  anatomy of, 546*f*
  anterior pain, 594–595
  congenital dislocations, 283–284, 284*f*

contractures, 158
deformities, 146
disarticulation, 159*f*
flexion contractures, 146, 182, 193
fractures, 491–492
ligamentous injuries to, 521–536
osteochondritis dissecans, 555–559
Knee-ankle-foot orthoses (KAFOs), 183
Knee valgus stress, 146
Kniest syndrome, 86
Knudson two-hit theory, 93
Köhler disease, 309
Kugelberg-Welander syndrome, 188
Kyphectomy, 375
Kyphosis, 385–394
assessment of, 387
cervical, 405–406
classification of, 389–390, 390*f*
congenital, 389–390, 391*f*
focal, 514
hamstring tightness and, 416
iatrogenic, 391
junctional, 343
myelomeningocele and, 137, 144–145, 145*f*
paraplegia in, 100
physiologic consequences of, 386–387
postural, 388
presentation, 387
progressive, 390–391
related conditions, 390–392
risk factors, 390–391
thoracic, 385, 386*f*

L

Lacertus fibrosus release, 127
Lachman test, 522
LaCroix, ring of, 523, 526
Lambrinudi triple arthrodesis, 197*f*
Laminectomy, multilevel, 403
Landis and Koch criteria, 20*t*
Langenskiöld classification, 290–291
Langerhans cell histiocytosis, 47, 47*t*, 51, 52*f*
Larsen syndrome, 154–156, 252, 283, 285, 370, 405
Lateral condyle fractures, 463, 463*f*, 464*f*
Lawnmower injuries, 434
LBX1 gene, 76, 353
Lean process, 4
Ledderhose fibromatosis, 53
Leechavengvongs procedure, 230
Lefunomide, 207
Leg pain, tibial stress injuries, 595–596
Legg-Calvé-Perthes disease, 84, 263, 269–282, 272*f*, 273*f*, 274*f*, 277*f*
Lenke classification of AIS, 351–352, 352*f*, 357
Leptin, 271
Léri-Weill dyschondrosteosis, 219
Lesser tubercle, 567, 570
Lethal multiple pterygium syndrome, 156
Leukemia, 47*t*, 423
Levels of evidence, in clinical practice guidelines, 14, 15*t*
Lever arm syndrome, 131
Li-Fraumeni syndrome, 45
Lidocaine, 26
Ligamentous laxity, 545
Ligamentum flavum, 402
Limb deficiencies, 327–330, 331*f*
Limb development, embryonic, 235–236, 237*f*
Limb-girdle muscular dystrophy, 177
Limb-length discrepancy (LLD), 62, 65, 323–327
Limb lengthening, 325–327
Limb Lengthening and Reconstruction Society index, 325, 326*f*
Limb patterning defects, 75–76
Limbus fractures. *See* Apophyseal ring fractures
Lipoblastoma, 53
Lipoblastomatosis, 53
Lipomas, 53
Lisch nodules, 100
Lisfranc fractures, 504
Little Leaguer's elbow, 594
Little Leaguer's shoulder, 571–572, 572*f*
LLRS AIM Index, 325, 326*f*
LMX1B gene, 89
Loeys-Dietz syndrome, 73
Loose bodies, imaging of, 547
Lovastatin, 100
Low ankle sprains, 579–580
Lower extremities
development of, 319
mechanical axes, 320*f*
normal alignment, 320*t*
overuse injuries, 595*t*
surgery in ambulatory children, 129–132
LTBP4 gene, 179
Lumbar lordosis, 385, 386*f*, 418
Lumbar pars interarticularis, 418
Lumbar Scheuermann disease, 418, 420*f*
Lumbar spine, growth of, 61
Lumbosacral junction, 422*f*
Lungs, development of, 339
Luque-Galveston fixation technique, 127
Luque trolley, 144–145, 373–374
Lyme arthritis, 41, 209, 209*t*
Lymphedema, 147
Lymphoma, 47, 47*t*, 423
Lysosomal storage disease, 390

M

Macrodactyly, 101
Macrogrowth, 59
Madelung deformity, 219, 219*f*
Maffucci syndrome, 46, 47*t*
Magnetic Expansion Control (MAGEC) system, 158, 189, 189*f*, 342, 373
Magnetic resonance imaging (MRI)
in bone neoplasms, 47
brain, 451
costs of sedation, 36
in evaluation of back pain, 416
physeal bars on, 441–442
Malignant fibrous histiocytoma, 46
Mallet scale, 229
Malunion, 458, 474, 490
Manual muscle test, 142*t*
MAPK2 mutations, 51
Marfan syndrome, 73, 99, 601
Marrow stimulation, 558
Masquelet technique, 293
Maxillary micrognathia, 89
McCune-Albright syndrome, 46
McGregor line, 397
McMurray test, 540
McRae line, 397, 398*f*
Meary angle, 194, 196*f*, 305
Medial epicondyle
apophysitis, 594
displaced, 466*f*
fractures of, 463–464
ossification of, 463
Medial femoral condyle, 557*f*, 558*f*
Medial femoral cutaneous nerve, 28
Medial malleolar osteotomy, 586*f*
Medial patellofemoral ligament (MPFL), 545–546, 546*f*, 549
Medial tibial stress syndrome (MTSS), 595–596
Median nerve injury, 463
Medical Outcomes Study 36-Item Short Form measures, 263
Megaspondylodysplasia, 93, 101
Mehta casts in spinal deformity, 367–368
Melanoma, imaging of, 47
Melorheostosis, 47*t*
Menarche, Risser grades and, 60
Mendelian genetic disorders, 72*t*
Meniscal compression tests, 537
Meniscal tears, 528, 537–544, 538*f*
Meniscectomies, 541–542
Meniscus, compression tests, 540
Meralgia paresthetica, 263
Metabolic bone disease, 169–171
Metaphyseal injuries, 451, 452, 453*f*
Metatarsus adductus, 308–309, 317
Methicillin-resistant *Staphylococcus aureus* (MRSA), 37, 112–113
Methicillin-sensitive *Staphylococcus aureus* (MSSA), 37, 112–113
Methotrexate (MTX), 51–54, 207

Meyer dysplasia, 84*f*
Microarray technology, 71
Microdeletions, 71, 72*t*
Microduplication, 72*t*
Micrognathia, 89
Microgrowth, 59
Midazolam, 437
Midline facial capillary malformation, 76*f*
Milch classification, 463
Milwaukee brace, 405
Minerva orthosis, 512
Minimum clinically important difference (MCID), 17, 18
Misoprostol, maternal ingestion of, 236
Missense mutations, de novo, 72
Möbius syndrome, 154, 235
Model for Improvement, 4
Monodactylous symbrachydactyly, 220
Monoplegia, 124
Monteggia fracture-dislocations, 475–477, 476*f*
Mood, overtraining and, 593
Morphine, 27
Morquio syndrome, 90, 92, 403
Mortality rates, as quality indicator, 4
Morton extension orthotic, 309
Mosaic, definition of, 72*t*
Moseley straight-line method, 62
MPK gene, 192
Mucopolysaccharidosis (MPS), 90–92, 91*t*, 390, 391*f*
Multidirectional instability, shoulder, 571
Multiple epiphyseal dysplasia (MED), 83–85, 99
Multiple hereditary exostoses, 46, 222–223, 423
Multiple organ failure, 439
Multiple pterygium syndromes, 156–157
Multiplier method, for growth remaining, 62
Multisystem failure, 439
Muscular dystrophies, 369
Musculoskeletal system
  classification of disorders, 81–82
  growth of, 59–68
  infections, 35–44
  neoplasms, 45–58
Mycobacterium tuberculosis, 423*f*
Myelodysplasia, 283, 373
Myelomeningocele, 137–152, 145*f*, 305, 318, 372*f*
  adult care, 147–148
  classification of, 138–141, 139*t*
  environmental factors in, 138
  etiology, 137–138
  fetal surgery for, 138
  orthopaedic treatment, 141–143
  prognosis for ambulation, 139
Myelopathy, kyphosis in, 387
Myers and McKeever classification system, 528
Myostatin inhibition, 186
Myotonic dystrophy, congenital, 191–193
Myxoid liposarcoma, 54*t*

N

Nail-patella syndrome, 89, 285
Nailing
  elastic, 489, 490
  intramedullary, 490*f*, 501
  PRECICE nails, 326
  rigid, 490
Naproxen, 206
Narakas classification, 227–228
Narakas Motor Scale, 229–230
National Action Plan for Combating Antibiotic-Resistant Bacteria, 114
National Electronic Surveillance System, 473
National Emergency X-radiography Utilization Study (NEXUS), 407
National Trauma Data Bank, 486
Nausea
  opioids and, 30
  sports participation and, 604
Navicular coalition, 306
Neck trauma, 510*f*
Necrotizing fasciitis, 41
Neer and Horowitz classification, 460
Negative pressure wound therapy, 440, 441
Neonates, bone infections in, 40
Neoplasms, musculoskeletal system, 45–58
Neostigmine, 108
Nerve compression, 101
Nerve injuries, classification of, 228*t*
Nerve transfers, 230
Neural arch ossification, 396
Neural tube defects, 137
Neurapraxia, 228*t*
Neurofibromas, 54
Neurofibromatosis, 100–101, 386–387, 405–406, 406*f*, 416
Neurofibromin, 100
Neurofibrosarcomas, 101
Neuromas, 54, 228*t*
Neuromonitoring, 371
Neuromuscular diseases, progressive, 177–201
Neuromuscular scoliosis, 27
Neuromuscular spinal deformity, 365–383
Neurotmesis, 228*t*
Neurotoxicity, anesthetic, 26
NF1 gene, 100
Night pain, 49
NIPBL gene, 89–90
Nitrate supplementation, 603
Nitrous oxide, 25, 437
Nonambulatory status, spinal deformity and, 365
Nonarthritic Hip scores, 263
Nonossifying fibromas, 47*t*
Nonsteroidal antiinflammatory drugs (NSAIDs), 30, 206. *See also* Ibuprofen
Noonan syndrome, 103, 103*t*
Nosology and Classification of Genetic Skeletal Disorders, 82
Nubbins, 330, 331*f*
Nursemaid's elbow, 465

O

Ober test, 593
Ober-Yount procedure, 189, 193
Oberg, Manske, and Tonkin (OMT) classification, 217
Oberlin procedure, 230
Obesity. *See also* Body mass index (BMI)
  fracture risk and, 433–434
  myelomeningocele patients and, 141
  rates in children, 59
  SCFE and, 259–260
  tibia vara and, 289–290
Obturator nerve branches, 28
Occipital condyle fractures, 511–512
Occipitocervical fusion, prophylactic, 403
Oculodentodigital dysplasia syndrome, 221–222, 222*f*
Odontoid fractures, 509, 512, 512*f*
Odontoid hypoplasia, 85, 92
Olecranon apophysis, 60, 64
Olecranon fractures, 465
  stress-related, 594
Olesoxime, 192
Olisthetic scoliosis, 419*f*
Ollier disease, 46, 47*t*
Omphalocele, 101
Online Mendelian Inheritance in Man, 82
Opioids
  adverse side effects of, 30
  dependence on, 109
  postoperative, 30
  withdrawal, 109
Optic nerve glioma, 101
Organomegaly, 101
Organ, regeneration, 238–239
Orthopaedics, medical therapy in, 107–119
Ortolani maneuver, 246
Os odontoideum, 400, 402*f*
Osgood-Schlatter disease, 498, 595
Ossification centers, 61
Osteoarthritis
  early onset, 246
  hip, 86

Osteoblastoma, 423
Osteochondral autograft transplantation (OAT), 276*f*, 558
Osteochondritis dissecans (OCD)
capitellar, 594
elbow, 555–565, 560*f*
knee, 555–559
talar, 584–586, 585
Osteochondritis Dissecans of the Knee Arthroscopy Classification System, 557*f*
Osteochondroma, spinal, 50
Osteochondromatosis, 222–223, 423
Osteochondroplasty, 275
Osteochondrosis, 309–310
Osteogenesis imperfecta, 109, 165–169, 166*f*, 166*t*
adult, 167
Bruck syndrome and, 157, 157*f*
extraskeletal manifestations, 165
fracture patterns, 168
inheritance of, 99
Osteoid osteoma, 49, 49*f*, 415, 423
Osteolysis of the distal clavicle, 574
Osteomalacia, 169
Osteomyelitis
bacteremia and, 36
chronic, 114–115
chronic recurrent multifocal, 39–40
evaluation, 36, 38*f*
infections and, 422
practice guidelines, 36–37
recurrent multifocal, 210*f*
severity of illness, 36–37
surgical interventions, 39
tibial, 39*f*
treatment, 37–39
vertebral, 422
Osteonecrosis
in DDH, 253–254
femoral head, 488, 490
Legg-Calvé-Perthes disease and, 269
musculoskeletal infections and, 36
phalangeal fractures and, 480
unstable SCFE and, 260
Osteopenia, 166, 369–370
Osteopoikilosis, 47*t*
Osteoporosis
etiologies of, 172*t*
female athlete triad, 603
glucocorticoid-induced, 165, 166, 171
medical treatment of, 109–113
secondary causes of, 171–172
Osteosarcoma, 74*f*
back pain and, 423
imaging, 51
incidence of, 51
McCune-Albright syndrome and, 46
presentation, 51
prognostic factors, 52
somatic mutations in, 73–75
survival rates, 74
TP53 mutations in, 45
treatment, 51–52
Otitis media, recurrent, 88
Ottawa Ankle Rules, 580
Outcome assessments, 17–18
Outcome measures, 7
Outcomes Data Collection Instrument, 20
Outtoeing, 318
Overgrowth syndrome, 73, 75, 76*f*
Overhead sports, 568
Overtraining syndrome, 592–593
Overuse conditions, 591–599
definition of, 591
epidemiology of, 591–592
overhead athletes, 571–574
in pediatric patients, 595*t*
prevention of, 593
risk factors, 591–592
shoulder, 567–568
stages of, 591
Oxford bone scores, modified, 261
Oxycodone, 30

P

Pain management
analgesia, 107–109
in fractures, 25–26, 436–437
ladder concept, 107
pediatric anesthesia and, 25–33
perioperative, 27–30
pharmacologic agents, 27
postoperative, 27–30, 108–109
Paley classification, 329*f*
Pamidronate, 185, 293
Parasol rib deformity, 374
Parenteral analgesics, 437
Parenteral hyperalimentation, 377
Pars interarticularis, 419–420
Patella, congenital dislocations, 283–287, 285*f*
Patella, dislocation of, 545
Patellar instability, 545–553, 547*f*
Patellar tendon shortening, 130
Patellar tendopathy, 595
Patellofemoral pain, 594–595
Patellofemoral stress syndrome, 594–595
Patient, intervention, comparison, and outcome (PICO) questions, 14
Patient-controlled analgesia, 108
Patient-Reported Outcome Measurement Information System (PROMIS), 7, 13, 18–21
Patient-reported outcome measures (PROMs), 236
Patient safety, 5–6
Pavlik harness, 251, 252, 284, 489
PAX3-FOXO1 translocations, 55
PAX7-FOXO1 translocations, 55
PAX1 gene, 76, 353
Peak height velocity (PHV), 59–68, 353
Pediatric Anesthesia and NeuroDevelopment Assessment study, 26
Pediatric Health Information Systems database, 26–27
Pediatric Orthopaedic Society of North America (POSNA), 3, 303, 354–355
Pediatric orthopaedics, medical therapy in, 107–119
Pediatric Outcomes Data Collection Instrument (PODCI), 18, 236
Pediatric Quality of Life (PedsQL)-15, 20, 236
Pediatric Quality of Life Inventory, 7
Pedicle subtraction osteotomy, 376*f*
Pedobarographs, 195
Pelvic binders, 486
Pelvic obliquity, spinal deformity and, 365
Pelvic osteotomy, 86
Pelvic ring fractures, 485, 486
Pelvic sheets, 486
Pelvis
crush injuries, 486
degloving, 485
fractures, 485–487
growth centers, 485
immature, 485
morphology of, 422*f*
Penicillin, 113
Performance-enhancing supplements, 602–603
Peripheral nerve blocks, continuous, 28
Peripheral nerve sheath tumors, 47, 55
Peripheral nerve tumors, 54
Peromelic symbrachydactyly, 220
Peroneal nerve, EMG changes, 327
Peroneal tendon
contracture, 131–132
injury to, 579, 582–584
Peroneus brevis, 196
Peroneus longus tendon
tears, 584
transfer, 196
Personalized medicine, genetics and, 71–80
Pes planus, 305–306
Peyronie disease, 53
Phalangeal fractures, 480, 504–505
Pharmacogenetic variants, 72*t*
Phemister technique, 325
PHEX mutations, 169–170
Phosphate homeostasis, 110*f*
Phosphopenic rickets, 169–171
Phosphorus, in osteoporosis, 109
Physeal arrest, 36, 478
Physeal bars, 442*f*, 592
Physeal fractures, 434–435
distal femur, 491–492
proximal tibia, 497
PICO questions, 14

Pigmented villonodular synovitis (PVS), 54
PI3K/mTOR gene pathway, 74
Piriformis syndrome, 416
PITX1/TBX4/HOXC gene pathway, 75–76
PITX1-TBX4 transcription factor, 303
Pivot shift test, 522
Plan-do-study-act cycle, 4, 4*f*
Platelet function, anticonvulsant drugs and, 369
Platyspondylia, progressive, 92
Platyspondyly, 86
Playground injuries, 433–434
Plexiform neurofibromas, 47
PMP gene, 194
POC5 gene, 76
Poland syndrome, 235
Polyarteritis nodosa, 210
Polyostotic fibrosis dysplasia, 46, 47*t*, 51*f*
Polysomnography, 181, 400–401
Polytrauma, 439–467.10
Ponseti treatment method, 193, 303–305
Ponte osteotomies, 375
Popliteal artery, tethering of, 497
Positron emission tomography (PET), 47
Postanesthesia care units (PACUs), 108
Posterior atlantodens interval (PADI), 397, 398*f*
Posterior drawer test, 522
Postoperative ileus, 369
Poststreptococcal arthritis, 209
Powers ratio, 397, 398*f*
Prader-Willi syndrome, 103
PRECICE nails, 326
Prednisone, 172, 184–185
Prenatal diagnoses, 188–189
Prenatal surgery, 138
Pressure sores, 147, 196–197
Prevent Injury and Enhance Performance program, 522
Primary nerve surgery, 227–234
Process measures, 5
Propofol, 26
Prostheses
  in limb deficiencies, 330–332
  management of, 331–332
  rejection of, 237
  sensory feedback from, 238
  upper limb, 236–239
Proteus syndrome, 75, 93–94, 101
Providence nighttime braces, 356
Proximal femoral focal deficiency (PFFD), 327–328
Proximal interphalangeal (PIP) joint arthritis, 204
Proximal phalanx phalangeal neck fractures, 479*f*
Proximal tibial metaphyseal fractures, 499
Pruritus, opioids and, 29
Pseudoachondroplasia, 85–86
Pseudoarthrosis, 100, 292–294
Pseudoparalysis, 40, 487
Pseudoxanthoma elasticum, 109
Psoas abscess, 422
Psoas muscle lengthening, 131
Psychometrics, 17
Pterygia, 156
Puberty, 59, 60
Pulmonary compromise
  age-related, 354
  osteogenesis imperfecta and, 167
  spinal deformity and, 369
  spinal muscular atrophy and, 191
Pyarthrosis, 41
Pyomyositis, 40, 41, 422
Pyrophosphates, 109, 112*f*

Q

Quadriceps (Q) angle, 546
Quadriceps contractures, 284
Quadriplegia, 124, 511
Quality, in healthcare
  definitions of, 3
  future directions in, 6
  improvement, 3–4, 5*t*
  indicators/measures of, 4–5
"Quality, Safety and Value Initiative" (POSNA), 3

R

Race, SCFE and, 259
Radial head fractures, 466
Radial hypoplasia, 344
Radial longitudinal deficiency (RLD), 218–220, 218*f*
Radial neck fractures, 466, 467*f*
Radial polydactyly, 220–221
Radiofrequency ablation, 49
Radius fractures, 436*f*, 473–475, 477–478
RAND/UCLA Appropriateness Method, 15–16
Randomized clinical trials, 15
Ras signaling, 100
Rasch analysis, 18
Rb1 suppressor gene, 46
Reactive arthritis, 208–210
Readmissions, as quality indicator, 4
Recreational injuries, 433–434
Regional anesthesia, 25–33
  postoperative, 31*t*
Regional anesthetics, 108
Regional nerve blocks, 436–437
Reimer migration index, 128, 128*f*
Relative energy deficiency in sport (RED-S), 596. *See also* Female athlete triad
Relative value units (RVUs), 7
Reliability, intrarater, 18
Renal tubular dysfunction, 169
Reoperations, as quality indicator, 4
Repetitive stress, 592
Resisted straight leg raises, 416
Respiratory depression, opioids and, 30
Rest, ice, compression, and elevation, 580
Resuscitation, multisystem failure in, 439
Retinoblastomas, 46
Rett syndrome, 366*t*, 369
Return to sports, 550
Rhabdomyolysis, anesthesia-induced, 184
Rhabdomyosarcomas, 45, 54–55, 54*t*, 101
Rheumatic diseases, systematic, 209–210
Rheumatoid factor, 204, 417
Rhizomelic, definition of, 82
Rib fractures, 451
Rib-vertebral angle difference (RVAD), 341, 341*f*
Ribbing disease, 84
Rickets, 169–171, 170*f*
Rigidity, in cerebral palsy, 124
Risser casts, 367–368
Risser progression, 60
Risser sign, 60
Rituximab, 207, 208
Rockwood classification, 458, 459*f*
Romberg test, 194
Ropivacaine, 30*t*
Rotational limb deformity, 315–322
Rotator cuff injuries, 572–573, 573*f*
Rotator cuff tendinitis, 572
Round-back deformity, 388
Rubinstein-Taybi syndrome, 285
Runners, stress injuries in, 595–596
RUNX2 gene, 102

S

SADDAN, 87
Safe Surgery Saves Lives initiative, 5
Safety, a culture of, 6
Safety, patient, 5–6
Sagittal spinal alignment, 385, 386*f*
Salter-Harris classification
  femoral physeal fractures, 491–492
  pediatric fractures, 435, 435*f*
  pelvic fractures, 486
  tibial fractures, 502
Salter osteotomy, 86
Salter-Thompson classification, 271
Sanfilippo syndrome, 90–92
Sarcoidosis, 209–210

Sauvegrain method, 60, 63, *64t*
Scaphoid fractures, 478–479
Scapular dyskinesis, 573–574
Scapulothoracic joint anatomy, 567
SCFE. *See* Slipped capital femoral epiphysis (SCFE)
Scheuermann kyphosis, 385–389, *388f*, 415, 418
Schmorl nodes, 388, 418, *420f*, 511
Schwannomas, 54
Sciatic nerve blockade, 28
Sciatic notch, palpation of, 416
SCIWORA, 511
Sclerosis, 85, *272f*
Sclerotomes, 395
Scoliosis
  arthrodesis for, 61
  in arthrogryposis, 157–158
  in cerebral palsy, 127
  in CMT disease, 197–198
  cost of treatment, 377
  curve magnitude, 366
  curve progression, 61, *61t*
  in DMD, 181
  early-onset, 339–349, *340f*
  ethics of treatment, 377
  growing rods, *373f*
  growth-friendly instrumentation, 342–343
  infantile, 341
  magnetic rods, 374
  myelomeningocele patients and, 143–144
  neuromuscular conditions and, *366t*, 377
  olisthetic, *419f*
  osteogenesis imperfecta and, 167, 168, *168f*
  outcomes, 377
  postoperative pain relief, 108
  progressive, 183–184
  sex and, 76
  spinal fusion in, 144
  in spinal muscular dystrophy, 189, *190f*
  spine growth and, 61
Scoliosis Research Society (SRS), 7, 354–355, 386
Scoliosis Research Society (SRS)-22, 17
Seat belt injuries, *516f*
Seddon and Sunderland classification, *228t*
SEDL gene, 86
Segmental overgrowth syndromes, *72t*, 75
Selective dorsal rhizotomy, 126–127
Septic arthritis, 36, 40–41, 113–114
Sever disease, 206, 310, 591. *See also* Calcaneal apophysitis
Sex. *See also* Female athlete triad
  femoroacetabular impingement and, 263
  overuse injuries and, 592
  spinal canal growth and, 398
Sheldon-Hall syndromes, 159
Shelf osteotomy, 276
SHILLA system, 342, 346, 373
Shin splints, 595–596
Shoe inserts, 318
Short-finger symbrachydactyly, 220
Short-trunk disproportionate dwarfism, 403
Shoulder
  anatomy of, 567–568
  dislocations, 459–460
  dystocia, 227
  fractures, 569
  injuries, 567–577
  internal rotation deformity, 159–160
  loss of passive external rotation, *232f*
  multidirectional instability, 571
  patient evaluation, 568–569
  pediatric injuries to, 457–460
  rotator cuff injury, 572–573
  sprains, 569
  strains, 569
  traumatic injuries, 569–571
SHOX (short stature homeobox gene) deficiency, 219
Shriners Hospital Upper Extremity Dynamic Positional Analysis, 127
Sickle cell disease, 37
Sillence classification, 165
Silfverskiöld test, 305
Silver-Russell syndrome, 93, 101
Simulation training, 5
Sinding-Larsen-Johanson disease, 595
Single-leg hop, 527
Single nucleotide polymorphisms (SNPs), 71, *72t*, 76–77
Single photon emission computed tomography (SPECT), 419–420
Sitting heights, 59, 60–61
Six Sigma methods, 4
Skeletal age, 62–64, *63t*, *64t*. *See also* Skeletal maturity
Skeletal degeneration, premature, 107
Skeletal dysplasia, 81–97, 390, 400–403
Skeletal maturity, 59–68
  Legg-Calvé-Perthes disease, 269
  meniscal tear patterns, 539
  progression of scoliosis in, 367
  residual deformity in LCPD, 276–277
Skeletal survey, complete, *451t*
Skeletal system, fracture patterns, 434–435
Skin hyperlaxity, 165
Skin rashes, sports participation and, 604–605
SLC26A2 gene, 84
Sleep deprivation, 433–434
Sleeper stretch, 594
Slipped capital femoral epiphysis (SCFE), 259–268, *262f*, 290
Smartphone applications, for growth assessment, 65
SmartTots, 26
Smith-Peterson intervals, modified, 263
Smith-Peterson osteotomies, 375, *376f*
SMN1 gene, 188, 191
SMN2 gene, 188, 191
Smoking cessation, in disk disease, 417
Snapping scapula syndrome, 573
Society for Pediatric Radiology, 451
Soft-tissue injuries, child abuse and, 450–451
Soft-tissue sarcomas, 47
Soft-tissue tumors, *49t*, 54–55
Solid ankle-foot orthoses, 131
Somatic mutations, *72t*, 73–75
Somatosensory-evoked potentials (SSEPs), 371
Somites, 395
Sonic Hedgehog morphogens, 217
Sorafenib, 53–54
SOX9 gene, 89, 102
SOX9 transcription factor, 76
Special Olympics screening, 403
Spica casts, 487
Spina bifida, *366t*, 367, *368f*, 373
Spinal canal growth, 61
Spinal column growth, 60–61
Spinal cord, cervical, 398, *398f*
Spinal cord infarct, posterior, 417
Spinal cord injuries, *366t*, 511
Spinal cord tumors, 423
Spinal deformity
  comorbidities, 369
  myelomeningocele patients and, 143
  neuromuscular, 365–383
  in nonambulatory children, 366–367
  nonsurgical interventions, 367–368
  patient assessment, 366–367
  progression of, 366
  quality of life assessments and, 365–366
  risk factors for, 365
  surgical interventions, 368–377
Spinal fusion, 27, 374–376, 391
Spinal muscular atrophy (SMA), 177, 187–191, *187t*, *190f*, *366t*, *371f*
Spinal sagittal alignment, *387f*
Spinal stenosis, 88, 417
Spine, 509–518. *See also specific* conditions
  anatomy, 509–510
  burst fractures, 514–515
  congenital disorders, 339–349
  development of, 395–397
  embryology of, 395–397
  growth, 60–61, 339
  overuse injuries, *595t*
  sagittal alignment, 385
  segmentation defects, *344f*
  subaxial fractures, 509

surgery, anesthetic considerations, 26–27
Spine osteotomies, 376*f*
SpineCor braces, 356
Spinopelvic transiliac fixation technique, 375*f*
Splinting, fractures, 438–439
Split-tibia coaptation technique, 292
Spondyloarthritis, 204
Spondyloarthropathy, 205
Spondyloepiphyseal dysplasia, 83*f*, 86*f*
Spondyloepiphyseal dysplasia congenita (SEDC), 403
Spondylolisthesis, 168, 168*f*, 415, 416, 421–422, 421*t*, 423*f*, 424*f*
Spondylolysis, 415, 416, 421*t*
Sports. *See also specific* athletes
concussion related to, 601–602
hyperextension-related injuries, 416
injury prevention programs, 602
overuse injuries and, 591
preparticipation screening, 602, 604
scaphoid fractures and, 478–479
screening before, 601
shoulder injuries, 567–568
specialization in, 593
Sportsmetrics program, 522
SPP1 gene, 179
Sprains, 569, 579–581
SSX gene, 55
STAG2 tumor suppressor gene, 74
Standardized clinical assessment and management plans (SCAMP), 8
Standing heights, 59
Staphylococcus aureus, 37, 112–113, 358
Statin inhibitors, 100
Statins, 102
Steindler flexorplasty, 160
Step-down tests, 527
Sterility, male, 193
Sternal fractures, 451
Sternoclavicular (SC) joint, 457, 567
Steroids, toxicity of, 208
Stickler syndrome, 87
Stimulants, performance and, 602
STOP Sports Injuries campaign, 593
Straight leg test, positive, 418*f*
Strains, shoulder, 569
Strayer technique, 130
Strength training in children, 602
Streptococcus agalactiae, 40
Streptococcus pneumoniae, 40
Stress fractures, 592, 596
Structural proteins, 83–87, 99
Stubby feet, 159*f*
Stulberg classification, 272
Subaxial cervical trauma, 407–408, 513
Subischial heights, 59
Subischial limb lengths, 60
Subtrochanteric femoral fractures, 491
Sudden cardiac death, 193, 604
Sulfasalazine, 207
Sulfate transport protein defects, 92
Sulfate transporter genes, 405
Superior labrum anterior to posterior (SLAP) tears, 573
Superior peroneal retinaculum (SPR), 583–584
Supracondylar extension osteotomy, 146
Supracondylar humerus fractures, 19*f*, 461–463, 463*f*, 464
Supraspinatus muscle, 230
Surgical Safety Checklist (WHO), 5
Surgical site infections, incontinence and, 370
Swan-Ganz catheter, preoperative, 369
Swanson classification, 217
Swelling, lateral ankle, 579
Swimmers, shoulder injuries, 572
Symbrachydactyly, 217, 220, 236
Syme ankle disarticulation, 330
Synchondroses, 395–396
Syndactyly, 221–222
Syndesmotic sprains, 581
Syndromes, orthopaedic-related, 99–106
Synephrine, 602
Synovial sarcoma, 54*t*, 55
Syringomyelia, 89
Systematic review process, 14–15
Systemic inflammatory response syndrome, 439
Systemic lupus erythematosus, 209–210
SYT gene, 55

T

Tadalafil, 187
Talar dome, blood supply to, 584
Talar neck fractures, 504
Talectomy, 305
Talonavicular arthrodesis, 305
Talipes equinovarus contractures, 158–159
Talus, 504–505, 584–586
Tamoxifen, 53–54
Tanner classification, 60
Tanner staging, 522
Tanner-Whitehouse scoring, 61, 64
TARDBP gene, 74
Tarsal coalition, 306–307
Taylor Spatial Frame, 171
Team Strategies and Tools to Enhance Performance and Patient Safety (TeamSTEPPS), 6
Teamwork, evidence-based system, 6
Telangiectatic osteosarcoma, 49, 50*f*
Temtamy and McKusick classification, 221–222
Tenotomy, 127
Tensor fasciae femoris release, 189, 193
Teres minor muscles, 230
Teriparatide therapy, 168
Tethered cord syndrome, 137, 141, 416
Tetralogy of Fallot, 344
Tetraplegia, 124
Thanatophoric dysplasia, 88
Thessaly tests, 540
Thigh-foot axis, 316
Thomas test, 593
Thoracic compression fractures, 514
Thoracic insufficiency syndrome, 339–349
Thoracic spine, growth of, 61
Thoracolumbar junction, 87, 385
Thoracolumbar kyphosis, 88, 185
Thoracolumbar spine, 513–516
Thoracolumbosacral orthoses (TLSO), 189, 190*f*, 356, 367–368
Thrombocytopenia, 218
Throwing athletes, 593–594, 595*t*
Thumb hypoplasia, 220
Thumb-in-palm deformity, 161, 161*f*
Thurston Holland fragments, 492*f*
Tibia
congenital pseudoarthrosis of, 292–294, 294*f*, 295*f*
deformities, 289–297
MRI, 291*f*
normal development, 316
Tibia, distal aspect
growth arrest, 441
physeal fractures, 501–502
Salter-Harris classification, 502*f*
Tibia, proximal aspects
fractures, 497–499
growth arrest, 441
Tibia vara, 289–291, 290*f*
Tibial deficiencies, 329–330
Tibial dysplasia, 100
Tibial nerve, EMG changes, 327
Tibial osteotomy, 295*f*
Tibial shaft fractures, 499–501, 501*t*
Tibial spine, fractures of, 527–531, 528, 529*f*
Tibial stress injuries, 595–596
Tibial torsion, 317*f*
Tibial tubercle avulsion fractures, 497–499
Tibial tubercle-trochlear groove (TT-TG) distance, 547–548
Tibiofibular diastasis, 581
Tibiofibular joint arthrodesis, 293
Tillaux fractures, 502–503, 503*f*, 581, 582*f*
Time-driven activity-based costing (TDABC), 7–8
Tinea, sports participation and, 605
Tocilizumab, 207, 208
Toddlers, fractures in, 451
Tofacitinib, 207
Tongue, fasciculations, 187
Tönnis system, 249, 250*f*, 263–264
Torode and Zieg system, 486

Torsional malalignment syndrome, 318
Torticollis, 401*f*
Torus fractures, 434–435
Total hip arthroplasty (THA), 276
TP53 tumor suppressor gene, 45, 74
Tracheostomy, prophylactic, 369
Training regimens, overuse injuries and, 592
Tramadol, 108
Tranexamic acid (TXA), 26–27
Transcervical fractures, 487–488
Transesophageal echocardiography, preoperative, 369
Transforming growth factor-β antagonism, 168
Transient synovitis, 35, 208
Transmalleolar axis, 316, 317
Transposition of the great vessels, 344
Transscaphoid perilunate fractures, 479*f*
Transverse deficiency, 330
Trapezoid ligaments, 458
Trauma
  damage control, 439
  growth disturbances, 441–442
  high-energy injuries, 434, 485
  mechanisms of injury, 433–434
  musculoskeletal infections and, 40
  nonaccidental, 453*f*
  principles in children, 433–447
Trendelenburg gait, 89
Trephination, 539
Trevor disease, 47*t*
Triamcinolone hexacetonide, 207
Trichorhinophalangeal syndrome, 103
Triplane fractures, 503, 504*f*, 582
Triple-hop distance, 527
Triple innominate osteotomy of Steel, 86
Triradiate cartilage, 61
Trisomy 21, 404*f*. *See also* Down syndrome
Trochanter palpation test, 316
Trochlear groove, 546
Trochleoplasty, 550
TRSP1 gene, 103
True equinus gait, 130–131
Truncal hypotonia, 365
Tumor necrosis factor (TNF) inhibitors, 207
Tumor suppressor genes, 92–94
Tumors, back pain in, 415
Turner syndrome, 103

U

UHMWPE sutures, 529
Ulnar collateral ligament injuries, 594
Ulnar fractures, 473–475
Ulnar longitudinal deficiency (ULD), 220
Ulnar nerve, iatrogenic injury to, 461–462
Ulnar polydactyly, 221
Ultrarapid metabolizers, 72*t*, 73
Ultrasonography, 204, 246–250, 248*f*, 249*f*
Upper extremities
  amyoplasia, 159–161, 160*f*, 161*f*
  arthrogryposis, 159–162, 162*f*
  in cerebral palsy, 127
  congenital differences, 217–226
  congenital transverse deficiency of, 235–241
  contractures, 127
  embryology of, 217
  function of, 236
  malformations, 217–222
  overuse injuries, 595*t*
  prostheses, 236–239, 238
  quality of life and, 236
  radial longitudinal deficiency, 218–219, 218*f*
  transverse deficiency of, 236*f*
  truncated, 218
Urinary incontinence, surgical site infections and, 370
Urinary retention, opioids and, 30
Ustekinumab, 207, 208
Utrophin, 186

V

V-Y quadricepsplasty, 284, 286
Vacuum delivery, brachial plexus palsy and, 227
Valgus femoral osteotomy (VFO), 276
Validity, dimensions of, 17–18
Valproic acid, 369, 372
Value, in healthcare, definition of, 7
Van Nes rotationplasty, 329
Vancomycin, 39
Varus derotation osteotomy, 129
Vastus medialis, nerve to, 28
Vastus medialis obliquus, 546, 549
Velpeau radiographs, 459–460, 460*f*
Velpeau splinting, 458, 460
Vemurafenib, 51
Ventilator support, 191, 192
Verocay bodies, 54
Vertebra plana, 424*f*
Vertebral-anal-cardiac-tracheal-esophageal-renal-limb (VACTERL) syndrome, 218, 344
Vertebral column resection, 27, 376*f*
Vertebral fractures, 171, 451
Vertebral osteomyelitis, 422
Vertical Expandable Prosthetic Titanium Rib (VEPTR), 144, 158, 346, 346*f*, 373–374, 374*f*
Vertical talus, 147, 148*f*
Vickers ligament, 219
Vitamin B_{12} deficiency, 138
Vitamin D, 109–111, 110*f*. *See also* 1,25-hydroxyvitamin D
  deficiency, 109–110, 165, 169, 370
  dietary allowance, 111
  high-dose therapy, 169
  homeostasis, 110*f*
  role in bone, 289
VNT-7a signaling, 217
Volkmann ischemia, 461
Vulpius technique, 130

W

Wackenheim clivus baseline, 397, 398*f*
Wagstaffe tubercle, 580
Wake-up tests, 371
Waldenström classification, 271–273, 272*f*
Walking boots, 306
Wallace technique, 466
Waste, prevention for healthcare improvement, 6
Watanabe classification, 540
Watson-Jones classification, 498, 499*f*, 500*f*
Weber-type ankle fractures, 580
Weight gain, in musculoskeletal growth, 59
Welcher basal angle, 397, 398*f*
Werdnig-Hoffman disease, 187
Western Ontario and McMaster Universities Index (WOMAC), 263
Wheelchair modifications, 367–368
Wilms tumors, 101
Wilson sign, 556
Wiltse-Neuman classification, 421*t*
Wolff law, 435
World Health Organization, 236
  Surgical Safety Checklist, 5
Wrist, arthrogryposis, 160–161, 161*f*

X

X-linked hypophosphatemia, 165, 169–171, 171*f*

Z

Z-lengthening, 130
Zinc deficiencies, 138
Zoledronate, 370
Zoledronic acid, 185, 293